MANUAL OF NEONATAL CARE

Sixth Edition

Editors

John P. Cloherty, MD

Associate Neonatologist
Neonatology Program at Harvard
Brigham and Womens Hospital
Beth-Israel Deaconess Medical Center
Children's Hospital, Boston
Associate Clinical Professor of Pediatrics
Harvard Medical School
Boston, Massachusetts

Eric C. Eichenwald, MD

Associate Professor of Pediatrics
Baylor College of Medicine
Medical Director, Newborn Center
Texas Children's Hospital
Houston, Texas

Ann R. Stark, MD

Professor of Pediatrics
Head, Section of Neonatology
Baylor College of Medicine
Chief of Neonatology
Texas Children's Hospital
Houston, Texas

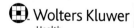 Wolters Kluwer | Lippincott Williams & Wilkins
Health

Philadelphia · Baltimore · New York · London
Buenos Aires · Hong Kong · Sydney · Tokyo

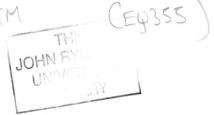
Acquisitions Editor: Sonya Seigafuse
Managing Editor: Ryan Shaw
Project Manager: Alicia Jackson
Manufacturing Coordinator: Kathleen Brown
Marketing Manager: Kimberley Schonberger
Design Coordinator: Terry Mallon
Cover Designer: Becky Baxendell
Production Services: Laserwords Private Limited, Chennai, India

530 Walnut Street
Philadelphia, PA 19106 USA
LWW.com

Fifth edition, © 2004 Lippincott Williams & Wilkins

Printed in the USA

Library of Congress Cataloging-in-Publication Data

Manual of neonatal care / editors, John P Cloherty, Eric C. Eichenwald, Ann R. Stark.—6th ed.
   p. ; cm.
  Includes bibliographical references and index.
  ISBN-13: 978-0-7817-6984-6
  1. Neonatology—Handbooks, manuals, etc. I. Cloherty, John P. II. Eichenwald, Eric C. III. Stark, Ann R.
  [DNLM: 1. Infant, Newborn, Diseases—Handbooks. 2. Infant Care—Handbooks. 3. Neonatology—methods—Handbooks. WS 39 M2945 2008]
  RJ251.M26 2008
  618.92′.01—dc22

                         2007025180

10 9 8 7 6 5 4 3 2 1

We dedicate this edition

to our spouses: Ann, Caryn, and Peter

to our children: Maryann, David, Joan, Neil, Danny, Monica, Tom, Victoria, Anne, Tim, Zachary, Taylor, Connor, Laura, and Gregory

to our grandchildren: Chrissy, Elizabeth, Daniel, Patrick, John, Tom, Ryan, Catherine, Sophie, Jack, Eva, Jane, Nora and Peter

to the many babies and parents we have cared for, and

to our long standing mentor, Dr. Mary Ellen Avery

Elisa Abdulhayoglu, MD, MS
Instructor in Pediatrics
Harvard Medical School
Boston, Massachusetts;
Neonatologist
Newton-Wellesley Hospital
Newton, Massachusetts

Steven A. Abrams, MD
Professor
Department of Pediatrics
Section of Neonatology
Baylor College of Medicine;
Neonatologist
Department of Pediatrics
Texas Children's Hospital
Houston, Texas

James M. Adams, MD
Professor
Department of Pediatrics
Baylor College of Medicine;
Neonatologist
Section of Neonatology
Department of Pediatrics
Texas Children's Hospital
Houston, Texas

Lisa M. Adcock, MD
Associate Professor
Department of Pediatrics
Section of Neonatology
Baylor College of Medicine;
Neonatologist
Texas Children's Hospital
Houston, Texas

Diane M. Anderson, PhD, RD
Associate Professor
Department of Pediatrics
Section of Neonatology
Baylor College of Medicine
Houston, Texas

Jennifer L. Anderson, MD
Fellow
Neonatology Program at Harvard
Harvard Medical School
Boston, Massachusetts

John H. Arnold, MD
Associate Professor
Department of Anaesthesia (Pediatrics)
Harvard Medical School;
Senior Associate
Department of Anesthesia and Critical
  Care Medicine
Children's Hospital
Boston, Massachusetts

Kushal Y. Bhakta, MD
Assistant Professor
Department of Pediatrics
Section of Neonatology
Baylor College of Medicine;
Attending Neonatologist
Section of Neonatal-Perinatal Medicine
Texas Children's Hospital
Houston, Texas

Diana W. Bianchi, MD
Natalie V. Zucker Professor of Pediatrics
Department of Obstetrics and Gynecology
Tufts University School of Medicine;
Vice Chair for Research
Department of Pediatrics
Floating Hospital for Children
Boston, Massachusetts

Dara Brodsky, MD
Instructor
Department of Pediatrics
Harvard Medical School;
Neonatologist
Department of Neonatology
Beth Israel Deaconess Medical Center
Boston, Massachusetts

Sandra K. Burchett, MD, MS
Assistant Professor
Department of Pediatrics
Harvard Medical School;
Clinical Director
Division of Infectious Diseases
Department of Medicine
Children's Hospital, Boston
Boston, Massachusetts

Sule U. Cataltepe, MD
Assistant Professor
Department of Pediatrics
Division of Newborn Medicine
Harvard Medical School;
Staff Neonataologist
Division of Newborn Medicine
Brigham and Women's Hospital
Boston, Massachusetts

Kimberlee Chatson, MD, BSN
Instructor of Pediatrics
Department of Newborn Medicine
Children's Hospital
Boston, Massachusetts
Associate Director
Special Care Nursery
Winchester Hospital
Winchester, Massachusetts

Helen A. Christou, MD
Assistant Professor
Department of Pediatrics
Harvard Medical School;
Attending Neonatologist
Department of Newborn Medicine
Brigham and Women's Hospital
Boston, Massachusetts

John P. Cloherty, MD
Associate Clinical Professor of Pediatrics
Department of Newborn Medicine
Harvard Medical School;
Associate Neonatologist
Department of Newborn Medicine
Childrens Hospital
Boston, Massachusetts

William D. Cochran, MD
Senior Associate in Medicine (emeritus)
Newborn Intensive Care Unit
Beth-Israel Deaconess Medical Center;
Associate Clinical Professor of Pediatrics
   (emeritus)
Harvard Medical School
Boston, Massachusetts

Nazan Dalgic, MD
Department of Infectious Diseases
Harvard Medical School;
Research Fellow
Department of Infectious Diseases
Children's Hospital Boston
Boston, Massachusetts

Elizabeth G. Doherty, MD
Instructor
Department of Pediatrics
Harvard Medical School;
Attending Neonatologist
Brigham and Women's Hospital,
   Winchester Hospital
Boston, Massachusetts

Caryn E. Douma, MS, RN
Clinical Specialist
NICU Level 3
Texas Children's Hospital
Houston, Texas

Adré J. du Plessis, MBChB, MPH
Associate Professor
Department of Neurology
Harvard Medical School;
Senior Associate
Department of Neurology
Children's Hospital
Boston, Massachusetts

Tola Dawodu, PharmD
Adjunct Professor
College of Pharmacy
Northeastern University
Bouve College of Health Sciences;
Clinical Pharmacist
Pharmacy
Brigham & Women's Hospital
Boston, Massachusetts

Eric C. Eichenwald, MD
Associate Professor
Department of Pediatrics
Section of Neonatology
Baylor College of Medicine;
Medical Director
Newborn Center
Department of Pediatrics/Neonatology
Texas Children's Hospital
Houston, Texas

Deirdre Ellard, MSRD, LDN, CNSP
Neonatal Nutritionist
Brigham and Women's hospital
Boston, Massachusetts

Josephine M. Enciso, MD
Assistant Professor
Department of Pediatrics
Section of Neonatology
Baylor College of Medicine;
Attending Neonatologist
Department of Pediatrics
Texas Children's Hospital
Houston, Texas

Regine M. Fortunov, MD
Neonatologist
Neonatology Associates Ltd.;
Neonatologist
Department of Pediatrics
Maricopa Medical Center
Phoenix, Arizona

Joseph A. Garcia-Prats, MD
Professor
Department of Pediatrics and Center for
   Ethics
Section of Neonatology
Baylor College of Medicine;
Medical Director
Arnold J. Rudolph Memorial Newborn
   Intensive Care Unit
Department of Pediatrics
Ben Taub General Hospital
Houston, Texas

Allen M. Goorin, MD
Associate Professor
Department of Pediatrics
Harvard Medical School
Boston, Massachusetts

James E. Gray, MD, MS
Assistant Professor
Department of pediatrics
Division of Newborn Medicine
Harvard Medical School;
Neonatologist
Department of Neonatology
Beth-Israel Deaconess Medical Center
Boston, Massachusetts

Munish Gupta, MD
Neonatologist
Department of Neonatology
Beth Israel Deaconess Medical Center
Boston, Massachusetts

Anne R. Hansen, MD, MPH
Assistant Professor
Department of Pediatrics
Harvard Medical School;
Medical Director MCU
Department of Medicine
Division of New Medicine
Children Hospital Boston
Boston, Massachusetts

Sandra L. Harmon, RN, BSN
Assistant Nurse Manager,
Neonatal Intensive Care Unit,
Brigham and Women's Hospital
Boston, Massachusetts

Leslie L. Harris, MD
Assistant Professor
Department of pediatrics
Section of Neonatology
Baylor College of Medicine;
Texas Children's Hospital
Houston, Texas

Linda J. Heffner, MD, PhD
Professor and Chair
Department of Obstetrics and Gynecology
Boston University School of Medicine;
Chief
Division of Obstetrics and Gynecology
Boston Medical Center
Boston, Massachusetts

John T. Herrin, MBBS, FRACP
Associate Clinical Professor
Department of Pediatrics
Harvard Medical School;
Attending Nephrologist
Division of Nephrology
Department of Medicine
Childrens Hospital Boston
Boston, Massachusetts

Nancy M. Hurst, RN, DSN, IBCLC
Assistant Professor
Department of Pediatrics
Section of Gastroenterology
Baylor College of Medicine;
Assistant Director
Lactation Program/Milk Bank
Texas Children's Hospital
Houston, Texas

Robert M. Insoft, MD
Assistant Professor
Department of Pediatrics
Harvard Medical School;
Medical Director
NICU & Neonatal Respiratory Services
Brigham & Women's Hospital
Boston, Massachusetts

Marsha R. Joselow, MSW LICSW
Social Worker
Infant Follow-Up Program;
Assistant Director
Pediatric Advanced Care Team
Children's Hospital Boston
Boston, Massachusetts

James R. Kasser, MD
John E. Hall Professor of Orthopaedic
    Surgery
Deparment of Orthopaedic Surgery
Harvard Medical School;
Orthopaedic Surgeon in Chief
Deparment of Orthopaedic Surgery
Childrens Hospital Boston
Boston, Massachusetts

Melanie S. Kim, MD
Associate Professor
Department of Pediatrics
Boston University School of Medicine;
Boston Medical Center
Boston, Massachusetts

Stella Kourembanas, MD
Clement A. Smith Chair of Pediatrics
Department of Pediatrics
Harvard Medical School;
Chair of Neonatology
Neonatology Program at Harvard
Children's Hospital Boston
Brigham & Women's Hospital
Beth Israel Deaconess Medical Center
Children's Hospital Boston
Boston, Massachusetts

Kimberly G. Lee, MD, MSc, IBCLC
Associate Professor
Department of Pediatrics
Division of Neonatology
Medical University of South Carolina;
Attending Neonatologist
Department of Pediatrics
Medical University of South Carolina
    Children's Hospital
Charleston, South Carolina

Harvey L. Levy, MD
Professor
Department of Pediatrics
Harvard Medical School;
Senior Associate
Department of Medicine
Children's Hospital Boston
Boston, Massachusetts

Nancy A. Louis, MD
Instructor in pediatrics
Harvard Medical School;
Neonatologist
Brigham and Women's Hospital
Boston, Massachusetts

Camilia R. Martin, MD, MS
Instructor in Pediatrics
Department of Medicine
Harvard Medical School;
Associate Director
Neonatal Intensive Care Unit
Department of Neonatology
Beth Israel Deaconess Medical Center
Boston, Massachusetts

Ginny May, RNC, BSN
Clinical Nurse
Neonatal Intensive Care Unit
Beth-Israel Deaconess Medical Center
Boston, Massachusetts

Thomas F. McElrath, MD, PhD
Assistant Professor
Department of Obstetrics, Gynecology and
    Reproductive Biology
Harvard Medicine School;
Director
Department of Obstetrical Reserch
Division of Maternal-Fetal Medicine
Brigham & Women's Hospital
Boston, Massachusetts

Tiffany M. McKee-Garrett, MD, FAAP
Assistant Professor
Department of Pediatrics
Section of Neonatology
Baylor College of Medicine
Assistant Director of Nurseries
The Methodist Hospital
Houston, Texas

Beth M. McManus, PT, ScD (c)
Neonatal Developmental Specialist
Newborn Intensive Care Unit
Brigham and Women's Hospital
Boston, Massachusetts

Ellis J. Neufeld, MD
Director
Department of Hematology;
Director
Boston Center for Genetic Blood Diseases
Children's Hospital;
Associate Professor
Department of Pediatrics
Harvard Medical School
Boston, Massachusetts

Rita Patnode, MSN, PNP
Nursing Clinical Educator
Newborn Intensive Care Unit
Brigham and Women's Hospital
Boston, Massachusetts

Karen M. Puopolo, MD, PhD
Assistant Professor
Department of Pediatrics
Harvard Medical School;
Attending Physician
Department of Newborn Medicine
Brigham and Women's Hospital
Boston, Massachusetts

Aviva Lee-Parritz, MD
Associate Professor and Vice Chair
Department of Obstetrics and Gynecology
Boston Medical Center
Boston University School of Medicine
Boston, Massachusetts

Lu-Ann Papile, MD
Professor
Department of Pediatrics
Baylor College of Medicine;
Attending Neonatologist
Division of Neonatology
Texas Children's Hospital
Houston, Texas

Karen M. Puopolo, MD, PhD
Assistant Professor
Department of Pediatrics
Harvard Medical School;
Attending Physician
Department of Newborn Medicine
Brigham and Women's Hospital
Boston, Massachusetts

Corinne Cyr Pryor, RNC, BA, IBCLC
Senior Staff Nurse
Newborn Intensive Care Unit
Brigham and Women's Hospital
Boston, Massachusetts

Steven A. Ringer, MD, PhD
Assistant Professor
Department of Pediatrics
Harvard Medical School;
Chief
Department of Newborn Medicine
Brigham and Women's Hospital
Boston, Massachusetts

David H. Rowitch, MD, PhD
Professor
Pediatrics and Neurological Surgery
University of California, San Francisco;
Chief
Division of Neonatology
UCSF Children's Hospital
San Francisco, California

Elizabeth T. Rosolowsky, MD
Fellow
Department of Medicine
Division of Endocrinology
Children's Hospital Boston;
Clinical Fellow
Department of Medicine
Children's Hospital Boston
Boston, Massachusetts

Sylvia Schechner, MD, MPH
Harvard Vanguard Medical Associate
  Neonatologist
Brigham and Woman's Hospital
Children's Hospital
Beth-Israel Deaconess Medical Center;
Assistant Clinical Professor of Pediatrics
Harvard Medical School
Boston, Massachusetts

Kevin Shannon, MD
Auerback Distinguished Professor of
  Molecular Oncology
Department of Pediatrics
University of California
San Francisco, California

Lori A. Sielski, MD
Assistant Professor
Department of Pediatrics
Baylor College of Medicine;
Medical Director Newborn Nursery
Department of Pediatrics
Ben Taub General Hospital
Houston, Texas

Charles F. Simmons, Jr., MD
Ruth and Harry Roman Chair
Department of Neonatology
Chairman
Department of Pediatrics
Cedars-Sinai Medical Center;
Professor
Department of Pediatrics
David Geffen School of Medicine at UCLA
Los Angeles, California

Steven R. Sloan, MD, PhD
Assistant Professor
Department of Pathology
Harvard Medical School;
Blood Bank Medical Director,
Laboratory Medicine & Joint Program in
   Transfusion Medicine
Children's Hospital Boston
Boston, Massachusetts

Janet S. Soul, MD, CM, FRCPC
Assistant Professor
Department of Neurology
Harvard Medical School;
Associate Director
Neonatal Neurology Program
Department of Neurology
Children's Hospital Boston
Boston, Massachusetts

Norman P. Spack, MD
Clinical Director
Endocrine Division
Children's Hospital;
Assistant Professor
Department of Pediatrics
Harvard Medical School
Boston, Massachusetts

Ann R. Stark, MD
Professor
Department of Pediatrics
Head
Section of Neonatology
Baylor College of Medicine;
Cheif of Neonatology
Texas Children's Hospital
Houston, Texas

Jane E. Stewart, MD
Co-Director
Infant Follow-up Program
Beth Israel Deaconess Medical Center;
Instructor
Department of Pediatrics
Harvard Medical School
Boston, Massachusetts

Jeffrey W. Stolz, MD, MPH
Chief
Department of Pediatrics
Swedish Medical Center
Seattle, Washington

Linda J. Van Marter, MD
Neonatologist
Brigham and Women's Hospital;
Associate Professor
Department of Pediatrics
Harvard Medical School
Boston, Massachusetts

Deborah K. VanderVeen, MD
Assistant Professor
Department of Ophthalmology
Harvard Medical School;
Associate
Department of Ophthalmology
Children's Hospital Boston
Boston, Massachusetts

**Mohan Pammi Venkatesh, MBBS,
MD, MRCPCH**
Assistant Professor
Department of Pediatrics
Section of Neonatology
Baylor College of Medicine;
Neonatologist
Department of Pediatrics
Section of Neonatology
Texas Children's Hospital
Houston, Texas

Louis Vernacchio, MD, MSc
Assistant Professor
Epidemiology and Pediatrics
Boston University School of Medicine;
Attending Physician
Department of Medicine
Children's Hospital
Boston, Massachusetts

Stephanie Burns Wechsler, MD
Associate Professor
Department of Pediatrics
Children's Heart Program
Duke University Medical Center
Durham, North Carolina

Gil Wernovsky, MD, FACC, FAPP
Director
Program Development
Staff Cardiologist
Cardiac Intensive Care Unit
Cardiac Center at the Children's Hospital
    of Philadelphia;
Associate Professor
Department of Pediatrics
University of Pennsylvania School of
    Medicine
Philadelphia, Pennsylvania

Richard E. Wilker, MD
Instructor
Department of Pediatrics
Harvard Medical School;
Chief
Department of Neonatology,
Newton-Wellesley Hospital,
Newton, Massachusetts

Louise E. Wilkins-Haug, MD, PhD
Associate Professor
Department of Obstetrics and Gynecology
Harvard Medical School;
Director
Division of Maternal Fetal Medicine and
    Reproductive Genetics
Brigham and Women's Hospital
Boston, Massachusetts

Gerhard K. Wolf, MD
Instructor
Department of Anesthesia
Harvard Medical School;
Assistant
Division of Critical Care Medicine
Department of Anesthesia;
Pediatric Medical Director
Boston Medflight
Boston, Massachusetts

Linda Zaccagnini, RN, NNP
Advanced Fetal Care Center
Children's Hospital
Boston, Massachusetts

John A. F. Zupancic, MD, ScD
Assistant Professor
Department of Pediatrics
Director
Harvard Neonatal-Perinatal Medicine
    Fellowship Program
Division of Newborn Medicine
Harvard Medical School
Children's Hospital Boston;
Associate Director
Neonatal Intensive Care Unit
Beth Israel Deaconess Medical Center
Boston, Massachusetts

$\mathcal{T}$his edition of the Manual has been completely updated and extensively revised to reflect the changes in fetal, perinatal, and neonatal care that have occurred since the fifth edition. In the Manual, we describe our current and practical approaches to evaluation and management of conditions encountered in the fetus and the newborn. We recognize that many areas of controversy exist, that there is often more than one approach to a problem, and that our knowledge continues to grow. In addition, this edition is the first collaborative effort with authors from two major neonatology programs, reflecting the move of two of the editors, Eric Eichenwald and Ann Stark, from Harvard to Baylor College of Medicine in Houston, Texas, and their ongoing collaboration with their colleague and co-editor John Cloherty.

The Children's Hospital Boston Neonatology Program at Harvard has grown to 56 attending neonatologists and 18 fellows who care for more than 28,000 newborns delivered annually at the Beth Israel Deaconess Medical Center (BIDMC), the Brigham and Women's Hospital (BWH) (formerly the Boston Lying-In Hospital and the Boston Hospital for Women), Beverly Hospital, Metro West Medical Center, Saint Elizabeth's Hospital, South Shore Hospital and Winchester Hospital. They also care for the 650 neonates transferred annually to the NICU at Children's Hospital Boston for management of complex medical and surgical problems. Fellows in the Harvard Neonatal–Perinatal Fellowship Program train in addition to Children's Hospital, at Beth Israel Deaconess Medical Center, Brigham and Women's Hospital and Massachusetts General Hospital.

The Neonatology Program at the Baylor College of Medicine includes 33 attending neonatologists, 12 pediatrician hospitalists, and 16 fellows who care for approximately 19,000 newborns delivered each year at Saint Luke's Episcopal Hospital, The Methodist Hospital, Ben Taub General Hospital, Saint Luke's Community Medical Center at the Woodlands, Methodist Willowbrook Hospital, Twelve Oaks Medical Center, and East Houston Regional Medical Center. They also care for the approximately 2,200 infants admitted annually to the Newborn Center at Texas Children's Hospital for management of complex medical and surgical problems, including congenital heart disease. Fellows in the Baylor College of Medicine Neonatal-Perinatal Fellowship Program train at Texas Children's Hospital, Ben Taub General Hospital, and Saint Luke's Episcopal Hospital.

Programs in both institutions, The Children's Hospital Boston Advanced Fetal Care Center (in collaboration with the obstetrical programs of Beth Israel Deaconess Medical Center and Brigham and Women's Hospital) and The Texas Children's Fetal Center (in collaboration with the Texas Children's Hospital/Baylor College of Medicine obstetric program at Saint Luke's Episcopal Hospital) provide evaluation, genetic and obstetric fetal imaging and invasive diagnostics, and *in utero* or peripartum therapy to mother and child. Using interventional techniques, some problems are treated *in utero* to prevent neonatal disease.

Our commitment to values including clinical excellence, collaboration with colleagues, and support of families is evident throughout our book. The hospitals mentioned earlier are referral centers for pregnancies complicated by maternal illness, fetal abnormalities, and anticipated neonatal problems. Obstetricians and neonatologists work together to provide prenatal, perinatal, and neonatal care. This perinatal experience is reflected in the chapters on Fetal Assessment and Prenatal Diagnosis, Maternal Conditions that Affect the Fetus, and Genetic Issues Presenting in the Nursery.

The neonatal intensive care units (NICUs) at Children's Hospital Boston and Texas Children's Hospital provide telephone consultation to pediatricians at local community hospitals and facilitate advanced care for patients cared for by neonatologists at referring NICUs. Both programs transport and care for critically ill newborns throughout New England and Texas and the surrounding states. Frequent problems in this outborn population include perinatal asphyxia, congenital heart disease, severe respiratory disorders, malformations, surgical emergencies, and metabolic disorders. The practical approaches we have developed to address these problems are described in the Manual.

Close involvement with the families is valued in our NICUs. This is reflected in the chapters on Breast Feeding, Developmentally Supportive Care, Management of Neonatal Death and Bereavement Follow Up, and Decision Making and Ethical Dilemmas.

We acknowledge the efforts of many individuals to advance the care of newborns and the training of physicians in newborn medicine. We are indebted to Clement Smith and Nicholas M. Nelson for their insights into newborn physiology and to Stewart Clifford, William D. Cochran, John Hubbell, and Manning Sears for their contributions to the care of infants at the Boston Lying-in Hospital. We thank the former and current directors of the Newborn Medicine Program at Harvard, H. William Taeusch Jr, Barry T. Smith, Michael F. Epstein, Merton Bernfield, Ann R. Stark, Gary A. Silverman, and Stella Kourembanas, and the former directors of the Baylor College of Medicine Neonatology Program, Murdina M. Desmond, Arnold J. Rudolph, Thomas N. Hansen, and Leonard E. Weisman, for their dedication to the training of physicians in the care of newborns.

We appreciate our many colleagues for their contribution of chapters or for permission to use data, illustrations, or tables. We thank the fellows of the Newborn Medicine Program at Harvard and Baylor College of Medicine Newborn Program for their hard work caring for infants and families and their field testing of the approaches to care discussed in the Manual. We thank Mica Astion and LaToya Graves for their secretarial work and administrative assistance without which this would have been an impossible task. We also thank Ryan Shaw, Alicia Jackson, and Sonya Seigafuse of Lippincott Williams and Wilkins for their invaluable help.

We dedicate this book to Mary Ellen Avery for her contributions to the care of infants all over the world and to the personal support and advice she has provided to so many, including the editors. Finally, we gratefully acknowledge the nurses, residents, parents, and babies who provide the inspiration for and measure the usefulness of the information contained in this book.

John P. Cloherty, MD
Eric C. Eichenwald, MD
Ann R. Stark, MD

CONTENTS

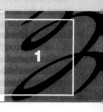

FETAL ASSESSMENT AND PRENATAL DIAGNOSIS

Louise E. Wilkins-Haug and Linda J. Heffner

1

I. **GESTATIONAL-AGE ASSESSMENT** is important to both the obstetrician and pediatrician and must be made with a reasonable degree of precision. Elective obstetric interventions such as chorionic villus sampling (CVS) and amniocentesis must be timed appropriately. When premature delivery is inevitable, gestational age is important with regard to prognosis, the management of labor and delivery, and the initial neonatal treatment plan.

   A. The clinical estimate of gestational age is usually made on the basis of the first day of the last menstrual period. Accompanied by physical examination, auscultation of fetal heart sounds and maternal perception of fetal movement can also be helpful.

   B. Ultrasonic estimation of gestational age. During the first trimester, fetal crown-rump length can be an accurate predictor of gestational age. Crown-rump length estimation of gestational age is expected to be within 7 days of the true gestational age. During the second and third trimesters, measurements of the biparietal diameter (BPD) and the fetal femur length best estimate gestational age. Strict criteria for measuring the cross-sectional images through the fetal head ensure accuracy. Nonetheless, owing to normal biologic variability, the accuracy of gestational age estimated by BPD decreases with increasing gestational age. For measurements made at 14 to 20 weeks of gestation, the variation is up to 11 days; at 20 to 28 weeks, the variation is up to 14 days; and at 29 to 40 weeks, the variation can be up to 21 days. The length of the calcified fetal femur is often measured and used in validating BPD measurements or used alone in circumstances where BPD cannot be measured (e.g., deeply engaged fetal head) or is inaccurate (e.g., hydrocephalus).

II. **PRENATAL DIAGNOSIS OF FETAL DISEASE** continues to improve. The genetic or developmental basis for many disorders is emerging, along with increased test accuracy. Two types of tests are available: screening tests and diagnostic procedures. Screening tests, such as a sample of the mother's blood or an ultrasonography, are safe but relatively nonspecific. A positive serum screening test, concerning family history, or a questionable ultrasonic examination may lead patient and physician to consider a diagnostic procedure. Diagnostic procedures, which necessitate obtaining a sample of fetal material, pose a small risk to both mother and fetus but can confirm or rule out the disorder in question.

   A. Screening by maternal serum analysis during pregnancy individualizes a woman's risk of carrying a fetus with a neural tube defect (NTD) or an aneuploidy such as trisomy 21 (Down syndrome) or trisomy 18 (Edward syndrome).

      1. Maternal serum alpha-fetoprotein (MSAFP) measurement between 15 and 22 weeks' gestation screens for NTDs. MSAFP elevated above 2.5 multiples of the median for gestation age occurs in 70% to 85% of fetuses with open spina bifida and 95% of fetuses with anencephaly. In half of the women with elevated levels, ultrasonic examination reveals another cause, most commonly an error in gestational age estimate. Ultrasonography will often detect an NTD if present.

      2. MSAFP/triple panel/quad panel. Low levels of MSAFP are associated with chromosomal abnormalities. Altered levels of human chorionic gonadotropin (hCG), unconjugated estriol (UE3), and inhibin are also associated with fetal chromosomal abnormalities. On average, in a pregnancy with a fetus with trisomy 21, hCG levels are higher than expected and UE3 levels are decreased. A serum panel in combination with maternal age can estimate the risk of trisomy 21 for an individual woman. For women younger than 35 years, 5% will have a positive serum screen, but the majority (98%) will not have a fetus with aneuploidy. However, only approximately 70% of fetuses with trisomy 21 will have a "positive" maternal triple screen (MSAFP, hCG, UE3) compared with 80% with a positive quad screen (MSAFP, hCG, UE3, inhibin).

3. **First trimester serum screening.** Maternal levels of two analytes, pregnancy-associated plasma protein-A (PAPP-A) and hCG (either free or total) are altered in pregnancies with an aneuploid conception, especially trisomy 21. Similar to second trimester serum screening, these values can individualize a woman's risk of pregnancy complicated by aneuploidy. However, these tests need to be drawn early in pregnancy (optimally at 9–10 weeks) and even if abnormal, detect less than half of the fetuses with trisomy 21.

4. **First trimester nuchal lucency screening.** Ultrasonographic assessment of the fluid collected at the nape of the fetal neck is a sensitive marker for aneuploidy. With attention to optimization of image and quality control, studies indicate a 70% to 80% detection of aneuploidy in pregnancies with an enlarged nuchal lucency on ultrasonography. In addition, many fetuses with structural abnormalities such as cardiac defects will also have an enlarged nuchal lucency.

5. **Combined first trimester screening.** Combining two maternal serum markers and the nuchal lucency measurements in addition to the maternal age detects 80% of trisomy 21 fetuses with a low screen positive rate (5% in women younger than 35 years). Other approaches to first- and second-trimester screening that use a variety of maternal serum markers and ultrasonography findings are currently under investigation.

B. In women with a **positive family history of genetic disease,** a positive screening test, or at-risk ultrasonographic features, diagnostic tests are considered. When a significant malformation or a genetic disease is diagnosed prenatally, the information gives the obstetrician and pediatrician time to educate parents, discuss options, and establish an initial neonatal treatment plan before the infant is delivered. In some cases, treatment may be initiated *in utero* (see Chap. 8).

1. **Chorionic villus sampling (CVS).** Under ultrasonic guidance, a sample of placental tissue is obtained through a catheter placed either transcervically or transabdominally. Performed at or after 10 weeks' gestation, CVS provides the earliest possible detection of a genetically abnormal fetus through analysis of trophoblast cells. Transabdominal CVS can also be used as late as the third trimester when amniotic fluid is not available or fetal blood sampling cannot be performed. Technical improvements in ultrasonographic imaging and in the CVS procedure have brought the pregnancy loss rate very close to the loss rate after second-trimester amniocentesis, 0.5 to 1.0%. The possible complications of amniocentesis and CVS are similar. CVS, if performed before 10 weeks of gestation, can be associated with an increased risk of fetal limb-reduction defects and oromandibular malformations.

    a. Direct preparations of rapidly dividing cytotrophoblasts can be prepared, making a full karyotype analysis available in 2 days. Although direct preparations minimize maternal cell contamination, most centers also analyze cultured trophoblast cells, which are embryologically closer to the fetus. This procedure takes an additional 8 to 12 days.

    b. In approximately 2% of CVS samples, both karyotypically normal and abnormal cells are identified. Because CVS-acquired cells reflect placental constitution, in these cases amniocentesis is typically performed as a follow-up study to analyze fetal cells. Approximately one-third of CVS mosaicisms are confirmed in the fetus through amniocentesis.

2. **Amniocentesis.** Amniotic fluid is removed from around the fetus through a needle guided by ultrasonic images. The removed amniotic fluid (~20 mL) is replaced by the fetus within 24 hours. Amniocentesis can technically be performed as early as 10 to 14 weeks' gestation, although early amniocentesis (<13 weeks) is associated with a pregnancy loss rate of 1% to 2%, and an increased incidence of clubfoot. Loss of the pregnancy following an ultrasonograph-guided second-trimester amniocentesis (16–20 weeks) occurs

V. ASSESSMENT OF FETAL WELL-BEING. Acute compromise is detected by studies that assess fetal function. Some are used antepartum, whereas others are used to monitor the fetus during labor.

A. Antepartum tests generally rely on biophysical studies, which require a certain degree of fetal neurophysiologic maturity. The following tests are not used until the third trimester; fetuses may not respond appropriately earlier in gestation.

    1. Fetal movement monitoring is the simplest method of fetal assessment. The mother lies quietly for an hour and records each perceived fetal movement. Although she may not perceive all fetal movements that might be noted by ultrasonic observation, she will record enough to provide meaningful data.

    Fetuses normally have a sleep–wake cycle, and mothers generally perceive a diurnal variation in fetal activity. Active periods average 30 to 40 minutes. Periods of inactivity >1 hour are unusual in a healthy fetus and should alert the physician to the possibility of fetal compromise.

    2. The **nonstress test (NST)** is a reliable means of fetal evaluation. It is simple to perform, relatively quick, and noninvasive, with neither discomfort nor risk to mother or fetus.

    The NST is based on the principle that fetal activity results in a reflex acceleration in heart rate. The required fetal maturity is typically reached by approximately 32 weeks of gestation. Absence of these accelerations in a fetus who previously demonstrated them may indicate that hypoxia has sufficiently depressed the central nervous system to inactivate the cardiac reflex.

    The test is performed by monitoring fetal heart rate (FHR) either through a Doppler ultrasonographic device or through skin-surface electrodes on the maternal abdomen. Uterine activity is simultaneously recorded through a tocodynamometer, palpation by trained test personnel, or the patient's report. The test result may be reactive, nonreactive, or inadequate. The criteria for a reactive test are as follows: (i) heart rate between 110 and 160, (ii) normal beat-to-beat variability (5 beats/minute), and (iii) two accelerations of at least 15 beats/minute lasting for not less than 15 seconds each within a 20-minute period. A nonreactive test fails to meet the three criteria. If an adequate fetal heart tracing cannot be obtained for any reason, the test is considered inadequate.

    Statistics show that a reactive result is reassuring, with the risk of fetal demise within the week following the test at approximately 3 in 1,000. A nonreactive test is generally repeated later the same day or is followed by another test of fetal well-being.

    3. The **contraction stress test (CST)** may be used as a backup or confirmatory test when the NST is nonreactive or inadequate.

    The CST is based on the idea that uterine contractions can compromise an unhealthy fetus. The pressure generated during contractions can briefly reduce or eliminate perfusion of the intervillous space. A healthy fetoplacental unit has sufficient reserve to tolerate this short reduction in oxygen supply. Under pathologic conditions, however, respiratory reserve may be so compromised that the reduction in oxygen results in fetal hypoxia. Under hypoxic conditions, the FHR slows in a characteristic way relative to the contraction. FHR begins to decelerate 15 to 30 seconds after onset of the contraction, reaches its nadir after the peak of the contraction, and does not return to baseline until after the contraction ends. This heart-rate pattern is known as a *late deceleration* because of its relationship to the uterine contraction. Synonyms are type II deceleration or deceleration of uteroplacental insufficiency.

    Similar to the NST, the CST monitors FHR and uterine contractions. A CST is considered completed if uterine contractions have spontaneously occurred within 30 minutes, lasted 40 to 60 seconds each, and occurred at a frequency of three within a 10-minute interval. If no spontaneous contractions occur, they can be induced with intravenous oxytocin, in which case the test is called an *oxytocin challenge* test.

    A CST is positive if late decelerations are consistently seen in association with contractions. A CST is negative if at least three contractions of at

least 40 seconds each occur within a 10-minute period without associated late decelerations. A CST is suspicious if there are occasional or inconsistent late decelerations. If contractions occur more frequently than every 2 minutes or last longer than 90 seconds, the study is considered a hyperstimulated test and cannot be interpreted. An unsatisfactory test is one in which contractions cannot be stimulated or a satisfactory fetal heart-rate tracing cannot be obtained.

A negative CST is even more reassuring than a reactive NST, with the chance of fetal demise within a week of a negative CST being approximately 0.4 per 1,000. If a positive CST follows a nonreactive NST, however, the risk of stillbirth is 88 per 1,000, and the risk of neonatal mortality is also 88 per 1,000. Statistically, about one-third of patients with a positive CST will require cesarean section for persistent late decelerations in labor.

4. The **biophysical profile** combines an NST with other parameters determined by real-time ultrasonic examination. A score of 0 or 2 is assigned for the absence or presence of each of the following: a reactive NST, adequate amniotic fluid volume, fetal breathing movements, fetal activity, and normal fetal musculoskeletal tone. The total score determines the course of action. Reassuring tests (8–10) are repeated at weekly intervals, whereas less-reassuring results (4–6) are repeated later the same day. Very low scores (0–2) generally prompt delivery. The likelihood that a fetus will die *in utero* within 1 week of a reassuring test is approximately the same as that for a negative CST, which is approximately 0.6 to 0.7 per 1,000.

5. Doppler ultrasonography of **fetal umbilical artery blood flow** is a noninvasive technique to assess downstream (placental) resistance. Poorly functioning placentas with extensive vasospasm or infarction have an increased resistance to flow that is particularly noticeable in fetal diastole. Umbilical artery Doppler flow velocimetry may be used as part of fetal surveillance based on characteristics of the peak systolic frequency shift (S) and the end-diastolic frequency shift (D). The two commonly used indices of flow are the systolic:diastolic ratio (S/D) and the resistance index (S-D/S). Umbilical artery Doppler velocimetry measurements have been shown to improve perinatal outcome only in pregnancies with a presumptive diagnosis of IUGR and should not be used as a screening test in the general obstetric population. Absent or reversed end-diastolic flow is seen in the most extreme cases of IUGR and is associated with a high mortality rate. The use of umbilical artery Doppler velocimetry measurements, in conjunction with other tests of fetal well-being, can reduce the perinatal mortality in IUGR by almost 40%. Doppler measurements of the **middle cerebral artery** can also be used in the assessment of the fetus that is at risk for IUGR and anemia.

B. **Intrapartum assessment of fetal well-being** is important in the management of labor.

1. **Continuous electronic fetal monitoring** is widely used despite the fact that it has not been shown to reduce perinatal mortality or asphyxia relative to auscultation by trained personnel but has increased the incidence of operative delivery. When used, the monitors simultaneously record FHR and uterine activity for ongoing evaluation.

a. The **fetal heart rate (FHR)** can be monitored in one of three ways. The noninvasive methods are ultrasonic monitoring and surface-electrode monitoring from the maternal abdomen. The most accurate but invasive method is to place a small electrode into the skin of the fetal presenting part to record the fetal electrocardiogram directly. Placement requires rupture of the fetal membranes. When the electrode is properly placed, it is associated with a very low risk of fetal injury. Approximately 4% of monitored babies develop a mild infection at the electrode site, and most respond to local cleansing.

b. **Uterine activity** can also be recorded either indirectly or directly. A tocodynamometer can be strapped to the maternal abdomen to record the timing and duration of contractions as well as crude relative intensity. When a

more precise evaluation is needed, an intrauterine pressure catheter can be inserted following rupture of the fetal membranes to directly and quantitatively record contraction pressure. Invasive monitoring is associated with an increased incidence of chorioamnionitis and postpartum maternal infection.

c. Parameters of the fetal monitoring record that are evaluated include the following:

i. Baseline heart rate is normally between 110 and 160 beats/minute. The baseline must be apparent for a minimum of 2 minutes in any 10-minute segment and does not include episodic changes, periods of marked FHR variability or segments of baseline that differ by more than 25 bpm. Baseline fetal bradycardia, defined as a FHR <110 bpm may result from congenital heart block associated with congenital heart malformation or maternal systemic lupus erythematosus. Baseline tachycardia, defined as an FHR >160 bpm, may result from a fetal dysrhythmia, hyperthyroidsim, maternal fever, or chorioamnionitis.

ii. Beat-to-beat variability is recorded from a calculation of each RR interval. The autonomic nervous system of a healthy, awake term fetus constantly varies the heart rate from beat to beat by approximately 5 to 25 beats/minute. Reduced beat-to-beat variability may result from depression of the fetal central nervous system due to fetal immaturity, hypoxia, fetal sleep, or specific maternal medications such as narcotics, sedatives, β-blockers and intravenous magnesium sulfate.

iii. Accelerations of the FHR are reassuring, as they are during an NST.

iv. Decelerations of the FHR may be benign or indicative of fetal compromise depending on their characteristic shape and timing in relation to uterine contractions.

  a) Early decelerations are symmetric in shape and closely mirror uterine contractions in time of onset, duration, and termination. They are benign and usually accompany good beat-to-beat variability. These decelerations are more commonly seen in active labor when the fetal head is compressed in the pelvis, resulting in a parasympathetic effect.

  b) Late decelerations are visually apparent decreases in the FHR in association with uterine contractions. The onset, nadir, and recovery of the deceleration occur after the beginning, peak, and end of the contraction, respectively. A fall in the heart rate of only 10 to 20 beats/minute below baseline (even if still within the range of 110–160) is significant. Late decelerations are the result of uteroplacental insufficiency and possible fetal hypoxia. As the uteroplacental insufficiency/hypoxia worsens, (i) beat-to-beat variability will be lost, (ii) decelerations will last longer, (iii) they will begin sooner following the onset of a contraction, (iv) they will take longer to return to baseline, and (v) the rate to which the fetal heart slows will be lower. Repetitive late decelerations demand action.

  c) Variable decelerations vary in their shape and in their timing relative to contractions. Usually they result from fetal umbilical cord compression. Variable decelerations are a cause for concern if they are severe (down to a rate of 60 beats/minute or lasting for 60 seconds or longer, or both), associated with poor beat-to-beat variability, or mixed with late decelerations. Umbilical cord compression secondary to a low amniotic fluid volume (oligohydramnios) may be alleviated by amnioinfusion of saline into the uterine cavity during labor.

2. A **fetal scalp blood sample for blood gas** analysis may be obtained to confirm or dismiss suspicion of fetal hypoxia. An intrapartum scalp pH above 7.20 with a base deficit <6 mmol/L is normal. Many obstetric units have replaced fetal scalp blood sampling with noninvasive techniques to assess fetal status. FHR accelerations in response to mechanical stimulation of the fetal scalp or to vibroacoustic stimulation are reassuring.

Suggested Readings

American College of Obstetricians and Gynecologists (ACOG). *ACOG practice bulletin no. 62: intrapartum fetal heart rate monitoring.* Washington, DC: American College of Obstetricians and Gynecologists, 2005.

Creasy RK, Resnik R, eds. *Maternal–fetal medicine: principles and practice*, 4th ed. Philadelphia: WB Saunders, 1999.

Hay WW Jr, Catz CS, Grave GD, et al. Fetal growth: its regulation and disorders. *Pediatrics* 1997;99:585.

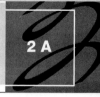

DIABETES MELLITUS

Aviva Lee-Parritz and John P. Cloherty

2 A

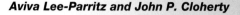

I. DIABETES AND PREGNANCY OUTCOME. Improved management of diabetes mellitus and advances in obstetrics, such as ultrasonography and measurement of fetal lung maturity (FLM), have reduced the incidence of adverse perinatal outcome in infants of diabetic mothers (IDMs). With appropriate management, women with good glycemic control and minimal microvascular disease can expect pregnancy outcomes comparable to the general population. Women with advanced microvascular disease, such as hypertension, nephropathy, and retinopathy, have a 25% risk of preterm delivery as a result of worsening maternal condition or preeclampsia. Pregnancy does not have a significant impact on the progression of diabetes. In women who begin pregnancy with microvascular disease, diabetes often worsens, but in most the levels return to baseline. Preconception glucose control may reduce the rate of complications to as low as that seen in the general population.

II. DIABETES IN PREGNANCY

A. General principles

1. Definition. Diabetes that antedates the pregnancy is rated according to the length of disease and presence of vascular complications using the White classification (see Table 2A.1). Gestational diabetes mellitus (GDM) is defined as carbohydrate intolerance of variable severity first diagnosed during pregnancy, and it affects 3% of pregnancies.

2. Epidemiology. Approximately 3% to 5% of patients with GDM actually have underlying type 1 or type 2 diabetes, but pregnancy is the first opportunity for testing. Risk factors for GDM include advanced maternal age, multifetal gestation, increased body mass index, and strong family history of diabetes. Certain ethnic groups, such as Native Americans, southeast Asians, and African Americans, have an increased risk of developing GDM.

3. Pathophysiology. In the first half of pregnancy, as a result of nausea and vomiting, **hypoglycemia** is more common than **hyperglycemia**. Hypoglycemia, followed by hyperglycemia from counter-regulatory hormones, can complicate diabetic control. Maternal hyperglycemia leads to fetal hyperglycemia and fetal hyperinsulinemia, which results in fetal overgrowth. Gastroparesis from long-standing diabetes may be a factor as well. There does not appear to be a direct relation between hypoglycemia alone and adverse perinatal outcome. Throughout pregnancy, **insulin requirements** increase because of placental hormones that antagonize the action of insulin. This is most prominent in the mid–third trimester and requires intensive blood glucose monitoring and frequent adjustment of insulin dosage.

B. Diagnosis. GDM is typically diagnosed during the third trimester of pregnancy and is classified as either diet-controlled (White class A1) or insulin-requiring (White class A2).

1. Differential diagnosis

a. Ketoacidosis is an uncommon complication during pregnancy. However, ketoacidosis carries a 50% risk of fetal death, especially if it occurs before the third trimester. Ketoacidosis can be present in the setting of even mild hyperglycemia (200 mg/dL) and should be excluded in any patient who presents with hyperglycemia or symptoms consistent with ketoacidosis.

b. Stillbirth remains an uncommon complication of diabetes in pregnancy. It is most often associated with poor glycemic control, fetal anomalies, severe

TABLE 2A.1	White Classification of Maternal Diabetes (Revised*)
Gestational diabetes (GD):	Diabetes not known to be present before pregnancy
	Abnormal glucose tolerance test in pregnancy
GD diet	Euglycemia maintained by diet alone
GD insulin	Diet alone insufficient; insulin required
Class A:	Chemical diabetes; glucose intolerance before pregnancy; treated by diet alone; rarely seen
	Prediabetes; history of large babies >4 kg or unexplained stillbirths after 28 weeks
Class B:	Insulin-dependent; onset after 20 years of age; duration <10 years
Class C:	C_1: Onset at 10–19 years of age
	C_2: Duration 10–19 years
Class D:	D_1: Onset before 10 years of age
	D_2: Duration 20 years
	D_3: Calcification of vessels of the leg (macrovascular disease)
	D_4: Benign retinopathy (microvascular disease)
	D_5: Hypertension (not preeclampsia)
Class F:	Nephropathy with >500 mg per day of proteinuria
Class R:	Proliferative retinopathy or vitreous hemorrhage
Class RF:	Criteria for both classes R and F coexist
Class G:	Many reproductive failures
Class H:	Clinical evidence of arteriosclerotic heart disease
Class T:	Prior renal transplantation

Note: All classes below A require insulin. Classes R, F, RF, H, and T have no criteria for age of onset or duration of disease but usually occur in long-term diabetes.
Modified from Hare JW. Gestational diabetes. In: *Diabetes complicating pregnancy: the Joslin clinic method.* New York: Alan R. Liss, 1989.

vasculopathy, and intrauterine growth restriction (IUGR), as well as severe preeclampsia. Shoulder dystocia that cannot be resolved can also result in fetal death.

   c. Polyhydramnios is not an uncommon finding in pregnancies complicated by diabetes. It may be secondary to osmotic diuresis from fetal hyperglycemia. Careful ultrasonographic examination is required to rule out structural anomalies, such as esophageal atresia, as an etiology, when polyhydramnios is present.

   d. Severe maternal vasculopathy especially nephropathy and hypertension, is associated with uteroplacental insufficiency, which can result in IUGR, fetal intolerance of labor, and neonatal complications.

III. MANAGEMENT OF DIABETES DURING PREGNANCY

   A. General principles. Management of type 1 or type 2 diabetes during pregnancy begins before conception. Tight glucose control is paramount during the periconceptional period and throughout pregnancy. Such control requires coordinated care between endocrinologists, maternal–fetal medicine specialists, diabetes nurse educators, and nutritionists. Preconception glycemic control has been shown to decrease the risk of congenital anomalies to close to that of the general population. However, <30% of pregnancies are planned. Physicians should discuss pregnancy planning or recommend contraception for all diabetic women of childbearing age until glycemic control is optimized.

B. Diagnosis. Most women are screened for GDM between 24 and 28 weeks' gestation by a 50-g, 1-hour glucose challenge. A positive result is a blood glucose equal to or greater than 140 mg/dL. The diagnosis of GDM is made by two or more elevated values on a 100-g oral glucose tolerance test. Uncontrolled GDM can lead to fetal macrosomia and concomitant risk of fetal injury at delivery. GDM shares many features with type 2 diabetes. Women diagnosed with GDM have a 50% lifetime risk of developing overt type 2 diabetes.

1. **Testing (first trimester)**
   a. **Measurement of glycosylated hemoglobin** in the first trimester can give a risk assessment for congenital anomalies by reflecting ambient glucose concentrations during the period of organogenesis.
   b. **Accurate dating of the pregnancy** is obtained by ultrasonography.
   c. **Ophthalmologic examination** is mandatory, because retinopathy may progress as a result of the rapid normalization of glucose concentration in the first trimester. Women with retinopathy need periodic examinations throughout pregnancy, and they are candidates for laser photocoagulation as indicated.
   d. **Renal function** is assessed by 24-hour urine collection for protein excretion and creatinine clearance. Patients with recent diagnosis of diabetes can have screening of renal function with urine microalbumin, followed by a 24-hour collection if abnormal.
   e. **Thyroid function** should be evaluated.

2. **Testing (second trimester)**
   a. **Maternal serum screening** for neural tube defects and Down syndrome screening is performed between 15 and 19 weeks' gestation. (Serum screening and nuchal translucency scanning for Down syndrome can also be performed in the first trimester.)
   b. All patients undergo a thorough **ultrasonography survey,** including fetal echocardiography for structural anomalies.
   c. Women older than 35 years of age or with other risk factors for fetal aneuploidy are offered **chorionic villus sampling** or **amniocentesis** for karyotyping.

3. **Testing (third trimester)**
   a. **Ultrasonographic examinations** are performed periodically through the third trimester for fetal growth measurement.
   b. **Weekly fetal surveillance** using nonstress testing or biophysical profiles are implemented between 28 and 32 weeks' gestation, depending on glycemic control and other complications (see Chap. 1).

C. Treatment.

Strict **diabetic control** is achieved with nutritional modification and insulin therapy, with the traditional goals of fasting glucose concentration <95 mg/dL and postprandial values <140 mg/dL for 1 hour and 120 mg/dL for 2 hours. Recent data have suggested that in pregnant women euglycemia may be even lower, with fasting glucose levels in the 60 mg/dL range and postmeal glucose levels <105 mg/dL. In addition, the oral hypoglycemic agent glyburide has been shown to be effective in the management of GDM, but it remains untested in pregestational diabetes.

IV. LABOR AND DELIVERY IN DIABETES

A. General principles. The **risk of preterm labor** is not increased in patients with diabetes, although the risk of iatrogenic preterm delivery is increased for patients with microvascular disease as a result of IUGR, nonreassuring fetal testing, and maternal hypertension. Antenatal corticosteroids for induction of FLM should be employed for the usual obstetric indications. Corticosteroids can cause temporary hyperglycemia; therefore, patients may need to be managed with continuous intravenous (IV) insulin infusions until the effect of the steroids wear off. **Delivery is planned** for 39 to 40 weeks, unless other pregnancy complications dictate earlier delivery. Elective delivery after 39 weeks does not require FLM testing. Nonemergent delivery before 39 weeks requires documentation of FLM testing

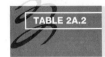

TABLE 2A.2 Lecithin-Sphingomyelin Ratio, Saturated Phosphatidylcholine Level, and Respiratory Distress Syndrome in Infants of Diabetic Mothers at the Boston Hospital for Women during 1977–1980

SPC level (mg/dL)	L/S ratio			Mild, moderate, or severe RDS/total
	<2.0:1.0	2.0–3.4:1	≥3.5:1.0	
Not done	0/1	0/12	0/13	0/26 (0%)
≤500	6/6	1/9	1/2	8/17 (47%)
501–1,000	0/2	3/20	1/15	4/37 (11%)
>1,000	0/0	2/22	0/142	2/164 (1.2%)
Total (RDS)	6/9 (67%)	6/63 (10%)	2/172 (1.2%)	14/244 (5.7%)

SPC = saturated phosphatidylcholine; L/S = lecithin/sphingomyelin; RDS = respiratory distress syndrome.

using the lecithin-sphingomyelin (L/S) ratio greater than 3.5:1, positive Amniostat (phosphatidyglycerol present), saturated phosphatidylcholine (SPC) greater than 1,000 µg/dL, or mature FLM (see Table 2A.2 and Fig. 2A.1). Emergent delivery should be carried out without FLM testing. **Route of delivery** is determined by ultrasonography-estimated fetal weight, maternal and fetal conditions, and previous obstetric history. The ultrasonography-estimated weight at which an elective cesarean delivery is recommended is a controversial issue.

B. Treatment. Blood glucose concentration is tightly controlled during labor and delivery. If an induction of labor is planned, patients are instructed to take one-half of their usual intermediate-acting insulin on the morning of induction. During spontaneous or induced labor, blood glucose concentration is measured

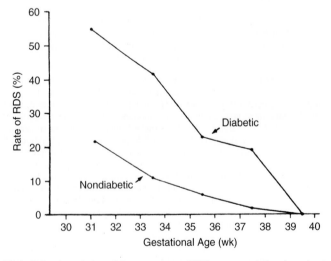

Figure 2A.1. Rate of respiratory distress syndrome (RDS) versus gestational age in nondiabetic and diabetic pregnancies at the Boston Hospital for Women from 1958 TO 1968. (Reprinted with permission from Robert M. Association between maternal diabetes and the respiratory distress syndrome in the newborn. *N Engl J Med* 1976;294:357.)

every 1 to 2 hours. Blood glucose concentration higher than 120 to 140 mg/dL is treated with an infusion of IV short-acting insulin. IV insulin is very short acting, allowing for quick response to changes in glucose concentration. Active labor may also be associated with hypoglycemia, because the contracting uterus uses circulating metabolic fuels. **Continuous fetal monitoring** is mandatory during labor. Cesarean delivery is performed for obstetric indications. The risk of cesarean section for obstetric complications is approximately 50%. Patients with **advanced microvascular disease** are at increased risk of cesarean delivery because of the increased incidence of IUGR, preeclampsia, and nonreassuring fetal status. A history of retinopathy that has been treated in the past is not necessarily an indication for cesarean delivery. Patients with active proliferative retinopathy that is unstable or active hemorrhage may benefit from elective cesarean delivery. **Postpartum,** patients are at increased risk of hypoglycemia, especially in the postoperative setting with minimal oral intake. Patients with pregestational diabetes may also experience a "honeymoon" period immediately after delivery, with greatly reduced insulin requirements that can last up to several days. Insulin is adjusted to approximate the prepregnancy dose. For women with type 2 diabetes, the use of oral hypoglycemic agent metformin is compatible with breast-feeding, and insulin management may need to be continued in some patients.

V. EVALUATION OF INFANTS OF DIABETIC MOTHERS (IDMs)
   A. General principles. The evaluation of the infant begins **before actual delivery**. If pulmonary maturity is not certain, amniotic fluid can be obtained before delivery through amniocentesis. Fluid may be evaluated by the shake test, L/S ratio, FLM testing, or saturated SPC content (see IV.A. and Chap. 24).
   B. Treatment
      1. After the infant is born, assessment is made on the basis of Apgar scores to determine the need for any resuscitative efforts (see Chap. 4). The infant should be dried and placed under a warmer. The airway is bulb suctioned for mucus, but the stomach is not aspirated because of the risk of reflex bradycardia and apnea from pharyngeal stimulation in the first 5 minutes of life. A screening physical examination for the presence of major congenital anomalies should be performed, and the placenta should be examined. Glucose level and pH may be determined on cord blood. In the nursery, **supportive care** should be given while a continuous evaluation of the infant is made. This includes providing warmth, suction, and oxygen as needed while checking vital signs (e.g., heart and respiratory rates, temperature, perfusion, color, and blood pressure). Cyanosis should make one consider cardiac disease, respiratory distress syndrome (RDS), transient tachypnea of the newborn, or polycythemia. An examination should be repeated for possible anomalies because of the 6% to 9% incidence of major congenital anomalies in IDMs. Special attention should be paid to the brain, heart, kidneys, and skeletal system. Reports indicate that IDMs have a 47% risk of significant hypoglycemia, 22% risk of hypocalcemia, 19% risk of hyperbilirubinemia, and a 34% risk of polycythemia; therefore, the following studies are performed:
         Blood glucose levels are checked at 1, 2, 3, 6, 12, 24, 26, and 48 hours. Glucose is measured with Chemstrip B-G (Bio-Dynamics, BMC, Indianapolis, Indiana). Readings <40 mg/dL should be checked rapidly by a clinical laboratory or by Ames eyetone instrument (Ames Company, Division of Miles Laboratories, Inc., Elkhart, Indiana). The infant is fed orally or given IV glucose by 1 hour of age (see VI. and Chap. 29A). **Hematocrit levels** are checked at 1 and 24 hours (see Chap. 26C). **Calcium levels** are checked if the infant appears jittery or is sick for any reason (see VIII.A.1 and Chap. 29). **Bilirubin levels** are checked if the infant appears jaundiced (see Chap. 18). Every effort is made to involve the parents in infant care as early as possible.

VI. HYPOGLYCEMIA IN INFANTS OF DIABETIC MOTHERS (IDMs)
   A. General principles
      1. Definition. Hypoglycemia is defined as a blood glucose level <40 mg/dL in any infant, regardless of gestational age and whether or not symptoms are present.

(Previously, we used a level of <30 mg/dL as the definition of hypoglycemia (see Chap. 29A).

2. **Epidemiology.** With <30 mg/dL as the definition, the **incidence of hypoglycemia** in IDMs is 30% to 40%. The onset is frequently within 1 to 2 hours of age and is most common in macrosomic infants.

3. **Pathophysiology.** The pathogenetic basis of **neonatal hypoglycemia in IDMs** is explained by the Pederson maternal hyperglycemia–fetal hyperinsulinism hypothesis. The correlation among fetal macrosomia, elevated HbA_1 in maternal and cord blood, and neonatal hypoglycemia, as well as between elevated cord blood C-peptide or immunoreactive insulin levels and hypoglycemia, suggests that control of maternal blood sugar in the last trimester may decrease the incidence of neonatal hypoglycemia in IDMs. Mothers should not receive large doses of glucose before or at delivery, because this may stimulate an insulin response in the hyperinsulinemic offspring. We attempt to keep maternal glucose level at delivery at approximately 120 mg/dL.

4. Hypoglycemia in small-for-gestational-age (SGA) infants born to mothers with vascular disease may be due to inadequate glycogen stores; it may also present later (e.g., at 12–24 hours of age). Other factors that may cause hypoglycemia in IDMs are decreased catecholamine and glucagon secretion as well as inadequate substrate mobilization (diminished hepatic glucose production and decreased oxygenation of fatty acids).

B. **Diagnosis**

1. **Clinical presentation. Symptomatic, hypoglycemic IDMs** are usually quiet and lethargic rather than jittery. Symptoms such as apnea, tachypnea, respiratory distress, hypotonia, shock, cyanosis, and seizures may occur. If symptoms are present, the infant is probably at greater risk for sequelae. The significance of asymptomatic hypoglycemia is unclear, but conservative management to maintain the blood sugar level in the normal range (>40 mg/dL) appears to be indicated.

2. **Laboratory studies.** Our neonatal protocol is explained in V.B.1. The blood glucose level is measured more often if the infant is symptomatic or has had a low level previously. The blood glucose level is also measured to see the response to therapy.

C. **Treatment**

1. **Asymptomatic infants with normal blood glucose levels.** In our nursery, we begin **feeding "well" IDMs** by bottle or gavage with dextrose 10% (5 mL/kg body weight) at or before 1 hour of age. Infants weighing <2 kg should have parenteral dextrose starting in the first hour of life. Larger infants can be fed hourly for three or four feedings until the blood sugar determinations are stable; infants should be switched to formula feeding (20 cal/oz) if the feedings are 2 hours apart or more. This schedule prevents some of the insulin release associated with oral feeding of pure glucose. The feedings can then be given every 2 hours and later every 3 hours and as the interval between feedings increases, the volume is increased. If by 2 hours of age the blood glucose level is <40 mg/dL despite feeding, or if feedings are not tolerated, as indicated by large volumes retained in the stomach, **parenteral treatment** is necessary.

2. **Symptomatic infants, infants with a low blood glucose level after enteral feeding, sick infants, or infants <2 kg in weight.** The basic treatment element is **IV glucose administration** through reliable access. Administration is usually by **peripheral IV catheter**. Peripheral lines may be difficult to place in obese IDMs, and sudden interruption of the infusion may cause a reactive hypoglycemia in such hyperinsulinemic infants. Rarely, in emergency situations, we have used umbilical venous catheters in the inferior vena cava until a stable peripheral line is placed. Specific treatment is determined by the infant's condition. If the infant is in **severe distress** (e.g., seizure or respiratory compromise), 0.5 to 1.0 g of glucose per kg of body weight is given by an IV push of 2 to 4 mL/kg 25% dextrose in water (D/W) at a rate of

1 mL/min/kg. For example, a 4-kg infant would receive 8 to 16 mL of 25% D/W over 2 to 4 minutes. This is followed by a continuous infusion at a rate of 4 to 8 mg of glucose per kg of body weight per minute. The concentration of dextrose in the IV fluid depends on the total daily fluid requirement. For example, on day 1, the usual fluid intake is 65 mL/kg, or 0.045 mL/kg/minute. Therefore, 10% D/W would provide 4.5 mg of glucose per kg per minute, and 15% D/W would provide 6.75 mg of glucose per kg per minute. In other words, 10% D/W at a standard IV fluid maintenance rate usually supplies sufficient glucose to raise the blood glucose level above 40 mg/dL. However, the concentration of dextrose and the infusion rates are increased as necessary to maintain the blood glucose level in the normal range (Fig. 29A.1). The **usual method** in an infant not in severe distress is to give 200 mg of glucose per kg of body weight (2 mL/kg 10% dextrose) over 2 to 3 minutes. This is followed by a maintenance drip of 6 to 8 mg of glucose per kg per minute (10% dextrose at 80 to 120 mL/kg/day) (Fig 29-1). **If the infant is asymptomatic** but has a blood glucose level in the hypoglycemic range, an initial push of concentrated sugar should not be given in order to avoid a hyperinsulinemic response. Rather, an initial infusion of 5 to 10 mL of 10% D/W at 1 mL/min is followed by continuous infusion at 4 to 8 mg/kg per minute. Blood glucose levels must be carefully monitored at frequent intervals after beginning IV glucose infusions, both to be certain of adequate treatment of the hypoglycemia and to avoid hyperglycemia and the risk of osmotic diuresis and dehydration. Parenteral sugar should never be abruptly discontinued, because of the risk of a **reactive hypoglycemia.** As oral feeding progresses, the rate of the infusion can be decreased gradually, and the concentration of glucose infused can be reduced by using 5% D/W. It is vital to measure blood glucose levels during tapering of the IV infusion. **In difficult cases,** hydrocortisone (5 mg/kg/day intramuscularly in two divided doses) has occasionally been helpful. In our experience, other drugs (epinephrine, diazoxide, or growth hormone) have not been necessary in the treatment of the hypoglycemia of IDMs. In a hypoglycemic infant, **if difficulty is experienced in achieving vascular access,** we may administer crystalline glucagon intramuscularly or subcutaneously (300 mg/kg to a maximum dose of 1.0 mg), which causes a rapid rise in blood glucose levels in large IDMs who have good glycogen stores; the response is not reliable in smaller infants of maternal classes D, E, F, and others. The rise in blood glucose may last 2 to 3 hours and is useful until parenteral glucose can be started. This method is rarely used. The hypoglycemia of most IDMs usually responds to the treatment mentioned earlier and resolves by 24 hours. **Persistent hypoglycemia** is usually due to a continued hyperinsulinemic state and may be manifested by glucose use of >8 mg of glucose/kg/minute (Fig. 29A.1). Efforts should be made to decrease islet cell stimulation (e.g., keeping blood glucose adequate but not high, moving a high umbilical artery line to a low line). **If the hypoglycemia lasts >7 days,** consider other etiologies (see Chap. 29A).

VII. RESPIRATORY DISTRESS IN INFANTS OF DIABETIC MOTHERS (IDMs)
  A. General principles
    1. Epidemiology. With changes in pregnancy management resulting in longer gestations and more vaginal deliveries, the incidence of RDS in IDMs has fallen from 28% during 1950 to 1960 to 4% in 1990, with the major difference in the incidence of RDS between diabetics and nondiabetics occurring in infants born before 37 weeks' gestation. Most of the deaths from RDS also occur at <35 weeks' gestation in infants who were delivered by cesarean section because of fetal distress or maternal indications.
    2. Etiology. Besides RDS, causes of respiratory distress are cardiac or pulmonary anomalies (4%), hypertrophic cardiomyopathy, transient tachypnea of the newborn, and polycythemia. Pneumonia, pneumothorax, and diaphragmatic hernia should also be considered. Delayed lung maturity may occur in IDMs because hyperinsulinemia blocks cortisol induction of lung maturation.

B. Diagnosis
   1. Laboratory studies
      a. Blood gas analysis should be performed to evaluate gas exchange and the presence of right-to-left shunts.
      b. Blood cultures, with spinal-fluid examination and culture should be taken if the infant's condition permits and infection is a possibility. (See Chap. 24 for the differential diagnosis and management of respiratory disorders.)
   2. Imaging
      a. A **chest x-ray** should be viewed to evaluate aeration, presence of infiltrates, cardiac size and position, and the presence of pneumothorax or anomalies.
      b. An **electrocardiogram** and an **echocardiogram** should be taken if **hypertrophic cardiomyopathy** or **a cardiac anomaly** is thought to be present.

VIII. OTHER PROBLEMS FREQUENTLY OBSERVED IN INFANTS OF DIABETIC MOTHERS (IDMs)
   A. Congenital anomalies. Congenital anomalies occur more frequently in IDMs than in infants of nondiabetic mothers. As mortality from other causes such as prematurity, stillbirth, asphyxia, and RDS falls, malformations become the major cause of perinatal mortality in IDMs. Infants of diabetic fathers show the same incidence of anomalies as the normal population; therefore, the maternal environment may be the important factor. Approximately 6% to 10% of pregnancies complicated with diabetes demonstrate a structural abnormality directly related to glycemic control in the period of organogenesis, compared with a usual major anomaly rate of 2% for the general population (see Chap. 8). The most common fetal structural defects associated with maternal diabetes are cardiac malformations, neural tube defects, renal agenesis, and skeletal malformations. Situs inversus also occurs. The central nervous system (anencephaly, meningocele syndrome, holoprosencephaly) and cardiac anomalies make up two-thirds of the malformations seen in IDMs. Although there is a general increase in the anomaly rate in IDMs, no anomaly is specific for IDMs, although half of all cases of caudal regression syndrome (sacral agenesis) are seen in IDMs. There have been several studies correlating poor metabolic control of diabetes in early pregnancy with **malformations in the IDMs.** Among the more recent studies, that performed by the Joslin Clinic showed a relation between elevated HbA$_1$ in the first trimester and major anomalies in IDMs. The data are consistent with the hypothesis that poor metabolic control of maternal diabetes in the first trimester is associated with an increased risk of major congenital malformations.
   1. Hypocalcemia (see Chap. 29B). This condition, which is found in 22% of IDMs, is not related to hypoglycemia. The nadir in calcium levels occurs between 24 and 72 hours, and 20% to 50% of IDMs become hypocalcemic, as defined by a total serum calcium level <7 mg/dL. Hypocalcemia in IDMs may be caused by a delay in the usual postnatal rise of parathyroid hormone or vitamin D antagonism at the intestinal level from elevated cortisol and hyperphosphatemia that is due to tissue catabolism.
      There is no evidence of elevated serum calcitonin concentrations in these infants in the absence of prematurity or asphyxia. Other causes of hypocalcemia, such as asphyxia and prematurity, may be seen in IDMs. Hypocalcemia in "well" IDMs usually resolves without treatment, and we do not routinely measure serum calcium levels in asymptomatic IDMs. Infants who are sick for any reason—prematurity, asphyxia, infection, respiratory distress—or IDMs with symptoms of lethargy, jitteriness, or seizures that do not respond to glucose should have their serum calcium levels measured. If an infant has symptoms that coexist with a low calcium level, has an illness that delays onset of calcium regulation, or is unable to feed, treatment with calcium may be necessary (see Chap. 29B). Hypomagnesemia should be considered in hypocalcemia in IDMs because the hypocalcemia may not respond until the hypomagnesemia is treated.

2. **Polycythemia** (see Chap. 26C). This condition is common in IDMs. It may be due to reduced oxygen delivery secondary to elevated HbA_1 in both maternal and fetal serum. In SGA infants, polycythemia may be related to placental insufficiency, causing fetal hypoxia and increased erythropoietin. If fetal distress has occurred, there may be a shift of blood from the placenta to the fetus.

3. **Jaundice.** Hyperbilirubinemia (bilirubin >15 mg/dL) is seen with increased frequency in IDMs. Bilirubin production is increased in IDMs as compared with infants of nondiabetic mothers. Bilirubin levels higher than 16 mg/dL were seen in 19% of IDMs at the Brigham and Women's Hospital. Mild hemolysis is compensated for but may cause increased bilirubin production. Insulin causes increased erythropoietin. When measurement of carboxyhemoglobin production is used as an indicator of increased heme turnover, IDMs are found to have increased production as compared with controls. There may be decreased erythrocyte life span because of less deformable cell membranes, possibly related to glycosylation of the erythrocyte cell membrane. Other factors that may account for jaundice are prematurity, impairment of the hepatic conjugation of bilirubin, and an increased enterohepatic circulation of bilirubin as a result of poor feeding. Infants born to well-controlled diabetic mothers have fewer problems with hyperbilirubinemia. The increasing gestational age of IDMs at delivery has contributed to the decreased incidence of hyperbilirubinemia. Hyperbilirubinemia in IDMs is diagnosed and treated as in any other infant (see Chap. 18).

4. **Poor feeding.** This condition is a major problem in IDMs, occurring in 37% of a series of 150 IDMs at the Brigham and Women's Hospital. In our most recent experience (unpublished), it was found in 17% of infants born to mothers with class B to class D diabetes and in 31% of infants born to women with class F diabetes. Infants born to women with class F diabetes are often preterm. There was no difference in the incidence of poor feeding in large-for-gestational-age infants versus appropriate-for-gestational-age infants, and there was no relation to polyhydramnios.

   Sometimes poor feeding is related to prematurity, respiratory distress, or other problems; however, it is often present in the absence of other problems. Poor feeding is a major reason for prolonged hospital stays and parent–infant separation.

5. **Macrosomia.** Macrosomia is defined as a birth weight higher than the 90th percentile or a weight of >4,000 g. The incidence of macrosomia was 28% at the Brigham and Women's Hospital from 1983 to 1984. Macrosomia is not usually seen in infants born to women with class F diabetes. Macrosomia may be linked with an increased incidence of primary cesarean section or obstetric trauma, such as fractured clavicle, Erb palsy, or phrenic nerve palsy as a result of shoulder dystocia. Associations have been found between macrosomia and the following:
   a. Third-trimester elevated maternal blood sugar
   b. Hyperinsulinemia
   c. Hypoglycemia

6. **Myocardial dysfunction.** In IDMs, transient hypertrophic subaortic stenosis resulting from ventricular septal hypertrophy has been reported. Infants may present with heart failure, poor cardiac output, and cardiomegaly. The cardiomyopathy may complicate the management of other illnesses such as RDS. The diagnosis is made using echocardiography, which shows hypertrophy of the ventricular septum, the right anterior ventricular wall, and the left posterior ventricular wall in the absence of chamber dilation. Cardiac output decreases with increasing septal thickness. Most symptoms resolve by 2 weeks of age, and septal hypertrophy resolves by 4 months. Most infants respond to supportive care. Oxygen and furosemide (Lasix) are often needed. Inotropic drugs are contraindicated unless myocardial dysfunction is seen on echocardiography. Propranolol is the most useful agent. The differential diagnosis of myocardial

dysfunction that is due to diabetic cardiomyopathy of the newborn includes the following:

a. Postasphyxial cardiomyopathy

b. Myocarditis

c. Endocardial fibroelastosis

d. Glycogen storage disease of the heart

e. Aberrant left coronary artery coming off the pulmonary artery (see Chap. 25)
There is some evidence that good diabetic control during pregnancy may reduce the incidence and severity of hypertrophic cardiomyopathy (see Chap. 25).

7. Renal vein thrombosis. Renal vein thrombosis may occur *in utero* or postpartum. Intrauterine and postnatal diagnosis may be made by ultrasonographic examination. Postnatal presentation may include hematuria, flank mass, hypertension, or embolic phenomena. Most renal vein thrombosis can be managed conservatively, allowing preservation of renal tissue (see Chaps. 26, 31, and 33).

8. Other thromboses (see Chap. 26F).

9. Small left colon syndrome. Small left colon syndrome presents as generalized abdominal distension because of inability to pass meconium. Meconium is obtained by passage of a rectal catheter. An enema performed with meglumine diatrizoate (Gastrografin) makes the diagnosis and often results in evacuation of the colon. The infant should be well hydrated before Gastrografin is used. The infant may have some difficulties with passage of stool in the first week of life, but this usually resolves after treatment with half-normal saline enemas (5 mL/kg) and glycerine suppositories. Other causes of intestinal obstruction should be considered (see Chap. 33).

IX. TOPICS OF CONCERN TO PARENTS

A. Genetics. The parents of IDMs are often concerned about the eventual development of diabetes in their children. There are conflicting data on the incidence of insulin-dependent diabetes in IDMs.

1. In type 1 diabetes, a person in the general population has a <1% chance of developing the disease. If the mother has type 1 diabetes, the risk of the offspring developing the disease is 1% to 4%. If the father has type 1 diabetes, the risk to the offspring is 10%. If both parents have the disease, the risk is approximately 20%.

2. In type 2 diabetes, the average person has a 12% to 18% chance of developing the disease. If one parent has the disease, the risk to offspring is 30%; if both parents have it, the risk is 50%to 60%.

B. Perinatal survival. Despite all problems, a diabetic woman has a 95% chance of having a healthy child if she is willing to participate in a program of pregnancy management and surveillance at an appropriate perinatal center. In a series of 215 IDMs at the Brigham and Women's Hospital from 1983 to 1984, the total perinatal mortality, from 23 weeks of gestation to 28 days postpartum, was 28 per 1,000. There was one intrauterine demise of a singleton near term.

Suggested Readings

American College of Obstetricians and Gynecologists (ACOG). ACOG practice bulletin no. 30. *Obstet Gynecol* 2001;89:525.

American Diabetes Association. Gestational diabetes mellitus. *Diabetes Care Suppl* 2002;25 (Suppl 1):S94–S96.

Buchanan TA, Metzger BE, Freinkel N, et al. Insulin sensitivity and B-cell responsiveness to glucose during late pregnancy in lean and moderately obese women with normal glucose tolerance or mild gestational diabetes. *Am J Obstet Gynecol* 1990;162: 1008.

Cloherty JP. Neonatal management. In: Brown F, ed. *Diabetes complicating pregnancy: the Joslin clinic method*, 2nd ed. New York: Wiley-Liss, 1995:169–186.

Kitzmiller JL, Gavin LA, Gin GD, et al. Preconception care of diabetes: glycemic control prevents congenital anomalies. *JAMA* 1991;265:731.

Landon MB. Diabetes in pregnancy. *Clin Perinatol* 1993;20:507.

Landon MB, Langer O, Gabbe SG, et al. Fetal surveillance in pregnancies complicated by insulin-dependent diabetes mellitus. *Am J Obstet Gynecol* 1992;167:617.

Langer O, Berkus MD, Huff RW, et al. Shoulder dystocia: should the fetus weighing >4000 grams be delivered by cesarean section? *Am J Obstet Gynecol* 1991;165:831–837.

Reece EA, Homko CJ. Infant of the diabetic mother. *Semin Perinatol* 1994;18:459.

THYROID DISORDERS
Camilia R. Martin

2 B

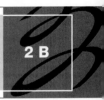

I. THYROID METABOLISM IN PREGNANCY. Multiple changes occur in maternal thyroid physiology during pregnancy.

A. Increased uptake and clearance of iodine. Increased renal glomerular filtration rate, a by-product of an enhanced hemodynamic state during pregnancy (increased cardiac output, increased stroke volume, increased heart rate, and decreased systemic vascular resistance), and increased placental transfer of iodide and iodothyronines promote accelerated iodine turnover.

B. Thyroid gland volume may enlarge in regions deficient in iodine, yet remains stable in iodine-sufficient areas (e.g., the USA).

C. Increased thyroxine-binding globulin (TBG) levels. Elevated estrogen levels lead to an increase in TBG levels. Estrogen stimulates TBG hepatic synthesis. In addition, estrogen promotes sialylation of the protein, which, in turn, increases the half-life and reduces hepatic clearance. Elevated TBG levels are evident very early in gestation and plateau midway through the pregnancy.

D. Increased total T_4 and T_3 levels. An increase in TBG results in an increase in total T_4 and T_3 levels. Free hormone concentrations, however, remain relatively unchanged. There may be a slight increase in free T_4 and T_3 early in pregnancy and then a decline to low-normal levels late in pregnancy. Throughout these changes, levels should remain within normal reference ranges and the woman should remain euthyroid.

E. Human chorionic gonadotropin (hCG) has thyrotropin(TSH)-like activity because of its structural similarity. There is a linear relationship between the rise in hCG and the rise in free T_4 levels and the fall in TSH levels. Once again, the rise in free T_4 levels to toxic ranges would be unusual.

F. There is minimal difference in the **hypothalamic–pituitary–thyroid (HPT) axis response** to thyrotropin-releasing hormone (TRH) between nonpregnant and pregnant women. First-trimester TSH response is more blunted (when free T_4 levels are the highest) compared with the second trimester; however, the TSH response is not flat, as seen in hyperthyroidism.

G. The **negative feedback control mechanisms of the HPT axis** remain intact.

H. Transplacental passage. Iodide and TRH readily cross the placenta. Transplacental passage of T_4, T_3, and rT_3 occur in limited but critical amounts. Maternal thyroid hormones are important for fetal development in the first trimester before establishment of the fetal HPT axis. Late transfer of maternal thyroid hormones is not as important to the fetus but may be neuroprotective for a fetus with congenital hypothyroidism (CH). Maternal thyroid-stimulating immunoglobulins (TSI) and thyrotropin-binding inhibitory immunoglobulins (TBII) also cross the placenta and can cause transient hyper- or hypothyroidism in the newborn. The placenta is impermeable to TSH.

II. MATERNAL HYPOTHYROIDISM. The incidence of maternal hypothyroidism is 3 in 1,000.

A. **Common causes** of hypothyroidism include autoimmune (Hashimoto) and previous treatment for hyperthyroidism that included radioiodine ablation or thyroidectomy. Less common causes include thyroiditis, external radiation, drug-induced hypothyroidism, and CH.

B. **Recognizing the typical symptoms** of hypothyroidism during pregnancy may be difficult because of the hypermetabolic state that normally occurs.

C. **Unrecognized or untreated maternal hypothyroidism** may result in an increased frequency of maternal and neonatal complications. Maternal complications include first-trimester miscarriages, preeclampsia, placental abruption, preterm delivery, and postpartum hemorrhage. Neonatal complications include intrauterine growth restriction (IUGR) and poor neurodevelopmental outcome. Treatment includes L-thyroxine replacement with the goal of maintaining TSH levels in the normal range. Thyroid function tests should be monitored every 4 weeks until this goal is achieved.

D. **Women with a prenatal diagnosis of hypothyroidism** who are appropriately treated typically deliver normal infants. Pregnant women who have primary hypothyroidism should have thyroid function tests as soon as pregnancy is confirmed and again at 6 weeks' gestation, 16 to 20 weeks' gestation, and 28 to 32 weeks' gestation. The thyroxine dose may need to be increased during pregnancy to keep TSH in the normal range and should be adjusted to normalize TSH as rapidly as possible.

E. **There is limited transfer of L-thyroxine into breast milk.** There is no contraindication to taking thyroxine while breast-feeding.

F. **In women who make TBII** placental transfer of the immunoglobulins may cause fetal hypothyroidism (VI.E.2.a.). TBII and TSI screening in the last trimester may aid in determining the risk to the fetus for altered thyroid physiology.

III. MATERNAL HYPERTHYROIDISM. Graves disease complicates 1 in 1,000 to 2,000 pregnancies.

A. **Untreated** maternal hyperthyroidism carries a significant risk to the mother and fetus. Potential maternal risks include miscarriage, pregnancy-induced hypertension, preterm delivery, congestive heart failure, thyroid storm, and placental abruption. Risks to the fetus include hyperthyroidism and IUGR.

B. **Treatment and obstetric monitoring.** Once maternal hyperthyroidism is diagnosed, prompt treatment should be commenced. Antithyroid drugs, including propylthiouracil (PTU) and methimazole (MMI), are the treatments of choice. There is some preference for PTU because of the reduced passage across the placenta and limited excretion into breast milk. In addition, small case series have suggested an association between MMI and aplasia cutis congenita, a focal scalp lesion. However, this has not been consistently proved in larger studies. β-adrenergic blocking agents may be added to aid in controlling hypermetabolic symptoms. However, long-term use should be avoided because of potential neonatal morbidities. Iodides are generally contraindicated because of secondary neonatal goiter and hypothyroidism. However, brief exposure to control hyperthyroid symptoms or to prepare for surgery seems to be well tolerated. Radioactive iodine is contraindicated, especially after the 12th week of gestation when the fetal thyroid develops iodine concentration abilities. Pregnant women with Graves disease should have regular monitoring of thyroid function and fetal well-being. The goal of treatment is to maintain free thyroxine levels in the upper third of the normal range.

C. **Thyroid function in neonates.** All fetuses of pregnant women with Graves disease should be monitored for intrauterine hyperthyroidism. Transplacental passage of TSI and TBII does occur and may be significant enough to alter neonatal thyroid function. However, neonatal hyperthyroidism occurs in only 1% to 5% of infants born to mothers with Graves disease. Fetal thyroid dysfunction is related to the duration of thyrotoxicosis in pregnancy, dosage levels of maternal antithyroid drugs, and maternal antibody levels at delivery. Measurements of TSI and TBII levels in the last trimester may be helpful in determining the risk of neonatal thyrotoxicosis. TSI values >300% or TBII values >30% of control values can be predictive of neonatal thyrotoxicosis. If values are elevated, neonates should be closely monitored for the development of thyrotoxicosis in the first 2 weeks of life.

D. Maternal medications, complications, and breast-feeding

1. **Antithyroid** drugs cross the placenta, are associated with fetal goiters (see IV.A), and are excreted into breast milk. As stated, transplacental passage of PTU and excretion into breast milk are less compared with that for MMI. Excretion into breast milk is limited and it is considered safe to breast-feed while receiving either PTU or MMI. Complications in breast-feeding newborns are rare with maternal doses <450 mg/day of PTU and <20 mg/day of MMI. Within these ranges, the infant does not require more than routine thyroid function testing if somatic and mental development are normal.

2. **Propranolol** can cause impaired responses to hypoxia, bradycardia, and hypoglycemia in the fetus. There is limited transfer of propranolol into breast milk. It is considered safe to breast-feed while taking propranolol. However, studies are lacking regarding long-term exposure.

IV. FETAL AND NEONATAL GOITER

A. PTU-induced fetal goiter can be seen, although the occurrence does not always correlate with level of maternal dosing. Transient neonatal hypothyroidism also may be evident. After delivery, neonates eliminate PTU in 2 to 4 weeks, with normal thyroid function tests obtained by 4 to 6 weeks (see Table 2B.1). Newborns with PTU-induced goiter should be treated with thyroxine for approximately 1 month. Enlarging fetal goiters in PTU-treated pregnant women may be due to either TSI-induced hyperthyroidism or PTU-induced hypothyroidism. Fetal blood sampling is diagnostic (see Chap. 1, II.B.3). Third-trimester goitrous fetal hypothyroidism has been successfully treated with weekly intra-amniotic injections of 250 to 500 mg of L-thyroxine.

B. Other forms of goiter. Neonatal goiter may be seen in inherited hypothyroidism or after maternal ingestion of iodine. The differential diagnosis includes hemangiomas or lymphangiomas. Iodine-induced goiter resolves over 2 to 3 months, with resolution accelerated by thyroxine treatment. T_4, T_3, and TSH determinations should be obtained from the infant before treatment to exclude permanent defects in T_4 synthesis.

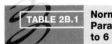

TABLE 2B.1	Normal Thyroid Function Parameters in Infants Aged 2 to 6 Weeks*

Serum constituent	Concentration
T_4	84–210 nmol/L (6.5–16.3 μg/dL)
T_3	1.5–4.6 nmol/L (100–300 ng/dL)
Free T_4[†]	12–28 pmol/L (0.9–2.2 ng/dL)
TSH	1.7–9.1 mU/L (1.7–9.1 U/mL)
TBG	160–750 nmol/L (1.0–4.5 mg/dL)
Thyroglobulin[‡]	15–375 pmol/L (10–250 ng/mL)

T_4 = thyroxine; T_3 = triiodothyronine; TSH = thyroid-stimulating hormone; TBG = thyroxine-binding globulin.
*Data from Nichols Institute reference values unless indicated otherwise.
[†]Measured by direct dialysis.
[‡]Thyroglobulin from Vulsma et al. *N Engl J Med* 1989;321:13.
Source: Fisher DA. Management of congenital hypothyroidism. *J Clin Endocrinol Metab* 1991;72:523–529.

V. NEONATAL HYPERTHYROIDISM. Neonatal hyperthyroidism is uncommon, accounting for approximately 1% of hyperthyroidism seen during childhood. Most often infants are born to mothers with Graves disease. A rare, autosome-dominant, nonimmune cause of neonatal hyperthyroidism is characterized by an activating mutation of the TSH receptor. This condition results in permanent hyperthyroidism and may require thyroid gland ablation. *Autoimmune, transient* neonatal hyperthyroidism is discussed in subsequent text.

A. Incidence. Out of infants born to mothers with Graves disease, 1% to 5% will go on to develop hyperthyroidism.

B. Pathogenesis
   1. **Altered thyroid function** results from transplacental passage of TSI and TBII. Because both stimulating and blocking antibodies are made and cross the placenta, infants may initially present with hypothyroidism or have a delay in the development of thyrotoxicosis. Initial hypothyroidism may also be present as a result of the transplacental passage of PTU or MMI.
   2. **Neonatal hyperthyroidism** usually occurs with active maternal disease. However, hyperthyroidism may also occur with inactive maternal disease because of the continued presence of thyroid autoantibodies.
   3. Measurements of maternal TSI and TBII levels may be predictive for the likelihood of **neonatal thyrotoxicosis.** Maternal TSI activity >300% or TBII levels >30% of control values are likely to result in thyrotoxicosis. Symptoms may persist for 2 to 4 months.

C. Clinical findings. Thyrotoxic newborns may present within 24 hours to 6 weeks of life. Usual clinical manifestations include microcephaly, low birth weight, prematurity, irritability, fever, tachycardia, heart failure, goiter, vomiting, diarrhea, hepatosplenomegaly, failure to thrive despite hyperphagia, flushing, hypertension, exophthalmos, and craniosynostosis. Arrhythmias and cardiac failure may be fatal. Measurements of TSI, TBII, T_4, free T_4, and TSH can be diagnostic.

D. Treatment.
   1. **In severe cases, PTU** (5–10 mg/kg/day in three divided doses) or **MMI** (0.5–1 mg/kg/day in three divided doses) may be used. If there is no response in 36 to 48 hours, the drug dose is increased by 50%.
   2. An **iodine preparation** such as Lugol (or strong iodine) solution containing 4.5 to 5.5 g of elemental iodine and 9.5 to 10.5 g of potassium iodide per dL is given in a dose of 1 drop three times a day. If there is no response in 48 hours, the dose is increased by 25% per day until control is obtained. Iopanoic acid (Telepaque) or sodium ipodate (Oragrafin) at 600 mg/m^2/day may be preferable to iodine solutions. Sodium ipodate decreases serum T_3 by 50% within 24 hours and appears to be safe and effective in newborns.
   3. Approximately 2 mg/kg/day of **propranolol** (range 1–3.5 mg/kg/day) in three divided doses is used to control tachycardia and congestive heart failure.
   4. Additional therapy may include **prednisone** at 1 to 2 mg/kg/day.
   5. **Supportive care** maintains adequate oxygenation, positive fluid balance, sufficient caloric intake and growth, and temperature regulation.
   6. **Treatment may be required for 4 to 12 weeks.** Once control is gained, the infant can be discharged with close follow-up. Iodine solutions are given for only 10 to 14 days. Infants are weaned off propranolol as indicated by heart rate, and then the dose of PTU is tapered as allowed by T_4 level and clinical situation.

E. Prognosis. Most newborns have rapid improvement and are able to withdrawn from treatment over several months. Rarely, the disease persists for >6 months. Mortality can be as high as 15%. Long-term morbidities include retarded growth, craniosynostosis, hyperactivity, and intellectual and developmental impairment.

VI. CONGENITAL HYPOTHYROIDISM (CH)
   A. Thyroid embryogenesis occurs during the first trimester. By 10 to 12 weeks, the fetal thyroid gland demonstrates the ability to concentrate iodide and synthesize iodothyronines. TRH, somatostatin, and TSH are also detectable by this age. However, activity of the HPT axis is low, and circulating TSH and T_4 levels are minimal until approximately 18 to 20 weeks. After 20 weeks, there is a progressive increase

| TABLE 2B.2 | Reference Ranges for Serum Free T_4 and Thyrotropin in Premature and Term Infants During the First Week of Life |

Age groups	Age (wk)	Weight, g (SD)	Free T_4 ng/dL (mean)	Thyrotropin (mU/L)
Premature infants*	25–27	772 (233)	0.6–2.2 (1.4)	0.2–30.3
	28–30	1,260 (238)	0.6–3.4 (2.0)	0.2–20.6
	31–33	1,786 (255)	1.0–3.8 (2.4)	0.7–27.9
	34–36	2,125 (376)	1.2–4.4 (2.8)	1.2–21.6
Term infants†	37–42	>2,500	2.0–5.3 (3.8)	1.0–39

T_4 = thyroxine; SD = standard deviation.
*Data from Adams LM, Emery JR, Clark SJ. Reference ranges for newer thyroid function test in premature infants. *J Pediatr* 1995;126:122;
†Nelson JC, Clark SJ, Borut DL, et al. Age-related change in serum free thyroxine during childhood and adolescence. *J Pediatr* 1993;123:899–905.
Source: Fisher DA. Thyroid function in premature infants: The hypothyroxinemia of prematurity. *Clin Perinatol* 1998;25:999–1014.

in TSH and free T_4 levels. There is also an increase in the T_4:TSH ratio, suggesting maturation of the negative feedback control of the HPT axis. T_3 levels also progressively increase, although later, after approximately 30 weeks of gestation.
B. Neonatal physiology. At birth there is a sharp increase in TSH as a result of neonatal cooling. This surge peaks at 30 minutes and declines over the next few days. The increased TSH results in a concomitant sharp rise in T_4 and T_3 levels, peaking at 36 to 48 hours of life, and then steadily declining to adult values over 4 to 5 weeks. Preterm infants demonstrate similar changes in thyroid hormone levels as full-term newborns. However, quantitatively the response is blunted because of axis immaturity, resulting in overall lower levels of total T_4, free T_4, and T_3. This attenuation increases with decreasing gestational age and in the extremely preterm infant (<28 weeks' gestation) the normal postnatal surge in free T_4 levels may be absent. Thyroid hormone levels are related to gestational age and birth weight (see Table 2B.2). Hypothyroxinemia of prematurity is discussed further in VI.E.2.c.
C. Screening. Screening of newborns for CH is routine in developed countries. Most North American programs use a spot T_4 measurement and TSH confirmation of low T_4 values.
    1. Screening and early discharge. With many neonates discharged on day 1 of life, obtaining early TSH measurements has increased the false-positive rate for CH screening. Because T_4 is also elevated on days 1 and 2 of life, mild cases of CH may be missed if T_4 is within the low-normal range. If the infant is tested before 24 hours of age, he or she should be retested 24 to 48 hours after discharge.
    2. Prematurity and low birth weight. Total T_4 levels are related to gestational age and birth weight. A majority of preterm, low–birth weight infants may have T_4 levels in the hypothyroid range. In addition, truly hypothyroid, low–birth weight infants may demonstrate a delayed rise in TSH 2.5 to 7 weeks after birth (see VI.E.1.d). These factors make the diagnosis of hypothyroidism more challenging in this group. As a result, it is recommended to repeat state newborn screening specimens at 2, 6, and 10 weeks of life for all newborns weighing <1,500 g.
    3. If signs of hypothyroidism appear (prolonged jaundice, delayed passage of stools, hypothermia, poor tone, mottled skin, poor feeding), screening should be repeated even if the original screening result was normal. Screening programs miss some cases of CH as a result of early discharge, laboratory error, improper or no specimen collection, hospital transfers, sick neonates, prematurity, low birth weight, and home deliveries.

D. **CH is seen more frequently** in infants with Down syndrome, trisomy 18, neural tube defects, congenital heart disease, metabolic disorders, familial autoimmune thyroid disorders, and Pierre Robin syndrome.

E. **Etiologies of CH**

1. **Permanent conditions.** The overall incidence of conditions leading to permanent hypothyroidism is 1 in 3,500 to 4,000 live births.

   a. **Thyroid dysgenesis** (aplasia, hypoplasia, ectopic thyroid) is the most common cause of permanent CH with an incidence of 1 in 4,000 births (~80% of cases). Thyroid dysgenesis is least common in blacks (1:32,000) and most common in Hispanic infants (1:2,000). It is usually sporadic, but may be familial if the cause is cytotoxic antibodies crossing the placenta in pregnant women with autoimmune thyroid disease. The female-to-male ratio is 2:1. Infants have no goiter, low T_4 and free thyroxine (T_4), low triiodothyronine (T_3), elevated thyroid-stimulating hormone (TSH), normal TBG, no or ectopic radioactive iodine uptake (RAIU), and an increased response to TRH at 30 minutes.

   b. **Thyroid hormone synthetic defects** (autosomal recessive) have an incidence of 1 in 30,000 (~10% of permanent CH cases). Synthetic defects may be anywhere along the synthetic pathway, including abnormalities in trapping, organification, deiodination, storage, or release. **Pendred syndrome** is an organification defect coupled with sensorineural deafness. Check for family history of deafness or goiter or for consanguinity. RAIU scans are typically normal, and a gland is present on ultrasonography. Thyroglobulin may be low; T_3, T_4, and free T_4 are low; TSH is high; TBG is normal; and there is an increased response to TRH at 30 minutes. Goiter is usually present.

   c. **Hypothalamic-pituitary hypothyroidism.** The incidence is 1 in 100,000. T_4, free T_4, and T_3 are low, with low-to-normal TSH, normal TBG, and a low or delayed response to TRH infusion. Infants with suspected hypothalamic or pan-hypopituitarism may also have hypoglycemia and microphallus. Cortisol and growth hormone measurements should be obtained and a magnetic resonance imaging scan done to visualize the hypothalamus and pituitary. Goiter is not present.

   d. **Hypothyroxinemia with delayed TSH elevation.** The incidence is 1 in 100,000 of all newborns, but 1 in 300 in very low birth weight infants. On initial screening, TSH is found to be normal, with low T_4, low free T_4, low T_3, and normal TBG. On subsequent testing 2.5 to 7 weeks later, TSH levels are found to be elevated with a pattern typical of primary hypothyroidism. Etiology remains unclear, with possibilities including an abnormality of the pituitary-thyroid feedback mechanism or a type of acquired hypothyroidism.

2. **Transient conditions** are seen frequently in sick or preterm neonates.

   a. **Thyroid-blocking antibodies.** Transient hypothyroidism that is due to thyroid-blocking antibodies has an incidence of 1 in 50,000. This is seen in maternal autoimmune thyroid disease. Antibodies freely cross the placenta and are secreted in breast milk. Antibodies may inhibit TSH binding to the receptors TSH-binding inhibitory immunoglobulins (TBII), inhibit TSH-mediated thyroid growth inhibitory immunoglobulin (TGII), or block the effects of TSH on cell function. Antibodies with blocking or stimulating properties may be found in the same pregnant woman and may have different or subsequent effects on the fetus, exerting their influence for as long as 9 months after birth. Hypothyroidism may persist for that length of time. T_4, free T_4, and T_3 are low, TSH is increased, TBG is normal, and antibodies are present in both mother and infant. TRH test shows an increased TSH response. RAIU may be absent, but a gland will be present on ultrasonography.

   b. **Iodine exposure.** Sick and preterm infants are at risk for transient hypothyroxinemia because of the exposure to iodine-containing disinfectant solutions. Exposed infants may demonstrate depressed free T_4 levels and elevated TSH and urinary iodine levels. Use of iodine-containing disinfectant solutions should be avoided or minimized in preterm, low–birth weight newborns.

  c. **Transient hypothyroxinemia of prematurity.** Transient hypothyroxinemia of prematurity is a poorly understood disorder, affecting as many as 85% of preterm infants. Typically, total T_4 levels are low, but free T_4, T_3, and TSH values are normal. Most values normalize within a few months. Previously, this transient phenomenon was attributed to a normal adaptive response of an immature hypothalamic-pituitary axis or to sick euthyroid syndrome and was considered clinically insignificant. However, more recently, hypothyroxinemia during the neonatal period in the preterm infant has been linked with significant postneonatal morbidities. Decreased total thyroxine levels are associated with intraventricular hemorrhage, white matter damage, cerebral palsy, poor neurodevelopment, and death. Treatment considerations are discussed under VI.G.2–3.

F. **Diagnosis.** Infants with abnormal newborn state screen thyroid-function results ($T_4 < 6$, TSH >20) should have the tests repeated by venipuncture (see Fig. 2B.1). In addition to TSH and total T_4 levels, free T_4, T_3 resin uptake, TBG, and thyroglobulin

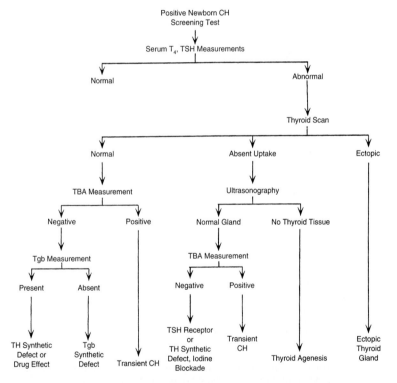

Figure 2B.1. Possible initial approaches to a newborn infant with presumptive positive test results for congenital hypothyroidism (CH) from a screening laboratory. All such infants require measurements of serum thyroxine (T_4) and serum thyroglobulin (Tgb) concentrations. Those infants with low T_4 and elevated TSH concentrations can be further screened by a thyroid scan using technetium or radioiodine 123. Finding an ectopic gland provides a definitive diagnosis. Infants with absent uptake or a normally appearing thyroid gland by scan can be evaluated further by ultrasound scanning and measurements of TBA and serum thyroglobulin (Tgb) concentrations. Infant with TBA-induced transient CH may have a normal scan if their CH is partially compensated. This initial evaluation should be accomplished within 2 to 5 days. (From Fisher DA. Management of congenital hypothyroidism. *J Clin Endocrinol Metab* 1991;72:525.)

levels should be considered to aid in diagnosis. Bone age evaluation (e.g., knee, foot) may show delay in epiphyseal maturation. RAIU with iodine-123 may be helpful in differentiating aplasia from synthetic defects. Absent uptake may also be seen in TSH receptor defects and iodide-trapping defects. TSH receptor blockade by maternal TSH receptor–blocking antibodies (TBA in figure) in maternal autoimmune thyroid disease may also cause absent RAIU. Thyroglobulin levels will be low in agenesis or thyroxine synthetic defects and elevated in thyroid dysgenesis, depending on the quantity of thyroid tissue and degree of TSH stimulation. TRH testing (7 mg/kg given intravenously; TSH release measured at 30 minutes and 1–2 hours) will show a subnormal response in pituitary CH (<10 mU/mL) and a delayed response in hypothalamic CH.

G. Treatment and monitoring of CH

1. **Preterm and term infants with low T$_4$ and elevated TSH** must be treated as primary hypothyroidism. All infants with an uncertain diagnosis or suspected transient disease should have a brief trial off medication between 3 and 4 years of age to determine whether they have transient disease or if permanent thyroxine replacement is necessary.

2. **Treatment with L-thyroxine** should be initiated at 10 to 15 μg/kg/day, using the highest dose for infants with the lowest T$_4$, highest TSH values, and most delayed bone ages. A term infant receiving 50 μg/day will have normal T$_4$ and TSH levels within 2 weeks. Keeping T$_4$ in the upper half of the normal range (10–16 μg/dL) should keep TSH levels <20 mU/mL in most of the infants, but as many as 20% of infants with CH will continue to have abnormal T$_4$-to-TSH feedback for the first decade of life. Thyroxine doses should be adjusted at 6-week intervals for the first 6 months of life and at 2-month intervals during the next 12 months to keep T$_4$ in the 10 to 16 μg/dL range and TSH <5 mU/L. Thyroxine must be crushed and fed directly to the infant. It cannot be made into a liquid or added to breast milk or formula in a bottle. Soy-based formulas and ferrous sulfate interfere significantly with L-thyroxine absorption. Soy-based formula and/or ferrous sulfate should be administered at least 2 hours apart from the L-thyroxine dose.

3. The question of whether **T$_4$ supplementation in preterm infants (<30 weeks' gestation) with low T$_4$ and *normal* TSH levels** might improve outcome remains controversial. Recent studies have suggested that supplementation in extremely preterm infants (<28 weeks' gestation) may demonstrate long-term benefit. However, present opinion, including that of the *New England Hypothyroid Collaborative and the Cochrane Neonatal Collaborative Review*, is that there is no clear benefit to routine T$_4$ supplementation in these infants. Larger clinical trials, especially among the most vulnerable preterm infants born at <28 weeks' gestation, are needed.

H. Prognosis. Prompt, early thyroxine replacement, close monitoring, and maintenance of T$_4$ levels in the upper half of reference range has significantly improved neurodevelopment, even in the most severe cases of CH. Although mental retardation can be avoided with early treatment, subtle neurocognitive deficits may persist, including poor visuospatial abilities, attention, and memory skills.

Suggested Readings

Azizi F, Khoshniat M, Bahrainian M, et al. Thyroid function and intellectual development of infants nursed by mothers taking methimazole. *J Clin Endocrinol Metab* 2000;85:3233–3238.

Berghout A, Wiersinga W. Thyroid size and thyroid function during pregnancy: An analysis. *Eur J Endocrinol* 1998;138:536–542.

Biswas S, Buffery J, Enoch H, et al. A longitudinal assessment of thyroid concentration in preterm infants younger than 30 weeks' gestation during the first two weeks of life and their relationship to outcome. *Pediatrics* 2002;109(2):222–227.

Briet JM, van Wassenaer AG, Dekkar FW et al. Neonatal thyroxine supplementation in very preterm children: Developmental outcome evaluated at early school age. *Pediatrics* 2001;107:712–718.

Buckingham B. The hyperthyroid fetus and infant. *NeoReviews* 2000;1:e103–e109.

Burrow GN, Fisher DA, Larsen PR. Maternal and fetal thyroid function. *N Engl J Med* 1994;331:1072–1078.

Den Ouden AL, Kok JH, Verkerk PH et al. The relation between neonatal thyroxine levels and neurodevelopmental outcome at age 5 and 9 years in a national cohort of very preterm and/or very low birth weight infants. *Pediatr Res* 1996;39:142–145.

Dubuis JM, Glorieux J, Richer F et al. Outcome of severe congenital hypothyroidism: Closing the developmental gap with early high dose levothyroxine treatment. *J Clin Endocrinol Metab* 1996;81:222–227.

Fantz CR, Dagogo-Jack S, Ladenson JH et al. Thyroid function during pregnancy. *Clin Chem* 1999;45:2250–2258.

Fisher DA. Hypothyroidism. *Pediatr Rev* 1994;15:227–232.

Fisher DA. Thyroid function in premature infants: The hypothyroxinemia of prematurity. *Clin Perinatol* 1998;25:999–1014,viii.

Haddow JE, Palomaki GE, Allan WC, et al. Maternal thyroid deficiency during pregnancy and subsequent neuropsychological development of the child. *N Engl J Med* 1999;341:549–555.

Kaplan MM. Monitoring thyroxine treatment during pregnancy. *Thyroid* 1992;2:147–152.

Larson C, Hermos R, Delaney A, et al. Risk factors associated with delayed thyrotropin elevations in congenital hypothyroidism. *J Pediatr* 2003;143:587–591.

Leviton A, Paneth N, Reuss ML, et al. Hypothyroxinemia of prematurity and the risk of cerebral white matter damage. *J Pediatr* 1999;134:706–711.

Lucas A, Morley R, Fewtrell MS. Low triiodothyronine concentration in preterm infants and subsequent intelligence quotient (IQ) at 8 year follow up. *Br Med J* 1996;312:1132–1133, discussion 1133–1134.

Mandel SJ, Cooper DS. The use of antithyroid drugs in pregnancy and lactation. *J Clin Endocrinol Metab* 2001;86:2354–2359.

Meijer WJ, Verloove-Vanhorick SP, Brand R et al. Transient hypothyroxinaemia associated with developmental delay in very preterm infants. *Arch Dis Child* 1992;67:944–947.

Mestman JH. Hyperthyroidism in pregnancy. *Endocrinol Metab Clin North Am* 1998;27:127–149.

Mitchell ML. Potential pitfalls in screening programs for congenital hypothyroidism. *NeoReviews* 2000;1:e110–e115.

Montoro MN. Management of hypothyroidism during pregnancy. *Clin Obstet Gynecol* 1997;40:65–80.

Murphy N, Hume R, van Toor H, et al. The hypothalamic-pituitary-thyroid axis in preterm infants: Changes in the first 24 hours of postnatal life. *J Clin Endocrinol Metab* 2004;89(6):2824–2831.

Parravicini E, Fontana C, Paterlini GL, et al. Iodine, thyroid function, and very low birth weight infants. *Pediatrics* 1996;98:730–734.

Paul DA, Leef KH, Stefano JL, et al. Low serum thyroxine on initial newborn screening is associated with intraventricular hemorrhage and death in very low birth weight infants. *Pediatrics* 1998;101:903–907.

Rapaport R, Rose SR, Freemark M. Hypothyroxinemia in the preterm infant: The benefits and risks of thyroxine treatment. *J Pediatr* 2001;139:182–188.

Reuss ML, Leviton A, Paneth N, et al. The relation of transient hypothyroxinemia in preterm infants to neurologic development at two years of age. *N Engl J Med* 1996;334:821–827.

Reuss ML, Paneth N, Lorenz JM, et al. Correlates of low thyroxine values at newborn screening among infants born before 32 weeks' gestation. *Early Hum Dev* 1997;47:223–233.

Reuss ML, Paneth N, Pinto-Martin JA, et al. Thyroxine values from newborn screening of 919 infants born before 29 weeks' gestation. *Am J Public Health* 1997;87:1693–1697.

Rovet JF, Ehrlich R. Psychoeducational outcome in children with early-treated congenital hypothyroidism. *Pediatrics* 2000;105:515–522.

Smit BJ, Kok JH, Vulsma T, et al. Neurologic development of the newborn and young child in relation to maternal thyroid function. *Acta Paediatr* 2000;89:291–295.

Toft AD. Thyroxine therapy. *N Engl J Med* 1994;331:174–180.

van Wassenaer AG, Kok JH, de Vijlder JJ, et al. Effects of thyroxine supplementation on neurologic development in infants born at less than 30 weeks' gestation. *N Engl J Med* 1997;336:21–26.

van Wassenaer AG, Westera J, Houtzager BA, et al. Ten-year follow-up of children born at <30 weeks' gestational age supplemented with thyroxine in the neonatal period in a randomized, controlled trial. *Pediatrics* 2005;116(5):e613–e618.

Wing DA, Millar LK, Koonings PP, et al. A comparison of propylthiouracil versus methimazole in the treatment of hyperthyroidism in pregnancy. *Am J Obstet Gynecol* 1994;170:90–95.

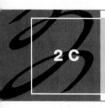

PREECLAMPSIA AND RELATED CONDITIONS

2 C

Thomas F. McElrath

I. **CATEGORIES OF PREGNANCY ASSOCIATED HYPERTENSIVE DISORDERS**
   A. **Chronic hypertension.** Hypertension preceding pregnancy or first diagnosed before 20 weeks gestation.
   B. **Chronic hypertension with superimposed preeclampsia.** Worsening hypertension and new onset proteinuria, in addition to possible concurrent hyperuricemia, thrombocytopenia, or transaminase derangements after the 20th week of pregnancy in a woman with known chronic hypertension.
   C. **Pregnancy-induced hypertension.** Hypertension without proteinuria after 20 weeks gestation.
   D. **Preeclampsia.** Hypertension with proteinuria after 20 weeks gestation.
   E. **Eclampsia.** Preeclampsia with generalized tonic–clonic seizure activity in a woman with no prior history of a seizure disorder.
II. **INCIDENCE AND EPIDEMIOLOGY.** Hypertensive disorders are a major cause of maternal morbidity and mortality, accounting for 15% to 20% of maternal deaths worldwide. In the United States, hypertensive disorders are the second leading cause of maternal mortality. Preeclampsia complicates 8% of pregnancies beyond 20 weeks gestation; severe preeclampsia, <1%. Eclampsia itself is much less frequent, occurring in 0.1% of pregnancies. Several risk factors have been identified (see Table 2C.1).
III. Preeclampsia has been called the "disease of theories" and many **etiologies** have been proposed. However, recent innovative work suggests that the increases in the soluble receptors for both vascularendothelial growth factor (VEGF) and transforming growth factor-beta (TGF-β), named *sFLT1* and *endoglin* respectively, within the maternal circulation are associated with preeclamptic pathology. Higher circulating levels of these soluble receptors reduce the bioavailable levels of both VEGF and TGF-β resulting in endothelial dysfunction within the maternal circulatory system. This dysfunction can manifest as both increased arterial tone (hypertension) and increased capillary leak (edema/proteinuria/pulmonary congestion). It is unclear what insult prompts the initial increase in sFLT1 and endoglin in some women versus others. One suggestion has been that abnormal trophoblastic invasion of both the maternal decidual arteries with an accompanying abnormal maternal immune response is at the root of this condition. This abnormal placentation is believed to lead to a reduction in placental perfusion and relative placental ischemia. Both sFLT1 and endoglin are proangiogenic proteins and may represent a placental compensatory response.

TABLE 2C.1	Risk Factors for Hypertensive Disorders	
Risk factor		**Risk ratio**
Nulliparity		3
Age >40		3
African-American race		1.5
Family history of PIH		5
Chronic HTN		10
Chronic renal disease		20
Antiphospholipid antibody syndrome		10
Diabetes		2
Twin gestation		4
Angiotensinogen gene T235		
Homozygous		20
Heterozygous		4

HTN = hypertension; PIH = pregnancy-induced hypertension.
Source: ACOG. Hypertension in pregnancy. Technical Bulletin # 219, January 1996.

IV. DIAGNOSIS. The classic triad defining preeclampsia is hypertension, proteinuria, and nondependent edema. The clinical spectrum of preeclampsia ranges from mild to severe. Most patients have mild disease that develops late in the third trimester.

A. Criteria for the diagnosis of mild preeclampsia

1. **Hypertension** defined as a blood pressure elevation to 140 mm Hg systolic or 90 mm Hg diastolic over two measurements at least 6 hours apart. Measurements should be taken in the sitting position, and proper cuff size should be ensured.

2. **Proteinuria** defined as at least 300 mg of protein in a 24-hour period.

3. **Nondependent edema** (e.g., facial or upper extremity) is also noted in many but not all cases of preeclampsia.

B. Criteria for the diagnosis of severe preeclampsia

1. **Blood pressure** >160 mm Hg systolic or 110 mm Hg diastolic with the diagnostic readings taken twice at least 6 hours apart.

2. **Proteinuria** >5 g per 24-hour collection.

3. **Symptoms suggestive of end-organ dysfunction.** Visual disturbances such as scotomata, diplopia or blindness, persistent severe headache, and epigastric pain.

4. **Pulmonary edema.**

5. **Oliguria** defined as <500 mL of urine per 24-hour collection.

6. **Microangiopathic hemolysis.**

7. **Thrombocytopenia.** Defined as a platelet count of <100,000.

8. **Hepatocellular dysfunction.** Elevated transaminases.

9. **Intrauterine growth restriction (IUGR) or oligohydramnios.**

C. HELLP syndrome (hemolysis, elevated liver enzymes, and low platelets) represents an alternative presentation of preeclampsia associated with disseminated intravascular coagulation (DIC) and reflects systemic end-organ damage. HELLP syndrome often appears without hypertension or proteinuria and may, in fact, have a separate pathologic origin from that of preeclampsia.

V. Complications of preeclampsia result in a **maternal mortality rate** of 3 per 100,000 live births in the United States. Maternal morbidity may include central nervous system complications (e.g., seizures, intracerebral hemorrhage, and blindness), DIC, hepatic failure or rupture, pulmonary edema, and *abruptio placentae* leading to maternal hemorrhage and/or acute renal failure. Fetal mortality markedly increases with rising maternal diastolic blood pressure and proteinuria. Diastolic blood pressures >95 mm Hg are associated with a threefold rise in the fetal death rate. Fetal morbidity may include IUGR, fetal acidemia, and complications from prematurity.

VI. CONSIDERATIONS IN MANAGEMENT

   A. The definitive treatment for preeclampsia is delivery. However, the severity of disease, dilatation/effacement of the maternal cervix, gestational age at diagnosis, and pulmonary maturity of the fetus influence obstetric management. Delivery is usually indicated if there is nonreassuring fetal testing in a viable fetus or if the maternal status becomes unstable regardless of gestational age or fetal pulmonary maturity.

   B. Delivery should be considered for all term patients with any degree of preeclampsia. Patients with mild disease and an unfavorable cervix can be closely monitored to await a more favorable cervix.

   C. For patients with **preterm gestation and mild preeclampsia,** their pregnancies may continue with close observation as outlined in section VII until 37 weeks gestation or some other ominous development such as the progression to severe preeclampsia, nonreassuring fetal testing, or maternal instability.

   D. Consideration for delivery should be made in all patients with severe preeclampsia. Conservative therapy of severe preeclampsia early in gestation has been suggested, with one study showing that in pregnancies between 28 and 32 weeks, conservative management resulted in a mean prolongation of pregnancy of 2 weeks. However, conservative management of severe preeclampsia may be associated with serious sequelae, such as acute renal failure, DIC, HELLP syndrome, *abruptio placentae*, eclampsia, and intrauterine fetal death. Patients should be counseled that prolongation of pregnancy in the setting of severe preeclampsia is for fetal benefit only as the mother assumes risk to her own well-being. Conservative management should only be undertaken in centers where there is rapid availability of immediate obstetrical and neonatal care.

   E. Conservative management entails hospitalization and frequent maternal and fetal surveillance. This should only be undertaken in carefully selected patients after an initial period of observation to ensure stability of the pregnant woman. Women with uncontrolled hypertension, thrombocytopenia, hepatocellular dysfunction, pulmonary edema, compromised renal function, or persistent headache or visual changes are not candidates for conservative management of severe preeclampsia.

   F. Although a trial of labor induction is not contraindicated in patients with severe preeclampsia, the success rate is low. The managing team must balance the risks of progression of the disease against the time required to induce labor.

VII. CLINICAL MANAGEMENT OF MILD PREECLAMPSIA

   A. Antepartum management. Conservative management of mild preeclampsia generally includes hospitalization with bed rest and close maternal and fetal observation. Outpatient management is an option only for a few carefully selected, well-supported and reliable patients after a period of initial observation to assess maternal and fetal status.

   1. Fetal evaluation

      a. An initial **ultrasound** should be performed at the time of diagnosis to rule out IUGR and/or oligohydramnios. A **nonstress test** or **biophysical profile** should also be performed.

      b. Betamethasone to accelerate fetal maturity should be administered if <34 weeks of gestation and no maternal contraindications exist.

      c. If the fetus is appropriately grown with reassuring fetal testing, **testing should be at regular intervals.**

      d. If the estimated fetal weight is <10th percentile or there is oligohydramnios (amniotic fluid index of 5 cm), then **testing should be performed at frequent regular intervals** (consider daily) after consideration of delivery.

      e. Any **change in maternal status** should prompt evaluation of fetal status.

    f. Fetal indications for delivery include severe fetal growth restriction, non-reassuring fetal testing, and oligohydramnios.

  2. Maternal evaluation

    a. Women should be **evaluated for signs and symptoms** of preeclampsia and severe preeclampsia.

    b. Laboratory evaluation includes hematocrit, platelet count, and quantification of protein excretion in the urine, serum creatinine, transaminases, and uric acid level in addition to prothrombin time/partial thromboplastin time.

    c. If criteria for mild preeclampsia are met laboratory studies should be performed at frequent intervals. At Brigham and Women's Hospital, women with mild preeclampsia have laboratory testing twice weekly.

    d. Maternal indications for delivery include gestational age ≥ 37 weeks, thrombocytopenia ($<100,000$), progressive deterioration in hepatic or renal function, *abruptio placentae*, and persistent severe headaches, visual changes, or epigastric pain.

    e. Antihypertensive agents are not routinely given to the mother because they have not been shown to improve outcome in cases of mild preeclampsia.

    f. When early delivery is indicated it is our practice to induce labor. Cesarean delivery should be performed in cases of suspected fetal distress, when further fetal evaluation is not possible, or when a rapidly deteriorating maternal condition mandates expeditious delivery (e.g., HELLP with decreasing platelet counts, abruption).

B. Intrapartum management of preeclampsia

  1. Magnesium sulfate (6 g intravenous [IV] load followed by 2 g/h infusion), used as seizure prophylaxis, is started when the decision to proceed with delivery is made and continued for at least 24 hours postpartum or until symptoms are resolving in the mother. Magnesium sulfate has been shown to be the agent of choice for seizure prophylaxis in randomized double blind comparisons both against placebo and against conventional antiepileptics. In patients with a contraindication to magnesium sulfate (e.g., myasthenia gravis, hypocalcemia), other antiseizure agents such as Dilantin may be used. The kidneys clear magnesium sulfate, therefore urine output should be carefully monitored. Signs and symptoms of maternal toxicity include loss of deep tendon reflexes, somnolence, respiratory depression, cardiac arrhythmia, and, in extreme cases, cardiovascular collapse.

  2. Careful monitoring of fluid balance is critical because preeclampsia is associated with endothelial dysfunction leading to decreased intravascular volume, pulmonary edema, and oliguria.

  3. Severe hypertension may be controlled with agents including hydralazine, labetalol, or nifedipine. Sodium nitroprusside should be avoided before delivery because of potential fetal cyanide toxicity. It is important to avoid large or abrupt reductions in blood pressure because decreased intravascular volume and poor uteroplacental perfusion can lead to acute placental insufficiency.

  4. Continuous electronic fetal monitoring is recommended given the risk of fetal compromise. Patterns that suggest fetal compromise include persistent tachycardia, minimal or absent variability, and recurrent late decelerations not responsive to standard resuscitative measures. Reduced fetal heart rate variability may also result from maternal administration of magnesium sulfate.

  5. Patients may be safely administered **epidural anesthesia** if the platelet count is $>70,000$ and there is no evidence of DIC. Consideration should be given for early epidural catheter placement when the platelet count is reasonable and there is concern that it is decreasing. Any anesthesia should be carefully administered by properly trained personnel experienced in the care of women with preeclampsia given the hemodynamic changes associated with the condition. Adequate preload should be ensured to minimize the risk of hypotension.

  6. Invasive central monitoring of the mother is rarely indicated, even in the setting of severe preeclampsia.

C. **Postpartum management.** The mother's condition may worsen immediately after delivery. Signs and symptoms usually begin to resolve within 24 to 48 hours postpartum, however, and completely resolve within 1 to 2 weeks. Because postpartum eclamptic seizures generally occur within the first 48 hours and usually within the first 24 hours after delivery, magnesium sulfate is continued for at least 24 hours. Close monitoring of fluid balance is continued. Once a spontaneous maternal diuresis has begun, recovery can be hastened by the administration of oral diuretics.

VIII. **MANAGEMENT OF ECLAMPSIA**

A. Approximately half of **eclamptic seizures** occur before delivery, 20% occur during delivery, and another 30% occur in the postpartum period. Although there is no clear constellation of symptoms that will accurately predict those patients who will have an eclamptic seizure, headache is a frequently reported heralding symptom.

B. **Basic principles of maternal resuscitation** should be followed in the initial management of an eclamptic seizure: airway protection, oxygen, left lateral displacement to prevent uterine compression of vena cava, intravenous access, and blood pressure control.

C. Magnesium sulfate should be initiated for **prevention of recurrent seizures**. If untreated, 10% of women with eclamptic seizures will have a recurrent seizure.

D. A **transient fetal bradycardia** is usually seen during the seizure followed by a **transient fetal tachycardia** with loss of variability. Ideally, the fetus should be resuscitated *in utero*.

E. **Eclampsia is an indication for delivery but not necessarily an indication for cesarean delivery.** No intervention should be initiated until maternal stability is ensured and the seizure is over. Because of the risk of DIC, coagulation parameters should be assessed and appropriate blood products should be set up if necessary.

F. A **neurologic exam** should be performed once the patient recovers from the seizure. If the seizure is atypical or any neurologic deficit persists, **brain imaging** is indicated.

IX. **RECURRENCE RISK.** Patients who have a history of preeclampsia are at increased risk for hypertensive disease in a subsequent pregnancy. Recurrence risk is as high as 40% in women with preeclampsia before 30 weeks of gestation in contrast to 10% or less in women with mild preeclampsia near term. Severe disease and eclampsia are also associated with recurrence. Racial differences exist, with African-American women having higher recurrence rates. The recurrence rate for HELLP syndrome is approximately 5%. The presence of a thrombophilia also confers an increase risk.

X. **RISK OF CHRONIC HYPERTENSION.** Preeclampsia may be linked to the development of chronic hypertension later in the mother's life. Women with recurrent preeclampsia, women with early-onset preeclampsia, and multiparas with a diagnosis of preeclampsia (even if not recurrent) are at an increased risk.

XI. **INNOVATIONS AND PROPOSED TREATMENTS**

A. Several analytic assays based on sFLT1 and related protein levels are currently in trial and may represent an additional diagnostic modality in the near future.

B. **Low-dose aspirin** has been evaluated as a possible prophylactic. However, no clear benefit has been shown. In fact, there is some suggestion of an increased risk of placental abruption in the patients receiving low-dose aspirin.

C. Although earlier studies suggested that **antenatal calcium supplementation** may reduce the incidence of hypertensive disorders of pregnancy, a large National Institutes of Health–sponsored placebo-controlled trial did not show any benefit when given to healthy nulliparous women.

D. Recent enthusiasm for antioxidant therapy has also been dulled after a well executed trial found vitamin E supplementation during pregnancy to be associated with an increased risk of adverse outcome compared with placebo.

E. The efficacy of **heparin therapy** for the prevention of preeclampsia in women with a genetic thrombophilia is unknown.

XII. **IMPLICATIONS FOR THE NEWBORN**

A. Infants born to mothers with moderate or severe preeclampsia may show evidence of **IUGR** (see Chaps. 1 and 3) and are frequently delivered prematurely. They may tolerate labor poorly and require resuscitation.

B. Medications used ante- or intrapartum may affect the fetus.

    1. Short-term sequelae of hypermagnesemia such as hypotonia and respiratory depression, are sometimes seen (see Chap. 29B). Long-term maternal administration of magnesium sulfate has rarely been associated with neonatal parathyroid abnormalities and other abnormalities of calcium homeostasis.

    2. Antihypertensive medications including calcium-channel blockers, may have fetal effects, including hypotension in the infant. Antihypertensive medications and magnesium sulfate generally are not contraindications to breastfeeding.

    3. Low-dose aspirin therapy does not appear to increase the incidence of intracranial hemorrhage, asymptomatic bruising, bleeding from circumcision sites, or persistent pulmonary hypertension.

    4. Approximately one-third of infants born to mothers with preeclampsia have **decreased platelet counts at birth,** but the counts generally increase rapidly to normal levels. Approximately 40% to 50% of newborns have neutropenia that generally resolves before 3 days of age. These infants may be at increased risk of neonatal infection.

Suggested Readings

American College of Obstetricians and Gynecologists. Practice Bulletin 33: Diagnosis and Management of Preeclampsia and Eclampsia. January 2002.

Levine RJ, Maynard SE, Qian C, et al. Circulating angiogenic factors and the risk of preeclampsia. *N Engl J Med* 2004;350:672–83.

Roberts JM. Pregnancy-related hypertension. In: Creasy RK, Resnik R, eds. *Maternal-fetal medicine*, 5th ed, Philadelphia: WB Saunders, 2004.

Sibai BM, Mercer BM, Schiff E, et al. Aggressive versus expectant management of severe preeclampsia at 28 to 32 weeks gestation: A randomized controlled trial. *Am J Obstet Gynecol* 1994;171:818–822.

Sibai BM, Taslimi M, Abdella TN, et al. Maternal and perinatal outcome of conservative management of severe preeclampsia in midtrimester. *Am J Obstet Gynecol* 1985;152:32–37.

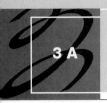

ASSESSMENT OF THE NEWBORN HISTORY AND PHYSICAL EXAMINATION OF THE NEWBORN

3 A

William D. Cochran and Kimberly G. Lee

I. **HISTORY.** The family, maternal, pregnancy, and perinatal history should be reviewed (see Table 3A.1).

II. **ROUTINE PHYSICAL EXAMINATION OF THE NEONATE.** Although no statistics are available, the first routine examination probably reveals more abnormalities than any other routine examination.

  A. General examination. At the initial examination, attention should be directed to determine (i) whether any congenital anomalies are present, (ii) whether the infant has made a successful transition from fetal life to air breathing, (iii) to what extent gestation, labor, delivery, analgesics, or anesthetics have affected the neonate, and (iv) whether he or she has any sign of infection or metabolic disease.

    1. The baby should be naked. Naked newborns are easily chilled, so they should not be kept uncovered for a long time unless they are in or under a warming device. A general appraisal of a naked newborn allows one to assess quickly whether any major anomalies are present, whether jaundice or meconium staining is present, and whether the infant is having trouble making the adjustment to breathing air. At least half of all infants will exhibit jaundice, although usually only at its peak on the third or fourth day of life. Visible jaundice usually means the bilirubin level is at least 5 mg/dL.

    2. It is usually wise to examine infants in the order listed because they will be quieter at the beginning, when you most need their cooperation. If the infant being examined is fretful, offer the baby a gloved finger.

  B. Cardiorespiratory system

    1. Color. Skin color is probably the single most important index of cardiorespiratory function. Good color in white infants means an overall reddish pink hue, except for possible cyanosis of the hands, feet, and occasionally the lips (acrocyanosis). The mucous membranes of dark-skinned infants are more reliable indicators of cyanosis than skin. Infants of diabetic mothers and premature infants are pinker than average, and postmature infants are paler.

    2. Respiratory rate is usually 40 to 60 breaths/minute. All infants are **periodic** rather than regular breathers, and premature infants are more so compared with term infants. Therefore, babies may breathe at a fairly regular rate for a minute or so and then have a short period of no breathing (usually 5–10 seconds). **Apnea,** often defined as periods of no breathing during which an infant's color changes from normal to grades of cyanosis, is not normal, whereas periodic breathing is. Apnea is therefore an abnormal prolongation of periodic breathing (see Chap. 24I).

    3. In a warm infant, there should be no expiratory grunting and little or no flaring of the nostrils. When crying, infants (especially premature infants) exhibit mild chest retraction; if unaccompanied by grunting, such retraction may be considered normal.

    4. When an infant is pink and breathing without retractions or grunting at a rate of <60 breaths/minute, the respiratory system is usually intact. Significant respiratory disease in the absence of tachypnea is rare unless the infant also has severe central nervous system (CNS) depression. Rales, decreased heart or breath sounds, or asymmetry of breath sounds are occasionally found in an asymptomatic infant and may reveal occult disease that is confirmed by chest x-ray (e.g., dextrocardia, pneumothorax, pneumomediastinum).

TABLE 3A.1   Important Aspects of Maternal and Perinatal History

FAMILY HISTORY

   Inherited diseases (e.g., metabolic disorders, hemophilia, cystic fibrosis, polycystic kidneys, history of perinatal deaths)

MATERNAL HISTORY

   Age

   Blood type

   Transfusions

   Blood group sensitizations

   Chronic maternal illness

   Diabetes

   Hypertension

   Renal disease

   Cardiac disease

   Bleeding disorders

   Sexually transmitted diseases, including herpes and HIV/AIDS

   Infertility IVF

   Recent infections or exposures

PREVIOUS PREGNANCIES: PROBLEMS AND OUTCOMES

   Abortions

   Fetal demise

   Neonatal deaths

   Prematurity

   Postmaturity

   Malformations

   Respiratory distress syndrome

   Jaundice

   Apnea

DRUG HISTORY

   Medications

   Drug abuse

   Alcohol

   Tobacco

CURRENT PREGNANCY

   Probable gestational age

   Quickening (normally 16–18 wk)

   Fetal heart heard with fetoscope (normally 18–20 wk)

   Results of any fetal testing (e.g., amniocentesis, ultrasound examination, estriols, fetal monitoring, tests of fetal lung maturity, and prenatal infection screening [hepatitis, group B streptococci, syphilis, etc.])

   Preeclampsia

   Bleeding

   Trauma

(continued)

TABLE 3A.1	*(Continued)*

Infection
Surgery
Polyhydramnios
Oligohydramnios
Glucocorticoids
Labor suppressant
Antibiotics

LABOR AND DELIVERY (PERINATAL)
Presentation
Onset of labor
Rupture of membranes
Duration of labor
Fever
Fetal monitoring
Amniotic fluid (blood, meconium, volume)
Analgesic
Anesthesia
Maternal oxygenation and perfusion
Method of delivery
Initial delivery room assessment (shock, asphyxia, trauma, anomalies, temperature, infection)
Apgar scores
Resuscitation
Placental examination

HIV = human immunodeficiency virus; AIDS = acquired immunodeficiency syndrome; IVF = *in vitro* fertilization.

5. The **heart** should be examined. The examiner should observe precordial activity, rate, rhythm, the quality of the heart sounds, and the presence or absence of murmurs.

   a. It should be determined whether the heart is on the right side or left side. This is done by auscultation and by palpation.

   b. The **heart rate** is normally 120 to 160 beats/minute. It varies with changes in the infant's activity, increasing when the baby is crying, active, or breathing rather rapidly, and decreasing when the baby is quiet and breathing slowly. To some, this physiologic slowing provides an important indicator that there is no significant cardiac stress. An occasional term or postmature infant may, at rest, have a heart rate well below 100. In a normal infant, the heart rate will increase if the baby is stimulated.

   c. **Murmurs** mean less in the newborn period than at any other time. Infants can have extremely serious heart anomalies without any murmurs. On the other hand, a closing ductus arteriosus may cause a murmur that is only transient, but at the time is very loud and worrisome. Gallop sounds may be an ominous finding, whereas the presence of a split S_2 may be reassuring.

   d. If there is any doubt after auscultation and observation that the heart is abnormally placed, abnormally large, or overactive, a **chest x-ray** is the best means of further assessment. Distant heart sounds, especially if accompanied by respiratory symptoms, are often secondary to pneumothorax or pneumomediastinum.

e. The **femoral pulses** should be felt, although often they are weak in the first day or two. If there is doubt about the femoral pulses by time of discharge, the blood pressure in the upper and lower extremities should be checked. In infants with coarctation, pulses and pressures may be normal in the first few days of life while the ductus is still open (see Chap. 25).

C. Abdomen. The abdominal examination of a newborn differs from that of older infants in that observation can again be used to greater advantage.

1. The anterior abdominal organs (e.g., liver, spleen, bowel) can often be seen through the abdominal wall, especially in thin or premature infants. The edge of the liver is occasionally seen, and intestinal pattern is easily visible. Asymmetry due to congenital anomalies or masses is often first appreciated by observation.

2. When palpating the abdomen, start with gentle pressure or stroking, moving from lower to upper quadrants to reveal the edges of the liver or spleen. Try to appreciate mushiness when palpating over the intestine compared with the firmer feel over the liver or other organs or masses. The normal newborn liver extends 2 to 2.5 cm below the costal margin. The spleen is usually not palpable. Remember there may be situs inversus.

3. After the abdomen has been gently palpated, **deep palpation** is possible, not only because of the lack of developed musculature but also because there is no food and there is little air in the intestine. Abnormal, absent, or misplaced kidneys and other deep masses should be felt. Only during the first day or two of life it is possible for the kidneys to be routinely palpated with relative ease and reliability (see Chap. 31).

D. Genitalia and rectum

1. Male

a. Male babies almost invariably have marked **phimosis.**

b. The **scrotum** is often quite large, because it is an embryonic analog of the female labia and has therefore responded to maternal hormones.

c. **Hydroceles** are not uncommon, but unless they are of communicating type, they will disappear in time without being the forerunner of an inguinal hernia.

d. The **testes** should be palpated, with the epididymis and vas identified. The testis is best found by running a finger from the internal ring down on either side of the upper shaft of the penis, thereby pushing and trapping the testes in the scrotum. Each testis should be the same size, and they should not appear blue (a sign of torsion) through the scrotal skin.

e. If present, the degree of **hypospadias** should be noted.

f. The length and width of the penis should be measured. Length under 2.5 cm is abnormal and requires evaluation (see Chap. 30). Torsion of the penis is seen in 1.5% of normal male babies.

2. Female

a. Female genitalia at term are most noticeable for their enlarged **labia majora.**

b. Occasionally, a **mucosal tag** from the wall of the vagina is noted.

c. A **discharge** from the vagina, usually creamy white in color, is commonly found and, on occasion, replaced after the second day by pseudomenses.

d. The **labia** should always be spread, and cysts of the vaginal wall, imperforate hymen, or other less common anomalies should be sought.

3. The **anus** and **rectum** should be checked carefully for patency, position, and size (normal diameter is 10 mm). Occasionally, large fistulas are mistaken for a normal anus, but if one checks carefully, it will be noted that a fistula will be either anterior or posterior to the usual location of a normal anus.

E. Skin (see Chap. 34). The epidermis of a newborn (especially a premature infant) is thin; therefore, the oxygenated capillary blood makes it very pink. Common abnormalities include tiny **milia** (plugged sweat glands) on the nose, unusually brown-pigmented nevi scattered around any body part, and what are referred to as **mongolian spots.** Mongolian spots are bluish, often large areas most commonly seen on the back, buttocks, or thighs that fade slightly over the first year of life.

Erythema toxicum may be noted occasionally at birth, although it is more common in the next day or two. These papular lesions with an erythematous base are found more on the trunk than on the extremities and fade without treatment by 1 week of age.

Look for **jaundice.**

F. Palpable **lymph nodes** are found in approximately one-third of normal neonates. They are usually under 12 mm in diameter and are often found in the inguinal, cervical, and occasionally the axillary area.

G. **Extremities, spine, and joints** (see Chap. 28)

1. **Extremities.** Anomalies of the digits (too few, too many, syndactyly, or abnormal placement), club feet, and hip dislocation are the common problems. Because of fetal positioning, many infants have forefoot adduction, tibial bowing, or even tibial torsion. Forefoot adduction, if correctable with stretching, will often correct itself in weeks and is no cause for concern. Mild degrees of tibial bowing or torsion are also normal. Decreased motion of an arm should make one consider **Erb palsy** or a **fracture** of a clavicle or other bone (see Chap. 20).

2. To check for **hip dislocation** (if present, remember that the head of the femur would most often have been displaced superiorly and posteriorly), place the infant's legs in the frogleg position. With the third finger on the greater trochanter and the thumb and index finger holding the knee, attempt to relocate the femoral head in the acetabulum by pushing upward away from the mattress with the third finger and toward the mattress and laterally with the thumb at the knee. If there has been a dislocation, a distinct upward movement of the femoral head will be felt as it relocates in the acetabulum. Hip "clicks," due to movement of the ligamentum teres in the acetabulum, are much more common than dislocated hips (hip "clunks") and are not a cause for concern. It has been shown that not all dislocated hips are present at birth, and hence the recent designation "developmental dysplasia of the hip."

3. **Back.** The infant should be turned over and held face down on your hand. The back, especially the lower lumbar and sacral areas, should be examined. Special care should be taken to look for pilonidal sinus tracts and small soft midline swellings that might indicate a small meningocele or other anomaly (see Chap. 27D).

H. **Head, neck, and mouth**

1. **Head**

a. The average full-term **head circumference** is 33 to 38 cm.

b. The infant's **scalp** should be inspected for cuts or bruises due to application of the forceps or fetal monitor leads. Check laterally for erosions from the bony spines of the maternal pelvis, which may be difficult to see under hair. Scalp aplasia may also be present.

c. **Caput succedaneum** (edema of the scalp from labor pressure) should be checked to see if there are underlying early cephalohematomas; **cephalo-hematomas** usually do not become full-blown until the third or fourth day.

d. **Mobility of the suture lines** will rule out **craniosynostosis.** Mobility is checked by putting each thumb on opposite sides of the suture and then pushing in alternately while feeling for motion. The skull should be observed for **deformational plagiocephaly.**

e. The degree of **molding of the skull bones** themselves should be noted, and it may be considerable. Usually, such molding will subside within 5 days.

f. Occasionally infants have **craniotabes,** a soft ping-pong ball effect of the skull bones (usually the parietal bones). It is most common in postmature or dysmature infants. If present, craniotabes is usually only an incidental finding that disappears in a matter of weeks, even if marked at birth.

g. **Fontanelles.** As long as the circumference of the head is within normal limits and there is motion of the suture lines, one need pay little attention to the size (large or small) of the fontanelles. Very large fontanelles reflect a delay in bone ossification and may be associated with hypothyroidism (see

Chap. 2B), trisomy syndromes, intrauterine malnutrition, hypophosphatasia, rickets, and osteogenesis imperfecta. Normal tension is that in which the fontanelle softens when the infant is raised to the sitting position.

   h. Ears. Note size, shape, position, and presence of auditory canals as well as preauricular sinus, pits, or skin tags.

2. The **neck** should be checked for range of motion, goiter, and thyroglossal or branchial-arch sinus tracts. Occasionally, marked asymmetry is noted with a deep concavity on one side. Although the uninitiated might interpret this as possible agenesis of a muscle or muscle group, it is most commonly due to persistent fetal posture with the head tilted to one side **(asynclitism).** This is most easily confirmed by noting that the mandibular gum line is not parallel to the maxillary line—further evidence of unequal pressure on the jaw as a result of the head being held tilted *in utero* over time (see Chap. 28).

3. The **mouth** should be checked to ensure that there are neither hard nor soft palatal clefts, no gum clefts, and no deciduous teeth present. Rarely, cysts appear on the gum or under the tongue. **Epstein pearls** (small white inclusion cysts clustered about the midline at the juncture of the hard and soft palate) are normal.

I. Neurologic examination. Much has been written about neonatal neurologic examinations, but more will have to be learned before the examination becomes an accurate evaluation—especially one with prognostic significance—when done at birth. A carefully performed, detailed examination will reveal more than a superficial one. Many senior physicians can recall an infant with hydranencephaly or a similar gross internal neurologic lesion that was completely missed by careful neurologic examination, only to be found later by ultrasonography of the head or even simple transillumination.

1. Probably the most reliable information that can be obtained quickly is while handling the infant during the preceding parts of the examination. With experience, the examiner is able to carry out at least two examinations concurrently, that is, the examination of organ and physiologic systems and a simultaneous neurologic evaluation. Symmetry of movement and posturing, body tone, and response to being handled and disturbed (i.e., crying appropriately and quieting appropriately) can all be evaluated while other body parts are being tested.

2. The amount of crying should be carefully noted, as well as the pitch. When the infant is crying, seventh nerve weaknesses should be sought (the affected side of the mouth does not pull down). **Erb palsy,** if present, will usually be revealed by lack of motion of the shoulder and arm; the arm will lie beside the body in repose rather than being normally flexed with fist near mouth. Jitteriness that is present but disappears in the prone position is usually benign (see Chap. 27A). Persistent crying should make one search for the cause of pain (e.g., fracture).

3. The essentials of a neurologic examination (beyond that acquired while carrying out other components of the physical examination) may be covered by doing the following:

   a. Put your index fingers in the infant's palms to obtain the Palmer grasp. Then hold the infant's fingers between your thumb and forefinger and pull him or her to a sitting position. Note the degrees of head lag and head control; remember a crying infant often throws the head back in anger. The infant should be held in a sitting position and the trunk moved forward and back enough to test head control again. Then let the trunk and head slowly fall back.

   b. To test the Moro reflex, pull your fingers quickly from his or her grasp just before the head touches the mattress, allowing the infant to fall onto the back. Usually the Moro reflex will result, although a "complete" Moro is demonstrable only in approximately 20% of cases.

   c. Touching the upper lip laterally will cause most infants to turn toward the touch and open their mouths; the hungrier and more vigorous the infant, the more intense is the rooting response. Placing a nipple in the mouth will initiate a sucking response.

4. Stepping (and placing) can be elicited by holding the infant upright with the feet on the mattress and then making the baby lean forward. This forward motion often sets off a slow alternate stepping action. However, frequently a normal infant will not perform the reflex.

5. The complete **behavioral examination** is more dependent on infant–examiner interaction. Much depends on the infant's relative wakefulness, whether the baby has just been fed or not, and to a degree, on the analgesia and anesthesia used during delivery. Eye opening is elicited when the infant is sucking or being held vertically. Some infants will appear alert and listen when they are spoken to in a pleasant voice. Almost all infants enjoy being cuddled. If some of these behavioral responses cannot be elicited, they may indicate either temporary or permanent problems. The more detailed behavioral examination also involves habituation to repeated stimuli of various types (noxious and otherwise) that will not be discussed here.

J. Head circumference and length. These measurements are usually done last in the examination. The head circumference of a term (38- to 40-week) infant of normal weight (2.7–3.6 kg, or 6–8 lb) is usually 33–38 cm (13–15 in.). Crown-foot length is 48 to 53 cm (19–21 in.).

K. Eye examination. The eyes should be examined for the presence of scleral hemorrhages, icterus, conjunctival exudate, iris coloring, and pupillary size, equality, extraocular muscle movement, and centering. The red reflex should be obtained, and cataracts sought. Glaucoma is manifest by a large cloudy cornea. The normal cornea in a neonate measures <10.5 mm in horizontal diameter. In the first 2 days of life, puffy eyelids sometimes make examination of the eyes impossible. If so, this fact should be noted so that the eyes will be examined upon follow-up.

III. DISCHARGE EXAMINATION. At discharge, the infant should be reexamined with the following points considered:

A. Heart. Development of murmur, cyanosis, failure, femoral pulses.

B. CNS. Fullness of fontanelles, sutures, activity.

C. Abdomen. Any masses previously missed, stools, urine output.

D. Skin. Jaundice, pyoderma.

E. Cord. Infection.

F. Infection. Signs of sepsis.

G. Feeding. Spitting, vomiting, distension, degree of weight loss (or gain), dehydration.

H. Parental competence. To provide adequate care.

I. Follow-up. Arrangements made with infant's primary physician.

Suggested Readings

Bamji M, Stone RK, Kaul A, et al. Palpable lymph nodes in healthy newborns and infants. *Pediatrics* 1986;78:573.

Ben-Ari J, Merlob P, Mimouni F, et al. Characteristics of the male genitalia in the newborn. *J Urol* 1985;135:521.

Brazelton TB. *Neurobehavioral assessment scale*. Philadelphia: JB Lippincott Co, 1973.

El-Haddao M, Corkery JJ. The anus in the newborn. *Pediatrics* 1985;76:927.

Faix RG. Fontanelle size in black and white term newborn infants. *J Pediatr* 1982;100:304.

Nelson LB. *Pediatric ophthalmology*. Philadelphia: WB Saunders, 1984.

Scanlon JW. *A system of newborn physical examination*. Baltimore: University Park Press, 1979.

IDENTIFYING THE HIGH-RISK NEWBORN AND EVALUATING GESTATIONAL AGE, PREMATURITY, POSTMATURITY, LARGE-FOR-GESTATIONAL-AGE, AND SMALL-FOR-GESTATIONAL-AGE INFANTS

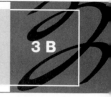

Kimberly G. Lee

I. **High-risk newborns** are associated with certain conditions; when one or more of these are present, nursery staff should be aware and prepared for possible difficulties. The cord blood and placenta should be saved after delivery in all cases of high-risk delivery, including cases that involve transfer from the birth hospital, since an elusive diagnosis such as toxoplasmosis may be made on the basis of placental pathology.

The following factors are associated with high-risk newborns:

A. **Maternal characteristics and associated risk for fetus or neonate**

   1. **Age at delivery**

      a. **Over 40 years.** Chromosomal abnormalities, macrosomia, intrauterine growth restriction (IUGR), blood loss (abruption, previa).

      b. **Under 16 years.** IUGR, prematurity, child abuse/neglect (mother herself may be abused).

   2. **Personal factors**

      a. **Poverty.** Prematurity, infection, IUGR.

      b. **Smoking.** IUGR, increased perinatal mortality.

      c. **Drug/alcohol use.** IUGR, fetal alcohol syndrome, withdrawal syndrome, sudden infant death syndrome, child abuse/neglect.

      d. **Poor diet.** Mild IUGR to fetal demise in severe malnutrition.

      e. **Trauma (acute, chronic).** Abruptio placentae, fetal demise, prematurity.

   3. **Maternal medical conditions and associated risk for fetus or neonate**

      a. **Diabetes mellitus.** Congenital anomalies, stillbirth, respiratory distress. syndrome (RDS), hypoglycemia, macrosomia/birth injury (see Chap. 2A).

      b. **Thyroid disease.** Goiter, hypothyroidism, hyperthyroidism (see Chap. 2B).

      c. **Renal disease.** IUGR, stillbirth, prematurity.

      d. **Urinary tract infection.** Prematurity, sepsis.

      e. **Heart, lung disease.** IUGR, stillbirth, prematurity.

      f. **Hypertension (chronic or pregnancy-related).** IUGR, stillbirth, asphyxia, prematurity.

      g. **Anemia.** IUGR, stillbirth, asphyxia, prematurity, hydrops.

      h. **Isoimmunization (red cell antigens).** Stillbirth, anemia, jaundice, hydrops.

      i. **Isoimmunization (platelet antigens).** Stillbirth, bleeding.

      j. **Thrombocytopenia.** Stillbirth, bleeding.

   4. **Obstetric history and associated risk for fetus or neonate**

      a. **Past history of infant with prematurity, jaundice, RDS, or anomalies.** Same with current pregnancy.

      b. **Maternal medications.** See Appendix B and C.

      c. **Bleeding in early pregnancy.** Stillbirth, prematurity.

      d. **Hyperthermia.** Fetal demise, fetal anomalies.

      e. **Bleeding in third trimester.** Stillbirth, anemia.

      f. **Premature rupture of membranes.** Infection/sepsis.

      g. **TORCH infections.** See Chapter 23.

      h. **Trauma.** Fetal demise, prematurity.

B. **Fetal conditions and associated risk for fetus or neonate**

   1. **Multiple gestation.** Prematurity, twin–twin transfusion syndrome, IUGR, asphyxia, birth trauma.

   2. **IUGR.** fetal demise, congenital anomalies, asphyxia, hypoglycemia, polycythemia.

   3. **Macrosomia.** Congenital anomalies, birth trauma, hypoglycemia.

   4. **Abnormal fetal position/presentation.** Congenital anomalies, birth trauma, hemorrhage.

5. **Abnormality of fetal heart rate or rhythm.** Hydrops, asphyxia, congestive heart failure, heart block.
6. **Decreased activity.** Fetal demise, asphyxia.
7. **Polyhydramnios.** Anencephaly, other central nervous system (CNS) disorders, neuromuscular disorders, problems with swallowing (e.g., agnathia, esophageal atresia), chylothorax, diaphragmatic hernia, omphalocele, gastroschisis, trisomy, tumors, hydrops, isoimmunization, anemia, cardiac failure, intrauterine infection, inability to concentrate urine, maternal diabetes. (May also be associated with large but otherwise well infant.)
8. **Oligohydramnios.** IUGR, placental insufficiency, postmaturity, fetal demise, intrapartum distress, renal agenesis, pulmonary hypoplasia, deformations.

C. **Conditions of labor and delivery and associated risk for fetus or neonate**
1. **Premature labor.** RDS, other issues of prematurity (see Chap. 6).
2. **Post-term labor (occurring more than 2 weeks after term).** Stillbirth, asphyxia, meconium aspiration (see VI).
3. **Maternal fever.** Infection/sepsis.
4. **Maternal hypotension.** Stillbirth, asphyxia.
5. **Rapid labor.** Birth trauma, intracranial hemorrhage (ICH), retained fetal lung fluid/transient tachypnea.
6. **Prolonged labor.** Stillbirth, asphyxia, birth trauma.
7. **Abnormal presentation.** Birth trauma, asphyxia.
8. **Uterine tetany**
9. **Meconium-stained amniotic fluid.** Stillbirth, asphyxia, meconium aspiration syndrome, persistent pulmonary hypertension.
10. **Prolapsed cord**
11. **Cesarean section.** RDS, retained fetal lung fluid/transient tachypnea, blood loss.
12. **Obstetric analgesia and anesthesia.** Respiratory depression, hypotension, hypothermia.
13. Placental anomalies.
   a. **Small placenta.** IUGR.
   b. **Large placenta.** Hydrops, maternal diabetes, large infant.
   c. **Torn placenta and/or umbilical vessels.** Blood loss.
   d. **Abnormal attachment of vessels to placenta.** Blood loss.

D. **Immediately evident neonatal conditions and associated risk for fetus or neonate**
1. **Prematurity.** RDS, other sequelae of prematurity (further elaborated in subsequent chapters).
2. **Low 5-minute Apgar score.** Prolonged transition (especially respiratory).
3. **Low 15-minute Apgar score.** Cardiac failure, renal failure, severe neurologic damage.
4. **Pallor or shock.** Blood loss.
5. **Foul smell of amniotic fluid or membranes.** Infection.
6. **Small size for gestational age (GA).** See IV.
7. **Postmaturity.** See VI.

II. **GA and birth weight classification** Neonates should be classified by GA if at all possible, as this is more meaningful than that based on birth weight.
A. **GA classification**
1. Assessment based on **obstetric information** is covered in Chapter 1. Note that GA estimates by first-trimester ultrasonography are accurate within 4 days.
2. To confirm or supplement obstetric dating, the modified Dubowitz (Ballard) examination for newborns (see Fig. 3B.1) may be useful in GA estimation. There are limitations to this method, especially with use of the neuromuscular component in sick newborns.
3. **Infant classification by gestational (postmenstrual) age**
   a. **Preterm.** Less than 37 completed weeks (259 days).
   b. **Term.** Thirty-seven to 41 6/7 weeks (260–294 days).
   c. **Post-term.** Forty-two weeks (295 days) or more.

Neuromuscular Maturity

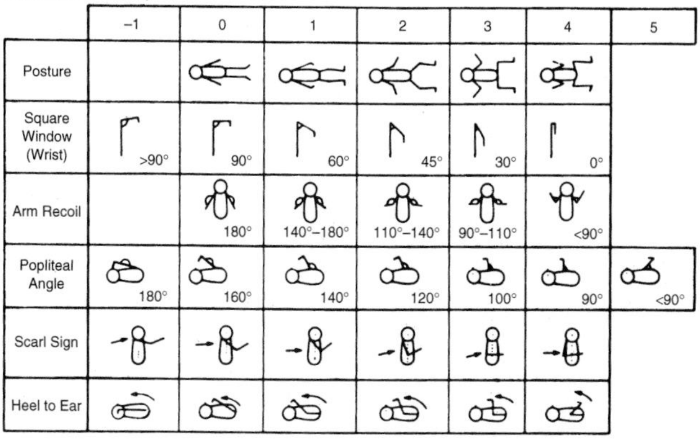

Physical Maturity

									Maturity Rating	
									Score	Weeks
Skin	Sticky Friable, Transparent	Gelatinous, Red, Translucent	Smooth Pink, Visible Veins	Superficial Peeling and/or Rash, Few Veins	Cracking, Pale Areas, Rare Veins	Parchment, Deep Cracking, No Vessels	Leathery, Cracked, Wrinkled		−10	20
									−5	22
Lanugo	None	Sparse	Abundant	Thinning	Bald Areas	Mostly Bald			0	24
Plantar Surface	Heel-Toe 40-50 mm:−1 <40 mm:−2	>50mm No Crease	Faint Red Marks	Anterior Transverse Crease Only	Creases Anterior 2/3	Creases Over Entire Sole			5	26
									10	28
Breast	Imperceptible	Barely Perceptible	Flat Areola No Bud	Stippled Areola 1–2 mm Bud	Raised Areola 3–4 mm Bud	Full Areola 5–10 mm Bud			15	30
									20	32
Eye/Ear	Lids fused Loosely:−1 Tightly:−2	Lids Open Prima Flat Stays Folded	Sl. curved pinna; soft; slow recoil	Well–Curved Pinna; Soft but Ready Recoil	Formed and Firm Instant Recoil	Thick Cartilage Car Stiff			25	34
									30	36
Genitals (Male)	Scrotum Flat, Smooth	Scrotum Empty Faint Rugae	Testes in Upper Canal Rare Rugae	Testes in Descending Lew Rugae	Testes Down, Good Rugae	Testes Pendulous, Deep Rugae			35	38
									40	40
Genitals (Female)	Clitoris Prominent, Labia Flat	Prominent Clitoris, Small Labia Minora	Prominent Clitoris, Enlarging Minora	Majora and Minora Equally Prominent	Majora Large, Minora Small	Majora Cover Clitoris and Minora			45	42
									50	44

Expanded NBS Includes Etremely Premature Infants and Has Been Refined to Improve Accuracy in More Mature Infant.

Figure 3B.1. New Ballard score. (From Ballard JL, Khoury JC, Wedig K, et al. New Ballard Score, expanded to include extremely premature infants. *J Pediatr* 1991;119:417.)

    d. Late preterm is an emerging classification referring to subgroups of infants between 34 and 38 weeks gestation; it is not yet used consistently for a single age range.

B. Birth weight classification. Although there is no universal agreement, the commonly accepted definitions are as follows:

    1. Normal birth weight (NBW). From 2,500 to 3,999 g.

    2. Low birth weight (LBW). Less than 2,500 g. Note that, while most LBW infants are preterm, some are term but small for gestational age (SGA). LBW infants can be further subclassified as follows:

        a. Very low birth weight (VLBW). Less than 1,500 g.

        b. Extremely low birth weight (ELBW). Less than 1,000 g.

III. Prematurity. As noted above, a **preterm neonate** is one whose birth occurs through the end of the last day of the 37th week (259th day; i.e., 366/7 weeks) following onset of the last menstrual period.

   A. Incidence. Approximately 12% of all births in the United States are premature, and approximately 2% are of <32 weeks' gestation. The incidence has been increasing in recent years, especially among later-gestation preterms or "late preterms." In some population segments, demographics play a major role in the incidence of prematurity.

   B. Etiology is unknown in most cases. Preterm and/or LBW delivery is associated with the following conditions:

   1. **Low socioeconomic status** (SES), whether measured by family income, educational level, geographic area/ZIP code, social class, and/or occupation.

   2. **African American** women's rate of very premature (<32 weeks' gestation) delivery is almost three times that of white women, and their rate of moderately premature (32–36 weeks) delivery is approximately one and a half times that of white women. Disparities persist even when SES is taken into account.

   3. Women **younger than 16 or older than 35** are more likely to deliver LBW infants; the association with age is more significant in whites than in African Americans.

   4. **Maternal activity** requiring long periods of standing or substantial amounts of physical stress may be associated with IUGR and prematurity. This is not significant in mothers from higher-SES groups, possibly because they are less likely to continue working in such jobs once they encounter pregnancy complications.

   5. **Acute or chronic maternal illness** is associated with early delivery, whether spontaneous or, not infrequently, induced.

   6. **Multiple-gestation births** frequently occur prematurely (57% of twins and 93% of triplets in the United States in 2000). In such births, higher rate of neonatal mortality is primarily due to prematurity.

   7. **Prior poor birth outcome** is the single strongest predictor of poor birth outcome. A preterm first birth is the best predictor of a preterm second birth.

   8. **Obstetric factors** such as uterine malformations, uterine trauma, placenta previa, abruptio placentae, hypertensive disorders, preterm cervical shortening, previous cervical surgery, premature rupture of membranes, and amnionitis also contribute to prematurity.

   9. **Fetal conditions** such as nonreassuring testing (see Chap. 1), IUGR, or severe hydrops may require preterm delivery.

   10. **Inadvertent early delivery** because of incorrect estimation of GA is now less common.

   C. Problems of prematurity, which are related to difficulty in extrauterine adaptation due to immaturity of organ systems, are noted here but discussed in greater detail in other chapters.

   1. **Respiratory.** Premature infants may experience the following:

      a. **Perinatal depression** in the delivery room due to poor adaptation to breathing (see Chap. 4).

      b. **RDS** due to surfactant deficiency (see Chap. 24A).

      c. **Apnea** due to immaturity in mechanisms controlling breathing (see Chap. 24I).

      d. **Bronchopulmonary dysplasia (BPD)** variously described/classified as chronic lung disease (CLD), Wilson-Mikity disease, and chronic pulmonary insufficiency of prematurity (see Chap. 24J).

   2. **Neurologic.** Premature infants have a higher risk for neurologic problems including the following:

      a. Perinatal depression.

      b. ICH (see Chap. 27B).

      c. Periventricular white-matter and other neural injury (see Chap. 27C).

   3. **Cardiovascular.** Premature infants may present with cardiovascular problems including the following:

   a. Hypotension. This may be due to the following:
      i. Hypovolemia.
      ii. Cardiac dysfunction.
      iii. Vasodilation due to sepsis.
   b. Patent ductus arteriosus is common and may lead to congestive heart failure (see Chap. 25).
4. Hematologic conditions for which premature infants are at higher risk include the following:
   a. Anemia (see Chap. 26A).
   b. Hyperbilirubinemia (see Chap. 18).
5. Nutritional. Premature infants require specific attention to the content, amount, and route of feeding (see Chap. 10).
6. Gastrointestinal. Prematurity is the single greatest risk factor for necrotizing enterocolitis; formula feeding is also a significant risk factor; breast milk appears to be protective (see Chap. 32).
7. Metabolic problems, especially in glucose and calcium metabolism, are more common in premature infants (see Chap. 29).
8. Renal. Immature kidneys are characterized by low glomerular filtration rate and an inability to handle water, solute, and acid loads; fluid and electrolyte management can be difficult (see Chaps. 9 and 31).
9. Temperature regulation. Premature infants are especially susceptible to hypothermia and hyperthermia (see Chap. 12).
10. Immunologic. Because of deficiencies in both humoral and cellular response, premature infants are at greater risk for infection than are term infants.
11. Ophthalmologic. Retinopathy of prematurity may develop in the immature retina in infants <32 weeks or with birth weight <1,500 g (see Chaps. 35A and 35B).
D. Management of the premature infant (see also Chap. 6).
   1. Immediate postnatal management
      a. Delivery in an appropriately equipped and staffed hospital is most important. Risks to the very premature or sick preterm infant are greatly increased by delays in initiating necessary specialized care.
      b. Resuscitation and stabilization require the immediate availability of qualified personnel and equipment. Anticipation and prevention are always preferred over reaction to problems already present. Adequate oxygen delivery and maintenance of proper temperature are immediate postnatal goals (see Chap. 4).
   2. Neonatal management
      a. Thermal regulation should be directed toward achieving a neutral thermal zone, that is, environmental temperature sufficient to maintain body temperature, yet with minimal oxygen consumption. For the small preterm infant, this will require either an overhead radiant warmer (with the advantages of infant accessibility and rapid temperature response) or a closed incubator (with the advantages of diminished insensible water loss) (see Chap. 12).
      b. Oxygen therapy and assisted ventilation (see Chap. 24).
      c. Patent ductus arteriosus in premature infants with birth weight >1,000 g usually requires only conservative management: adequate oxygenation, fluid restriction, and possibly intermittent diuresis. In smaller infants, a prostaglandin antagonist such as indomethacin may be necessary. In the most symptomatic infants or those for whom medical therapy fails to close the ductus, surgical ligation may become necessary. Prophylactic treatment for ELBW infants remains controversial (see Chap. 25).
      d. Fluid and electrolyte therapy must account for potentially high insensible water loss while maintaining proper hydration and normal glucose and plasma electrolyte concentrations (see Chap. 9).
      e. Nutrition, which may be limited by the inability of many preterm infants to suck and swallow effectively or to tolerate enteral feedings, may require

gavage feeding or parenteral nutrition. Mother's milk is the optimal primary source of enteral nutrition (see Chap. 10).

f. Hyperbilirubinemia, which is inevitable in the smallest infants, can be usually managed effectively by careful monitoring of bilirubin levels and judicious use of phototherapy. In the most severe cases, exchange transfusion may be necessary (see Chap. 18).

g. Infection is always possible after preterm delivery. Broad-spectrum antibiotics should be begun when suspicion is strong. Consider antistaphylococcal antibiotics for VLBW infants who have undergone multiple procedures or have remained for long periods in the hospital and are at increased risk of nosocomial infection (see Chap. 23).

h. Immunization. Diphtheria, tetanus, and acellular pertussis (DTaP) vaccine; inactivated polio vaccine (IPV); multivalent pneumococcal conjugate vaccine (PCV); and hemophilus influenzae type b (HIibvaccine are given in full doses to premature infants on the basis of their chronologic age (i.e., weeks after birth), and postmenstrual age. Hepatitis B (HepB) vaccine administration for medically unstable preterm infants of hepatitis B surface antigen (HBsAg)-negative mothers may be given on a modified schedule.

i. If the infant remains hospitalized at the appropriate chronologic age (usually at 2, 4, and 6 months), DTaP, PCV, IPV, and Hib should be given in the hospital. Pertussis vaccine remains contraindicated in infants with evolving or unstable neurologic disorders; these infants must receive pediatric DT, not adult DT vaccine. Infants with stable neurologic conditions may receive DTaP.

ii. HepB. Preterm infants whose mothers test positive for hepatitis B surface antigen (**HBsAg-positive**) should receive hepatitis B immune globulin (HBIG) within 12 hours of birth with the appropriate dose of HepB given concurrently at a different site (see Chap. 23). This dose should not be counted as part of the routine series of HepB; three subsequent doses should be given beginning at one month of age. Testing for HBsAg and antibody to HBsAg after completion of the vaccine series should be conducted at age 9 to 18 months.

Preterm infants whose mother's HBsAg status is **unknown** at the time of delivery should receive HepB within 12 hours of life. Those weighing <2 kg should also receive HBIG within 12 hours if the mother's HBsAg test results are not available by that time. For infants with birth weight over 2 kg, HBIG administration may be delayed up to 7 days while awaiting the mother's HBsAg results.

The optimal timing for HepB vaccination in preterm infants with birth weight <2 kg and whose mothers are HBsAg-**negative** is not clear. However, some studies have reported seroconversion rates in VLBW infants in whom vaccination was initiated shortly postpartum to be lower than in preterm infants vaccinated later or in term infants vaccinated shortly postpartum. The first vaccination in preterm infants with birth weight <2 kg and whose mothers are HBsAg-negative may therefore be delayed until just before hospital discharge or one month of age, whichever occurs first. Two subsequent doses of HepB are indicated, the first at 1 or 2 months and the second after 24 weeks of age. Administering four doses of HepB is permissible (e.g., when combination vaccines are administered after the birth dose); however, if monovalent HepB is used, a dose at four months is not needed.

iii. All infants 6 to 23 months of age, especially those with chronic respiratory disease, should receive **influenza immunization** annually. To protect infants younger than 6 months, their family and other caretakers should be immunized against influenza. Children aged 8 years or younger who are receiving influenza vaccine for the first time should receive two doses separated by at least 4 weeks.

iv. **Respiratory syncytial virus (RSV) prophylaxis**. Intramuscular immune globulin, palivizumab, is usually preferred over intravenous immune globulin respiratory syncytial virus immune globulin intravenous (RSV-IGIV). The following text is from the American Academy of Pediatrics Redbook 2006:

Palivizumab, a humanized mouse monoclonal antibody that is administered intramuscularly, is available to reduce the risk of RSV hospitalization in high-risk children. RSV-IGIV, a hyperimmune, polyclonal globulin prepared from donors selected for high serum titers of RSV neutralizing antibody, is no longer available. Palivizumab is licensed for prevention of RSV lower respiratory tract disease in selected infants and children with CLD of prematurity (formerly called *bronchopulmonary dysplasia*) or with a history of preterm birth (<35 weeks' gestation) or with congenital heart disease. Palivizumab is administered every 30 days, beginning in early November, with 4 subsequent monthly doses (total of 5 doses). The dose of palivizumab is 15 mg/kg, administered intramuscularly. Palivizumab is not effective in the treatment of RSV disease, and it is not approved for this indication.

Recommendations by the American Academy of Pediatrics for the use of palivizumab are as follows:

Palivizumab prophylaxis should be considered for infants and children younger than 24 months with CLD or prematurity who have required medical therapy (supplemental oxygen, bronchodilator or diuretic or corticosteroid therapy) for CLD within 6 months before the start of the RSV season. Patients with more severe CLD who continue to require medical therapy may benefit from prophylaxis during a second RSV season. Data are limited regarding the effectiveness of palivizumab during the second year of life. Individual patients may benefit from decision made in consultation with neonatologists, pediatric intensivists, pulmonologists, or infectious disease specialists.

Infants born at 32 weeks of gestation or earlier may benefit from RSV prophylaxis, even if they do not have CLD. For these infants, major risk factors to be considered include their GA and chronologic age at the start of the RSV season. Infants born at 28 weeks of gestation or earlier may benefit from prophylaxis during their first RSV season, whenever that occurs during the first 12 months of life. Infants born at 29 to 31 weeks of gestation may benefit most from prophylaxis up to 6 months of age. For the purpose of this recommendation, 32 weeks' gestation refers to an infant born on or before the 32nd week of gestation (i.e., 32 weeks, 0 day). Once a child qualifies for initiation of prophylaxis at the start of the RSV season, administration should continue throughout the season and not stop at the point an infant reaches either 6 months or 12 months of age.

Although palivizumab has been shown to decrease the likelihood of hospitalization in infants born between 32 and 35 weeks of gestation (i.e., between 32 weeks, 1 day and 35 weeks, 0 day), the cost of administering prophylaxis to this large group of infants must be considered carefully. Therefore, most experts recommend that prophylaxis should be reserved for infants in this group who are at greatest risk of severe infection and who are younger than 6 months at the start of RSV season. Epidemiologic data suggest that RSV infection is more likely to lead to hospitalization for these infants when the following risk factors are present: child care attendance, school-aged siblings, exposure to environmental air pollutants, congenital abnormalities of the airways, or severe neuromuscular disease. However, no single risk factor causes a very large increase in the rate of hospitalization, and the risk is additive as the number of risk factors for an individual infant increases. Therefore, prophylaxis should be considered for infants between 32 and 35 weeks of gestation only if two or more of these risk factors are present. Passive household exposure to tobacco smoke has not been associated with an increased risk of RSV hospitalization on a consistent basis. Furthermore, exposure to tobacco smoke is a risk factor that can be controlled by the family of an infant at increased risk of severe RSV disease, and preventive measures will be far less costly than palivizumab prophylaxis. High-risk infants should never be exposed to tobacco smoke. In contrast to the well-documented beneficial effect of breast-feeding against many viral illnesses, existing data are conflicting regarding the specific protective effect of breast-feeding against RSV infection. High-risk infants should be kept away from crowds and from situations in which exposure to infected individuals cannot be controlled. Participation in group child care should be restricted during the RSV season for high-risk infants whenever feasible. Parents should be instructed on the importance of meticulous hand hygiene. In addition, all high-risk infants and their contacts should be immunized against influenza beginning at 6 months of age.

In the Northern hemisphere and particularly within the United States, RSV circulates predominantly between November and March. The inevitability of the RSV season is predictable, but the severity of the season, the time of onset, the peak of activity, and the end of the season cannot be predicted precisely. There can be substantial variation in the timing of the community outbreaks of RSV disease from year to year in the same community and between communities in the same year, even in the same region. These variations, however, occur within the overall pattern of RSV outbreaks, usually beginning in November or December, peaking in January or February, and ending by the end of March or sometime in April. Communities in the southern United States tend to experience the earliest onset of RSV activity, and midwestern states tend to experience the latest. The duration of the season for western and northwest regions is typically between that noted for the south and the midwest. In recent years, the national median duration of the RSV season has been 15 weeks and even in the south, with a seasonal duration of 16 weeks, the range is 13 to 20 weeks. Results from clinical trials indicate that palivizumab trough serum concentrations >30 days after the fifth dose will be well above the protective concentration for most infants. If the first dose is administered in November, five monthly doses of palivizumab will provide substantially >20 weeks of protective serum antibody concentrations for most of the RSV season, even with variation in onset and end of season. Changes from this recommendation of 5 monthly doses require careful consideration of the benefits and costs.

Children who are 24 months or younger with hemodynamically significant cyanotic and acyanotic congenital heart disease will benefit from palivizumab prophylaxis. Decisions regarding prophylaxis with palivizumab in children with congenital heart disease should be made on the basis of the degree of physiologic cardiovascular compromise. Children younger than 24 months with congenital heart disease who are most likely to benefit from immunoprophylaxis include the following:

- Infants who are receiving medication to control congestive heart failure
- Infants with moderate to severe pulmonary hypertension
- Infants with cyanotic heart disease

Because a mean decrease in palivizumab serum concentration of 58% was observed after surgical procedures that use cardiopulmonary bypass, for children who still require prophylaxis, a postoperative dose of palivizumab (15 mg/kg) should be considered as soon as the patient is medically stable.

The following groups of infants are not at increased risk of RSV and generally should not receive immunoprophylaxis.

■ Infants and children with hemodynamically insignificant heart disease (e.g., secundum atrial septal defect, small ventricular septal defect, pulmonic stenosis, uncomplicated aortic stenosis, mild coarctation of the aorta, and patent ductus arteriosus)

■ Infants with lesions adequately corrected by surgery, unless they continue to require medication for congestive heart failure

■ Infants with mild cardiomyopathy who are not receiving medical therapy

Dates for initiation and termination of prophylaxis should be on the basis of the same considerations as for high-risk preterm infants.

Palivizumab prophylaxis has not been evaluated in randomized trials in immunocompromised children. Although specific recommendations for immunocompromised patients cannot be made, children with severe immunodeficiencies (e.g., severe combined immunodeficiency or advanced acquired immunodeficiency syndrome) may benefit from prophylaxis.

Limited studies suggest that some patients with cystic fibrosis may be at increased risk of RSV infection. However, insufficient data exist to determine the effectiveness of palivizumab in the use of this patient population.

If an infant or child who is receiving palivizumab immunoprophylaxis experiences a breakthrough RSV infection, monthly prophylaxis should continue through the RSV season. This recommendation is based on the observation that high-risk infants may be hospitalized more than once in the same season with RSV lower respiratory tract disease and the fact that more than one RSV strain often cocirculates in a community.

Physicians should arrange for drug administration within 6 hours after opening a vial of palivizumab, because this biological product does not contain a preservative.

RSV is known to be transmitted in the hospital setting and to cause serious disease in high-risk infants. In high-risk hospitalized infants, the major method of preventing RSV disease is strict observance of infection control practices, including prompt isolation of RSV-infected infants. If an RSV outbreak occurs in a high-risk unit (e.g., pediatric intensive care unit), primary emphasis should be placed on proper infection control practices, especially hand hygiene. No data exist to support palivizumab use in controlling outbreaks of nosocomial disease.

Palivizumab does not interfere with response to vaccines.

Isolation of the hospitalized patient. In addition to standard precautions, contact precautions are recommended for the duration of RSV-associated illness among infants and young children, including patients treated with ribavirin. The effectiveness of these precautions depends on compliance and necessitates scrupulous adherence to appropriate hand hygiene practices. Patients with RSV infection should be cared for in single rooms or placed in a cohort.

Control measures. The control of nosocomial RSV transmission is complicated by the continuing chance of introduction through infected patients, staff, and visitors. During the peak of the RSV season, many infants and children hospitalized with respiratory tract symptoms will be infected with RSV and should be cared for with contact precautions. Early identification of RSV-infected patients is important so that appropriate precautions can be instituted promptly. During large outbreaks, a variety of measures have been demonstrated to be effective, including the following: (i) laboratory screening of symptomatic patients for RSV infection; (ii) cohorting infected patients and staff; (iii) excluding visitors with respiratory tract infections; (iv) excluding staff with respiratory tract illness or RSV infection from providing care to susceptible infants; and (v) use of gowns, gloves, goggles, and perhaps masks.

A critical aspect of RSV prevention among high-risk infants is education of parents and other caregivers about the importance of decreasing exposure to and transmission of RSV. Preventative measures include limiting, where feasible, exposure to contagious settings (e.g., child care centers) and emphasis on hand hygiene in all setting, including the home, especially during periods when contacts of high-risk infants have respiratory infections.

The 2006 American Academy of Pediatrics Guidelines for palivizumab prophylaxis (Synagis) are as follows:

- Between 32 and 35 weeks gestation who are less than six months of age (chronological) by the start of RSV season with additional risk factors.

    Siblings.

    Child care center attendance

    Exposure to tobacco smoke in the home

    Underlying conditions that predispose to respiratory complications

    Anticipated cardiac surgery during the RSV season

    Distance to and availability of hospital care for severe respiratory illness

- Between 29 and 32 weeks gestation who are less than six months of age (chronological) by the start of RSV season.

- Twenty-eight weeks of gestation or less and who are <1 year of age (chronological) by the start of RSV season.

- CLD—infants and children younger than 2 years of age with BPD/CLD who have required medical therapy for their BPD/CLD within the past 6 months before the anticipated RSV season.

v. Rotavirus vaccine(RV)
   a) Since it is a live vaccine it is not given until after discharge.
   b) Premature Infants (e.g., those born at <37 weeks' gestation): Premature infants can be immunized if they (i) are at least 6 weeks of age, (ii) are being or have been discharged from the hospital nursery, or (iii) are clinical stable and are not immunocompromised.
   c) Small prematures (26- to 28-week infants) may not be home at 90 days and since the vaccine is not to be given after 90 days of age, they would not get it.
   d) Currently the vaccine is recommended to infants born at 35 weeks GA or greater who are home and are not immunocompromised.
   e) This is a new vaccine, so recommendations may change.
   vi. Immunizations except RV should be given at least 48 hours before discharge so that any febrile response will occur in the hospital.
   vii. All Advisory Committee on Immunization Practices of the Center of Disease control (CDC) (ACIP) recommendations can be found at http://www.cdc.gov/acip.

E. Survival of premature infants. For many reasons survival statistics vary by institution as well as geographic region and country. Figures 3B.2 and 3B.3 show survival rates of 42,935 premature infants from 557 hospitals enrolled in the Vermont Oxford Network in 2005. The network maintains data on survival, intraventricular hemorrhage, retinopathy of prematurity, CLD, and many other problems of premature infants.

F. Long-term problems of prematurity. Premature infants are vulnerable to a wide spectrum of morbidities. The risk of morbidity, like that of mortality, declines markedly with increasing GA. Although severe impairment occurs in a small population, the prevalence of lesser morbidities is less clearly defined, and large

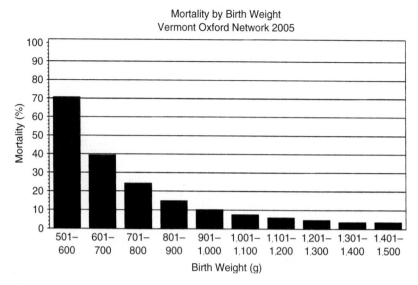

Figure 3B.2. Mortality by birth weight. Vermont Oxford Network 2005 with permission of Jeffery D. Horbar, MD, Editor of 2005 Database Summary. Vermont Oxford Network, 33 Kilburn Street, Burlington, VT 05401. Email: Lynn@vtoxford.org. Website: www.vtoxford.org.

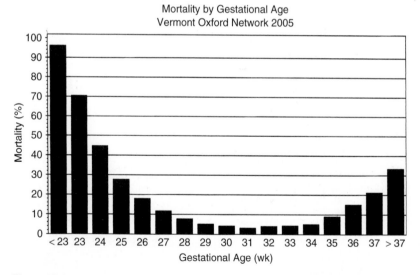

Figure 3B.3. Mortality by gestational age. Vermont Oxford Network 2005 with permission of Jeffery D. Horbar, MD, Editor of 2005 Database Summary. Vermont Oxford Network, 33 Kilburn Street, Burlington, VT 05401. Email: Lynn@vtoxford.org. Website: www.vtoxford.org.

controlled multicenter trials are now providing a more comprehensive picture both of these sequelae and of the effects of intervention.

1. **Developmental disability**
   a. **Major handicaps** (cerebral palsy, mental retardation).
   b. **Sensory impairments** (hearing loss, visual impairment) (see Chaps. 35A and 35B).
   c. **Minimal cerebral dysfunction** (language disorders, learning disability, hyperactivity, attention deficits, behavior disorders).
2. **Retinopathy of prematurity** (see Chap. 35A).
3. **CLD** (see Chap. 24).
4. **Poor growth** (see Chap. 10).
5. **Increased rates of postneonatal illness and rehospitalization.**
6. **Increased frequency of congenital anomalies.**

IV. **Infants who are SGA** (see Chap. 1)
   A. **Definition.** There is no uniform definition of SGA, although most reports define it as two standard deviations below the mean for GA or as below the tenth percentile. For practical purposes, infants with birth weights less than the third percentile for GA are at the greatest risk of perinatal morbidity and mortality. Further, babies who are constitutionally SGA are at lower risk compared with those who have experienced IUGR due to some pathologic process. Numerous "normal birth curves" have been defined using studies of large infant populations (see Fig. 3B.4); it should be noted that over the past 30 years birth weight has increased in the general population.
   B. **Etiology.** Approximately one-third of LBW infants are SGA. There is an association between the following factors and SGA infants:
      1. **Maternal factors**
         a. Genetic size.
         b. Demographics.
            i. Age (extremes of reproductive life).
            ii. Race.
            iii. SES.
         c. Underweight before pregnancy (e.g., malnutrition).
         d. Chronic disease.
         e. Factors interfering with placental flow and oxygenation.
            i. Heart disease.
            ii. Renal disease.
            iii. Hypertension (chronic or preeclampsia).
            iv. Tobacco use.
            v. Cocaine use.
            vi. Sickle-cell anemia and other hemoglobinopathies.
            vii. Pulmonary disease.
            viii. Collagen-vascular disease.
            ix. Diabetes (e.g., classes D, E, F, and R) (see Chap. 1).
            x. Postmaturity.
            xi. Multiple gestation/placentation.
            xii. Uterine anomalies.
            xiii. Thrombotic disease.
            xiv. High-altitude environment.
         f. Parity (nulliparity, grand multiparity).
         g. Malnutrition.
         h. Exposure to teratogens such as alcohol, drugs, and radiation.
      2. **Placental anatomical factors**
         a. Malformations (e.g., vascular malformations, velamentous cord insertion).
         b. Chorioangioma.
         c. Infarction.
         d. Abruption.
         e. Previa.
         f. Abnormal trophoblast invasion.

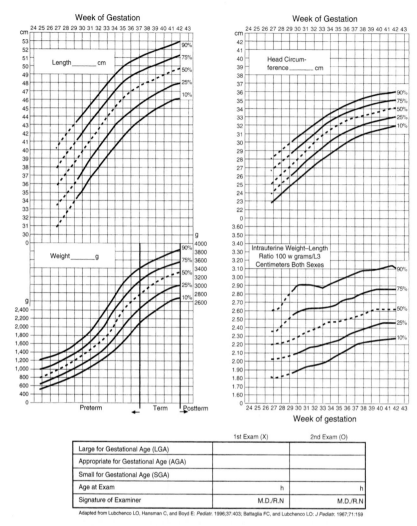

Figure 3B.4. Sample of a form used to classify newborns on the basis of maturity and intrauterine growth. (Reproduced with permission from a form developed by Kay J. L., Seton Medical Center, Austin, TX, with Mead Johnson & Co., Evansville, IN.)

3. **Fetal factors**
   a. **Constitutional**—most of SGA infants: normal, "genetically small."
   b. **Chromosomal abnormality**—under 5% of SGA infants; more likely in the presence of malformation.
   c. **Malformations,** especially abnormalities of CNS and skeletal system.
   d. **Congenital infection,** especially rubella and cytomegalovirus (see Chap. 23).
   e. **Multiple gestation.**
C. **Management of IUGR**
   1. **Pregnancy** (see Chap. 1).

    a. Attempt to determine the cause of IUGR. The investigation includes a search for relevant factors (listed in IV.B) and includes thorough ultrasonic examination.

    b. Assess and monitor fetal well-being. Antepartum fetal monitoring, including nonstress testing, oxytocin challenge testing, a biophysical profile, and serial ultrasonic examinations, is generally used (see Chap. 1). Doppler evaluation of placental flow may be used to evaluate uteroplacental insufficiency.

    c. Treat any underlying cause (e.g., hypertension) when possible.

    d. Consider the issue of fetal lung maturity if early delivery is contemplated (see Chaps. 1 and 24).

2. Delivery. Early delivery is necessary if the risk to the fetus of remaining *in utero* is considered greater than the risks of prematurity.

    a. Generally, indications for delivery are arrest of fetal growth, fetal distress, and pulmonary maturity near term, especially in a mother with hypertension.

    b. Acceleration of pulmonary maturity with glucocorticoids administered to the mother should be considered if amniotic fluid analyses suggest pulmonary immaturity, or delivery is anticipated remote from term.

    c. If there is poor placental blood flow, the fetus may not tolerate labor and may require cesarean delivery.

    d. As noted in IV.A, infants with extreme IUGR are at risk for perinatal problems and often require specialized care in the first few days of life. Therefore, if possible, delivery should occur at a center with a special care nursery. The delivery team should be prepared to manage fetal distress, perinatal depression, meconium aspiration, hypoxia, hypoglycemia, and heat loss.

3. In the nursery

    a. If not yet known, the cause of IUGR should be investigated; in many cases the etiology will remain unclear.

        i. Newborn examination. The infant should be evaluated for signs of any of the previously listed causes of poor fetal growth, especially chromosomal abnormalities, malformations, and congenital infection.

            a) Infants with growth restriction due to factors active during the phase of cellular hypertrophy in the last part of pregnancy (e.g., preeclampsia) will have a relatively normal head circumference, some reduction in length, but a more profound reduction in weight (see Figs. 3B.5 and 3B.6). This is thought to be due to the redistribution of fetal blood flow preferentially to vital organs, mainly the brain; hence the term "head-sparing IUGR." Use of the ponderal index (cube root of birth weight in grams × 100/[length in centimeters]) or the weight–length ratio will quantify weight loss. These infants may have little subcutaneous tissue, peeling loose skin, a wasted appearance, and meconium staining. The usual physical markers of GA (e.g., vernix, breast buds) may not be reliable owing to the "head-sparing" redistribution of perfusion.

            b) Infants whose growth restriction began in early pregnancy, during the phase of early fetal cellular hyperplasia, will have proportionally small head circumference, length, and weight. These infants are sometimes referred to as *symmetrically IUGR* and their ponderal index may be normal. As compared with infants whose IUGR began in late pregnancy, symmetrically IUGR infants are more likely to have significant intrinsic fetal problems (e.g., chromosomal defects, malformations, and/or congenital infection).

        ii. **Pathologic examination of the placenta** for infarction or congenital infection may be helpful.

        iii. Generally, **serologic screening** for congenital infection is not indicated unless history or examination suggests infection as a possible cause.

    b. Potential complications related to IUGR:

        i. Congenital anomalies.

        ii. Perinatal depression.

        iii. Meconium aspiration.

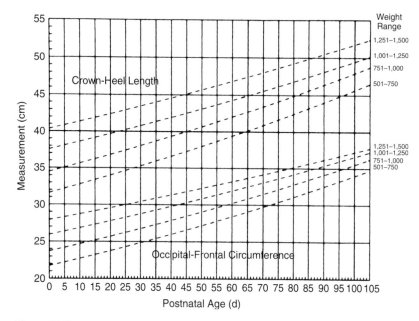

Figure 3B.5. Average crown–heel length and occipital-frontal circumference (centimeters) versus postnatal age (days) for infants with birth weight ranges 501 to 750 g, 751 to 1,000 g, 1,001 to 1,250 g, and 1,251 to 1,500 g. (Reproduced with permission from Wright K, Dawson JP, Fallis D, et al. New postnatal growth grids for very low birth weight infants. *Pediatrics* 1993;91:922–926, Copyright © 1993 by the AAP.)

      iv. Pulmonary hemorrhage.
      v. Persistent pulmonary hypertension.
      vi. Hypothermia.
      vii. Hypoglycemia.
      viii. Hypocalcemia.
      ix. Acute tubular necrosis/renal insufficiency.
      x. Polycythemia.
      xi. Thrombocytopenia.
      xii. Neutropenia.
  c. Specific management considerations
      i. SGA infants in general require **more calories per kilogram** than appropriate for gestational age (AGA) infants for "catch-up" growth; term SGA infants will often regulate their intake accordingly.
      ii. Blood glucose level should be monitored every 2 to 4 hours until it is in the normal range and stable.
      iii. Serum calcium levels may be significantly depressed in preterm SGA infants and/or those who have experienced hypoperfusion.
      iv. The **serum sodium concentration** may also be low (see Chap. 9).
D. Long-term issues of SGA infants. As noted in IV.A., most SGA infants have not experienced IUGR and are at low risk. However, it is difficult to determine specific effects of IUGR because of the multifactorial etiologies involved. Further, not all studies control well for parental height and SES, and there are often overlapping effects from prematurity and asphyxia. The comparison groups vary as well: while SGA infants have a lower risk of neonatal death compared with premature AGA infants of the same birth weight, they have a higher perinatal

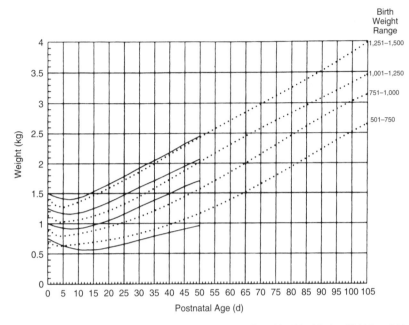

Figure 3B.6. Average daily weight (grams) versus postnatal age (days) for infants with birth weight ranges 501 to 701 g, 751 to 1,000 g, 1,001 to 1,250 g, and 1,250 to 1,500 g (dotted lines), plotted with the curves of Dancis et al. for infants with birth weights 750, 1,000, 1,250, and 1,500 g (solid lines.)

mortality rate than AGA infants of the same GA. They also have a greater risk of morbidity at 1 year of age. In general, SGA infants are at higher risk for poor postnatal growth. Those who are preterm and/or from disadvantaged socioeconomic environments may also be at increased risk for adverse cognitive outcomes. Finally, some adults who were SGA at birth appear to have a higher risk of coronary heart disease and related health problems, including hypertension, non–insulin-dependent diabetes, and stroke.

    E. Management of subsequent pregnancies is important because commonly IUGR recurs. Specific recommendations include the following:

        1. The mother should be cared for by personnel experienced in handling high-risk pregnancies.

        2. The health of mother and fetus should be assessed throughout pregnancy by ultrasonography and nonstress tests (see Chap. 1).

        3. Early delivery should be considered if fetal growth is poor.

V. Infants who are large for gestational age (LGA) (see Chap. 1)

    A. Definition. As with SGA, there is no uniform definition of LGA, although most reports define it as two standard deviations above the mean for GA or as above the 90th percentile.

    B. Etiology

        1. Constitutionally large infants (large parents).

        2. Infants of diabetic mothers (e.g., classes A, B, and C).

        3. Some post-term infants.

        4. Beckwith-Wiedemann and other syndromes.

    C. Management

        1. Evaluate for evidence of problems listed in V.B.

2. Look for evidence of birth trauma, including brachial plexus injury and perinatal depression (see Chaps. 20 and 27).
3. Allow the infant to feed early, and monitor the blood sugar level. Some LGA infants may have hyperinsulinism and may hence be prone to hypoglycemia (especially infants of diabetic mothers, infants with Beckwith-Wiedemann syndrome, or infants with erythroblastosis [see Chaps. 2A and 29A]).
4. Consider the possibility of polycythemia (see Chap. 26).

VI. Post-term infants
A. **Definition.** The newborn's gestation exceeds 42 completed weeks. Fewer than 12% of pregnancies reach this point; obstetric intervention often occurs earlier.
B. **Etiology.** The cause of prolonged pregnancy is unknown in most cases. The following are known associations:
   1. **Anencephaly.** An intact fetal pituitary–adrenal axis appears to be necessary for the initiation of labor.
   2. **Trisomies 16 and 18.**
   3. **Seckel syndrome** (bird-headed dwarfism).
   4. **Erroneous estimation of GA.**
C. **Syndrome of postmaturity.** These infants usually have normal length and head circumference. If they have postmaturity syndrome, however, they would have begun to lose weight. SGA infants also may have these signs and symptoms, and postmature infants may also be SGA. Postmature infants may be classified as follows:
   1. **Stage 1**
      a. Dry, cracked, peeling, loose, and wrinkled skin.
      b. Malnourished appearance.
      c. Decreased subcutaneous tissue.
      d. Skin "too big" for baby.
      e. Open-eyed and alert baby.
   2. **Stage 2**
      a. All features of stage 1.
      b. Meconium staining of amniotic fluid.
      c. Perinatal depression (in some cases).
   3. **Stage 3**
      a. The findings in stages 1 and 2.
      b. Meconium staining of cord and nails.
      c. A higher risk of fetal, intrapartum, or neonatal death.
D. **Management**
   1. **Antepartum management**
      a. Careful estimation of true GA, including ultrasonographic data.
      b. Antepartum assessments by cervical examination and monitoring of fetal well-being (see Chap. 1) should be initiated between 41 and 42 weeks on at least a weekly basis. If fetal testing is not reassuring, delivery is usually indicated. In most instances, a patient is a candidate for induction of labor if the pregnancy is at >41 weeks of gestation and the condition of the cervix is favorable.
   2. **Intrapartum management** involves use of fetal monitoring and preparation for possible perinatal depression and meconium aspiration.
   3. **Postpartum management**
      a. **Evaluation for complications related to postmaturity.** The following conditions occur more frequently in postmature infants:
         i. Congenital anomalies.
         ii. Perinatal depression.
         iii. Meconium aspiration.
         iv. Persistent pulmonary hypertension.
         v. Hypoglycemia.
         vi. Hypocalcemia.
         vii. Polycythemia.
      b. **Attention to proper nutritional support.**

Suggested Readings

American Academy of Pediatrics. *Report of Committee on Infectious Disease: The Redbook*, 27th ed. Evanston: American Academy of Pediatrics, 2006.

American Academy of Pediatrics and American College of Obstetricians and Gynecologists. *Guidelines for perinatal care*, 5th ed. Elk Grove Village, IL; Washington, DC: American Academy of Pediatrics and American College of Obstetricians and Gynecologists, 2002.

American Academy of Pediatrics Committee on Infectious Diseases and Committee on Fetus and Newborn. Revised indications for the use of palivizumab and respiratory syncytial virus immune globulin intravenous for the prevention of respiratory syncytial virus infections: Policy statement. *Pediatrics* 2003;112(6):1442–1446

Barker DJ. Early growth and cardiovascular disease. *Arch Dis Child* 1999;80:305.

Centers for Disease Control and Prevention. Recommended childhood and adolescent immunization schedule—United States, 2006. *MMWR* 2005;54(51,52):Q1–Q4.

Dancis J, O'Connell JR, Holt LE. A grid for recording the weight of premature infants. *J Pediatr* 1948;33:570–572.

Horbar JD, Badger GJ, Carpenter JH, et al. Trends in mortality and morbidity for very low birth weight infants, 1991–1999. *Pediatrics* 2002;110:143–151.

Lee S, McMillan DD, Ohlsson A, et al. Variations in practice and outcomes in the Canadian NICU Network: 1996–97. *Pediatrics* 2000;106:1070.

McCormick M, McCarton C, Tonascia J, et al. Early educational intervention for very low birth weight infants: Results from the infant health and development program. *Pediatrics* 1993;123:527.

National Center for Health Statistics. Births: Final data for 2000. *Natl Vital Stat Rep* 2002;50(5):15,16.

Saari TN. The American Academy of Pediatrics Committee on Infectious Diseases. Immunization of preterm and low birth weight infants. *Pediatrics* 2003;112(1):193–198.

Vohr BR, Wright LL, Dusick AM, et al. Neurodevelopmental and functional outcomes of extremely low birth weight infants in the National Institute of Child Health and Human Development Neonatal Research Network, 1993–1994. *Pediatrics* 2000;105:1216.

RESUSCITATION IN THE DELIVERY ROOM
Steven A. Ringer

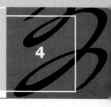

4

I. **GENERAL PRINCIPLES.** A person skilled in basic neonatal resuscitation should be present at every delivery. Delivery of all high-risk infants should be attended by skilled personnel whose sole responsibility is the newborn.

The highest standard of care requires the following: (i) knowledge of perinatal physiology and principles of resuscitation; (ii) mastery of the technical skills required; and (iii) a clear understanding of the roles of other team members, which allows accurate anticipation of each person's reactions in a specific instance. Certification of each caregiver by the Newborn Resuscitation Program (NRP) of the American Academy of Pediatrics/American Heart Association ensures that each employs a consistent approach to resuscitations. NRP provides an approach to resuscitation that is succesful in a very high percentage of cases and aids clinicians in more rapidly identifying those unusual cases in which specialized interventions may be required.

A. **Perinatal physiology.** Resuscitation efforts at delivery are designed to help the newborn make the respiratory and circulatory transitions that must be accomplished immediately after birth: the lungs expand, clear fetal lung fluid, and establish effective air exchange, and the right-to-left circulatory shunts terminate. The critical period for these physiologic changes is during the first several breaths, which result in lung expansion and elevation of the partial pressure of oxygen (Po_2) in both the alveoli and the arterial circulation. Elevation of the Po_2 from the fetal level of approximately 25 mm Hg to values of 50 to 70 mm Hg is associated with (i) decrease in pulmonary vascular resistance, (ii) decrease in right-to-left shunting through the ductus arteriosus, (iii) increase in venous return to the left atrium, (iv) rise in left atrial pressure, and (v) cessation of right-to-left shunt through the foramen ovale. The end result is conversion from fetal to transitional to neonatal circulatory pattern. Adequate systemic arterial oxygenation results from perfusion of well-expanded, well-ventilated lungs and adequate circulation.

Conditions at delivery may compromise the fetus's ability to make the necessary transitions. Alterations in tissue perfusion and oxygenation ultimately result in depression of cardiac function, but human fetuses initially respond to hypoxia by becoming apneic. Even a relatively brief period of oxygen deprivation may result in this **primary apnea.** Rapid recovery from this state is generally accomplished with appropriate stimulation and oxygen exposure. If the period of hypoxia continues, the fetus will irregularly gasp and lapse into **secondary apnea.** This state may occur remote from birth or in the peripartum period. Infants born during this period require resuscitation with assisted ventilation and oxygen (see III.B).

B. **Goals of resuscitation** are the following:
   1. **Minimizing immediate heat loss** by drying and providing warmth, thereby decreasing oxygen consumption by the neonate.
   2. **Establishing normal respiration and lung expansion** by clearing the upper airway and using positive-pressure ventilation if necessary.
   3. **Increasing arterial Po_2** by providing adequate alveolar ventilation. The **routine** use of added oxygen is not warranted, but this therapy may be necessary in some situations.
   4. **Supporting adequate cardiac output.**

II. **PREPARATION.** Anticipation is key to ensuring that adequate preparations have been made for a neonate likely to require resuscitation at birth. It is estimated that as many as 10% of neonates require some assistance at birth for normal transition.

A. Perinatal conditions associated with high-risk deliveries. Ideally, the obstetrician should notify the pediatrician well in advance of the actual birth. The pediatrician may then review the obstetric history and events leading to the high-risk delivery and prepare for the specific problems that may be anticipated. If time permits, the problems should be discussed with the parent(s). The following antepartum and intrapartum events warrant the presence of a resuscitation team at delivery.

1. **Evidence of nonreassuring fetal status**
   a. Serious fetal heart-rate abnormalities, for example, sustained bradycardia.
   b. Scalp pH of 7.20 or less.
   c. Nonreassuring fetal heart-rate pattern (see Chap. 1).

2. **Evidence of fetal disease or potentially serious conditions (see Chap. 3)**
   a. Meconium staining of the amniotic fluid and other evidence of possible fetal compromise (see Chap. 24).
   b. Prematurity (<36 weeks), postmaturity (>42 weeks), anticipated low birth weight (<2.0 kg), or high birth weight (>4.5 kg).
   c. Major congenital anomalies diagnosed prenatally.
   d. Hydrops fetalis.
   e. Multiple gestation (see Chap. 7).
   f. Cord prolapse.
   g. Abruptio placentae.

3. **Labor and delivery conditions**
   a. Significant vaginal bleeding.
   b. Abnormal fetal presentation.
   c. Prolonged, unusual, or difficult labor.
   d. Suspicion about a possible shoulder dystocia.

B. The following conditions do not require a pediatric team to be present, but personnel should be available for assessment and triage.

1. **Neonatal conditions**
   a. Unexpected congenital anomalies.
   b. Respiratory distress.
   c. Unanticipated neonatal depression, for example, Apgar score of <6 at 5 minutes.

2. **Maternal conditions**
   a. Signs of maternal infection.
      i. Maternal fever.
      ii. Membranes ruptured for >24 hours.
      iii. Foul-smelling amniotic fluid.
      iv. History of sexually transmitted disease.
   b. Maternal illness or other conditions
      i. Diabetes mellitus.
      ii. Rh or other isoimmunization without evidence of hydrops fetalis.
      iii. Chronic hypertension or pregnancy-induced hypertension.
      iv. Renal, endocrine, pulmonary, or cardiac disease.
      v. Alcohol or other substance abuse.

C. Necessary equipment must be present and operating properly. Each delivery room should be equipped with the following:

1. **Radiant warmer** with procedure table or bed. The warmer must be turned on and checked before delivery. Additional heat lamps for warming a very low-birth-weight (VLBW) infant should be available.

2. **Oxygen source (100%)** with adjustable flowmeter and adequate length of tubing. A humidifier and heater may be desirable. Pulse oximetry and a system for providing an air–oxygen mixture of adjustable content should be available for treatment of premature infants (<30–32 weeks' gestation).

3. Flow-through **anesthesia bag** with adjustable pop-off valve or self-inflating bag with reservoir. The bag must be appropriately sized for neonates (generally about 750 mL) and capable of delivering 100% oxygen.

4. **Face mask(s)** of appropriate size for the anticipated infant.

5. **A bulb syringe** for suctioning.
6. **Stethoscope** with infant- or premature-sized head.
7. **Equipped emergency box**
   a. Laryngoscope with no. 0 and no. 1 blades.
   b. Extra batteries.
   c. Uniform diameter endotracheal (ET) tubes (2.5-, 3.0-, and 3.5-mm internal diameters), two of each.
   d. Drugs, including epinephrine (1:10,000), sodium bicarbonate (0.50 mEq/mL), naloxone, and NaCl 0.9%.
   e. Umbilical catheterization tray with 3.5 and 5F catheters.
   f. Syringes (1.0, 3.0, 5.0, 10.0, and 20.0 mL), needles (18–25 gauge), T-connectors, and stopcocks.
8. Transport incubator with battery-operated heat source and portable oxygen supply should be available if delivery room is not close to the nursery.
9. The utility of equipment for continuous monitoring of cardiopulmonary status in the delivery room is hampered by difficulty in effectively applying monitor leads. Pulse oximetry can usually be applied quickly and successfully to provide information on oxygen saturation and heart rate, and should be available for premature infants.
10. End Tidal CO_2 monitor/indicator to confirm ET tube position after intubation.

D. **Preparation of equipment.** Upon arrival in the delivery room, check that the transport incubator is plugged in and warm, and has a full oxygen tank. The specialist should introduce himself or herself to the obstetrician and anesthesiologist, the mother (if she is awake), and the father (if he is present). While the history or an update is obtained, the following should be done:
1. Ensure that the radiant warmer is on, and that dry, warm blankets are available.
2. Turn on the oxygen source or air–oxygen blend and adjust the flow to 5 to 8 L/minute.
3. Test the anesthesia bag for pop-off control and adequate flow. Be sure the proper-sized mask is present.
4. Make sure the laryngoscope light is bright and has an appropriate blade (no. 1 for full-term neonates, no. 0 for premature neonates, no.00 for extremely low-birth-weight neonates).
5. Set out an appropriate ET tube for the expected birth weight (3.5 mm for full-term infants, 3.0 mm for premature infants >1,250 g, and 2.5 mm for smaller infants). The NRP recommends a 4.0-mm tube for larger babies, but this is rarely necessary. For all babies, the tube should be 13 cm long. An intubation stylet may be used, if the tip is kept at least 0.5 cm from the distal end of the ET tube.
6. If the clinical situation suggests that extensive resuscitation may be needed, the following actions may be required:
   a. Set up an umbilical catheterization tray for venous catheterization.
   b. Draw up 1:10,000 epinephrine and sodium bicarbonate (0.5 mEq/mL) solution, and isotonic saline for catheter flush solution and volume replacement.
   c. Check that other potentially necessary drugs are present and ready for administration.

E. **Universal precautions.** Exposure to blood or other body fluids is inevitable in the delivery room. Universal precautions must be practiced by wearing caps, goggles or glasses, gloves, and impervious gowns until the cord is cut and the newborn is dried and wrapped.

III. **DURING DELIVERY,** the team should be aware of the type and duration of anesthesia, extent of maternal bleeding, and newly recognized problems such as a nuchal cord or meconium in the amniotic fluid.
A. **Immediately following delivery, begin a process of evaluation, decision, and action (resuscitation)**
1. Place the newborn on the warming table.
2. Dry the infant completely and discard the wet linens, including those upon which the infant is lying. Drying should be thorough but gentle, avoid vigorous rubbing or attempts to clean all blood or vernix from the baby. Make sure the infant

| TABLE 4.1 | Apgar Scoring System | | |

	Score		
Sign	**0**	**1**	**2**
Heart rate	Absent	<100 bpm	>100 bpm
Respiratory effort	Absent	Slow (irregular)	Good crying
Muscle Tone	Limp	Some flexion of extremities	Active motion
Reflex irritability	No response	Grimace	Cough or sneeze
Color	Blue, pale	Pink body, blue extremities	All pink

Source: Adapted from Apgar V. A proposal for a new method of evaluation of the newborn infant. *Anesth Analg* 1953;32:260.

is warm. Extremely small infants may require extra warming lamps. Quickly placing the body and extremities of these small infants in a plastic wrap or bag will maintain warmth and reduce fluid losses(see Chap. 6).

3. Place the infant with head in midline position, with slight neck extension.

4. Suction the mouth, oropharynx, and nares thoroughly with a suction bulb. Deep pharyngeal stimulation with a suction catheter may cause arrhythmias that are probably of vagal origin, and should be avoided. A suction bulb should be used instead. If meconium-stained amniotic fluid is present and the infant is not vigorous, suction the oropharynx and trachea as quickly as possible (see **IV.A** and Chap. 24K).

B. Sequence of intervention. While Apgar scores (see Table 4.1) are assigned at 1 and 5 minutes, resuscitative efforts should begin during the initial neonatal stabilization period. The NRP recommends that at the time of birth, the baby should be assessed by posing five questions: (i) is the baby or amniotic fluid clear of meconium?; (ii) is the baby crying or breathing?; (iii) does the baby have good muscle tone?; (iv) is the baby centrally pink?; (v) is it a term gestation? If the answer to any of these questions is "no," the intial steps of resuscitation should commence.

First, assess whether the infant is **breathing spontaneously.** Next, assess whether the **heart rate is >100 beats per minute (bpm).** Finally, evaluate whether the infant's overall color is pink (acrocyanosis is normal). If any of these three characteristics is abnormal, take immediate steps to correct the deficiency, and reevaluate every 15 to 30 seconds until all characteristics are present and stable. In this way, adequate support will be given while overly vigorous interventions are avoided when newborns are making adequate progress on their own. This approach will help avoid complications such as laryngospasm and cardiac arrhythmias from excessive suctioning or pneumothorax from injudicious bagging. Some interventions are required in specific circumstances.

1. Infant breathes spontaneously, heart rate is >100 bpm, and color is becoming pink (Apgar score of 8–10). This situation is found in over 90% of all term newborns, with a median time to first breath of approximately 10 seconds. Following (or during) warming, drying, positioning, and oropharyngeal suctioning, the infant should be assessed. If respirations, heart rate, and color are normal, the infant should be wrapped and returned to the parents.

Some newborns do not immediately establish spontaneous respiration but will rapidly respond to tactile stimulation, including vigorous flicking of the soles of the feet or rubbing the back (e.g., cases of **primary apnea**). More vigorous or other techniques of stimulation have no therapeutic value and are potentially harmful. If breathing does not start after **two** attempts at tactile stimulation, the baby should be considered to be in **secondary apnea,** and respiratory support should be initiated. It is better to overdiagnose secondary apnea in this situation than to continue attempts at stimulation that are not successful.

2. **Infant breathes spontaneously, heart rate is >100 bpm, but the overall color remains cyanotic (Apgar score of 5–7).** This situation is not uncommon and may follow primary apnea. The term newborn should be given blow-by oxygen (100%) at a rate of 5 L/minute by mask or by tubing held approximately 1 cm from the face. If color improves, oxygen should be gradually withdrawn while color is reassessed. If cyanosis recurs, the oxygen source should be moved closer to the infant. There is evidence that resuscitaion with room air alone may be as effective as providing additional oxygen, and the use of an oxygen–air blend may also be effective. If resuscitation is started using an oxygen concentration <100%, the concentration should be increased if there is no improvement in color within 90 seconds of birth.

   For infants born at less than 30 to 32 weeks, blended oxygen should be used for resuscitation in conjunction with monitoring of blood oxygen saturation (pulse oximetry). In lieu of any data to guide the initial concentration of oxygen, it makes sense to start at 60% oxygen and wean up or down to keep the oxygen saturation in a normal range of 85% to 93% for the premature baby.

   Independent of oxygen concentration or gestational age, the use of unregulated continuous positive airway pressure by face mask has no role in resuscitation.

3. **The infant is apneic despite tactile stimulation or has a heart rate of <100 bpm despite apparent respiratory effort (Apgar score of 3–4).** This represents **secondary apnea** and requires treatment with bag-and-mask ventilation. When starting this intervention, call for assistance if your team is not already present.

   A bag of approximately 750 mL volume should be connected to oxygen (100%) or an air-oxygen blend (depending on gestational age as in III.B.2.) at a rate of 5 to 8 L/minute and to a mask of appropriate size. The mask should cover the chin and nose but leave eyes uncovered. After positioning the newborn's head in the midline with slight extension, the initial breath should be delivered at a peak pressure that is adequate to produce appropriate chest rise, which may be as high as 30 to 40 cm H_2O in the term infant. This will establish functional residual capacity, and subsequent inflations will be effective at lower inspiratory pressures.

   The inspiratory pressures for subsequent breaths should again be chosen to result in adequate chest rise. In infants with normal lungs, this inspiratory pressure is usually no more than 15 to 20 cm H_2O. In infants with known or suspected disease causing decreased pulmonary compliance, continued inspiratory pressures in excess of 20 cm H_2O may be required. Especially in premature infants, every effort should be made to use the minimal pressures necessary for chest rise and the maintenance of normal oxygen saturation levels. A rate of 40 to 60 breaths per minute should be used, and the infant should be reassessed in 15 to 30 seconds. It is usually preferable to aim for a rate closer to 40 bpm, as many resuscitators deliver less adequate breaths at higher rates. Support should be continued until respirations are spontaneous, and the heart rate is >100 bpm, but effectiveness can also be gauged by improvements in color and tone before spontaneous respirations are established.

   Such moderately depressed infants will be acidotic but generally able to correct this respiratory acidosis spontaneously after respiration is established. This process may take up to several hours, but unless the pH remains <7.25, acidosis does not need further treatment.

4. **The infant is apneic, and the heart rate is below 100 bpm despite 30 seconds of assisted ventilation (Apgar score of 0–2).** If the heart rate is >60, positive-pressure ventilation should be continued, and the heart rate rechecked in 30 seconds. It is appropriate to carefully assess the effectiveness of support during this time period using the following steps.

a. **Adequacy of ventilation** is most important, and should be assessed by observing chest-wall motion at the cephalad portions of the thorax and listening for equal breath sounds laterally over the right and left hemithoraces at the midaxillary lines. The infant should be ventilated at 40 to 60 breaths per minute using the minimum pressure that will move the chest and produce audible breath sounds. Infants with respiratory distress syndrome, pulmonary hypoplasia, or ascites may require higher pressures. The equipment itself should be checked, and the presence of a good seal between the mask and the infant's face should be quickly ascertained. At the same time, the position of the infant's head should be checked and returned as needed to midline and slight extension. The airway should be cleared as needed.

b. **Increase the oxygen concentration to 100%** for infants of any gestational age, if the resuscitation was started using an air–oxygen blend.

   Continue bag-and-mask ventilation and reassess in 15 to 30 seconds. The most important measure of ventilation adequacy is infant response. If, despite good air entry, the heart rate fails to increase and color remains poor, intubation may be considered (see Chap. 36). Air leak (e.g., pneumothorax) should be ruled out.

c. **Intubation is absolutely indicated** only when a diaphragmatic hernia or similar anomaly is suspected or known to exist. It may be warranted when bag-and-mask ventilation is ineffective, when an ET tube is needed for emergency administration of drugs, or when the infant requires transportation for more than a short distance after stabilization. Even in these situations, effective ventilation with a bag and mask may be done for long periods, and it is preferred over repeated unsuccessful attempts at intubation or attempts by unsupervised personnel unfamiliar with the procedure.

   Intubation should be accomplished rapidly (limiting each attempt to 20 seconds with intervening bag-and-mask ventilation) by a skilled person. If inadequate ventilation was the sole cause of the bradycardia, intubation will result in an increase in heart rate to over 100 bpm, and a rapid improvement in color. Intubation skills can be readily learned and maintained through practice utilizing one of several commercially available models or through humane use of ketamine-anesthetized kittens.

   The key to successful intubation is to correctly position the infant and laryngoscope and to know the anatomic landmarks. If the baby's chin, sternum, and umbilicus are all lined up in a single plane, and if, after insertion into the infant's mouth, the laryngoscope handle and blade are aligned in that plane and held at approximately a 60-degree angle to the baby's chest, only one of four anatomic landmarks will be visible to the intubator: from cephalad to caudad these include the posterior tongue, the vallecula and epiglottis, the larynx (trachea and vocal cords), or the esophagus. The successful intubator will view the laryngoscope tip and a landmark, and should then know whether the landmark being observed is cephalad or caudad to the larynx. The intubator can adjust the position of the blade by several millimeters and locate the vocal cords. The ET tube can then be inserted under direct visualization.

d. **Circulation.** If, after intubation and 30 seconds of ventilation with 100% oxygen, the heart rate remains below 60 bpm, **cardiac massage** should be instituted. The best technique is to stand at the foot of the infant and place both thumbs at the junction of the middle and lower thirds of the sternum, with the fingers wrapped around and supporting the back. Alternatively, one can stand at the side of the infant and compress the lower third of the infant's sternum with the index and third fingers of one hand. In either method, compress the sternum about one-third the diameter of the chest at a rate of 90 times per minute in a ratio of three compressions for each breath. Positive-pressure ventilation should be continued at a rate of 30 breaths per minute, interspersed in the period following every third compression. Determine effectiveness of compressions by palpating the femoral, brachial, or umbilical cord pulse.

After 30 seconds, suspend both ventilation and compression for 6 seconds as heart rate is assessed. If the rate is >60 bpm, chest compression should be discontinued and ventilation continued until respiration is spontaneous. If no improvement is noted, compression and ventilation should be continued for successive periods of 30 seconds interposed with 6-second periods of assessment.

Infants requiring ventilatory and circulatory support are markedly depressed and require immediate, vigorous resuscitation. Resuscitation may require at least three trained people working together.

e. Medication. If, despite adequate ventilation with 100% oxygen and chest compressions, a heart rate of >60 bpm has not been achieved by 1 to 2 minutes after delivery, medications such as chronotropic and inotropic agents should be given to support the myocardium, ensure adequate fluid status, and in some situations to correct acidosis. (See Table 4.2 for drugs, indications, and dosages.) Medications provide substrate and stimulation for the heart so that it can support circulation of oxygen and nutrients to the brain. For rapid calculations, use 1, 2, or 3 kg as the estimate of birth weight.

   i. The most accessible intravenous route for neonatal administration of medications is catheterization of the umbilical vein (see Chap. 36), which can be done rapidly and aseptically. Although the saline-filled catheter can be advanced into the inferior vena cava (i.e., 8–10 cm), in 60% to 70% of neonates the catheter may become wedged in an undesirable or dangerous location (e.g., hepatic, portal, or pulmonary vein). Therefore, insertion of the catheter approximately 2 to 3 cm past the abdominal wall (4–5 cm total in a term neonate), just to the point of easy blood return, is safest before injection of drugs. In this position, the catheter tip will be in or just below the ductus venosus; it is important to flush all medications through the catheter because there is no flow through the vessel after cord separation.

  ii. Drug therapy as an adjunct to oxygen is to support the myocardium and correct acidosis. Continuing bradycardia is an indication for **epinephrine** administration, once effective ventilation has been established. Epinephrine is a powerful adrenergic agonist, and works in both adults and neonates by inducing an intense vasoconstriction and improved coronary (and cerebral) artery perfusion. The recommended dose is extrapolated from the apparently efficacious dose in adults, and is based on both measured responses and empiric experience. The intravenous dose of 0.1 to 0.3 mL/kg (up to 1.0 mL) of a 1:10,000 epinephrine solution should ideally be given through the umbilical venous catheter and flushed into the central circulation. This dose may be repeated every 3 to 5 minutes if necessary, and there is no apparent benefit to higher doses.

      When access to central circulation is difficult or delayed, epinephrine may be delivered through an ET tube for transpulmonary absorption. Studies in asphyxiated animals have demonstrated the rapid absorption and action of endotracheally administered epinephrine, leading to increased heart rate and arterial blood pressure even in the presence of severe acidosis. Case reports support the same effect in newborns, although larger experiences and controlled studies are lacking. When given through this route, doses of 0.1 to 0.3 mL/kg of 1:10,000 (0.01–0.03 mg/kg) will likely be ineffective, and higher doses of 0.3 to 1.0 mL/kg of 1:10,000 dilution (0.03–0.1 mg/kg) should be considered. These larger doses need not be diluted to increase the total volume. However, because of limited effectiveness of the intratracheal route, the intravenous route for epinephrine is preferred.

TABLE 4.2 Neonatal Resuscitation

Drug/therapy	Dose/kg	Weight (kg)	Volume IV	Volume IT	Method	Indication
Epinephrine 1:10,000 0.1 mg/mL	0.01–0.03 mg/kg IV 0.03–0.1 mg/kg IT	1 2 3 4	0.2 0.4 0.6 0.8	0.6 1.2 1.8 2.4	Give IV push or IT push. The current IT doses do not require dilution or flushing with saline. DO not give into an artery; **do not mix** with bicarbonate; repeat in 5 min PRN	Asystole or severe bradycardia
Volume expanders Normal saline 5% Albumin plasma Whole blood	– 0.1–0.2 mg/kg	1 2 3 4	10 mL 20 mL 30 mL 40 mL		Give IV over 5–10 min Slower in premature infants	Hypotension because of intravascular volume loss (see Chap. 17)
Naloxone (Narcan) 0.4 mg/mL	0.1–0.2 mg/kg	1 2 3 4	0.25–0.5 0.50–1.0 0.75–1.5 1.0–2.0		Give IV push, IM, SQ, or IT; repeat PRN 3 times if no response, **if material narcotic addiction is suspected do not give;** do not mix with bicarbonate (see Chap. 19)	Narcotic depression

	Dose	Weight			Indication
Sodium bicarbonate 0.5 mEq/mL	2 mEq/kg IV	1 2 3 4	2 mL 4 mL 6 mL 8 mL	Give IV over 2 min; do not mix with epinephrine, calcium, or phosphate; assure adequate ventilation; repeat in 5–10 min PRN	Metabolic acidosis, **rarely** needed in delivery room. Better to wait for proved acidosis
Dopamine	30/60/90 mg/100 ml of solution			Give as continuous infusion	Hypotension because of poor cardiac output (see Chap. 17)
Cardioversion/defibrillation (see Chap. 25)	1 to 4 J/kg increase 50% each time	—	—	—	Ventricular fibrillation, ventricular tachycardia
ET tube (see Chap. 36)	—	<1,000 g 1,000–2,000 g 2,000–4,000 g >4,000 g	Internal diameter (mm) 2.5 uncuffed 3.0 uncuffed 3.5 uncuffed 3.5–4.0 uncuffed		Distance of tip of ET tube 7 cm (for nasal 8 cm intubation 9 cm add 2 cm) 10 cm
Laryngoscope blades (see Chap. 36)	—	<2,000 g >2,000 g			0 (straight) 1 (straight)

IM = intramuscular; IT = intratracheal; IV = intravenous; SQ = subcutaneous; ET = endotracheal.

If two doses of epinephrine do not produce improvement, additional doses may be given, but one should consider other causes for continuing depression.

iii. **Volume expansion.** If ventilation and oxygenation have been established but blood pressure is still low or the peripheral perfusion is poor, volume expansion may be indicated through the use of normal saline, 5% albumin, packed red blood cells, or whole blood, starting with 10 mL/kg (see IV.B and Chap. 17). Additional indications for volume expansion include evidence of acute bleeding or poor response to resuscitative efforts. Volume expansion should be carried out cautiously in newborns in whom hypotension may be caused by asphyxial myocardial damage rather than hypovolemia. It is important to use the appropriate gestational age–and birth weight–related blood pressure norms to determine volume status (see Chap. 26B).

In most situations, there is no need for the rapid correction of acidosis as part of the initial resuscitation. In the absence of a response to epinephrine and volume expansion, documented or suspected acidosis should be treated with 2 mEq of bicarbonate per kilogram body weight. The **bicarbonate** should be given as **4 mL/kg of 0.5 mEq/mL of sodium bicarbonate** administered over 2 to 4 minutes through the umbilical vein.

Because there are potential risks as well as benefits for all medications (Table 4.2), drug administration through the umbilical vein should be reserved for those newborns in whom bradycardia persists despite adequate oxygen delivery and ventilation. If an adequate airway has been established, adequate ventilation achieved, and the heart rate exceeds 100 bpm, the infant should be moved to the neonatal intensive care unit (NICU), where physical examination, determination of vital signs, and test results such as chest radiographic appearance will more clearly identify needs for specific interventions.

iv. **Reversal of narcotic depression is rarely necessary** during the primary steps of a resuscitation, and is not recommended. If the mother has received narcotic analgesia within a few hours of delivery, the newborn may manifest respiratory depression because of transplacental passage. The depression usually presents as apnea that persists even after bradycardia and cyanosis have been easily corrected with bag-and-mask ventilation. These infants should be treated with naloxone (0.4 mg/mL), in a dose of 0.25 mL/kg (e.g., 0.1 mg/kg). Naloxone should not be used if the mother is a chronic user of narcotics because of the risk of acute withdrawal in the infant. Respiratory support should be maintained until spontaneous respirations occur.

IV. SPECIAL SITUATIONS

A. Meconium aspiration (see Chap. 24B)

1. In the presence of any meconium staining of the amniotic fluid, the obstetrician should quickly assess the infant during the birth process for the presence of secretions or copious amniotic fluid. **Routine suctioning** of all meconium-stained infants is not recommended, but in the presence of significant fluid or secretions, the mouth and pharynx should be aspirated with a bulb syringe after delivery of the head and before breathing begins.

2. The newborn should immediately be assessed to determine whether it is vigorous, as defined by strong respiratory effort, good muscle tone, and a heart rate >100 bpm. Infants who are vigorous should be treated as normal, despite the presence of meconium-stained fluid. If both the obstetric provider and the pediatric team in attendance agree that the infant is vigorous, it is not necessary to take the infant from his/her mother after birth. Infants who are not clearly vigorous should be rapidly intubated and their trachea suctioned for meconium, preferably before the first breath. In many cases, even if the infant has gasped, some meconium may still be removed with direct tracheal suction. Suctioning is accomplished through adapters that allow connection of the ET tube to the

suction catheter. The resuscitator should avoid suction techniques that could allow self-contamination with blood or vaginal contents.

3. For infants at risk of meconium aspiration syndrome who show initial respiratory distress, care should be taken at all times in the delivery room and NICU to provide adequate oxygen and prevent even transient hypoxemia.

B. Shock. Some newborns present with pallor and shock in the delivery room (see Chaps. 17 and 26B). Shock may result from significant intrapartum blood loss because of placental separation, fetal-maternal hemorrhage, avulsion of the umbilical cord from the placenta, vasa or placenta previa, incision through an anterior placenta at cesarean section, twin–twin transfusion, or rupture of an abdominal viscus (liver or spleen) during a difficult delivery. It may also result from vasodilation or loss of vascular tone because of septicemia or hypoxemia and acidosis. These newborns will be pale, tachycardic (over 180 bpm), tachypneic, and hypotensive with poor capillary filling and weak pulses.

After starting respiratory support, immediate transfusion with O-negative packed red blood cells and 5% albumin may be necessary if acute blood loss is the underlying cause. A volume of 20 mL/kg can be given through an umbilical venous catheter. If clinical improvement is not seen, causes of further blood loss should be sought, and more vigorous blood and colloid replacement should be continued. It is important to remember that the hematocrit may be normal immediately after delivery if the blood loss was acute during the intrapartum period.

Except in cases of massive acute blood loss, the emergent use of blood replacement is not necessary and acute stabilization can be achieved with crystalloid solutions. Normal saline is the primary choice of replacement fluid. This allows time to obtain proper products from the blood bank, if blood replacement is subsequently needed.

Except in the most extreme emergency situation where no other therapeutic option exists, the use of autologous blood from the placenta is not recommended.

C. Air leak. If an infant fails to respond to resuscitation despite apparently effective ventilation, chest compressions, and medications, consider the possibility of air-leak syndromes. Pneumothoraces (uni- or bilateral) and pneumopericardium should be ruled out by transillumination or diagnostic thoracentesis (see Chap. 24A).

D. Prematurity. Premature infants require additional special care in the delivery room, including the use of oxygen–air mixtures and oximetry monitoring, and precautions such as plastic wraps or bags to prevent heat loss because of thinner skin and an increased surface-area-to-body-weight ratio. Apnea because of respiratory insufficiency is more likely at lower gestational ages, and support should be provided. Surfactant-deficient lungs are poorly compliant, and higher ventilatory pressures may be needed for the first and subsequent breaths. Depending on the reason for premature birth, perinatal infection is more likely in premature infants, which increases their risk of perinatal depression.

V. APGAR SCORES. Evaluation and decisions regarding resuscitation measures should be guided by assessment of respiration, heart rate, and color. Apgar scores are conventionally assigned after birth and recorded in the newborn's chart. The Apgar score consists of the total points assigned to five objective signs in the newborn. Each sign is evaluated and given a score of 0, 1, or 2. Total scores at 1 and 5 minutes after birth are usually noted. If the 5-minute score is 6 or less, the score is then noted at successive 5-minute intervals until it is >6 (Table 4.1). A score of 10 indicates an infant in perfect condition; this is quite unusual because most babies have some degree of acrocyanosis. The scoring, if done properly, yields the following information:

A. One-minute Apgar score. This score generally correlates with umbilical cord blood pH and is an index of intrapartum depression. It does not correlate with outcome. Babies with a score of 0 to 4 have been shown to have a significantly lower pH, higher partial pressure of carbon dioxide ($Paco_2$), and lower buffer base than those with Apgar scores >7. In the VLBW infant a low Apgar may not indicate severe depression. As many as 50% of infants with gestational ages of 25 to 26 weeks and Apgar scores of 0 to 3 have a cord pH of >7.25. Therefore, a VLBW infant with a low Apgar score cannot be assumed to be severely depressed. Nonetheless, such infants should be resuscitated actively and will usually respond more promptly and to less invasive measures than newborns whose low Apgar scores reflect acidemia.

B. Apgar scores beyond 1 minute are reflective of the infant's changing condition and the adequacy of resuscitative efforts. Persistence of low Apgar scores indicates need for further therapeutic efforts and usually the severity of the baby's underlying problem. In assessing the adequacy of resuscitation, the most common problem is inadequate pulmonary inflation and ventilation. It is important to verify a good seal with the mask, correct placement of the ET tube, and adequate peak inspiratory pressure applied to the bag if the Apgar score fails to improve as resuscitation proceeds.

The more prolonged the period of severe depression (i.e., Apgar score 3), the more likely is an abnormal long-term neurologic outcome. Nevertheless, many newborns with prolonged depression (>15 minutes) are normal in follow-up. Moreover, most infants with long-term motor abnormalities such as cerebral palsy have not had periods of neonatal depression after birth, and have normal Apgar scores (see Chap. 27C). Apgar scores were designed to monitor neonatal transition and the effectiveness of resuscitation, and their utility remains essentially limited to this important role. The American Academy of Pediatrics is currently recommending an expanded Apgar score reporting form which details both the numeric score as well as concurrent resuscitative interventions.

VI. EVOLVING PRACTICES. The practice of neonatal resuscitation continues to evolve with the availablity of new devices and enhanced understanding of the best approach to resuscitation.

A. Laryngeal mask airways. Masks that fit over the laryngeal inlet have been developed and are effective for ventilating newborn infants. Ease of insertion and the ability to maintain a stable airway with these devices without the need for skill at intubation may make these a preferred method of airway support in many instances. These airways have been most widely studied in full-term infants, but there have been case reports of their utility in ventilating even small premature infants for extended periods of time. However, these masks have not been evaluated in small, preterm infants, and relative effectiveness for the suctioning of meconium has not been reported.

B. The Neopuff Infant Resuscitator (Fisher & Paykel, Inc.). This is a manually triggered, pressure-limited, and manually cycled device that is pneumatically powered by a flowmeter. This device offers greater control over manual ventilation by delivering breaths of reproducible size (peak and end-expiratory pressures) and a simplified method to control breath rate. One important use for this device is to transport preterm infants requiring supported ventilation, when the use of a powered mechanical ventilator may not be possible.

C. Room-air resuscitation. The NRP continues to recommend the use of oxygen in the conduct of neonatal resuscitation, but there is evidence that room air resuscitation is equally effective and potentially safer. Animal studies have shown that neither hyperbaric nor normobaric oxygen is more efficient in the resuscitation of newborn rabbits, and that high oxygen levels may result in increased mortality and worse neurologic outcome among survivors. In studies of term human infants, the groups treated with oxygen and room air had equal time to the normalization of heart rate after birth, and similar Apgar scores at 1 and 5 minutes. Blood gases normalized at the same rate in both groups, except for higher carbon dioxide tensions in the oxygen-treated group. The time until first cry was prolonged in the oxygen-treated group, and neonatal mortality was similar in both groups. As better understanding of the normal changes in oxygen saturation after birth develops, and more data accumulated about the effectiveness of room air resuscitation, it is likely that respiratory support in the delivery room with 100% oxygen will be replaced by regulated blended oxygen or room air.

D. Withholding or withdrawing resuscitation. Resuscitation at birth is indicated for those babies likely to have a high rate of survival and a low likelihood of severe morbidity, including those with a gestational age of 25 weeks or greater. In those situations where survival is unlikely or associated morbidity is very high, the wishes of the parents as the best spokespeople for the newborn should guide decisions about initiating resuscitation.

If there are no signs of life in an infant after 10 minutes of aggressive resuscitative efforts with no evidence for other causes of newborn compromise, discontinuation of resuscitation efforts may be appropriate.

Suggested Readings

Burchfield DJ. Medication use in neonatal resuscitation. *Clin Perinatol* 1999;26:683.

Davis PG, Tan A, O'Donnell CP, et al. Resuscitation of newborn infants with 100% ocxygen or air: A systemic review and meta-analysis. *Lancet* 2004;364:1329–1333.

Kattwinkel J, ed. *Textbook of neonatal resuscitation*, 5th ed. Dallas: American Academy of Pediatrics and American Heart Association, 2006.

Ostrea EM, Odell GB. The influence of bicarbonate administration on blood pH in a "closed system": Clinical implications. *J Pediatr* 1972;80:671.

Perlman JM, Rissewr R. Cardiopulmonary resuscitation in the delivery room. *Arch Pediatr Adolesc Med* 1995;149:20.

Saugstad OD. Resuscitation of newborn infants with room air or oxygen. *Semin Neonatol* 2001;6:233.

Saugstad OD, Rootwelt T, Aalen O. Resuscitation of asphyxiated newborn infants with room air or oxygen: An international controlled trial. *Pediatrics* 1998;102:e1.

Vain NE, Szyld EG, Prudent LM, et al. Oropharyngeal and nasopharyngeal suctioning of meconium stained neonates before delivery of their shoulders: Multicentre, randomised controlled trial. *Lancet* 2004;364:597–602.

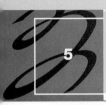

NURSERY CARE OF THE WELL NEWBORN

Lori A. Sielski and Tiffany M. McKee-Garrett

I. ADMISSION TO THE NEWBORN NURSERY. Healthy newborns should remain in the delivery room with their mother as long as possible to promote immediate initiation of breast-feeding and early bonding (see Chap. 11). Every effort should be made to avoid separation of mother and infant.

  A. Criteria for admission to the newborn nursery vary among hospitals. The minimum requirement typically is a well-appearing infant of at least 35 weeks gestational age, although some nurseries may specify a minimum birth weight, for example, 2 kg.

  B. Impeccable **security** in the nursery is necessary to protect the safety of families and to prevent the abduction of newborns.

    1. Many nurseries use electronic security systems to track newborns.

    2. Identification bands with matching numbers are placed on the newborn and mother as soon after birth as possible. Transport of infants between areas should not occur if identification banding has not been done.

    3. All staff are required to wear a picture identification (ID) badge and parents should be instructed to allow the infant to be taken only by someone wearing an ID badge.

II. TRANSITIONAL CARE

  A. The transitional period is usually defined as the first 4 to 6 hours after birth. During this period, the infant's pulmonary vascular resistance decreases, blood flow to the lungs is greatly increased, overall oxygenation and perfusion improve, and the ductus arteriosus begins to constrict or close.

  B. Interruption of normal transitioning, usually due to complications occurring in the peripartum period, will cause signs of distress in the newborn.

  C. Common signs of disordered transitioning are (i) respiratory distress, (ii) poor perfusion with cyanosis or pallor, or (iii) need for supplemental oxygen.

  D. Transitional care of the newborn can take place in the mother's room or in the nursery.

    1. Infants are evaluated for problems that may disqualify their admission to the normal nursery, such as gross malformations and disorders of transition.

    2. The infant should be evaluated every 30 to 60 minutes during this period including assessment of heart rate, respiratory rate, and axillary temperature; assessment of color and tone; and observation for signs of withdrawal from maternal medications.

    3. When disordered transitioning is suspected, a hemodynamically stable infant can be observed closely in the nursery setting for a brief period of time. Infants with persistent signs of disordered transitioning require transfer to a higher level of care.

III. ROUTINE CARE

  A. Healthy newborns should be with their mothers all or nearly all the time. When possible, physical assessments, administration of medications, and bathing should occur in the mother's room. Nursing ratio of 1:6–8 is recommended for routine newborn care.

    1. Upon admission to the nursery, an assessment of gestational age is performed on all infants using the expanded Ballard score (see Chap. 3B).

    2. The infant's weight, frontal-occipital circumference (FOC), and length are recorded. On the basis of these measurements, the infant is classified as average for gestational age (AGA), small for gestational age (SGA), or large for gestational age (LGA) (see Chap. 3).

B. The infant's temperature is stabilized with one of three possible modalities:
1. Open radiant warmer on servo control.
2. Incubator on servo control.
3. Skin-to-skin contact with the mother.

C. Universal precautions should be used with all patient contact.

D. The first **bath** is given with nonmedicated soap and warm tap water after an axillary temperature >97.5°F has been recorded.

E. Acceptable practices for **umbilical cord care** include exposure to air, or application of topical antiseptics, such as triple dye, or topical antibiotics, such as bacitracin. The use of topical antiseptics or antibiotics appears to reduce bacterial colonization of the cord, although no single method of cord care has proved to be superior in preventing colonization and disease. Keeping the cord dry promotes earlier detachment of the umbilical stump.

IV. ROUTINE MEDICATIONS

A. All newborns should receive prophylaxis against gonococcal ophthalmia neonatorum within 1 hour of birth, regardless of mode of delivery. Prophylaxis is administered as single ribbon of erythromycin ointment (0.5%) bilaterally in the conjunctival sac; alternatively, 1% silver nitrate drops are used if concern exists for erythromycin-resistant gonococci.

B. A single, intramuscular dose of 0.5 to 1 mg of vitamin K_1 oxide (phytonadione) should be given to all newborns before 6 hours of age to prevent vitamin K deficient bleeding (VKDB). Oral vitamin K preparations are **not** recommended because late VKDB (2–12 weeks of age) is best prevented by the administration of parenteral vitamin K.

C. Administration of the first dose of preservative-free hepatitis B vaccine is recommended for all infants during the newborn hospitalization, even if the mother is HepBsAg negative.
1. Hepatitis B vaccine is administered by 12 hours of age when the maternal HepBsAg is positive or unknown. Infants of HepBsAg positive mothers also require hepatitis B immune globulin (see Chap. 23).
2. The vaccine is given after parental consent as a single intramuscular injection of 0.5 mL of either Recombivax HB (5 µg) (Merck & Co., Inc., Whitehouse Station, New Jersey) or Engerix-B (10 µg) (GlaxoSmithKline Biologicals, Rixensart, Belgium).
3. Parents must be given a vaccine information statement at the time the vaccine is administered. This is available at www.cdc.gov/nip/publications.

V. SCREENING

A. Prenatal screening test results should be reviewed and documented on the infant's chart at the time of delivery. Maternal prenatal screening tests typically include the following:
1. Blood type, Rh, antibody screen.
2. Hemoglobin or hematocrit.
3. Rubella antibody.
4. Hepatitis B surface antigen.
5. Serologic test for syphilis (Venereal Disease Research Laboratory [VDRL] or rapid plasmin reagin [RPR]).
6. Human immunodeficiency virus (HIV).
7. Gonorrhea and chlamydia cultures.
8. Serum α-fetoprotein/triple panel.
9. Glucose tolerance test.
10. Group B streptococcus (GBS) culture.

B. Cord blood is saved up to 14–21 days, depending on blood bank policy.
1. A blood type and direct Coombs should be performed on any infant born to a mother who is Rh-negative, has a positive antibody screen, or who has had a previous infant with Coombs positive hemolytic anemia.
2. A blood type and direct Coombs should be obtained on any infant if jaundice is noted within the first 24 hours of age or there is unexplained hyperbilirubinemia (see Chap. 18).

    C. Newborn metabolic screen (see Chap. 29)

       1. All 50 states and the District of Columbia universally screen for four core metabolic conditions including congenital hypothyroidism, phenylketonuria, galactosemia, and hemoglobinopathies.

       2. Newborn screening programs vary considerably among states. The National Newborn Screening and Genetics Resource Center (http://genes-r-us.uthscsa.edu/) lists currently screened conditions, by state.

       3. Routine collection of the specimen is between 24 and 72 hours of life. In some states, a second screen is routinely performed at 2 weeks of age.

    D. Group B streptococcal disease

       1. All newborns should be screened for the risk of perinatally acquired GBS disease as outlined by the Centers for Disease Control (http//www.cdc.gov/groupbstrep/hospitals/hospitals_guidelines_summary.htm).

       2. Penicillin is the preferred intrapartum chemotherapeutic agent. Intravenous administration to the mother at >4 hours or earlier before delivery provides adequate neonatal prophylaxis.

       3. Newborns should be managed according to the management algorithm (see Chap. 23).

    E. Glucose screening

       1. Infants should be fed early and frequently to prevent hypoglycemia.

       2. Infants of diabetic mothers (see Chap. 2) and SGA and LGA infants should be screened for hypoglycemia in the immediate neonatal period (see Chap. 29).

    F. Bilirubin screening

       1. Before discharge, all newborns should be screened for the risk of subsequent, significant hyperbilirubinemia. This can be done using a serum bilirubin measurement from a sample obtained at the time of the metabolic screen or a transcutaneous bilirubin measurement. The value should be plotted and interpreted on an hour-specific nomogram (see Chap. 18).

       2. Provide parents with verbal and written information about newborn jaundice.

    G. Routine hearing screen for congenital hearing loss is mandated in most states (see Chap. 35). Verbal and written documentation of the hearing screen results should be provided to the parents with referral information if needed.

VI. ROUTINE ASSESSMENTS

    A. The infant's physician should perform a complete physical examination within 24 hours of birth.

    B. Vital signs, including respiratory rate, heart rate, and axillary temperature are recorded every 8 to 12 hours.

    C. Each urine and stool output is recorded in the baby's chart. The first urination should occur by 30 hours of life. The first passage of meconium is expected by 48 hours of life. Delayed urination or stooling is cause for concern and must be investigated.

    D. Daily weights are recorded in the infant's chart. Weight loss in excess of 7% is cause for concern and must be investigated. Excessive weight loss is usually due to insufficient caloric intake (see Chap. 11). If caloric intake is thought to be adequate, organic etiologies should be considered, that is, metabolic disorders, infection, or hypothyroidism.

VII. FAMILY AND SOCIAL ISSUES

    A. Sibling visitation is encouraged and is an important element of family-focused care. However, siblings with fever, signs of acute respiratory or gastrointestinal illness, or a history of recent exposure to communicable diseases, such as chicken pox, are discouraged from visiting.

    B. Social service involvement is helpful in circumstances such as teenaged mothers; lack of, or limited, prenatal care; history of domestic violence; maternal substance abuse; history of previous involvement with Child Protective Services, or similar agency.

VIII. FEEDINGS. The frequency, duration, and volume of each feed will depend on whether the infant is breast-feeding or bottle-feeding.

A. The **breast-fed** infant should feed as soon as possible after delivery, preferably in the delivery room and feed 8 to 12 times/day during the newborn hospitalization. Consultation with a lactation specialist during the postpartum hospitalization is strongly recommended for all breast-feeding mothers (see Chap. 11).

B. Standard 20 cal/oz, iron-containing infant formula is offered to infants for whom breast-feeding is contraindicated, or at the request of a mother who desires to bottle-feed. Unless contraindicated by a strong family history, lactose-containing formulas with milk protein (whey and casein) can be given to all newborns.

  1. Infants are fed at least every 3 to 4 hours.

  2. During the first few days of life, the well newborn should consume at least 0.5 to 1 oz/feed.

  3. The frequency and volume of each feed is recorded in the baby's chart.

IX. NEWBORN CIRCUMCISION

A. The American Academy of Pediatrics (AAP) states that scientific evidence exists that demonstrates potential medical benefits of newborn male circumcision; however, these data are not sufficient to recommend routine neonatal circumcision. Potential benefits are decreased incidence of urinary tract infection in the first year of life; decreased risk for the development of squamous cell carcinoma of the penis; decreased risk of acquiring sexually transmitted diseases, particularly HIV infection.

B. Informed consent is obtained before performing the procedure. The potential risks and benefits of the procedure are explained to the parents.

  1. The overall complication rate for newborn circumcision is approximately 0.5%.

  2. The most common complication is bleeding (~0.1%) followed by infection. A family history of bleeding disorders, such as hemophilia or von Willebrand disease, needs to be explored with the parents when consent is obtained. Appropriate testing to exclude a bleeding disorder must be done before the procedure if the family history is positive.

  3. The parents should understand newborn circumcision is an elective procedure; the decision to have their son circumcised is voluntary and not medically necessary.

  4. Contraindications to circumcision in the newborn period include the following:

  a. Sick or unstable clinical status.

  b. Diagnosis of a congenital bleeding disorder. Circumcision can be performed if the infant receives appropriate medical therapy before the procedure (i.e., infusion of factor VIII, or IX).

  c. Inconspicuous or "buried" penis.

  d. Anomalies of the penis, including hypospadias, ambiguity, chordee, or micropenis.

  e. Circumcision should be delayed in infants with bilateral cryptorchidism.

C. Adequate analgesia must be provided for neonatal circumcision. Acceptable methods of analgesia are dorsal penile nerve block, subcutaneous ring block, and eutectic mixture of local anesthetics (EMLA ccream): 2.5% prilocaine and 2.5% lidocaine.

D. In addition to analgesia, other methods of comfort are provided to the infant during circumcision.

  1. Twenty-four percent sucrose on a pacifier, per nursery protocol, should be given to all infants as an adjunct to analgesia.

  2. The infant's upper extremities should be swaddled, and the infant placed on a padded circumcision board with restraints on the lower extremities only.

  3. Administration of acetaminophen before the procedure is not an effective adjunct to analgesia.

E. Circumcision in the newborn can be performed using one of three different methods:

  1. Gomco clamp.

  2. Mogen clamp.

  3. Plastibell device.

F. Oral or written instructions explaining postcircumcision care should be given to all parents.

X. DISCHARGE PREPARATION

A. Parental education on routine newborn care should be initiated at birth and continued until discharge. Written information in addition to verbal instruction may be helpful and in some cases it is mandated. A review of the following newborn issues should be done at discharge:

1. Observation for neonatal jaundice.
2. Routine cord and skin care.
3. Routine postcircumcision care (when indicated).
4. Back to sleep positioning.
5. Subtle signs of infant illness including fever, irritability, lethargy, or a poor feeding pattern.
6. Adequacy of oral intake, particularly for breast-fed infants (see Chap. 11). This includes minimum of eight feeds per day; one wet diaper per day of age, constant at the sixth day of life; two stools in a 24-hour period.
7. Appropriate installation and use of an infant car seat.
8. Smoke detectors.
9. Lowering of hot water temperature.
10. Avoidance of second-hand smoke.

B. The discharge examination is reviewed in Chapter 3.

C. Discharge readiness

1. Each mother–infant dyad should be evaluated individually to determine the optimal time of discharge.
2. The AAP recommends that minimum discharge criteria be met before any newborn is discharged from the hospital. It is unlikely that fulfillment of these criteria can be accomplished with a postnatal stay of <48 hours.
3. Discharge before 48 hours of age should be limited to infants who are of singleton birth, at least 38 weeks' gestational age, and who have a birth weight that is appropriate for gestational age. Early discharge criteria include the following:
   a. Uncomplicated antepartum, intrapartum, and postpartum courses for both mother and infant.
   b. Vaginal delivery.
   c. Normal, stable vital signs in an open crib for at least 12 hours preceding discharge.
   d. Passage of first urine and stool.
   e. Completion of at least two successful feedings.
   f. Unremarkable physical examination, absence of abnormalities that would require continued hospitalization.
   g. Assessment of risk for hyperbilirubinemia.
   h. Maternal competence in routine newborn care.
   i. Assessment of maternal support.
   j. Assessment of family, environmental, and social risk factors.
   k. Review of maternal and infant blood tests.
   l. Administration of initial hepatitis B vaccine.
   m. Completion of hearing and metabolic screen per state regulations.
   n. No excessive bleeding at the circumcision site for at least two hours
   o. Definitive follow-up arrangements for both mother and infant

XI. FOLLOW-UP

A. For newborns discharged within 48 hours after delivery, outpatient follow-up should be within 48 hours of discharge. If early follow-up cannot be ensured, early discharge should be deferred.

B. For newborns discharged between 48 and 72 hours of age, outpatient follow-up should be within 2 to 3 days of discharge. Timing will depend on the risk for subsequent hyperbilirubinemia, feeding issues, or other concerns.

C. The follow-up visit is designed to perform the following functions:

1. Assess the infant's general state of health including weight, hydration, and degree of jaundice.
2. Identify any new problems.

3. Perform screening tests in accordance with state regulations.
4. Review adequacy of oral intake and assess elimination patterns.
5. Assess quality of mother–infant bonding.
6. Reinforce parental education.
7. Review results of any outstanding laboratory tests.
8. Provide anticipatory guidance and health care maintenance

Suggested Readings

American Academy of Pediatrics. American College of Obstetricians and Gynecologists. *Guidelines for Perinatal Care*, 6th ed. Elk Grove Village, IL, 2007.

CDC National Immunization Program http://www.cdc.gov/nip/recs/Child_schedule.htm

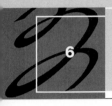

CARE OF THE EXTREMELY LOW-BIRTH-WEIGHT INFANT

Steven A. Ringer

6

I. INTRODUCTION. Extremely low-birth-weight (ELBW, birth weight <1,000 g) infants are a unique group of patients in the Newborn Intensive Care Unit (NICU). Because these infants are so physiologically immature, they are extremely sensitive to small changes in respiratory management, blood pressure, fluid administration, nutrition, and virtually all other aspects of care. The optimal way to care for these infants ultimately will be established by ongoing research. However, the most effective care based on currently available evidence is best ensured through the implementation of standardized protocols for the care of the ELBW infant within individual NICUs. Our approach is outlined in Table 6.1. Uniformity of approach within an institution and a commitment to provide and evaluate care in a collaborative manner may be the most important aspects of such protocols.

II. PRENATAL CONSIDERATIONS. If possible, extremely premature infants should be delivered in a facility with a high-risk obstetrical service and a level III NICU. The safety of maternal transport must be weighed against the risks of infant transport (see Chap. 13). Prenatal administration of glucocorticoids to the mother, even if there is not time for a full course, reduces the risk of respiratory distress syndrome (RDS) and the other sequelae of prematurity.

A. Neonatology consultation. If delivery of an extremely premature infant is threatened, a neonatologist should consult with the parents with the obstetrician present if possible. The consultation should address the following issues:

1. Survival. To most parents, the impending delivery of an extremely premature infant is frightening, and their initial concern is the chance for infant survival. In our consultations, we use survival data from our experience based on the best obstetrical estimate of gestational age. Most published data on survival is based on birth weight because it can be determined with greater accuracy than gestational age. However, birth weight is not available until after birth, it does not account for the impact of intrauterine growth restriction, and gestational maturity is usually the more important factor in determining survival and outcome. One recent study reported that the survival rate for infants at <23 weeks' gestational age was 0 and at 23, 24, and 25 weeks the rates were 15%, 55%, and 79%, respectively. Published data are helpful in counseling, but the importance of local results should not be underestimated, especially in antenatal counseling. The best obstetrical estimate of gestational age may vary between institutions, and local practices and capabilities may significantly affect both mortality and morbidity in ELBW infants. For this reason, a general assessment of the gestational age at which an infant has any hope of survival should be agreed upon by all caregivers within an institution. If only birth weight–stratified data are available, gestational age estimates for appropriate for gestational age (AGA) fetuses can be roughly converted as follows: 600 g = 24 weeks; 750 g = 25 weeks; 850 g = 26 weeks; 1,000 g = 27 weeks.

In discussions with parents, we advocate attempting resuscitation of all newborns who are potentially viable, but recognize that in individual cases parents may reasonably choose otherwise. Realistically, the lower gestational age limit is between 232/7 and 235/7 weeks, since at lower gestations efforts at support are usually futile. The addition of medical problems other than prematurity may result in extremely low survival even at higher gestational ages,

TABLE 6.1   **Elements of a Protocol for Standardizing Care of the Extremely low-Birth-Weight (ELBW) Infant**

Prenatal consultation
- Parental education
- Determining parental wishes when viability is questionable
- Defining limits of parental choice; need for caregiver–parent teamwork

Delivery room care
- Define limits of resuscitative efforts
- Respiratory support
- Low tidal volume ventilation strategy
- Prevention of heat and water loss
- Early surfactant therapy

Ventilation strategy
- Low tidal volume, short inspiratory time
- Avoid hyperoxia and hypocapnia
- Early surfactant therapy as indicated
- Define indications for high-frequency ventilation

Fluids
- Early use of humidified incubators to limit fluid and heat losses
- Judicious use of fluid bolus therapy for hypotension
- Careful monitoring of fluid and electrolyte status
- Use of double-lumen umbilical venous catheters for fluid support

Nutrition
- Initiation of parenteral nutrition shortly after birth
- Early initiation of trophic feeding. with maternal milk
- Advancement of feeding density to provide adequate calories for healing and growth

Cardiovascular support
- Maintenance of blood pressure within standard range
- Use of dopamine for support as indicated
- Corticosteroids for unresponsive hypotension

PDA
- Avoidance of excess fluid administration
- Early medical therapy when hemodynamically significant PDA is present
- Surgical ligation after failed medical therapy

Infection control
- Scrupulous hand washing, use of bedside alcohol gels
- Limiting blood drawing, skin punctures
- Protocol for CVL care, acceptable dwell time
- Minimal entry into CVLs, no use of fluids prepared in NICU

PDA = patent ductus arteriosus; CVL = central venous line; NICU = Newborn Intensive Care Unit.

and parents are told that the risks of morbidity are high at lowest gestational ages. Parents are counseled that delivery room resuscitation has a high (but not absolute) chance of success, unless the infant appears more immature than the estimated gestational age would suggest, or weighs <500 g. We not only wish to stress that the moments following delivery are inappropriate for making reliable decisions about viability or long-term outcome but also that the initiation of support in no way mandates that it be continued if it is later determined to be futile, or very likely to result in a poor long-term outcome. We assure parents that initial resuscitation is always followed by frequent reassessment in the NICU. Intensive support may be withdrawn if the degree of immaturity results in no response to therapy, or if a catastrophic and irreversible complication occurs. Parents are counseled that the period of highest vulnerability may last several weeks in infants of lowest gestational ages. If parents disagree with our recommended approach to resuscitation and care, we first attempt to resolve differences directly. Almost always, a consensus on a plan of care is reached, but if an impasse continues, we seek consultation from the institutional Ethics service.

2. **Morbidity.** We try to inform parents as fully as possible about short- and long-term prognosis. Before delivery, particular attention is paid to the problems that might appear at birth or shortly thereafter. We explain the risk of RDS and the potential need for ventilatory support. In our NICU, all infants of 24 weeks' gestation require some ventilatory support; at 25 to 26 weeks, this proportion drops to 80% to 90%; at 27 to 28 weeks, approximately 50% to 60% of infants require ventilatory support. We also inform parents of the likelihood of infection at birth as well as our plan to screen for it and begin prophylactic antibiotic therapy while final culture results are pending.

3. **Potential morbidity.** We avoid giving parents long lists of potential sequelae because they may be too overwhelmed to process extensive information during the period surrounding premature birth. However, we do discuss problems that are either likely to occur in many ELBW infants or will be specifically screened for during hospitalization. These include apnea of prematurity, intraventricular hemorrhage (IVH), nosocomial sepsis (or evaluations for possible sepsis), and feeding difficulties, as well as long-term sensory disabilities. We specifically discuss retinopathy of prematurity and subsequent visual deficits, and the need for hearing screening and the potential for hearing loss.

4. **Parents' desires.** In most instances, parents are the best surrogate decision makers for their child. We believe that, within each institution, there should be a uniform approach to parental demands for attempting or withholding resuscitation at very low gestational ages. The best practice is to formulate decisions in concert with parents, after providing them with clear, realistic, and factual information about the possibilities for success of therapy and its long-term outcome.

During the consultation, the neonatologist should try to understand parental wishes about resuscitative efforts and subsequent support especially when chances for infant survival are slim. When counseling parents around an expected birth at <24 weeks, we specifically tell them that they might choose to forgo resuscitation of the baby, if the prognosis appears too bleak for their child, and encourage them to voice their understanding of the planned approach and their expectations for their soon-to-be born child. We reassure them that the strength of their wishes does help guide caregivers in determining whether and how long to continue resuscitation attempts. Through this approach, we clarify for parents their role in decision making as well as the limitations of that role. In practice, parents' wishes about resuscitation predominate when the gestational age is <242/7 weeks, and we very strongly advocate for resuscitation at gestational age >244/7, in the absence of other factors.

III. **DELIVERY ROOM CARE.** The pediatric team should include an experienced pediatrician or neonatologist, particularly when the fetus is of <26 weeks' gestational age. The approach to resuscitation is similar to that in more mature infants (see Chap. 4). Special attention should be paid to the following:

A. Warmth and drying. The ELBW neonate is at particular risk for hypothermia. Conventional practice has been to place the infant under a preheated warmer, quickly dry the baby, and remove the wet toweling. Care should be taken minimize rubbing so as to limit damage to immature skin. Alternatively, the infant's body can be placed (undried) directly into polyethylene bag to maintain warmth until the baby can be moved to a prewarmed isolette and then patted dry. It is helpful to place additional warming lights near the radiant warmer.

B. Respiratory support. Most ELBW infants require some degree of ventilatory support because of pulmonary immaturity and limited respiratory muscle strength. Blended oxygen should be available to help avoid prolonged hyperoxia after the initial resuscitation; our initial resuscitation usually starts with 60% oxygen and is titrated to response. We place an oximeter probe on the infant within the first minute after birth to help target oxygen saturations during the initial resuscitation. If the neonate cries vigorously, we administer blow-by blended oxygen as required and observe the infant for signs of distress. Many of these infants require bag-and-mask ventilation because of apnea or ineffective respiratory drive. The resolution of bradycardia is the best indicator of adequate response to resuscitation. If the infant's lungs are deficient in surfactant, moderately high inflating pressures may be necessary for the initial breaths, but the peak pressure should be rapidly lowered to minimize lung injury. Because these infants generally require continued respiratory support and benefit from early application of end-expiratory pressure, we generally perform endotracheal intubation and ventilation shortly after birth. After initial lung inflation, the use of a Neopuff Infant Resuscitator (Fisher and Paykel) is preferred over hand-bagging because it ensures uniform breaths, adequate positive end-expiratory pressure, and regulated inflation pressures. The goal is to use the lowest tidal volumes possible while still adequately ventilating the infant. Initiation of exogenous surfactant therapy before the first breath has not yet been proved to be more beneficial than administration after initial stabilization of the infant. Exogenous surfactant may be safely administered in the delivery room once correct endotracheal tube position has been confirmed clinically.

The pediatrician should assess the response to resuscitation and gauge the need for further interventions. If the infant fails to respond, the team should recheck that all support measures are being effectively administered. Support for apnea or poor respiratory effort must include intermittent inflating breaths or regulated nasal continuous positive airway pressure (CPAP). Face-mask CPAP alone is not adequate support for an apneic baby, and failure to respond to this limited intervention does not mean that the infant is too immature to be resuscitated. If no positive response to resuscitation occurs after a reasonable length of time, we consider withdrawing support.

C. Care after resuscitation. Immediately after resuscitation, the plastic-wrapped infant should be placed in a prewarmed transport incubator for transfer to the NICU. We always show the baby to the parents in the delivery room (while in the transport incubator) to enhance the beginning of parent–infant interaction. In the NICU, the infant is moved to an incubator/radiant warmer combination unit (Giraffe Bed, Ohmeda Medical) where a complete assessment is done and treatment initiated. The infant's temperature should be rechecked at this time and closely monitored. As soon as possible, the unit is closed to function as an incubator for continued care. Humidity is maintained at 70% for the first week of life, and 50% to 60% thereafter up to 32 weeks corrected gestation. In addition to reducing insensible fluid losses and thereby simplifying fluid therapy, the use of incubators aids in reducing unnecessary stimulation and noise experienced by the baby.

IV. CARE IN THE INTENSIVE CARE UNIT. Careful attention to detail and frequent monitoring are the basic components of care of the ELBW infant, because critical changes can occur rapidly. Large fluid losses, balances between fluid intake and blood glucose levels, delicate pulmonary status, and the immaturity and increased sensitivity of several organ systems all require close monitoring. Monitoring itself, however, may pose increased risks because of small blood volumes, tiny-caliber vessels, and limited skin integrity. Issues in routine care that require special attention in ELBW infants include the following:

A. Survival. The first 24 to 48 hours are the most critical for survival. Infants who require significant respiratory, cardiovascular, and/or fluid support are assessed continuously, and their chances for survival are estimated. If caregivers and the parents determine that death is imminent, continued treatment is futile, or treatment is likely to result in survival of a neurologically devastated infant, we recommend the withdrawal of ventilator support and redirection of care to comfort measures only.

B. Respiratory support. Most ELBW infants require initial respiratory support.

   1. Conventional ventilation. We generally use conventional pressure-limited synchronized intermittent mandatory ventilation (SIMV) as our primary mode of mechanical ventilation (see Chap. 24B). The lowest possible tidal volume to provide adequate ventilation and oxygenation and a short inspiratory time should be used. Special effort should be made to avoid hyperoxia by targeting oxygen saturations at lower levels than have been used in the past. Recent reports suggest that setting oximeter alarm limits at 85% to 93% and training staff to reduce the number of hypoxia–hyperoxia fluctuations may reduce the severity of retinopathy of prematurity. It is hypothesized that limiting hyperoxia may also reduce the incidence or severity of chronic lung disease. It is important as well to avoid hypocapnia, although the potential benefit of permissive hypercapnia as a ventilatory strategy remains a subject of debate.

   2. Surfactant therapy (see Chap. 24A). We administer surfactant to infants with RDS who are ventilated with a mean airway pressure of at least 7 cm H_2O and an inspired oxygen concentration (F_{IO2}) of 0.3 or higher in the first 2 hours after birth. We give the first dose as soon as possible after birth, preferably within the first hour.

   3. High-frequency oscillatory ventilation (HFOV) is used in infants who fail to improve after surfactant administration and require conventional ventilation at high peak inspiratory pressures. For infants with air leak, especially pulmonary interstitial emphysema (see Chap. 24E), high-frequency jet ventilation may be the preferred mode of ventilation.

   4. Vitamin A supplementation. All infants with birth weight of 1,000 g and less should receive 5,000 IU of vitamin A intramuscularly 3 times a week for the first 4 weeks. This therapy has been shown to slightly reduce the incidence of chronic lung disease.

   5. Caffeine citrate administered within the first 10 days after birth at standard doses (see Appendix A) may reduce the risk of developing bronchopulmonary dysplasia (BPD).

C. Fluids and electrolytes (see Chaps. 9 and 31). Fluid requirements increase tremendously as gestational age decreases <28 weeks, owing to both an increased surface area–body weight ratio and immaturity of the skin. Renal immaturity may result in large losses of fluid and electrolytes that must be replaced. Early use of humidified incubators significantly reduces insensible fluid losses and therefore the total administered volume necessary to maintain fluid balance.

   1. Route of administration. Whenever possible, an umbilical arterial line and a double-lumen umbilical venous line are placed shortly after birth. Arterial lines are maintained for 7 to 10 days and then replaced by peripheral arterial lines if needed. Umbilical venous catheters (UVC) may be used for as long as 7 to 14 days, and are often replaced by percutaneously inserted central venous catheters (PICC) when the UVC is removed.

   2. Rate of administration. Table 6.2 presents initial rates of fluid administration for different gestational ages and birth weights. We monitor weight, blood pressure, urine output, and serum electrolyte levels frequently. Fluid rate is adjusted to avoid dehydration or hypernatremia. We generally measure electrolytes before the age of 12 hours (6 hours for infants <800 g), and repeat as often as every 6 hours until the levels are stable. By the second to third day, many infants have a marked diuresis and natriuresis and require continued frequent assessment and

		Fluid rate	Frequency of
Birth weight (g)	Gestational age (wk)	(mL/kg/d)	electrolyte testing
500–600	23	140–200	q6h
601–800	24	120–130	q8h
801–1,000	25–26	90–110	q12h

TABLE 6.2 Fluid Administration Rates for the First 2 Days of Life for Infants on Radiant Warmers*

*Rates should be 20%–30% lower when a humidified incubator is used. Urine output and serum electrolytes should be closely monitored to determine the best rates.

adjustment of fluids and electrolytes. Insensible water loss diminishes as the skin thickens and dries over the first few days of life.

3. **Fluid composition.** Initial intravenous (IV) fluids should consist of dextrose solution in a concentration sufficient to maintain serum glucose levels >45 to 50 mg/dL. Often immature infants do not tolerate dextrose concentrations >10% at high fluid rates, so we generally use dextrose 7.5% or 5% solutions. Usually, a glucose administration rate of 4 to 10 mg/kg/minute is sufficient. If hyperglycemia results, we lower dextrose concentrations, but avoid hypoosmolar solutions (dextrose <5%). If hyperglycemia persists at levels above 180 mg/dL with glycosuria, we begin an insulin infusion at a dose of 0.05 to 0.1 unit/kg/hour and adjust as required (see Chap. 29A).

ELBW infants begin losing protein and develop negative nitrogen balance soon after birth. To avoid this, we start parenteral nutrition immediately upon admission to the NICU, using a premixed solution of amino acids and trace elements in dextrose 5%. Multivitamin solutions are not included in this initial parenteral nutrition because of shelf-life issues, but are added within 24 hours after delivery. No electrolytes are added to the initial solution other than the small amount of potassium phosphate needed to buffer the amino acids. The solution is designed so that the administration of 60 mL/kg/day (the maximum infusion rate used) provides 1.5 g of protein/kg/day. Additional fluid needs are met by the solutions described earlier. Customized parenteral nutrition, including lipid infusion, is begun as soon as it is available, generally within the first day.

4. **Skin care.** Immaturity of skin and susceptibility to damage requires close attention to maintenance of skin integrity (see Chap. 34). Topical emollients or petroleum-based products are not used except under extreme situations, but semipermeable coverings (Tegaderm and Vigilon) are used over areas of skin breakdown.

D. **Cardiovascular support**

1. **Blood pressure.** There is disagreement over acceptable values for blood pressure in extremely premature infants and some suggestion that cerebral perfusion may be adversely affected at levels below a mean blood pressure of 30 mm Hg. In the absence of data demonstrating an impact on long-term neurologic outcome, we accept mean blood pressures of 26 to 28 mm Hg for infants of 24 to 26 weeks' gestational age if the infant appears well perfused and has a stable heart rate. Early hypotension is more commonly due to altered vasoreactivity than hypovolemia, so therapy with fluid boluses is limited to 10 to 20 mL/kg, after which pressor support, initially with dopamine, is begun. Stress dose hydrocortisone (1 mg/kg every 12 hours for two doses) may be useful in infants with hypotension refractory to this strategy (see Chap. 17).

2. **Patent ductus arteriosus (PDA).** The incidence of symptomatic PDA is as high as 70% in infants with a birth weight <1,000 g. The natural timing of presentation has been accelerated by exogenous surfactant therapy, so that a symptomatic PDA now commonly occurs between 24 and 48 hours after birth, manifested by

an increasing need for ventilatory support or an increase in oxygen requirement. A murmur may be absent or difficult to hear, and the physical signs of increased pulses or an active precordium may be difficult to discern. PDA has been associated with most of the serious complications of prematurity, but it has not been proved to be responsible for these comorbidities. As a result, it is prudent to delay indomethacin or ibuprofen therapy (see Chap. 25) until the PDA has been evaluated by echocardiography, including the effect on left ventricular function and distal flow in the descending aorta. Therapy may also be initiated when overt clinical signs of cardiorespiratory compromise are present, and echocardiography is not readily available. Prophylactic treatment with indomethacin has been demonstrated to reduce the incidence and severity of PDA, and the need for subsequent ligation. However, it has not been demonstrated to result in a change in long-term neurologic or respiratory outcome, and has not become routine therapy. Persistent or recurrent confirmed PDA is treated with a second course of indomethacin or ibuprofen. Recurrence of a PDA with a significant left to right shunt after a second treatment course is generally an indication for surgical ligation.

E. Blood transfusions. These are often necessary in small infants because of large obligatory phlebotomy losses. Infants who weigh <1,000 g at birth and are moderately or severely ill may receive as many as eight or nine transfusions in the first few weeks of life. Donor exposure can be limited by reducing laboratory testing to the minimum necessary level, employing strict uniform criteria for transfusion, and by identifying a specific unit of blood for each patient likely to need several transfusions (see Chap. 26). Each such unit can be split to provide as many as eight transfusions for a single patient over a period of 21 days with only a single donor exposure. Erythropoietin therapy in conjunction with adequate iron therapy will result in accelerated erythropoiesis, but it has not been shown to reduce the need for transfusion. It is not routinely used in these patients.

F. Infection and infection control (see Chap. 23B). In general, premature birth is associated with an increased incidence of early-onset sepsis, with an incidence of 1.5% of infants having birth weight <1,500 g. Group B streptococcus (GBS) remains an important pathogen, but gram-negative organisms now account for most of early-onset sepsis in infants weighing <1,500 g. We almost always screen for infection immediately after birth, and treat with prophylactic antibiotics (ampicillin and gentamicin) pending culture results. ELBW infants are also particularly susceptible to nosocomial infections (occurring at >72 hours after birth). Approximately one-third of infants weighing <1,000 g at birth will have at least one episode of late-onset sepsis, although wide variations in its incidence between centers is observed. Almost half of late-onset infections are due to coagulase-negative staphylococcus, 18% due to gram-negative organisms, and 12% due to fungi. Mortality is higher among infants who develop these late-onset infections, particularly in those with gram-negative infections. Risk factors for late-onset infection include longer duration of mechanical ventilation, umbilical and central venous lines, and parenteral nutrition support.

Comparison of practices among institutions with different rates of nosocomial infection has led to a number of recommendations that we have employed to potentially reduce the incidence within our NICUs. Foremost among these is meticulous attention to hand washing. We use alcohol-based gels that are available at every bedside for hand hygiene, and have a strict policy for its use before touching every patient. In-line suctioning is used in respiratory circuits to minimize disruption, and every effort is made to minimize the duration of mechanical ventilation. We only use hyperalimentation solutions that have been prepared under laminar flow, and never alter them after preparation. The early introduction of feedings, preferably with human milk, minimizes the need for central lines and provides the benefits of milk-borne immune factors. Laboratory testing is kept to a minimum, and tests clustered whenever possible, to reduce the number of skin punctures and to reduce patient handling. These practices are part of a standardized protocol for skin care for all neonates born with weight of <1,000 g. Finally, the establishment of a uniform NICU culture that encompasses pride in care and cooperation has fostered an environment of blameless questioning between practitioners.

G. Nutritional support

1. **Initial management.** In all infants who weigh <1,200 g at birth, parenteral nutrition is begun shortly after birth using a standard solution administered at a rate of 60 mL/kg/day (see IV. C.), resulting in protein administration of 1.5 g/kg/day. On subsequent days, customized parenteral solutions are formulated to increase the protein administration rate by 1 g/kg/day up to a maximum of 3.5 g/kg/day. Parenteral lipids are begun on day 2 and advanced each day to a maximum of 3 g/kg/day. Enteral feeding is begun as soon as the patient is clinically stable, and is not receiving indomethacin or pressor therapy.

2. The safe initiation of enteral feeds begins with the introduction of small trophic amounts of breast milk (10 to 20 mL/kg/day), with the goal of priming the gut by inducing local factors necessary for normal function. This amount may be started even in the presence of an umbilical arterial line, and are continued for 3 to 4 days without a change in volume. Feedings of 20 cal/30 mL breast milk or formula are then slowly advanced (10–20 mL/kg/day) while monitoring for signs of feeding intolerance such as abdominal distention, vomiting (which is rare), and increased gastric residuals. It is important but often difficult to differentiate the characteristically poor gastrointestinal motility of ELBW infants from signs of a more serious gastrointestinal disorder such as necrotizing enterocolitis (see Chap. 32). At least two-thirds of our ELBW infants have episodes of feeding intolerance that result in interruption of feeds. Once successful tolerance of feedings is established at 90 to 100 mL/kg/day, caloric density is advanced to 24 cal/30 mL, and then the volume is advanced (see Chap. 10). This eliminates a drop in caloric intake as parenteral nutrition is weaned while feedings advance. Once tolerance of full feedings of 24 cal/30 mL is established, the density of feedings may be advanced by 2 cal/30 mL/day up to a maximum of 30 to 32 cal/30 mL. Protein powder is added to a total protein content of 4 g/kg/day, as this promotes improved somatic and head growth over the first several weeks of life. Many extremely small infants benefit from restriction of total fluids to 130 to 140 mL/kg/day. This minimizes problems with fluid excess while still providing adequate caloric intake.

Suggested Readings

El-Metwally D, Vohr B, Tucker RB. Survival and neonatal morbidity at the limits of viability in the mid 1990s: 22 to 25 weeks. *J Pediatr* 2000;137(5):616–622.

Horbar JD, Rogowski J, Plsek P, et al. Collaborative quality improvement for neonatal intensive care. *Pediatrics* 2001;107:14–22.

Laughton MM, Simmons MA, Bose CL. Patency of the ductus arteriosus in the premature infant: Is it pathologic? Should it be treated? *Curr Opin Pediatr* 2004;16:146–151.

Schmidt B, Davis P, Moddeman D, et al. Long-term effects of indomethacin prophylaxis in extremely low birth weight infants. *N Engl J Med* 2001;344:1966–1972.

Seri I. Management of management of hypotension and low systemic blood flow in the very low birth weight neonate during the first postnatal week. *J Perinatol* 2006;26: (Suppl 1):S8–13.

Stoll BJ, Hansen N, Fanaroff AA, et al. Late-onset sepsis in very low birth weight neonates: The experience of the NICHD Neonatal Research Network. *Pediatrics* 2002; 110:285–291.

Vohra S, Roberts RS, Zhang B, et al. Heat loss prevention (HeLP) in the delivery room: A randomized controlled trial of polyethylene occlusive skin wrapping in very preterm infants. *J Pediatr* 2004;145:750–753.

Wood NS, Marlow N, Costeloe K, et al. The EPICure Study Group. Neurologic and developmental disability after extremely preterm birth. *N Engl J Med* 2000;343:378–384.

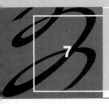

MULTIPLE BIRTHS
Josephine M. Enciso

I. CLASSIFICATION

A. Zygosity. Monozygotic (MZ) twins originate and develop from a single fertilized egg (zygote) as a result of division of the inner cell mass of the blastocyst. MZ twins are of the same sex and are genetically identical. Dizygotic (DZ) or fraternal twins originate and develop from two separately fertilized eggs. Triplets and higher-order pregnancies (quadruplets, quintuplets, sextuplets, septuplets, etc.) can be mutizygotic, MZ and identical, or rarely, a combination of both.

B. Placenta and fetal membranes. A major portion of the placenta and the fetal membranes originate from the zygote. The placenta consists of two parts: (i) a larger fetal part derived form the villous chorion and (ii) a smaller maternal part derived from the deciduas basalis. The chorionic and amniotic sacs surround the fetus. The chorion begins to from at day 3 after fertilization, and the amnion begins to form between day 6 and day 8. The two membranes eventually fuse to form the amniochorionic membrane.

   1. MZ twins commonly have one placenta with one chorion and two amnions (**monochorionic diamniotic**) or rarely, one placenta with one chorion and one amnion (**monochorionic monoamniotic**).

   2. If early splitting occurs before the formation of the chorion and amnion (day 0–3), MZ twins can end up having two placentas with two chorions and two amnions (**dichorionic diamniotic**).

   3. DZ twins always have two placentas with two chorions and two amnions (dichorionic diamniotic); however the two placentas and chorions may be fused (see Fig. 7.1).

II. EPIDEMIOLOGY

A. Incidence. The twin birth rate increased by approximately 67% from 1980 to 2003 (18.9–31.5 twin births per 1,000 total live births).

   1. The rate of MZ twinning has remained relatively constant (3.5 per 1,000).

   2. The rate of DZ twinning is approximately 1 in 100 births. This rate is influenced by several factors such as ethnicity (1 in 500 Asians, 1 in 125 in whites, and as high as 1 in 20 in African populations) and maternal age. The frequency of DZ twinning has a genetic tendency that is affected by the genotype of the mother and not that of the father. In the United States, approximately two-thirds of twins are DZ.

   3. The birth rate of triplet and higher-order multiples in 1980 was 0.37 per 1,000 live births. This rate increased dramatically after 1993 and peaked at 1.9 per 1,000 live births in 1998. Since then the rate has remained stable at approximately 1.8 per 1,000 live births.

B. Causative factors. Two main factors account for the increase in multiple births over the last two decades: one factor is the increasing use of ovulation-inducing drugs and intrauterine insemination and artificial reproductive technologies (ARTs) such as *in vitro* fertilization (IVF), although the number of ART procedures involving the transfer of three or more embryos has declined between 1997 and 2000. A second factor is the trend toward **older maternal age** at childbearing (peak at 35–39 years), which is associated with an increase in multiples.

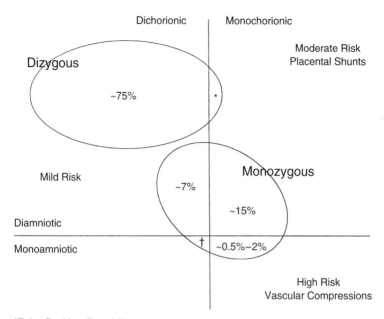

Dichorionic | Monochorionic

Dizygous

Monozygous

~75%

~7%

~15%

~0.5%–2%

Moderate Risk
Placental Shunts

Mild Risk

Diamniotic

Monoamniotic

High Risk
Vascular Compressions

*False Positive: Fused Placentas

†False Positive: Ruptured Septum

Figure 7.1. Distribution of zygosity according to the type of placentation. (With permission from Bernischke K. Multiple pregnancy. In: Polin RA, Fox WW, eds. *Fetal and neonatal physiology,* 2nd ed. Philadelphia: Saunders, 1998:115–123.)

III. ETIOLOGY

A. MZ pregnancies result from the splitting of a single egg anywhere from day 0 to day 14 postfertilization, and therefore a spectrum of placentas can form depending on the day of embryo splitting.

1. A **dichorionic diamniotic** placenta can result when early splitting occurs at day 0 to day 3 before chorion formation (which usually occurs around day 3) and before implantation. A **monochorionic diamniotic** placenta results if splitting occurs around day 4 to day 7, at which time the blastocyst cavity has developed and the chorion has formed. Amnion formation occurs at day 6 to day 8, and splitting of the egg after this time (day 4–7) can result in a **monochorionic monoamniotic** placenta. At day 14 and thereafter, the primitive streak begins to form and late splitting of the embryo at this time results in **conjoined twins**.

2. **DZ or multizygous pregnancies** result when more than one dominant follicle has matured during the same menstrual cycle and multiple ovulations occur. Increased levels of follicle stimulating hormone (FSH) in the mother have been associated with spontaneous DZ twinning. FSH levels increase with advanced maternal age (peak at age ~37). A familial tendency toward twinning has also been shown to be associated with increased levels of FSH.

IV. DIAGNOSIS. Multiple gestational sacs can be detected by ultrasonography as early as 5 weeks and cardiac activity can be detected from more than one fetus at 6 weeks.

A. Placentation. First-trimester ultrasonography can best determine the chorionicity of a multiple gestation; chorionicity is more difficult to determine in the second trimester. From week 10 to week 14, a fused dichorionic placenta may often be distinguished from a true monochorionic placenta by the presence of an internal dividing membrane or ridge at the placental surface (lambda sign). The dividing septum of a dichorionic placenta appears thicker and includes two amnions and two chorionic layers. In contrast, the dividing septum of a monochorionic placenta consists of two thin amnions. One placenta, same-sex fetuses, and absence of a dividing septum suggests monoamniotic twins, but absence of a dividing septum may also be due to septal disruption. Both conditions have a poor prognosis.

B. Zygosity. Deoxyribonucleic acid (DNA) typing can be used to determine zygosity in same-sex twins. Prenatally, DNA can be obtained by chorionic villus sampling (CVS) or amniocentesis. Postnatally, DNA typing should optimally be performed on umbilical cord tissue, buccal smear, or a skin biopsy specimen instead of blood. There is evidence that DZ twins, even in the absence of vascular connections, can also carry hematopoietic stem cells (HSCs) derived from their twin. HSCs are most likely transferred from one fetus to the other through maternal circulation.

C. Pathological examination of the placenta(s) at birth is important in establishing and verifying chorionicity.

V. PRENATAL SCREENING AND DIAGNOSIS

A. Zygosity determines the degree of risk of chromosomal abnormalities in each fetus of a multiple gestation. The risk for aneuploidy in each fetus of an MZ pregnancy is the same as a singleton pregnancy, and except for rare cases of genetic discordancy, both fetuses are affected. In a DZ pregnancy, each twin has an independent risk for aneuploidy, and therefore has twice the risk of having a chromosomal abnormality compared with a singleton.

B. Second-trimester maternal serum screening for women with multiples is limited because each fetus contributes variable levels of these serum markers. When levels are abnormal, there is difficulty in identifying which fetus is affected.

C. First-trimester ultrasonography to assess for **nuchal translucency** is a more sensitive and specific test to screen for chromosomal abnormalities. A **second-trimester ultrasonography exam** is important in surveying each fetus for **anatomic defects. Second-trimester amniocentesis** and **first-trimester CVS** can be safely performed on multiples and are both accurate diagnostic procedures for determining aneuploidy.

VI. MATERNAL COMPLICATIONS

A. Gestational diabetes has been shown in some studies to be more common in twin pregnancies.

B. Spontaneous abortion occurs in 8% to 36% of multiple pregnancies with reduction to a singleton pregnancy by the end of the first trimester **("vanishing twin").** Possible causes include abnormal implantation, early cardiovascular developmental defects, and chromosomal abnormalities. Before fetal viability, the management of the surviving cotwin in a dichorionic pregnancy includes expectant management until term or close to term, in addition to close surveillance for preterm labor, fetal well-being, and fetal growth. The management of a single fetal demise in a monochorionic twin pregnancy is more complicated. The surviving cotwin is at high risk for ischemic multiorgan and neurological injury that is thought to be secondary to hypotension or thromboembolic events. Fetal imaging by ultrasonography or magnetic resonance imaging (MRI) may be useful in detecting neurological injury. Termination of pregnancy may be offered as an option when single fetal demise occurs in a previable monochorionic twin pregnancy.

C. Incompetent cervix occurs in up to 14% of multiple gestations.

D. Placental abruption risk rises as the number of fetuses per pregnancy increases. In a large retrospective cohort study, the incidence of placental abruption was 6.2, 12.2, and 15.6 per 1,000 pregnancies in singletons, twins, and triplets, respectively.

E. Preterm premature rupture of membranes complicates 7% to 10% of twin pregnancies compared with 2% to 4% of singleton pregnancies. **Preterm labor and birth** occur in approximately 57% of twin pregnancies and in 76% to 90% of higher-order multiple gestations.

F. Pregnancy-induced hypertension (PIH) and preeclampsia are 2.5 times more common in multifetal pregnancies compared with singleton pregnancies.

G. Cesarean delivery. Approximately 66% of patients with twins and 91% of patients with triplets have cesarean delivery. Breech position of one or more fetuses, cord prolapse, and placental abruption are factors that account for the increased frequency of cesarean deliveries for twin and multiple gestations.

VII. FETAL AND NEONATAL COMPLICATIONS

A. Prematurity and low birth weight. The average duration of gestation is shorter in multifetal pregnancies, and further shortens as the number of fetuses increases. The mean gestational age at birth is 36, 33, and 29 1/2 weeks, respectively, for twins, triplets, and quadruplets. In developed countries, the incidence of preterm birth in twins was 53% in 1997, compared with 9% to 10% in singletons. Although most of this increased incidence is due to mild prematurity, multifetal pregnancy increases the risk of severe prematurity and very low birth weight (VLBW). The likelihood of a birth weight <1,500 g is 8 and 33 times greater in twins and triplets or higher-order multiples, respectively, compared with singletons. In two multicenter surveys, multiples occurred in 21% to 24% of births <1,500 g and in 30% of births <1,000 g.

B. Intrauterine growth restriction (IUGR). Fetal growth is independent of the number of fetuses until approximately 30 weeks' gestation, after which growth of multiples gradually falls off compared with singletons (see Fig. 7.2). IUGR is defined as an estimated fetal weight (EFW) less than the third percentile for gestational age or an EFW <10th percentile for gestational age in addition to evidence of fetal compromise. The mechanisms are likely uterine crowding, limitation of placental perfusion, and anomalous umbilical cord insertion. Monochorionic twins are more

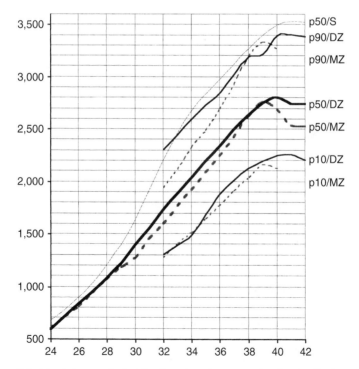

Figure 7.2. Intrauterine growth chart for dizygotic and monozygotic twins. S = Singleton; DZ = Dizygotic; MZ = Monozygotic. (From Naeye R, Bernischke K, Hagstrom J, et al. Intrauterine growth of twins as estimated from liveborn birth-weight data. *Pediatrics* 1966;37:409.)

likely to be IUGR compared with dichorionic twins and have higher perinatal mortality. Neonatal morbidities that are seen in 50% of neonates with IUGR that complicate management of these infants include hypoglycemia, polycythemia, and pulmonary hemorrhage.

C. Fetal growth discordance is expressed as a percentage of the larger twin's weight and can be mild (<15%), moderate (15%–30%), or severe (>30%). Risk factors for discordant growth include monochorionic placentation associated with velamentous cord insertion, placental dysfunction, preeclampsia, antepartum bleeding, twin-to-twin transfusion syndrome (TTTS), fetal infection, and fetal structural and chromosomal abnormalities. The smaller twin has an increased risk of fetal demise, perinatal death, and preterm birth. Five percent to 15% of twins and 30% of triplets will have fetal growth discordance that is associated with a sixfold increase in perinatal morbidity and mortality.

D. Intrauterine fetal demise (IUFD) refers to fetal demise after 20 weeks' gestation but before delivery and can be confirmed by ultrasonographic evidence of absent fetal cardiac activity. The death of one twin, which occurs in 9% of multiple pregnancies, is less common in the second and third trimesters. The risk of IUFD is 4 to 6 times greater in MZ pregnancies. Since almost all MZ twins have placental vascular connections with resulting shared circulations, there is a significant risk (20%–40%) of neurological injury (multicystic encephalomalacia) to the surviving cotwin as a result of associated severe hypotension or thromboembolic events upon death of the cotwin. Owing to the lack of a shared circulation, the death of one DZ twin usually has minimal adverse effect on the surviving cotwin. In this case, the cotwin is either completely resorbed if death occurs in the first trimester or is compressed between the amniotic sac of its cotwin and the uterine wall (fetus papyraceous). Other complications involving the surviving cotwin include antepartum stillbirth, preterm birth, placental abruption, and chorioamnionitis. In the event of a demise of one monochorionic twin, immediate delivery of the surviving cotwin should be considered after fetal viability. However, this does not seem to change the outcome as neurologic injury is thought to occur at the time of death of the cotwin. Disseminated intravascular coagulopathy is a complication seen in 20% to 25% of women who retain a dead fetus for >3 weeks. Monitoring of maternal coagulation profiles is recommended and delivery within this time frame should be considered.

E. Congenital malformations occur in approximately 6% of twin pregnancies, or 3% of individual twins. The risk in MZ twins is approximately 2.5-fold greater than in DZ twins or singletons. Structural defects specific to MZ twins include (i) early malformations that share a common origin with the twinning process, (ii) vascular disruption syndromes, and (iii) deformations.

1. **Early structural defects** include the following:
   a. Caudal malformations (sirenomelia, sacrococcygeal teratoma).
   b. Urological malformations (cloacal or bladder exstrophy).
   c. The VATER spectrum (vertebral anomalies, anal atresia, tracheoesophageal fistula, renal agenesis, cardiac defects).
   d. Neural tube defects (anencephaly, encephalocele, or holoprosencephaly).
   e. Defects of laterality (situs inversus, polysplenia, or asplenia).
2. **Vascular disruption syndromes** may occur early or late in gestation.
   a. The presence of large anastomoses between two embryos early in development may cause unequal arterial perfusion resulting in **acardia**. One embryo receives only low-pressure blood flow through the umbilical artery and preferentially perfuses its lower extremities. Profound malformations can result ranging from complete amorphism to severe upper body abnormalities such as anencephaly, holoprosencephaly, rudimentary facial features and limbs, and absent thoracic or abdominal organs. The cotwin is usually well formed. Acardia is rare with an incidence of 1 in 35,000. In acardiac twin pregnancies, the incidence of spontaneous abortion and prematurity is 20% and 60%, respectively. Perinatal mortality in the donor twin is 40%.

    b. Vascular disruptions that occur later in gestation are due to embolic events or the exchange of tissue between twins through placental anastomoses. Late vascular disruptions often occur after the demise of one fetus. Resulting malformations include cutis aplasia, limb interruption, intestinal atresia, gastroschisis, anorchia or gonadal dysgenesis, hemifacial microsomia, Goldenhar syndrome (facioauriculovertebral defects), or Poland sequence. Cranial abnormalities include porencephalic cysts, hydranencephaly, microcephaly, and hydrocephalus.

  3. Deformations such as clubfoot, dislocated hips, and cranial synostosis are more frequent in multiple pregnancies as a result of overcrowding of the intrauterine environment.

  4. Surveillance. Twin pregnancies should be evaluated for anomalies by fetal ultrasonography or more invasive procedures if indicated. Congenital anomalies are concordant only in a minority of cases, even in MZ twins. Whether assisted reproductive techniques result in an increased incidence in congenital birth defects is uncertain.

F. Chromosomal anomalies occur at a higher frequency in offspring of multiple gestations. **Advanced maternal age** contributes to the increased risk in chromosomal anomalies seen in multiple gestations. The risk in MZ twins is equivalent to that of a singleton. The risk in DZ twins is independent for each fetus, so the risk of chromosomal abnormality in at least one DZ twin is twice that of a singleton fetus.

G. Conjoined twins result when incomplete embryonic division occurs late after day 14 postconception. At this time, differentiation of the chorion and amnion has occurred, and therefore conjoined twins are seen only in monochorionic monoamniotic twins. Conjoined twins are rare and occur in approximately 1 in 50,000 to 100,000 births. The most common sites of fusion are the chest and/or abdomen. Survival is rare when there is cardiac or cerebral fusion. In one small case series of conjoined twins, 28% died *in utero*, 54% died immediately after birth, and only 18% survived. Serial ultrasonography can define the fetal anatomy and help determine management options. Polyhydramnios can affect as many as 50% of cases of conjoined twins and may require amnioreduction. Elective cesarean delivery close to term is recommended, and in cases wherein one twin is not likely to survive, delivery of the cotwin by an ex utero intrapartum treatment (EXIT) procedure should be considered. Surgical separation should be performed emergently in the event that one twin dies, and survival of the cotwin in these cases is 30% to 50%. Survival is 80% to 90% in twins that undergo elective separation, which is usually performed at 2 to 4 months of age.

H. TTTS occurs only in monochorionic gestations and complicates 5% to 15% of such pregnancies.

  1. The **pathophysiology** of TTTS is not completely understood, but anomalous placental vascular connections between twins are necessary for it to occur. Eight-five percent of monochorionic placentas have vascular connections that include superficial arterial-to-arterial (AA) and venous-to-venous (VV) anastomoses that are potentially bidirectional and deep interfetal artery-to-vein (AV) communications located in the placental cotyledons that are supplied by one fetus and drained by the other. AA connections are thought to be protective whereas AV anastomoses lead to shunting of blood from one twin to the other. TTTS results when the superficial network of anastomoses does not compensate for the intertwin AV shunts. Five percent to 10% of monochorionic placentas have sufficient circulatory imbalance to produce TTTS. One fetus (**the donor**) slowly pumps blood into the cotwin's circulation (**the recipient**). Complications in the donor include anemia, hypovolemia, growth restriction, brain ischemic lesions, renal insufficiency, oligohydramnios ("stuck twin"), lung hypoplasia, limb deformation, and high risk for fetal demise. Complications in the recipient include polycythemia, thrombosis, cerebral emboli, disseminated intravascular coagulation (DIC), polyhydramnios, progressive cardiomyopathy due to volume overload, and fetal hydrops. Newer evidence suggests that the pathophysiology of TTTS involves changes in the renin-angiotensin system and increased levels of human brain natriuretic peptide (hBNP) and endothlin-1. Vasoactive mediators produced in the donor are shunted to the recipient resulting in hypertension, contributing to the development of hypertensive cardiomyopathy.

2. Diagnosis is usually made between 17 and 26 weeks' gestation, but the process may occur as early as 13 weeks. Severe cases of TTTS have signs before 20 weeks' gestation and have a mortality of 60% to 100%. **Diagnostic criteria** for TTTS include monochorionicity, polyhydramnios in the sac of one twin (the recipient) and oligohydramnios in the sac of the other twin (the donor), umbilical cord size discrepancy, cardiac dysfunction in the polyhydramniotic twin, abnormal umbilical artery and/or ductus venosus Doppler velocimetry, and significant growth discordance (>20%).

3. **Fetal treatment** interventions include serial amnioreduction, microseptostomy of the intertwin membrane, fetoscopic laser photocoagulation, and selective feticide. A randomized clinical trial comparing amnioreduction and septostomy showed that only one procedure was required with septostomy whereas serial amnioreduction required multiple procedures. Results from the Eurofoetus Trial serial found that laser photocoagulation improved both perinatal survival and short-term neurologic outcome at 6 months of life compared with serial amnioreduction. However, the selection of patients most likely to benefit, the best intervention for a particular patient, and the optimal timing of intervention remain uncertain. In addition, data on long-term neurodevelopmental outcome in surviving infants of TTTS (i.e., the incidence of cerebral palsy [CP]) are needed.

4. **Neonatal management** may include **resuscitation** at birth and need for continued ventilatory and cardiovascular support; rapid establishment of **intravascular access** for volume expansion to treat hypotension, correct hypoglycemia, and transfuse "packed red blood cells" to treat anemia; **partial exchange transfusion** in the recipient to treat significant polycythemia; and **neuroimaging** to detect central nervous system (CNS) injury.

I. **Velamentous cord insertion and vasa previa** occur 6 to 9 times more often in twins than in singletons, and even more often in higher-order gestations. Probable factors contributing to this higher risk include placental crowding and abnormal blastocyst implantation. All types of placentation can be affected. With velamentous cord insertion, vessels are unprotected by Wharton jelly and are more prone to compression, thrombosis, or disruption, leading to fetal distress or hemorrhage.

J. **Cord blood flow interruption** due to cord accidents (i.e., cord entanglement or compression) accounts for the reported high rate of intrauterine death of one or both twins. The period of highest risk is 26 to 32 weeks. The overall perinatal mortality in monochorionic monoamniotic twins is reported to be in the range of 12% to 60%. More recent literature reports lower rates of perinatal mortality due to umbilical cord accidents. This reduction may be attributable to improved prenatal diagnosis of monochorionic monoamniotic pregnancies, closer fetal surveillance, and increased delivery of multiples by cesarean section.

VIII. **OUTCOMES**

A. **Neonatal mortality.** Rates of neonatal mortality are gestational age specific and are similar for singletons, twins, and triplets. Prematurity and low birth weight are the predominating factors that increase the rates of mortality and morbidity for multiple births. Assisted reproduction has contributed to the increased incidence of multifetal pregnancies, and preterm birth is strongly correlated with the number of fetuses. Therefore, techniques that limit the number of reimplanted eggs or transferred embryos, or selective reduction of higher-order multiples may improve the likelihood of a successful outcome.

B. **Morbidity. Prematurity and growth restriction** are associated with an increased risk of morbidities such as bronchopulmonary dysplasia, necrotizing enterocolitis, retinopathy of prematurity, and intraventricular hemorrhage. These are discussed in more detail elsewhere (see chaps. 24, 27, 32, and 35).

C. **Long-term morbidity** such as **CP** and other neurological handicaps affect more twins and multiples than singletons. There is a 5- to10-fold increased risk of CP in multiples compared with singleton gestations. Twins account for 5% to 10% of all cases of CP in the United States. The prevalence of CP in twins is 7.4%, compared with 1% in singletons. This is related to a number of factors including increased risk of prematurity and low birth weight in multiple births and high risk for cerebral injury in twins with monochorionic placentation and in those with TTTS.

D. Economic impact. Hospital stays for mothers and babies are typically longer for multiple gestations. One study showed that, compared with singletons, average hospital costs were estimated to be 3 and 6 times higher for twins and triplets, respectively; total family costs were 4 and 11 times higher, respectively. The increase in multiple births due to the use of assisted reproductive technologies has made an impact on overall medical costs. Thirty-five percent of twins and 75% of triplets resulted from assisted reproduction techniques. In another study, medical costs from induction of IVF pregnancy until the end of the neonatal period for a twin pregnancy were found to be more than 5 times higher than in a singleton pregnancy.

E. Social and family impact. Caring for twins or higher-order multiples contributes to increased marital strain, financial stress, parental anxiety, and depression, and has a greater influence on the professional and social life of mothers of these infants, particularly first-time mothers, compared with mothers of singletons. In one study, IVF twin parents were found to have a lower risk (7.3%) of divorce/separation compared with parents of control twins (13.3%) suggesting that IVF twin parents were able to better cope with the increased stress of twins. Multiples are more likely to have medical complications (i.e., prematurity, congenital defects, IUGR) that result in prolonged hospital stays that contribute further to a family's emotional and financial stress. Social services, lactation support, and assistance from additional caregivers and family members can help parents cope with the increased amount of care required by multiples. Organizations of parents of multiples can provide advice and emotional support that can further help new parents of multiples cope.

Suggested Readings

Cleary-Goldman J, D'Alton ME, Berkowitz RL. Prenatal diagnosis and multiple pregnancy. *Semin Perinatol* 2005;29:312–320.

Cordero I, Franco A, Joy SD. Monochorionic monoamniotic twins: Neonatal outcome. *J Perinatol* 2006;26:170–175.

Garite TJ, Clark RH, Elliott JP, et al. Twins and triplets: The effect of plurality and growth on neonatal outcome compared with singleton infants. *Am J Obstet Gynecol* 2004;191:700–707.

Moise KJ Jr, Dorman K, Lamvu G, et al. A randomized trial of amnioreduction versus septostomy in the treatment of twin-twin transfusion syndrome. *Am J Obstet Gynecol* 2005;193:701–707.

Senat MV, Deprest J, Boulvain M, et al. Endoscopic laser surgery versus serial amnioreduction for severe twin-to-twin transfusion syndrome. *N Engl J Med* 2004;351:136–144.

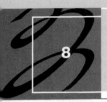

GENETIC ISSUES PRESENTING IN THE NURSERY
Diana W. Bianchi

I. GENERAL PRINCIPLES
  A. Introduction. Although as many as 40% of pediatric hospital admissions have a genetic basis, it is usually the infant with major malformations or an inborn error of metabolism who presents in the nursery setting. Furthermore, many newborns with genetic problems present to the special care nursery because of a suspected malformation noted on a prenatal sonographic examination.
  B. Major malformations are defined as anomalies that are prenatal in origin and have cosmetic, medical, or surgical significance. The birth of an infant with major malformations, whether diagnosed antenatally or not, evokes an emotional parental response. The medical staff must ensure that the affected infant has an expedient but thorough evaluation so appropriate diagnostic procedures and therapy may proceed.
II. INCIDENCE. Major malformations occur in 2% to 3% of live births and have surpassed prematurity as the leading cause of neonatal death. For a twin the incidence of congenital anomalies is double that of the general population. Infants who are conceived by *in vitro* **fertilization** also have an increased incidence of anomalies.
III. ETIOLOGY. The etiologies of congenital anomalies are shown in Table 8.1. Note that the cause is unknown in most cases. Approximately 10% are associated with a chromosomal abnormality.
IV. APPROACH TO THE INFANT
  A. History
    1. Prenatal. The obstetric chart should be reviewed for the presence or absence of the following:
      a. Chronic maternal illness, for example, diabetes, phenylketonuria, Graves' disease, myasthenia gravis, myotonic dystrophy, or systemic lupus erythematosus (see Table 8.2).
      b. Specific exposure to drugs or alcohol during pregnancy (Table 8.2).
      c. Infections during pregnancy.
      d. Abnormal uterine shape or the presence of large fibroids.
      e. Multiple gestations.
      f. Fetal growth pattern (e.g., relationship of uterine size to gestational age).
      g. Results of antenatal ultrasonographic examinations (were anomalies, polyhydramnios, or oligohydramnios diagnosed?).
      h. Results of first and second trimester maternal serum screening (see Chap. 1). A **low alpha-fetoprotein** (AFP) level may be present if the fetus has trisomy 18 or 21. A **high AFP** level may indicate a multiple gestation, impending fetal demise, open neural tube defect, abdominal wall defect, congenital nephrosis, epidermolysis bullosa, or Turner syndrome. A **high human chorionic gonadotropin (hCG)** level is also associated with trisomy 21. An **increased nuchal translucency measurement** may indicate a fetal chromosomal abnormality or an increased risk for congenital heart disease.
      i. Quality and frequency of fetal movements.
    2. Family history. The parents and, if possible, the grandparents should be asked the following:
      a. What is the ethnic background of both mother and father?
      b. Have there been any prior affected infants in the family?

TABLE 8.1 **Etiology of Congenital Anomalies: Brigham and Women's Hospital Malformations Surveillance Data from 69,227 Newborns**

	Number	Percentage (%)
Single gene (Mendelian inheritance)	48	3.1
Chromosome abnormality	157	10.1
Familial	225	14.5
Multifactorial	356	23.0
Teratogens	49	3.2
Uterine factors	39	2.5
Twinning	6	0.4
Unknown	669	43.2
Total	1,549	100

Source: Adapted from Nelson K, Holmes LB. Malformations due to presumed spontaneous mutations in newborn infants. *N Engl J Med* 1989;320:19. Copyright © 1989 Massachusetts Medical Society. All rights reserved.

 TABLE 8.2 **Known Human Teratogens**

DRUGS
Aminopterin/amethopterin
Androgenic hormones
Busulfan
Chlorobiphenyls
Cocaine
Cyclophosphamide
Diethylstilbestrol
Iodide
Isotretinoin (13-*cis*-retinoic acid)
Lithium
Phenytoin
Propylthiouracil
Tetracycline
Trimethadione
Valproic acid
Warfarin

HEAVY METALS
Lead
Mercury

RADIATION
Cancer therapy

MATERNAL CONDITIONS
Alcoholism
Graves disease
Insulin-dependent diabetes mellitus
Maternal phenylketonuria
Myasthenia gravis
Myotonic dystrophy
Systemic lupus erythematosus

INTRAUTERINE INFECTIONS
Cytomegalovirus
Herpes simplex
Rubella
Syphilis
Toxoplasmosis
Varicella
Venezuelan equine encephalitis virus

OTHER EXPOSURES
Gasoline fumes
Heat
Hypoxia
Maternal smoking

   c. Is there a history of infertility, multiple miscarriages, neonatal death, new-borns with other malformations, or children with developmental delay?

   d. Is there consanguinity in the family?

3. **Perinatal events**

   a. What was the fetal position *in utero*?

   b. Was there fetal distress during labor? How did delivery occur?

   c. What was the umbilical cord length (e.g., a positive association exists between fetal motor activity and cord length)?

   d. What was the placental appearance?

4. **Neonatal course**

   a. Did the infant breathe spontaneously? Have there been difficulties feeding? Is the baby hypo- or hypertonic?

B. **Physical examination.** A complete physical examination is essential to making an accurate diagnosis. Often, however, the critically ill neonate is partially hidden by monitoring equipment. Beware of making a definitive diagnosis when (i) the midface is obscured by adhesive tape securing endotracheal and nasogastric tubes, (ii) the extremities cannot be visualized because there are peripheral intravenous (IV) lines in place, or (iii) the infant is hydropic.

   1. **Anthropometrics.** Specific physical parameters that should be measured include length, head circumference, outer and inner canthal distance, palpebral fissure length, interpupillary distance, ear length, philtrum length, internipple distance, chest circumference, upper–lower segment ratio, and hand and foot length. Normal standards exist for all these measurements in infants of 27 to 41 weeks' gestation.

   2. The physical examination should include a thorough inspection of the skin; note the position of the hair whorls on the scalp, the head shape and facial characteristics, and a description of the extremities. The dermatoglyphic pattern of low-arch dermal ridges is particularly useful in the bedside diagnosis of trisomy 18 (see Table 8.3).

   3. **Ophthalmologic examination** should be performed.

   4. **Auditory screening** should be performed.

   5. Examine both parents, if possible.

C. **Laboratory studies**

   1. **Chromosome studies.** Skin and peripheral blood are the most available sources of cells for chromosome analysis. Generally, 1 mL of peripheral blood is collected in a green-top tube (sodium heparin being the anticoagulant). The sample should be kept at room temperature. For chromosomal analysis, it does not matter if the infant has received transfusions, because blood for neonates is generally irradiated. Irradiation prevents cell division; therefore the dividing cells in the karyotype originate from the newborn. Results of chromosome analysis are usually available within 48 hours. Although 0.6% of newborns have abnormal chromosomes, only a third of these have serious malformations. (See Table 8.3 for a summary of physical findings in the three major live-born autosomal trisomies.)

   2. **Fluorescence *in situ* hybridization (FISH) analysis.** For all newborns with **conotruncal heart malformations** (e.g., interrupted aortic arch, truncus arteriosus, tetralogy of Fallot), particularly in the setting of additional malformations such as cleft palate or single kidney, FISH studies should be performed, with specific emphasis on using probes that recognize long-arm deletions of chromosome 22. The FISH test is the diagnostic test of choice for DiGeorge syndrome. Similarly, for newborns with severe unexplained hypotonia and oral feeding difficulties, consider a diagnosis of Prader-Willi syndrome. The FISH test detects long-arm deletions of chromosome 15. If negative, it should be followed by a DNA methylation test. Other disorders that present in the newborn period that may be diagnosed by FISH are listed in Table 8.4. Clinical applications of FISH include: rapid screening for aneuploidy, identification of microdeletion syndromes, and cancer cytogenetics. FISH studies are not automatically

TABLE 8.3 Physical Findings in the Three Major Live-born Autosomal Trisomies

	Trisomy 13	Trisomy 18	Trisomy 21
Birth weight:	Normal range	Growth retarded	Normal range
Skin:	Scalp defects	—	—
CNS:	Major malformations	Microcephaly	—
	Holoprosencephaly	—	—
	Neural tube defects	—	—
Facies:	Abnormal midface	Micrognathia	Upslanting eyes
	Microphthalmia	—	Flattened facies
	Cleft lip/palate	—	Epicanthal folds
			Prominent tongue
			Small ears
Heart:	VSD, PDA, ASD	VSD, ASD, PDA,	AV canal
	Dextrocardia	—	VSD, PDA
Abdomen:	Polycystic kidneys	Omphalocele	—
Extremities:	Polydactyly	Camptodactyly	Brachydactyly
		Overlapping fingers	Simian crease in 45%
		Abnormal dermato-glyphics	Fifth finger clinodactyly
		Nail hypoplasia	Wide space between first and second toe
Neurologic:	—	Hypertonic	Muscular hypotonia
			Weak Moro reflex

CNC = central nervous system; VSD = ventricular septal defect; PDA = patent ductus arteriosus; ASD = atrial septal defect; AV = atrioventricular.

 TABLE 8.4 FISH Tests Commonly Ordered in the Newborn Setting

	Chromosome	
Condition	**Location**	**Symptoms**
DiGeorge syndrome	22q11	Congenital heart disease, cleft palate, other malformations, hypocalcemia
Miller-Dieker syndrome	17p13	Lissencephaly
Prader-Willi syndrome	15q11–13	Hypotonia, feeding problems
Steroid sulfatase deficiency (X-linked ichthyosis)	Xp22	Skin rash, low maternal estriol
Williams syndrome	7q11	Hypercalcemia, aortic stenosis

TABLE 8.5	DNA Mutations Presenting as Serious Neonatal Illness

Hemophilia

Ornithine transcarbamylase deficiency

Autosomal dominant polycystic kidney disease

α-1-Antitrypsin deficiency

Chronic granulomatous disease

21-OH deficiency (congenital adrenal hyperplasia)

Cystic fibrosis

Phenylketonuria

Myotonic dystrophy

Osteogenesis imperfecta

Spinal muscular atrophy

performed when a chromosome analysis is ordered; the particular probe for the condition being sought must be specified.

3. **Array comparative genomic hybridization (CGH)** is becoming increasingly used to diagnose submicroscopic deletions, unbalanced translocations, and interindividual copy number variation of genomic segments.

4. **DNA-based diagnosis and/or banking.** An increasing number of diseases presenting in the nursery result from single-gene mutations. Many are potentially lethal. The relevant disorders are listed in Table 8.5. Obtaining blood or skin fibroblasts for DNA studies may facilitate genetic counseling and prenatal diagnosis in future pregnancies. Note that if an infant has been transfused, the donor white blood cells will contribute DNA to the sample. Therefore, in infants who have received transfusions, a fibroblast culture obtained from a skin biopsy is preferable. DNA mutation analysis for infants suspected to have cystic fibrosis is recommended for premature infants, who cannot have a sweat test. DNA studies are also useful in the determination of twin zygosity and paternity.

5. **Infectious diseases.** Determination of toxoplasmosis, rubella, cytomegalovirus, herpes simplex (TORCH) titers, and "other," which may include parvovirus, syphilis, and human immunodeficiency virus (HIV) is indicated if the physical findings are suggestive of congenital infection (see Chap. 23A).

6. **Metabolic testing.** Results of state-mandated newborn metabolic screening should be verified. Measurement of urinary organic acids is useful to diagnose metabolic disease in the dysmorphic newborn with metabolic acidosis (see Chap. 29D).

7. **Other blood tests.** Serum cholesterol level (if low) may diagnose Smith-Lemli-Opitz syndrome.

D. Imaging

1. **Ultrasonographic examinations** can detect cranial malformations, congenital heart disease, and liver and renal anomalies.

2. **Radiographs** can define bony malformations or skeletal dysplasias.

3. **Magnetic resonance imaging (MRI) and computed tomographic (CT) imaging** may be helpful in defining brain and abdominal anatomy.

E. Pathologic findings

1. **Placental pathology** should be requested if the placenta is available

V. **DIFFERENTIAL DIAGNOSIS.** After the physical examination, history, and all test results are known, a diagnosis may be possible. In many cases it is not possible to make a diagnosis in the neonatal setting. Because of major changes in facial features over the first year after birth, as well as subsequent information that an infant failed to achieve certain developmental milestones, the true diagnosis may only become apparent later. Careful follow-up is vitally important.

VI. MANAGEMENT

A. Genetic consultation. If a diagnosis is made, consultation with a medical geneticist should be offered to discuss prognosis and potential therapy.

B. Follow-up. If the infant is otherwise stable, an appointment with a medical geneticist should be made for approximately 3 months of age.

C. A future genetic counseling session with the parents can be scheduled to provide recurrence risk and give information about the possibility of prenatal and/or preimplantation diagnosis in a subsequent pregnancy.

VII. SPECIAL CONSIDERATIONS

A. Perinatal death of an infant with malformations

1. Have a complete **autopsy** performed, including radiographs and photographs.

2. Obtain a sterile **skin biopsy specimen** for tissue culture. Cultured fibroblasts may serve as a source of chromosomes, enzymes, or DNA (see Chap. 29D). The umbilical cord or placenta can serve as an alternate source of fetal cells for study.

3. Arrange a follow-up meeting with the family to summarize the results of studies.

 ONLINE RESOURCES

GENE TESTS (www.GeneTests.org) Provides updated summaries of known single gene disorders. Also provides helpful information as to whether DNA mutation testing is available for the condition.

ONLINE MENDELIAN INHERITANCE IN MAN [OMIM] (http://www3.ncbi.nlm .nih.gov) Allows one to search for a diagnosis of a Mendelian disorder based on shared terms such as "cleft lip AND club foot." Provides a summary of causative gene, type of inheritance pattern, and gene map location.

Suggested Readings

Baraitser M, Winter R. *A colour atlas of clinical genetics*. London: Wolfe Medical Publications, 1983.

Bianchi DW, Crombleholme TM, D'Alton ME, et al. *Fetology:Diagnosis and management of the fetal patient*. New York: McGraw-Hill, 2000.

Jones KL. *Smith's recognizable patterns of human malformation*, 6th ed. Philadelphia: Elsevier Science, 2006.

Merlob P, Sivan Y, Reisner SH, et al. Arthropometric measurements of the newborn infant (27 to 41 gestational weeks). *Birth Defects* 1984;20:1.

Taybi H, Lachman RS. *Radiology of syndromes and metabolic disorders*, 4th ed. St. Louis: Mosby-Year Book, 1996.

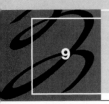

FLUID AND ELECTROLYTE MANAGEMENT
Elizabeth G. Doherty and Charles F. Simmons, Jr.

$\mathcal{C}$ areful fluid and electrolyte management in term and preterm infants is an essential component of neonatal care. Developmental changes in body composition in conjunction with functional changes in skin, renal, and neuroendocrine systems account for the fluid balance challenges faced by neonatologists on a daily basis. Fluid management requires the understanding of several physiologic principles.

I. DISTRIBUTION OF BODY WATER
A. General principles.
Transition from fetal to newborn life is associated with major changes in water and electrolyte homeostatic control. Before birth, the fetus has constant supply of water and electrolytes from the mother across the placenta. After birth, the newborn assumes responsibility for its own fluid and electrolyte homeostasis. The body composition of the fetus changes during gestation with a smaller proportion of body weight being composed of water as gestation progresses.
B. Definitions
- Total body water (TBW) = intracellular fluid (ICF) + extracellular fluid (ECF) (see Fig. 9.1).
- ECF is composed of intravascular and interstitial fluid.
- Insensible water loss (IWL) = fluid intake − urine output + weight change.
C. Perinatal changes in TBW.
A proportion of diuresis in both term and preterm infants during the first days of life should be regarded as physiologic. This diuresis results in a weight loss of 5% to 10% in term infants and up to 15% in preterm infants. At lower gestational ages, ECF accounts for a greater proportion of birth weight (Fig. 9.1). Therefore, very low birth weight (VLBW) infants must lose a greater percentage of birth weight to maintain ECF proportions equivalent to those of term infants. Larger weight loss is possibly beneficial to the preterm infant, as administration of excessive fluid and Na may increase risk of chronic lung disease (CLD) and patent ductus arteriosus (PDA).
D. Sources of water loss
1. **Renal losses.** Renal function matures with increasing gestational age (GA). Immature Na and water homeostasis is common in the preterm infant. Contributing factors leading to varying urinary water and electrolyte losses include the following:
   a. Decreased glomerular filtration rate (GFR).
   b. Reduced proximal and distal tubule Na reabsorption.
   c. Decreased capacity to concentrate or dilute urine.
   d. Decreased bicarbonate and potassium (K) and hydrogen ion secretion.
2. **Extra renal losses.** In VLBW infants IWL can exceed 150 mL/kg/day owing to increased environmental and body temperatures, skin breakdown, radiant warmers, phototherapy, and extreme prematurity (see Table 9.1). Respiratory water loss increases with decreasing GA and with increasing respiratory rate; in intubated infants, inadequate humidification of the inspired gas may lead to increased IWL. Other fluid losses that should be replaced if amount is deemed significant include stool (diarrhea or ostomy drainage), cerebrospinal fluid (from ventriculotomy or serial lumbar punctures), and nasogastric tube or thoracostomy tube drainage.

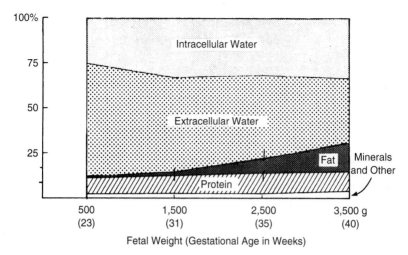

Figure 9.1. Body composition in relation to fetal weight and gestational age. (From Dweck HS. Feeding the prematurely born infant. Fluids, calories, and methods of feeding during the period of extrauterine growth retardation. *Clin Perinatol* 1975;2:183. Data from Widdowson EM. Growth and composition of the fetus and newborn. In: Assali NS, ed. *Biology of gestation,* Vol. 2. New York: Academic Press, 1968).

Incubators for newborn infants are being designed to improve maintenance of warmth and humidity and may lead to decreased IWL (e.g., the Giraffe Isolette).

II. ASSESSMENT OF FLUID AND ELECTROLYTE STATUS
A. History
1. **Maternal.** The newborn's fluid and electrolyte status partially reflects maternal hydration status and drug administration. Excessive use of oxytocin, diuretics, or hyponatremic intravenous (IV) fluid can lead to maternal and fetal hyponatremia. Antenatal steroids may increase skin maturation, subsequently decreasing IWL and the risk of hyperkalemia.
2. **Fetal/perinatal.** The presence of oligohydramnios may be associated with congenital renal dysfunction, including renal agenesis, polycystic kidney disease,

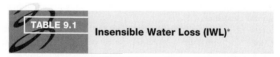

Birth weight (g)	IWL (mL/kg/d)
750–1,000	82
1,001–1,250	56
1,251–1,500	46
>1501	26

*Values represent mean IWL for infants in incubators during the first week of life. IWL is increased by phototherapy (up to 40%), radiant warmers (up to 50%), and fever. IWL is decreased by the use of humidified gas with respirators and heat shields in incubators Bell et al. 1980, Bell et al. 1980, Fanaroff et al. 1972 and Okken et al. 1979.

or posterior urethral valves. Severe in utero hypoxemia or birth asphyxia may lead to acute tubular necrosis.

B. Physical examination

1. **Change in body weight.** Acute changes in an infant's weight generally reflect a change in TBW. The compartment affected will depend on the gestational age and clinical course of the infant. For example, long-term use of paralytic agents and peritonitis may lead to increased interstitial fluid volume and increased body weight but decreased intravascular volume. Therefore, weight should be measured at least daily.

2. **Skin and mucosal manifestations.** Altered skin turgor, sunken anterior fontanelle, and dry mucous membranes are not sensitive indicators of fluid or electrolyte balance.

3. **Cardiovascular.** Tachycardia can result from ECF excess (e.g., heart failure) or hypovolemia. Capillary refill time can be delayed with reduced cardiac output or peripheral vasoconstriction and hepatomegaly can occur with increased ECF volume. Blood pressure changes occur late in the sequence of responses to reduced cardiac output.

C. Laboratory studies

1. **Serum electrolytes and plasma osmolarity** reflect the composition and tonicity of the ECF. Frequent monitoring, every 4 to 6 hours, should be done in the extremely low birth weight (ELBW) infants during the first few days of life owing to high IWL.

2. **Fluid balance** with input and output measurements should be monitored. Normal urine output is 1 to 3 mL/kg/hour. With ECF depletion (dehydration), urine output may fall to <1 mL/kg/hour. However, in neonates with immature renal function, urine output may not decrease despite ECF volume depletion.

3. **Urine electrolytes and specific gravity (SG)** can reflect renal capacity to concentrate or dilute urine and reabsorb or excrete Na. Increases in SG can occur when the infant is receiving decreased fluids, has decreased urine output, or is spilling glucose. Neither urine electrolytes nor SG is very helpful when infant is on diuretics.

4. **Fractional excretion of Na (FE-Na)** reflects the balance between glomerular filtration and tubular reabsorption of Na.

   FE-Na = (urine Na × plasma creatinine)/(plasma Na × urine creatinine) × 100

   ■ Level of <1% indicates prerenal factors reducing renal blood flow.
   ■ Level of 2.5% occurs with acute renal failure (ARF).
   ■ Level of >2.5% is frequently seen in infants of <32 weeks' gestation.

5. **Blood urea nitrogen (BUN) and serum Cr** values provide indirect information about ECF volume and GFR. Values in the early postnatal period reflect placental clearance.

6. **Arterial pH, carbon dioxide tension (PCO_2), and Na bicarbonate** determinations can provide indirect evidence of intravascular volume depletion because poor tissue perfusion leads to high-anion-gap metabolic acidosis (lactic acidosis).

III. MANAGEMENT OF FLUIDS AND ELECTROLYTES. The goal of early management is to allow initial ECF loss over the first 5 to 6 days as reflected by weight loss, while maintaining normal tonicity and intravascular volume as reflected by blood pressure, heart rate, urine output, serum electrolyte levels, and pH. Subsequent fluid management should maintain water and electrolyte balance, including requirements for body growth.

A. The term infant. Body weight decreases by 3% to 5% over the first 5 to 6 days. Subsequently, fluids should be adjusted so that changes in body weight are consistent with caloric intake. Clinical status should be monitored for maldistribution of water (e.g., edema). Na supplementation is not usually required in the first 24 hours unless ECF expansion is necessary. Small-for-gestational-age term infants may require early Na supplementation to maintain adequate ECF volume.

| **TABLE 9.2** | Initial Fluid Therapy* | | | |

		Fluid rate (mL/kg/d)		
Birth weight (kg)	Dextrose (g/100 mL)	<24 h	24–48 h	>48 h
<1	5–10	100–150†	120–150	140–190
1–1.5	10	80–100	100–120	120–160
>1.5	10	60–80	80–120	120–160

*Infants in humidified incubators. Infants under radiant warmers usually require higher initial fluid rates.
†Very low birth weight (VLBW) infants frequently require even higher initial rates of fluid administration, and frequent reassessment of serum electrolytes, urine output, and body weight.

B. The premature infant. Allow a 5% to 15% weight loss over the first 5 to 6 days. Table 9.2 summarizes initial fluid therapy. Then, adjust fluids to maintain stable weight until an anabolic state is achieved and growth occurs. Frequently assess response to fluid and electrolyte therapy during the first 2 days of life. **Physical examination and urine output and SG and serum electrolyte determinations may be required initially as frequently as every 6 to 8 hours in infants <1,000 g** (see VIII.A).

Water loss through skin and urine may exceed 200 mL/kg/day, which can represent up to **one-third of TBW.** IV Na supplementation is not required for the first 24 hours unless ECF volume loss exceeds 5% of body weight/day (see Chap. 6). If ECF volume expansion is necessary, **normal saline (NS) is preferred over 5% albumin solutions** in order to reduce risk of CLD.

IV. APPROACH TO DISORDERS OF NA AND WATER BALANCE. Abnormalities can be grouped into disorders of **tonicity** or **ECF volume.** The conceptual approach to disorders of tonicity (e.g., hyponatremia) depends on whether the newborn exhibits normal ECF (euvolemia), ECF depletion (dehydration), or ECF excess (edema).

A. Isonatremic disorders

   1. Dehydration

      a. Predisposing factors frequently involve equivalent losses of Na and water (through thoracostomy, nasogastric, or ventriculostomy drainage) or third-space losses that accompany peritonitis, gastroschisis, or omphalocele. Renal Na and water losses in the VLBW infant can lead to hypovolemia despite normal body tonicity.

      b. Diagnosis. Dehydration is usually manifested by weight loss, decreased urine output, and increased urine SG. However, infants of <32 weeks' gestation may not demonstrate oliguria in response to hypovolemia. Poor skin turgor, tachycardia, hypotension, metabolic acidosis, and increasing BUN may coexist. A low FE-Na (<1%) is usually only seen in infants of >32 weeks' gestational age (see II.C.4).

      c. Therapy. Administer Na and water to first correct deficits and then adjust to equal maintenance needs plus ongoing losses. Acute isonatremic dehydration may require IV infusion of 10 mL/kg of NS if acute weight loss is >10% of body weight with signs of poor cardiac output.

   2. Edema

      a. Predisposing factors include excessive isotonic fluid administration, heart failure, sepsis, and neuromuscular paralysis.

      b. Diagnosis. Clinical signs include periorbital and extremity edema, increased weight, and hepatomegaly.

TABLE 9.3   Hyponatremic Disorders

Clinical diagnosis	Etiology	Therapy
Factitious hyponatremia	Hyperlipidemia	
Hypertonic hyponatremia	Mannitol	
	Hyperglycemia	
ECF volume normal	Syndrome of inappropriate antidiuretic hormone (SIADH)	Restrict water intake
	Pain	
	Opiates	
	Excess intravenous fluids	
ECF volume deficit	Diuretics	Increase Na intake
	Late-onset hyponatremia of prematurity	
	Congenital adrenal Hyperplasia	
	Severe glomerulotubular imbalance (immaturity)	
	Renal tubular acidosis	
	Gastrointestinal losses	
	Necrotizing enterocolitis (third-space loss)	
ECF volume excess	Heart failure	Restrict water intake
	Neuromuscular blockade (e.g., pancuronium)	
	Sepsis	

ECF = extracellular fluid.

    c. Therapy includes **Na restriction** (to decrease total-body Na) and water restriction (depending on electrolyte response).
  B. Hyponatremic disorders (see Table 9.3). Consider **factitious hyponatremia** due to hyperlipidemia or **hypoosmolar hyponatremia** due to osmotic agents. True hyposmolar hyponatremia can then be evaluated.
    1. Hyponatremia due to ECF volume depletion
      a. Predisposing factors include diuretic use, osmotic diuresis (glycosuria), VLBW with renal water and Na wasting, adrenal or renal tubular salt-losing disorders, gastrointestinal losses (vomiting, diarrhea), and third-space losses of ECF (skin sloughing, early necrotizing enterocolitis [NEC]).
      b. Diagnosis. Decreased weight, poor skin turgor, tachycardia, rising BUN, and metabolic acidosis are frequently observed. If renal function is mature, the newborn may develop decreased urine output, increased urine SG, and a low FE-Na.
      c. Therapy. If possible, reduce ongoing Na loss. Administer Na and water to replace deficits and then adjust to match maintenance needs plus ongoing losses.
    2. Hyponatremia with normal ECF volume
      a. Predisposing factors include excess fluid administration and the syndrome of inappropriate antidiuretic hormone (SIADH) secretion. Factors that cause SIADH include pain, opiate administration, intraventricular hemorrhage (IVH), asphyxia, meningitis, pneumothorax, and positive-pressure ventilation.

b. **Diagnosis of SIADH.** Weight gain usually occurs without edema. Excessive fluid administration without SIADH results in low urine SG and high urine output. In contrast, SIADH leads to **decreased urine output** and **increased urine osmolarity.** Urinary Na excretion in infants with SIADH varies widely and reflects Na intake. The diagnosis of SIADH presumes no volume-related stimulus to antidiuretic hormone (ADH) release, such as reduced cardiac output or abnormal renal, adrenal, or thyroid function.

c. **Therapy. Water restriction** is therapeutic unless (i) serum Na concentration is less than approximately 120 mEq/L or (ii) neurologic signs such as obtundation or seizure activity develop. In these instances, **furosemide** 1 mg/kg IV q6h can be initiated while replacing urinary Na excretion with **hypertonic NaCl (3%) (1–3 mL/kg initial dose).** This strategy leads to loss of free water with no net change in total-body Na. Fluid restriction alone can be utilized once serum Na concentration is >120 mEq/L and neurologic signs abate.

3. **Hyponatremia due to ECF volume excess**

a. **Predisposing factors** include sepsis with decreased cardiac output, late NEC, heart failure, abnormal lymphatic drainage, and neuromuscular paralysis.

b. **Diagnosis.** Weight increase with edema is observed. Decreasing urine output, increasing BUN and urine SG, and a low FE-Na are often present in infants with mature renal function.

c. **Therapy.** Treat the underlying disorder and **restrict water** to alleviate hypotonicity. Na restriction and improving cardiac output may be beneficial.

C. **Hypernatremic disorders**

1. **Hypernatremia with normal or deficient ECF volume**

a. **Predisposing factors** include increased renal and IWL in VLBW infants. Skin sloughing can accelerate water loss. ADH deficiency secondary to IVH can occasionally exacerbate renal water loss.

b. **Diagnosis.** Weight loss, tachycardia and hypotension, metabolic acidosis, decreasing urine output, and increasing urine SG may occur. Urine may be dilute if the newborn exhibits central or nephrogenic diabetes insipidus.

c. **Therapy.** Increase **free water administration** to reduce serum Na no faster than 1 mEq/kg/hour. If signs of ECF depletion or excess develop, adjust Na intake. **Hypernatremia does not necessarily imply excess total-body Na.** For example, **in the VLBW infant, hypernatremia in the first 24 hours of life is almost always due to free water deficits** (see VIII.A.1).

2. **Hypernatremia with ECF volume excess**

a. **Predisposing factors** include excessive isotonic or hypertonic fluid administration, especially in the face of reduced cardiac output.

b. **Diagnosis** Weight gain associated with edema is observed. The infant may exhibit normal heart rate, blood pressure, and urine output and SG, but an elevated FE-Na.

c. **Therapy. Restrict Na** administration.

V. **OLIGURIA** exists if urine flow is <1 mL/kg/hour. Although delayed micturition in a healthy infant is not of concern until 24 hours after birth, urine output in a critically ill infant should be assessed by 8 to 12 hours of life, using urethral catheterization if indicated. Diminished urine output may reflect abnormal prerenal, renal parenchymal, or postrenal factors (see Table 9.4). The most common causes of neonatal ARF are asphyxia, sepsis, and severe respiratory illness. It is important to exclude other potentially treatable etiologies (see Chap. 31). In VLBW infants oliguria may be normal in the first 24 hours of life (see VIII.A.1).

A. **History and physical examination.** Screen the maternal and infant history for maternal diabetes (renal vein thrombosis), birth asphyxia (acute tubular necrosis), and oligohydramnios (Potter syndrome). Force of the infant's urinary stream (posterior urethral valves), rate and nature of fluid administration and urine

TABLE 9.4 Etiologies of Oliguria

Prerenal	Renal parenchymal	Postrenal
Decreased inotropy	Acute tubular necrosis	Posterior urethral valves
	Ischemia (hypoxia, hypo volemia)	
Decreased preload	Disseminated intravascular coagulation	
	Renal artery or vein thrombosis	Neuropathic bladder
Increased peripheral resistance	Nephrotoxin	
	Congenital malformation	Prune-belly syndrome
	Polycystic disease	
	Agenesis	
	Dysplasia	Uric acid nephropathy

output, and nephrotoxic drug use (aminoglycosides, indomethacin, furosemide) should be evaluated. **Physical examination** should determine blood pressure and ECF volume status; evidence of cardiac disease, abdominal masses, or ascites; and the presence of any congenital anomalies associated with renal abnormalities (e.g., Potter syndrome, epispadias).

B. Diagnosis
1. **Initial laboratory examination** should include urinalysis, BUN, Cr, and FE-Na determinations. These aid in diagnosis and provide baseline values for further management.
2. **Fluid challenge** consisting of a total of 20 mL/kg of NS, is administered as two infusions at 10 mL/kg/hour if no suspicion of structural heart disease or heart failure exists. Decreased cardiac output not responsive to ECF expansion may require the institution of inotropic/chronotropic pressor agents. Dopamine at a dose of 1 to 5 μg/kg/minute may increase renal blood flow and a dose of 2 to 15 μg/kg/minute may increase total cardiac output. These effects may augment GFR and urine output (see Chap. 17).
3. **If no response to fluid challenge occurs** one may induce diuresis with **furosemide** 2 mg/kg IV.
4. Patients who are unresponsive to increased cardiac output and diuresis should be evaluated with an **abdominal ultrasonography** to define renal, urethral, and bladder anatomy. IV pyelography, renal scanning, angiography, or cystourethrography may be required (see Chap. 31).

C. Management. Prerenal oliguria should respond to increased cardiac output. **Postrenal** obstruction requires urologic consultation, with possible urinary diversion and surgical correction. If parenchymal **ARF** is suspected, minimize excessive ECF expansion and electrolyte abnormalities. If possible, eliminate reversible causes of declining GFR, such as nephrotoxic drug use.
1. **Monitor** daily weight, input and output, and BUN, Cr, and serum electrolytes.
2. **Fluid restriction.** Replace insensible fluid loss plus urine output. **Withhold K supplementation** unless hypokalemia develops. Replace urinary Na losses unless edema develops.
3. **Adjust dosage and frequency of drugs** eliminated by renal excretion. Monitor serum drug concentrations to guide drug-dosing intervals.
4. **Peritoneal or hemodialysis** may be indicated in patients whose GFR progressively declines causing complications related to ECF volume or electrolyte abnormalities (see Chap. 31).

VI. METABOLIC ACID–BASE DISORDERS

A. Normal acid–base physiology. Metabolic acidosis results from excessive loss of buffer or from an increase of volatile or nonvolatile acid in the extracellular space. Normal sources of acid production include the metabolism of amino acids containing sulfur and phosphate, as well as hydrogen ion released from bone mineralization. Intravascular buffers include bicarbonate, phosphate, and intracellular hemoglobin. Maintenance of normal pH depends on excretion of volatile acid (e.g., carbonic acid) from the lungs, skeletal exchange of cations for hydrogen, and renal regeneration and reclamation of bicarbonate. Kidneys contribute to maintenance of acid–base balance by reabsorbing the filtered load of bicarbonate, secreting hydrogen ions as titratable acidity (e.g., H_2PO_4), and excreting ammonium ions.

B. Metabolic acidosis (see Chap. 29D)

1. Anion gap. Metabolic acidosis can result from accumulation of acid or loss of buffering equivalents. Anion gap determination will suggest mechanism. Na, Cl, and bicarbonate are the primary ions of the extracellular space and exist in approximately electroneutral balance. The **anion gap,** calculated as the difference between the Na concentration and sum of the Cl and bicarbonate concentrations, reflects the unaccounted-for anion composition of the ECF. An increased anion gap indicates an accumulation of organic acid whereas a normal anion gap indicates a loss of buffer equivalents. Normal values for the neonatal anion gap are 5 to 15 mEq/L and vary directly with serum albumin concentration.

2. Metabolic acidosis associated with an increased anion gap (>15 mEq/L). Disorders (see Table 9.5) include renal failure, inborn errors of metabolism, lactic acidosis, late metabolic acidosis, and toxin exposure. Lactic acidosis results from diminished tissue perfusion and resultant anaerobic metabolism in infants with asphyxia or severe cardiorespiratory disease. Late metabolic acidosis typically occurs during the second or third week of life in premature infants who ingest high casein-containing formulas. Metabolism of sulfur-containing amino acids in casein and increased hydrogen ion release due to the rapid mineralization of bone cause an increased acid load. Subsequently, inadequate hydrogen ion excretion by the premature kidney results in acidosis.

3. Metabolic acidosis associated with a normal anion gap (<15 mEq/L) results from buffer loss through the renal or gastrointestinal systems (Table 9.5). Premature infants <32 weeks' gestation frequently manifest a proximal or distal renal tubular acidosis (RTA). Urine pH persistently >7 in an infant

TABLE 9.5	Metabolic Acidosis

Increased anion gap (>15 mEq/L)	Normal anion gap (<15 mEq/L)
Acute renal failure	Renal bicarbonate loss
Inborn errors of metabolism	Renal tubular acidosis
Lactic acidosis	Acetazolamide
Late metabolic acidosis	Renal dysplasia
Toxins (e.g., benzyl alcohol)	Gastrointestinal bicarbonate loss
	Diarrhea
	Cholestyramine
	Small-bowel drainage
	Dilutional acidosis
	Hyperalimentation acidosis

TABLE 9.6   **Metabolic Alkalosis**

Low urinary Cl (<10 mEq/L)	High urinary Cl (>20 mEq/L)
Diuretic therapy (late)	Barters syndrome with mineralocorticoid excess
Acute correction of chronically compensated respiratory acidosis	Alkali administration
Nasogastric suction	Massive blood product transfusion
Vomiting	Diuretic therapy (early)
Secretory diarrhea	Hypokalemia

CI = confidence interval.

with metabolic acidosis suggests a distal RTA. Urinary pH <5 documents normal distal tubule hydrogen ion secretion but proximal tubular bicarbonate resorption could still be inadequate (proximal RTA). IV Na bicarbonate infusion in infants with proximal RTA will result in a urinary pH >7 before attaining a normal serum bicarbonate concentration (22–24 mEq/L).

4. **Therapy.** Whenever possible, **treat the underlying cause.** Lactic acidosis due to low cardiac output or due to decreased peripheral oxygen delivery should be treated with specific measures. The use of a low-casein formula may alleviate late metabolic acidosis. Treat normal anion gap metabolic acidosis by decreasing the rate of bicarbonate loss (e.g., decreased small-bowel drainage) or providing buffer equivalents. **IV Na bicarbonate or Na acetate** (which is compatible with Ca salts) is most commonly used to treat arterial pH <7.25. Oral buffer supplements can include citric acid (Bicitra) or Na citrate (1–3 mE/kg/day). Estimate bicarbonate deficit from the following formula:

Deficit = 0.4× body weight × (desired bicarbonate—actual bicarbonate)

The premature infant's acid–base status can change rapidly, and frequent monitoring is warranted. The infant's ability to tolerate an increased Na load and to metabolize acetate is an important variable that influences acid–base status during treatment.

C. **Metabolic alkalosis.** The etiology of metabolic alkalosis can be clarified by determining urinary Cl concentration. Alkalosis accompanied by ECF depletion is associated with decreased urinary Cl, whereas states of mineralocorticoid excess are usually associated with increased urinary Cl (see Table 9.6). Treat the underlying disorder.

VII. **DISORDERS OF K BALANCE.** K is the fundamental intracellular cation. Serum K concentrations do not necessarily reflect total-body K because extracellular and intracellular K distribution also depends on the pH of body compartments. **An increase of 0.1 pH unit in serum results in approximately a 0.6 mEq/L fall in serum K concentration due to an intracellular shift of K ions.** Total-body K is regulated by balancing K intake (normally 1–2 mEq/kg/day) and excretion through urine and the gastrointestinal tract.

A. **Hypokalemia** can lead to arrhythmias, ileus, renal concentrating defects, and obtundation in the newborn.

1. **Predisposing factors** include nasogastric or ileostomy drainage, chronic diuretic use, and renal tubular defects.

2. **Diagnosis.** Obtain serum and urine electrolytes, pH, and an electrocardiogram (ECG) to detect possible conduction defects (prolonged QT interval and U waves).

3. **Therapy** Reduce renal or gastrointestinal losses of K. Gradually increase intake of K as needed.

B. Hyperkalemia. The normal serum K level in a nonhemolyzed blood specimen at normal pH is 3.5 to 5.5 mEq/L; symptomatic hyperkalemia may begin at a serum K level >6 mEq/L.

    1. Predisposing factors. Hyperkalemia can occur unexpectedly in any patient but should be **anticipated** and **screened** for in the following scenarios:

        a. Increased K release secondary to tissue destruction, trauma, cephalhematoma, hypothermia, bleeding, intravascular or extravascular hemolysis, asphyxia/ischemia, and IVH.

        b. Decreased K clearance due to renal failure, oliguria, hyponatremia, and congenital adrenal hyperplasia.

        c. Miscellaneous associations including dehydration, birth weight <1,500 g (see VIII.A.2), blood transfusion, inadvertent excess (KCl) administration, CLD with KCl supplementation, and exchange transfusion.

        d. Up to 50% of VLBW infants born before 25 weeks' gestation manifest serum K levels >6 mEq/L in the first 48 hours of life (see VIII.A.2). **The most common cause of sudden unexpected hyperkalemia in the neonatal intensive care unit (NICU) is medication error.**

    2. Diagnosis. Obtain serum and urine electrolytes, serum pH, and Ca concentrations. The hyperkalemic infant may be asymptomatic or may present with a spectrum of signs including bradyarrhythmias or tachyarrhythmias, cardiovascular instability or collapse. The ECG findings progress with increasing serum K from peaked T waves (increased rate of repolarization), flattened P waves and increasing PR interval (suppression of atrial conductivity), to QRS widening and slurring (conduction delay in ventricular conduction tissue as well as in the myocardium itself), and finally supraventricular/ventricular tachycardia, bradycardia, or ventricular fibrillation. The ECG findings may be the first indication of hyperkalemia (see Chap. 25).

        Once hyperkalemia is diagnosed, remove all sources of exogenous K (change all IV solutions and analyze for K content, check all feedings for K content), rehydrate the patient if necessary, and eliminate arrhythmia-promoting factors. The pharmacologic therapy of neonatal hyperkalemia consists of three components:

        a. Goal 1: stabilization of conducting tissues. This can be accomplished by Na or Ca ion administration. **Ca gluconate (10%) given carefully at 1 to 2 mL/kg IV (over 0.5–1 hour)** may be the most useful in the NICU. Treatment with hypertonic NaCl solution is not done routinely. However, if the patient is both hyperkalemic and hyponatremic, NS infusion may be beneficial. Use of antiarrhythmic agents such as lidocaine and bretylium should be considered for refractory ventricular tachycardia (see Chap. 25).

        b. Goal 2: dilution and intracellular shifting of K. Increased serum K in the setting of dehydration should respond to fluid resuscitation. Alkalemia will promote intracellular K-for-hydrogen-ion exchange. **Na bicarbonate 1 to 2 mEq/kg/hour IV** may be used, although the resultant pH change may not be sufficient to markedly shift K ions. Na treatment as described in goal 1 may be effective. **In order to reduce risk of IVH, avoid rapid Na bicarbonate administration, especially in infants born before 34 weeks' gestation and younger than 3 days.** Respiratory alkalosis may be produced in an intubated infant by hyperventilation, although the risk of hypocarbia-diminishing cerebral perfusion may make this option more suited to emergency situations. Theoretically, every 0.1 pH unit increase leads to a decrease of 0.6 mEq/L in serum K.

        Insulin enhances intracellular K uptake by direct stimulation of the membrane-bound Na–K ATPase. Insulin infusion with concomitant glucose administration to maintain normal blood glucose concentration is relatively safe as long as serum or blood glucose levels are frequently monitored. **This therapy may begin with a bolus of insulin and glucose (0.05 unit/kg of human regular insulin with 2 mL/kg of dextrose 10% in water [D10W]) followed by continuous infusion of D10W at 2 to 4 mL/kg/hour and**

human regular insulin (10 units/100 mL) at 1 mL/kg/hour. To minimize the effect of binding to IV tubing, insulin diluted in D10W may be flushed through the tubing. Adjustments in infusion rate of either glucose or insulin in response to hyperglycemia or hypoglycemia may be simplified if the two solutions are prepared individually (see Chap. 29A).

β-2-Adrenergic stimulation enhances K uptake, probably through stimulation of the Na−K ATPase. The immaturity of the β-receptor response in preterm infants may contribute to nonoliguric hyperkalemia in these patients (see VIII.A.2). To date, β stimulation is not primary therapy for hyperkalemia in the pediatric population. However, if cardiac dysfunction and hypotension are present, use of dopamine or other adrenergic agents could, through β-2 stimulation, lower serum K.

c. **Goal 3: enhanced K excretion.** Diuretic therapy (e.g., **furosemide 1 mg/kg IV**) may increase K excretion by increasing flow and Na delivery to the distal tubules. In the clinical setting of inadequate urine output and reversible renal disease (e.g., indomethacin-induced oliguria), **peritoneal dialysis** and **double volume exchange transfusion** are potentially life-saving options. Peritoneal dialysis can be successful in infants weighing <1,000 g and should be considered if the patient's clinical status and etiology of hyperkalemia suggest a reasonable chance for good long-term outcome. **Use fresh whole blood (<24 hours old) or deglycerolized red blood cells reconstituted with fresh-frozen plasma for double volume exchange transfusion.** Aged, banked blood may have K levels as high as 10 to 12 mEq/L; aged, washed packed red blood cells will have low K levels (see Chap. 26E).

Enhanced K excretion using cation exchange resins such as Na or Ca polystyrene sulfonate has been studied primarily in adults. The resins can be administered orally per gavage (PG) or rectally. A study involving uremic and control rats demonstrated that Na polystyrene sulfonate (Kayexalate) administered by rectum with sorbitol was toxic to the colon, but rectal administration after suspension in distilled water produced only mild mucosal erythema in 10% of animals. Another possible complication of resins is bowel obstruction secondary to bezoar or plug formation.

The reported experience with resin use in neonates covers those born at 25 to 40 weeks' gestation. **PG administration of Kayexalate is not recommended in preterm infants because they are prone to hypomotility and are at risk for NEC. Rectal administration of Kayexalate (1 g/kg at 0.5 g/mL of NS) with a minimum retention time of 30 minutes should be effective in lowering serum K levels by approximately 1 mEq/L. The enema should be inserted 1 to 3 cm using a thin silastic feeding tube.** Published evidence supports the efficacy of this treatment in infants. Kayexalate prepared in water or NS (eliminating sorbitol as a solubilizing agent) and delivered rectally should be a therapeutic agent with an acceptable risk–benefit ratio.

The clinical condition, ECG, and actual serum K level all affect the choice of therapy for hyperkalemia. Figure 9.2 contains guidelines for treatment of hyperkalemia.

VIII. COMMON CLINICAL SITUATIONS

A. VLBW infant

1. **VLBW infants undergo three phases of fluid and electrolyte homeostasis** prediuretic (first day of life), diuretic (second to third day of life), and postdiuretic (fourth to fifth day of life). Marked diuresis and natriuresis can occur during the diuretic phase leading to **hypernatremia** and the need for frequent serum electrolyte determinations (q6–8h) and increased rates of parenteral fluid administration. Increased free water loss through skin and dopamine-associated natriuresis (due to increased GFR) can further complicate management. Hypernatremia often occurs despite a total-body Na deficit. Lack of a brisk diuretic phase has been associated with increased CLD incidence.

Remove All Sources of Exogenous Potassium

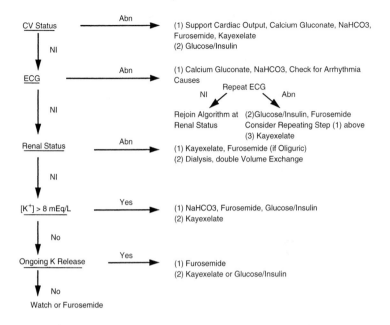

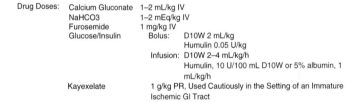

In General, if [K$^+$] Acceptable for 6 h Cease Therapy but Continue Monitoring

Drug Doses:
Calcium Gluconate	1–2 mL/kg IV	
NaHCO3	1–2 mEq/kg IV	
Furosemide	1 mg/kg IV	
Glucose/Insulin	Bolus:	D10W 2 mL/kg
		Humulin 0.05 U/kg
	Infusion:	D10W 2–4 mL/kg/h
		Humulin, 10 U/100 mL D10W or 5% albumin, 1 mL/kg/h
Kayexelate	1 g/kg PR, Used Cautiously in the Setting of an Immature Ischemic GI Tract	

Figure 9.2. Treatment of hyperkalemia (CV = cardiovascular; NI = normal; Abn = abnormal; ECG = electrocardiogram; GI = gastrointestinal). For a given algorithm outcome proceed by administering the entire set of treatments labeled (1). If unsuccessful in lowering [K$^+$] or improving clinical condition, proceed to the next set of treatments, for example, (2) and then (3).

In addition, **impaired glucose tolerance** can lead to hyperglycemia, requiring reduced rates of parenteral glucose infusion (see Chap. 29A). This combination frequently leads to administration of reduced dextrose concentrations (<5%) in parenteral solutions. Avoid the infusion of parenteral solutions containing <200 mOsmol/L (i.e., D3W), to minimize local osmotic hemolysis and thereby reduce renal K load.

2. **VLBW infants often develop a nonoliguric hyperkalemia** in the first few days of life. This is caused by a relatively low GFR combined with an intracellular to extracellular K shift due to decreased Na, K ATPase activity. Postnatal glucocorticoid use may further inhibit Na, K ATPase activity. Insulin infusion to treat hyperkalemia may be necessary but elevates the risk of iatrogenic hypoglycemia. Treatment with Kayexalate (see VII.B.2.c) can occasionally be beneficial in infants born before 32 weeks' gestation despite the obligate Na

load and potential irritation of bowel mucosa by rectal administration. Na restriction can reduce the risk of CLD.

3. Late-onset hyponatremia of prematurity often occurs 6 to 8 weeks postnatally in the growing premature infant. Failure of the immature renal tubules to reabsorb filtered Na in a rapidly growing infant often causes this condition. Other contributing factors include the low Na content in breast milk and diuretic therapy for CLD. Infants at risk should be monitored with periodic electrolytes measurements and if affected, treated with simple Na supplementation (start with 2 mEq/kg/day).

B. Severe chronic lung disease (CLD) (see Chap. 24J). CLD requiring **diuretic** therapy often leads to **hypokalemic, hypochloremic metabolic alkalosis.** Affected infants frequently have a chronic respiratory acidosis with partial metabolic compensation. Subsequently, vigorous diuresis can lead to total-body K and ECF volume depletion, causing a superimposed metabolic alkalosis. If the alkalosis is severe, alkalemia (pH >7.45) can supervene and result in central hypoventilation. If possible, gradually reduce urinary Na and K loss by reducing the diuretic dose, and/or increase K intake by administration of KCl (starting at 1 mEq/kg/day). Rarely, administration of ammonium chloride (0.5 mEq/kg) is required to treat the metabolic alkalosis. Long-term use of loop diuretics such as furosemide promotes excessive urinary Ca losses and nephrocalcinosis. Urinary Ca losses may be reduced through concomitant thiazide diuretic therapy (see Chap. 24J).

Suggested Readings

Anand SK. Acute renal failure in the neonate. *Pediatr Clin North Am* 1982;29:791.

Baumgart S, Costarino AT. Water and electrolyte metabolism of the micropremie. *Clin Perinatol* 2000;27(1):131.

Bell EF, Warburton D, Stonestreet BS, et al. Effect of fluid administration on the development of symptomatic patent ductus arteriosus and congestive heart failure in premature infants. *N Engl J Med* 1980;302:598.

Bell EF, Weinstein MR, Oh W. Heat balance in premature infants: Comparative effects of convectively heated incubator and radiant warmer, with or without plastic heat shield. *J Pediatr* 1980;96:460.

Bell EF, Gray JC, Weinstein MR, et al. The effects of thermal environment on heat balance and insensible water loss in low-birth-weight infants. *J Pediatr* 1980;96:452.

Bhatia J. Fluid and electrolyte management in the very low birth weight neonate. *J Perinatol* 2006;26:S19–S21.

Brown ER, Stark A, Sosenko I, et al. Bronchopulmonary dysplasia: Possible relationship to pulmonary edema. *J Pediatr* 1978;92:982.

Celsi G, Wang ZM, Akusjarvi G, et al. Sensitive periods for glucocorticoids' regulation of Na+, K(+)-ATPase mRNA in the developing lung and kidney. *Pediatr Res* 1993;33(1):5.

Cheek DB, Maddison TG, Malinek M, et al. Further observations on the corrected bromide space of the neonate and investigation of water and electrolyte status in infants born of diabetic mothers. *Pediatrics* 1961;28:861.

Costarino AT Jr, Gruskay JA, Corcoran L, et al. Sodium restriction versus daily maintenance replacement in very low birth weight premature neonates: A randomized, blind therapeutic trial. *J Pediatr* 1992;120:99.

Fanaroff AA, Wald M, Gruber HS, et al. Insensible water loss in low birth weight infants. *Pediatrics* 1972;50:236.

Fink CW, and Cheek DB. The corrected bromide space (extracellular volume) in the newborn. *Pediatrics* 1960;26:397.

Fisher DA, Pyle HR Jr, Porter JC, et al. Control of water balance in the newborn. *Am J Dis Child* 1963;106:137.

Gruskay J, Costarino AT, Polin RA, et al. Nonoliguric hyperkalemia in the premature infant weighing less than 1000 grams. *J Pediatr* 1988;113:381.

Leake RD. Perinatal nephrobiology: A developmental perspective. *Clin Perinatol* 1977;4:321.

Lorenz JM, Kleinman LI, Kotagal UR, et al. Water balance in very low-birth-weight infants: Relationship to water and sodium intake and effect on outcome. *J Pediatr* 1982;101:423.

Lorenz JM, Kleinman LI, Ahmed G, et al. Phases of fluid and electrolyte homeostasis in the extremely low birth weight infant. *Pediatrics* 1995;96(3 Pt 1):484.

Norman ME, and Asadi FK. A prospective study of acute renal failure in the newborn infant. *Pediatrics* 1979;63:475.

Okken A, Jonxis JH, Rispens P, et al. Insensible water loss and metabolic rate in low birth weight newborn infants. *Pediatr Res* 1979;13:1072.

Rahman N, Boineau FG and Lewy JE. Renal failure in the perinatal period. *Clin Perinatol* 1981;8:241.

Shaffer SG, Kilbride HW, Hayen LK, et al. Hyperkalemia in very low birth weight infants. *J Pediatr* 1992;121:275.

Skorecki KL, and Brenner BM. Body fluid homeostasis in man. A contemporary overview. *Am J Med* 1981;70:77.

Stefano JL, and Norman ME. Nitrogen balance in extremely low birth weight infants with nonoliguric hyperkalemia. *J Pediatr* 1993;123:632.

Stevenson JG. Fluid administration in the association of patent ductus arteriosus complicating respiratory distress syndrome. *J Pediatr* 1977;90:257.

Wu PYK, and Hodgman JE. Insensible water loss in pre-term infants: Changes with postnatal development and non-ionizing radiant energy. *Pediatrics* 1974;54:704.

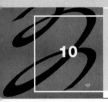

NUTRITION
Deirdre Ellard and Diane M. Anderson

$\mathcal{F}$ollowing birth, term infants rapidly adapt from a relatively constant intrauterine supply of nutrients to intermittent feedings of milk. Preterm infants, however, are at increased risk of potential nutritional compromise. These infants are born with limited nutrient reserves, immature metabolic pathways, and increased nutrient demands. In addition, medical and surgical conditions commonly associated with prematurity have the potential to alter nutrient requirements and complicate adequate nutrient delivery. As survival for these high-risk newborns continue to improve, current data suggest that early, aggressive nutrition intervention is advantageous.

I. GROWTH

A. Fetal body composition changes throughout gestation, with accretion of most nutrients occurring primarily in the late second and throughout the third trimester. Term infants will normally have sufficient glycogen and fat stores to meet energy requirements during the relative starvation of the first days of life. In contrast, preterm infants will rapidly deplete their limited nutrient reserves, becoming both hypoglycemic and catabolic unless appropriate nutritional therapy is provided. In practice, it is generally assumed that the severity of nutrient insufficiency is inversely related to gestational age at birth and birth weight.

B. Postnatal growth varies from intrauterine growth in that it begins with a period of weight loss, primarily through the loss of extracellular fluid. The typical loss of 5% to 10% of birth weight for a full-term infant may increase to as much as 15% of birth weight in infants born preterm. The nadir in weight loss usually occurs by 4 to 6 days of life, with birth weight being regained by 14 to 21 days of life in most preterm infants. Currently, there is no widely accepted measure of neonatal growth that captures both the weight loss and subsequent gain characteristic of this period. Our goals are to limit the degree and duration of initial weight loss in preterm infants and to facilitate regain of birth weight within 7 to 14 days of life.

C. After achieving birth weight, intrauterine growth and nutrient accretion rate data are widely accepted as reference standards for assessing growth and nutrient requirements. We use goals of: 10 to 20 g/kg/day weight gain (15 to 20 g/kg/day for infants <1,500 g), approximately 1 cm/week in length, and 0.5 to 1 cm/week in head circumference. Although these goals are not initially attainable in most preterm infants, replicating growth of the fetus at the same gestational age remains an appropriate goal as recommended by the American Academy of Pediatrics (AAP).

D. Along with monitoring rates of growth, serial measurements of weight, head circumference, and length plotted on growth curves provide valuable information in the nutritional assessment of the preterm infant. The Lubchenco intrauterine growth curves (1966) (see Fig. 10.1A) have been widely used because the chart is based on a reasonable sample size, provides curves to monitor weight, length and head circumference, and is easy to use and interpret. Recently the Fenton (2003) (see Fig. 10.1B) fetal-infant chart has become available. Weight, length and head circumference curves are given from 22 to 50 weeks postmenstrual age. The chart is based on a larger number of infants from a wider geographic location and reflects infants born more recently. Postnatal growth curves are also available, but we do not recommend their use in the neonatal intensive care unit (NICU). Postnatal

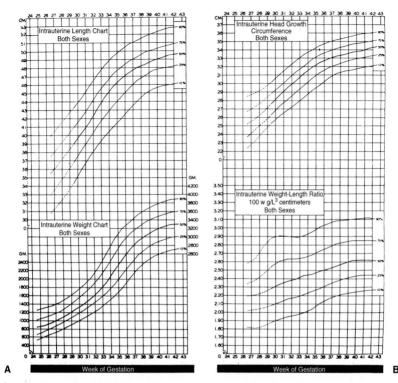

Figure 10.1. **(A)** Lubchenco intrauterine growth curves. From Lubchenco LO, Hansman C, Boyd E, et al. Intrauterine growth in length and head circumference as estimated from live births at gestational ages from 26 to 42 weeks. *Pediatrics* 1966;37:403; **(B)** Fetal-Infant Growth Chart for Preterm Infants. From Fenton TR. A new growth chart for preterm babies; Babson and Benda's chart updated with recent data and a new format. *BMC Pediatr* 2003;3:13. Chart may be downloaded from: http://members.shaw.ca/growthchart.

growth curves follow the same infants over time (i.e., longitudinal growth curves), and are available from a number of single-NICU studies and more recently from the National Institute for Child Health and Human Development (NICHD) multicenter study (2000). The problem with these curves, however, is that they show **actual,** not ideal growth. Although these curves provide interesting information by allowing comparison of the growth of infants in one NICU to those in another, they do not indicate if either group of infants is growing adequately. Intrauterine growth remains the gold standard for comparison.

E. When an infant is full-term-corrected gestational age, monitoring of growth should use the 2,000 Centers for Disease Control (CDC) United States Growth Charts (formerly, the National Center for Health Statistics, [NCHS], growth curves). Alternatively, the Infant Health and Development Program (IHDP) growths curves, based on a sample of low-birth-weight infants (1,501–2,500 g at birth) and very-low-birth-weight (VLBW) infants (<1,500 g at birth), are also available for this age group. However, these curves are subject to the same criticisms as the postnatal growth curves. These curves represent average premature infant growth and not the growth achieved by term infants. We do not recommend their use in former preterm infants, because these infants should still be striving to achieve catch-up growth as assessed on the CDC charts.

II. NUTRIENT RECOMMENDATIONS

A. Sources for nutrient recommendations for preterm infants include the American Academy of Pediatrics Committee on Nutrition (AAP-CON), the European Society of Paediatric Gastroenterology and Nutrition Committee on Nutrition (ESPGAN-CON), and the Reasonable Ranges of Nutrient Intakes published by Tsang and colleagues (see Table 10.1). These recommendations are based on: (i) intrauterine accretion rate data, (ii) the nutrient content of human milk, (iii) the assumed decreased nutrient stores and higher nutritional needs in preterm infants, and (iv) the available data on biochemical measures reflecting adequate intake. However, due to the limitations of the currently available data, the goals for nutrient intake for preterm infants are considered to be recommendations only.

B. Fluid (see Chap. 9). The initial step in nutritional support is to determine an infant's fluid requirement, which is dependent on gestational age, postnatal age, and environmental conditions. Generally, baseline fluid needs are inversely related to gestational age at birth and birth weight. During the first week of life, VLBW infants are known to experience increased water loss because of the immaturity of their skin, which has a higher water content and increased permeability, and the immaturity of their renal function with a decreased ability to concentrate urine. Environmental factors, such as radiant warmers, phototherapy, and low humidity, also increase insensible losses and raise fluid requirements. Conversely, restriction of fluid intake may be necessary to assist with the prevention and/or treatment of patent ductus arteriosus, renal insufficiency, and chronic lung disease (CLD). Fluid requirements in the first weeks of life are, therefore, continually reassessed, as the transition is made from fetal to neonatal life, and at least daily afterward.

C. Energy. Estimates suggest that preterm infants in a thermoneutral environment require approximately 40 to 60 kcal/kg/day for maintenance of body weight, assuming adequate protein is provided. Additional calories are needed for growth, with the smallest neonates tending to demonstrate the greatest need, as their rate of growth is highest (see Table 10.2). In practice, we generally strive for energy intakes of 120 to 130 kcal/kg/day. Infants with severe and/or prolonged illness may require up to 130 to 150 kcal/kg/day. Lesser intakes (90 to 120 kcal/kg/day) may sustain intrauterine growth rates, if energy expenditure is minimal or if parenteral nutrition (PN) is used.

III. PN

A. Nutrient goals. The practice of withholding nutrition support for the first weeks of life has changed as research suggests that earlier nutritional intervention is desirable. Our initial goal for PN is to provide adequate calories and amino acids to prevent negative energy and nitrogen balance. Goals thereafter include the promotion of appropriate weight gain and growth, while awaiting the attainment of adequate enteral intake.

B. Indications for initiating PN

1. Infants with a birth weight <1,500 g. For these infants, this is often done in conjunction with slowly advancing enteral nutrition.

2. Infants with a birth weight of ≥1,501 g for whom significant enteral intake is not expected for >3 days.

C. Peripheral versus central PN

1. Parenteral solutions may be infused through peripheral veins or a central vein, usually the superior or inferior vena cava. The AAP recommends that peripheral solutions maintain an osmolarity between 300 and 900 mOsm/L. Because of this limitation, peripheral solutions often cannot adequately support growth in extremely low-birth-weight (ELBW) infants. Central PN allows for the use of more hypertonic solutions but also incurs greater risks, particularly catheter-related sepsis.

2. We consider central PN to be warranted under the following conditions:

a. Nutritional needs exceed the capabilities of peripheral PN.

TABLE 10.1 Comparison of Enteral Intake Recommendations of the Preterm Infant per Kilogram per Day*

Nutrient	Unit	Summary of reasonable nutrient intakes [3]	AAP-CON[1]†	Mature human milk¶	Mature human milk plus 4 packets enfamil HMF/dl	Mature human milk plus 4 packets similac HMF/dl	24 kcal/oz enfamil premature LIPIL w/Iron	24 kcal/oz Similac special care advance w/Iron
Protein								
ELBW infants	gm/kg/day	3.8–4.4	3.5–4	1.6	3.2	3	3.6	3.6
VLBW infants	gm/kg/day	3.4–4.2						
Carbohydrate	gm/kg/day		10–14	10.8	11.4	13.2	13.4	12.5
ELBW infants	gm/kg/day	9–20						
VLBW infants	gm/kg/day	7–17						
Fat	gm/kg/day		5–7	5.9	7.4	6.2	6.2	6.6
ELBW infants	gm/kg/day	6.2–8.4						
VLBW infants	gm/kg/day	5.3–7.2						
Docosahexaenoic Acid	mg/kg/day						20.7	17.1
ELBW infants	mg/kg/day	≥21						
VLBW infants	mg/kg/day	≥18						
Arachidonic Acid	mg/kg/day						42	26.9
ELBW infants	mg/kg/day	≥28						

(continued)

117

TABLE 10.1 *(Continued)*

Nutrient	Unit	Summary of reasonable nutrient intakes [3]	AAP-CON[1]†	Mature human milk¶	Mature human milk plus 4 packets enfamil HMF/dl	Mature human milk plus 4 packets similac HMF/dl	24 kcal/oz enfamil premature LIPIL w/Iron	24 kcal/oz Similac special care advance w/Iron
VLBW infants	mg/kg/day	≥ 24						
Vitamin A	IU/kg/day	700–1500	90–270	338	1763	1,228	1,515	1,521.6
Vitamin D	IU/day	150–400‡	400§	3	228	178	292.5	182.6
Vitamin E	IU/kg/day	6–12	>1.3	0.6	7.5	5.3	7.7	4.9
Vitamin K	µg/kg/day	8–10	4.8	0.3	6.9	12.4	9.8	14.6
Ascorbate (Vitamin C)	mg/kg/day	18–24	42	6.1	24	42.3	24.3	45
Thiamine	µg/kg/day	180–240	>48	32	256.7	370	243	304.3
Riboflavin	µg/kg/day	250–360	>72	52	382	659	360	755
Pyridoxine	µg/kg/day	150–210	>42	30.6	203	338	183	304.3
Niacin	mg/kg/day	3.6–4.8	>0.3	0.2	4.7	5.4	4.8	6.1
Pantothenate	mg/kg/day	1.2–1.7	>0.36	0.27	1.4	2.5	1.5	2.3
Biotin	µg/kg/day	3.6–6	>1.8	0.6	4.7	38.5	4.8	45
Folate	µg/kg/day	25–50	39.6	7.2	44.7	40.6	48	45
Vitamin B$_{12}$	µg/kg/day	0.3	>0.18	0.07	0.3	1	0.3	0.67

Sodium	mEq/kg/day	3–5	2–3	1.2	2.2	2.1	3.1	2.3
Potassium	mEq/kg/day	2–3	1.7–2.5	2	3.2	4.3	3.1	4
Chloride	mEq/kg/day	3–7	2–3	1.8	2.3	3.3	3.1	2.8
Calcium	mg/kg/day	100–220	210	42	176.9	212	201	219
Phosphorus	mg/kg/day	60–140	110	21	96.5	118.8	100.5	121.8
Magnesium	mg/kg/day	7.9–15		5.2	6.7	15.3	11	14.6
Iron	mg/kg/day	2–4	2–3	0.04	2.2	0.5	2.2	2.2
Zinc	µg/kg/day	1,000–3,000	>600	183	1263	1,630.5	1,830	1825.5
Copper	µg/kg/day	120–150	108	38	103.8	283.6	145.5	304.4
Selenium	µg/kg/day	1.3–4.5		2.3	2.3	2.9	3.5	2.2
Chromium	µg/kg/day	0.1–2.25						
Manganese	µg/kg/day	0.7–7.5	>6	1	16	11.6	7.7	14.6
Molybdenum	µg/kg/day	0.3						
Iodine	µg/kg/day	10–60	6	16	16	16	30	7.3
Taurine	mg/kg/day	4.5–9					7.3	
Carnitine	mg/kg/day	~2.9					2.9	
Inositol	mg/kg/day	32–81		22.5	22.5	27.5	54	48.8
Choline	mg/kg/day	14.4–28		14.3	14.3	16.5	24.3	12.2

ELBW = Extremely low-birth-weight; VLBW = very-low-birth-weight.
HMF = human milk fortifier.
*Recommendations and calculated intakes of formulas and human milk are based on 150 mL/kg/day.
†Recommendations per 100 calories were converted to 120 kcal/kg/day values for comparison with the exception of the values for carbohydrate, fat, and sodium.
‡Total recommended vitamin D is IU/day.
§Aim for 400 IU/day.
¶Denotes milk of mothers of preterm infants post the first 21 days of lactation.

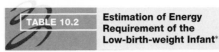

	Average estimation, kcal/kg/d
Energy expended	40–60
Resting metabolic rate	40–50[†]
Activity	0–5[†]
Thermoregulation	0–5[†]
Synthesis	15[‡]
Energy stored	20–30[‡]
Energy excreted	15
Energy intake	90–120

*From: American Academy of Pediatrics, Committee on Nutrition (AAP-CON). *Pediatric nutrition handbook,* 5th ed. Elk Grove Village: American Academy of Pediatrics, 2004.
[†] Energy for maintenance.
[‡] Energy cost of growth.

    b. An extended period (e.g., >7 days) of inability to take enteral feedings, such as in infants with necrotizing enterocolitis (NEC) and in some postoperative infants.
    c. Imminent lack of peripheral venous access.
 D. Carbohydrate. Dextrose (D-glucose) is the carbohydrate source in intravenous solutions.
    1. The caloric value of dextrose is 3.4 kcal/g.
    2. Because dextrose contributes to the osmolarity of a solution, it is generally recommended that the concentration administered through peripheral veins be limited to $\leq 12.5\%$ dextrose. We do not infuse dextrose containing solutions through umbilical arterial catheters (UACs), however, if UACs are employed in this manner, the dextrose concentration should be limited to $\leq 12.5\%$ dextrose. We will use up to 25% dextrose for central venous infusions. In unusual circumstances, higher concentrations have been used, if the fluid volume must be severely restricted.
    3. Dextrose infusions are typically referred to in terms of the milligrams of glucose per kilogram per minute (mg/kg/min) delivered, which expresses the total glucose load and accounts for infusion rate, dextrose concentration, and patient weight (see Fig. 10.2).
    4. The initial glucose requirement for term infants is defined as the amount that is necessary to avoid hypoglycemia. In general, this may be achieved with initial infusion rates of approximately 4 mg/kg/minute.
    5. Preterm infants usually require higher rates of glucose, as they have a higher brain-to-body weight ratio and higher total energy needs. Initial infusion rates of 4 to 8 mg/kg/minute are generally required to maintain euglycemia.
    6. Initial rates may be advanced, as tolerated, by 1 to 2 mg/kg/minute daily to a maximum of 11 to 12 mg/kg/minute. This may be accomplished by increasing dextrose concentration, by increasing infusion rate, or by a combination of both. Infusion rates above 11 to 12 mg/kg/minute may exceed the infant's oxidative capacity and are generally not recommended, as this may cause the excess glucose to be converted to fat, particularly in the liver. This conversion may also increase oxygen consumption, energy expenditure, and CO_2 production.

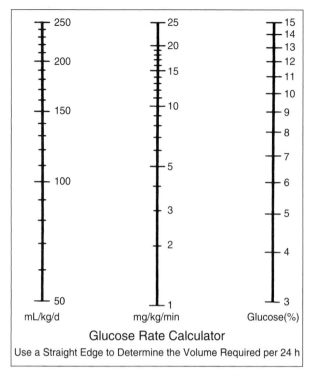

Figure 10.2. Interconversion of glucose infusion units. From Klaus MH, Faranoff AA, eds. *Care of the high-risk neonate*, 2nd ed. Philadelphia: WB Saunders, 1979:430.

    7. The quantity of dextrose that an infant can tolerate will vary with gestational and postnatal age. Signs of glucose intolerance include hyperglycemia and secondary glucosuria with osmotic diuresis.

E. Protein. Crystalline amino acid solutions provide the nitrogen source in PN.

    1. The caloric value of amino acids is 4 kcal/g.

    2. At present, three pediatric amino acid formulations are commercially available in the United States: TrophAmine, B. Braun, Aminosyn-PF, Abbott Laboratories, and PremaSol, Baxter. In theory, these products are better adapted to the needs of newborns than are standard adult formulations, as they have been modified for improved tolerance and contain conditionally essential amino acids. However, the optimal amino acid composition for neonatal PN has not yet been defined, and there are no products currently available that are specifically designed for preterm infants.

    3. It has been demonstrated that VLBW infants who do not receive amino acids in the first days of life catabolize body protein at a rate of at least 1 g/kg/day. Studies investigating the use of early amino acids have consistently shown a reversal of this catabolism without adverse metabolic consequences. Current recommendations support the infusion of amino acids in a dose of at least 1.5–2 g/kg/day beginning in the first 24 hours of life.

    4. We provide all infants with a birth weight <1,250 g with 2 g/kg/day beginning immediately after birth. Infants with a birth weight between 1,250 and 1,500 g are initiated on 2 g/kg/day within the first 24 hours of life. Infants >1,500 g are only initiated on 2 g/kg/day if indicated; depending on their size, clinical condition, and estimated time to achieve significant enteral volumes.

   5. Protein infusion rates are generally advanced to a target of 3.5 g/kg/day for all infants weighing <1,500 g at birth and 3 g/kg/day for neonates weighing >1,500 g at birth.

F. Lipid. Soybean oil, or a combination of soybean and safflower oil, provides the fat source for intravenous fat emulsions.

   1. The caloric value of 20% lipid emulsions is 2 kcal/mL (approximately 10 kcal/g). The use of 20% emulsions is preferred over 10% because the higher ratio of phospholipids to triglyceride in the 10% emulsion interferes with plasma triglyceride clearance. Twenty percent emulsions also provide a more concentrated source of calories. For these reasons, we only use 20% lipid emulsions.

   2. Current data suggest that preterm infants are at risk of essential fatty acid (EFA) deficiency within 72 hours of life, if an exogenous fat source is not delivered. This deficiency state can be avoided by the administration of 0.5 to 1 g/kg/day of lipid emulsion. Therefore, in our institutions, all infants are initiated on 0.5 to 1 g/kg/day within the first 24 to 48 hours of life. This rate is advanced by approximately 0.5 to 1 g/kg/day, as tolerated, to a target of 3 g/kg/day.

   3. Tolerance also correlates with hourly infusion rate, and no benefit to a rest period has been identified. We, therefore, infuse lipid emulsions over 24 hours for optimal clearance. However, due to sepsis risk factors, syringes may be changed every 12 hours.

G. Electrolytes

   1. Sodium and potassium concentrations are adjusted daily based on individual requirements (see Chap. 9). Maintenance requirements are estimated at approximately 2 to 4 mEq/kg.

   2. Increasing the proportion of anions provided as acetate aids in the treatment of metabolic acidosis in VLBW infants.

H. Vitamins. The current vitamin formulation (MVI Pediatric, Astra Pharmaceuticals) does not maintain blood levels of all vitamins within an acceptable range for preterm infants. However, there are no products currently available that are specifically designed for preterm infants. Table 10.3 provides guidelines for the use of the available formulations for term and preterm infants. We typically add 1.5 mL MVI Pediatric/100 mL PN administered at a rate of 150 mL/kg. For those infants receiving <150 mL/kg, the AAP guideline of 2 mL/kg/d of the currently available single dose vial per kg (not to exceed 5 mL/day) may need to be considered. Vitamin A is the most difficult to provide in adequate amounts to the VLBW infant without providing excess amounts of the other vitamins, as it is subject to losses through photodegradation and absorption to plastic tubing and solution-containing bags. B vitamins may also be affected by photodegradation. This is of particular concern with long-term PN use and for this reason PN-containing plastic bags and tubing should be shielded from light.

I. Minerals. The amount of calcium and phosphorus that can be administered through IV is limited by the precipitation of calcium phosphate. Unfortunately, the variables that determine calcium and phosphate compatibility in PN are complex and what constitutes maximal safe concentrations is controversial. The aluminum content of these preparations should also be considered.

   1. We aim for calcium to phosphorus ratios of approximately 1.3:1 to 1.7:1 by weight (1:1 to 1.3:1 molar). However, despite efforts to optimize mineral intake, preterm infants receiving prolonged PN remain at increased risk for metabolic bone disease (see Chap. 29C).

   2. We do not use 3-in-1 PN solutions (dextrose, amino acid, and lipid mixed in single bag) for the following reasons:

   a. The pH of lipid emulsions is more basic and increases the pH of the total solution, which decreases the solubility of calcium and phosphorus and limits the amount of these minerals in the solution.

   b. If the calcium and phosphorus in a 3-in-1 solution did precipitate, it would be difficult to detect, as the solution is already cloudy.

| TABLE 10.3 | Suggested Intakes of Parenteral Vitamins in Infants |

| Vitamins | Estimated needs | | 2 mL/kg of a Single dose vial MVI pediatric (Astra) | 1.5 mL MVI pediatric per 100 mL PN administered at a rate of 150 mL/kg/day† |
	Term infants (≥2.5 kg) (dose/day)	Preterm infants (≤ 2.5 kg) (dose/day)*		
Lipid Soluble				
A (μg)‡	700	280	280	315
D (IU)‡	400	160	160	180
E (IU)‡	7	2.8	2.8	3.2
K (μg)	200	80	80	90
Water Soluble				
Thiamine (mg)	1.2	0.48	0.48	0.54
Riboflavin (mg)	1.4	0.56	0.56	0.63
Niacin (mg)	17	6.8	6.8	7.65
Pantothenate (mg)	5	2	2	2.25
Pyridoxine (mg)	1	0.4	0.4	0.45
Biotin (μg)	20	8	8	9
Vitamin B_{12} (μg)	1	0.4	0.4	0.45
Ascorbic Acid (mg)	80	32	32	36
Folate (μg)	140	56	56	63

*Maximum not to exceed term dose.
†Assumes 150 mL/kg is the maximum PN administration rate.
‡700 MCG Retinol equivalent = 2,300 IU; 7 MG Alpha-tocopherol = 7 IU; 10 MG Vitamin D = 400 IU.

    c. 3-in-1 solutions require either a larger-micron filter or no filter, which may pose a greater sepsis risk.
J. Trace elements
    1. We currently add 0.2 mL/dL of NeoTrace and 1.5 μg/dL of selenium beginning in the first days of PN. However, when PN is supplementing enteral nutrition or limited to <2 weeks, only zinc may be needed.
    2. As copper and manganese are excreted in bile, we routinely reduce or omit these trace elements if impaired biliary excretion and/or cholestatic liver disease is present.
K. General PN procedures
    1. If possible, the continuity of a central line should not be broken for blood drawing or blood transfusion because of the risk of infection.
    2. Most medications are not given in PN solutions. If necessary, the PN catheter may be flushed with saline solution and a medication then infused in a compatible IV solution. Refer to the table in Appendix A for our guidelines for PN/IL and medication compatibility.
    3. Heparin is added to all central lines at a concentration of 0.5 unit/mL of solution.
L. Metabolic monitoring for infants receiving PN. All infants receiving PN are typically monitored according to the schedule indicated in Table 10.4.
M. Potential complications associated with PN
    1. Cholestasis (see Chap. 18) may be seen and is more often transient than progressive. Experimentally, even short-term PN can reduce bile flow and bile salt formation.

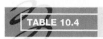

TABLE 10.4	**Schedule for Metabolic Monitoring of Infants Receiving Parenteral Nutrition**

Measurement	Frequency of measurement
BLOOD	
Glucose, electrolytes, including total carbon dioxide or pH	Daily until stable, then approximately twice weekly
Blood urea nitrogen, creatinine, calcium, phosphorus, magnesium, ALT, AST, total and direct bilirubin, alkaline phosphatase, triglycerides, Hematocrit	Weekly or every other week
URINE	
Total volume	Daily

ALT = alanine aminotransferase; AST = aspartate aminotransferase.

    a. Risk factors include:
      i. Prematurity
      ii. Duration of PN administration
      iii. Duration of fasting (lack of enteral feeding also produces bile inspissation and cholestasis)
      iv. Infection
      v. Narcotic administration
    b. Recommended management:
      i. Attempt enteral feeding. Even minimal enteral feedings may stimulate bile secretion.
      ii. Avoid overfeeding of PN.
      iii. Provision of a mixed fuel source may be helpful.
  2. Metabolic bone disease (see Chap. 29C). The use of earlier enteral feedings and central PN, with higher calcium and phosphorus ratios, has reduced the incidence of metabolic bone disease. However, this continues to be seen with the prolonged use of PN in place of enteral nutrition.
  3. Metabolic abnormalities. Azotemia, hyperammonemia, and hyperchloremic metabolic acidosis have become uncommon since introduction of the current crystalline amino acid solutions. These complications may occur, however, with amino acid intakes exceeding 4 g/kg/day.
  4. Metabolic abnormalities related to lipid emulsions
    a. Hyperlipidemia/hypertriglyceridemia. The incidence tends to be inversely related to gestational age at birth and postnatal age. A short-term decrease in the lipid infusion rate usually is sufficient to normalize serum lipid levels. We typically aim to maintain serum triglyceride levels below 200 mg/dL.
    b. Indirect hyperbilirubinemia. Because free fatty acids can theoretically displace bilirubin from albumin-binding sites, the use of lipid emulsions during periods of neonatal hyperbilirubinemia has been questioned. Recent research, however, suggests that infusion of lipid at rates up to 3 g/kg/day is unlikely to displace bilirubin. However, during periods of extreme hyperbilirubinemia (e.g., requiring exchange transfusion), rates <3 g/kg/day should be provided.
    c. Sepsis has been associated with decreased lipoprotein lipase activity and impaired triglyceride clearance. Therefore, during a sepsis episode, it may be necessary to temporarily limit the lipid infusion to—approximately 2 g/kg/day if the triglyceride level is > 150 mg/dL.
    d. The potential adverse effects of lipid emulsions on pulmonary function, the risk of CLD, and impaired immune function remain subjects of debate.

Because of the concern about toxic products of lipid peroxidation, lipid emulsions should also be protected from both ambient and phototherapy lights.

N. Current controversies

1. **Carnitine** facilitates the transport of long-chain fatty acids into the mitochondria for oxidation. However, this nutrient is not routinely added to PN solutions. Preterm infants who receive prolonged, unsupplemented PN are at risk of carnitine deficiency due to their limited reserves and inadequate rates of carnitine synthesis. For those infants who are able to tolerate enteral nutrition, we assume their needs are met by the use of human milk and/or carnitine-containing infant formula. However, for infants requiring prolonged (e.g., >4 weeks) PN, we will routinely supplement carnitine at an initial dose of approximately 10 to 20 mg/kg/day until enteral nutrition can be established.

2. **Cysteine** is not a component of current crystalline amino acid solutions, as it is unstable over time and will form a precipitate. Cysteine is ordinarily synthesized from methionine and provides a substrate for taurine. However, this may be considered an essential amino acid for preterm infants due to low activity of the enzyme hepatic cystathionase, which converts methionine to cysteine. Supplementation with L-cysteine hydrochloride lowers the pH of the PN solution and may necessitate the use of additional acetate to prevent acidosis. However, the lower pH also enhances the solubility of calcium and phosphorus and allows for improved mineral intake. We routinely supplement cysteine at a rate of approximately 30 to 40 mg/g protein.

3. **Glutamine** is an important fuel for intestinal epithelial cells and lymphocytes, however, due to its instability, it is presently not a component of crystalline amino acid solutions. Recent studies did not prove its addition to PN as helpful for the neonate.

4. **Insulin** is not routinely added to PN. Its use must be weighed against the risk of wide swings in blood glucose levels, as well as the concerns surrounding the overall effects of the increased uptake of glucose. When hyperglycemia is severe or persistent, an insulin infusion may be useful. We initiate an infusion of regular insulin at a rate of 0.05 unit/kg per hour, with the dose titrated to maintain blood glucose concentrations of 100 to 200 mg/dL. A convenient initial solution is 10 units of insulin per 100 mL of fluid (0.1 unit/mL). The IV tubing should first be thoroughly flushed with the solution (see Chap. 29A).

5. **Vitamin A** is important for normal growth and differentiation of epithelial tissue, particularly the development and maintenance of pulmonary epithelial tissue. ELBW infants are known to have low vitamin A stores at birth, minimal enteral intake for the first several weeks after birth, poor enteral absorption of vitamin A, and unreliable parenteral delivery. Studies have suggested that vitamin A supplementation can reduce the risk of bronchopulmonary dysplasia (BPD). At present, we supplement infants weighing <1,000 g at birth with 5,000 IU vitamin A intramuscularly three times per week for the first 4 weeks of life, beginning in the first 72 hours of life (see Chap. 24J).

IV. ENTERAL NUTRITION

A. Early enteral feeding

1. The structural and functional integrity of the gastrointestinal (GI) tract is dependent upon the provision of enteral nutrition. Withholding enteral feeding after birth places the infant at risk for all the complications associated with luminal starvation, including mucosal thinning, flattening of the villi, and bacterial translocation. **Trophic feedings** (also referred to as "gut priming" or "minimal enteral feedings") may be described as feedings that are delivered in very small volumes (approximately 10 to 20 mL/kg/day) for the purpose of induction of gut maturation rather than nutrient delivery.

2. **Benefits associated with trophic feedings include:**

   a. Improved levels of gut hormones

   b. Less feeding intolerance

   c. Earlier progression to full enteral feedings

   d. Improved weight gain

e. Improved calcium and phosphorus retention

f. Fewer days on PN.

3. **We adhere to the following guidelines for the use of trophic feedings:**

a. Begin as soon after birth as possible, ideally by day of life 2 to 3.

b. Use full-strength colostrum/human milk or full-strength 20 kcal/oz preterm formula at a volume of 10 to 20 mL/kg/day. We administer trophic feedings every 3, 4, 6, or 8 hours.

c. We do not use trophic feedings in infants with severe hemodynamic instability, suspected or confirmed NEC, evidence of ileus, or clinical signs of intestinal pathology. We also do not provide topics to infants who are undergoing treatment with indomethacin for patent ductus arteriosus.

d. Controlled trials of gut priming with UACs in place have not shown an increased incidence of NEC. We do not consider the presence of a UAC to be a contraindication to trophic feeding. However, the clinical condition accompanying the prolonged use a UAC may serve as a contraindication.

B. Preterm infants

1. **Fortified human milk.** Human milk provides the gold standard for feeding term infants, and although there is no such gold standard for preterm infants, we consider the use of fortified human milk to be the most nutritionally optimal diet for preterm infants.

a. Preterm human milk contains higher amounts of protein, sodium, chloride, and magnesium than term milk. However, the levels of these nutrients remain below preterm recommendations, the differences only persist for the first 21 days of lactation, and composition is known to vary.

b. For these reasons, we routinely supplement human milk for preterm infants with human milk fortifier (HMF). The addition of HMF to human milk (see Table 10.1) increases energy, protein, vitamin, and mineral contents to levels more appropriate for preterm infants.

c. HMF is added to the milk once the infants are tolerating approximately 100 mL/kg of human milk.

d. When human milk is fed through continuous infusion, incomplete delivery of nutrients may occur, in particular, the nonhomogenized fat and nutrients in the HMF may cling to the tubing. Small, frequent bolus feedings may result in improved nutrient delivery and absorption compared with continuous feedings.

e. Our protocols for the collection and storage of human milk are outlined in Chapter 11.

2. **Preterm formulas** (see Tables 10.1 and 10.6) are designed to meet the nutritional and physiologic needs of preterm infants and have some common features:

a. Whey-predominant, taurine-supplemented protein source, which is better tolerated and produces a more normal plasma amino acid profile than casein-predominant protein.

b. Carbohydrate mixtures of 40% to 50% lactose and 50% to 60% glucose polymers to compensate for preterm infants' relative lactase deficiency.

c. Fat mixtures containing approximately 50% medium-chain triglycerides (MCTs), to compensate for limited pancreatic lipase secretion and small bile acid pools, as well as 50% long-chain triglycerides to provide a source of EFAs.

d. Higher concentrations of protein, vitamins, minerals, and electrolytes to meet the increased needs associated with rapid growth, decreased intestinal absorption, and limited fluid tolerance.

3. **Feeding advancement.** When attempting to determine how best to advance a preterm infant to full enteral nutrition, there is very limited data to support any one method as optimal. The following guidelines reflect our current practice:

a. We use full-strength, 20 kcal/oz human milk or preterm formula and advance feeding volume according to the guidelines in Table 10.5 for any infant being fed by tube feedings.

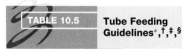

TABLE 10.5	Tube Feeding Guidelines[*],[†],[‡],[§]	

Birth weight (g)	Initial rate (mL/kg/day)	Volume increase (mL/kg/day)
<800	10	10–20
800–1,000	10–20	10–20
1,001–1,250	20	20–30
1,251–1,500	30	30
1,501–1,800	30–40	30–40
1,801–2,500	40	40–50
>2,500	50	50

[*]This table does not apply to infants capable of PO feeding.
[†]The above guidelines must always be individualized based on the infant's clinical status/severity of illness.
[‡]Consider advancing feeding volume more rapidly than the above guidelines once tolerance of >100 mL/kg/day is established, but do not exceed increments of 30 mL/kg/day in most infants weighing <1,500 g.
[§]The recommended volume goal for feedings is 140–160 mL/kg/day.

  b. For those infants receiving 20 kcal/oz premature infant formula, the caloric density is advanced from 20 to 24 kcal/oz at 100 mL/kg of volume. As previously discussed, in the case of human milk–fed infants, this is accomplished through the addition of HMF. This volume is then maintained for approximately 24 hours before the advancement schedule is resumed.

  c. As enteral volumes are increased, the rate of any IV fluid is reduced accordingly so that the total daily fluid volume remains the same. Enteral nutrients are taken into account when administering any supplemental PN.

C. Term Infants

 1. Human milk is considered the preferred feeding choice for term infants.

 2. Term formulas. The AAP provides specific guidelines for the composition of infant formulas so that term infant formulas approximate human milk in general composition. Table 10.6 describes the composition of commonly available formulas, many of which are derived from modified cow's milk.

D. Specialized formulas have been designed for a variety of congenital and neonatal disorders, including milk protein allergy, malabsorption syndromes, and several inborn errors of metabolism. Indications for the most commonly used of these specialized formulas are briefly reviewed in Table 10.7, whereas composition is outlined in Table 10.6. However, it is important to note that **these formulas were not designed to meet the special nutritional needs of preterm infants.** Preterm infants who are fed these formulas require vigilant nutritional assessment and monitoring for protein, mineral, and multivitamin supplementation.

E. Caloric-enhanced feedings. Many ill and preterm infants require increased energy/nutrient intakes in order to achieve optimal rates of growth.

 1. As previously discussed, we first increase the caloric density of human milk by concentrating feedings to 24 kcal/oz with HMF. If needed, formula powder, MCT or corn oil and/or Polycose are then added in increments of 2 to 3 kcal/oz (typically not to exceed a maximum caloric density of 30 kcal/oz). Adjustments should be made gradually with feeding tolerance assessed after each change. If the mother's milk production is greater than her infant's intake, the use of

TABLE 10.6 Human Milk and Formula Composition

Formula (distributor)	kcal/ 30 mL	Protein (gm/dL)	Fat (gm/dL)	DHA (mg/dL)	ARA (mg/dL)	Carbohydrate* (gm/dL)	Minerals (mg/dL)			Electrolytes (mEq/dL)			Vitamins (IU/dL)			Folate (µg/dL)	Osmolality (mOsmol/kg)	PRSL (mOsmol/L)
							Ca	P	Fe†	Na	K	Cl	A	D	E			
Term Human Milk (composition varies)	20	1	3.9			7.2	28	14	0.03	0.8	1.3	1.2	225	2	0.4	4.8	286	97.6
Standard Cow's Milk Based Formula																		
Enfamil LIPIL (Mead Johnson)	20	1.4	3.6	11.5	23	7.4	53	29	1.22	0.8	1.9	1.2	200	41	1.35	10.8	300	130
Similac Advance (Ross)	20	1.4	3.6	5.4	14.9	7.3	53	28	1.2	0.7	1.8	1.2	203	41	1	10	300	126.8
Enfamil LIPIL (Mead Johnson)	24	1.7	4.3	13.8	28	8.8	63	35	1.46	1	2.3	1.4	240	49	1.62	13	360	156
Milk Protein, Lactose Free																		
Lactofree LIPIL (Mead Johnson)	20	1.4	3.6	11.5	23	7.4	55	31	1.22	0.9	1.9	1.3	200	41	1.35	10.8	200	132
Similac Lactose Free Advance (Ross)	20	1.4	3.6	5.4	14.9	7.2	57	38	1.2	0.9	1.8	1.2	203	41	2	10.1	200	134.7
Soy Formulas																		
Isomil Advance (Ross)	20	1.7	3.7	5.4	14.9	7	71	51	1.2	1.3	1.9	1.2	203	41	1	10.1	200	154.5
Prosobee LIPIL (Mead Johnson)	20	1.7	3.6	11.5	23	7.2	71	47	1.22	1	2.1	1.5	200	41	1.35	10.8	Liquid 200, Powder 170	161

Preterm Formulas

Enfamil Premature LIPIL (Mead Johnson)	20	2	3.4	11.5	23	7.4	112	56	1.22	1.7	1.7	1.7	850	162	4.3	27	240	181
Similac Special Care Advance (Ross)	20	2	3.7	9.5	14.9	7	122	68	1.2	1.3	2.2	1.5	845	101	2.7	25	235	188
Enfamil Premature LIPIL (Mead Johnson)	24	2.4	4.1	13.8	28	8.9	134	67	1.46	2	2.1		1,010	195	5.1	32	300	220
Similac Special Care Advance (Ross)	24	2.4	4.4	11.4	17.9	8.4	146	81	1.5	1.5	2.7	1.9	1,014	122	3.3	30	280	226
Similac Special Care Advance (Ross)	30	3	6.7	14.2	22.3	7.8	183	101	1.8	1.9	3.4	2.3	1,268	152	4.1	37.5	325	282

Nutrient-enriched Postdischarge Formulas

EnfaCare LIPIL (Mead Johnson)	22	2.1	3.9	12.6	25	7.7	89	49	1.33	1.1	2	1.6	330	59	3	19.2	Liquid 250,	181
Similac NeoSure Advance (Ross)	22	2.1	4.1	5.4	14.9	7.5	78	46	1.3	1.1	2.7	1.6	342	52	2.7	18.6	250	187.4

Specialized Formulas

Alimentum Advance (Ross)	20	1.9	3.7	5.4	14.9	6.9	71	51	1.2	1.3	2	1.5	203	30	2	10.1	370	171.3

(continued)

TABLE 10.6 *(Continued)*

Formula (distributor)	kcal/ 30 mL	Protein (gm/dL)	Fat (gm/dL)	DHA (mg/dL)	ARA (mg/dL)	Carbo- hydrate* (gm/dL)	Minerals (mg/dL)			Electrolytes (mEq/dL)			Vitamins (IU/dL)			Folate (µg/dL)	Osmolality (mOsmol/kg)	PRSL (mOsmol/L)
							Ca	P	Fe†	Na	K	Cl	A	D	E			
Nutramigen LIPIL (Mead Johnson)	20	1.9	3.6	11.5	23	7	64	35	1.22	1.4	1.9	1.6	200	34	1.35	10.8	Liquid 320, Powder 300	171
Pregestimil LIPIL (powder) (Mead Johnson)	20	1.9	3.8	11.5	23	6.9	64	35	1.22	1.4	1.9	1.6	260	34	2.7	10.8		168
Pregestimil RTF (Mead Johnson)	20	1.9	3.8	11.5	23	6.9	78	51	1.27	1.4	1.9	1.6	260	34	2.6	10.8	280	174
Pregestimil RTF (Mead Johnson)	24	2.3	4.5			8.3	93	61	1.53	1.6	2.3	2	310	41	3.1	13	330	210
Elecare (Ross)	20	2	3.2			7.2	73	55	1.2	1.3	2.6	1.2	185	28	1.4	20	335	184.6
Neocate (Nutricia)	20	2.1	3.1	5.75	10.14	7.9	83	62	1.2	1.1	2.6	1.5	275	40	0.5	6.9	375	192.7
Portagen (Mead Johnson)	20	2.4	3.2			7.7	63	47	1.3	1.6	2.2	1.7	529	53	2.1	10.6	230	204
Similac PM 60/40 (Ross)	20	1.5	3.8			6.9	38	19	0.5	0.7	1.4	1.1	203	41	1.7	10.1	280	124.1

DHA = docosahexaenoic acid; ARA = arachidonic acid; Ca = calcium; P = phosphorus; Fe = iron; Na = sodium; K = potassium; Cl = chloride; RTF = Ready-to-feed.
*See text for types of carbohydrates used in formulas.
† In instances where high and low Fe formulations are available, the iron-fortified value appears.

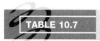

TABLE 10.7 Indications for Use of Infant Formulas

Clinical condition	Suggested formula	Rationale
Allergy to cow's milk protein or soy protein	Protein hydrolysate (Pregestimil, Nutramigen LIPIL, Alimentum Advance) Or Free amino acids (Elecare, Neocate	Impaired digestion/utilization of intact protein
Bronchopulmonary dysplasia	High-energy, nutrient dense	Increased energy requirement, fluid restriction
Biliary atresia	Pregestimil	Impaired intraluminal digestion and absorption of long-chain fats
Chylothorax (persistent)	Portagen	Decrease lymphatic absorption of fats
Congestive heart failure	High-energy formula	Lower fluid and sodium intake; increased energy requirement
Cystic fibrosis	Pregestimil or standard formula with pancreatic enzyme supplementation	Impaired intraluminal digestion and absorption of long-chain fats
Diarrhea		
Chronic nonspecific	Standard formula	
	Low lactose formula (Lactofree LIPIL, Lactose Free Advance	If malabsorbing lactose
Intractable	Pregestimil	Impaired digestion of intact protein, long-chain fats, and disaccharides
Galactosemia	Soy formula	Lactose- free
Gastroesophageal reflux	Standard formula, Enfamil AR LIPIL	Consider small, frequent feedings
Hepatic insufficiency	Pregestimil	Impaired intraluminal digestion and absorption of long-chain fats
Hypoparathyroidism, late-onset hypocalcemia	Similac PM 60/40	Low phosphate content
Lactose intolerance	Low lactose formula (Lactofree LIPIL, Lactose Free Advance	Impaired digestion or utilization of lactose
Lymphatic anomalies	Portagen	Impaired absorption of long-chain fats
Necrotizing enterocolitis	Preterm formula or Pregestimil (once feeding is resumed)	Impaired digestion
Renal insufficiency	Standard formula	
	Similac PM 60/40	Low phosphate content, low renal solute load

TABLE 10.8	Oral Dietary Supplements Available for Use in Infants		
Nutrient	**Product**	**Source**	**Energy content**
Fat	MCT oil (Novartis)	Medium-chain triglycerides	8.3 kcal/g
			7.7 kcal/mL
	Microlipid (Novartis)	Long-chain triglycerides	4.5 kcal/mL
	Corn oil	Long-chain triglycerides	8.6 kcal/gm
			8 kcal/mL
Carbohydrate	Polycose (Ross)	Glucose polymers	4 kcal/gm
			8 kcal/tsp (powder)
Protein	Beneprotein (Novartis)	Whey	3.6 kcal/g
		Protein isolates	5.5 kcal/tsp

MCT = medium-chain triglyceride.

hindmilk may be employed to enhance caloric intake. However, this should not replace the use of HMF. Fat modulars may be added to the feeding as a bolus or in the 24 hour supply, however, it should be noted that fat added to the 24 hour supply is subject to adherence to the storage container.

2. Formula-fed, fluid-restricted preterm infants may be switched to a 27 or 30 kcal/oz premature infant formula once they are tolerating appropriate volumes of 24 kcal/oz feedings.

3. Human milk-fed term infants requiring caloric enhancement may also utilize formula powder, MCT or corn oil and/or Polycose, added in increments of 2 to 3 kcal/oz (typically not to exceed a maximum caloric density of 30 kcal/oz). As with preterm infants, adjustments should be made gradually with feeding tolerance assessed after each change. Hindmilk may also be used.

4. For term infants receiving standard formula, the formula density may be increased as needed by the use of standard formula concentrate diluted to a more calorically dense feeding.

5. We may also consider protein supplementation with a whey protein modular for all VLBW infants in order to increase the protein content to approximately 4 g/kg/day, as indicated.

6. These supplements are further described in Table 10.8.

7. Growth patterns of infants receiving these supplements are monitored closely and the nutritional care plan is adjusted accordingly.

F. Feeding method. These should be individualized based on gestational age, clinical condition, and feeding tolerance.

1. **Nasogastric/orogastric feedings.** We utilize nasogastric tube feedings more frequently, as orogastric tubes tend to be more difficult to secure.

   a. **Candidates**

   i. Infants <34 weeks' gestation, as most do not yet have the ability to coordinate suck-swallow-breathe patterns.

   ii. Infants with impaired suck/swallow coordination due to conditions such as encephalopathy, hypotonia and maxillofacial abnormalities.

   b. **Bolus versus continuous.** Studies may be found in support of either method and, in practice, both are utilized. We usually initiate with bolus feedings divided every 3 to 4 hours. If difficulties with feeding tolerance occur, we will lengthen the amount of time over which a feeding is given by placing on a syringe pump for 30 to 120 minutes.

   2. Transpyloric feedings
   a. Candidates. There are only a few indications for transpyloric feedings.
      i. Infants intolerant to nasogastric/orogastric feedings.
      ii. Infants at increased risk for aspiration.
      iii. Severe gastric retention or regurgitation.
      iv. Anatomic abnormalities of the GI tract such as microgastria.
   b. Other considerations
      i. Transpyloric feedings should be delivered continuously, as the small intestine does not have the same capacity for expansion as does the stomach.
      ii. There is an increased risk for fat malabsorption, as lingual and gastric lipase secretions are bypassed.
      iii. These tubes are routinely placed under guided fluoroscopy.
   3. Transition to breast/bottle feedings is a gradual process. Infants who are approximately 34 weeks' gestation who have coordinated suck-swallow-breathe patterns and respiratory rates <60 per minute are appropriate candidates for introducing breast/bottle feedings.
   4. Gastrostomy feedings
   a. Candidates
      i. Infants with neurological impairment and/or those who are unable to take sufficient volumes through breast/bottle feeding to maintain adequate growth/hydration status.
G. Iron. The AAP recommends that preterm infants receive a source of iron, provided at 2 mg/kg/day for human milk-fed preterm infants, by the time they are 1 month of age. The AAP further suggests that formula-fed infants may benefit from 1 mg/kg in addition to that provided by iron-fortified formula. The Summary of Reasonable Nutrient Intakes continue to recommend 2–4 mg/kg/day for VLBW and ELBW infants. Iron supplementation is recommended until the infant is 12 months of age. Iron-fortified formulas and iron-fortified HMF provide approximately 2.2 mg/kg/day when delivered at a rate of 150 mL/kg/day. Low iron formulas are not recommended for use.
   1. Vitamin E is an important antioxidant that acts to prevent fatty acid peroxidation in the cell membrane. The recommendation for preterm infants is 6 to 12 IU vitamin E/kg/day, with the upper limit being desirable. Preterm infants are not initiated on iron supplements until they are tolerating full enteral volumes of 24 kcal/oz feedings, which provides vitamin E at the low to midrange of the recommendations. An additional vitamin E supplement would be required to meet the upper end of the recommendation.
H. Current controversies
   1. Glutamine. As with parenteral glutamine supplementation, there are presently no recommendations for enteral glutamine supplementation in preterm infants.
   2. Long-chain polyunsaturated fatty acids (LCPUFAs). The inclusion of LCPUFAs, specifically docosahexaenoic acid (DHA) and arachidonic acid (ARA), in infant formulas has been the subject of much debate. These LCPUFAs are derivatives of the EFAs, linoleic acid and alpha-linolenic acid, and they are important in cognitive development and visual acuity. Human milk contains these LCPUFAs but, until recently, standard infant formula did not. Controlled trials investigating the effects of LCPUFA-supplemented formula on cognitive development in preterm infants have been inconclusive. The effects on visual acuity have more consistently suggested an advantage. Furthermore, no adverse effects were noted.
V. SPECIAL CONSIDERATIONS
   A. Gastroesophageal reflux (GER). Episodes of GER, as monitored by esophageal pH probes, are common in both preterm and full-term infants. The majority of infants, however, do not exhibit clinical compromise from GER.
      1. Introduction of enteral feeds. Emesis can be associated during the introduction and advancement of enteral feeds in preterm infants. These episodes are most

commonly related to intestinal dysmotility secondary to prematurity and will respond to modifications of the feeding regimen.

   a. Temporary reductions in the feeding volume, removal of nutritional additives, lengthening the duration of the feeding (sometimes to the point of using continuous feeding), and temporary cessation of enteral feeds are all possible strategies depending upon the clinical course of the infant.

   b. Rarely, specialized formulas are used when all other feeding modifications have been tried without improvement. In general, these formulas should only be used for short periods of time with close nutritional monitoring.

   c. Infants who have repeated episodes of symptomatic emesis that prevent achievement of full-volume enteral feeds may require evaluation for anatomic problems such as malrotation or Hirschsprung's disease. In general, radiographic studies are not undertaken unless feeding problems have persisted for 2 or more weeks, or unless bilious emesis occurs.

2. Established feeds. Preterm infants on full-volume enteral feeds will have occasional episodes of symptomatic emesis. If these episodes do not compromise the respiratory status or growth of the infant, no intervention is required other than continued close monitoring of the infant. If symptomatic emesis is associated with respiratory compromise, repeated apnea, or growth restriction, therapeutic maneuvers are indicated.

   a. Positioning. Reposition the infant to elevate the head and upper body, in either a prone or right side down position.

   b. Feeding intervals. Shortening the interval between feeds to give a smaller volume during each feed may sometimes improve signs of GER. Infants fed by gavage may have the duration of the feed increased.

   c. Metoclopramide. Infants who remain clinically compromised from GER after positioning and feeding interval changes can have a therapeutic trial of metoclopramide. The metoclopramide should be discontinued after 1 week if there is no improvement in clinical status.

3. Apnea. Studies using pH probes and esophageal manometry have not shown an association between GER and apnea episodes. Treatment with promotility agents should not be used for uncomplicated apnea of prematurity.

B. NEC (see Chap. 32). Nutritional support of the patient with NEC focuses around providing complete PN during the acute phase of the disease, followed by gradual introduction of feeds after the patient has stabilized and the gut has been allowed to heal.

1. PN. For at least 2 weeks after the initial diagnosis of NEC, the patient is kept NPO and receives total PN. The goals for PN were delineated previously in section III.

2. Initiation of feeds. If the patient is clinically stable after a minimum 2 weeks of bowel rest, feeds are introduced at approximately 10 to 20 mL/kg/day, preferably with human milk, although a standard formula appropriate for the gestational age of the patient may also be used (i.e., preterm formula for the typical NICU infant). More specialized formulas containing elemental proteins are rarely indicated.

3. Feeding advancement. If trophic feedings (10 to 20 mL/kg/day) are tolerated for 24 to 48 hours, gradual advancement of feeding volume is continued at approximately 10 mL/kg every 12 to 24 hours for the next 2 to 3 days. If this advancement is tolerated, further advancement proceeds according to the guidelines in Table 10.5. Supplemental PN is continued until enteral feeds are providing ≥75% of goal volume.

4. Feeding intolerance. Signs of feeding intolerance include large gastric residuals, emesis, abdominal distension, and increased numbers of apnea episodes. Reduction of feeding volume or cessation of feeding is usually indicated. If these clinical signs prevent attainment of full-volume enteral feeds despite several attempts to advance feeds, radiographic contrast studies may be indicated to rule out intestinal strictures. This type of evaluation would typically take place after 1 to 2 weeks of attempting to achieve full-volume enteral feeds.

5. **Enterostomies.** If one or more enterostomies are created as a result of surgical therapy for NEC, it may be difficult to achieve full nutritional intake by enteral feeds. Depending on the length and function of the upper intestinal tract, increasing feeding volume or nutritional density may result in problems with malabsorption, dumping syndrome, and poor growth.

   a. **Refeeding.** Output from the proximal intestinal enterostomy can be refed into the distal portion(s) of the intestine through the mucous fistula(s). This may improve the absorption of both fluid and nutrients.

   b. **PN support.** If growth targets cannot be achieved using enteral feeds, continued use of supplemental PN may be indicated depending on the patient's overall status and liver function. Enteral feeding should be continued at the highest rate and nutritional density tolerated, and supplemental PN should be given to achieve the nutritional goals and growth outcomes as previously outlined.

C. **BPD.** Preterm infants who have BPD have increased caloric requirements due to their increased metabolic expenditure, and at the same time have a lower tolerance for excess fluid intake.

   1. **Fluid restriction.** Total fluid intake is typically restricted from the usual 150 mL/kg/day to 140 mL/kg/day. In cases of severe CLD, further restriction to 130 and, rarely, 120 mL/kg/day may be required. Careful monitoring is required when fluid restrictions are implemented to ensure adequate caloric and micronutrient intake. Growth parameters must also be monitored so that continued growth is not compromised.

   2. **Caloric density.** Infants with CLD will commonly require up to 30 kcal/oz feeds in order to achieve the desired growth targets. In fluid-restricted infants with severe CLD, the maximum density of 32 kcal/oz is used on an infrequent basis.

VI. **NUTRITIONAL CONSIDERATIONS IN DISCHARGE PLANNING.** Recent data describing postnatal growth in the United States suggest that a significant number of VLBW and ELBW infants continue to have catch-up growth requirements at the time of discharge from the hospital.

A. **Human milk.** The use of human milk and efforts to transition to full breastfeeding in former preterm infants who continue to require enhanced caloric density feedings poses a unique challenge. We plan individualized care in order to support the transition to full breastfeeding while continuing to allow for optimal rates of growth. Usually this is accomplished by a combination of a specified number of nursing sessions per day, supplemented by feedings of calorically enhanced breast milk or nursing on demand supplemented by several feeds per day of nutrient-enriched postdischarge formula. Growth rate data obtained in the hospital may be forwarded to infant follow-up clinics and the private pediatrician for VLBW and ELBW infants.

B. **Formula choices**

   1. **Nutrient-enriched postdischarge formulas.** Preterm infants fed nutrient-enriched postdischarge formulas grow better than infants fed standard term formulas. The AAP suggests these nutrient-enriched formulas may be used to a postnatal age of 9 months. Additionally, ESPGAN recently suggested that preterm infants who demonstrate subnormal weight for age at discharge should be fed with fortified human milk or special formula fortified with high contents of protein, minerals and trace elements, as well as LCPUFAs until at least 40 weeks postconceptual age, but possibly for another 3 months thereafter. We consider preterm infants to be appropriate candidates for the use of these formulas, either as an additive to human milk or as a sole formula choice, once they are >2,000 g and 35 weeks corrected.

   2. **Term formulas** may also be utilized; however, careful attention must be paid to ensure adequate caloric and micronutrient intake.

C. **Vitamin supplementation.** We presently adhere to the following vitamin supplementation guidelines:

   1. The AAP recommends 200 IU vitamin D per day for all human milk-fed infants unless they are weaned to at least 500 mL/day of vitamin D-fortified formula. The

American Academy of Breastfeeding Medicine suggests up to 400 IU vitamin D per day for the NICU graduate. Preterm infants who are >2,000 g and 35 weeks corrected gestational age, and human milk-fed, are supplemented daily with approximately 0.5 mL of pediatric MVI with iron. Alternatively, pediatric MVI without iron may be provided with ferrous sulfate drops administered separately.

   2. Iron supplementation is recommended as previously described.

Suggested Readings

American Academy of Pediatrics, Committee on Nutrition (AAP-CON). *Pediatric nutrition handbook*, 5th ed. Elk Grove Village: American Academy of Pediatrics, 2004.

European Society of Paediatric Gastroenterology and Nutrition, Committee on Nutrition of the Preterm Infant (ESPGAN-CON). *Nutrition and feeding of preterm infants*. Oxford: Blackwell Science, 1987.

Fenton TR. A new growth chart for preterm babies; Babson and Benda's chart updated with recent data and a new format. *BMC Pediatr* 2003;3:13. Chart may be downloaded from: http://members.shaw.ca/growthchart.

Tsang RC, Uauy R, Koletzko B, et al, eds. *Nutritional needs of the premature infant: Scientific basis and practical guidelines*, 3rd ed. Baltimore: Lippincott Williams & Wilkins, 2005.

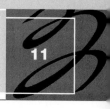
I. RATIONALE FOR BREASTFEEDING. Breastfeeding enhances maternal involvement, interaction and bonding; provides species-specific nutrients to support normal infant growth; provides nonnutrient growth factors, immune factors, hormones, and other bioactive components that can act as biological signals; and can decrease the incidence and severity of infectious diseases, enhance neurodevelopment, decrease the incidence of childhood obesity and some chronic illnesses, and decrease the incidence and severity of atopic disease. Breastfeeding is beneficial for the mother's health because it increases maternal metabolism; has maternal contraceptive effects with exclusive, frequent breastfeeding; is associated with a decreased incidence of maternal premenopausal breast cancer and osteoporosis; and imparts community benefits by decreasing health care costs and economic savings related to commercial infant formula expenses.

II. RECOMMENDATIONS ON BREASTFEEDING FOR HEALTHY TERM INFANTS INCLUDE THE FOLLOWING GENERAL PRINCIPLES
  A. Exclusive breastfeeding for the first 6 months
  B. When direct breastfeeding in not possible, expressed breast milk should be provided
  C. Place infants skin-to-skin with their mothers immediately after birth and encourage frequent feedings (8 to 12 feeds/24 hour)
  D. Supplements (i.e., water or formula) and pacifiers should not be given unless medically indicated
  E. Complementary foods should be introduced around 6 months with continued breastfeeding up to and beyond the first year
  F. Oral vitamin D drops (100 IU/daily) should be given to the infant beginning at 2 months
  G. Supplemental fluoride should not be provided during the first 6 months of life

III. MANAGEMENT AND SUPPORT ARE NEEDED FOR SUCCESSFUL BREAST-FEEDING
  A. Early postpartum period. All mothers should be instructed before discharge from the hospital about:
    1. Basic positioning of infant to allow correct infant attachment at the breast
    2. Minimum anticipated feeding frequency (8 times/24 hour period)
    3. Infant signs of hunger and adequacy of milk intake
    4. Common breast conditions experienced during early breastfeeding and basic management strategies
    5. Proper referral sources when indicated
  B. All breastfeeding infants should be seen by a pediatrician or other health care provider at 3 to 5 days of age to ensure that the infant has stopped losing weight and has lost no more than 7% birth weight; has yellow, seedy stools (approximately 3/d)—no more meconium stools; and has at least six wet diapers per day.
    1. At 3 to 5 days postdelivery, the mother should experience some breast fullness, and notice some dripping of milk from opposite breast during breastfeeding; demonstrate ability to latch infant to breast; understand infant signs of hunger and satiety; understand expectations and treatment of minor breast/nipple conditions
    2. Expect a return to birth weight by 12–14 days of age and a continued rate of growth of at least 1/2 ounce per day during the first month.
      a. If infant growth is inadequate, after ruling out any underlying health conditions in the infant, breastfeeding assessment should include adequacy of

infant attachment to the breast; presence or absence of signs of normal lactogenesis (i.e., breast fullness, leaking); maternal history of conditions (i.e., endocrine, breast surgery) that may effect lactation.

b. The ability of infant to transfer milk at breast can be measured by weighing the infant before and after feeding using the following guidelines:

i. Weighing the diapered infant before and immediately after (without changing the diaper) the feeding

ii. 1 gram infant weight gain equals 1 mL milk intake

c. If milk transfer is inadequate, supplementation (preferably with expressed breast milk) may be indicated

d. Instructing the mother to express her milk with a mechanical breast pump following feeding will allow additional breast stimulation to increase milk production

IV. MANAGEMENT OF BREASTFEEDING PROBLEMS

A. Sore, tender nipples. Most mothers will experience some degree of nipple soreness most likely a result of increased surface tension caused by the infant's sucking action. A common description of this soreness includes an intense onset at the initial latch-on with a rapid subsiding of discomfort as milk flow increases. Nipple tenderness should diminish during the first few weeks until no discomfort is experienced during breastfeeding. Purified lanolin and/or expressed breast milk applied sparingly to the nipples following feedings may hasten this process.

B. Traumatized, painful nipples (may include bleeding, blisters, cracks). Nipple discomfort associated with breastfeeding that does not follow the scenario described in the preceding text requires immediate attention to determine cause and develop appropriate treatment modalities. Possible causes include: ineffective, poor latch-on to breast, improper infant sucking technique, removing infant from breast without first breaking suction, underlying nipple condition or infection (i.e., yeast, eczema). Management includes: (i) assessment of infant positioning and latch-on with correction of improper techniques. Ensure that the mother can duplicate positioning technique and experiences relief with adjusted latch-on. (ii) Diagnose any underlying nipple condition and prescribe appropriate treatment (iii) In cases of severely traumatized nipples, temporary cessation of breastfeeding may be indicated to allow for healing. It is important to instruct the mother to maintain lactation with mechanical/hand expression until direct breastfeeding is resumed.

C. Engorgement usually presents on day 3–5 postpartum signaling the onset of copious milk production resulting in swollen, hard breasts that are warm to the touch. The infant may have difficulty latching to the breast until the engorgement is resolved. Treatment includes: (i) Application of warm, moist heat to the breast alternating with cold compresses to relieve edema of the breast tissue (ii) Gentle hand-expression of milk to soften areola to facilitate infant attachment to the breast (iii) Gentle massage of the breast during feeding and/or milk expression (iv) Mild analgesic (acetaminophen) or anti-inflammatory (ibuprofen) for pain relief and/or reduction of inflammation

D. Plugged ducts usually present as a palpable lump or area of the breast that does not soften during a feeding or pumping session. It may be the result of an ill-fitting bra, tight, constricting clothing, or a missed or delayed feeding/pumping. Treatment includes: (i) Frequent feedings or pumping sessions beginning with the affected breast (ii) Application of moist heat and breast massage before and during feeding (iii) Positioning infant during feeding to locate the chin toward the affected area to allow for maximum application of suction pressure to facilitate breast emptying

E. Mastitis is an inflammatory and/or infectious breast condition—usually affecting only one breast. Signs and symptoms include: rapid onset of fatigue, body aches, headache, fever and tender, reddened breast area. Treatment includes: (i) Immediate bed rest concurrent with continued breastfeeding (ii) Frequent and efficient milk removal—using an electric breast pump when necessary (iii) Appropriate antibiotics for a sufficient period (10–14 days) (iv) Comfort measures to relieve breast discomfort and general malaise (i.e., analgesics, moist heat/massage to breast).

V. SPECIAL SITUATIONS. Certain conditions in the infant, mother, or both may indicate specific strategies that require a delay and/or modification of the normal breastfeeding relationship. Whenever breastfeeding is delayed or suspended for a period of time, frequent breast emptying with an electric breast pump is recommended to ensure maintenance of lactation.

A. Infant conditions. Hyperbilirubinemia is not a contraindication to breastfeeding. Special attention should be given to ensuring infant is breastfeeding effectively in order to enhance gut motility and facilitate bilirubin excretion.

1. Congenital anomalies may require special management.

a. Craniofacial anomalies (i.e., cleft lip/palate, Pierre-Robin) present challenges to the infant's ability to latch effectively to the breast. Modified positioning and special devices (i.e., obturator, nipple shield) may be utilized to achieve an effective latch.

b. Cardiac disease/defects may require fluid restriction status of the infant and special attention to pacing of feeds to minimize fatigue during feeding.

c. Ankyloglossia (tongue tie) may interfere with the infant's ability to effectively breastfeed. The inability of the infant to extend the tongue over the lower gum line and lift the tongue to compress the underlying breast tissue may compromise effective milk transfer. Frenulotomy is often the treatment of choice.

2. Premature infants receive profound benefits from breastfeeding and the receipt of mother's own milk. Mothers should be encouraged to express their milk (See breast milk collection and storage in the subsequent text)—even if they do not plan on direct breastfeeding—in order to provide their infant with the special nutritional and nonnutritional human milk components.

a. Special attention should be given to late preterm infants (35–37 weeks) who are often discharged from the hospital before they are breastfeeding effectively. Management should include: (i) Mechanical milk expression concurrent with breastfeeding until the infant is breastfeeding effectively (ii) Weighing the infant before and after breastfeeding to evaluate adequacy of milk intake and determine need for supplementation.

b. For premature infants less than 35 weeks, mothers should be encouraged to practice early and frequent skin-to-skin holding and suckling at the emptied breast to facilitate early nipple stimulation/milk volume and infant oral feeding assessment.

B. Maternal conditions

1. Endocrine diseases have the potential to affect lactation and milk production.

a. Women with diabetes should be encouraged to breastfeed and many find an improvement in their glucose metabolism during lactation. Early, close monitoring to ensure the establishment of lactation and adequacy of infant growth are recommended due to a well-documented delay (1 to 2 days) in the onset of lactogenesis II.

b. Thyroid disease does not preclude breastfeeding, although without proper treatment of the underlying thyroid condition, poor milk production (hypothyroidism) or maternal loss of weight, nervousness, heart palpitations (hyperthyroidism) may negatively effect lactation. With proper pharmacologic treatment, the ability to lactate does not appear to be affected.

c. Women with a history of breast surgery should be able to breastfeed successfully. Prenatal assessment should include documenting the type of procedure (i.e., augmentation, reduction mammoplasty) and surgical approach (i.e., submammary, periareolar, free nipple transplantation) used to evaluate the level of follow-up indicated in the early postpartum period to monitor the progress of breastfeeding and adequacy of milk production and infant growth.

VI. CARE AND HANDLING OF EXPRESSED BREAST MILK. When possible, direct breastfeeding provides the greatest benefit for mother and infant, especially in terms of provision of specific human milk components and maternal-infant interaction. However, when direct breastfeeding is not possible, expressed breast milk should be encouraged with special attention to milk expression and storage techniques. Mothers separated from their infants immediately following delivery due to infant prematurity or illness must initiate lactation by mechanical milk expression. Milk expression and storage techniques can affect the composition and bacterial content of mother's own milk.

A. Breast milk expression and collection. Recommendations for initiation and maintenance of mechanical milk expression for pump-dependent mothers of hospitalized infants include: (i) Milk expression within the first few hours following delivery with a hospital-grade electric breast pump (ii) Frequent pumping (8 to 10 times daily) during the first 2 weeks following birth theoretically stimulates mammary alveolar growth and maximizes potential milk yield (iii) Pumping 10 to 15 minutes per session during the first few days until the onset of increased milk flow at which time pumping time per session can be modified to continue 1 to 2 minutes beyond a steady milk flow (iv) A target daily milk volume of 800 to 1,000 mL at the end of the second week following delivery is optimal

B. Guidelines for **breast milk collection** include: (i) Instructing the mother to wash hands and scrub under fingernails before each milk expression (ii) All milk collection equipment coming in contact with the breast and breast milk should be thoroughly cleaned before and following each use (iii) Sterilizing milk collection equipment once a day (iv) Collect milk in sterile glass or hard plastic containers. Plastic bags are not recommended for milk storage for preterm infants (v) Label each milk container with infant's identifying information, date and time of milk expression

C. Guidelines for **breast milk storage** include: (i) Use fresh, unrefrigerated milk within 1 hour of milk expression (ii) Refrigerate milk immediately following expression when the infant will be fed within 48 hours (iii) Freeze milk when infant is not being fed or the mother is unable to deliver the milk to the hospital within 24 hours of expression (iv) In the event that frozen milk completely/partially thaws, either feed the milk to the infant or discard; do not refreeze

VII. Contraindications and conditions **not** contraindicated to breastfeeding.

A. There are a few contraindications to breastfeeding or expressed breast milk feeding. Maternal health conditions should be evaluated and appropriate treatments prescribed in order to support continued breastfeeding and/or minimal interruption of feeding when possible. Most maternal medications enter breast milk to some degree, however, with few exceptions, the concentrations of most are relatively low, and the dose delivered to the infant often subclinical.

B. Contradictions to breastfeeding

    1. An infant with **galactosemia** will be unable to breastfeed or receive breast milk.

    2. A mother with **active tuberculosis** will be isolated from her newborn for initial treatment. She can express her milk to initiate and maintain her milk volume during this period and once it is deemed safe for her to have contact with her infant she can begin breastfeeding.

    3. The Center for Disease Control recommends that **women who test positive for human immunodefiency virus (HIV)** in the United States should avoid breastfeeding.

    4. Some maternal medications are contraindicated during breastfeeding. Clinicians should maintain reliable resources for information on the transfer of drugs into human milk (see Appendix C)

C. Conditions that are **not** contraindications to breastfeeding

    1. Mothers who are hepatitis B surface antigen positive. Infants should receive hepatitis B immune globulin and hepatitis B vaccine to eliminate risk of transmission.

    2. Hepatitis C virus transmission through breastfeeding has not been shown.

    3. In full term infants, the benefits of breastfeeding appear to outweigh the risk of transmission from cytomegalovirus (CMV) positive mothers. The extremely preterm infant is at increased risk or perinatal CMV acquisition. Frozen milk or pasteurization may reduce the risk of transmission in human milk.

    4. Mothers who are febrile

5. Mothers exposed to low-level environmental chemical agents
6. Although tobacco smoking is not contraindicated, mothers should be advised to avoid smoking in the home and make every effort to stop smoking while breastfeeding.

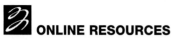 **ONLINE RESOURCES**

The Academy of Breastfeeding Medicine; http://www.bfmed.org.

International Lactation Consultants Association; http://www.ilca.org.

LactMed—drugs and lactation database; http://toxnet.nlm.nih.gov/cgi-bin/sis/htmlgen? LACT.

La Leche League International; www.lalecheleague.org.

Suggested Readings
American Academy of Pediatrics. Breastfeeding and the use of human milk. *Pediatrics* 2005;115(2):496–506.
Hale T. *Medications and mother's milk*, 12th ed. Amarillo: Pharmasoft Medical, 2006.
Hurst NM, Meier PP. Breastfeeding the preterm infant. In: Riordan J, ed. *Breastfeeding and human lactation*. Boston: Jones & Bartlett, 2005:367–408.
Lawrence RA. *Breastfeeding: A guide for the medical profession*, 6th ed. St. Louis: Mosby, 2005.

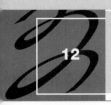

TEMPERATURE CONTROL
Kimberlee Chatson

12

I. HEAT PRODUCTION. Thermoregulation in adults is achieved by both metabolic and muscular activity (e.g., shivering). During pregnancy, maternal mechanisms maintain intrauterine temperature. After birth, newborns must adapt to their relatively cold environment by the metabolic production of heat because they are not able to generate an adequate shivering response.

Term newborns have a source for thermogenesis in brown fat, which is highly vascularized and innervated by sympathetic neurons. When these infants face cold stress, norepinephrine levels increase and act in the brown-fat tissue to stimulate lipolysis. Most of the free fatty acids (FFAs) are re-esterified or oxidized; both reactions produce heat. Hypoxia or β-adrenergic blockade decreases this response.

II. TEMPERATURE MAINTENANCE

   A. Premature infants have special problems in temperature maintenance that put them at a disadvantage compared with term infants. These include the following:

   1. A higher ratio of skin surface area to weight.

   2. Highly permeable skin leads to increased transepidermal water loss.

   3. Decreased subcutaneous fat, with less insulative capacity.

   4. Less-developed stores of brown fat.

   5. The inability to take in enough calories to provide nutrients for thermogenesis and growth.

   6. Limitation of oxygen consumption in some preterm infants because of pulmonary problems.

   B. Cold stress. Premature infants subjected to acute hypothermia respond with peripheral vasoconstriction, causing anaerobic metabolism and metabolic acidosis, which can cause pulmonary vessel constriction, leading to further hypoxemia, anaerobic metabolism, and acidosis. Hypoxemia further compromises the infant's response to cold. Premature infants are therefore at great risk for hypothermia and its sequelae (i.e., hypoglycemia, metabolic acidosis, increased oxygen consumption). The more common problem facing premature infants is caloric loss from unrecognized chronic cold stress, resulting in excess oxygen consumption and inability to gain weight.

   C. Neonatal cold injury occurs in low-birth-weight (LBWs) infants and term infants with central nervous system (CNS) disorders. It occurs more often in home deliveries, emergency deliveries, and settings where inadequate attention is paid to the thermal environment and heat loss. These infants may have a bright red color because of the failure of oxyhemoglobin to dissociate at low temperature. There may be central pallor or cyanosis. The skin may show edema and sclerema. Core temperature is often <32.2°C (90°F). Signs may include the following: (i) hypotension, (ii) bradycardia, (iii) slow, shallow, irregular respiration, (iv) decreased activity, (v) poor sucking reflex, (vi) decreased response to stimulus, (vii) decreased reflexes, and (viii) abdominal distention or vomiting. Metabolic acidosis, hypoglycemia, hyperkalemia, azotemia, and oliguria are present. Sometimes there is generalized bleeding, including pulmonary hemorrhage. It is uncertain whether warming should be rapid or slow. Setting the abdominal skin temperature to 1°C higher than the core temperature in a radiant warmer will produce slow rewarming and setting it to 36.5°C will also result in slow rewarming. If the infant is hypotensive, normal saline (10–20 mL/kg) should be given; sodium bicarbonate is used to correct metabolic acidosis. Infection, bleeding, or injury should be evaluated and treated.

D. Hyperthermia defined as an elevated core body temperature, may be caused by a relatively hot environment, infection, dehydration, CNS dysfunction, or medications. Placing newborns in sunlight to control bilirubin is hazardous and may be associated with significant hyperthermia.

If environmental temperature is the cause of hyperthermia, the trunk and extremities are the same temperature and the infant appears vasodilated. In contrast, infants with sepsis are often vasoconstricted and the extremities are 2°C to 3°C colder than the trunk.

III. MECHANISMS OF HEAT LOSS

A. Radiation. Heat dissipates from the infant to a colder object in the environment.

B. Convection. Heat is lost from the skin to moving air. The amount lost depends on air speed and temperature.

C. Evaporation. The amount of loss depends primarily on air velocity and relative humidity. Wet infants in the delivery room are especially susceptible to evaporative heat loss.

D. Conduction. This is a minor mechanism of heat loss that occurs from the infant to the surface on which he or she lies.

IV. NEUTRAL THERMAL ENVIRONMENTS minimize heat loss. Thermoneutral conditions exist when heat production (measured by oxygen consumption) is minimum and core temperature is within the normal range (see Table 12.1).

V. MANAGEMENT TO PREVENT HEAT LOSS

A. Healthy infant

1. Newborns should be dried and wrapped in a warmed blanket after delivery.
2. Examination in the delivery room should be done with the infant under a radiant warmer. A skin probe with servocontrol to keep skin temperature at 36.5°C (97.7°F) should be used for prolonged examinations.
3. A cap is very useful in preventing significant heat loss through the scalp.
4. If the temperature is stable, the infant can be placed in a crib with blankets.

B. Sick infant

1. The infant should be dried.
2. A heated incubator should be used for transport.
3. A radiant warmer should be used during procedures.
4. Sick or premature infants require a thermoneutral environment to minimize energy expenditure; the incubator should be kept at an appropriate temperature on air mode (Table 12.1) if a skin probe cannot be used because of the potential damage to skin in small premature infants. Alternatively, skin mode or servocontrol can be set so that the incubator's internal thermostat responds to changes in the infant's skin temperature to ensure a normal temperature despite any environmental fluctuation.
5. Humidification of incubators has been shown to reduce evaporative heat loss and decrease insensible water loss. Risks and concerns for possible bacterial contamination have been addressed in current incubator designs that include heating devices that elevate the water temperature to a level that destroys most organisms. Also, the water transforms into a gaseous vapor and not a mist eliminating the airborne water droplet as a medium for infection.
6. Servocontrolled open warmer beds may be used for very sick infants when access is important. The use of a tent made of plastic wrap is effective in preventing both convection heat loss and insensible water loss (see Chap. 9).
7. Double-walled incubators limit radiant heat loss and decreases convective and evaporative losses as well.
8. Current technology includes the development of hybrid devices such as the Versalet Incuwarmer (Hill-Rom Air-Shields) and the Giraffe Omnibed (Ohmeda Medical). They offer the combined features of a traditional radiant warmer bed and an incubator in a single device. This allows for the seamless conversion between modes, which minimizes thermal stress and allows for ready access to the infant for routine and emergency procedures.
9. Premature infants in relatively stable condition can be dressed in clothes and caps and covered with a blanket. We try to do this as soon as possible even if

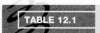

TABLE 12.1   Neutral Thermal Environmental Temperatures

	Temperature*	
Age and weight	**At start (°C)**	**Range (°C)**
0–6 h		
Under 1,200 g	35.0	34.0–35.4
1,200–1,500 g	34.1	33.9–34.4
1,501–2,500 g	33.4	32.8–33.8
Over 2,500 g (and >36 wk gestation)	32.9	32.0–33.8
6–12 h		
Under 1,200 g	35.0	34.0–35.4
1,200–1,500 g	34.0	33.5–34.4
1,501–2,500 g	33.1	32.2–33.8
Over 2,500 g (and >36 wk gestation)	32.8	31.4–33.8
12–24 h		
Under 1,200 g	34.0	34.0–35.4
1,200–1,500 g	33.8	33.3–34.3
1,501–2,500 g	32.8	31.8–33.8
Over 2,500 g (and >36 wk gestation)	32.4	31.0–33.7
24–36 h		
Under 1,200 g	34.0	34.0–35.0
1,200–1,500 g	33.6	33.1–34.2
1,501–2,500 g	32.6	31.6–33.6
Over 2,500 g (and >36 wk gestation)	32.1	30.7–33.5
36–48 h		
Under 1,200 g	34.0	34.0–35.0
1,200–1,500 g	33.5	33.0–34.1
1,501–2,500 g	32.5	31.4–33.5
Over 2,500 g (and >36 wk gestation)	31.9	30.5–33.3
48–72 h		
Under 1,200 g	34.0	34.0–35.0
1,200–1,500 g	33.5	33.0–34.0
1,501–2,500 g	32.3	31.2–33.4
Over 2,500 g (and >36 wk gestation)	31.7	30.1–33.2
72–96 h		
Under 1,200 g	34.0	34.0–35.0
1,200–1,500 g	33.5	33.0–34.0
1,501–2,500 g	32.2	31.1–33.2
Over 2,500 g (and >36 wk gestation)	31.3	29.8–32.8

(continued)

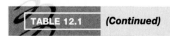

TABLE 12.1 *(Continued)*

| Age and weight | Temperature* | |
	At start (°C)	Range (°C)
4–12 d		
Under 1,500 g	33.5	33.0–34.0
1,501–2,500 g	32.1	31.0–33.2
Over 2,500 g (and >36 wk gestation)	—	—
4–5 d	31.0	29.5–32.6
5–6 d	30.9	29.4–32.3
6–8 d	30.6	29.0–32.2
8–10 d	30.3	29.0–31.8
10–12 d	30.1	29.0–31.4
12–14 d		
Under 1,500 g	33.5	32.6–34.0
1,501–2,500 g	32.1	31.0–33.2
Over 2,500 g (and >36 wk gestation)	29.8	29.0–30.8
2–3 wk		
Under 1,500 g	33.1	32.2–34.0
1,501–2,500 g	31.7	30.5–33.0
3–4 wk		
Under 1,500 g	32.6	31.6–33.6
1,501–2,500 g	31.4	30.0–32.7
4–5 wk		
Under 1,500 g	32.0	31.2–33.0
1,501–2,500 g	30.9	29.5–35.2
5–6 wk		
Under 1,500 g	31.4	30.6–32.3
1,501–2,500 g	30.4	29.0–31.8

*Generally speaking, the smaller infants in each weight group will require a temperature in the higher portion of the temperature range. Within each time range, the younger infants require the higher temperatures.
Source: Klaus M, Fanaroff A. The physical environment. In: *Care of the high risk neonate,* 5th ed. Philadelphia: WB Saunders, 2001.

the infant is on a ventilator. Heart rate and respiration should be continuously monitored because the clothing may limit observation.

VI. HAZARDS OF TEMPERATURE CONTROL METHODS

A. Hyperthermia. A servocontrolled warmer can generate excess heat, causing severe hyperthermia if the probe becomes detached from the infant's skin. Temperature alarms are subject to mechanical failure.

B. Undetected infections. Servocontrol of temperature may mask the hypothermia or hyperthermia associated with infection. A record of both environmental and core temperatures, along with observation for other signs of sepsis, will help detect this problem.

C. Volume depletion. Radiant warmers can cause increased insensible water loss. Body weight and input and output should be closely monitored in infants cared for on radiant warmers.

Suggested Readings

Klaus MA, Martin RJ, Fanaroff AA, eds. The physical environment. In: *Care of the high risk neonate*, 5th ed. Philadelphia: WB Saunders, 2001.

Sherman T. Optimizing the neonatal thermal environment. *Neonatal Netw* 2006;25(4): 251–258.

Sinclair JC. Servo-control for maintaining abdominal skin temperature at 36°C in low-birth-weight infants. *Cochrane Database Syst Rev* 2002;1:CD001074.

13

NEONATAL TRANSPORT
Robert M. Insoft

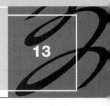

I. INDICATIONS

A. Interhospital transport should be considered if the medical resources or personnel needed for a high-risk infant are not available at the hospital currently providing care. Ideally, the pregnant woman should be transferred before delivery to a high-risk perinatal center capable of caring for both her and her newborn when a problem is known or arises in early labor. If a high-risk newborn is delivered at a hospital without advanced services, a medical team that is capable of performing the initial stabilization should be available.

B. Transfer to the regional neonatal tertiary center should be expedited following initial stabilization. Medical personnel from the referring center should contact their affiliated neonatal intensive care unit (NICU) transport service to arrange transfer and agree upon a treatment plan to optimize patient care before the transport team's arrival at the referring center.

C. Criteria for neonatal transfer depend on the capability of the referring hospital as defined by the American Academy of Pediatrics policy statement on levels of neonatal care and as dictated by local and state public health guidelines. Conditions that require transfer to a center that provides neonatal intensive care include the following:

1. Prematurity and/or birth weight <1,500 g.

2. Gestational age <32 weeks.

3. Respiratory distress requiring ventilatory support (continuous positive airway pressure [CPAP], ventilation).

4. Seizures.

5. Congenital anomalies and/or inborn errors of metabolism.

6. Congenital heart disease or cardiac arrhythmias requiring cardiac services.

7. Severe hypoxic-ischemic injury.

8. Other conditions requiring neonatology consultation and consideration of transfer.

   a. Severe hyperbilirubinemia possibly requiring exchange transfusion.

   b. Infant of diabetic mothers.

   c. Severe intrauterine growth restriction.

   d. Birth weight between 1,500 and 2,000 g and gestational age between 32 and 36 weeks.

   e. Procedures unavailable at referring hospital.

II. ORGANIZATION OF TRANSPORT SERVICES

A. All hospitals with established maternity services and level I or II neonatal care services should have **agreements** with regional perinatal centers outlining criteria for perinatal consultations and neonatal transfer.

B. The regional NICU transport team should have an appointed **medical director.** Neonatologists should monitor the protocols and procedures carried out by the team.

C. Transport teams consist of a combination of at least two or three trained personnel. Advanced practice nurses, neonatal nurse practitioners, respiratory therapists, and physicians may be team members. Senior pediatric residents and subspecialty fellows provide the physician component for some teams. Skills of team members must be assessed and arrangements made for advice and supervision.

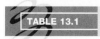

TABLE 13.1	Transport Team Equipment

Transport incubator equipped with monitors for heart rate, vascular pressures, oxygen saturation, temperature

Suction device

Infusion pumps

Gel-filled mattress

Adaptors to plug into both hospital and vehicle power

Airway equipment

Anesthesia bag with manometer

Laryngoscopes with no. 0 and no. 1 blades

Magill forceps

Instrument tray for chest tubes and vascular catheters

Stethoscope

Tanks of oxygen and compressed air oxygen, compressed air, heat, light, and a source of electrical power

Each transport should be supervised by a medical control officer, who may be the attending neonatologist.

D. Modes of transport include ambulance, fixed-wing aircraft, or helicopter depending on distance, acuity, and geography. Some hospitals own, maintain, and insure ambulances or helicopters. Other hospitals contract with commercial ambulance or fixed- or rotor-wing services that can accommodate a transport incubator and appropriate equipment.

E. Equipment. The team should be self-sufficient in terms of equipment, medications, and other supplies. Packs especially designed for neonatal transport are commercially available. These packs or other containers should be stocked by members of the transport team. The weight of the stocked packs should be documented for air transport (see Tables 13.1–13.3).

F. Legal issues. The transport process may raise legal issues, which vary among states. We periodically review all routine procedures and documentation forms with hospital legal counsel and provide the team with access to legal advice by phone when problems occur.

G. Malpractice insurance coverage is required for all team members. The tertiary hospital should decide whether transport is considered as an off-site or extended on-site activity because this can affect the necessary coverage.

H. Carrier regulations vary from state to state and may conflict with transport goals. For example, some states require that an ambulance stop at the scene of an unattended accident until a second ambulance arrives. If this is an issue, it should be reviewed with the medical director of the commercial carrier.

III. REFERRING HOSPITAL RESPONSIBILITIES

A. Documentation. A complete transfer note should be available at time of transfer. Initial transport consent should be obtained by the referring hospital staff and documented in the patient's medical record. Any risk to the patient for communicable diseases must be disclosed to the tertiary center. We recommend that a senior pediatric clinician remain in attendance until the patient leaves the referring hospital with the transport team.

B. If the patient is known before transfer to require a specialized medical and/or surgical service (e.g., surfactant, nitric oxide, surgery, extracorporeal membrane oxygenation [ECMO]), the referring hospital and transport team staff should ensure that the service is available at the referral center. If it is not available, alternative tertiary centers should be considered for that patient.

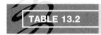

TABLE 13.2	Supplies Used by Transport Teams

Airways	Kelly clamp
Alcohol swabs	Lubricating ointment
Armboards	Monitor leads and transducers
Batteries	Needles: 18, 20, 26 gauge
Benzoin	Oxygen tubing
Betadine* swabs	Replogle nasogastric tube
Blood culture bottles	Scalpel blades, no. 11
Blood pressure cuff	Sterile gown
Butterfly needles: 23 and 25 gauge	Stopcocks
Chest tubes: 10 and 12 F, and connectors	Stylus
Chemstrip*	Suction catheters: 6, 8, and 10 F and traps
Clipboard with transport data forms, permission forms, progress notes, and booklet for parents	Suture material (silk 3–0, 4–0, on curved needle)
Culture tubes	Syringes: 1, 3, 10, 50 mL
Endotracheal tubes: 2.5, 3, 3.5, 4 mm	Tape
Face mask, term and premature	T-connectors
Feeding tubes: 5 and 8 F	Thermometer
Gauze pads	Tubes for blood specimens
Gloves, sterile and examination	Umbilical catheters: 3.5 and 5 F (double lumen)
Heimlich valves	Urine collection bags
Intravenous tubing	Xeroform* gauze
Intravenous catheters: 22 and 24 gauge	

*These are trademark items

C. The speed of the transfer should never take precedence over ensuring the correct level of transport staff and accepting facilities for a critically ill neonatal patient.

IV. TRANSPORT TEAM RESPONSIBILITIES

A. The referral center should provide a team of skilled personnel and appropriate equipment.

TABLE 13.3	Medications Used on Transport

Adenosine	Furosemide
Albumin 5%	Gentamicin
Ampicillin	Heparin
Atropine	Lidocaine
Calcium	Midazolan
Calcium gluconate	Morphine
Dexamethasone	Naloxone
Dextrose 50% in water	Normal saline
Dextrose 10% in water	Pancuronium
Diphenylhydantoin	Phenobarbital
Digoxin	Potassium chloride
Dobutamine	Prostaglandin E_1 (refrigerated)
Dopamine	Sodium bicarbonate
Epinephrine	Sterile water for injection
Erythromycin eye ointment	Sucrose oral solution
Fentanyl	Vitamin K_1

B. The medical control officer or attending neonatologist should discuss the patient's condition and potential therapies with team members before departure. Recommendations should focus on respiratory, cardiovascular, and metabolic stabilization. Interventions concerning airway management and vascular access should be specific. All recommendations should be documented.

C. The team should obtain consent for transfer as well as any other anticipated procedures upon arrival at the NICU.

D. Team members should introduce themselves clearly and politely to the staff of the referring hospital and family members. Appropriate photo identification should be worn.

E. Transfer of patient information (handoff) should be clear and there should be agreement on when the transport team assumes responsibility for management.

F. The team should work collegially with the referring hospital staff and be objective in their assessment and stabilization. The referring staff should be included in as much of the care as appropriate.

G. The referring and primary physicians should be identified and their names documented.

H. The parents should have time to see their newborn before the team leaves the referring hospital. We take instant photos for the benefit of the parents.

I. The team's policy regarding parents traveling with their newborn on transport should be reviewed with the family. The team should have policies regarding the presence of parents during ground or air transport. We allow one parent to travel with the patient as long as all team members agree that the family member will not interfere with medical care.

J. The team should call back the referring hospital staff after the transport is complete with pertinent follow-up while respecting the confidentiality of the patient and family.

K. Outreach education should be provided to the referring hospital staff. This could be in the form of transport conferences, in-service presentations, and case reviews.

V. MEDICAL MANAGEMENT BEFORE TRANSPORT

A. The tertiary center should mobilize their transport team as soon as possible. While the transport team is *en route*, the neonatologist responsible should discuss additional treatment strategies with the referring hospital staff.

B. The referring staff should stabilize the patient in conjunction with recommendations from the transport medical control officer or neonatologist. While awaiting the transport team, the referring staff should perform the following functions:

1. Maintain airway, oxygenation, and thermal stability.
2. Normalize circulatory deficits.
3. Maintain adequate blood glucose concentration.
4. Secure umbilical venous access, if appropriate.
5. Secure umbilical arterial access, if appropriate.
6. Obtain appropriate cultures and give first doses of antibiotics.
7. Insert a nasogastric tube and decompress the stomach.
8. Have a recent chest radiograph and other applicable studies available.
9. Obtain initial transport consent from parents.
10. Maximize the parents' ability to be near their newborn.
11. Obtain copies of obstetric and neonatal charts for the transport team.

VI. RETURNING TO THE NICU. If the patient has been stabilized, most return trips are uneventful. Continuous direct observation of the infant is one of the most important forms of monitoring. During the transport, the benefit of handling the patient and taking vital signs must be weighed against the possibility of an accidental extubation or thermal loss incurred by opening the transport incubator. We prepare all medications and intravenous fluids that may be needed during the transport in advance. Teams should use wireless telephones or direct radios to maintain contact with the NICU and seek advice for unexpected events.

VII. ARRIVAL AT THE NICU

A. The team should give the NICU caregivers complete clinical information (handoff) and copies of charts, consents, and radiographs.

B. A team member should telephone the parents to tell them their child has arrived safely.

C. All transport medications should be immediately restocked and all equipment checked and secured for subsequent calls.

D. A team member should telephone the referring and primary physicians to inform them of the patient's status and who will be providing further communication.

E. Quality assurance documentation used to monitor transport activities should be done immediately and the team's medical director notified of any issues that require follow-up.

VIII. SPECIAL MEDICAL CONDITIONS AND THERAPIES

A. Most infants with **congenital diaphragmatic hernia** (CDH) require immediate intubation and mechanical ventilation. Placement of a nasogastric tube prevents gaseous distention of herniated viscera during respiratory support.

B. When **cyanotic congenital heart disease** is a possible diagnosis, prostaglandin E_1 (PGE_1) must be available during transport. Ideally, treatment should be initiated at the referring hospital and administered through a central venous catheter, such as an umbilical venous catheter. Apnea, hypothermia, and hypotension are common side effects of PGE_1. Endotracheal intubation is usually warranted for transport of an infant requiring PGE_1 infusion.

C. Anemia may result from a variety of conditions, including fetal–maternal hemorrhage, abruption, hydrops fetalis, and twin-to-twin transfusion. Acute blood loss may not be reflected in a hematocrit drop for several hours but may be suggested by the history and clinical presentation. In such cases, cross-matching of blood should begin at the referring hospital while the transport team is *en route*. Infants in urgent need of a transfusion can be given non–cross-matched type O-negative packed cells until matched blood is available.

D. Abdominal wall defects. Both gastroschisis and omphalocele are treated by placing a nasogastric tube and immediately wrapping exposed abdominal contents with warm, sterile, saline-soaked (noncling) gauze. We use an outer wrapping with a plastic bag or plastic wrap to decrease heat and insensible water losses.

E. Tracheoesophageal fistula and esophageal atresia. A Replogle-type (sump) tube should be placed gently in the esophageal pouch to minimize the risk of aspiration. Positive-pressure ventilation should be avoided if possible in order to avoid overdistention of the gastrointestinal (GI) tract.

F. Neural tube defects should be wrapped in warm, sterile, saline-soaked noncling gauze and plastic wrap for protection and to minimize heat and fluid loss, as well as to prevent contamination with stool.

G. Premature infants with respiratory distress syndrome (RDS) and newborns with other disorders may require **surfactant administration.** The transport team should consult the medical control physician before surfactant administration, and the consultation should be documented. After administration, we wait for at least 30 minutes before moving the newborn to the transport incubator. This provides time for direct observation and initial ventilatory changes, thereby minimizing the risk of morbidity such as a plugged endotracheal tube or a pneumothorax from acute changes in compliance.

IX. AIR TRANSPORTS

A. Changes in barometric pressure. Barometric pressure decreases as altitude increases, leading to a decrease in oxygen tension. This is important even in aircraft with pressurized cabins because pressure is usually maintained at a level equal to 8,000 to 10,000 ft above sea level. To correct for this, Fio_2 must be increased to result in an adequate Pao_2. Oxygen saturation should be continuously monitored and Fio_2 adjusted as needed. If oxygen saturation monitoring is unavailable, Pao_2 can be estimated using the alveolar gas equation. Values of Fio_2 needed to maintain a constant Pao_2 at any altitude are shown in Table 13.4.

B. Gas expansion. As barometric pressure decreases with increasing altitude, gases trapped in closed spaces will expand. Even a small pneumothorax or the normal gaseous distention of the GI tract may result in clinical deterioration and should be drained or vented with a nasogastric tube before an air transport.

TABLE 13.4 Fio$_2$ Required to Maintain a Constant Pao$_2$ at Increasing Altitude

Sea level	Fio$_2$ at altitude (ft) of									
	2,000	4,000	6,000	8,000	10,000	12,000	14,000	16,000	18,000	20,000
0.21	0.23	0.24	0.27	0.29	0.29	0.34	0.37	0.41	0.45	0.49
0.03	0.32	0.35	0.38	0.41	0.45	0.49	0.53	0.59	0.64	0.71
0.04	0.43	0.47	0.51	0.55	0.60	0.65	0.71	0.78	0.85	0.94
0.50	0.54	0.58	0.63	0.69	0.75	0.81	0.89	0.98	—	—
0.60	0.65	0.70	0.76	0.83	0.99	0.98	—	—	—	—
0.70	0.76	0.82	0.89	0.96	—	—	—	—	—	—
0.80	0.86	0.94	—	—	—	—	—	—	—	—
0.90	0.97	—	—	—	—	—	—	—	—	—
1.00	—	—	—	—	—	—	—	—	—	—

Fio$_2$ = fractional concentration of inspired oxygen; Pao$_2$ = arterial oxygen tension.

X. NITRIC OXIDE ON TRANSPORTS

A. Inhaled nitric oxide (iNO) reduces the need for ECMO in critically ill-term or near-term infants with pulmonary hypertension and hypoxemic respiratory failure. In some cases (e.g., anticipated prolonged transport time or rapid deterioration of the patient), it may be appropriate to begin iNO treatment on transport. In patients already receiving iNO, treatment should be continued if transfer to an ECMO center is required.

B. Protocols should be developed by each transport team for the use of iNO. The protocol should be acceptable to all associated ambulance and aircraft vendors and referral hospital staff.

C. A certified neonatal respiratory therapist or other appropriately trained team member should be responsible for the administration of iNO on transport, including management of the needed equipment. Initiation of iNO at the referring hospital or during the transport should be done with the supervision of the responsible transport medical control physician or neonatologist.

D. If feasible, we document the presence of pulmonary hypertension by echocardiogram or a difference in preductal and postductal oxygen saturation before initiating iNO therapy (see Chap. 24F). Nitric oxide should not be used for newborns who have or are highly suspected to have certain congenital heart disease.

Suggested Readings

Woodward A, Insoft R, Kleinman M, eds. *Guidelines for air and ground transport of neonatal and pediatric patients*, 3rd ed. Elk Grove Village: American Academy of Pediatrics, 2007.

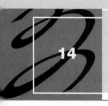

14 DEVELOPMENTALLY SUPPORTIVE CARE
Sandra L. Harmon and Beth M. McManus

I. **INTRODUCTION.** The incidence of cognitive, neuromotor, sensory, and feeding delays and disabilities is substantially higher among infants born preterm compared with their healthy, full-term counterparts (1–7). Our challenge, as neonatal caregivers is to foster a culture that respects the personhood of premature infants and optimizes the care and environment in which health care is delivered to this fragile, neurodevelopmentally vulnerable population. Developmentally supportive care (DSC) effectively meets this challenge. The pioneering work of Als and others (8–10) has provided a greater understanding of preterm infant brain development and neurobehavior, and the importance of individualized DSC to promote both. Implementing the principles of family-focused DSC in a neonatal intensive care unit (NICU) environment is associated with improved neurodevelopmental outcomes in the preterm infant population (11,12) and promotes the family adaptation process (13).

II. **NEUROBEHAVIORAL ASSESSMENT.** Neonatal developmental specialists conduct neurobehavioral assessment to identify infant's level of behavioral organization and state regulation, assess muscle tone and movement patterns, and evaluate autonomic stability (14,15). Accurate identification of infants' stress responses and self-regulating behaviors at rest and during routine care and procedures facilitates creation and modification of developmental plans of care to promote infants' neurodevelopment.

A. **Stress responses.** Autonomic, motoric, state organizational behavior, and attentional/interactive signs of stress combine to provide a baseline profile of an infant's overall tolerance to various stimuli. Autonomic signs of stress include changes in color, heart rate, and respiratory patterns as well as visceral changes such as gagging, hiccuping, vomiting, and stooling. Motoric signs of stress include facial grimacing, gaping mouth, twitching, hyperextension of limbs, finger splaying, back arching, flailing, and generalized hyper- or hypotonia. State alterations suggesting stress include rapid state transitions, diffuse sleep states, irritability, and lethargy. Changes in attention or the interactional availability of preterm infants, exhibited by covering eyes/face, gaze aversion, frowning, and hyperalert or panicky facial presentation, represent signs of stress in premature infants (14,15).

B. **Self-regulating behavior.** Preterm infants elicit a number of self-consoling behaviors that facilitate their coping responses to stress. Self-regulating behaviors commonly include hand or foot bracing, sucking, bringing hands to face, flexed positioning, cooing, and grasping of linens or own body parts (14,15).

III. **DEVELOPMENTALLY SUPPORTIVE EXTRAUTERINE ENVIRONMENT.** Preterm infants' exposure to the extrauterine environment during a period of rapid brain growth may adversely affect their neurodevelopmental outcomes (11). The goal of DSC is to mitigate the gap between a mother's womb and the high-technology environment of the NICU (8,16). Neonatal caregivers can potentially minimize negative outcomes by providing a modified extrauterine environment designed to support neurologic and sensory development.

A. **Structuring the physical environment.** Increased noise levels in the NICU are associated with infant's physiologic stress and autonomic instability (17). Therefore, the American Academy of Pediatrics (AAP) recommends that NICU sound levels not exceed 50 A-weighted decibels (dBA) (18). Installation of sound-absorbing walls and ceilings, individual curtains, and implementation of a DSC program including sound management (care in opening and closing portholes, refraining from placing items or writing on top of incubators, and reducing use of metal trash cans and running water near incubators) is associated with a significant reduction in noxious ambient noise levels (17). The relationship between ambient light and neurodevelopment is less clear. Reduced illumination (i.e., dark incubator covers and eye patches during phototherapy) appears to be associated with increased autonomic stability and more frequent eye opening among preterm infants (19). Reduction of light in the NICU does not appear to affect incidence or progression of retinopathy of prematurity (20) or follow-up pattern evoked potential measured during later infancy and toddler years (17). However, reduced light is associated with reduced noise and handling of infants, which may have beneficial developmental sequelae. Thus, the 1992 AAP Guidelines for Perinatal Care suggest illumination parameters of 650 lux for observation, and 1080 lux for procedures (21,22). Further, during procedures, the infant's eyes should be protected from direct light with use of protective patches.

IV. **DEVELOPMENTALLY SUPPORTIVE DIRECT INFANT CARE PRACTICES.** Developmental specialists devise care plans to meet both the medical and developmental needs of the preterm infant. This entails a coordinated, primary team effort designed to cluster care and interventions around the infant's state of alertness, sleep cycles, and family visits. The goal is to maximize rest, minimize stress, and optimize healing and growth.

A. **Positioning.** The goals of positioning of preterm infants are to facilitate flexed, midline positioning of extremities, improve respiration, and reduce physiologic stress. The use of "nesting materials" such as sheepskin, soft blanket rolls, and commercially available devices, as well as swaddling, assists the infant in maintaining softly flexed posturing (i.e., reduces lower extremity abduction, scapular retraction, and cervical hyperextension prevalent in the preterm population) (22). Further, hands-on "containment" reduces excessive motor activity and behavioral distress in preterm infants (23).

B. **Feeding.** Oral feeding is a complex task for the preterm infant that requires physiologic maturation, coordination of suck–swallow–breathe mechanics, and development of oral motor skills (24–26). Progression to oral feeds is highly contingent upon elements of DSC and occurs predictably in several phases. Pre–non-nutritive suck (NNS) is characterized by weak suck and poor motor, autonomic and state regulation stability; NNS is characterized by more optimal suck patterns and should be encouraged during gavage feeds, and nutritive suck, typically beginning at 33 weeks, progresses from minimal to full oral intake as autonomic stability and oral motor coordination improve. Strategies to promote successful progression through these phases include identifying and minimizing signs of physiologic stress, environmental modification to promote autonomic stability, feeding in a flexed, midline position, pacing techniques, and use of slow-flow nipples (26,27,40).

C. **Skin to skin care.** Also called *Kangaroo care*, this technique has consistently been associated with improved infant outcomes (i.e., fewer respiratory complications, improved weight gain, and temperature regulation) and maternal outcomes (i.e., improved maternal competence and longer breast-feeding duration) (28). Kangaroo care should be initiated as soon as infants are medically stable for transfer out of the incubator.

V. **COMFORT AND PAIN RELIEVING MEASURES.** Preterm infants must endure many uncomfortable/painful procedures necessary to meet their medical needs. Freedom from pain is a basic right of *all* patients. Research suggests that providing a continuous infusion of morphine to preterm infants requiring ventilatory support may decrease the incidence of poor neurologic outcomes (29). Effective nonpharmacologic interventions include swaddling, pacifiers, and administration of a 20% sucrose solution orally (30) (see Chap. 37).

VI. **PARENT SUPPORT/EDUCATION.** Effective DSC and family adaptation is dependent on adequate implementation of principles of family-centered care during NICU stay as well as upon transition to home.

A. **In the NICU.** Premature birth and NICU hospitalization negatively impact parent–infant interactions, which is associated with long-term adverse developmental sequelae (8). Individual family-centered interactions (i.e., family-based developmental evaluations, support, and education) have been associated with reduced parent stress and more positive parent–infant interactions (31). Family-centered NICU policies include welcoming families 24 hours/day, promotion of family participation in infant care, creation of parent advisory boards, implementation of parent support groups, and comfortable rooming-in areas for parents (32).

B. Discharge teaching. Because brain growth and maturation occurs at a slower rate in the extrauterine environment (3), parents must be prepared for the fact that their baby is not likely to behave as a term baby would even after he/she has actually reached 40 weeks postmenstrual age (PMA) (33). Research suggests that most of NICU parents report being ill-prepared for discharge with respect to recognizing signs of illness, employing effective calming strategies, being aware of typical and delayed development, and using strategies to promote infant development (34).

C. Postdischarge family supports. Many parents of preemies report feeling frightened and alone following discharge from the NICU even when sent home with services from a visiting nurse and early intervention (EI) specialists (35). Various support groups that are designed to provide long-term emotional and educational support needed by the parents of preterm and near-term infants are available in most communities. Additionally, the availability of magazines, books, and web-based materials related to parenting premature infants has increased dramatically in recent years (36–38). A promising approach to facilitating seamless transition to community-based services includes initiation of an EI referral before the infant's discharge and collaboration between NICU and EI professionals to create a developmentally supportive transition plan (39,40).

D. Infant follow-up and EI programs. Close follow-up is paramount to maximizing developmental outcome. At Brigham and Women's Hospital, all infants born at <32 weeks PMA, as well as those with complex medical issues, are referred to state run EI programs. Infants born at <1,500 g or having risk factors for long-term morbidity meet the criteria for the infant follow-up program. Both of these programs aim to prevent or minimize developmental delay through early identification of risk factors and referral to appropriate treatment programs.

References

1. Huppi PS, Warfield S, Kikinis R, et al. Quantitative magnetic resonance imaging of brain development in premature and mature newborns. *Ann Neurol* 1998;43:224.
2. Huppi PS, Maier SE, Peled S, et al. Microstructural development of human newborn cerebral white matter assessed *in vivo* by diffusion tensor magnetic resonance imaging. *Pediatr Res* 1998;44:584.
3. Huppi PS, Schuknecht B, Boesch C, et al. Structural and neurobehavioral delay in postnatal brain development of preterm infants. *Pediatr Res* 1996;39:895.
4. Hintz SR, Kendrick DE, Vohr BR, et al. Improved survival rates with increased neurodevelopmental disabilities of extremely low birth weight infants in 1990's. *Pediatrics* 2005;115(4):997–1003.
5. Wilson-Costello D, Friedman H, Minich N, et al. Changes in neurodevelopmental outcomes at 18–22 months' corrected age among infants less than 25 weeks' gestational age born 1993–1999. *Pediatrics* 2005;115(6):1645–1651.
6. Thoyre S, Shaker C, Pridham K. The early feeding skills assessment for preterm infants. *Neonatal Netw* 2004;24(3):7–16.
7. Peterson B, et al. Regional brain volume abnormalities and long-term cognitive outcome in preterm infants. *JAMA* 2000;284:1939.
8. Als H, et al. Individualized developmental care for the very low birth weight preterm infant. *JAMA* 1994;272:853.
9. McGrath J. Developmental physiology of the neurological system. *Cent Lines* 2000; 16:1.
10. Vandenberg K. Basic principles of developmental caregiving. *Neonatal Netw* 1997; 16:69.

11. Buehler D, et al. Effectiveness of individualized developmental care for low-risk preterm infants: Electrophysiologic evidence. *Pediatrics* 1995;96:923.
12. Als H, et al. Early experience alters brain function and structure. *Pediatrics* 2004;113: 846–857.
13. Aita M, et al. The art of developmental care in the NICU: A concept analysis. *J Adv Nurs* 2003;41:223.
14. Brazelton TB. *Neonatal behavioral assessment scale.* Philadelphia: JB Lippincott, 1973.
15. Als H, Butler S, Kosta S, et al. The Assessment of Preterm Infants' Behavior (APIB): Furthering the understanding and measurement of neurodevelopmental competence in preterm and full-term infants. *Ment Retard Dev Disabil Res Rev* 2005;11(1): 94–102.
16. Robison L. An organizational guide for an effective developmental program in the NICU. *J Obstet Gynecol Neonatal Nurs* 2003;32:379.
17. Fowler Byers J. Components of developmental care and the evidence for their use in the NICU. *Matern Child Nurs* 2003;28:174.
18. Byers J, Waugh WR, Lowman L. Sound level exposure of high-risk infants in different environmental conditions. *Neonatal Netw* 2006;25(1):25–32.
19. American Academy of Pediatrics, Committee on Environmental Health. Noise: A hazard for the fetus and newborn. *Pediatrics* 1997;100(4):724–727.
20. Phelps DL, Watts JL. Early light reduction for preventing retinopathy of prematurity in very low birth weight infants. *Cochrane Database Syst Rev* 2001;1:CD0001222.
21. Fielder A, Moseley M. Environmental light and the preterm infant. *Semin Perinatol* 2000;24(4):291–298.
22. Graven SN. Sound and the developing infant in the NICU: conclusions and recommendations for care. *Journal of Perinatology.* 2000;20:588–593.
23. Monterosso L, Kristjanson L, Cole J. Neuromotor development and the physiologic effects of positioning in very low birth weight infants. *J Obstet Gynecol Neonatal Nurs* 2002;31:138–146.
24. Harrison L, Williams A, Berbaum M, et al. Physiologic and behavioral effects of gentle human touch on preterm infants. *Res Nurs Health* 2000;23:435–446.
25. Shaker C. Nipple feeding preterm infants: An individualized, developmentally supportive approach. *Neonatal Netw* 1999;18(3):15–22.
26. Premji S, McNeil D, Scotland J. Regional neonatal oral feeding protocol changing the ethos of feeding preterm infants. *J Perinat Neonatal Nurs* 2004;18(4):371–384.
27. Ross E, Browne J. Developmental progression of feeding skills: An approach to supporting feeding in preterm infants. *Semin Neonatol* 2002;7:469–475.
28. Conde-Agudelo A, Diaz-Rossello JL, Belizan JM. Kangaroo mother care to reduce morbidity and mortality in low birth weight infants. *Cochrane Database Syst Rev* 2003;2:CD002771.
29. Anand KJ, Coskun V, Thrivikraman KV, et al. Analgesia and sedation in preterm neonates who require ventilatory support. *Arch Pediatr Adolesc Med* 1999;153:331.
30. American Academy of Pediatrics Committee on Fetus and Newborn and Section on Surgery. Prevention and Management of Pain in the Neonate: An Update. *Pediatrics* 2006;18(5):2234.
31. Browne J, Talmi A. Family-based intervention to enhance infant-parent relationships in the neonatal intensive care unit. *J Pediatr Psychol* 2005;30(8):667–677.
32. Cisneros Moore K, Coker K, DuBuisson A, et al. Implementing potentially better practices for improving family-centered care in neonatal intensive care units: Successes and challenges. *Pediatrics* 2003;111:e450–e460.
33. Vandenberg K. What to tell parents about the developmental needs of their baby at discharge. *Neonatal Netw* 1999;18:57.
34. Sheikh L, Obrien M. Parent preparation for the NICU-to-home transition: Staff and parent perceptions. *Child Health Care* 1993;22(3):227–239.
35. Bakewell-Sachs S. Parenting the post-NICU premature infant. *Matern Child Nurs* 2004;29:398.
36. March of Dimes Prematurity education for parents and caregivers. Online @ http://www .marchofdimes.com/prematurity/prematurity.asp. Accessed 2006.

37. March of Dimes Share Site: Support for parents of premature infants. Online @ http://www.shareyourstory.org. Accessed 2006.

38. Association of Women's Health, Obstetric and Neonatal Nurses, Near Term Infant Initiative: What parents need to know. Online @ http://www.awhonn.org/awhonn/?pg =872-2100-16920-18010. Accessed 2006.

39. Browne J, Langlois A, Ross E, et al. Beginnings: An interim individualized family service plan for use in the intensive care nursery. *Infants Young Child* 2001;14(2):19–32.

40. Hussey-Gardner B, McNinch A, Anastasi J, et al. Early interevention best practice: Collaboration among an NICU, an early intervention program, and an NICU follow-up program. *Neonatal Netw.* 2002;21(3):15–22.

FOLLOW-UP CARE OF VERY LOW BIRTH WEIGHT INFANTS

Jane E. Stewart, Camilia R. Martin, and Marsha R. Joselow

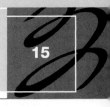

15

I. **INTRODUCTION.** The number of surviving preterm infants who are <32 weeks gestational age has increased steadily over the last 15 years and was 2.01% in 2004. Although these infants are a small percentage of total births, there were 82,652 very preterm infants born in 2004. The rise in the incidence of premature birth has been attributed in part to the increased number of multiple births associated with fertility therapies. In 2004 the rate of twin births was 32.2 per 1,000 total births; a 42% increase from the rate in 1990. Of the twins born in 2004, 11.8% were born <32 weeks' gestational age. However, the rate of triplets and higher order multiple births has decreased after a peak in 1998 (193.5 per 100,000 live births) and was 176.9 per 100,000 live births in 2004.

    Infants <32 weeks' gestational age have a high rate of medical and developmental sequelae related to prematurity. The survival rate of extremely low birth weight infants (ELBW; birth weight <1,000 g), the subset of premature infants who are at highest risk of long-term morbidity, has increased to 40% to 55%. As the survival rate of these extremely premature infants continues to improve, the total number of infants with unique follow-up needs, including the utilization of special medical and educational resources, will continue to grow.

II. **MEDICAL CARE ISSUES**
    A. Respiratory issues. (see Chaps. 3B and 24J). on Bronchopulmonary dysplasia,). Approximately 23% of very low birth weight (VLBW; birth weight <1,500 g) infants and 35% to 46% of ELBW infants develop bronchopulmonary dysplasia (BPD) (defined as O_2 dependent at 36 weeks' post menstrual age). Infants with BPD have a twofold increase in the risk of developing reactive airway disease particularly in the setting of viral respiratory infection, than do infants with birth weights >1,500 g. Infants with severe BPD may require treatment with tracheostomy and long-term ventilator support. More commonly, infants with significant BPD require supplemental oxygen therapy at home as well as bronchodilator or diuretic therapy. Infants with BPD are also at increased risk of feeding problems, gastroesophageal reflux, poor weight gain, and delays in achieving early developmental milestones.

        1. VLBW infants are four times more likely to be rehospitalized during the first year than are higher birth weight infants; up to 60% are rehospitalized at least once by the time they reach school age. Admissions during the first year of life are most commonly for complications of respiratory infections. The increased risk of hospitalization persists into early school age; 7% of VLBW children are hospitalized in a given year, compared with 2% of higher birth weight children.

        2. Respiratory syncytial virus (RSV) is the most important cause of bronchiolitis and pneumonia in premature infants, particularly in those with chronic lung disease. To prevent illness caused by RSV, VLBW infants should receive prophylactic treatment with palivizumab (Synagis) monoclonal antibody. The American Academy of Pediatrics (AAP) recommends treatment during RSV season for at least the first year of life for infants born ≤28 weeks' gestation and for at least the first 6 months of life for those born between 28 and 32 weeks' gestation. Likewise, good hand hygiene by all those in close contact with infants, avoidance of exposure to others with respiratory infections (especially young children during the winter season) and avoidance of cigarette smoke exposure to prevent illness caused by respiratory viruses should be recommended to families. The influenza vaccine is also recommended for VLBW infants when they are older than 6 months; until then, care providers in close contact with the infant should consider receiving the influenza vaccine.

   3. Air travel. In general, air travel is not recommended for infants with BPD because of the increased risk of exposure to infection and because of the lowered cabin pressure resulting in lower oxygen content in the cabin air. If an infant's PaO_2 is ≤ 80 mm Hg, supplemental oxygen will be needed while flying.

B. Immunizations. VLBW infants should receive their routine pediatric immunizations on the same schedule as term infants with the exception of Hepatitis B vaccine. Medically stable, thriving infants should receive the Hepatitis B vaccine as early as 30 days of age regardless of gestational age or birth weight. If the baby is doing well enough medically to go home before 30 days of age, it can be given at the time of discharge to home. Although studies evaluating the long-term immune response to routine immunizations have shown antibody titers to be lower in preterm infants, most achieve titers in the therapeutic range.

C. Growth. VLBW infants have a high incidence of feeding and growth problems for multiple reasons. Infants with severe BPD have increased caloric needs for appropriate weight gain. Many of these infants also have abnormal or delayed oral motor development and have oral aversion because of negative oral stimulation during their early life. Growth should be followed carefully on standardized growth curves using the child's age corrected for prematurity for at least the first 2 years of life. Supplemental caloric density is commonly required to optimize growth. Specialized premature infant formulas with increased protein, calcium, and phosphate (either added to human milk or used alone) should be considered in infants who have borderline growth for the first 6 to 12 months of life. ELBW infants commonly demonstrate growth that is close to or below the fifth percentile. However, if their growth runs parallel to the normal curve, they are usually demonstrating a healthy growth pattern. Infants whose growth curve plateaus or whose growth trajectory falls off warrant further evaluation to assess caloric intake. If growth failure persists, consultation with a gastroenterologist or endocrinologist to rule out gastrointestinal pathology such as severe gastroesophageal reflux disease or endocrinologic problems such as growth hormone deficiency should be considered.

   Gastrostomy tube placement may be necessary in a small subset of patients with severe feeding problems. Long-term feeding problems are frequent in this population of children and they usually require specialized feeding and oral motor therapy to ultimately wean from gastrostomy tube feedings.

   1. Anemia. VLBW infants are at risk for iron deficiency anemia and should receive supplemental iron for the first 12 to 15 months of life.

   2. Rickets. VLBW infants who have had nutritional deficits in calcium, phosphorous, or vitamin D intake are at increased risk for rickets. Infants who are at highest risk are those treated with long-term parenteral nutrition, furosemide, and those with decreased vitamin D absorption due to fat malabsorption. Infants with rickets diagnosed in the neonatal intensive care unit (NICU) may need continued supplementation of calcium, phosphorous, and vitamin D during the first year of life. Supplemental vitamin D (400 IU/day) should also be provided to all infants discharged home on human milk.

D. Sensory issues that need follow-up include vision and hearing.

   1. Ophthalmologic follow-up (see Chap. 35A). Infants with severe retinopathy of prematurity (ROP) are at increased risk of significant vision loss or blindness, if retinal detachment occurs. The risk of severe ROP is highest in the ELBW population in whom the incidence of blindness is 2% to 9%. Preterm infants with mild or moderately severe ROP that has regressed and even those with no ROP are at increased risk of ophthalmologic problems including refractive error (myopia most commonly), strabismus (both esotropia and exotropia), amblyopia, and glaucoma. All VLBW infants should have follow-up with an ophthalmologist who has experience with ophthalmologic problems related to prematurity. This should occur by 8 months of age and then according to the ophthalmologist's recommendation, usually again at 3 years of age at the latest.

2. **Hearing follow-up.** Hearing loss occurs in approximately 2% to 11% of VLBW infants. Prematurity increases the risk of both sensorineural and conductive hearing loss. All VLBW infants should be screened both in the neonatal period and again at 1 year of age (earlier if parental concerns are noted or if the infant has additional risk factors for hearing loss) (see Chap. 35B). There is also evidence that VLBW infants are at increased risk for central auditory processing problems.

E. **Dental problems.** VLBW infants have been noted to have an increased incidence of enamel hypoplasia and discoloration. Long-term oral intubation in the neonatal period may result in palate and alveolar ridge deformation affecting tooth development. Referral to a pediatric dentist in the first 18 months of life is recommended, as is routine supplemental fluoride.

III. **NEURODEVELOPMENTAL OUTCOMES.** Infants with intracranial hemorrhage, in particular parenchymal hemorrhage, or periventricular white matter injury are at increased risk of neuromotor and cognitive delay. Infants with white matter injury are also at increased risk of visuomotor problems, as well as visual field deficits. Among ELBW infants with neonatal complications including BPD, brain injury (defined on ultrasonographic imaging as intraparenchymal echodensity, periventricular leukomalacia, porencephalic cyst, grade 3 or 4 intraventricular hemorrhage (IVH) and severe ROP (threshold or stage 4 or 5 ROP in one or both eyes), 88% had poor neurosensory outcomes at 18 months of age with either cerebral palsy, cognitive delay, severe hearing loss, or bilateral blindness. Infants with cerebellar hemorrhage are at increased risk for motor development as well as cognitive, behavioral, functional, and social development.

A. **Neuromotor problems.** The incidence of cerebral palsy is 7% to 12% in VLBW infants and 11% to 15% in ELBW infants. The most common type of cerebral palsy is spastic diplegia. This correlates to the anatomic location of the corticospinal tracts in the periventricular white matter. VLBW infants are also at risk for other types of abnormal motor development including motor coordination problems and later problems with motor planning.

1. Both transient and long-term motor problems in infants require assessment and treatment by physical therapists and occupational therapists. These services are usually provided at home through local programs. Infants with sensorineural handicaps require coordination of appropriate clinical services and developmental programs. For older children, consultation with the schools and participation in an educational plan are important.

2. Early diagnosis and referral to a neurologist and orthopedic surgeon will prompt referral for appropriate early intervention services such as physical and occupational therapy. Some infants with cerebral palsy are candidates for treatment with orthotics or other adaptive equipment. Others with significant spasticity are candidates for treatment with botulinum-A toxin (Botox) injections. In the case of severe spasticity, treatment with baclofen (oral or through an intrathecal catheter with a subcutaneous pump) may be helpful. Older children are candidates for surgical procedures.

B. **Cognitive delay.** Progress is typically assessed by use of some form of intelligence quotient (IQ) or development quotient (DQ) on an established scale such as the Bayley Scales of Infant Development or the Mullen Scales of Early Learning.

1. VLBW infants tend to have average scores somewhat lower on such scales than term infants, but many still fall within the normal range. The percentage of VLBW infants with scores >2 standard deviations below the mean is between 5% and 20% and between 14% and 40% for ELBW infants. Most studies reflect the status of children younger than age 2. Among older children, the percentage of children who are severely affected appears to be the same, but the percentage with school failure or school problems is as high as 50%, with rates of 20% even among children with average IQ scores. When children were tested at ages 8 to 11, learning disabilities particularly related to visual spatial and visual motor abilities, written output and verbal functioning were more common in ELBW infants (without neurologic problems diagnosed) compared to term infants of similar sociodemographic status. More than 50% of ELBW infants require some

type of special education assistance compared to <15% of healthy term infants. However, children who were ELBW assessed in the teenage years with measures of self esteem do not differ from term infants.

2. Referral to early intervention programs at the time of discharge from the NICU allows early identification of children with delays and referral for therapy from educational specialists and speech therapists when appropriate. Children with severe language delays may also benefit from referral to special communication programs that utilize adaptive technology to enhance language and communication.

C. Emotional and behavioral health

1. **Sleep problems** are more common in preterm than term infants. The cause is frequently multifactorial with medical and behavioral components. Parents may benefit from books on sleep training or in more severe cases, referral to a sleep specialist.

2. **Behavior problems.** VLBW children are at increased risk for behavior problems related to hyperactivity and/or attention deficit. The risk factors for behavioral problems also include stress within the family, maternal depression, and smoking. Behavior problems can contribute to school difficulties. In relation to both school problems and other health issues, VLBW children are seen as less socially competent than normal BW children. Detection of behavioral problems is achieved most commonly using scales developed to elicit parental and teacher concerns. The youngest children for whom such standardized scales are available are 2 years old. Management depends on the nature of the problem and the degree of functional disruption. Some problems may be managed with special educational programs; others may involve referral to appropriate psychotherapy services.

IV. DEVELOPMENTAL FOLLOW-UP PROGRAMS support optimization of health outcomes for NICU graduates and provide feedback information for improvement of medical care. Activities can include the following:

A. Management of sequelae associated with prematurity. As ever smaller infants survive, the risk of chronic sequelae increases.

B. Consultative assessment and referral. Regardless of specific morbidity at the time of discharge, NICU graduates require surveillance for the emergence of a variety of problems that may require referral to and coordination of multiple preventive and rehabilitative services.

C. Monitoring outcomes. Information on health problems and use of services by NICU graduates is integral to both the assessment of the effect of services and the counseling of parents regarding an individual child's future.

D. Program structure

1. The population requiring follow-up care differs with each NICU and the availability and quality of community resources. Most programs use as criteria some combination of birth weight and specific complications. The criteria must be explicit and well understood by all members of the NICU team, with mechanisms developed for identifying and referring appropriate children.

2. Visits depend on the infant's needs and community resources. Some programs recommend a first visit within a few weeks of discharge to assess the transition to home. If not dictated by acute problems, future visits are scheduled to assess progress in key activities. In the absence of acute care needs, we assess patients routinely at 6-month intervals.

3. Because the focus of follow-up care is enhancement of individual and family function, personnel must have breadth of expertise, including (i) clinical skill in the management of sequelae of prematurity; (ii) the ability to perform neurologic and cognitive diagnostic assessment;(iii) familiarity with general pediatric problems presenting in premature infants; (iv) the ability to manage children with complex medical, motor, and cognitive problems; and (v) knowledge of the availability of and access to community programs.

4. Methods for assessing an individual's progress depend on the need for direct assessment by health professionals and the quality of primary care and early

intervention services. A variety of indirect approaches including parental surveys now exist for children with few problems and access to adequate community resources that provide information needed by NICU programs. Recommended staff team members and consultants include pediatrician (developmental specialist or neonatologist), neonatology fellows or pediatric residents (for training), pediatric neurologist, physical therapist, psychologist, occupational therapist, dietician, speech and language specialist, and social worker.

5. **Family/parent function and support.** Having a premature infant is often the most stressful experience parents have had. Providing specialized care in assessment, supportive counselling and resources to families caring for the VLBW infant is essential and includes special attention to issues of postpartum affective conditions and anxiety following the potentially traumatic experience of having a critically ill infant. Provision of specialized behavioral guidance and supportive counseling in addition to facilitating referrals to community providers for additional care should be provided by the team. Attending to the basic needs of families including health insurance issues, respite, advocating for services in the community, financial resources, and marital stress are also important.

Suggested Readings

Johnson S, Marlow N. Developmental screen or developmental testing? *Early Hum Dev* 2006;82(3):173–83.

Wilson-Costello D, Friedman H, Minich N, et al. Improved neurodevelopmental outcomes for extremely low birth weight infants in 2000–2002. *Pediatrics* 2007;119(1):37–45.

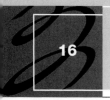

16 DISCHARGE PLANNING*
Ginny May and Linda Zaccagnini

$\mathcal{T}$he survival rate for low-birth-weight (<2,500 g), moderately low-birth-weight (1,500–2,500 g), very low birth weight (<1,500 g), and extremely low-birth-weight (<1,000 g) infants has increased in the past three decades. The infant who weighs <750 g has a >30% chance of survival, while survival rates for the infant weighing >1,000 g are 90% (see Fig. 3B.2 and 3B.3 in Chap. 3). Greater survival rates for preterm infants have created a population with unique long-term health-care needs. Changes in the health-care system in the United States are encouraging earlier discharge and more out-of-hospital care.

Effective discharge planning promotes continuity of care from hospital to home. The plan must provide for individualized family and infant needs and prepare family members and health-care providers for infant care requirements.

I. FEATURES OF A COMPREHENSIVE DISCHARGE PLAN
  A. Individualized to meet infant and family needs and resources.
  B. Begins early—planning can begin with a prenatal diagnosis or upon admission to the neonatal intensive care unit (NICU).
  C. Includes ongoing assessment and clearly identified goals.
  D. Anticipates potential delays in development and directs care toward prevention and early intervention.
  E. Community-based, with early identification of a primary pediatrician.
  F. Decreases delays in accessing care and progressing through the provider system.
  G. Decreases fragmentation of care and duplication of services.
  H. Decreases the possibility of readmission.
  I. Increases the quality of care.
II. SYSTEM ASSESSMENT. It is important to know how your facility functions, who assumes responsibility for various components of discharge planning, and how communication is carried out. Assigning a consistent team of caregivers assists the family in developing trusting relationships with staff, enhances communication with care providers, and minimizes the number of staff with whom the family would need to interact. Early and ongoing planning will expedite discharge, can prevent costly delays, and helps to prevent readmissions that are traumatic to both the infant and the family. Identifying payer coverage early promotes timely assessment of contractual requirements.
  A. A **physician** or **nurse practitioner** is responsible for daily management of care. In teaching institutions where staff rotate, families may need to adjust to many different providers. For those infants with complex issues, identifying a primary attending physician or practitioner provides the family with more continuity.
  B. **The infant's primary nurse and nursing team** follows the family through the NICU stay coordinating, implementing, and evaluating the developed care plan.
  C. **Respiratory, physical, and occupational therapists** teach families skills and assist in transitioning care to community resources.
  D. **Social workers** support the family in crisis and assist in locating available financial and emotional resources.

*This is a revision of a chapter in the 4th edition originally written by Kimberly Cox and Linda Zaccagnini. Thanks also to Theresa Andrews, RN at Children's Hospital Boston.

E. The role of **discharge coordinator** varies from institution to institution, and as input on the discharge plan is provided, the coordinator organizes the various aspects of care.

F. **Interpreters** assist in communication with families when indicated.

G. **Payer resources such as** health maintenance organization (HMOs) and third-party payers, often have case managers to assist in the coordination of services. Use of preferred providers may be contractually required. Case managers can clarify issues of coverage and resource availability.

III. **FAMILY ASSESSMENT** may begin before admission. Ongoing communication between professionals and the family will allow providers to develop a multidisciplinary, individualized care plan that includes discharge planning. Involving the family in developing the plan optimizes its success by individualizing the plan and enhancing the parents' feeling of control. The transition to home can go smoothly, even in the most complex cases, with early planning, ongoing teaching, and attention to the family's needs and resources.

A. **Family dynamics.** Include the following issues when assessing the family's readiness for discharge:

1. Willingness to assume responsibility for care.
2. Previous or present experiences with infant care and medical procedures.
3. Actual as well as perceived complexity of the skills required to care for the infant.
4. Family structure.
5. Financial concerns.
6. Home setting.
7. Coping skills.
8. Supports.
9. Medical and psychological history (ongoing illness may impact caretaking needs).
10. Cultural beliefs (bonding, roles, and available supports).
11. Language barriers (may require an interpreter).

B. **Home environment.** Structural components of the home may need alteration. Confirm electrical, water, heating, cooling, and communication (telephone) resources.

C. **Stress and coping.** In the NICU, discuss what it will be like to have the infant at home. Consider who will be involved and available for support. Referral to a parent group or specialized support group may be helpful. Explore the availability of community services for counseling and social needs. The following are common issues:

1. **Grief.** Parents need to cope with the loss of their "perfect" infant. The four psychological effects of a high-risk pregnancy are denial, blame and guilt, feelings of failure, and ambivalence.
2. **Abandonment and isolation.** Much attention and support are available while the infant is hospitalized. After discharge, parents may feel alone and abandoned.
3. **Siblings.** Other children in the family may delay reacting until the new baby comes home and then respond with regressive or acting-out behaviors.
4. **Parenting disorders.** When the child is well, parents may be so overburdened with the memories of severe illness that they never treat the infant as a healthy child.
5. **Privacy.** Infants requiring complex care at home may require "blocks" of nursing or ancillary care at home; these disrupt space and privacy. An array of "strangers" in the home adds stress to the family.

D. **Financial resources.** Complete a financial assessment early. Early delivery or complex care can alter the family's plans for work and child care. Loss of work, income changes, cost of copayments, and inability to make career moves because of insurance coverage all impact the family's financial stability.

IV. **INFANT'S READINESS FOR DISCHARGE**

A. **Healthy growing preterm infants** are considered ready for discharge when they meet the following criteria:

1. Ability to maintain temperature in an open crib.
2. Ability to take all feedings by bottle or breast without respiratory compromise.
3. No apnea or bradycardia for 5 days (see Chap. 24i).
4. Steady weight gain.

B. Infants with specialized needs require a complex, flexible, ongoing discharge, and teaching plan. Discharge specifics may not be identified until just before discharge. Medications and special formulas or dietary supplements should be obtained as early as possible to optimize teaching. It is important to consider the relative fragility and stability of various systems and the complexity of interventions. Include assessment of behavioral and developmental issues, and evaluate parental recognition and response.

C. Discharge screening. Complete routine screening tests and immunizations according to individual institutional guidelines (see Table 16.1).

1. **Hearing screening** (see Chap. 35B and Table 16.1).
2. **Eye examinations** (see Chap. 35A and Table 16.1).
3. **Cranial ultrasonography** (see Chap. 27B and Table 16.1) screening for intraventricular hemorrhage and periventricular leukomalacia for all infants who satisfy the following criteria:
   a. Weigh <1,500 g or are under 32 weeks gestational age.
   b. Are under 34 weeks gestational age if mechanically ventilated.
      Perform head ultrasonography at day of life 1 to 3 if results alter clinical management, day of life 7 to 10, and then day of life 21 to 28.
4. **Immunizations.** Administer according to American Academy of Pediatrics guidelines based on chronologic, not postconceptional, age (see Chap. 3B).

V. FOLLOW-UP CARE. The infant with special needs may require many different services and providers to meet all of the child's needs.

A. Primary care is usually provided through a pediatrician, family practitioner, or nurse practitioner. Ongoing communication between NICU staff and the primary-care provider begins long before discharge. This maintains continuity and improves the infant's chances of receiving appropriate medical care after discharge.

B. Specialty services may be required.

C. Infant follow-up programs affiliated with many Level III nurseries offer multidisciplinary services including developmental assessments, hearing and visual screening, physical therapy assessments, and referrals to community-based providers and support groups (see Chap. 15).

D. Early intervention programs are community-based and offer multidisciplinary services for children from birth to age 3. Children deemed at biological, environmental, or emotional risk are eligible. Programs are partially federally funded and are offered free or on a sliding scale. They provide multidisciplinary services including physical therapy, early childhood education, social services, and parental support groups. Services may be home-based or center-based. Make referrals early in the child's hospital stay, as some centers have long waiting lists.

VI. PREPARING HOME SERVICES FOR THE INFANT'S DISCHARGE

A. Home-care services are becoming more widely available; however, their ability to provide specialized pediatric or neonatal services is variable. Assess individual programs separately before making a referral.

B. Skilled nursing care

1. **Public health nurses** may do home visits before discharge to assess the family's readiness and the home situation. They may also do well-baby and basic health-care teaching.
2. **Visiting nurse associations** provide home visits for reinforcement of teaching, health and psychosocial assessments, and short-term treatments or nursing care. Usually they charge service fees.
3. **Home health-care agencies** provide skilled nursing care, home health aids, physical and/or occupational therapy, and medical equipment and supplies. Fees for service and insurance coverage are highly variable.

C. Respite care. Many parents do not realize how emotionally and physically draining it can be to care for a child with complex medical needs. The usual

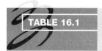

| TABLE 16.1 | Guidelines for Routine Screening, Testing, Treatment, and Follow-up at Neonatal Intensive Care Unit (NICU), Beth Israel Deaconess Medical Center |

Newborn state screening for metabolic disease (see Chap. 29D)

Criteria

■ All infants admitted to the NICU

Initial

■ Day 3 or discharge (D/C) date (whichever comes first)

Follow-up

■ Day 14 or D/C date (whichever comes first)
■ Week 6 (if BW <1,500 g)
■ Week 10 (if BW <1,500 g)

Head ultrasonography (see Chap. 27B)

Criteria

■ All infants with gestational age (GA) <32 wk (an ultrasonography would be done at any GA at any time if thought to be clinically indicated)

Initial

■ Day 7–10 (in the case of critically ill infants, when results of an earlier ultrasonography may alter clinical management, an ultrasonography should be performed at the discretion of the clinician)

Follow-up (minimum if no abnormalities noted)

■ If no hemorrhage or germinal matrix hemorrhage
  ■ If <28 wk: week 4 *and* at 36 wk corrected age (or discharge if <36 wk)
  ■ If <28 and 0/7–31 and 6/7 wk: week 4 *or* at 36 wk corrected age (or discharge if <36 wk)
■ If intraventricular (grade 2+) or intraparenchymal hemorrhage: follow-up at least weekly until stable (more frequently if unstable posthemorrhagic hydrocephalus and clinically indicated)

Ophthalmologic examination (see Chap. 35A)

Criteria

■ All infants with BW <1,500 g or GA <32 wk

Initial

■ If <27 wk: week 6
■ If 27–28 wk: week 5
■ If 29–30 wk: week 4
■ If 31–316/7 wk: week 3

Note

■ If the infant is transferred to another nursery before 4 wk of age, recommend examination at the receiving hospital
■ If the infant is discharged home before 4 wk of age, examine before discharge

Follow-up (based on initial examination findings)

■ Immature retina zone 1 or zone 2, or low-grade ROP: follow-up every 2 wk
■ Immature retina zone 3: follow-up in 4–10 wk
■ Prethreshold ROP: follow-up weekly
■ Regressing ROP: follow-up every 1–10 wk depending on zone

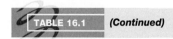

TABLE 16.1   *(Continued)*

Audiology screening (see Chap. 35B)

Criteria

■ All infants to be discharged home from NICU

Timing

■ Examine at 34 wk gestation or greater

Car seat screening

Criteria

■ All infants to be discharged from NICU **and** born at <37 wk or with other conditions that may compromise respiratory status (we also screen **ALL** infants <2,500 g)

Timing

■ Screen before discharge home

Hepatitis B vaccination (see Chap. 3B)

Criteria

■ All infants to be discharged home from NICU or at 2 mo of age

Initial

■ If weight >2,000 g: vaccinate before discharge home or at 2 mo
■ If weight <2,000 g: vaccinate at 2 mo of age

Follow-up (dose 2)

■ Vaccinate 2 mo after initial vaccine dose

Occupational therapy consultation

Criteria

■ All infants meeting one of the following conditions:
　■ Birth at or <28 wk gestation
　■ BW <1,000 g
　■ Neurological insults including IVH, PVL, seizure disorder
　■ Genetic syndromes that affect quality of movement or state regulation
　■ Symptoms associated with neonatal abstinence syndrome
　■ Orthopaedic or musculoskeletal impairments
　■ Born to parents with physical disabilities
　■ Brachial plexus palsy (Erb or Klumpke palsy)
　■ Critically ill term infants

Social security

Criteria

■ All infants meeting one of the following conditions:
　■ BW <1,200 g
　■ BW 1,200–2,000 g and at least 4 wk small for gestational age (GA) (refer to growth curve)
　■ Any infant with serious handicapping conditions

Timing

■ Application completed during first week of life

Follow-up

■ Parent notifies social security intake (SSI) office of baby's discharge through form letter

(continued)

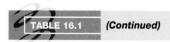

TABLE 16.1   *(Continued)*

Infant follow-up program (IFUP)
Criteria

- All infants meeting one of the following conditions:
  - BW <1,000 g
  - BW 1,000–1,499 g with one of the following:
  - Maternal age <20
  - IVH (note grade)
  - PVL
  - Surgical NEC
  - ROP
  - Psychosocial concerns

Timing

- Referral completed before discharge

Neonatal neurology program
Criteria

- All infants meeting one of the following conditions:
  - Neurologic disorders (e.g., stroke, intracranial hemorrhage, and neonatal seizures)
  - Neuromuscular disorders
  - BW <1,500 g with IVH (grades 2–4) or PVL (referral to infant follow-up program also)

Timing

- Referral completed before discharge

Early intervention program (EIP)
Criteria

- Infant meeting **four** or more of the following criteria:
  - BW <1,200 g
  - GA <32 wk
  - NICU admission >5 d
  - Apgar <5 at 5 min
  - Intrauterine growth restriction (IUGR) or small for gestational age (SGA) (refer to growth curves)
  - Hospital stay >25 d
  - Chronic feeding difficulties
  - Insecure attachment
  - Suspected central nervous system abnormality
  - Maternal age <17 *or* 3 or more births at maternal age <20
  - Maternal education <10 yr
  - Parental chronic illness or disability affecting caregiving
  - Lack of family supports
  - Inadequate food, shelter, and clothing
  - Open or confirmed protective service investigation ("51-A")
  - Substance abuse in the home
  - Domestic violence in the home

Timing

- Referral completed before discharge

ROP = retinopathy of prematurity; IVH = intraventricular hemorrhage; PVL = periventricular leukomalacia; BW = birth weight; GA = gestational age.

support people, such as relatives, friends, and baby-sitters, may be uncomfortable or unable to deal with the added responsibility. Explore resources for respite care before discharge.

D. **Notify emergency care providers** including community hospital emergency wards and local Emergency medical technician (EMT) or fire responders of the child's presence, medical needs, and possible problems. This will assure appropriate emergency response.

E. **Local utility companies** (telephone, electricity, fuel) should be notified in writing of the child's presence in the home so they will assign priority resumption of services if there is an interruption.

F. **Structural modifications** may be required to support access and/or support mechanical equipment

G. **Supplies and equipment**
1. Order **equipment** well before discharge to ensure availability. Have caregivers care for their child using the home monitors and oxygen equipment in the NICU. This increases their skill and confidence.
2. **Supplies, medications, and special formulas** or dietary supplements should also be specified and ordered as early as possible. Many preparations vary in the community; obtaining and utilizing these items during hands-on teaching in the NICU increases the family's understanding and promotes safety.

VII. **PREPARING THE FAMILY FOR DISCHARGE**
A. **Simplify care** by thoroughly reviewing the infant's care regimen. Alter medication schedules to fit the family's schedule. Eliminate unnecessary medications. Formulas and additives can be changed to less-expensive or more easily obtained products. Get the infant used to the daily schedule that will be followed at home.
B. Begin **teaching** early to allow the caregivers adequate time to process information, practice skills, and formulate questions. Make teaching protocols detailed and thorough. Include written information for the family to take home to use as reference (see Fig. 16.1 and Table 16.2). Standardize information to ensure that every family member receives the same essential information. Address well-baby care, developmental issues, and necessary medical information. Include several family members in the learning process so that the parents can get needed support.
C. **Provide transitional programs for parents.** Schedule blocks of hands-on care or have the parents room in with the infant in the NICU. This maximizes parental confidence and competence and helps strengthen the parent–infant bond.
D. **Retrotransfer** to a Level II nursery in the community. This may allow the family to spend more time with the infant, and facilitate learning in a less-acute environment.
E. It is vital to **include the family** in formulating all plans and, whenever possible, choosing care providers.

VIII. **COMMUNICATION WITH COMMUNITY PROVIDERS** is essential for a smooth transition to home. Identification of the primary-care provider early allows for ongoing updates in complex situations. Utilizing the primary-care providers network along with insurance guidelines will avoid confusion for an already anxious family. A verbal conversation before discharge promptly followed up with the faxed dictated summary (Table 16.3) and copies of in-house studies will allow for optimal communication. A dictated summary may need to be also faxed to follow-up programs as deemed appropriate.

IX. **ALTERNATIVES TO HOME DISCHARGE** may be temporary or permanent. Integrating the child into the home may be difficult because of medical needs or family dynamics. Decisions regarding alternative placement may be painful for the family. Alternatives vary widely from community to community.
A. **Specialized foster care** places the special-needs infant in a home setting with specially trained caregivers. The ultimate goal is to place the infant back with the family.
B. **Pediatric rehabilitation hospitals** can be used for the high-risk infant who requires ongoing but less-acute hospital care.
C. **Pediatric nursing homes** provide extended care at a skilled level.

BETH ISRAEL DEACONESS MEDICAL CENTER
A member of CAREGROUP
Boston, MA 02215

NEONATAL INTENSIVE CARE UNIT
DISCHARGE INSTRUCTION SHEET

Baby's Caregivers:
Attending Neonatologist at Discharge: _____
Primary Nurse & Team: _____
Social Worker: _____

PARENT INFORMATION

	Reviewed	N/A	RN Signature	Date
NICU parent packet	☐		_____	__/__/__
WIC form	☐	☐	_____	__/__/__
Immunization booklet	☐	☐	_____	__/__/__
Synagis information sheet	☐	☐	_____	__/__/__
Hepatitis B information sheet	☐	☐	_____	__/__/__
Other _____	☐	☐	_____	__/__/__

PREPARATION FOR DISCHARGE

	Reviewed	RN Signature	Date
Feeding: breast milk or formula	☐	_____	__/__/__
Bowel and bladder pattern	☐	_____	__/__/__
Bulb syringe use	☐	_____	__/__/__
Bathing, skin care, cord care	☐	_____	__/__/__
Temperature taking	☐	_____	__/__/__
Circumcision care (if applicable)	☐	_____	__/__/__
CPR instruction	☐	_____	__/__/__
When to call your baby's doctor	☐	_____	__/__/__
Car seat instruction	☐	_____	__/__/__
Car seat screening	☐	_____	__/__/__
Protection from infection	☐	_____	__/__/__
Other _____	☐	_____	__/__/__

DATE OF DISCHARGE: __/__/__

Discharge Measurements: RN Signature   Date
Weight _____ gms (___ lbs ___ oz) _____ __/__/__
Length _____ cm (___ in) _____ __/__/__
Head Circumference _____ cm (___ in) _____ __/__/__

STATE NEWBORN SCREENING: Most recent test: __/__/__

NEWBORN HEARING SCREEN: ☐Pass ☐Refer (see follow-up care)

ADDITIONAL NOTES:

BABY'S FOLLOW UP CARE

Primary Pediatric Provider: ☐N/A
Name: _____
Telephone: _____
Appt. Date: __/__/__   Time: _____
Early Intervention: ☐N/A
Center Name/Town: _____
Telephone: _____
Initial Contact: __/__/__ Date Confirmed: __/__/__
Visiting Nurse: ☐N/A
Center Name/Town: _____
Telephone: _____
Date Contacted: __/__/__   ☐ referral faxed
Infant Follow-up Program: (617) 667-1330 ☐N/A
(<1500g-see criteria on referral sheet)
Date Contacted: __/__/__   ☐ referral faxed
Neonatal Neurology Program: (617) 355-6388 ☐N/A
Children's Hospital
(see criteria on referral sheet)
Date Contacted: __/__/__
Lactation Consultant: ☐N/A
Name: _____
Telephone: _____
Ophthalmologist: ☐N/A
Name: _____
Telephone: _____
Date: __/__/__   Time: _____
☐ Recommended Follow-up at 8 months
Follow-up Hearing Screen: ☐N/A
Date: __/__/__   Time: _____
Location:
☐ Children's Hospital - Fegan 11   (617) 355-6461
☐ Children's Hospital - Lexington (781) 672-2000
☐ HVMA - Kenmore   (617) 421-8888
☐ Other: _____   ( ) ___ - _____
Other:

Medication/Feeding Additives	Reason	Amount to give	When to give	How to give
☐ Check medroom for stored breastmilk				

This information has been reviewed with me, and my questions have been answered. I authorize the NICU staff to provide necessary information from my child's medical record to the above named providers/services.

_____   ☐ Copy given to parent   _____   __/__/__
Parent Signature   RN Signature   Date

MC0104   Revised 5/00   White - Medical Record   Yellow - Parent   *Note: This is a general guideline, and it does not represent a professional standard of care governing providers' obligations to patients. Care is revised to meet individual patient needs.*   ©Beth Israel Deaconess Medical Center

Figure 16.1. Newborn discharge instruction sheet.

    D. Hospice care may be institutional or home-based. It focuses on maximizing the quality of life when cure is no longer possible.

X. FINANCIAL CONCERNS

    A. Neonatal intensive care, especially for very low birth weight infants, ranks among the most costly of all hospital admissions. Health insurance may not cover 100% of costs.

    B. Home-care benefits are often limited. Prior authorization is almost universally required. Services may be restricted to a particular provider or to a finite period.

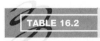

| TABLE 16.2 | Additional Discharge Instruction Sheet |

Beth Israel Deaconess Medical Center, Boston, MA

Parent resources

At Beth Israel Deaconess Medical Center

- Neonatal Intensive Care Unit ⋯⋯⋯⋯⋯⋯⋯⋯⋯⋯⋯⋯⋯ (617) 667–4042
- Social Work Office ⋯⋯⋯⋯⋯⋯⋯⋯⋯⋯⋯⋯⋯⋯⋯⋯⋯ (617) 667–3421
- Birth Certificate Office ⋯⋯⋯⋯⋯⋯⋯⋯⋯⋯⋯⋯⋯⋯⋯ (617) 667–4167
- Learning Center ⋯⋯⋯⋯⋯⋯⋯⋯⋯⋯⋯⋯⋯⋯⋯⋯⋯⋯ (617) 667–9100

Community resources

- **Poison Control Center** ⋯⋯⋯⋯⋯⋯⋯⋯⋯ (617) 232-2120/(800) 682–9211
- **Children's Hospital (Boston) Emergency Room** ⋯⋯⋯⋯⋯ (617) 355–6611
- **Parental Stress Line** ⋯⋯⋯⋯⋯⋯⋯⋯⋯⋯⋯⋯⋯⋯⋯ (800) 632–8188
- **Battered Women's Hotline** (24 h) ⋯⋯⋯⋯⋯⋯⋯⋯⋯⋯ (617) 661–7203
- **Statewide Alcohol and Drug Hotline** ⋯⋯⋯⋯⋯⋯⋯⋯⋯ (800) 327–5050
- **Mother of Twins Association** ⋯⋯⋯⋯⋯⋯⋯⋯⋯⋯⋯⋯ (781) 646–TWIN
- **Triplets, Moms, and More** ⋯⋯⋯⋯⋯⋯⋯⋯⋯⋯⋯⋯⋯ (339) 449–3261

Breast-feeding

- BI-Deaconess Lactation Program ⋯⋯⋯⋯⋯⋯⋯⋯⋯⋯⋯ (617) 667–5765
- La Leche League of Mass ⋯⋯⋯⋯⋯⋯⋯⋯⋯⋯⋯⋯⋯⋯ (800) 525–3243
- Women, Infants, and Children (WIC) Office ⋯⋯⋯⋯⋯ (617) 624-6100/(800) 942–1007
- Nursing Mother's Council of Boston Area Childbirth Education (BACE) ⋯⋯ (617) 244–5102

When to call your baby's doctor

Any sudden changes in baby's usual patterns of behavior:

- Increased sleepiness
- Increased irritability
- Feeding poorly

Any of the following:

- Breathing difficulties
- Blueness around lips, mouth, or eyes
- Fever (by rectal temperature) over 100°F or 99.6°F under the arm or low temperature under 97°F (rectal)
- Vomiting or diarrhea
- Dry diapers for >12 h
- No bowel movement for >4 d
- Black or bright red color seen in stool

Protecting your baby from infection

Your baby's immune system is still quite immature. This makes him/her especially vulnerable to colds and other communicable diseases. To protect your baby from infections we advise that you do the following:

- Avoid taking your baby to crowded indoor places
- Avoid contact with anyone who has a cold, flu, or other active infection
- Do not allow anyone to smoke around baby
- Encourage anyone who comes into close contact with your baby to wash their hands

(continued)

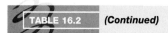

TABLE 16.2   *(Continued)*

Safety

The Commonwealth of Massachusetts requires the use of car seats for all infants and children until they are at least 5-yr-old and weigh over 40 lb. A federally approved infant car seat is required at discharge for any infant leaving the hospital in a private motor vehicle.

TABLE 16.3   **Neonatal Intensive Care Unit (NICU) Discharge/Interim Summary Dictation Guideline**

NICU Discharge/Interim Summary Dictation Guideline

Department of Neonatology Beth Israel Deaconess Medical Center (BIDMC)

Begin dictation when you hear the tone

1. Name of dictator (spell name).
2. Name of attending physician (spell name).
3. Patient's name (spell name). *Use **only** "Boy" or "Girl" for first name.*
4. Service ("neonatology").
5. Patient unit number.
6. Date of birth and sex of patient.
7. Date of admission.
8. Date of discharge. *Use the best estimate. A date **must** be entered.* If interim summary, state "interim date."
9. History.
    a. If interim summary, specify dates covered and author/date of prior summary.
    b. Include reason for admission, birth weight, gestational age.
    c. Maternal history — including prenatal labs, pregnancy, labor, and birth history.
10. Physical examination on admission.
    a. Include weight head circumference, and length — note percentile.
11. Summary of hospital course by systems (concise). Include pertinent lab results
    a. **Respiratory** — Initial impression. Surfactant given? Maximum level of support. Days on ventilation, continuous positive airway pressure (CPAP), supplemental oxygen. If apnea, report how patient was treated, when treatment ended, and condition resolved (levels if still on therapy).
    b. **Cardiovascular** — Diagnoses/therapies in summary form. Echo/electrocardiogram (ECG) results.
    c. **Fluids, electrolytes, nutrition** — Brief feeding history. Include recent weight, length, and head circumference.
    d. **Gastrointestinal (GI)** — Pertinent diagnoses and treatment. Maximum bilirubin and therapy used.
    e. **Hematology** — Patient blood type, brief transfusion summary, recent hematocrit (Hct).
    f. **Infectious disease** — Cultures, antibiotic courses.
    g. **Neurology** — Describe ultrasonographic findings.
    h. **Sensory** —
        i. *Audiology* — "Hearing screening was performed with automated auditory brain stem responses." Results. (If baby didn't pass or testing not performed, indicated date/location of follow-up test or recommend test before discharge.)

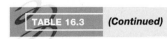

TABLE 16.3 *(Continued)*

     ii. Ophthalmologic findings
- **Not examined:** patient is due for a first examination on.
- **Immature:** eyes examined most recently on revealing immaturity of the retinal vessels but no ROP as of yet. A follow-up examination should be scheduled for the week of.
- **ROP eyes:** examined most recently on, revealing ROP. A follow-up examination by a pediatric ophthalmologist should be scheduled for.
- **Mature:** eyes were examined most recently on, revealing mature retinal vessels. A follow-up exam is recommended in 6 months.

    i. **Psychosocial** — BIDMC Social Work involved with family. The contact social worker is (name), and she can be reached at 667–4700. Follow-up will be provided by (name of agency/social worker and telephone number). (If applicable, "A 51-A has been filed.")

12. Condition at discharge.

13. Discharge disposition (e.g., home, [Level II], [Level III], chronic care]).

14. Name of primary pediatrician (spell name). Phone #: Fax #:.

15. Care/recommendations (quick summary for those assuming care of the infant).
- **a.** Feeds at discharge *(if Neosure, recommend until 6 to 9 months corrected age)*
- **b.** Medications.
- **c.** Car seat screening.
- **d.** State newborn screening status.
- **e.** Immunizations received.
- **f.** Immunizations recommended (dictate verbatim).
  - **i.** "Synagis RSV prophylaxis should be considered from November through March for infants who meet any of the following three criteria: (i) born at <32 wk; (ii) born between 32 and 35 wk with two of the following: daycare during RSV season, a smoker in the household, neuromuscular disease, airway abnormalities, or school age siblings; or (iii) with chronic lung disease."
  - **ii.** "Influenza immunization should be considered annually in the fall for all infants once they reach 6 mo of age. Before this age (and for the first 24 mo of the child's life), immunization against influenza is recommended for household contacts and out-of-home caregivers."
- **g.** Follow-up appointments scheduled/recommended.

16. Discharge diagnoses list.

ROP = retinopathy of prematurity; RSV = respiratory syncytial virus.

C. Alternative funding

    1. Social security. Several states have programs that waive parental income criteria and provide medicaid benefits to infants and children or to those whose hospitalization may be extended if home-care services are not provided.

    2. State government financial assistance. The maternal and child health agencies in most state governments will provide some financial assistance for follow-up of certain infants whose families meet state-established financial criteria. Services vary from state to state but may include physical therapy services, equipment, and diagnostic and treatment services.

    3. Private charities can be explored. Many have local chapters that provide specialized services and supports on an ability to pay or free basis.

    4. Public health departments may offer immunizations and well-child clinics at no cost or very low cost.

    5. Women, Infants, and Children (WIC) Program is federally funded and provides nutrition education and supplemental formula to financially eligible pregnant women and to children up to 5 years of age who are assessed as being at risk.

D. Social services or continuing-care departments are invaluable in determining existing coverage and in accessing alternative sources of financial support.

Suggested Readings

American Academy of Pediatrics, Committee on Fetus and Newborn. Hospital discharge of the high risk neonate-proposed guidelines (RE9812). *Pediatrics* 1998;102:411–441.

American Academy of Pediatrics, Committee on Children With Disabilities. Pediatric services for infants and children with special health care needs. *Pediatrics* 1993;92: 163–165.

American Academy of Pediatrics, Committee on Practice and Ambulatory Medicine. The role of the primary care pediatrician in the management of high-risk newborn infants. *Pediatrics* 1996;98(4 PT 1):786–788.

American Academy of Pediatrics, Task force on Infant Positioning and SIDS Positioning and SIDS. Changing concepts of sudden infant death syndrome: Implications for infant sleep environment and sleep position. *Pediatrics.* 2000;105:650–656.

Damato E. Discharge planning from the neonatal intensive care unit. *J Perinat Neonatal Nurs* 1991;5(1):43.

Hulseman ML, Lee N. The neonatal ICU graduate: Part I. Common problems. *Am Fam Physician* 1992;45(3):1301.

Hulseman ML, Lee N. The neonatal ICU graduate: Part II. Fundamentals of outpatient care. *Am Fam Physician* 1992;45(4):1696.

Hummell P, Cronin J. Home care of the high-risk infant. *Adv Neonatal Care* 2004;4(6): 354–364.

Hutt HL. Home care. In: Kenner C, Brueggemeyer A, Gunderson LP, eds. *Comprehensive neonatal nursing.* Philadelphia: WB Saunders, 1991.

Kenner C, Bagwell G. Assessment and management of the transition to home. In: Kenner C, Brueggemeyer A, Gunderson LP, eds. *Comprehensive neonatal nursing.* Philadelphia: WB Saunders, 1991.

Leonard C. High-risk infant follow-up programs. In: Ballard R, ed. *Pediatric care of the ICN graduate.* Philadelphia: WB Saunders, 1988.

Sherman Michael P, et al. http://www.emedicine.com/pedi/topic2600.htm.

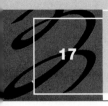

17 SHOCK
Stella Kourembanas

I. **DEFINITION.** Shock is an acute, complex state of circulatory dysfunction resulting in insufficient oxygen and nutrient delivery to satisfy tissue requirements. Systemic hypotension is the key presenting sign of uncompensated shock that eventually progresses to metabolic acidosis. However, the lowest acceptable normal blood pressure (BP) is not well established in newborns, particularly in preterm infants. As a result, the BP that triggers a decision to treat infants who do not have acidosis is somewhat arbitrary. One study reported continuous arterial BP measurements in 103 neonates between 23 and 43 weeks' gestation. On the basis of these data, the statistically defined lower limit of mean arterial pressure during the first postnatal day roughly equals the gestational age of the infant. However, by the third day, >90% of preterm infants <26 weeks' gestation have a mean arterial BP >30 mm Hg. More than 90% of term infants have a mean BP of >45 mm Hg immediately after birth with a rise to >50 mm Hg by the third postnatal day.

II. **ETIOLOGY.** In the immediate postnatal period, abnormal regulation of peripheral vascular resistance with or without myocardial dysfunction is the most frequent cause of hypotension underlying shock, especially in preterm infants. Hypovolemia must also be considered as an underlying cause of shock in the setting of fluid loss (blood, plasma, excessive urine, or transepidermal water losses).

A. **Abnormal peripheral vasoregulation** may be due to (i) increased or dysregulated endothelial nitric oxide (NO) production in the perinatal transitional period, particularly in the preterm neonate; (ii) immature neurovascular pathways; or (iii) proinflammatory cascades that lead to vasodilation

B. **Hypovolemia.** Common scenarios of fluid loss in the neonatal period include the following:
1. Placental hemorrhage, as in abruptio placentae or placenta previa.
2. Fetal-to-maternal hemorrhage (diagnosed by the Kleihauer-Betke test of the mother's blood for fetal erythrocytes).
3. Twin-to-twin transfusion.
4. Intracranial hemorrhage.
5. Massive pulmonary hemorrhage (i.e., patent ductus arteriosus, [PDA]).
6. Disseminated intravascular coagulation (DIC) or other severe coagulopathies.
7. Plasma loss into the extravascular compartment, as seen with low oncotic pressure states or capillary leak syndrome (e.g., sepsis).
8. Excessive extracellular fluid losses, as seen with volume depletion from insensible water loss or inappropriate diuresis, commonly seen in extremely low birth weight infants.

C. **Myocardial dysfunction.** Although an infant's myocardium normally exhibits good contractility, various perinatal insults, congenital abnormalities, or arrhythmias can result in heart failure:
1. Intrapartum asphyxia can cause poor contractility and papillary muscle dysfunction with tricuspid regurgitation, resulting in low cardiac output.
2. Myocardial dysfunction can occur secondary to infectious agents (bacterial or viral) or metabolic abnormalities such as hypoglycemia. Cardiomyopathy can be seen in infants of diabetic mothers (IDMs) with or without hypoglycemia.
3. Obstruction to blood flow resulting in decreased cardiac output can be seen with many congenital heart defects.

a. **Inflow obstructions**
   i. Total anomalous pulmonary venous return.
   ii. Cor triatriatum.
   iii. Tricuspid atresia.
   iv. Mitral atresia.
   v. Acquired inflow obstructions can occur from intravascular air or thrombotic embolus, or from increased intrathoracic pressure caused by high airway pressures, pneumothorax, pneumomediastinum, or pneumopericardium.

b. **Outflow obstructions**
   i. Pulmonary stenosis or atresia.
   ii. Aortic stenosis or atresia.
   iii. Hypertrophic subaortic stenosis seen in IDMs with compromised left ventricular outflow, particularly when cardiotonic agents are used.
   iv. Coarctation of the aorta or interrupted aortic arch.
   v. Arrhythmias, if prolonged. Supraventricular arrhythmias such as paroxysmal atrial tachycardia are most common.

III. DIAGNOSIS

A. Clinical presentation. In addition to hypotension and tachycardia (the latter is not always present in very premature infants), shock is manifested principally by (i) pallor and poor skin perfusion, (ii) cool extremities, (iii) central nervous system signs of lethargy, and (iv) decreased urine output. Organ dysfunction occurs because of inadequate blood flow and oxygenation, and cellular metabolism becomes predominantly anaerobic, producing lactic and pyruvic acid. Hence, metabolic acidosis often indicates inadequate circulation. In preterm infants, the associated decrease in brain blood flow and oxygen supply during severe hypotension predisposes to intraventricular hemorrhage and periventricular leukomalacia with long-term neurodevelopmental abnormalities. In addition, in extremely low birth weight infants, the vasculature of the cerebral cortex may respond with vasoconstriction to transient myocardial dysfunction/shock rather than vasodilation, further diminishing cerebral perfusion and increasing the risk for neurologic injury.

IV. TREATMENT.

Volume, pressors, and inotropes are used to treat shock in the neonate.

A. Volume. Small randomized controlled trials support the usefulness of isotonic crystalloid rather than albumin-containing solutions for acute volume expansion as they are more readily available, have lower cost, and lesser risk of infectious complications. Importantly, albumin has not been shown to be more efficacious than saline in treating hypotension. An infusion of 10 to 20 mL/kg isotonic saline solution is used to treat suspected hypovolemia. Blood cell transfusions or fresh frozen plasma are recommended in cases of blood loss or DIC.

B. Measurement of **central venous pressure** (CVP) may help management, especially in term or late preterm infants. CVP is measured using a catheter with its tip in the right atrium or in the intrathoracic superior vena cava. The catheter can be placed through the umbilical vein or percutaneously through the external or internal jugular or subclavian vein. In many infants, maintaining CVP at 5 to 8 mm Hg with volume infusions is associated with improved cardiac output. If CVP exceeds 5 to 8 mm Hg, additional volume will usually not be helpful. CVP is influenced by noncardiac factors such as ventilator pressures and by cardiac factors such as tricuspid valve function. Both types of factors may affect the interpretation and usefulness of CVP measurements.

C. Correction of negative inotropic factors such as hypoxia, acidosis, hypoglycemia, and other metabolic derangements will improve cardiac output. In addition, hypocalcemia frequently occurs in infants with circulatory failure, especially if they have received large amounts of volume resuscitation; this must be corrected. In this setting, calcium frequently produces a positive inotropic response. Calcium gluconate 10% (1 mL/kg) can be infused slowly if ionized calcium levels are low.

D. Positive inotropic agents
   1. Sympathomimetic amines are commonly used in infants. The advantages include rapidity of onset, ability to control dosage, and ultrashort half-life.

a. **Dopamine** is a naturally occurring catecholamine. Exogenous dopamine activates receptors in a dose-dependent manner. At low doses (0.5 to 2 μg/kg/minute), dopamine stimulates peripheral dopamine receptors (DA_1 and DA_2) and increases renal, mesenteric, and coronary blood flow with little effect on cardiac output. In intermediate doses (2 to 6 μg/kg/minute), dopamine has positive inotropic and chronotropic effects (β-1 and β-2). At high doses (6 to 10 μg/kg/minute), dopamine stimulates α-1 and α-2 adrenergic receptors and serotonin receptors, resulting in vasoconstriction and increased peripheral vascular resistance. High-dose dopamine also increases venous return. In preterm infants, dopamine may stimulate the α receptors at lower doses. The increase in myocardial contractility depends in part on myocardial norepinephrine stores. Dopamine has been used at high infusion rates (>25 μg/kg/minute) to normalize BP in preterm newborns without detrimental vasoconstrictive effects, probably due to the decreased cardiovascular sensitivity to sympathomimetic agents that is prevalent in these infants.

b. **Dobutamine** is a synthetic catecholamine with relatively cardioselective inotropic effects. In doses of 5 to 15 μg/kg per minute, dobutamine increases cardiac output (α-1 receptors) with little effect on heart rate. Dobutamine can decrease systemic vascular resistance (SVR) (β-receptors). Dobutamine is often used with dopamine to improve cardiac output in cases of decreased myocardial function as its inotropic effects, unlike those of dopamine, are independent of norepinephrine stores. However, because hypotension is a result of decreased SVR in the majority of nonasphyxiated newborns, dopamine remains the first line of pressor therapy.

c. **Epinephrine** increases myocardial contractility and peripheral vascular resistance (β- and α-receptors). It is not a first-line drug in newborns; however, it may be effective in patients who do not respond to dopamine. Epinephrine may be helpful in conditions such as sepsis when low perfusion is due to peripheral vasodilatation. The starting dose is 0.05 to 0.1 μg/kg/minute and can be increased rapidly as needed while dopamine infusion rates are decreased. Epinephrine is an effective adjunct therapy to dopamine because cardiac norepinephrine stores are readily depleted with prolonged and higher rate dopamine infusions.

2. **Milrinone** is a phosphodiesterase-III inhibitor that enhances intracellular cyclic adenosine monophosphate (cAMP) content preferentially in the myocardium leading to increased cardiac contractility. It improves diastolic myocardial function more readily than dobutamine. Milrinone also lowers pulmonary vascular resistance (PVR) and SVR by increasing cAMP levels in vascular smooth muscle often necessitating the use of volume and dopamine to raise SVR.

3. **Other agents**

a. **Corticosteroids** may be useful in extremely premature infants with hypotension refractory to volume expansion and vasopressors, but their usage has not been adequately tested in clinical trials. Hydrocortisone stabilizes BP through multiple mechanisms. It induces the expression of the cardiovascular adrenergic receptors that are downregulated by prolonged use of sympathomimetic agents and also inhibits catecholamine metabolism. Moreover, some extremely preterm infants have adrenal insufficiency, especially in the setting of prolonged illness. After hydrocortisone administration, there is a rapid increase in intracellular calcium availability, resulting in enhanced responsiveness to adrenergic agents. The BP response is evident as early as 2 hours after hydrocortisone treatment. For refractory hypotension, hydrocortisone can be used at a dose of 1 mg/kg. If efficacy is noted, the dose can be repeated every 12 hours for 2 to 3 days, especially if low serum cortisol levels are documented before hydrocortisone treatment. High-dose steroids have been used in sepsis, but their efficacy remains controversial, perhaps because administration is initiated late in the clinical course after the cascade of inflammatory mediators has begun.

b. **Vasopressin** has been primarily studied in adults for the treatment of shock although recent reports suggest a therapeutic efficacy in the treatment of vasodilatory shock in children. Vasopressin is a hormone that is primarily involved in the postnatal regulation of fluid homeostasis but also plays an important role in maintaining vascular tone in the setting of hemodynamic instability. Vasopressin deficiency may occur in catecholamine-resistant hypotension in the evolution of sepsis, and hence its reported efficacy in vasodilatory shock. Vasopressin is not routinely used to treat shock in the neonate but may be a therapeutic option to consider in the setting of abnormal peripheral vasoregulation as occurs in sepsis. An added beneficial effect may be its inhibitory action on NO-induced increases in the second messenger cyclic guanosine monophosphate (cGMP), a potent vasodilatory signal that predominates in the setting of sepsis from the increased endotoxin/inflammation-induced NO synthesis.

V. TYPICAL CLINICAL SCENARIOS OF SHOCK IN THE NEONATE AND THEIR MANAGEMENT

A. Very low birth weight (VLBW) neonate in the immediate postnatal period
   1. Physiology includes poor vasomotor tone, immature myocardium that is more sensitive to changes in afterload, and dysregulated NO production.
   2. Recommended therapy is dopamine and judicious use of volume if hypovolemia is suspected. It is important not to give large volume infusions due to their association with increased risk of bronchopulmonary dysplasia reported in the premature infant.

B. Perinatal depression in preterm or full term neonate
   1. Physiology involves release of endogenous catecholamines leading to normal or increased SVR clinically manifested by pallor, mottled appearance, and poor perfusion and myocardial dysfunction. The baby is likely to be euvolemic and may have associated pulmonary hypertension.
   2. Recommended therapy is dopamine with or without dobutamine up to 10 μg/kg/minute. Milrinone can be used to provide afterload reduction and inotropy without risk of further myocardial injury due to excess catecholamine exposure. In cases with associated pulmonary hypertension, the use of inhaled NO is warranted for infants >34 weeks' gestation. Some infants may manifest vasodilatory shock and would benefit from increased doses of dopamine rather than milrinone. The patient's skin color and perfusion on physical examination can be used to guide therapy.

C. Preterm neonate with PDA
   1. Physiology includes ductal "steal" compromising vital organ perfusion and increase in left-to-right shunt with increased risk for pulmonary hemorrhage.
   2. Recommended therapy includes avoiding high dose dopamine (>10 μg/kg/minute) as its use will further increase left to right shunting and reduce vital organ perfusion. Use dobutamine or milrinone to enhance cardiac inotropy. Target ventilation management to increase PVR by increasing positive end-expiratory pressure (PEEP), maintaining permissive hypercarbia, and avoiding hyperoxygenation.

D. Septic shock
   1. Physiology involves relative hypovolemia, myocardial dysfunction, and peripheral vasodilation.
   2. Therapy includes volume resuscitation with crystalloid (10–30 mL/kg) which should be repeated as needed and administration of dopamine 5–40 μg/kg/minute with or without epinephrine 0.05 to 0.3 μg/kg/minute. A cardiac echocardiogram can be obtained to evaluate cardiac function, volume status, and intracardiac shunting. Consider extracorporeal membrane oxygenation (ECMO) in infants >34 weeks' gestation if they do not respond to these interventions.

E. Preterm neonates with "pressor-resistant" hypotension
   1. A proportion of VLBW infants become dependent on medium to high doses of pressors (usually dopamine) beyond the first postnatal days. Etiologies include

relative cortisol deficiency, adrenal insufficiency, and downregulation of adrenergic receptors.

2. Consider low-dose hydrocortisone (3 mg/kg/day for 3–5 days) after drawing serum cortisol level. Hydrocortisone may be preferable to equivalent steroid doses of dexamethasone due to the added mineralocorticoid effect of the former. Studies support the efficacy of hydrocortisone in raising BP within 2 hours of administration, yet the long-term neurologic effects of this treatment in the VLBW infant remain to be investigated. Additionally, due to one published report of possible increased incidence of intestinal perforation in infants treated with hydrocortisone that also received indomethacin, the concurrent use of these drugs cannot be recommended until larger trials are conducted.

Suggested Readings

Seri I, Noori S. Diagnosis and treatment of neonatal hypotension outside the transition period. *Early Hum Dev* 2005;81:405–411.

Short BL Van Meurs K, Evans JR, et al. Summary proceedings from the cardiology group on cardiovascular instability in preterm infants. *Pediatrics* 2006;117:S34–S39.

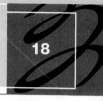
I. BACKGROUND. The normal adult serum bilirubin level is <1 mg/dL. Adults appear jaundiced when the serum bilirubin level is >2 mg/dL, and newborns appear jaundiced when it is >7 mg/dL. Between 25% and 50% of all term newborns and a higher percentage of premature infants develop clinical jaundice. Also, 6.1% of well term newborns have a maximal serum bilirubin level >12.9 mg/dL. A serum bilirubin level >15 mg/dL is found in 3% of normal term babies. **Physical examination is not a reliable measure of serum bilirubin.**

A. Source of bilirubin. Bilirubin is derived from the breakdown of heme-containing proteins in the reticuloendothelial system. The normal newborn produces 6 to 10 mg of bilirubin/kg/day, as opposed to the production of 3 to 4 mg/kg/day in the adult.

1. The major heme-containing protein is **red blood cell (RBC) hemoglobin.** Hemoglobin released from senescent RBCs in the reticuloendothelial system is the source of 75% of all bilirubin production. One gram of hemoglobin produces 34 mg of bilirubin. Accelerated release of hemoglobin from RBCs is the cause of hyperbilirubinemia in isoimmunization (e.g., Rh and ABO incompatibility), erythrocyte biochemical abnormalities (e.g., glucose-6-phosphate dehydrogenase [G6PD] and pyruvate kinase deficiencies), abnormal erythrocyte morphology (e.g., hereditary spherocytosis [HS]), sequestered blood (e.g., bruising and cephalohematoma), and polycythemia.

2. The other 25% of bilirubin is called **early-labeled bilirubin.** It is derived from hemoglobin released by ineffective erythropoiesis in the bone marrow, from other heme-containing proteins in tissues (e.g., myoglobin, cytochromes, catalase, and peroxidase), and from free heme.

B. Bilirubin metabolism. The heme ring from heme-containing proteins is oxidized in reticuloendothelial cells to **biliverdin** by the microsomal enzyme heme oxygenase. This reaction releases **carbon monoxide (CO)** (excreted from the lung) and **iron** (reutilized). Biliverdin is then reduced to bilirubin by the enzyme **biliverdin reductase.** Catabolism of 1 mol of hemoglobin produces 1 mol each of CO and bilirubin. Increased bilirubin production, as measured by CO excretion rates, accounts for the higher bilirubin levels seen in Asian, Native American, and Greek infants.

1. **Transport.** Bilirubin is nonpolar, insoluble in water, and is transported to liver cells bound to serum **albumin.** Bilirubin bound to albumin does not usually enter the central nervous system (CNS) and is thought to be nontoxic. Displacement of bilirubin from albumin by drugs, such as the sulfonamides, or by free fatty acids (FFAs) at high molar ratios of FFA: albumin, may increase bilirubin toxicity (see Table 18.1).

2. **Uptake.** Nonpolar, fat-soluble bilirubin (dissociated from albumin) crosses the hepatocyte plasma membrane and is bound mainly to cytoplasmic **ligandin** (Y protein) for transport to the smooth endoplasmic reticulum. Phenobarbital increases the concentration of ligandin.

3. **Conjugation.** Unconjugated (indirect) bilirubin (UCB) is converted to water-soluble conjugated (direct) bilirubin (CB) in the smooth endoplasmic reticulum by **uridine diphosphate glucuronyl-transferase (UDPG-T).** This enzyme is inducible by phenobarbital and catalyzes the formation of bilirubin monoglucuronide. The monoglucuronide may be further conjugated to bilirubin diglucuronide. Both mono- and diglucuronide forms of CB are able to be excreted into the bile canaliculi against a concentration gradient.

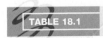

TABLE 18.1	Drugs That Cause Significant Displacement of Bilirubin from Albumin *In vitro*

Sulfonamides

Moxalactam

Fusidic acid

Radiographic contrast media for cholangiography (sodium iodipamide, sodium ipodate, iopanoic acid, meglumine loglycamate)

Aspirin

Apazone

Tolbutamide

Rapid infusions of albumin preservatives (sodium caprylate and *N*-acetyltryptophan)

Rapid infusions of ampicillin

Long-chain FFAs at high molar ratios of FFA:albumin

FFA = free fatty acid.
Source: From Roth P, Rolin RA. Controversial topics in kernicterus. *Clin Perinatol* 1988;15:970.

Inherited deficiencies and polymorphisms of the conjugating enzyme gene can cause severe hyperbilirubinemia in neonates. **Bilirubin uridine 5′-diphosphate-glucuronyltransferase gene (UGT1A1) polymorphisms** have been described which diminish the expression of the UDPG-T enzyme. The **TATA box mutation** is the most common mutation found and is implicated in Gilbert syndrome in the Western population. Instead of the usual six (TA) repeats in the promotor region, there is an extra two-base pair (TA) repeat resulting in seven (TA) repeats ([TA]7TAA). The estimated allele frequency among whites is 0.33 to 0.4 and among Asians it is less frequent at 0.15. Alone, this mutation may not result in significant neonatal hyperbilirubinemia; however, with other risk factors for hyperbilirubinemia present (G6PD deficiency, ABO incompatibility, HS, and breast milk jaundice), the presence of this mutation may confer a significant risk for neonatal hyperbilirubinemia. The **211G → A (G71R)** mutation has been found with increased frequency among the Japanese population and the presence of this mutation alone (homozygote or heterozygote) can result in reduced enzyme activity and neonatal hyperbilirubinemia. This mutation is also the most common mutation in Japanese patients with Gilbert syndrome. The G71R mutation has not been found in the white population. Other mutations have been described, such as **1456T → G** and the **CAT box mutation** (CCAAT → GTGCT); however, less is known about these mutations and further investigation is needed to determine their role in the development of nonphysiologic hyperbilirubinemia in the newborn. The population differences in allele frequencies may account for some of the racial and ethnic variation seen in the development of jaundice.

4. **Excretion.** CB in the biliary tree enters the gastrointestinal (GI) tract and is then eliminated from the body in the stool, which contains large amounts of bilirubin. CB is not normally resorbed from the bowel unless it is converted back to UCB by the intestinal enzyme β-**glucuronidase.** Resorption of bilirubin from the GI tract and delivery back to the liver for reconjugation is called **enterohepatic circulation.** Intestinal bacteria can prevent enterohepatic circulation of bilirubin by converting CB to **urobilinoids,** which are not substrates for β-glucuronidase. Pathologic conditions leading to increased enterohepatic circulation include decreased enteral intake, intestinal atresias, meconium ileus, and Hirschsprung disease.

5. **Fetal bilirubin metabolism.** Most UCB formed by the fetus is cleared by the placenta into the maternal circulation. Formation of CB is limited in the fetus

because of decreased fetal hepatic blood flow, decreased hepatic ligandin, and decreased UDPG-T activity. The small amount of CB excreted into the fetal gut is usually hydrolyzed by β-glucuronidase and resorbed. Bilirubin is normally found in amniotic fluid by 12 weeks' gestation and is usually gone by 37 weeks' gestation. Increased amniotic fluid bilirubin is found in hemolytic disease of the newborn and in fetal intestinal obstruction below the bile ducts.

II. **PHYSIOLOGIC HYPERBILIRUBINEMIA.** The serum UCB level of most newborn infants rises to >2 mg/dL in the first week of life. This level usually rises in full-term infants to a peak of 6 to 8 mg/dL by 3 days of age and then falls. A rise to 12 mg/dL is in the physiologic range. In premature infants, the peak may be 10 to 12 mg/dL on the fifth day of life, possibly rising >15 mg/dL without any specific abnormality of bilirubin metabolism. Levels <2 mg/dL may not be seen until 1 month of age in both full-term and premature infants. This "normal jaundice" is attributed to the following mechanisms:

A. **Increased bilirubin production** due to
  1. Increased RBC volume per kilogram and decreased RBC survival (90 day versus 120 day) in infants compared with adults.
  2. Increased ineffective erythropoiesis and increased turnover of nonhemoglobin heme proteins.

B. Increased enterohepatic circulation caused by high levels of intestinal β-glucuronidase, preponderance of bilirubin monoglucuronide rather than diglucuronide, decreased intestinal bacteria, and decreased gut motility with poor evacuation of bilirubin-laden meconium.

C. **Defective uptake** of bilirubin from plasma caused by decreased ligandin and binding of ligandin by other anions.

D. **Defective conjugation** due to decreased UDPG-T activity.

E. **Decreased hepatic excretion** of bilirubin.

III. **NONPHYSIOLOGIC HYPERBILIRUBINEMIA.** Nonphysiologic jaundice may not be easy to distinguish from physiologic jaundice. The following situations suggest nonphysiologic hyperbilirubinemia and require investigation (see Fig. 18.1 and Table 18.2):

A. **General conditions** (see Tables 18.3 and 18.4)
  1. Onset of jaundice before 24 hours of age.
  2. Any elevation of serum bilirubin that requires phototherapy (see Figs. 18.2–18.4 and VI.D).
  3. A rise in serum bilirubin levels of >0.5 mg/dL/hour.
  4. Signs of underlying illness in any infant (vomiting, lethargy, poor feeding, excessive weight loss, apnea, tachypnea, or temperature instability).
  5. Jaundice persisting after 8 days in a term infant or after 14 days in a premature infant.

B. **History**
  1. A family history of jaundice, anemia, splenectomy, or early gallbladder disease suggests hereditary hemolytic anemia (e.g., spherocytosis, G6PD deficiency).
  2. A family history of liver disease may suggest galactosemia, α₁-antitrypsin deficiency, tyrosinosis, hypermethioninemia, Gilbert disease, Crigler-Najjar syndrome types I and II, or cystic fibrosis.
  3. Ethnic or geographic origin associated with hyperbilirubinemia (East Asian, Greek, and American Indian) (see I.B.3 for potential genetic influences).
  4. A sibling with jaundice or anemia may suggest blood group incompatibility, breast-milk jaundice, or Lucey-Driscoll syndrome.
  5. Maternal illness during pregnancy may suggest congenital viral or toxoplasmosis infection. Infants of diabetic mothers tend to develop hyperbilirubinemia (see Chap. 2A).
  6. Maternal drugs may interfere with bilirubin binding to albumin, making bilirubin toxic at relatively low levels (sulfonamides) or may cause hemolysis in a G6PD-deficient infant (sulfonamides, nitrofurantoin, antimalarials).
  7. The labor and delivery history may show trauma associated with extravascular bleeding and hemolysis. Oxytocin use may be associated with neonatal

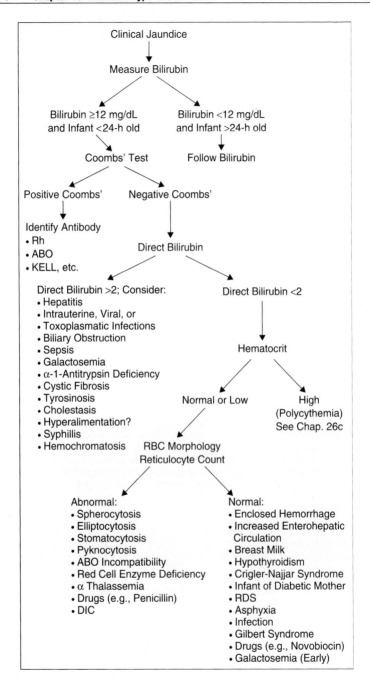

Figure 18.1. Diagnosis of the etiology of hyperbilirubinemia. Rh = rhesus factor; RBCs = red blood cells; DIC = disseminated intravascular coagulation; RDS = respiratory distress syndrome.

TABLE 18.2 Causes of Neonatal Hyperbilirubinemia

Overproduction	Undersecretion	Mixed	Uncertain mechanism
Fetomaternal blood group incompatibility (e.g., Rh, ABO)	**Metabolic and endocrine conditions**	Sepsis	Chinese, Japanese, Korean, and American Indian infants (see polymorphism discussion, section I.B.3)
Hereditary spherocytosis, eliptocytosis, somatocytosis	Galactosemia	Intrauterine infections	
	Familial nonhemolytic jaundice types 1 and 2 (Crigler-Najjar syndrome)	Toxoplasmosis	Breast-milk jaundice
Nonspherocytic hemolytic anemias		Rubella	
G6PD deficiency and drugs	Gilbert disease	CID	
Pyruvate-kinase deficiency	Hypothyroidism	Herpes simplex	
Other red cell enzyme deficiencies	Tyrosinosis	Syphilis	
α Thalassemia	Hypermethioninemia	Hepatitis	
δ–β Thalassemia	Drugs and hormones	Respiratory distress syndrome	
Acquired hemolysis due to vitamin K, nitrofurantonin, sulfonamides, antimalarials, penicillin, oxytocin, bupivacaine, or infection	Novobiocin	Asphyxia	
	Pregnanediol	Infant of diabetic mother	
	Lucy-Driscoll syndrome	Severe erythroblastosis fetalis	
	Infants of diabetic mothers		
	Prematurity		
Extravascular blood	Hypopituitarism and anencephaly		
Petechiae	**Obstructive disorders**		
Hematomas	Biliary atresia*		
Pulmonary, cerebral, or occult hemorrhage	Dubin-Johnson and Rotor syndrome*		
	Choledochal cyst*		
Polycythemia	Cystic fibrosis (inspissated bile)*		
Fetomaternal or fetofetal transfusion	Tumor* or band* (extrinsic obstruction)		
Delayed clamping of the umbilical cord			

(continued)

185

TABLE 18.2 (Continued)

Overproduction	Undersecretion	Mixed	Uncertain mechanism
Increased enteropathic circulation	α-1-antitrypsin deficiency*		
Pyloric stenosis*	Parenteral nutrition		
Intestinal atresia or stenosis including annular pancreas			
Hirschsprung disease			
Meconium ileus and/or meconium plug syndrome			
Fasting or hypoperistalsis from other causes			
Drug-induced paralytic ileus (hexamethonium)			
Swallowed blood			

G6PD = glucose-6-phosphate dehydrogenase; CID = cytomegalovirus inclusion disease, as in TORCH (toxoplasmosis, other, rubella, cytomegalovirus, herpes simplex).
*Jaundice may not be seen in the neonatal period.
Source: Modified from Odell GB, Poland RL, Nostrea E Jr. Neonatal hyperbilirubinemia. In: Klaus MH, Fanaroff A, eds. *Care of the high risk neonate.* Philadelphia: WB Saunders, 1973, Chapter 11.

| TABLE 18.3 | Timing of Follow-up |

Infant discharged	Should be seen by age
Before age 24 h	72 h
Between 24 and 47.9 h	96 h
Between 48 and 72 h	120 h

For some newborns discharged before 48 h, two follow-up visits may be required, the first visit between 24 and 72 h and the second between 72 and 120 h. Clinical judgment should be used in determining follow-up. Earlier or more frequent follow-up should be provided for those who have risk factors for hyperbilirubinemia (Table 18.4), whereas those discharged with few or no risk factors can be seen after longer intervals.
Source: Reprinted with permission from the Subcommittee on Hyperbilirubinemia. Management of hyperbilirubinemia in the newborn infant 35 or more weeks of gestation. *Pediatrics* 2004;114:297–316.

hyperbilirubinemia, although this is controversial. Asphyxiated infants may have elevated bilirubin levels caused either by inability of the liver to process bilirubin or by intracranial hemorrhage. Delayed cord clamping may be associated with neonatal polycythemia and increased bilirubin load.

8. The infant's history may show delayed or infrequent stooling, which can be caused by poor caloric intake or intestinal obstruction and lead to increased enterohepatic circulation of bilirubin. Poor caloric intake may also decrease bilirubin uptake by the liver. Vomiting can be due to sepsis, pyloric stenosis, or galactosemia.

9. **Breast-feeding.** A distinction has been made between breast-milk jaundice, in which jaundice is thought to be due to the breast milk itself, and breast-feeding jaundice, in which low caloric intake may be responsible.

   a. **Breast-milk jaundice** is of late onset and has an incidence in term infants of 2% to 4%. By day 4, instead of the usual fall in the serum bilirubin level, the bilirubin level continues to rise and may reach 20 to 30 mg/dL by 14 days of age. If breast-feeding is continued, the levels will stay elevated and then fall slowly at 2 weeks of age, returning to normal by 4 to 12 weeks of age. If breast-feeding is stopped, the bilirubin level will fall rapidly in 48 hours. If nursing is then resumed, the bilirubin may rise 2 to 4 mg/dL but usually will not reach the previous high level. These infants show good weight gain, have normal liver function test (LFT) results, and show no evidence of hemolysis. Mothers with infants who have breast-milk jaundice syndrome have a recurrence rate of 70% in future pregnancies (see I.B.3 for potential genetic influences). The mechanism of true breast-milk jaundice is unknown but is thought to be due to an unidentified factor (or factors) in breast milk interfering with bilirubin metabolism. Additionally, compared with formula-fed infants, breast-fed infants are more likely to have increased enterohepatic circulation because they ingest the β-glucuronidase present in breast milk, are slower to be colonized with intestinal bacteria that convert CB to urobilinoids, and excrete less stool. There are reports of kernicterus in otherwise healthy, breast-fed, term newborns.

   b. **Breast-feeding jaundice.** Infants who are breast-fed have higher bilirubin levels after day 3 of life compared to formula-fed infants. The differences in the levels of bilirubin are usually not clinically significant. The incidence of peak bilirubin levels >12 mg/dL in breast-fed term infants is 12% to 13%. The main factor thought to be responsible for breast-feeding jaundice is a decreased intake of milk that leads to increased enterohepatic circulation.

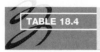

| TABLE 18.4 | Risk Factors for Development of Severe Hyperbilirubinemia in Infants of 35 or More Weeks' Gestation (in Approximate Order of Importance) |

Major risk factors

Predischarge TSB or TcB level in the high-risk zone (Fig. 18.3)

Jaundice observed in the first 24 h

Blood group incompatibility with positive direct antiglobulin test, other known hemolytic disease (e.g., G6PD deficiency), elevated ETCOc

Gestational age 35–36 wk

Previous sibling received phototherapy

Cephalohematoma or significant bruising

Exclusive breast-feeding, particularly if nursing is not going well and weight loss is excessive

East Asian race

Minor risk factors

Predischarge TSB or TcB level in the high intermediate-risk zone

Gestational age 37–38 wk

Jaundice observed before discharge

Previous sibling with jaundice

Macrosomic infant of a diabetic mother

Maternal age ≥25 y

Male gender

Decreased risk (these factors are associated with decreased risk of significant jaundice, listed in order of decreasing importance)

TSB or TcB level in the low-risk zone (Fig. 18.3)

Gestational age ≥41 wk

Exclusive bottle feeding

Black race*

Discharge from hospital after 72 h

*Race as defined by mother's description.
TSB = total serum bilirubin; TcB = transcutaneous bilirubin; G6PD = glucose-6-phosphate dehydrogenase; ETCOc = end-tidal carbon monoxide.
Source: Reprinted with permission from the Subcommittee on Hyperbilirubinemia. Management of hyperbilirubinemia in the newborn infant 35 or more weeks of gestation. *Pediatrics* 2004;114:297–316.

C. The physical examination. Jaundice is detected by blanching the skin with finger pressure to observe the color of the skin and subcutaneous tissues. Jaundice progresses in a cephalocaudal direction. The highest bilirubin levels are associated with jaundice below the knees and in the hands. However, visual inspection is not a reliable indicator of serum bilirubin levels.

Jaundiced infants should be examined for the following physical findings:
1. **Prematurity.**
2. **Small for gestational age (SGA),** which may be associated with polycythemia and in utero infections.
3. **Microcephaly,** which may be associated with *in utero* infections.
4. **Extravascular blood** bruising, cephalohematoma, or other enclosed hemorrhage.
5. **Pallor** associated with hemolytic anemia or extravascular blood loss.
6. **Petechiae** associated with congenital infection, sepsis, or erythroblastosis.

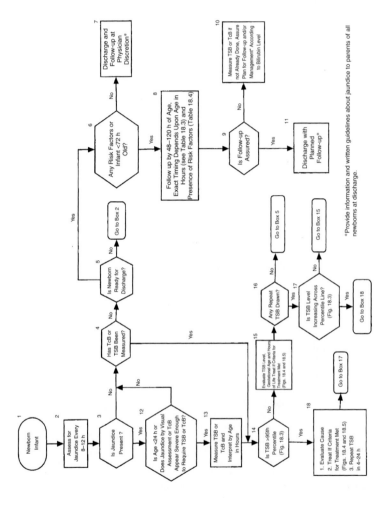

Figure 18.2. Algorithm for the management of jaundice in the newborn nursery. TSB = total serum bilirubin; TcB = transcutaneous bilirubin. (Reprinted with permission from the Subcommittee on Hyperbilirubinemia. Management of hyperbilirubinemia in the newborn infant 35 or more weeks of gestation. *Pediatrics* 2004;114:297–316.)

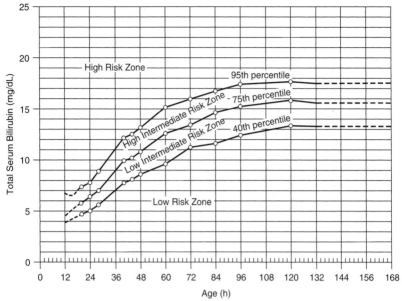

Risk designation of term and near-term well newborns based on their hour-specific serum bilirubin values. The high-risk zone is designated by the 95th percentile track. The intermediate-risk zone is subdivided to upper- and lower-risk zones by the 75th percentile track. The low-risk zone has been electively and statistically defined by the 40th percentile track. (Dotted extensions are based on <300 TSB values/epoch). This study is based on heel stick venous bilirubins and lower bilirubins.

Figure 18.3. Hour-specific bilirubin nomogram. G6PD = 'glucose-6-phosphate dehydrogenase; TSB = total serum bilirubin. (Reprinted with permission from Bhutani VK, et al. Predictive ability of a predischarge hour-specific serum bilirubin for subsequent significant hyperbilirubinemia in healthy term and near-term newborns. *Pediatrics* 1999;103:6–14.)

7. **Hepatosplenomegaly** associated with hemolytic anemia, congenital infection, or liver disease.
8. **Omphalitis.**
9. **Chorioretinitis** associated with congenital infection.
10. Evidence of **hypothyroidism** (see Chap. 2B).
   D. Prediction of nonphysiologic hyperbilirubinemia
   1. Physical examination is **not** a reliable measure of serum bilirubin.
   2. A **screening total serum bilirubin (TSB)** collected predischarge from the newborn nursery and plotted on an "hour-specific bilirubin nomogram" (Fig. 18.3) has been shown to be helpful in identifying infants at high risk of developing nonphysiologic hyperbilirubinemia.
   3. In infants >30 weeks' gestation, **transcutaneous bilirubin (TcB)** using multiple wavelength analysis (versus two-wavelength method) can reliably estimate serum bilirubin levels independent of skin pigmentation, gestational age, postnatal age, and weight of infant. Similar to TSB, TcB can be used as a screening tool to identify infants at high risk for severe hyperbilirubinemia by plotting obtained values on an hour-specific bilirubin nomogram. Despite advancements in transcutaneous technology, extrapolation to serum bilirubin levels from TcB should continue to be done with caution. We check TcB in all well term infants at discharge from the hospital. If the TcB is >8, we check a TSB. In addition, TcB monitoring is unreliable after phototherapy has begun due to bleaching

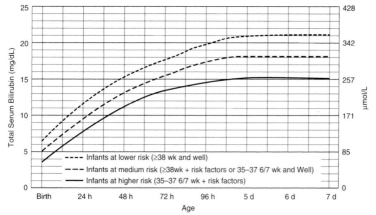

- Use total bilirubin. Do not subtract direct reacting or conjugated bilirubin.
- Risk factors = isoimmune hemolytic disease, G6PD deficiency, asphyxia, significant lethargy, temperature instability, sepsis, acidosis, or albumin <3.0 g/dL (if measured).
- For well infants 35–37 6/7 wk can adjust TSB levels for intervention around the medium risk line. It is an option to intervene at lower TSB levels for infants closer to 35 wks and at higer TSB levels for those closer to 37 6/7 wk.
- It is an option to provide conventional phototherapy in hospital or at home at TSB levels 2–3 mg/dL (35–50 mmol/L) below those shown but home phototherapy should not be used in any infant with risk factors.

Figure 18.4. Guidelines for phototherapy in hospitalized infants of 35 or more weeks' gestation. TSB = total serum bilirubin. (Reprinted with permission from the Subcommittee on Hyperbilirubinemia. Management of hyperbilirubinemia in the newborn infant 35 or more weeks of gestation. *Pediatrics* 2004;114:297–316.)

of the skin with treatment. TcB as a screening tool has the potential to reduce the number of invasive blood tests performed in newborns and reduce related health care costs.

4. Due to the production of CO during bilirubin metabolism (see I.B), **end-tidal carbon monoxide (ETCOc)** has been hypothesized as a potential screening tool. In a recent study, ETCOc was not shown to improve the sensitivity or specificity of predicting nonphysiologic hyperbilirubinemia over TSB or TcB alone. However, it may offer insight to the underlying pathologic process contributing to the hyperbilirubinemia (hemolysis versus conjugation defects).

E. **Clinical tests** (Figs. 18.1 and 18.2). The following tests are indicated in the presence of nonphysiologic jaundice:

1. TSB and/or TcB.

2. **Blood type, Rh, and direct Coombs test of the infant** to test for isoimmune hemolytic disease. Infants of women who are Rh-negative should have a blood type, Rh, and Coombs test performed at birth. Routine blood typing and Coombs testing of all infants born to O Rh-positive mothers to determine whether there is risk for ABO incompatibility is probably unnecessary. Such testing is reserved for infants with clinically significant jaundice, those in whom follow-up is difficult, or those whose skin pigmentation is such that jaundice may not be easily recognized. Blood typing and Coombs testing should be considered for infants who are to be discharged early, especially if the mother is type O (see Chap. 5).

3. **Blood type, Rh, and antibody screen of the mother** should have been done during pregnancy and the antibody screen repeated at delivery.

4. **Peripheral smear for RBC morphology and reticulocyte count** to detect causes of Coombs-negative hemolytic disease (e.g., spherocytosis).

5. **Hematocrit** will detect polycythemia or suggest blood loss from occult hemorrhage.

6. Identification of **antibody on infant's RBCs** (if result of direct Coombs test is positive).

7. **Direct bilirubin** determination is necessary when jaundice persists beyond the first 2 weeks of life or whenever there are signs of cholestasis (light-colored stools and bilirubin in urine). If elevated, a urinalysis and a urine culture should be obtained. Check state newborn screen for hythyroidism and galactosemia.

8. In prolonged jaundice, tests for liver disease, congenital infection, sepsis, metabolic defects, or hypothyroidism are indicated. Total parenteral nutrition (PN) is a well-recognized cause of prolonged direct hyperbilirubinemia.

9. **A G6PD screen** may be helpful, especially in male infants of African, Asian, southern European, and Mediterranean or Middle Eastern descent. The incidence of G6PD among African Americans is 11% to 13%, comprising the most affected subpopulation in America. Previously, term black infants with G6PD deficiency were not thought to be at significant risk for hyperbilirubinemia. However, recent literature suggests otherwise. Not all infants with G6PD deficiency will manifest neonatal hyperbilirubinemia. A combination of genetic and environmental risk factors will determine the individual risk (see I.B.3 for potential genetic influences). Screening the parents for G6PD deficiency is also helpful in making the diagnosis. Infants who had G6PD deficiency and were discharged early have been reported with severe hyperbilirubinemia and significant sequelae.

IV. DIAGNOSIS OF NEONATAL HYPERBILIRUBINEMIA (Table 18.2 and Fig. 18.1).

V. BILIRUBIN TOXICITY. This area remains highly controversial. The problem is that bilirubin levels that are toxic to one infant may not be toxic to another, or even to the same infant in different clinical circumstances. Currently, major debate surrounds the toxicity of bilirubin in otherwise healthy full-term infants and in premature, low birth weight infants.

Bilirubin levels refer to total bilirubin. Direct bilirubin is not subtracted from the total unless it constitutes >50% of total bilirubin.

A. Bilirubin entry into the brain occurs as free (unbound) bilirubin or as bilirubin bound to albumin in the presence of a disrupted blood–brain barrier. It is estimated that 8.5 mg of bilirubin will bind tightly to 1 g of albumin (molar ratio of 1), although this binding capacity is less in small and sick prematures. FFAs and certain drugs (Table 18.1) interfere with bilirubin binding to albumin, although acidosis affects bilirubin solubility and its deposition into brain tissue. Factors that disrupt the blood–brain barrier include hyperosmolarity, anoxia, and hypercarbia, and the barrier may be more permeable in premature infants.

B. **Kernicterus** is a pathologic diagnosis and refers to **yellow staining** of the brain by bilirubin together with evidence of **neuronal injury.** Grossly, bilirubin staining is most commonly seen in the basal ganglia, various cranial nerve nuclei, other brainstem nuclei, cerebellar nuclei, hippocampus, and anterior horn cells of the spinal cord. Microscopically, there is necrosis, neuronal loss, and gliosis. The use of the term **kernicterus** in the clinical setting should be used to denote the *chronic* and *permanent sequelae* of bilirubin toxicity.

C. **Acute bilirubin encephalopathy** is the clinical manifestation of bilirubin toxicity seen in the neonatal period. The clinical presentation of acute bilirubin encephalopathy can be divided into three phases:

1. **Early phase.** Hypotonia, lethargy, high-pitched cry, and poor suck.

2. **Intermediate phase.** Hypertonia of extensor muscles (with opisthotonus, rigidity, oculogyric crisis, and retrocollis), irritability, fever, and seizures. Many infants die in this phase. All infants who survive this phase develop chronic bilirubin encephalopathy (clinical diagnosis of kernicterus).

3. **Advanced phase.** Pronounced opisthotonus (although hypotonia replaces hypertonia after approximately 1 week of age), shrill cry, apnea, seizures, coma, and death.

D. **Chronic bilirubin encephalopathy** (kernicterus) is marked by athetosis, partial or complete sensorineural deafness, limitation of upward gaze, dental dysplasia, and intellectual deficits.

E. Bilirubin toxicity and hemolytic disease. There is general agreement that in Rh hemolytic disease there is a direct association between marked elevations of bilirubin and signs of bilirubin encephalopathy with kernicterus at autopsy. Studies and clinical experience have shown that in full-term infants with hemolytic disease, if the total bilirubin level is kept <20 mg/dL, bilirubin encephalopathy is unlikely to occur. Theoretically, this should apply to other causes of isoimmune hemolytic disease, such as ABO incompatibility, and to hereditary hemolytic processes such as HS, pyruvate kinase deficiency, or G6PD deficiency.

F. Bilirubin toxicity and the healthy full-term infant. In contrast to infants with hemolytic disease, there is little evidence showing adverse neurologic outcome in healthy term neonates with bilirubin levels <25 to 30 mg/dL. A large prospective cohort study failed to demonstrate a clinically significant association between bilirubin levels >20 mg/dL and neurologic abnormality, long-term hearing loss, or intelligence quotient (IQ) deficits. However, an increase in minor motor abnormalities of unclear significance was detected in those with serum bilirubin levels >20 mg/dL. Hyperbilirubinemia in term infants has been associated with abnormalities in brainstem audiometric-evoked responses (BAERs), cry characteristics, and neurobehavioral measures. However, these changes disappear when bilirubin levels fall and there are no measurable long-term sequelae. Kernicterus has been reported in jaundiced healthy, full-term, breast-fed infants. **All predictive values for bilirubin toxicity are based on heel stick values.**

G. Bilirubin toxicity and the low-birth-weight infant. Initial early studies of babies of 1,250 to 2,500 g and 28 to 36 weeks' gestational age showed no relation between neurologic damage and bilirubin levels >18 to 20 mg/dL. Later studies, however, began to report "kernicterus" at autopsy or neurodevelopmental abnormalities at follow-up in premature infants <1,250 g who had bilirubin levels previously thought to be safe (e.g., <10 to 20 mg/dL). Because kernicterus in preterm infants is now considered uncommon, hindsight suggests that this so-called "low bilirubin kernicterus" was largely due to factors other than bilirubin alone. For example, unrecognized intracranial hemorrhage, inadvertent exposure to drugs that displace bilirubin from albumin, or the use of solutions (e.g., benzyl alcohol) that can alter the blood–brain barrier may have accounted for developmental handicaps or kernicterus in infants with low levels of serum bilirubin. In addition, premature infants are more likely to suffer from anoxia, hypercarbia, and sepsis, which also open the blood–brain barrier and lead to enhanced bilirubin deposition in neural tissue. Finally, the pathologic changes seen in postmortem preterm infant brains has been more consistent with nonspecific damage than with true kernicterus. Therefore, bilirubin toxicity in low-birth-weight infants may not be a function of bilirubin levels *per se* but of their overall clinical status.

VI. MANAGEMENT OF UNCONJUGATED HYPERBILIRUBINEMIA. Given the uncertainty of determining what levels of bilirubin are toxic, these are general clinical guidelines only and should be modified in any sick infant with acidosis, hypercapnia, hypoxemia, asphyxia, sepsis, hypoalbuminemia (<2.5 mg/dL), or signs of bilirubin encephalopathy.

A. General principles. Management of unconjugated hyperbilirubinemia is clearly tied to the etiology. Early identification of known causes of nonphysiologic hyperbilirubinemia (see III. B, C, and D) should prompt close observation for development of jaundice, appropriate laboratory investigation, and timely intervention. Any medication (Table 18.1) or clinical factor that may interfere with bilirubin metabolism, bilirubin binding to albumin, or the integrity of the blood–brain barrier should be discontinued or corrected. Infants who are receiving inadequate feedings, or who have decreased urine and stool output, need increased feedings both in volume and in calories to reduce the enterohepatic circulation of bilirubin. Infants with hypothyroidism need adequate replacement of the thyroid hormone. If levels of bilirubin are so high that the infant is at risk for kernicterus, bilirubin may be removed mechanically by exchange transfusion, its excretion increased by alternative pathways using phototherapy, or its normal metabolism increased by drugs such as phenobarbital.

B. Infants with hemolytic disease (see XII)

1. In Rh disease we start intensive phototherapy immediately. An exchange transfusion is performed if the bilirubin level is predicted to reach 20 mg/dL (see Fig. 18.5A and B).

2. In ABO hemolytic disease we start phototherapy if the bilirubin level exceeds 10 mg/dL at 12 hours, 12 mg/dL at 18 hours, 14 mg/dL at 24 hours, or 15 mg/dL at any time. If the bilirubin reaches 20 mg/dL, an exchange transfusion is done.

3. In hemolytic disease of other causes we treat as if it were Rh disease (see Tables 18.5–18.7).

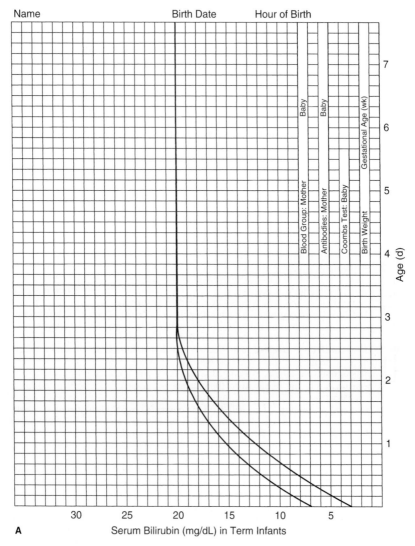

Figure 18.5. Serum bilirubin levels plotted against age in term infants **(A)** and premature infants **(B)** with erythroblastosis. TSB = total serum bilirubin; G6PD = glucose-6-phosphate dehydrogenase.

Name   Birth Date   Hour of Birth

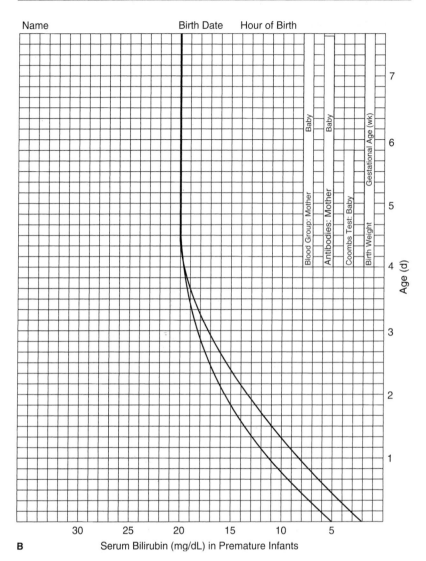

B   Serum Bilirubin (mg/dL) in Premature Infants

Figure 18.5. *(continued)*

C. Healthy late-preterm and term infants (Figs. 18.2–18.4 and 18.6). The American Academy of Pediatrics (AAP) has published a practice parameter for the treatment of unconjugated hyperbilirubinemia in healthy, newborn infants at 35 weeks' gestation and greater. This practice parameter rests on three general principles to reduce the occurrence of severe hyperbilirubinemia while also reducing unintended harm: universal systematic assessment, close follow-up, and prompt intervention when indicated.

1. In our nurseries, some have begun to use TcB (see III.D) measurements, whereas others have instituted universal TSB measurements usually taken at the same

| TABLE 18.5 | Common Antigens Other Than Rh Implicated in Hemolytic Diseases of the Newborn | |

Antigen	Alternative symbol or name	Blood group system
Do^a	—	Dombrock
Fy^a	—	Duffy
Jk^a	—	Kidd
Jk^b	—	Kidd
K	K:1	Kell
Lu^a	Lu:1	Lutheran
M	—	MNSs
N	—	MNSs
S	—	MNSs
s	—	MNSs

time as the state newborn screen. These bilirubin measurments are used in conjunction with an hour-specific bilirubin nomogram to identify infants at risk for significant hyperbilirubinemia.

2. Most of our healthy late-preterm and term infants are sent home by 24 to 48 hours of age; therefore, parents should be informed about neonatal jaundice before discharge from the hospital. **Arrangements should be made for follow-up within 1 or 2 days. This is especially true if the infant is <38 weeks' gestation, is the first child, is breast-feeding, or has any other risk factors for hyperbilirubinemia.**

(Additional information on jaundice and kernicterus can be found at http://www.aap.org/moc/docs/020707hyperb.cfm)

| TABLE 18.6 | Other Antigens Involved in Hemolytic Diseases of the Newborn | |

Antigen	Alternative symbol or name	Blood group system
Co^a	—	Colton
Di^b	—	Diego
Ge	—	Gerbich
Hy	Holley	—
Jr	—	—
Js^b	Matthews, K:7	Kell
K	Cellano, K:2	Kell
Kp^b	Rautenberg, K:4	Kell
Lan	Langereis	—
Lu^b	—	Lutheran
LW	Landsteinder-Weiner	—
P,P1,P^k	Tj^a	P
U	—	MNSs
Yt^a	—	Cartwright

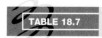

TABLE 18.7	Infrequent Antigens Implicated in Hemolytic Diseases of the Newborn

Antigen	Alternative symbol or name	Blood group system
Be^a	Berrens	Rh
Bi	Biles	—
By	Batty	—
C^w	Rh:8	Rh
C^x	Rh:9	Rh
Di^a*	—	Diego
Evans	—	Rh
E^w	Rh:11	Rh
Far	See Kam	—
Ga	Gambino	—
Go^a	Gonzales	Rh
Good	—	—
Heibel	—	—
Hil	Hill	MNSs Mi sub+
Ht^a	Hunt	—
Hut	Hutchinson	MNSs Mi sub
Js^a	Sutter	Kell
Kam (Far)	Kamhuber	—
Kp^a	Penney	Kell
Mit	Mitchell	—
Mt^a	Martin	MNSs#
Mull	Lu:9	Lutheran
Mur	Murrell	MNSs Mi sub
Rd	Radin	—
Re^a	Reid	—
R^N	Rh:32	Rh
Vw(Gr)	Verweyst (Graydon)	MNSs Mi sub
Wi^a	Wright	—
Zd	—	—

*This may not be a complete list. Any antigen that the father has and the mother does not have and that induces an immunoglobulin G (IgG) response in the mother may cause sensitization.

3. In healthy late-preterm and term infants who are jaundiced, we follow the guidelines published by the AAP (Fig. 18.2).
4. In **breast-fed infants** with hyperbilirubinemia, preventive measures are the best approach and include encouragement of frequent nursing (at least every 3 hours) and, if necessary, supplementation with expressed breast milk or formula (***not*** with water or dextrose water) (see III.B.9).
5. Guidelines for phototherapy and exchange transfusion are identical for breast-fed and formula-fed infants. However, in **breast-fed infants,** a decision is often made whether to discontinue breast-feeding. In a randomized controlled trial of breast-fed infants with bilirubin levels of at least 17 mg/dL, 3% of those who switched to formula and received phototherapy reached bilirubin levels

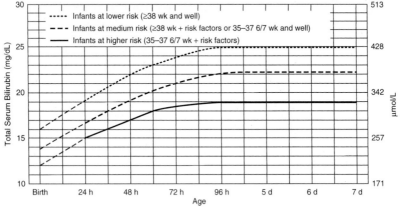

- The dashed lines for the first 24 h indicate uncertainty due to a wide range of clinical circumstances and a range of responses to phototherapy.
- Immediate exchange transfusion is recommended if infant shows signs of acute bilirubin encephalopathy (hypertonia, arching, retrocollis, opisthotonos, fever, high pitched cry) or if TSB is ≥5 mg/dL (85 μmol/L) above these lines.
- Risk factors–isoimmune hemolytic disease, G6PD deficiency, asphyxia, significant lethargy, temperature instability, sepsis, acidosis.
- Measure serum albumin and calculate B/A ratio (see legend)
- Use total bilirubin. Do not subtract direct reacting or conjugated bilirubin.
- If infant is well and 35–37 6/7 wk (median risk) can individualize TSB levels for exchange based on actual gestational age.

Figure 18.6. Guidelines for exchange transfusion in hospitalized infants of 35 or more weeks' gestation. TSB = total serum bilirubin; G6PD = glucose-6-phosphate dehydrogenase. (Reprinted with permission from the Subcommittee on Hyperbilirubinemia. Management of hyperbilirubinemia in the newborn infant 35 or more weeks of gestation. *Pediatrics* 2004;114:297–316.)

>20 mg/dL compared with 14% of those who continued nursing while they were receiving phototherapy. In infants not receiving phototherapy, 19% of those who switched to formula reached bilirubin levels >20 mg/dL compared with 24% of those who simply continued nursing. No infant in any group had a bilirubin >23 mg/dL, and none required exchange transfusion. However, discontinuing breast-feeding entirely may not be necessary. In a later prospective trial, breast-fed infants who continued to breast-feed and were supplemented with formula had a comparable response to treatment to infants who stopped breast-feeding and were fed formula alone.

In general, **our current practice** is that if the bilirubin reaches a level that would require phototherapy and is predicted to exceed 20 mg/dL, we will start phototherapy, and discontinue breast-feeding for 48 hours and supplement with formula. The mother requires much support through this process and is encouraged to pump her breasts until breast-feeding can be resumed.

6. Failure of bilirubin levels to fall after the interruption of breast-feeding may indicate other causes of prolonged indirect hyperbilirubinemia, such as hemolytic disease, hypothyroidism, and familial nonhemolytic jaundice (Crigler-Najjar syndrome).

D. **Premature infants.** There are no consensus guidelines for phototherapy and exchange transfusion in low birth weight infants. The following statement from the Guidelines for Perinatal Care from the AAP and the American Academy of Obstetricians and Gynecologists emphasize our current lack of knowledge in this area:

"Some pediatricians use guidelines that recommend aggressive treatment of jaundice in low-birth-weight neonates, initiating phototherapy early and performing exchange transfusions in certain neonates with very low bilirubin levels (<10 mg/dL). However, this approach will not prevent kernicterus consistently. Some pediatricians prefer to adopt a less-aggressive therapeutic stance and allow serum bilirubin concentrations in low-birth-weight neonates to approach 15 to 20 mg/dL (257 to 342 mmol/L), before considering exchange transfusions. At present, both of these approaches to treatment should be considered reasonable. In either case, the finding of low bilirubin kernicterus at autopsy in certain low-birth-weight neonates cannot necessarily be interpreted as a therapeutic failure or equivalent to bilirubin encephalopathy. Like retinopathy of prematurity, kernicterus is a condition that cannot be prevented in certain neonates, given the current state of knowledge. Although there is some evidence of an association between hyperbilirubinemia and neurodevelopmental handicap less severe than classic bilirubin encephalopathy, a cause-and-effect relationship has not been established. Furthermore, there is no information presently available to suggest that treating mild jaundice will prevent such handicaps."

Our current practice for treating jaundiced premature infants is as follows:

1. **Infants <1,000 g.** Phototherapy is started within 24 hours, and exchange transfusion is performed at levels of 10 to 12 mg/dL.

2. **Infants 1,000 to 1,500 g.** Phototherapy at bilirubin levels of 7 to 9 mg/dL and exchange transfusion at levels of 12 to 15 mg/dL.

3. **Infants 1,500 to 2,000 g.** Phototherapy at bilirubin levels of 10 to 12 mg/dL and exchange transfusion at levels of 15 to 18 mg/dL.

4. **Infants 2,000 to 2,500 g.** Phototherapy at bilirubin levels of 13 to 15 mg/dL and exchange transfusion at levels of 18 to 20 mg/dL.

VII. PHOTOTHERAPY. Although bilirubin absorbs visible light with wavelengths of approximately 400 to 500 nm, the most effective lights for phototherapy are those with high-energy output near the maximum adsorption peak of bilirubin (450 to 460 nm). Special blue lamps with a peak output at 425 to 475 nm are the most efficient for phototherapy. Cool white lamps with a principal peak at 550 to 600 nm and a range of 380 to 700 nm are usually adequate for treatment. Fiberoptic phototherapy (phototherapy blankets) have been shown to reduce bilirubin levels although less effectively for term infants; likely due to the limited skin exposure it can offer.

A. Photochemical reactions. When bilirubin absorbs light, three types of photochemical reactions occur.

1. **Photoisomerization** occurs in the extravascular space of the skin. The natural isomer of UCB (4Z,15Z) is instantaneously converted to a less-toxic polar isomer (4Z,15E) that diffuses into the blood and is excreted into the bile without conjugation. However, excretion is slow, and the photoisomer is readily converted back to UCB, which is resorbed from the gut if the baby is not having stools. After approximately 12 hours of phototherapy, the photoisomers make up approximately 20% of total bilirubin. Standard tests do not distinguish between naturally occurring bilirubin and the photoisomer, so bilirubin levels may not change much although the phototherapy has made the bilirubin present less toxic. Photoisomerization occurs at low-dose phototherapy (6 μW/cm^2/ nm) with no significant benefit from doubling the irradiance.

2. **Structural isomerization** is the intramolecular cyclization of bilirubin to **lumirubin.** Lumirubin makes up 2% to 6% of serum concentration of bilirubin during phototherapy and is rapidly excreted in the bile and urine without conjugation. Unlike photoisomerization, the conversion of bilirubin to lumirubin is irreversible, and it cannot be reabsorbed. It is the most important pathway for the lowering of serum bilirubin levels and is strongly related to the dose of phototherapy used in the range of 6 to 12 μW/cm^2/ nm.

3. The slow process of **photo-oxidation** converts bilirubin to small polar products that are excreted in the urine. It is the least important reaction for lowering bilirubin levels.

B. Indications for phototherapy

1. Phototherapy should be used when the level of bilirubin may be hazardous to the infant if it were to increase, although it has not reached levels requiring exchange transfusion (see VI).

2. Prophylactic phototherapy may be indicated in special circumstances, such as extremely low birth weight infants or severely bruised infants. In hemolytic disease of the newborn, phototherapy is started immediately while the rise in the serum bilirubin level is plotted (Fig. 18.6) and during the wait for exchange transfusion.

3. Phototherapy is usually contraindicated in infants with direct hyperbilirubinemia caused by liver disease or obstructive jaundice because indirect bilirubin levels are not usually high in these conditions and because phototherapy may lead to the **"bronze baby" syndrome.** If both direct and indirect bilirubin are high, exchange transfusion is probably safer than phototherapy because it is not known whether the bronze pigment is toxic.

C. Technique of phototherapy

1. We have found that **light banks** with alternating special blue (narrow-spectrum) and daylight fluorescent lights are effective and do not make the baby appear cyanotic. The irradiance can be measured at the skin by a radiometer and should exceed 5 $\mu W/cm^2$ at 425 to 475 nm. There is not much benefit in exceeding 9 $\mu W/cm^2/$ nm. In infants with severe hyperbilirubinemia we use Neo-Blue phototherapy lights (Natus, 1501 Industrial Park, San Carlos, CA 94070, natus.com). They do not cause overheating. Bulbs should be changed at intervals specified by the manufacturer. Our practice is to change all the bulbs every 3 months because this approximates the correct number of hours of use in our unit.

2. For infants under radiant warmers, we lay infants on fiberoptic blankets and/or use **spot phototherapy** overhead with quartz halide white light having output in the blue spectrum.

3. **Fiberoptic blankets** with light output in the blue-green spectrum have proved very useful in our unit, not only for single phototherapy but also for delivering **"double phototherapy"** in which the infant lies on a fiberoptic blanket with conventional phototherapy overhead.

4. Infants under phototherapy lights are kept naked except for eye patches and a face mask used as a diaper to ensure light exposure to the greatest skin surface area. We have recently been using eyecovers called *Biliband* (Natus, 1501 Industrial Park, San Carlos, CA 94070, natus.com). The infants are turned every 2 hours. Care should be taken to ensure that the eye patches do not occlude the nares, as asphyxia and apnea can result.

5. If an incubator is used, there should be a 5- to 8-cm space between it and the lamp cover to prevent overheating.

6. The infants' temperature should be carefully monitored and servocontrolled.

7. Infants should be weighed daily (small infants are weighed twice each day). Between 10% and 20% extra fluid over the usual requirements is given to compensate for the increased insensible water loss in infants in open cribs or warmers who are receiving phototherapy. Infants also have increased fluid losses caused by increased stooling (see Chap. 9).

8. Skin color is not a guide to hyperbilirubinemia in infants undergoing phototherapy; consequently, bilirubin level should be monitored at least every 12 to 24 hours.

9. Once a satisfactory decline in bilirubin levels has occurred (e.g., exchange transfusion has been averted), we allow infants to be removed from phototherapy for feedings and brief parental visits.

10. **Phototherapy is stopped** when it is believed that the level is low enough to eliminate concern about the toxic effects of bilirubin, when the risk factors for toxic levels of bilirubin are gone, and when the baby is old enough to handle the bilirubin load. A bilirubin level is usually checked 12 to 24 hours after phototherapy is stopped. In a recent study of infants with nonhemolytic

hyperbilirubinemia, phototherapy was discontinued at mean bilirubin levels of 13 ± 0.7 mg/dL in term and 10.7 ± 1.2 mg/dL in preterm infants. Rebound bilirubin levels 12 to 15 hours later averaged <1 mg/dL, and no infant required reinstitution of phototherapy.

11. **Home phototherapy** is effective and is cheaper than hospital phototherapy, and is easy to implement with the use of fiberoptic blankets. Most candidates for home phototherapy are breast-fed infants whose bilirubin problems can be resolved with a brief interruption of breast-feeding and increased fluid intake. Constant supervision is required, and all the other details of phototherapy, such as temperature control and fluid intake, are also required. The AAP has issued guidelines for the use of home phototherapy.

12. It is contraindicated to put jaundiced infants under direct sunlight, as severe hyperthermia may result.

D. **Side effects of phototherapy**

1. **Insensible water loss** is increased in infants undergoing phototherapy, especially those under radiant warmers. The increase may be as much as 40% for term and 80% to 190% in premature infants. Incubators with servocontrolled warmers will decrease this water loss. Extra fluid must be given to make up for these losses (see Chap. 9).

2. **Redistribution of blood flow.** In **term** infants, left ventricular output and renal blood flow velocity decrease, whereas left pulmonary artery and cerebral blood flow velocity increase. All velocities return to baseline after discontinuation of phototherapy. In the **preterm** infant, cerebral blood flow velocity also increases and renal vascular resistance increases with a reduction of renal blood flow velocity. In ventilated preterm infants the changes in blood flow velocities do not return to baseline even after discontinuation of phototherapy. In addition, in preterm infants under conventional phototherapy, it has been shown that the usual postprandial increase in superior mesenteric blood flow is blunted. Fiberoptic phototherapy did not seem to affect the postprandial response. Although, the changes in cerebral, renal, and superior mesenteric artery blood flow with phototherapy treatment in preterm infants is of potential concern, no detrimental clinical effects due to these changes have been determined.

3. **Watery diarrhea and increased fecal water loss** may occur. The diarrhea may be caused by increased bile salts and UCB in the bowel.

4. **Low calcium** levels have been described in preterm infants under phototherapy.

5. **Retinal damage** has been described in animals whose eyes have been exposed to phototherapy lamps. The eyes should be shielded with eye patches. Followup studies of infants whose eyes have been adequately shielded show normal vision and electroretinography.

6. **Tanning** of the skin of black infants. Erythemia and increased skin blood flow may also be seen.

7. **"Bronze baby" syndrome** (see VII.B.3).

8. **Mutations, sister chromatid exchange, and DNA strand breaks** have been described in cell culture. It may be wise to shield the scrotum during phototherapy.

9. **Tryptophan is reduced in amino acid solutions** exposed to phototherapy. Methionine and histidine are also reduced in these solutions if multivitamins are added. These solutions should probably be shielded from phototherapy by using aluminum foil on the lines and bottles.

10. **No significant long-term developmental differences** have been found in infants treated with phototherapy compared with controls.

11. Phototherapy upsets **maternal–infant interactions** and therefore should be used only with adequate thought and explanation.

VIII. **EXCHANGE TRANSFUSION**

A. **Mechanisms.** Exchange transfusion removes partially hemolyzed and antibody-coated RBCs as well as unattached antibodies and replaces them with donor

RBCs lacking the sensitizing antigen. As bilirubin is removed from the plasma, extravascular bilirubin will rapidly equilibrate and bind to the albumin in the exchanged blood. Within half an hour after the exchange, bilirubin levels return to 60% of preexchange levels, representing the rapid influx of bilirubin into the vascular space. Further increases in postexchange bilirubin levels are due to hemolysis of antibody-coated RBCs sequestered in bone marrow or spleen, from senescent donor RBCs, and from early labeled bilirubin.

B. Indications for exchange transfusion

1. When phototherapy fails to prevent a rise in bilirubin to toxic levels (see VI and Figs. 18.2–18.5).

2. Correct anemia and improve heart failure in hydropic infants with hemolytic disease.

3. Stop hemolysis and bilirubin production by removing antibody and sensitized RBCs.

4. Figure 18.6 shows the natural history of bilirubin rise in infants with Rh sensitization without phototherapy. In hemolytic disease, immediate exchange transfusion is usually indicated if:
   a. The cord bilirubin level is >4.5 mg/dL and the cord hemoglobin level is under 11 g/dL.
   b. The bilirubin level is rising >1 mg/dL/hour despite phototherapy.
   c. The hemoglobin level is between 11 and 13 g/dL and the bilirubin level is rising >0.5 mg/dL/hour despite phototherapy.
   d. The bilirubin level is 20 mg/dL, or it appears that it will reach 20 mg/dL at the rate it is rising (Fig. 18.6).
   e. There is progression of anemia in the face of adequate control of bilirubin by other methods (e.g., phototherapy).

5. Repeat exchanges are done for the same indications as the initial exchange. All infants should be under intense phototherapy while decisions regarding exchange transfusion are being made.

C. Blood for exchange transfusion

1. We use fresh (<7 days old) irradiated reconstituted whole blood (hematocrit 45 to 50) made from packed red blood cells (PRBCs) and fresh frozen plasma collected in citrate-phosphate-dextrose (CPD). Cooperation with the obstetrician and the blood bank is essential in preparing for the birth of an infant requiring exchange transfusion (see Chap. 26E).

2. **In Rh hemolytic disease,** if blood is prepared before delivery, it should be type O Rh-negative cross-matched against the mother. If the blood is obtained after delivery, it also may be cross-matched against the infant.

3. **In ABO incompatibility,** the blood should be type O Rh-negative or Rh-compatible with the mother and infant, be cross-matched against the mother and infant, and have a low titer of naturally occurring anti-A or anti-B antibodies. Usually, type O cells are used with AB plasma to ensure that no anti-A or anti-B antibodies are present.

4. In other isoimmune hemolytic disease, the blood should not contain the sensitizing antigen and should be cross-matched against the mother.

5. In nonimmune hyperbilirubinemia, blood is typed and cross-matched against the plasma and red cells of the infant.

6. Exchange transfusion usually involves double the volume of the infant's blood and is known as a two-volume exchange. If the infant's blood volume is 80 mL/kg, then a two-volume exchange transfusion uses 160 mL/kg of blood. This replaces 87% of the infant's blood volume with new blood.

D. Technique of exchange transfusion

1. Exchange is done with the infant under a servocontrolled radiant warmer and cardiac and blood pressure monitoring in place. Equipment and personnel for resuscitation must be readily available, and an intravenous line should be in place for the administration of glucose and medication. The infant's arms and legs should be properly restrained.

2. An assistant should be assigned to the infant to record volumes of blood, observe the infant, and check vital signs.

3. The glucose concentration of CPD blood is approximately 300 mg/dL. After exchange, we measure the infant's glucose to detect rebound hypoglycemia.

4. Measurement of potassium and pH of the blood for exchange may be indicated if the blood is >7 days old or if metabolic abnormalities are noted following exchange transfusion.

5. The blood should be warmed to 37°C.

6. Sterile techniques should be used. Old, dried umbilical cords can be softened with saline-soaked gauze to facilitate locating the vein and inserting the catheter. If a dirty cord was entered or there was a break in sterile technique, we treat with oxacillin and gentamicin for 2 to 3 days.

7. We do most exchanges by the **push-pull technique** through the umbilical vein inserted only as far as required to permit free blood exchange. A catheter in the heart may cause arrhythmias (see Chap. 36).

8. **Isovolumetric** exchange transfusion (simultaneously pulling blood out of the umbilical artery and pushing new blood in the umbilical vein) may be tolerated better in small, sick, or hydropic infants.

9. If it is not possible to insert the catheter in the umbilical vein, exchange transfusion can be accomplished through a central venous pressure line placed through the antecubital fossa or into the femoral vein through the saphenous vein.

10. In the push-pull method, blood is removed in aliquots that are tolerated by the infant. This usually is **5 mL** for infants <1,500 g, **10 mL** for infants 1,500 to 2,500 g, **15 mL** for infants 2,500 to 3,500 g, and **20 mL** for infants >3,500 g. The rate of exchange and aliquot size have little effect on the efficiency of bilirubin removal, but smaller aliquots and a slower rate place less stress on the cardiovascular system. The recommended time for the exchange transfusion is 1 hour.

11. The blood should be gently mixed after every deciliter of exchange to prevent the settling of RBCs and the transfusion of anemic blood at the end of the exchange.

12. After exchange transfusion, phototherapy is continued and bilirubin levels are measured every 4 hours.

13. When the exchange transfusion is finished, a silk purse-string suture should be placed around the vein; the tails of the suture material should be left. This localization of the vein will facilitate the next exchange transfusion.

14. When the catheter is removed, the tie around the cord should be tightened snugly for approximately 1 hour. It is important to remember to loosen the tie after 1 hour to avoid necrosis of the skin.

E. **Complications of exchange transfusions**

1. **Hypocalcemia and hypomagnesemia.** The citrate in CPD blood binds ionic calcium and magnesium. Hypocalcemia associated with exchange transfusion may produce cardiac and other effects (see Chap. 29B). We usually do not give extra calcium unless the electrocardiogram (ECG) and clinical assessment suggest hypocalcemia. The fall in magnesium associated with exchange transfusion has not been associated with clinical problems.

2. **Hypoglycemia.** The high glucose content of CPD blood may stimulate insulin secretion and cause hypoglycemia 1 to 2 hours after an exchange. Blood glucose is monitored for several hours after exchange and the infant should have an intravenous line containing glucose (see Chap. 29A).

3. **Acid–base balance.** Citrate in CPD blood is metabolized to alkali by the healthy liver and may result in a late metabolic alkalosis. If the baby is very ill and unable to metabolize citrate, the citrate may produce significant acidosis.

4. **Hyperkalemia.** Potassium levels may be greatly elevated in stored PRBCs, but washing the cells before reconstitution with fresh frozen plasma removes this excess potassium. Washing by some methods (IBM cell washer) may cause

hypokalemia. If blood is >24 hours old, it is best to check the potassium level before using it (see Chap. 9).

5. **Cardiovascular.** Perforation of vessels, embolization (with air or clots), vasospasm, thrombosis, infarction, arrhythmias, volume overload, and arrest.

6. **Bleeding.** Thrombocytopenia, deficient clotting factors (see Chap. 26B).

7. **Infections.** Bacteremia, hepatitis, cytomegalovirus (CMV), human immunodeficiency virus (HIV) (acquired immune deficiency syndrome [AIDS]), West Nile virus, and malaria (see Chap. 23A).

8. **Hemolysis.** Hemoglobinemia, hemoglobinuria, and hyperkalemia caused by overheating of the blood have been reported. Massive hemolysis, intravascular sickling, and death have occurred from the use of hemoglobin sickle cell (SC) donor blood.

9. **Graft-versus-host disease.** This is prevented by using **irradiated blood.** Before blood was irradiated, a syndrome of transient maculopapular rash, eosinophilia, lymphopenia, and thrombocytopenia without other signs of immunodeficiency was described in infants receiving multiple exchange transfusions. This did not usually progress to graft-versus-host disease.

10. **Miscellaneous.** Hypothermia, hyperthermia, and possibly necrotizing enterocolitis.

IX. OTHER TREATMENT MODALITIES

A. **Increasing bilirubin conjugation. Phenobarbital,** in a dose of 5 to 8 mg/kg every 24 hours, induces microsomal enzymes, increases bilirubin conjugation and excretion, and increases bile flow. It is useful in treating the indirect hyperbilirubinemia of Crigler-Najjar syndrome type II (but not type I) and in the treatment of the direct hyperbilirubinemia associated with hyperalimentation. Phenobarbital given antenatally to the mother is effective in lowering bilirubin levels in erythroblastotic infants, but concerns about toxicity prevent its routine use in pregnant women in the United States. Phenobarbital does not augment the effects of phototherapy.

B. **Decreasing enterohepatic circulation.** In breast-fed and formula-fed infants with bilirubins >15 mg/dL, oral agar significantly increases the efficiency and shortens the duration of phototherapy. In fact, oral agar alone was as effective as phototherapy in lowering bilirubin levels. Although oral agar may prove to be an economical therapy for hyperbilirubinemia, we have limited experience with its use in our nurseries.

C. **Inhibiting bilirubin production.** Metalloprotoporphyrins (e.g., tin and zinc protoporphyrins) are competitive inhibitors of heme oxygenase, the first enzyme in converting heme to bilirubin. They have been used to treat hyperbilirubinemia in Coombs-positive ABO incompatibility and in Crigler-Najjar type I patients. In addition, a single dose of tin mesoporphyrin given shortly after birth substantially reduced the incidence of hyperbilirubinemia and the duration of phototherapy in Greek preterm (30 to 36 weeks) infants. A follow-up study by the same research group demonstrated that a single dose of Sn-mesoporphyrin in G6PD-deficient newborns significantly reduced bilirubin levels and eliminated the need for phototherapy. However, these agents are still experimental and are not yet in routine use.

D. **Inhibiting hemolysis.** High-dose intravenous immune globulin (500–1,000 mg/kg IV >2 to 4 hours) has been used to reduce bilirubin levels in infants with isoimmune hemolytic disease. The mechanism is unknown, but theroetically the immune globulin acts by occupying the Fc receptors of reticuloendothelial cells, thereby preventing them from taking up and lysing antibody-coated RBCs.

X. DIRECT OR CONJUGATED HYPERBILIRUBINEMIA is due to failure to excrete CB from the hepatocyte into the duodenum. It is manifested by a CB level >2 mL/dL or a CB level >15% of the total bilirubin level. It may be associated with hepatomegaly, splenomegaly, pale stools, and dark urine. CB is found in the urine; UCB is not. The preferred term to describe it is cholestasis, which includes retention of CB, bile acids, and other components of bile.

A. Differential diagnosis
   1. Liver cell injury (normal bile ducts)
       a. Toxic. Intravenous hyperalimentation in low birth weight infants is a major cause of elevated CB in the neonatal intensive care unit (NICU). It appears to be unrelated to the parenteral use of lipid. Sepsis and ischemic necrosis may cause cholestasis.
       b. Infection. Viral: hepatitis (B, C), giant-cell neonatal hepatitis, rubella, CMV, herpes, Epstein–Barr virus, coxsackievirus, adenovirus, echoviruses 14 and 19. Bacterial: syphilis, *Escherichia coli*, group B β-hemolytic streptococcus, listeria, tuberculosis, staphylococcus. Parasitic: toxoplasma.
       c. Metabolic. α-1-Antitrypsin deficiency, cystic fibrosis, galactosemia, tyrosinemia, hypermethionemia, fructosemia, storage diseases (Gaucher, Niemann-Pick, glycogenosis type IV, Wolmans), Rotor syndrome, Dubin-Johnson syndrome, Byler disease, Zellweger syndrome, idiopathic cirrhosis, porphyria, hemochromatosis, trisomy 18.
   2. Excessive bilirubin load (inspissated bile syndrome). Seen in any severe hemolytic disease but especially in infants with erythroblastosis fetalis who have been treated with intrauterine transfusion. In addition, a self-limited cholestatic jaundice is frequently seen in infants supported on extracorporeal membrane oxygenation (ECMO) (see Chap. 24D). The cholestasis may last as long as 9 weeks and is thought to be secondary to hemolysis during ECMO.
   3. Bile flow obstruction (biliary atresia, extrahepatic or intrahepatic). The extrahepatic type may be isolated or associated with a choledochal cyst, trisomy 13 or 18, or polysplenia. The intrahepatic type may be associated with the Alagille syndrome, intrahepatic atresia with lymphedema (Aagenaes syndrome, nonsyndromic paucity of intrahepatic bile ducts, coprostanic acidemia, choledochal cyst, bile duct stenosis, rupture of bile duct, lymph node enlargement, hemangiomas, tumors, pancreatic cyst, inspissated bile syndrome, and cystic fibrosis).
   4. In the NICU, the most common causes of elevated CB, in decreasing order of frequency, are PN, idiopathic hepatitis, biliary atresia, α-1-antitrypsin deficiency, intrauterine infection, choledochal cyst, galactosemia, and increased bilirubin load from hemolytic disease.
B. Diagnostic tests and management
   1. Evaluate for hepatomegaly, splenomegaly, petechiae, chorioretinitis, and microcephaly.
   2. Evaluate liver damage and function by measurement of serum glutamic oxaloacetic transaminase (SGOT) level, serum glutamic pyruvic transaminase (SGPT) level, alkaline phosphatase level, prothrombin time (PT), partial thromboplastin time (PTT), and serum albumin level.
   3. Stop PN with amino acids. If this is the cause, the liver dysfunction will usually resolve.
   4. Test for bacterial, viral, and intrauterine infections (see Chap. 23A, B, D).
   5. Serum analysis for α-1-antitrypsin deficiency.
   6. Serum and urine amino acids determinations (see Chap. 29D).
   7. Urinalysis for glucose and reducing substances (see Chap. 29D).
   8. If known causes are ruled out, the problem is to differentiate idiopathic neonatal hepatitis from bile duct abnormalities such as intrahepatic biliary atresia or hypoplasia, choledochal cyst, bile plug syndrome, extrahepatic biliary atresia, hypoplasia, or total biliary atresia.
       a. Abdominal ultrasound should be done to rule out a choledochal cyst or mass.
       b. We use a hepatobiliary scan with technetium [Tc 99m]diisopropyliminodiacetic (DISIDA) as the next step to visualize the biliary tree.
       c. Iodine-131–rose bengal fecal excretion test may be useful if the [Tc 99m]DISIDA scan is not available.

d. A nasoduodenal tube can be passed and fluid collected in 2-hour aliquots for 24 hours. If there is no bile, treat with phenobarbital, 5 mg/kg/day for 7 days, and repeat the duodenal fluid collection.

e. If the duodenal fluid collections, scans, and ultrasonography suggest no extrahepatic obstruction, the child may be observed with careful follow-up.

f. If the ultrasonography scans, or fluid collections suggest extrahepatic obstruction disease, the baby will need an exploratory laparotomy, cholangiogram, and open liver biopsy to enable a definite diagnosis.

g. If the diagnosis of extrahepatic obstruction disease cannot be ruled out, the baby must have the studies outlined, because surgical therapy for choledochal cyst is curative if done early and hepatoportoenterostomy has better results if done early.

h. Most cholestasis in the NICU is due to prolonged exposure to PN. After ruling out other causes (sepsis, metabolic disorders, ultrasound for choledochal cyst, and the presence of a gallbladder) we institute the following:

i. Enteral feedings, even at "trophic" volumes of 10 ml/ kg/day should be initiated as soon as they can safely be introduced.

ii. Once enteral feedings are restarted, infants with persistently elevated direct bilirubin and LFTs should have fat-soluble vitamin supplements (ADEK).

iii. Patients on PN should have LFTs checked regularly (once a week) and if the direct bilirubin begins to rise, along with the alanine aminotransferase (ALT) and gamma-glutamyltransferase (GGT), the PN should be adjusted. Decrease mineral content to minimize toxic effects of mineral accumulation. Cycle PN, on for 18 to 20 hours, off of 6 to 4 hours. (Run dextrose solution when PN is off).

iv. Phenobarbital should not be used to treat cholestasis in this patient population.

v. Recommendations regarding routine use of ursodiol (Actigall) and intestinal decontamination cannot currently be recommended give the lack of safety data.

vi. Recently we have used parenteral fish oil (Omegaven 10% fish oil emulsion—Fresenius Kabi, Homburg, Germany) in infants with PN associated liver disease. The intralipid is discontinued and replaced with Omegaven. It is started at 1 g/kg/day for 2 days and then slowly advanced to 2 to 3 g/kg/day. Extra calories are given as glucose. So far 23 patients with PN associated liver disease (mostly infants with severe short gut syndromes) at Children's Hospital Boston have been treated with Omegaven with good results. It is not approved for use in the United States so one must apply to the U.S. Food and Drug Administration (FDA) for compassionate use and purchase it through an international pharmacy in Germany. This treatment shows promise but will need further study before it can be recommended.

XI. HYDROPS is a term used to describe generalized subcutaneous edema in the fetus or neonate. It is usually accompanied by ascites and often by pleural and/or pericardial effusions. Hydrops fetalis is discussed here, because in the past, hemolytic disease of the newborn was the major cause of both fetal and neonatal hydrops. However, because of the decline in Rh sensitization, nonimmune conditions are now the major causes of hydrops in the United States.

A. Etiology. The pathogenesis of hydrops includes anemia, cardiac failure, decreased colloid oncotic pressure (hypoalbuminemia), increased capillary permeability, asphyxia, and placental perfusion abnormalities. There is a general, but not a constant, relation between the degree of anemia, the serum albumin level, and the presence of hydrops. There is no correlation between the severity of hydrops and the blood volume of the infant. Most hydropic infants have normal blood volume (80 mg/kg).

1. Hematologic due to chronic *in utero* anemia (10% of cases). Isoimmune hemolytic disease (e.g., Rh incompatibility), homozygous α thalassemia, homozygous G6PD deficiency, chronic fetomaternal hemorrhage, twin-to-twin transfusion, hemorrhage, thrombosis, bone marrow failure (chloramphenicol, maternal parvovirus infection), and bone marrow replacement (Gaucher disease), leukemia.

2. **Cardiovascular** due to heart failure (20% of cases) (see Chap. 25).
   a. **Rhythm disturbances.** Heart block, supraventricular tachycardia, atrial flutter.
   b. **Major cardiac disease.** Hypoplastic left heart, Epstein anomaly, truncus arteriosus, myocarditis (coxsackievirus), endocardial fibroelastosis, cardiac neoplasm (rhabdomyoma), cardiac thrombosis, arteriovenous malformations, premature closure of foramen ovale, generalized arterial calcification, premature restructure of the foramen ovale.
3. **Renal** (5% of cases). Nephrosis, renal vein thrombosis, renal hypoplasia, urinary obstruction.
4. **Infection** (8% of cases). Syphilis, rubella, CMV, congenital hepatitis, herpes virus, adenovirus, toxoplasmosis, leptospirosis, Chagas disease, parvovirus (see Chap. 23).
5. **Pulmonary** (5% of cases). Congenital chylothorax, diaphragmatic hernia, pulmonary lymphangiectasia, cystic adenomatoid malformations, intrathoracic mass.
6. **Placenta or cord** (rare cause). Chorangioma, umbilical vein thrombosis, arteriovenous malformation, chorionic vein thrombosis, true knot in umbilical cord, cord compression, choriocarcinoma.
7. **Maternal conditions** (5% of cases). Toxemia, diabetes, thyrotoxicosis.
8. **GI** (5% of cases). Meconium peritonitis, *in utero* volvulus, and atresia.
9. **Chromosomal** (10% of cases). Turner syndrome; trisomy 13, 18, 21; triploidy; aneuploidy.
10. **Miscellaneous** (10% of cases). Cystic hygroma. Wilms tumor, angioma, teratoma, neuroblastoma, CNS malformations, amniotic band syndrome, lysosomal storage disorders, congenital myotonic dystrophy, skeletal abnormalities (osteogenesis imperfecta, achondrogenesis, hypophosphatasia, thanatophoric dwarf, arthrogryposis), Noonan syndrome, acardia, absent ductus venosus, renal venous thrombosis, and cystic hygroma.
11. **Unknown** (20% of cases).

B. **Diagnosis.** A pregnant woman with polyhydramnios, severe anemia, toxemia, or isoimmune disease should undergo ultrasonic examination of the fetus. If the fetus is hydropic, a careful search by ultrasonography and real-time fetal echocardiography may reveal the cause and may guide fetal treatment. The accumulation of pericardial or ascitic fluid may be the first sign of impending hydrops in a Rh-sensitized fetus. Investigations should be carried out for the causes of fetal hydrops mentioned in A. The usual investigation includes the following:

1. **Maternal** blood type and Coombs test as well as red cell antibody titers, complete blood count (CBC) and RBC indices, hemoglobin electrophoresis, Kleihauser-Betke stain of maternal blood for fetal red cells, tests for syphillis, studies for viral infection, and toxoplasmosis (see Chap. 23), sedimentation rate, and lupus tests.
2. **Fetal** echocardiography for cardiac abnormalities and ultrasonography for other structural lesions.
3. **Amniocentesis** for karyotype, metabolic studies, fetoprotein, cultures, and polymerase chain reaction (PCR) for viral infections and restriction endonucleases as indicated.
4. **Doppler** ultrasonographic measurments of peak velocity of blood flow in the fetal middle cerebral artery have had good correlation with fetal anemia.
5. **Fetal blood sampling–percutaneous umbilical blood sampling (PUBS)** (see Chap. 1). Karyotype, CBC, hemoglobin electrophoresis, cultures, and PCR, DNA studies, and albumin.
6. **Neonatal.** Following delivery, many of the same studies may be carried out on the infant. A CBC, blood typing, and Coombs test; ultrasonographic studies

of the head, heart, and abdomen; and a search for the causes listed in XI.A should be done. Examination of pleural and/or ascitic fluid, LFT, urinalysis, viral titers, chromosomes, placental examination, and x-rays may be indicated. If the infant is stillborn or dies, a detailed autopsy should be done.

C. Management

1. A hydropic fetus is at great risk for intrauterine death. A decision must be made about intrauterine treatment if possible, for example, fetal transfusion in isoimmune hemolytic anemia (see Chap. 1) or maternal digitalis therapy for supraventricular tachycardia (see Chap. 25). If fetal treatment is not possible, the fetus must be evaluated for the relative possibility of intrauterine death versus the risks of premature delivery. If premature delivery is planned, pulmonary maturity should be induced with steroids if it is not present (see Chap. 24A). Intrauterine paracentesis or thoracentesis just before delivery may facilitate subsequent newborn resuscitation.

2. Resuscitation of the hydropic infant is complex and requires advance preparation whenever feasible. Intubation can be extremely difficult with massive edema of the head, neck, and oropharynx and should be done by a skilled operator immediately after birth. (A fiberoptic scope may facilitate placement of the endotracheal tube.) A second individual should provide rapid relief of hydrostatic pressure on the diaphragm and lungs by paracentesis and/or thoracentesis with an 18- to 20-gauge angiocatheter attached to a three-way stopcock and syringe. After entry into the chest or abdominal cavity, the needle is withdrawn so that the plastic catheter can remain without fear of laceration. Cardiocentesis may also be required if there is electromechanical dissociation due to cardiac tamponade.

3. Ventilator management can be complicated by pulmonary hypoplasia, barotrauma, pulmonary edema, or reaccumulation of ascites and/or pleural fluid. If repeated thoracenteses cannot control hydrothorax, chest tube drainage may be indicated. Judicious use of diuretics (e.g., furosemide) is often helpful in reducing pulmonary edema. Arterial access is needed to monitor blood gases and acid–base balance.

4. Because hydropic infants have enormous quantities of extravascular salt and water, fluid intake is based on an estimate of the infant's "dry weight" (e.g., 50th percentile for gestational age). Free water and salt are kept at a minimum (e.g., 40 to 60 mL/kg/day as dextrose water) until edema is resolved. Monitoring the electrolyte composition of serum, urine, ascites fluid, and/or pleural fluid, and careful measurement of intake, output, and weight are essential for guiding therapy. Normoglycemia is achieved by providing glucose at a rate of 4 to 8 mg/kg/minute. Unless cardiovascular and/or renal function are compromised, edema will eventually resolve and salt and water intake can then be normalized.

5. If the hematocrit is <30%, a partial exchange transfusion with 50 to 80 mL/kg PRBCs (hematocrit 70%) should be performed to raise the hematocrit and increase oxygen-carrying capacity. If the problem is Rh isoimmunization, the blood should be type O Rh-negative. We often use O Rh-negative cells and AB serum prepared before delivery and cross-matched against the mother. An isovolumetric exchange (simultaneous removal of blood from the umbilical artery while blood is transfused in the umbilical vein at 2 to 4 mL/kg/minute) may be better tolerated in infants with compromised cardiovascular systems.

6. Inotropic support (e.g., dopamine) may be required to improve cardiac output. Central venous and arterial lines are needed for monitoring pressures. Most hydropic infants are normovolemic, but manipulation of the blood volume may be indicated after measurement of arterial and venous pressures and after correction of acidosis and asphyxia. If a low serum albumin level is contributing to hydrops, fresh-frozen plasma may help. Care must be taken not to volume overload an already failing heart, and infusions of colloid may need to be followed by a diuretic.

7. Hyperbilirubinemia should be treated as in VI.

8. Many infants with hydrops will survive if aggressive neonatal care is provided.

XII. ISOIMMUNE HEMOLYTIC DISEASE OF THE NEWBORN

A. **Etiology.** Maternal exposure (through blood transfusion, fetomaternal hemor-rhage, amniocentesis, or abortion) to foreign antigens on fetal RBCs causes the production and transplacental passage of specific maternal immunoglobulin G (IgG) antibodies directed against the fetal antigens, resulting in the immune destruction of fetal RBCs. The usual antigen involved prenatally is the Rh(D) antigen, and postnatally, the A and B antigens. A positive Coombs test result in an infant should prompt identification of the antibody. If the antibody is not anti-A or anti-B, then it should be identified by testing the mother's serum against a panel of red cell antigens or the father's red cells. This may have implications for subsequent pregnancies. Since the dramatic decline in Rh hemolytic disease with the use of RhoGAM, maternal antibody against A or B antigens (ABO incompatibility) is now the most common cause of isoimmune hemolytic disease. In addition, other relatively uncommon antigens (Kell, Duffy, E, C, and c) now account for a greater proportion of cases of isoimmune hemolytic anemia (Tables 18.5–18.7). The **Lewis antigen** is a commonly found antigen, but this antigen does not cause hemolytic disease of the newborn. Most Lewis antibodies are of the IgM class (which do not cross the placenta) and the Lewis antigen is poorly developed and expressed on the fetal and/or neonatal erythrocytes.

B. **Fetal management.** All pregnant women should have blood typing, Rh determi-nation, and an antibody screening performed on their first prenatal visit. This will identify the Rh-negative mothers and identify any antibody due to Rh or any rare antigen sensitization. In a white population in the United States, 15% of people lack the D antigen (dd). Of the remainder, 48% are heterozygous (dD) and 35% are homozygous (DD). Approximately 15% of matings in this population will result in a fetus with the D antigen and a mother without it.

1. If the mother is **Rh-positive** and her **antibody screening is negative,** it may be advisable to repeat the antibody screening later in pregnancy, but this will have a low yield.

2. If the mother is **Rh-negative/antibody screen negative** and the father of the fetus is Rh-negative, she should be retested at 28 and 35 weeks' gestation (see XII.D). If the father is Rh-positive, she should be retested at 18 to 20 weeks and monthly thereafter. If the paternal phenotype is heterozygous for Rh(O) amniocentesis is used to determine the fetal blood type by PCR.

3. If the mother is **Rh-negative/antibody screen positive,** the antibody titer is repeated at 16 to 18 weeks, at 22 weeks, and every 2 weeks thereafter. Amniocentesis is usually done for antibody titers >1:16 or at a level at which the local center has had a fetal demise (each center should have its own standards for action on various titers). Irrespective of antibody titers, if there is a prior history of a severely isoimmunized fetus, serial amniocentesis may be indicated beginning at 16 to 18 weeks to measure the optical density at a wavelength of 450 nm (bilirubin) to assess the risk for fetal death from hydrops. If the fetus is <24 weeks (optical density is less accurate) or if placental trauma is likely with amniocentesis, direct percutaneous fetal blood sampling for blood type, direct Coombs test, hematocrit, CBC, and blood gases may be preferable. Doppler assessment of fetal middle cerebral artery peak blood flow velocity is emerging as an accurate tool to predict fetal anemia and may replace amniocentesis for evaluation of fetal anemia. A recent editorial by Moise KJ. *N Engl J Med* 2006;355(2):192; discusses this further.

4. Fetuses at high risk for death may be treated by early delivery if the risk of fetal demise or intrauterine transfusion exceeds the risk of early delivery. In our institution, this is usually 30 weeks, but this requires careful fetal monitoring, induction of pulmonary maturity, and close cooperation between obstetrician and neonatologist. If the hydropic fetus is too immature for early delivery to be considered, **intrauterine transfusion is indicated.** Transfusion can be carried out by intraperitoneal or intravascular routes, although intravascular transfusion may be the only option in a moribund hydropic infant who has ascites, is not breathing, and is unable to absorb intraperitoneal blood.

Intrauterine transfusions are repeated whenever fetal hemoglobin levels fall below approximately 10 g/dL. Following transfusion, serial ultrasonography examinations are done to assess changes in the degree of hydrops and fetal well-being. Some infants who have undergone multiple intrauterine transfusions will be born with all adult O Rh-negative RBCs because all the fetal cells are destroyed. Although one should be prepared, not all infants will need postnatal exchange transfusion. These infants are at risk of developing conjugated hyperbilirubinemia. Intensive maternal plasma exchange is rarely done, but may be considered for the pregnant woman who has a history of hydropic fetal deaths before 28 weeks' gestation.

C. Neonatal management. About half the number of infants with a positive Coombs test result from Rh hemolytic disease will have minimum hemolysis and hyperbilirubinemia (cord bilirubin level <4 mg/dL and hemoglobin level >14 g/dL). These infants may require no treatment or only phototherapy. One-fourth of infants with Rh hemolytic disease present with anemia, hemoglobin level <14 g/dL, and hyperbilirubinemia (cord bilirubin >4 mg/dL). They have increased nucleated red cells and reticulocytes on blood smear. These infants may have thrombocytopenia and a very elevated white blood cell count. They have an enlarged liver and spleen, and require early exchange transfusion and phototherapy (see VI.B, VII, and VIII). Figure 18.6 and Tables 18.5–18.7 can be used in deciding what treatment to use. Infants with isoimmune hemolytic anemia may develop an exaggerated physiologic anemia at 12 weeks of age, requiring blood transfusion. Erythropoietin is currently being evaluated for use in preventing this late anemia. High-dose intravenous immune γ-globulin therapy 500 to 1,000 mg/kg IV is used for hemolytic disease (see IX.D).

D. Prevention. Eliminating exposure of women to foreign red cell antigens will prevent immune hemolytic disease of the newborn. Avoiding unnecessary transfusions and medical procedures that carry the risk of transplacental passage of blood will help decrease sensitization. Rh hemolytic disease is now being prevented by the administration of **Rho(D) immune globulin (RhoGAM)** to unsensitized Rh-negative mothers. This is usually done at 28 weeks' gestation and again within 72 hours after delivery. Other indications for Rho(D) immune globulin (or using larger doses) are prophylaxis following abortion, amniocentesis, chorionic villus sampling, and transplacental hemorrhage. Interestingly, ABO incompatibility between mother and fetus protects against sensitization of an Rh-negative mother, probably because maternal antibodies eliminate fetal RBCs from the maternal circulation before they can encounter antibody-forming lymphocytes.

XIII. ABO HEMOLYTIC DISEASE OF THE NEWBORN. Since the introduction of Rh immune globulin, ABO incompatibility has been the most common cause of hemolytic disease of the newborn in the United States.

A. Etiology. The cause is the reaction of maternal anti-A or anti-B antibodies to the A or B antigen on the RBCs of the fetus or newborn. It is usually seen only in type A or B infants born to type O mothers because these mothers make anti-A or anti-B antibodies of the IgG class, which cross the placenta, whereas mothers of type A or B usually make anti-A or anti-B antibodies of the immunoglobulin M (IgM) class, which do not cross the placenta. The combination of a type O mother and a type A or type B infant occurs in 15% of pregnancies in the United States. Only one-fifth of infants with this blood group setup (or 3% of all infants) will develop significant jaundice. Some bacterial vaccines, such as tetanus toxoid and pneumococcal vaccine, had A and B substance in the culture media and were associated with significant hemolysis in type A or type B neonates born to type O mothers who were given these vaccines. New preparations of the vaccine are said to be free of these A and B substances.

B. Clinical presentation. The situation is a type O mother with a type A or type B infant who becomes jaundiced in the first 24 hours of life. Approximately 50% of the cases occur in firstborn infants. There is no predictable pattern of recurrence in subsequent infants. **Most ABO-incompatible infants have anti-A or anti-B antibody on their RBCs, yet only a small number have significant ABO hemolytic disease of the newborn.** Infants may have a low concentration of antibody on their red cells; consequently, their antibody will not be demonstrated by elution techniques or by a positive direct antiglobulin test (Coombs test). As the antibody concentration increases, the antibody can be demonstrated first by elution techniques and then by the Coombs test. Although all ABO-incompatible infants have some degree of hemolysis, significant hemolysis is usually associated only with a positive direct Coombs test result on the infant's red cells. If there are other causes of neonatal jaundice, ABO incompatibility will add to the bilirubin production. In infants with significant ABO incompatibility, there will be many spherocytes on the blood smear and an elevated reticulocyte count. RBCs from infants with ABO incompatibility may have increased osmotic fragility and autohemolysis, as in HS. The autohemolysis is not corrected by glucose, as in HS. The family history and long-term course will usually help with the diagnosis of HS.

   C. Management. If blood typing and Coombs test are done on the cord blood of infants born to type O mothers, these infants can have bilirubin levels monitored and therapy instituted early enough to prevent severe hyperbilirubinemia. However, this approach may not be cost effective, because most infants do not develop significant jaundice and only 10% of infants with a positive direct Coombs test result for ABO incompatibility will need phototherapy. In the absence of a routine test on all infants born to type O mothers, one must rely on clinical observation to notice the jaundiced infants. This will depend on the observation of the caregivers and may not be reliable in infants whose skin pigmentation makes the diagnosis of jaundice difficult. A bilirubin level at 12 hours of age, or cord blood typing and a Coombs test on all black or Asian infants born to type O mothers, may be a reasonable compromise. Infants born to type O mothers who are to have an early discharge (within 24 hours) should be evaluated for ABO incompatibility, and the parents should be made aware of the possibility of jaundice. Many infants have an initial rise in bilirubin that quickly falls to normal levels. If the criteria for Rh disease are used, many will undergo unnecessary treatment. An approach to phototherapy and exchange transfusion management has been outlined in VI.B. IV γ globulin to inhibit hemolysis can be considered (see IX.D). Kernicterus has been reported in ABO incompatibility. If exchange transfusion is necessary, it should be with type O blood that is of the same Rh type as the infant with a low titer of anti-A or anti-B antibody. We often use type O cells resuspended in type AB plasma. There is no need for prenatal diagnosis or treatment and no need for early delivery.

Suggested Readings

American Academy of Pediatrics, Subcommittee on Hyperbilirubinemia. Practice parameter: Management of hyperbilirubinemia in the newborn infant 35 or more weeks of gestation. *Pediatrics* 2004;114:297–316.

Benders MJ, van Bel F, van de Bor M. The effect of phototherapy on cerebral blood flow velocity in preterm infants. *Acta Paediatr* 1998;87:786–791.

Benders MJ, van Bel F, van de Bor M. The effect of phototherapy on renal blood flow velocity in preterm infants. *Biol Neonate* 1998;73:228–234.

Bhutani VK, Johnson L, Sivieri EMJohnson. Predictive ability of a predischarge hour-specific serum bilirubin for subsequent significant hyperbilirubinemia in healthy term and near-term newborns. *Pediatrics* 1999;103:6–14.

Bhutani VK, Gourley GR, Adler S. Noninvasive measurement of total serum bilirubin in a multiracial predischarge newborn population to assess the risk of severe hyperbilirubinemia. *Pediatrics* 2000;106:E17.

Bhutani VK, Johnson LH. Jaundice technologies: Prediction of hyperbilirubinemia in term and near-term newborns. *J Perinatol* 2001;21(Suppl 1):S76–S82; discussion S83–S87.

Caglayan S, Candemir H, Aksit S, et al. Superiority of oral agar and phototherapy combination in the treatment of neonatal hyperbilirubinemia. *Pediatrics* 1993;92:86–89.

Dennery PA, Seidman DS, Stevenson DK. Neonatal hyperbilirubinemia. *N Engl J Med* 2001;344:581–590.

Gura KM, Duggan CP, Collier SB, et al. Reversal of parenteral nutrition-associated liver disease in two infants with short bowel syndrome using parenteral fish oil: Implications for future management. *Pediatrics* 2006;118:e197–201.

Gourley GR. Breastfeeding, diet, and hyperbilirubinemia. *NeoReviews* 2000;1:e25–e30.

Hammerman C, Kaplan M. Recent developments in the management of neonatal hyperbilirubinemia. *NeoReviews* 2000;1:e19–e24.

Iolascon A, Faienza MF, Moretti A, et al. UGT1 promoter polymorphism accounts for increased neonatal appearance of hereditary spherocytosis. *Blood* 1998;91:1093.

Kaplan M, Hammerman C, Renbaum P, et al. Gilbert's syndrome and hyperbilirubinaemia in ABO-incompatible neonates. *Lancet* 2000;356:652–653.

Kaplan M, Hammerman C. Glucose-6-phosphate dehydrogenase deficiency: A worldwide potential cause of severe neonatal hyperbilirubinemia. *NeoReviews* 2000;1:e32–e38.

Kaplan M. Genetic interactions in the pathogenesis of neonatal hyperbilirubinemia: Gilbert's Syndrome and glucose-6-phosphate dehydrogenase deficiency. *J Perinatol* 2001;21(Suppl 1):S30–S34; discussion S35–S39.

Kappas A, Drummond GS, Valaes T. A single dose of Sn-mesoporphyrin prevents development of severe hyperbilirubinemia in glucose-6-phosphate dehydrogenase-deficient newborns. *Pediatrics* 2001;108:25–30.

MacDonald MG. Hidden risks: Early discharge and bilirubin toxicity due to glucose 6-phosphate dehydrogenase deficiency. *Pediatrics* 1995;96:734–738.

Maisels MJ, Newman TB. Kernicterus in otherwise healthy, breastfed term newborns. *Pediatrics* 1995;96:730–733.

Maisels MJ, Kring E. Transcutaneous bilirubinometry decreases the need for serum bilirubin measurements and saves money. *Pediatrics* 1997;99:599–601.

Maisels MJ. Neonatal Jaundice. *Pediatr Rev* 2006;27:443–454.

Martinez JC, Maisels MJ, Otheguy L, et al. Hyperbilirubinemia in the breastfed newborn: A controlled trial of four interventions. *Pediatrics* 1993;91:470–473.

Maruo Y, Nishizawa K, Sato H, et al. Association of neonatal hyperbilirubinemia with bilirubin UDP-glucuronosyltransferase polymorphism. *Pediatrics* 1999;103:1224–1227.

Maruo Y, Nishizawa K, Sato H, et al. Prolonged unconjugated hyperbilirubinemia associated with breast milk and mutations of the bilirubin uridine diphosphate-glucuronosyltransferase gene. *Pediatrics* 2000;106:E59.

Monaghan G, McLellan A, McGeehan A, et al. Gilbert's syndrome is a contributory factor in prolonged unconjugated hyperbilirubinemia of the newborn. *J Pediatr* 1999;134:441–446.

Moise KJ. *Diagnosis and management of Rhesus (Rh) alloimmunization.* http://stone.utdol .com/APP/index.asp. December 2002.

Moise KJ. Diagnosing hemolytic disease of the fetus- time to put away the needles? *N Engl J Med* 2006;355(2):192–194.

Newman TB, Klebanoff MA, Neonatal hyperbilirubinemia and long-term outcome: Another look at the Collaborative Perinatal Project. *Pediatrics* 1993;92:651–657.

Newman TB, Xiong B, Gonzales VM, Prediction and prevention of extreme neonatal hyperbilirubinemia in a mature health maintenance organization. *Arch Pediatr Adolesc Med* 2000;154:1140–1147.

Newman TB, Liljestrand P, Jeremy RJ, Outcomes among newborns with total serum bilirubin levels of 25 mg per deciliter or more. *N Engl J Med* 2006;354:1889–900.

Peterec SM. Management of neonatal Rh disease. *Clin Perinatol* 1995;22:561–592.

Pezzati M, Biagiotti R, Vangi V, et al. Changes in mesenteric blood flow response to feeding: Conventional versus fiber-optic phototherapy. *Pediatrics* 2000;105:350–353.

Rubo J, Albrecht K, Lasch P, High-dose intravenous immune globulin therapy for hyperbilirubinemia caused by Rh hemolytic disease. *J Pediatr* 1992;121:93–97.

Stevenson DK, Fanaroff AA, Maisels MJ, et al. Prediction of hyperbilirubinemia in near-term and term infants. *Pediatrics* 2001;108:31–39.

Suchy FJ. Neonatal cholestasis. *Pediatr Rev* 2004;25:388–396.

Tan KL. Decreased response to phototherapy for neonatal jaundice in breast-fed infants. *Arch Pediatr Adolesc Med* 1998;152:1187–1190.

Watchko JF, Oski FA. Kernicterus in preterm newborns: Past, present, and future. *Pediatrics* 1992;90:707–715.

Wennberg RP, Ahlfors CE, Bhutani VK, et al. Toward understanding kernicterus: A challenge to improve the management of jaundiced newborns. *Pediatrics* 2006;117:474–485.

Zallen GS, Bliss DW, Curran TJ, et al. Bilary atresia. *Pediatr Rev* 2006;27:243–248.

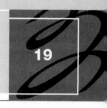

DRUG ABUSE AND WITHDRAWAL
Sylvia Schechner

19

I. MATERNAL SUBSTANCE ABUSE. In the epidemic of substance abuse in the United States, the drugs most often abused are cannabinoids, heroin, crystal meth, and cocaine. Cocaine is used probably because of its inexpensive alkaloidal free-base form, "crack." The high purity of heroin available makes snorting or smoking viable options and has thereby increased heroin consumption compared with years ago when injection was the only option. Methamphetamine can be smoked, snorted or ingested orally, and easily purchased on the street. There is a 15% overall prevalence of at least one of the illicit substances mentioned in the preceding text in urine samples obtained during pregnancy. Intrauterine exposure to alcohol occurs more often than all the illicit substances listed in the preceding text combined. Despite all the adverse publicity, tobacco use continues in approximately 17% of pregnancies and only 20% quit smoking when they become pregnant. We are seeing more women who are taking psychotropic medications during pregnancy. It is estimated that approximately 14% of pregnant women suffer from some form of mental illness and more than half take medications that are not recommended in pregnancy (1). Iatrogenic neonatal abstinence syndrome (NAS) may be seen in infants who required narcotics for sedation for surgery or other procedures.

II. DIAGNOSIS

A. Take a comprehensive medical and psychosocial history including a specific inquiry about maternal drug use as part of every prenatal and newborn evaluation, although accurate information regarding illicit drug use during pregnancy is often difficult to obtain.

1. Maternal associations with drug abuse
   a. Poor or no prenatal care.
   b. Preterm labor.
   c. Placental rupture.
   d. Precipitous delivery.
   e. Frequent demands or requests for large doses of pain medication.

2. Signs of maternal drug abuse in the infant
   a. Small for gestational age (SGA).
   b. Microcephaly.
   c. Neonatal stroke or any arterial infarction.
   d. Any of the symptoms listed in Table 19.1.

B. Diagnostic tests. Screen urine if drug withdrawal is a possibility. Meconium analysis by radioimmunoassay affords a longer view into the drug-use pattern, but is an expensive test. Hair analysis of the infant can reveal maternal drug use during the previous 3 months, but hair grows slowly and recent drug use may not be detected. Consider the implications of a positive test result. The following is our statement for testing:

Physician Guidelines for Testing, Reporting, and Care of Neonates Who May Have Been Exposed Prenatally to Controlled Substances
Brigham and Women's Hospital, Boston, MA

1. Testing
   a. Purpose. A positive urine test for controlled substances can serve several purposes: (i) it may help complete a diagnostic workup for an infant with symptoms of drug dependency or withdrawal (e.g., seizures or jitteriness), (ii) it may serve as a marker for an infant at risk for developmental delay, and (iii) it may indicate an at-risk family in need of social services. (A negative test result, however, cannot rule out any of these items.)

213

TABLE 19.1 — Reported Withdrawal Syndromes in Newborns After Maternal Drug Ingestion

	Lethargy	Poor state control	Fever	Diaphoresis	Tachycardia	Tachypnea	Cyanosis	High-pitched cry	Altered sleeping	Tremors	Hypotonicity	Hypertonicity	Hyperreflexia	Increased suck
Narcotics														
Heroin			X	X	X	X		X	X	X		X	X	X
Methadone			X	X	X	X		X	X	X		X	X	X
Propoxyphene				X	X	X		X		X		X	X	X
Pentazocine plus tripelennamine ("T's and Blues")					X	X		X		X	X	X		X
Codeine			X							X		X	X	
Sedatives														
Barbiturates				X				±	X	X	X	X	X	
Butalbital (Fiorinal, Esgic)														
Chlordiazepoxide										X				
Diazepam					X	X				X			X	X
Diphenhydramine										X				
Ethanol						X				X	X			
Ethchlorvynol (Placidyl) (plus propoxyphene plus diazepam)						X						X		
Glutethimide (plus heroin)			X			X		X		X		X	X	
Hydroxyzine (Vistaril) (600 mg/d plus Pb)						X		X		X			X	
Stimulants														
Methamphetamine	X	X						X				X		
Phencyclidine											X	X	X	
Cocaine	X	X						X	X	X		X	X	X
Antidepressants														
Tricyclics				X	X	X	X			X	X	X	X	
Antipsychotics														
Phenothiazines								X		X		X	X	X

X = symptom usually present; ± = symptom may be present, but not always; Pb = phenobarbital.

b. Symptomatic infants

    i. Performance of a toxic screen is recommended for infants with any of the following symptoms: (i) severe intrauterine growth retardation (IUGR), which is defined as a birth weight below the third percentile; (ii) symptoms consistent with neonatal drug dependency and withdrawal; (iii) central nervous system (CNS) irritability; and (iv) symptoms consistent with intracranial hemorrhage (ICH) such as focal seizures or paresis. These criteria are intended to serve as guidelines only. The

Ineffective suck	Irritability	Jitteriness	Seizures	Nasal congestion	Sneezing/yawning	Ravenous appetite	Vomitting	Excessive regurgitation	Diarrhea	Weight loss	Abdominal distention	Onset	Duration
	X	X	X	X	X	X	X	X	X	X		1–144 h	7–20 d
	X	X	X	X	X	X	X	X	X	X		1–14 d	20–45 d
	X	X	X	X	X	X		X	X	±		3–20 h	56 h–6 d
	X	X	X		X		X		X		X		
X	X	X											
X	X	X					X		X			0.5–30 h	4–17 d
X	X	X	X		X	X	X	X	X	X		0.5h–14 d	11 d–6 mo
X	X	X	?	X								2 d	24 d
	X											21 d	37 d
X		X						X		X		2–6 h	10 d–6 wk
							X					5 d	10 d–5 wk
	X	X	X		±				±	X		6–12 d	
X	X	X				X	X					24 h	9–10 d
	X							X				8 h	45 d
X	X	X	X									15 min	156 h
	X				X								5–24 h
		X					X		X			18–20 h	18 d–2 mo
X			X	X	X							1–3 d	
X	X	X	X									5–12 h	96 h–30 d
X	X	X								X		21 d	>11 d–4 mo

attending physician must decide on a case-by-case basis whether a toxic screen is indicated.

ii. It is hospital policy not to require a separate specific consent from the parents for a toxic screen on a symptomatic infant. As testing of symptomatic infants is done to assist in the medical diagnosis or treatment of the infant, the general parental consent obtained in the initial admission consent form is usually sufficient. Parents, however, should be informed by the responsible pediatrician (before the test if possible) of the purpose of the toxic screen, and that a positive test will be included in any report to the State Department of Social Services. This discussion should be documented in the medical record. In the event that the parents, when informed, object to the performance of the toxic screen, the legal office should be contacted for consultation. The results of the test and any follow-up or treatment should also be discussed with the parents. The obstetrician should also be notified of all positive test results.

c. Asymptomatic infants

i. Specific parental consent must be obtained in order to perform a toxic screen on an asymptomatic infant. (The general admission consent form is not sufficient.) As part of the process of seeking consent, the parent or parents should be advised by the attending physician or the physician designee of the purpose of the test and that a positive test will likely result in a referral to the Department of Social Services. Documentation of this discussion and the oral parental response should be made in the infant's medical record. (A separate written consent form signed by the parent is not required.) The obstetrician should also be notified of all positive test results.

ii. Testing of an asymptomatic infant may be indicated by the following circumstances: (i) lack of adequate prenatal care, (ii) past or present parental history or signs of substance abuse, or (iii) abruptio placenta. These criteria are simply guidelines. It is the responsibility of the attending physician to determine on a case-by-case basis whether testing of an asymptomatic infant may be beneficial.

2. Referral. Physicians, nurses, social workers, and other patient-care employees are required by the State of Massachusetts' Protection and Care of Children Act (commonly known as 51A) to report to the Massachusetts Department of Social Services cases of suspected child abuse and neglect, including all infants "determined to be physically dependent upon an addictive drug at birth." Reports generated by this hospital are usually filed by the hospital social services department. The hospital social services department should therefore be notified of all infants with symptoms of physical dependency to an addictive drug so that a 51A report can be filed as legally required.

The hospital social services department should also be notified of all asymptomatic infants with a positive toxic screen and all infants believed to be at risk owing to possible parental or family substance abuse. Such cases are not automatically required by law to be reported, and the hospital social services department will conduct a further evaluation to determine whether a potential abuse or neglect situation exists. If such situation is believed to exist, a report will be made. Prior experience indicated that most situations involving an infant with a positive screen (regardless of whether the infant is asymptomatic) will warrant the filing of a report.

Drugs administered during labor may cause difficulty in interpreting urine results. The length of time during which results may be positive varies with the drug.

a. Cocaine: up to 4 days

b. Heroin: 2 to 4 days

c. Phencyclidine (PCP): 2 to 4 days

d. Marijuana: 2 to 5 days

If the drugs were taken before these periods, negative results may be falsely reassuring.

C. A drug-addicted mother is at **increased risk for other diseases** such as sexually transmitted diseases, tuberculosis, hepatitis B and C, and acquired immunodeficiency syndrome (AIDS), especially if she involves herself in intravenous drug use or prostitution. Approximately 30% of pregnant intravenous drug users are seropositive for human immunodeficiency virus (HIV).

III. **WITHDRAWAL IN THE INFANT.** The onset of symptoms for acute narcotic withdrawal varies from shortly after birth to 2 weeks of age, but symptoms usually begin in 24 to 48 hours, depending on the type of drug and when the mother took the last dose. Table 19.1 shows the withdrawal symptoms in newborns. Methadone, heroin, and cocaine are the most common reasons for withdrawal seen in our nurseries.

A. **The severity of withdrawal** depends on the drugs used. Withdrawal from polydrug use is more severe than that from methadone, which is more severe than that from opiates alone or cocaine alone.

B. **Methadone** because of its ability to block the euphoric effects of heroin, is used in pregnancy to treat heroin addiction.

1. It can cause withdrawal in 75% to 90% of infants exposed *in utero*. Term infants have more severe abstinence symptoms than preterm infants.

2. The severity of the symptoms correlates with the maternal dose.

3. Maintaining a woman on <20 mg/day of methadone during pregnancy will minimize symptoms in the infant. Higher methadone doses may increase the severity and length of withdrawal. Higher doses have been used in the past few years, because better compliance was noted in heroin addicts maintained on methadone doses of >80 mg.

4. Some infants have late withdrawal, which may be of two types:
   a. Symptoms appear shortly after birth, improve, and recur at 2 to 4 weeks.
   b. Symptoms are not seen at birth but develop 2 to 3 weeks later.

5. Effects in the infant exposed to methadone during pregnancy:
   a. Lower birth weight, length, and head circumference.
   b. Sleep disturbances.
   c. Depressed interactive behavior.
   d. Poor self-calming.
   e. Tremors.
   f. Increased tone.
   g. Abstinence-associated seizures.
   h. Abnormal pneumograms.
   i. Increased incidence of sudden infant death syndrome (SIDS).
   j. Follow-up studies reveal a higher incidence of hyperactivity, learning and behavior disorders, and poor social adjustment. This may be due more to environmental factors than as a consequence of *in utero* methadone exposure.

C. **Differential diagnosis.** Consider hypoglycemia, hypocalcemia, hypomagnesemia, sepsis, and meningitis even if the diagnosis of drug-addicted mother is certain.

IV. **TREATMENT OF INFANT NARCOTIC WITHDRAWAL.** The goal is an infant who is not irritable, has no vomiting or diarrhea, can feed well and sleep between feedings, and yet is not heavy sedated (see Fig. 19.1). Never give **naloxone** (Narcan) to these infants nor to one whose mother was on methadone; it may precipitate immediate withdrawal or seizures.

A. **Symptomatic treatment.** Forty percent need no medication. Symptomatic care includes tight swaddling, holding, rocking, placing in a slightly darkened quiet area, and hypercaloric formula (24 cal/30 mL) as needed.

B. **Medication.** Infants who are unresponsive to symptomatic treatment will need medication. Base the decision to start medication on objective measurement of symptoms recorded on a withdrawal scoring sheet, such as the one shown in Fig. 19.2. A total abstinence score of 8 or higher for three consecutive scorings indicates a need for pharmacologic intervention. Once the infant scores 8 or higher, decrease the scoring interval from 4- to 2-hour intervals. Once the desired effect has been obtained for 72 hours, slowly taper the dose until it is discontinued. Observe the infant for 2 to 3 days before discharge. Currently there is very little evidence regarding the efficacy of different pharmacologic therapeutic regimes for treating NAS. More studies are required to produce the evidence to allow us a rational choice between treatment modalities (tincture of opium, morphine, phenobarbital,

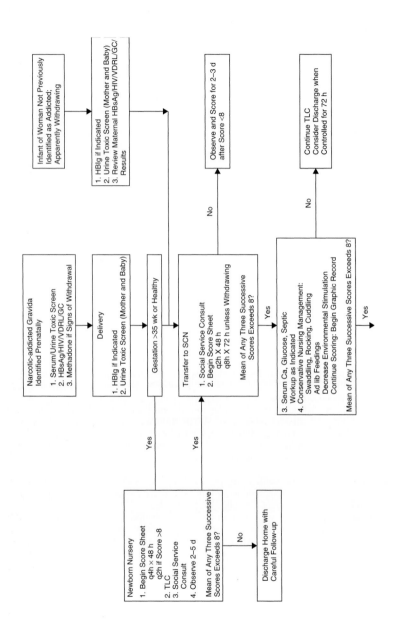

Narcotic-addicted Gravida Identified Prenatally

1. Serum/Urine Toxic Screen
2. HBsAg/HIV/VDRL/GC
3. Methadone if Signs of Withdrawal

Infant of Woman Not Previously Identified as Addicted; Apparently Withdrawing

1. HBIg if Indicated
2. Urine Toxic Screen (Mother and Baby)
3. Review Maternal HBsAg/HIV/VDRL/GC/ Results

Delivery

1. HBIg if Indicated
2. Urine Toxic Screen (Mother and Baby)

Gestation >35 wk or Healthy

Yes

Transfer to SCN

1. Social Service Consult
2. Begin Score Sheet
   q2h X 48 h
   q8h X 72 h unless Withdrawing

Mean of Any Three Successive Scores Exceeds 8?

No → Observe and Score for 2–3 d after Score <8

Yes

3. Serum Ca, Glucose, Septic Workup as Indicated
4. Conservative Nursing Management:
   Swaddling, Rocking, Cuddling
   Ad lib Feedings
   Decrease Environmental Stimulation
   Continue Scoring: Begin Graphic Record

Mean of Any Three Successive Scores Exceeds 8?

No → Continue TLC
Consider Discharge when Controlled for 72 h

Yes

Newborn Nursery

1. Begin Score Sheet
   q4h × 48 h
   q2h if Score >8
2. TLC
3. Social Service Consult
4. Observe 2–5 d

Yes

Mean of Any Three Successive Scores Exceeds 8?

No → Discharge Home with Careful Follow-up

218

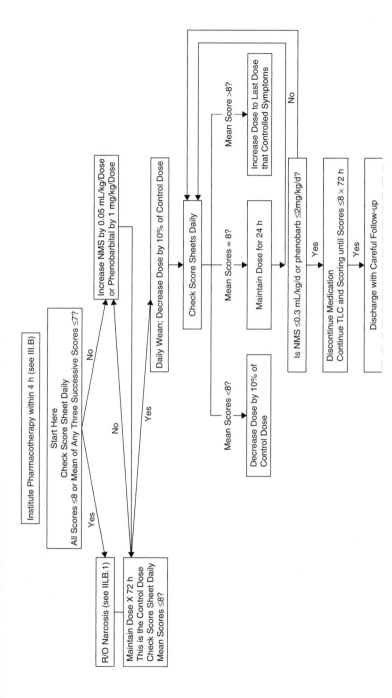

Figure 19.1. General approach to management of a narcotic-addicted gravida identified antenatally and of a withdrawing infant of a woman not previously identified as addicted. HBsAg = hepatitis B surface antigen; HIV = human immunodeficiency virus; VDRL = Venereal Disease Research Laboratory; GC = gonorrhea; HBIg = hepatitis B immune globulin; TLC = tender loving care; SCN = special care nursery; NMS = neonatal morphine solution; RR = respiratory rate; HR = heart rate; R/O = rule out.

DATE: _____

SYSTEM	SIGNS AND SYMPTOMS	SCORE	AM					PM						COMMENTS
CENTRAL NERVOUS SYSTEM DISTURBANCES	Excessive High-pitched (OR Other) Cry Continuous High-pitched (OR Other) Cry	2 3												Daily Weight:
	Sleeps < 1 Hour After Feeding Sleeps < 2 Hours After Feeding Sleeps < 3 Hours After Feeding	3 2 1												
	Hyperactive Moro Reflex Markedly Hyperactive Moro Reflex	2 3												
	Mild Tremors Disturbed Moderate-Severe Tremors Disturbed	1 2												
	Mild Tremors Undisturbed Moderate-Severe Tremors Undisturbed	3 4												
	Increased Muscle Tone	2												
	Excoriation (Specify Area):	1												
	Myoclonic Jerks	3												
	Generalized Convulsions	5												
METABOLIC/VASOMOTOR/RESPIRATORY DISTURBANCES	Sweating	1												
	Fever < 101 (99-100.8° F /37.2-38.2° C) Fever > 101 (38.4° C. and Higher)	1 2												
	Frequent Yawning (> 3-4 times/interval)	1												
	Mottling	1												
	Nasal Stuffiness	1												
	Sneezing (> 3-4 times/interval)	1												
	Nasal Flaring	2												
	Respiratory Rate > 60/Min. Respiratory Rate > 50/Min. with Retractions	1 2												

Guidelines for the use of neonatal abstinence scoring system

1. Record time of scoring (end of observation interval).
2. Give points for all behaviors or symptoms observed during the scoring interval, even though they may not be present at the time of recording. (For example, if the baby was diaphoretic at 11 A.M. and is "scored" at noon, when he or she is not, the baby still gets the "sweating" point.)
3. Awaken the baby to test reflexes. Calm before assessing muscle tone, respirations, or Moro reflex. Many of the signs of hunger can appear the same as withdrawal. Appearance after feeding gives a good idea of muscle activity.
4. Count respirations for a full minute. Always take temperature at the same site. The temperatures on the sheet are *rectal* levels; an axillary temperature that is 2 degrees cooler may also indicate withdrawal.
5. Do not give points for perspiration if it occurs due to swaddling.
6. A startle reflex should not be substituted for the Moro reflex.

220

Figure 19.2. Neonatal abstinence syndrome assessment and treatment. Guidelines for use of the neonatal abstinence scoring system are also included. (Adapted from Finnigan LP, et al. A scoring system for evaluation and treatment of neonatal abstinence syndrome: A new clinical and research tool. In: Morselli PL, Garattini S, Serini F, eds. *Basic and therapeutic aspects of perinatal pharmacology*. New York: Raven Press, 1975.)

morphine and phenobarbital, methadone). We use the following pharmacologic agents in our nurseries:

1. **Neonatal morphine solution (NMS).** This solution of morphine sulfate made up in a concentration of 0.4 mg/mL is our treatment of choice for narcotic withdrawal.
   a. It is a pharmacologic replacement.
   b. It controls all symptoms.
   c. It impairs sucking less than other medications do.
   d. It contains few additives.

   However, high doses are often necessary, and withdrawal is slow.

   This is the equivalent dose of morphine contained in neonatal opium solution (NOS). Because the only diluent is water, it avoids alcohol, preservatives, or camphor. NMS is made up in the hospital pharmacy. It has greater stability than deodorized tincture of opium (DTO), and if it is prepared properly there are no problems with overgrowth of mold or microorganisms.

   A dosing scheme for NMS or NOS according to abstinence score is as follows:

Score	NMS or NOS
8–10	0.8 mL/kg/d divided q4h
11–13	1.2 mL/kg/d divided q4h
14–16	1.6 mL/kg/d divided q4h
17 or greater	2.0 mL/kg/d divided q4h; increase by 0.4-mL increments until controlled

   Add phenobarbital to control irritability when the NMS or NOS dose is >2 mL/kg/day. Some babies will need medication more often than every 4 hours.

   Once an adequate dose has been found, and infant scores have been <8 for 72 hours, wean by 10% of total dose daily. If weaning results in scores >8, restart the last effective dose. Discontinue NMS or NOS when the daily dose is <0.3 mL/kg/day. The infant should be able to tolerate mild symptomatology during reduction.

   If the scores are low, make sure that the infant is not overdosed. Effects of overdosage include sleepiness, constipation, poor suck, hypothermia, respiratory depression, apnea, bradycardia, and ultimately profound narcosis with obtundation. If these symptoms occur, stop the medication until the abstinence scores are over 8. Use docusate

2. **NOS** (DTO). If NMS is not available, use neonatal opium solution (NOS) for treatment of narcotic withdrawal. Deodorized tincture of opium (DTO) is a hydroalcoholic solution containing 10% USP laudanum and is equal to morphine 1.0%. This is diluted 25-fold with sterile water to a concentration and potency equal to that of paregoric (0.4 mg of morphine/mL). The diluted mixture should be called *NOS*, as suggested in the Neonatal Drug Withdrawal Statement of the American Academy of Pediatrics (AAP) Committee on Drugs. The NOS dose is the same as that of NMS. This dilution is stable for 2 weeks. Keep the stock solution of tincture of opium in the pharmacy and dilute it there because of the possibility of giving the stronger mixture to the patient in error.

3. **Paregoric** contains opium 0.4%, equivalent to morphine 0.04% (0.4 mg/mL). It also contains anise oil, benzoic acid, camphor, and glycerin in an alcohol base. Dose as for NMS or NOS. Paregoric is readily available and has a long shelf life. Because of the unknown effects of many of the ingredients, we do not use it.

4. **Phenobarbital.** A loading dose of 20 mg/kg is given. If three consecutive scores are >8, or two consecutive scores or >12, may reload with 10 mg/kg/dose q8–12 h as needed until the cumulative total of all loading doses reaches a maximum of 40 mg/kg. A maintenance dose is given depending on the sum of the total loading doses. It is given q24h.

Cumulative sum of loading doses	Maintenance phenobarbital
20 mg/kg	5 mg/kg/d
30 mg/kg	6.5 mg/kg/d
40 mg/kg	8 mg/kg/d

Phenobarbital can be given PO or IM. It is usually given PO.

a. Serum levels

i. If a cumulative dose of 30 mg/kg or more of phenobarbital has been given, draw a serum level before giving any additional loading doses.

ii. Draw a serum level before the first maintenance dose to assess initial phenobarbital concentration.

iii. Draw trough levels weekly.

iv. Draw serum levels if the infant's scores remain >8 despite appropriate loading doses or repeat scores of <4 with clinical signs of sedation.

Taper by 10% each day after improvement of symptoms. Phenobarbital is the drug of choice if the infant is thought to be withdrawing from a nonnarcotic drug or from multiple drug use. In narcotic withdrawal, some prefer phenobarbital to NOS to discontinue exposing the developing neonatal brain to narcotics. The possible side effects of phenobarbital include sedation and poor sucking. It does not control the diarrhea that occurs with withdrawal. Using phenobarbital with NMS allows a lower dose of NMS and lessens the side effects. Phenobarbital elixir may contain 20% alcohol, and the parenteral form may contain propylene glycol, ethyl alcohol, and benzyl alcohol.

5. Morphine and phenobarbital can be initiated together for infants withdrawing from multiple drugs and may lessen the symptoms compared with single medical therapy.

Morphine starting dose (0.4 mg/mL) is 0.05 mL/kg q4h, increased by 0.1 mL/kg increments for scores >7. The morphine is reduced by 0.1 mL/kg for scores <5 for 24 hours. Phenobarbital is given in two doses of 10 mg/kg q12h followed by maintenance therapy of 5 mg/kg given twice a day 12 hours after the last loading dose. Serum phenobarbital levels of 20 to 30 mg/dL are ideal.

Morphine should be withdrawn first and the infant observed for 2 to 3 days off morphine and on phenobarbital alone.

This may allow the discharge of an infant home in the setting of an appropriate environment, with phenobarbital being prescribed. The infant can be allowed to outgrow the dose at home or the dose decreased under the care of the pediatrician. Because of recent literature reporting cognitive impairment and reduced brain mass associated with pre- or postnatal exposure of humans to antiepileptic therapy our first choice of drugs in treatment of NAS remains morphine.

Morphine in doses of 0.1 to 0.2 mg/kg can be effective in the emergency treatment of seizures or shock due to acute narcotic withdrawal.

6. Chlorpromazine is no longer used by us because of its unacceptable side effects, including tardive dyskinesia. It is useful to control the vomiting and diarrhea that sometimes occur in withdrawal. The dosage is 1.5 to 3 mg/kg/day, administered in four divided doses, initially IM, and then PO. Maintain this dose for 2 to 4 days and then taper as tolerated every 2 to 4 days.

7. Methadone is not routinely used by us for withdrawal from narcotics. Methadone is excreted in breast milk at a very low level. It is now considered safe for methadone-treated mothers to breast feed if there are no other contraindications. It has a prolonged plasma half-life (24 hours). Doses used are an initial loading dose of 0.1 mg/kg/dose with additional 0.025 mg/kg/doses given every 4 hours until symptoms are controlled. The maximum daily dose is 0.5 mg/kg/day. The maintenance dose is the total methadone dose given over the previous 24 hours divided by 2 and given every 12 hours. Weaning can then be attempted by giving methadone every 12 hours, and then every 24 hours at the last dose used. Once the dose reached is 0.05 mg/kg/day, it could be discontinued. The oral formulation of methadone contains 8% ethanol.

8. We do not recommend **diazepam** (Valium), but it has been used for control of symptoms. Some hospitals use it in doses of 0.1 to 0.3 mg/kg IM until symptoms are controlled, halve the dose, then change to every 12 hours, and lower the dose again. The major side effect is respiratory depression. Breakthrough symptoms, including seizures, respiratory depression, and bradycardia have been seen during use of diazepam. Withdrawal has recurred after termination of therapy. The sodium benzoate included in parenteral diazepam may interfere with the binding of bilirubin to albumin. The manufacturer warns that the safety and efficacy of injectable diazepam have not been established in the newborn (see Appendix A).

9. **Lorazepam** is often used for sedation either alone or with NMS or NOS. The parenteral preparation of lorazepam contains benzyl alcohol and polyethylene glycol. It is given as 0.05 to 0.1 mg/kg IV per dose. When used in conjunction with NOS, it may decrease the amount of NOS needed. Limited data are available about its use in newborns.

Closely monitor **fluid and electrolyte** intake and losses. Replace as needed.

The **narcotic abstinence scoring sheet** (see Fig. 19.2) will help establish objective criteria for weaning the infant from the medications. Irritability, tremors, and disturbance of sleeping patterns may last for up to 6 months and should not be a reason for continuing medication. For a general approach to management, see Fig. 19.1.

V. MATERNAL ADDICTION TO DRUGS OTHER THAN NARCOTICS. Infants born to mothers using drugs other than narcotics may be symptomatic.

A. **Cocaine** has a potent anorexic effect and may cause prenatal malnutrition, an increased rate of premature labor, spontaneous abortion, placental abruption, fetal distress, meconium staining, and low Apgar scores. Cocaine increases catecholamines, which can increase uterine contractility and cause maternal hypertension and placental vasoconstriction with diminished uterine blood flow and fetal hypoxia.

1. The following are **congenital anomalies** associated with cocaine use during pregnancy: cardiac anomalies; genitourinary malformations; intestinal atresias; microcephaly with or without growth retardation, perinatal cerebral infarctions, usually in the distribution of the middle cerebral artery with resultant cystic lesions; early-onset necrotizing enterocolitis; and retinal dysgenesis and retinal coloboma.

2. **Effects in the newborns.** Although cocaine-addicted infants do not show the classic signs of narcotic withdrawal, they demonstrate abnormal sleep patterns, tremors, poor organizational response, inability to be consoled, and transiently abnormal electroencephalograms (EEGs) and visual evoked potentials. Many of these findings are also true of tobacco use, and because many crack cocaine users also smoke cigarettes, it may be difficult to identify which defects are specific to cocaine.

3. **Treatment.** The newborn's withdrawal rarely requires pharmacologic treatment. When the pregnant cocaine abuser also uses other drugs, the neonate may have more severe withdrawal; in this case we use phenobarbital.

If symptomatic treatment is not adequate (see III.4), use phenobarbital or lorazepam for sedation.

4. **SIDS.** Cocaine-exposed infants appear to be at a 3 to 7 times higher risk for SIDS. This may be due to impaired regulation of respiration and arousal.

5. **Long-term disabilities** such as attention deficits, concentration difficulties, abnormal play patterns, and flat, apathetic moods have been reported. Some believe that the neurologic and cognitive outcomes of cocaine exposure are unclear because standard methods of measuring infant neurologic and behavioral functions are difficult to quantitate. It is also difficult to extricate the effects of cocaine use from the effects of lack of prenatal care, polydrug use, smoking,

and the increased risks associated with a drug-using lifestyle. Convulsions have been seen both in infants of breast-feeding mothers using cocaine and in infants exposed to passive crack smoke inhalation. Because cocaine and its metabolites can be found in breast milk for up to 60 hours after use, breast-feeding is not recommended.

B. PCP. A meta-analysis of 206 infants exposed to phencyclidine prenatally did not show any congenital anomalies. Infants of PCP-abusing mothers are of normal size. Most of the neonatal manifestations of *in utero* exposure center on neurobehavioral effects (irritability, jitteriness, hypertonicity). Because phencyclidine is excreted in breast milk, discourage breast-feeding if the mother uses this drug.

C. Marijuana. Prenatal use may result in shorter gestation with prolonged or arrested labor. There may be decreased fetal growth but no increase in major or minor morphologic anomalies. No reported adverse effects have been documented with breast-feeding. However, the drug may persist in milk for days after exposure and become concentrated with long-term use. Encourage abstinence if the infant is to be breast-fed. Some have found low Brazelton scores in these neonates and poor McCarthy scores on follow-up.

D. Ethanol. Teratogenic studies are confounded by other risk factors, but there is no established safe level of ethanol use in pregnancy. Symmetric growth retardation can occur *in utero*, the extent of which depends on the dose and duration of maternal use and on other factors such as concomitant tobacco or other drug use and overall nutrition. Although alcohol passes freely into breast milk, acetaldehyde, the toxic metabolite of ethanol, does not pass into milk. Therefore, the AAP considers moderate maternal ethanol use to be compatible with breast-feeding.

1. **Fetal alcohol syndrome (FAS)** includes the following features: microcephaly, growth retardation, dysmorphic facial features (such as hypoplastic midface, low nasal bridge, flattened philtrum, thinned upper vermilion, epicanthal fold, shortened palpebral fissure), cardiac problems, hydronephrosis, increased incidence of mental retardation, motor problems, and behavioral issues. Heavy prenatal alcohol exposure with or without physical features of FAS can lead to intelligence quotient (IQ) deficits. As is the case with other syndromes associated with craniofacial anomalies and hearing impairments, speech and language pathologies may also occur in FAS babies.

E. Tobacco. Smoking by pregnant women is associated with a higher rate of spontaneous abortions. Placental vascular resistance is increased as a consequence of the effects of nicotine, with resultant chronic ischemia and hypoxia. Nicotine can enter breast milk in relatively low levels and is not well absorbed by the infant's intestinal tract. This does not negate the risks to the infant from passive exposure to smoke.

1. **Effects on newborn infants of regular smokers (1 pack per day)**
   a. **Such infants** typically weigh 150 to 250 g less than the newborns of nonsmokers. The most pronounced effects of smoking on fetal growth occur after the second trimester. Fetuses may also be at risk by passive exposure.
   b. Increased tremors.
   c. Poor auditory responsiveness.
   d. Increased tone.
   e. No association has been found between maternal smoking during pregnancy and congenital anomalies.
   f. SIDS has been associated, in a dose–response manner, with maternal smoking, possibly secondary to passive exposure to smoke after birth.

F. Oxycodone (OxyContin) has been increasingly identified as a **potent narcotic** that can result in drug dependency and is becoming a popular street drug. We have occasionally been seeing its legal use in pregnant woman. There are no reports linking congenital defects with its use in the first trimester. The metabolites of OxyContin are excreted in the urine. At our institution levels <100 ng/mL in the urine are undetected and would not be picked up by our usual opiate screens. We have only encountered mild symptoms of withdrawal in the neonate. It is excreted in breast milk, the AAP has no current recommendations regarding breast-feeding.

G. **Psychotropic drugs.** Women who are on psychotropic medications and who decide to become pregnant have to think about whether they wish to continue their medications throughout pregnancy and the effects this decision would have on their health and the consequences of the potential risk profiles these medications have for their fetus. The withdrawal symptoms we have seen in the newborns of mothers only on a single psychotropic and no other narcotic or any non-narcotics listed in the preceding text, has been limited to transient symptoms of irritability, jitteriness, and mild respiratory distress.

Long-term developmental outcomes in children exposed to these selective serotonin-reuptake inhibitors (SSRIs) is unknown. Several of the most commonly used ones are indicated in the subsequent text. For a more complete review, please refer to the recommendations of the Fetus and Newborn Committee of the American Academy of Pediatrics on use of psychoactive medications during pregnancy. The most common SSRIs we encounter are as follows:

1. **Paroxetine hydrochloride (Paxil)** is commonly used to treat depression and anxiety attacks. It readily crosses the placenta and although it was originally thought that it does not increase teratogenic risk, more recent advisories indicate that infants of women receiving paroxetine in the first trimester had 1.5-fold increased risk for cardiac malformations and a 1.8-fold increased risk of congenital malformations as compared with women receiving other antidepressants. U.S. Food and Drug Administration (FDA) has changed paroxetine's pregnancy category from C to D. Lactation risk is Level II by FDA.

   Levels in breast milk are variable with concentrations higher in foremilk as compared with hind milk. Serum samples of breast-fed infants whose mothers are on Paxil have had minimal amounts of the drug with no untoward resultant symptoms. Therefore it appears that for healthy full term infants there may be no reason to discourage women on Paxil from breast-feeding.

2. **Sertraline (Zoloft).** Mean umbilical cord to maternal serum ratios appear to be significantly lower for sertraline than for fluoxetine (Prozac). It is categorized as pregnancy class C by the FDA.

   A recent study demonstrated detectable serum levels in breast-feeding infants of those mothers who took 100 mg or higher of sertraline. There were no significant adverse sequelae. Lactation risk is categorized as Level II by the FDA.

3. **Fluoxetine (Prozac)** is the SSRI that has been most studied in pregnancy. There does not appear to be an increased risk of fetal loss, major fetal anomalies, or any effect on global IQ or behavioral development. Cases of mild transient respiratory distress, persistent pulmonary hypertension of the newborn, feeding problems, and jitteriness have been reported in women who took fluoxetine late in the third trimester of pregnancy. It is categorized as pregnancy class C by the FDA.

   The level of fluoxetine in breast milk is the highest compared with other SSRIs. This amounted to 10.8% of the weight-adjusted maternal dose. Currently the AAP "considers the effects on the nursing infant unknown, but they may be of concern." For this reason, recommendation might be to consider treating the breast-feeding mother with other SSRIs post delivery, if an SSRI is required. It is classified Level III by the FDA for lactation risk. (See Appendices B and C for information on all these drugs.)

VI. **DISPOSITION.** The major problems with infants of a drug-addicted mother are proper disposition and follow-up. Studies show a high incidence of abuse and violence in the childhood and lives of drug-abusing women. This, combined with their own drug use and chaotic lifestyles, places them at risk for inadequate parenting. These factors may be more important to the outcome of the child than the drug abuse. The health of the mother, especially if she has AIDS, is significant for the ultimate well-being of the infant.

A. These infants are difficult to care for, as they are often irritable, have poor sleeping patterns, and will try the patience of any caregiver. They are at increased risk for child abuse. Infants of HIV-positive mothers should be followed up closely because of their increased risk of AIDS (see Chap. 23A).

B. Coordination of plans with social service agencies, drug treatment centers, and the courts, when necessary, is essential for proper follow-up and disposition.

C. Many states require that infants who show signs of withdrawal be reported as battered children.

Suggested Readings

American Academy of Pediatrics. Neonatal drug withdrawal. *Pediatrics* 1998;101(6):1079–1088.

Covington CY, et al. Birth to age 7 growth of children prenatally exposed to drugs: A prospective cohort study. *J Neurotoxicol Teratol* 2002;24(4):489–496.

Coyle Mara, et al. Diluted Tincture of Opium (DTO) and phenobarbital versus DTO alone for neonatal opiate withdrawal in term infants. *J Pediatr* 2002;140(5):561–564.

Frank DA, et al. Growth, development and behavior in early childhood following prenatal cocaine exposure: A systematic review. *JAMA* 2001;285(12):1613–1625.

Gentile S. The safety of newer antidepressants in pregnancy and breastfeeding. *Drug Saf* 2005;28(2):137–152.

Hale T, McAfee Ghia. *Medications for the breastfeeding mother*, 12th ed. Amarillo: Pharmasoft Publishing LP, 2005:378–1317.

McCarthy JJ, et al. High-dose methadone maintenance in pregnancy: Maternal and neonatal outcomes. *Am J Obstet Gynecol* 2005;193(3):606–610.

Mian Ayesha. Depression in pregnancy and the postpartum period: Balancing adverse effects of untreated illness with treatment risks. *J Psychiatr Pract* 2005;11(6):389–396.

Osborn DA, Jeffery HE, Cole M. Opiate treatment for opiate withdrawal in newborn infants. *Cochrane Database Syst Rev* 2005; 3:CDOO2059.

Philipp BL, et al. Methadone and breast feeding: New horizons. *Pediatrics* 2003;111:1429–1430.

Rosen TS, Bateman DA. Infants of addicted mothers. In: Fanaroff AA, Martin RJ, eds. *Neonatal-perinatal medicine*, 7th ed. St. Louis: WB Saunders, 2002;56:661–673.

Website for evidence-based information about the safety or risks of drugs, chemicals and disease during pregnancy and lactation from Hospital for Sick Children in Toronto, Ontario. http://www.motherisk.org. Accessed 2006.

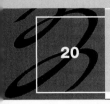

20 BIRTH TRAUMA
Elisa Abdulhayoglu

I. BACKGROUND. Birth injury is defined by the National Vital Statistics Report as "an impairment of the infant's body function or structure due to adverse influences that occurred at birth." Injury may occur antenatally, intrapartum, or during resuscitation, and may be avoidable or unavoidable.

A. Incidence. The morbidity rate due to birth trauma is 2.8 per 1,000 live births, and varies with the type of injury. Because cause-of-death coding has changed, the comparability of mortality rates from the year 2001 to 2004 is difficult. For 2005, the mortality rate in the United States for birth trauma was 0.6 per 100,000 live births.

B. Risk factors. When fetal size, immaturity, or malpresentation complicate delivery, the normal intrapartum compressions, contortions, and forces can lead to injury in the newborn, including hemorrhage and fracture. Obstetrical instrumentation may increase the mechanical forces, amplifying or inducing a birth injury. Breech presentation carries the greatest risk of injury. However, cesarean delivery without labor does not prevent all birth injuries. The following factors may contribute to an increased risk of birth injury:

1. Primiparity.
2. Small maternal stature.
3. Maternal pelvic anomalies.
4. Prolonged or unusually rapid labor.
5. Oligohydramnios.
6. Malpresentation of the fetus.
7. Use of mid-forceps or vacuum extraction.
8. Versions and extraction.
9. Very low birth weight or extreme prematurity.
10. Fetal macrosomia or large fetal head.
11. Fetal anomalies.

C. Evaluation. A newborn at risk for birth injury should have a thorough examination, including a detailed neurologic evaluation. Newborns who require resuscitation after birth should be evaluated, as occult injury may be present. Particular attention should be paid to symmetry of structure and function, cranial nerves, range of motion of individual joints, and integrity of the scalp and skin.

II. TYPES OF BIRTH TRAUMA

A. Head and neck injuries

1. **Injuries associated with intrapartum fetal monitoring.** Placement of an electrode on the fetal scalp or presenting part for fetal heart monitoring occasionally causes superficial abrasions or lacerations. These injuries require minimal local treatment, if any. Facial or ocular trauma may result from a malpositioned electrode. Rarely, abscesses form at the electrode site. Hemorrhage is a rare complication of fetal blood sampling.

2. **Extracranial hemorrhage**
   a. **Caput succedaneum**
      i. **Caput succedaneum** is a commonly occurring subcutaneous, extraperiosteal fluid collection that is occasionally hemorrhagic. It has poorly defined margins and can extend over the midline and across suture lines. It typically extends over the presenting portion of the scalp, and is usually associated with molding.

ii. The lesion usually resolves spontaneously without sequelae over the first several days after birth. It rarely causes significant blood loss or jaundice. There are rare reports of scalp necrosis with scarring.

iii. Vacuum caput is a *caput succedaneum* with margins well demarcated by the vacuum cup.

b. Cephalohematoma

i. A **cephalohematoma** is a subperiosteal collection of blood resulting from rupture of the superficial veins between the skull and periosteum. The lesion is always confined by suture lines. It may occur in as many as 2.5% of live births.

ii. An extensive cephalohematoma can result in significant hyperbilirubinemia. Hemorrhage is rarely serious enough to necessitate blood transfusion. Infection is also a rare complication, and usually occurs in association with septicemia and meningitis. Skull fractures have been associated with 5% to 20% of cephalohematomas. A head computed tomography (CT) scan should be obtained if neurologic symptoms are present. Most cephalohematomas resolve within 8 weeks. Occasionally, calcification may persist for several months or years.

iii. Management is limited to observation in most cases. Incision and aspiration of a cephalohematoma may introduce infection and is contraindicated. Anemia or hyperbilirubinemia should be treated as needed.

c. Subgaleal hematoma

i. Subgaleal hematoma is hemorrhage under the aponeurosis of the scalp. It is more often seen after vacuum- or forceps-assisted deliveries.

ii. Because the subgaleal or subaponeurotic space extends from the orbital ridges to the nape of the neck and laterally to the ears, the hemorrhage can spread across the entire calvarium.

iii. The initial presentation typically includes pallor, poor tone, and a fluctuant swelling on the scalp. The hematoma may grow slowly or increase rapidly and result in shock. With progressive spread, the ears may be displaced anteriorly and periorbital swelling can occur. Ecchymosis of the scalp may develop. The blood is resorbed slowly and swelling gradually resolves. The morbidity may be significant in infants with severe hemorrhage who require intensive care for this lesion.

iv. There is no specific therapy. The infant must be observed closely for signs of hypovolemia and blood volume should be maintained as needed with transfusions. Phototherapy should be provided for hyperbilirubinemia. An investigation for a bleeding disorder should be considered. Surgical drainage should be considered only for unremitting clinical deterioration. A subgaleal hematoma associated with skin abrasions may become infected; it should be treated with antibiotics and may need drainage.

3. Intracranial hemorrhage (see Chapter 27B)

4. Skull fracture

a. Skull fractures may be either linear, usually involving the parietal bone, or depressed, involving the parietal or frontal bones. The latter are often associated with forceps use. Occipital bone fractures are most often associated with breech deliveries.

b. Most infants with linear or depressed skull fractures are asymptomatic unless there is an associated intracranial hemorrhage (e.g., subdural or subarachnoid hemorrhage). Occipital osteodiastasis is a separation of the basal and squamous portions of the occipital bone that often results in cerebellar contusion and significant hemorrhage. It may be a lethal complication in breech deliveries. A linear fracture that is associated with a dural tear may lead to herniation of the meninges and brain, with development of a leptomeningeal cyst.

c. Uncomplicated linear fractures usually require no therapy. The diagnosis is made by taking a skull x-ray. Head CT scan should be obtained if intracranial injury is suspected. Depressed skull fractures require neurosurgical evaluation. Some may be elevated using closed techniques. Comminuted or large skull fractures associated with neurologic findings need immediate neurosurgical evaluation. If leakage of cerebrospinal fluid from the nares or ears is noted, antibiotic therapy should be started and neurosurgical consultation obtained. Follow-up imaging should be performed at 8 to 12 weeks to evaluate possible leptomeningeal cyst formation.

5. **Facial or mandibular fractures**
    a. Facial fractures can be caused by numerous forces including natural passage through the birth canal, forceps use, or delivery of the head in breech presentation.
    b. Fractures of the mandible, maxilla, and lacrimal bones warrant immediate attention. They may present as facial asymmetry with ecchymoses, edema, and crepitance, or respiratory distress with poor feeding. Untreated fractures can lead to facial deformities with subsequent malocclusion and mastication difficulties. Treatment should begin promptly because maxillar and lacrimal fractures begin to heal within 7 to 10 days and mandibular fractures start to repair at 10 to 14 days. Treated fractures usually heal without complication.
    c. Airway patency should be closely monitored. A plastic surgeon or otorhinolaryngologist should be consulted immediately and appropriate radiographic studies obtained. Head CT scan or magnetic resonance imaging (MRI) may be necessary to evaluate for retro-orbital or cribriform plate disruption. Antibiotics should be administered for fractures involving the sinuses or middle ear.

6. **Nasal injuries**
    a. Nasal fracture and dislocation may occur during the birth process. The most frequent nasal injury is dislocation of the nasal cartilage, which may result from pressure applied by the maternal symphysis pubis or sacral promontory. The incidence of dislocation is <1%.
    b. Infants with significant nasal trauma develop respiratory distress. Similar to facial fractures, nasal fractures begin to heal in 7 to 10 days and must be treated promptly. Rapid healing usually occurs once treatment is initiated. If treatment is delayed, deformities are common.
    c. A misshapen nose may appear dislocated. To differentiate dislocation from a temporary deformation, compress the tip of the nose. With septal dislocation, the nares collapse and the deviated septum is more apparent. With a misshapen nose, no nasal deviation occurs. Nasal edema from repeated suctioning may mimic partial obstruction. Patency can be assessed with a cotton wisp under the nares. Management involves protection of the airway and otorhinolaryngology consultation.
    d. If nasal dislocations are left untreated, there is an increased risk of long-term septal deformity.

7. **Ocular injuries**
    a. Retinal and subconjunctival hemorrhages are commonly seen after vaginal delivery. They result from increased venous congestion and pressure during delivery. Malpositioned forceps can result in ocular and periorbital injury including hyphema, vitreous hemorrhage, lacerations, orbital fracture, lacrimal duct or gland injury, and disruption of Descemet's membrane of the cornea (which can lead to astigmatism and amblyopia).
    b. Retinal hemorrhages usually resolve within 1 to 5 days. Subconjunctival hemorrhages resorb within 1 to 2 weeks. No long-term complications usually occur. For other ocular injuries, prompt diagnosis and treatment are necessary to ensure a good long-term outcome.
    c. Management. Prompt ophthalmologic consultation should be obtained.

8. **Ear injuries**
    a. Ears are susceptible to injury, particularly with forceps application. More significant injuries occur with fetal malposition. Abrasions, hematomas, and lacerations may develop.

b. Abrasions generally heal well with local care. Hematomas of the pinna may lead to the development of a "cauliflower" ear; lacerations may result in perichondritis. Temporal bone injury can lead to middle and inner ear complications, such as hemotympanum and ossicular disarticulation.

c. Hematomas of the pinna should be drained to prevent clot organization and development of cauliflower ear. If the cartilage and temporal bone are involved, an otolaryngologist should be consulted. Antibiotic therapy may be required.

9. Sternocleidomastoid

a. Sternocleidomastoid (SCM) injury is also referred to as congenital or muscular torticollis. The etiology is uncertain. The most likely cause is a muscle compartment syndrome resulting from intrauterine positioning. Torticollis can also arise during delivery as the muscle is hyperextended and ruptured, with development of a hematoma and subsequent fibrosis and shortening.

b. Torticollis may present at birth with a palpable 1 to 2 cm mass in the SCM region and head tilt to the side of the lesion. More often it is noted at 1 to 4 weeks of age. Facial asymmetry may be present along with hemihypoplasia on the side of the lesion. Prompt treatment may lessen or correct the torticollis.

c. Other conditions may mimic congenital torticollis and should be ruled out. These include cervical vertebral anomalies, hemangioma, lymphangioma, and teratoma.

d. Treatment is initially conservative. Stretching of the involved muscle should begin promptly and be performed several times per day. Recovery typically occurs within 3 to 4 months in approximately 80% of cases. Surgery is needed if torticollis persists after 6 months of physical therapy.

e. In up to 10% of patients with congenital torticollis, congenital hip dysplasia may be present. A careful hip examination is warranted with further evaluation as indicated.

10. Pharyngeal injury

a. Minor submucosal pharyngeal injuries can occur with postpartum bulb suctioning. More serious injury, such as perforation into the mediastinal or pleural cavity, may result from nasogastric or endotracheal tube placement. Affected infants may have copious secretions and difficulty swallowing, and it may be difficult to advance a nasogastric tube.

b. Mild submucosal injuries typically heal without complication. More extensive trauma requires prompt diagnosis and treatment for complete resolution.

c. The diagnosis of a retropharyngeal tear is made radiographically using water-soluble contrast material. Infants are treated with broad-spectrum antibiotics and oral feedings are withheld for 2 weeks. The contrast study is repeated to confirm healing before feeding is restarted. Infants with pleural effusions may require chest tube placement. Surgical consultation is obtained if the leak persists or the perforation is large.

B. Cranial nerve, spinal cord, and peripheral nerve injury

1. Cranial nerve injuries

a. Facial nerve injury (cranial nerve VII)

   i. Injury to the facial nerve is the most common peripheral nerve injury in neonates, occurring in up to 1% of live births. The exact incidence is unknown, as many cases are subtle and resolve readily. The etiology includes compression of the facial nerve by forceps (particularly midforceps), pressure on the nerve secondary to the fetal face lying against the maternal sacral promontory, or, rarely, from pressure of a uterine mass (e.g., fibroid).

   ii. Facial nerve injury results in asymmetric crying facies.

      a) Central facial nerve injury occurs less frequently than peripheral nerve injury. Paralysis is limited to the lower 1/2 to 2/3 of the contralateral side, which is smooth with no nasolabial fold present. The corner of the mouth droops. Movement of the forehead and eyelid is unaffected.

      b) **Peripheral injury** involves the entire side of face and is consistent with a lower motor neuron injury. The nasolabial fold is flattened and the mouth droops on the affected side. The infant is unable to wrinkle the forehead and close the eye completely. The tongue is not involved.

      c) **Peripheral nerve branch injury** results in paralysis that is limited to only one group of facial muscles: the forehead, eyelid, or mouth.

   iii. Differential diagnosis includes Mobius syndrome (nuclear agenesis), intracranial hemorrhage, congenital hypoplasia of the depressor anguli oris muscle, congenital absence of facial muscles or nerve branches.

   iv. The prognosis of acquired facial nerve injury is excellent with recovery usually complete by 3 weeks. Initial management is directed at prevention of corneal injuries by using artificial tears and protecting the open eye by patching. Electromyography may be helpful to predict recovery or potential residual effects. Because full recovery is likely, surgical intervention should not be considered within the first year.

b. Recurrent laryngeal nerve injury

   i. Unilateral abductor paralysis may be caused by recurrent laryngeal injury secondary to excessive traction on the fetal head during breech delivery or lateral traction on the head with forceps. The left recurrent laryngeal nerve is involved more often because of its longer course. Bilateral recurrent laryngeal nerve injury can be caused by trauma, but is usually due to hypoxia or brain-stem hemorrhage.

   ii. A neonate with unilateral abductor paralysis is often asymptomatic at rest, but has hoarseness and inspiratory stridor with crying. Unilateral injury is occasionally associated with hypoglossal nerve injury, and presents with difficulty with feedings and secretions. Bilateral paralysis usually results in stridor, severe respiratory distress, and cyanosis.

   iii. Differential diagnosis of symptoms similar to unilateral injury includes congenital laryngeal malformations. Particularly with bilateral paralysis, intrinsic central nervous system (CNS) malformations must be ruled out, including Chiari malformation and hydrocephalus. If there is no history of birth trauma, cardiovascular anomalies and mediastinal masses should be considered.

   iv. The diagnosis can be made using direct or flexible fiberoptic laryngoscopy. A modified barium swallow and speech pathology consultation may be helpful to optimize feeding. Unilateral injury usually resolves by 6 weeks of age without intervention and treatment. Bilateral paralysis has a variable prognosis; tracheostomy may be required.

2. Spinal cord injuries

  a. Vaginal delivery of an infant with a hyperextended head or neck, breech delivery, and severe shoulder dystocia are risk factors for spinal cord injury. However, significant spinal cord injuries are rare. Injuries include spinal epidural hematomas, vertebral artery injuries, traumatic cervical hematomyelia, spinal artery occlusion, and transection of the cord.

  b. Spinal cord injury presents in four ways:

   i. Some infants with severe high cervical or brain-stem injury present as stillborn or in poor condition at birth, with respiratory depression, shock, and hypothermia. Death generally occurs within hours of birth.

   ii. Infants with an upper or midcervical injury present with central respiratory depression. They have lower extremity paralysis, absent deep tendon reflexes and absent sensation in the lower half of the body, urinary retention, and constipation. Brachial plexus injury may be present.

   iii. Injury at the seventh cervical vertebra or lower may be reversible. However, permanent neurologic complications may result, including muscle atrophy, contractures, bony deformities, and constant micturition.

   iv. Partial spinal injury or spinal artery occlusions may result in subtle neurologic signs and spasticity.

   c. Differential diagnosis includes amyotonia congenita, myelodysplasia associated with spina bifida occulta, spinal cord tumors, and cerebral hypotonia.

   d. The prognosis depends on the severity and location of the injury. If a spinal injury is suspected at birth, efforts should focus on resuscitation and prevention of further damage. The head, neck, and spine should be immobilized. Neurology and neurosurgical consultations should be obtained. Careful and repeated examinations are necessary to help predict long-term outcome. Cervical spine radiographs, CT scan, and MRI may be helpful.

3. Cervical nerve root injuries

  a. Phrenic nerve injury (C3, 4, or 5)

    i. Phrenic nerve damage leading to paralysis of the ipsilateral diaphragm may result from a stretch injury due to lateral hyperextension of the neck at birth. Risk factors include breech and difficult forceps deliveries. Injury to the nerve is thought to occur where it crosses the brachial plexus. Therefore, approximately 75% of patients also have brachial plexus injury. Occasionally, chest tube insertion or surgery injures this nerve.

    ii. Respiratory distress and cyanosis are often seen. Some infants present with persistent tachypnea and decreased breath sounds at the lung base. There may be decreased movement of the affected hemithorax. Chest radiographs may show elevation of the affected diaphragm, although this may not be apparent if the infant is on continuous positive airway pressure (CPAP) or mechanical ventilation. If the infant is breathing spontaneously and not on CPAP, increasing atelectasis may develop. The diagnosis is confirmed by ultrasonography or fluoroscopy that shows paradoxical (upward) movement of the diaphragm with inspiration.

    iii. Differential diagnosis includes cardiac, pulmonary, and other neurologic causes of respiratory distress. These can usually be evaluated by a careful examination and appropriate imaging. Congenital absence of the nerve is rare.

    iv. The initial treatment is supportive. CPAP or mechanical ventilation may be needed, with careful airway care to avoid atelectasis and pneumonia. Most infants recover in 1 to 3 months without permanent sequelae. Diaphragmatic plication is considered in refractory cases. Phrenic nerve pacing is possible for bilateral paralysis.

  b. Brachial plexus injury

    i. The incidence of brachial plexus injury ranges from 0.1% to 0.2% of all births. The cause is excessive traction on the head, neck, and arm during birth. Risk factors include macrosomia, shoulder dystocia, malpresentation, and instrumented deliveries. Injury usually involves the nerve root, especially where the roots come together to form the nerve trunks of the plexus.

    ii. Duchenne-Erb palsy involves the upper trunks (C5, C6, and occasionally C7) and is the most common type of brachial plexus injury, accounting for approximately 90% of cases. Total brachial plexus palsy occurs in some cases and involves all roots from C5 to T1. Klumpke palsy involves C7/C8 to T1 and is the least common.

    a) Duchenne-Erb palsy. The arm is typically adducted and internally rotated at the shoulder. There is extension and pronation at the elbow and flexion of the wrist and fingers in the characteristic "waiter's tip" posture. The deltoid, infraspinatus, biceps, supinator and brachioradialis muscles, and the extensors of the wrist and fingers may be weak or paralyzed. The Moro, biceps, and radial reflexes are absent on the affected side. The grasp reflex is intact. Sensation is variably affected. Diaphragm paralysis occurs in 5% of cases.

    b) Total brachial plexus injury. Accounts for approximately 10% of all cases. The entire arm is flaccid. All reflexes, including grasp, and sensation, are absent. If sympathetic fibers are injured at T1, Horner syndrome may be seen.

c) Klumpke palsy. The rarest of the palsies, accounting for <1% of brachial plexus injuries. The lower arm paralysis affects the intrinsic muscles of the hand and the long flexors of the wrist and fingers. The grasp reflex is absent. However, the biceps and radial reflexes are present. There is sensory impairment on the ulnar side of the forearm and hand. Because the first thoracic root is usually injured, its sympathetic fibers are damaged, leading to an ipsilateral Horner syndrome.

iii. Differential diagnosis includes a cerebral injury, which usually has other associated CNS symptoms. Injury of the clavicle, upper humerus, and lower cervical spine may mimic a brachial plexus injury.

iv. Radiographs of the shoulder and upper arm should be performed to rule out bony injury. The chest should be carefully examined to detect diaphragm paralysis. Initial treatment is conservative. Physical therapy and passive range of motion exercises prevent contractures. These should be started at 7 to 10 days when the postinjury neuritis has resolved. "Statue of Liberty" splinting should be avoided as contractures in the shoulder girdle may develop. Wrist and digit splints may be useful.

v. The prognosis for full recovery varies with the extent of injury. If the nerve roots are intact and not avulsed, the prognosis for full recovery is excellent (>90%). Notable clinical improvement in the first 2 weeks after birth indicates that normal or near-normal function will return. Most infants recovery fully by 3 months of age. In those with slow recovery, electromyography and nerve-conduction studies may distinguish an avulsion from a stretch injury.

C. Bone injuries

1. Clavicular fracture is the most commonly injured bone during delivery, occurring in up to 3% newborns. Up to 40% of clavicular fractures are not identified until after discharge from the hospital.

a. These fractures are seen in vertex presentations with shoulder dystocia or in breech deliveries when the arms are extended. Macrosomia is a risk factor.

b. A greenstick or incomplete fracture may be asymptomatic at birth. The first clinical sign may be a callus at 7 to 10 days of age. Signs of a complete fracture include crepitus, palpable bony irregularity, and spasm of the SCM. The affected arm may have a pseudoparalysis because motion causes pain.

c. Differential diagnosis includes fracture of the humerus or a brachial plexus palsy.

d. A **clavicular fracture** is confirmed by chest x-ray. If the arm movement is decreased, the cervical spine, brachial plexus, and humerus should be assessed. Therapy should be directed at decreasing pain with analgesics. The infant's sleeve should be pinned to the shirt to limit movement until the callus begins to form. Complete healing is expected.

2. Long bone injuries

a. Humeral fractures

i. Humeral fractures typically occur during a difficult delivery of the arms in the breech presentation and/or of the shoulders in vertex. Direct pressure on the humerus may also result in fracture.

ii. A greenstick fracture may not be noted until the callus forms. The first sign is typically loss of spontaneous arm movement, followed by swelling and pain on passive motion. A complete fracture with displaced fragments presents as an obvious deformity. X-ray confirms the diagnosis.

iii. Differential diagnosis includes clavicular fracture and brachial plexus injury.

iv. The prognosis is excellent with complete healing expected. Pain should be treated with analgesics.

a) A fractured humerus usually requires splinting for 2 weeks. Displaced fractures require closed reduction and casting. Radial nerve injury may be seen.

b) Epiphyseal displacement occurs when the humeral epiphysis separates at the hypertrophied cartilaginous layer of the growth plate. Severe displacement may result in significant compromise of growth. The diagnosis can be confirmed by ultrasonography because the epiphysis is not ossified at birth. Therapy includes immobilization of the limb for 10 to 14 days.

b. Femoral fractures

i. Femoral fractures usually follow a breech delivery. Infants with congenital hypotonia are at increased risk.

ii. Physical examination usually reveals an obvious deformity of the thigh. In some cases, the injury may not be noted for a few days until swelling, decreased movement, or pain with palpation develop. The diagnosis is confirmed by x-ray.

iii. Complete healing without limb shortening is expected.

   a) Fractures, even if unilateral, should be treated with traction and suspension of both legs with a spica cast. Casting is maintained for approximately 4 weeks.

   b) Femoral epiphyseal separation may be misinterpreted as developmental dysplasia of the hip because the epiphysis is not ossified at birth. Pain and tenderness with palpation are more likely with epiphyseal separation than dislocation. The diagnosis is confirmed by ultrasonography. Therapy includes limb immobilization for 10 to 14 days and analgesics for pain.

D. Intra-abdominal Injuries. Intra-abdominal birth trauma is uncommon.

1. Hepatic injury

a. The liver is the most commonly injured solid organ during birth. Macrosomia, hepatomegaly, and breech presentation are risk factors for hepatic hematoma and/or rupture. The etiology is thought to be direct pressure on the liver.

b. Subcapsular hematomas are generally not symptomatic at birth. Nonspecific signs of blood loss such as poor feeding, pallor, tachypnea, tachycardia, and onset of jaundice develop during the first 1 to 3 days after birth. Serial hematocrits may suggest blood loss. Rupture of the hematoma through the capsule results in discoloration of the abdominal wall and circulatory collapse with shock.

c. Differential diagnosis includes trauma to other intra-abdominal organs.

d. Management includes restoration of blood volume, correction of coagulation disturbances, and surgical consultation for probable laparotomy. Early diagnosis and correction of volume loss increase survival.

2. Splenic injury

a. Risk factors for splenic injury include macrosomia, breech delivery, and splenomegaly (e.g., congenital syphilis, erythroblastosis fetalis).

b. Signs are similar to hepatic rupture. A mass is sometimes palpable in the left upper quadrant and the stomach bubble may be displaced medially on an abdominal radiograph.

c. Differential diagnosis includes injury to other abdominal organs.

d. Management includes volume replacement and correction of coagulation disorders. Surgical consultation should be obtained. Expectant management with close observation is appropriate if the bleeding has stopped and the patient has stabilized. If laparotomy is necessary, salvage of the spleen is attempted to minimize the risk of sepsis.

3. Adrenal hemorrhage

a. The relatively large size of the adrenal gland at birth may contribute to injury. Risk factors are breech presentation and macrosomia. Ninety percent of adrenal hemorrhages are unilateral; 75% occur on the right.

b. Findings on physical examination depend on the extent of hemorrhage. Classic signs include fever, flank mass, purpura, and pallor. Adrenal insufficiency may present with poor feeding, vomiting, irritability, listlessness, and shock. The diagnosis is made with abdominal ultrasound.

c. Differential diagnosis includes other abdominal trauma. If a flank mass is palpable, neuroblastoma and Wilms tumor should be considered.

d. Treatment includes blood volume replacement. Adrenal insufficiency may require steroid therapy. Extensive bleeding that requires surgical intervention is rare.

E. Soft tissue injuries

1. Petechiae and ecchymoses are commonly seen in newborns. The birth history, location of lesions, their early appearance without development of new lesions, and the absence of bleeding from other sites help differentiate petechiae and ecchymoses secondary to birth trauma from those caused by a vasculitis or coagulation disorder. If the etiology is uncertain, studies to rule out coagulopathies and infection should be performed. Most petechiae and ecchymoses resolve within 1 week. If bruising is excessive, jaundice and anemia may develop. Treatment is supportive.

2. Lacerations and abrasions may be secondary to scalp electrodes and fetal scalp blood sampling or injury during birth. Deep wounds (e.g., scalpel injuries during cesarean section) may require sutures. Infection is a risk, particularly with scalp lesions and an underlying ***caput succedaneum*** or hematoma. Treatment includes cleansing the wound and close observation.

3. Subcutaneous fat necrosis is not usually recognized at birth. It usually presents during the first 2 weeks after birth as sharply demarcated, irregularly shaped, firm, nonpitting subcutaneous plaques or nodules on the extremities, face, trunk, or buttocks. The injury may be colorless, or have a deep-red or purple discoloration. Calcification may occur. No treatment is necessary. Lesions typically resolve completely over several weeks to months.

Suggested Readings

Uhing MR. Management of birth injuries. *Clin Perinatol* 2005;32:19–38.
Rosenberg AA. Traumatic birth injury. *NeoReviews* 2003;4(10):e270–e276.

DECISION-MAKING AND ETHICAL DILEMMAS

Joseph A. Garcia-Prats

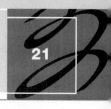

21

I. **BACKGROUND.** The practice of neonatology necessitates decision making in all aspects of care. Most neonatologists feel comfortable making routine clinical decisions regarding management of pulmonary or cardiac function, infection, nutrition, and neurodevelopmental care. On the other hand, clinical situations with ethical implications are less common and more difficult for professionals and families. These include decisions regarding instituting, withholding, or withdrawing life-supporting therapy in patients with irreversible or terminal conditions including extreme immaturity, severe hypoxic ischemic encephalopathy, certain congenital anomalies, or other conditions that are refractory to the best available treatments.

A. The **ethical principles** that must be considered in the decision-making process in neonatal intensive care unit (NICU) care include beneficence, nonmaleficence, respect for autonomy, and justice. Caregivers and parents must balance choices that are in the infant's best interest (beneficence) against choices that minimize harm to the infant (nonmaleficence).

1. Treatment decisions must be based on the infant's best interests, free from considerations of race, ethnicity, ability to pay, or other influences (justice).

2. The infant's parents serve as the legal and moral fiduciaires of their child. The relationship of parents to children is that of responsibility, not rights. Because infants are incapable of making decisions for themselves, the parents become their surrogate decision makers. Therefore, the parents are owed respect for autonomy in making decisions for their infants.

3. The physician serves as a fiduciary who acts in the best interest of the patient using the most current evidence-based medical information. In this role as patient advocates, physicians oversee the responses (decisions) of their patient's parents.

B. The debate between quality and sanctity of life enters into difficult decisions more frequently as it becomes technically possible to sustain smaller and sicker infants. Staff and parents often struggle with identifying the medical and moral choices and with making decisions based on those choices. These choices, including the understanding of what defines a fulfilling or adequate quality of life, vary substantially among families and professionals.

II. **DEVELOPING A PROCESS FOR ETHICAL DECISION MAKING.** It is important for an NICU to define the decision-making process and to identify those individuals (nursing staff, medical staff, social services, ethicists, hospital legal counsel) that may need to participate in that process. Developing this process allows for healthy discussions among NICU personnel that incorporate ethical knowledge and values at a time and place distant from a specific patient. Ideally, this preparation will ease the stress when an actual decision needs to be made.

A. **Develop an educational program to prepare the NICU caregivers to** address difficult decisions regarding patient care. Focus on process (who, when, where) as well as on substance (how). Identifying areas of frequent consensus and disagreement within an NICU and outlining a general approach to those situations can provide helpful guidance. The educational program should be available for NICU staff and discussed during the orientation of new personnel. The hospital ethics committee can serve as an educational resource in personnel regarding how to deal with ethical decision-making.

B. **Part of the educational program could be to identify common ethical situations** (e.g., extreme prematurity, multiple congenital anomalies, severe asphyxia) that might produce conflict and have a series of multidisciplinary discussions about these models. These conversations should include a review of the common underlying ethical principles likely to be in conflict and illuminate common areas of agreement or disagreement. These discussions help develop a consensus on group values, promote a tolerance for individual differences, and establish trust among professionals. The overall goal is to better prepare caregivers when actual situations arise.

C. **Define and support the role of the parents** who should be seen as the primary decision makers for their infant unless they have indicated otherwise. The parents' desired decision-making role should be explored with them in open and honest discussions. The ethical and legal presumption is that they will make decisions that are in the best interests of their child (best interests standard) and within the context of accepted legal and social boundaries. If the health care providers believe that the parental choice is not in the child's best interest, then they have an obligation as an advocate for the infant to override the parental decision. Although every effort must be made to align the views of the parents and medical team, in cases of continued disagreement by the parents with the course chosen by the physician to be in the best interests of their infant, the hospital ethics committee, hospital legal counsel, and social services should be consulted and the court system may need to be involved. In this case, the physician should continue to serve as the infant's advocate.

D. **Develop consensus among the primary clinical team** and consultants before meeting with the parents. Team meetings before family meetings provide the opportunity for caregivers to clarify the dilemmas and options that will be offered to the family and, hopefully, to reach a consensus regarding recommendations. It also allows the team to establish who will communicate with the family to help maintain consistency during the discussion of complicated medical and ethical issues.

E. **Identify available resources.** Determine the roles of social service, chaplain, hospital attorney, and the hospital ethics committee. Although a general knowledge of existing hospital policies on common situations such as "do not attempt resuscitation" orders or withdrawal of life support should be included in the multidisciplinary discussions mentioned in the preceding text, the NICU should identify one or two key resource people who are easily accessible. These professionals should be familiar with hospital policies, the ethics codes of the hospital as well as those of national organizations such as the American Academy of Pediatrics or the American Medical Association, and applicable federal and state laws. This key resource person is often a member of the hospital ethics committee who can be available without pursuing a formal ethics consult.

F. **Base decisions on the most accurate, up-to-date medical information.** Good ethics begin with good facts. Take the time to accumulate the relevant data. Consultation services are likely to provide valuable input. Be consistent in asking the same appropriate questions in each clinical setting. The answers to these questions may vary from case to case but the ethical questions regarding the ethical principles must always be asked. Be wary of setting certainty as a goal, as it is almost never achievable in the NICU. Instead, a reasonable degree of medical certainty is often more achievable. As the weight of a decision's consequences increases, so does the rigor of the requirement for a reasonable degree of certainty and the importance of parental involvement in the decision-making process.

G. **People of good conscience can disagree.** Individual caregivers must feel free to remove themselves from patient care if their ethical sense conflicts with the decision of the primary team and parents. This conflict should be handled with the director of nursing or medical director of the NICU. Parents and caregivers must be able to appeal decisions to an individual such as the NICU medical director or to the hospital's ethics committee. No system will provide absolute certainty that the "right" decision will always be made. However, a system that is inclusive, systematic, and built on an approach that establishes a procedure for handling these difficult issues is most likely to produce acceptable decisions.

III. **EXTREMELY PREMATURE INFANTS.** Almost all NICUs have struggled with decisions about infants at the threshold of viability and the question of "how small is too small."

The practice of resuscitating extremely preterm infants presents difficult medical and ethical challenges. Current technology allows some of these infants to survive, but with a high risk of substantial handicap. Parents may ask that neonatologists pursue aggressive therapies despite poor prognoses. Neonatologists are concerned that instituting those therapies may not be the most appropriate course of action. The American Academy of Pediatrics statement on perinatal care at the threshold of viability stresses several key areas: (i) parents must receive adequate and current information about potential infant survival and short- and long-term outcomes; (ii) physicians are obligated to be aware of the most current national and local survival data; and (iii) parental choice should be respected as much as possible with joint decision making by both the parents and the physicians as the standard. As more experience is gained with these very difficult situations, further debate and discussion are likely to lead to greater consensus in this area.

IV. THE DECISION TO REDIRECT LIFE-SUSTAINING CARE TO COMFORT MEA-SURES. One of the most difficult issues is deciding when to withhold or withdraw life-sustaining therapies. Philosophies and approaches vary among caregivers and NICUs. The American Academy of Pediatrics' statement on noninitiation or withdrawal of intensive care for high-risk newborns stresses several key areas: (i) decisions about noninitiation or withdrawal of intensive care should be made by the health care team in collaboration with the parents, who must be well informed about the condition and prognosis of their infant; (ii) parents should be active participants in the decision-making process; (iii) compassionate comfort care should be provided to all infants, including those for whom intensive care is not provided; (iv) it is appropriate to provide intensive care when it is thought to be of benefit to the infant, and not when it is thought to be harmful, of no benefit, or futile.

One model to consider emphasizes an objective interdisciplinary approach to determine the best course of action.

A. The goal of the process is to identify the action that is in the **baby's best interest.** The interests of others, including family and caregivers, are of less priority than are the baby's.

B. Decision making should be guided by data. Caregivers should explore every reasonable avenue to maximize collection of data relevant to the ethical question at hand. Information about alternative therapies and prognosis should be sought. The objective data are evaluated in the context of the primary team's meetings. Subspecialty consultations should be obtained when indicated and included in the primary team's deliberations. Often, these consultations may add extra input to assist in the questions that the primary team is trying to address. It is important that these consultants' input be reviewed with the primary team before discussing such findings with the parents.

C. Communication among caregivers and parents is completely open. The primary care team should meet daily with the parents to discuss the baby's progress, current status, plan of care, and to summarize the team's medical and ethical discussions.

D. As the decision to withhold or withdraw life-sustaining medical treatment becomes the focus, the team discusses the best data available, their implications, and their degree of certainty. The goal should be to build a **consensus** regarding the best plan of care for the baby and/or recommendations for the parents. Sometimes there will be strong scientific support for a particular option. In other instances, the best course of action must be estimated. During this time, it is especially important to actively seek feedback from the parents regarding their thoughts, feelings, and understanding of the clinical situation. It should be emphasized that different caregivers reach the consensus at different rates and times. It may be the nursing caregivers who understand and accept the futility of a patient's condition long before the physicians and parents or vice versa. Supporting each party of this process is important until all parties understand and accept the consensus issue whereupon a decision is then readily agreed upon.

E. The parents' role as surrogate decision makers is respected. Parental views are always considered; they are most likely to influence decisions when it remains unclear which option (e.g., continuing versus discontinuing life-sustaining treatment) is in the child's best interest. Parents are not expected to evaluate clinical data in isolation. Even in instances of medical uncertainty, the primary team objectively assesses what is known as well as what remains uncertain about the baby's condition and/or prognosis. The team should provide the parents with this information as well as their best assessment and recommendation. In the face of substantial medical uncertainty, parental wishes should be supported in deference to those of the primary medical team.

F. There is agreement among ethical and legal scholars that there is no important distinction between **withholding or withdrawing life-sustaining treatments.** Amendments to the Child Abuse and Neglect Prevention and Treatment Act of 1984 established that medically indicated treatment can be withheld or withdrawn under the following conditions: (i) ongoing treatment is prolonging the baby's death, (ii) the baby is in an irreversible coma, or (iii) the underlying condition is so significant as to render ongoing treatment futile and inhumane. It has been argued that these conditions both protect the rights of children to treatment despite underlying conditions or potential handicaps and support the importance of quality of life determinations in the provision of care. Substantial conflict can arise if the caregivers and parents disagree about the goals of care. An NICU must be prepared for these circumstances.

G. The **hospital ethics committee** is helpful when the primary team is unable to reach consensus or disagrees with the parents' wishes. In our experience, consultation with the ethics committee helps encourage communication among all involved parties and improve collaborative decision making. They can often ease tensions between parents and caregivers, allowing for a resolution to the dilemma.

Suggested Readings

Committee on the Fetus and Newborn. Noninitiation or withdrawal of intensive care for high-risk newborns. *Pediatrics* 2007;119:401–403.

Goldworth A, Silverman W, Stevenson DK, et al. eds. *Ethics and perinatology.* New York: Oxford University Press, 1995.

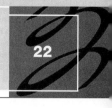

MANAGEMENT OF NEONATAL DEATH AND BEREAVEMENT FOLLOW-UP

Caryn E. Douma

22

I. INTRODUCTION

A. General principles

1. Neonatal death is traumatic for both families and caretakers. The goal of management is to establish and reinforce a memory of the infant to facilitate successful grieving.

2. It is important for families to be cared for by a compassionate, knowledgeable staff that can provide a dignified, pain-free death for their child.

3. Bereavement follow-up provides an important link that guides families toward recovery.

II. MANAGEMENT OF NEONATAL DEATH

A. Staff.
The primary team caring for an infant and the family usually consists of an attending physician, nurses, and a social worker. The team may also include a neonatology fellow, pediatric resident, respiratory therapist, and pediatric consultants. This multidisciplinary team supports the family and cares for the infant during the hospital course and bereavement period. End-of-life care is always challenging for caretakers. It is helpful to have guidelines that include a plan for discussing the withdrawal of life support, management of the dying infant, follow-up, and support for families and staff. Parents need consistent information presented in a concise, honest manner. It may be difficult for families to build close relationships with the entire team. Depending on individual circumstances, it may be more appropriate to choose one or two representatives to discuss the end-of-life decisions.

B. Relationship with family.
Developing an honest, trusting relationship with families is crucial to the management of neonatal death and bereavement. Staff can facilitate this relationship in the following ways:

1. Communicate with families through frequent meetings with the primary team.

2. Include obstetrical care team when appropriate.

3. Encourage sibling visitation and extended family support.

4. Encourage cultural and spiritual customs.

5. Provide an environment that allows parents to develop a relationship with their infant, visiting and holding as often as medically indicated.

C. Decision making.
End-of-life decisions are made collaboratively with parents through a series of meetings with the care team. Parents should not feel that they alone are responsible for any decisions made. When the primary team is in agreement that further intervention is not in the best interest of the infant, this information should be presented to the family. When meeting with the family it is important to take care of the following:

1. Meet in a quiet, private area and allow ample time for the family to understand the information presented and the recommendations of the team.

2. Refer to the baby by name.

3. Ask the parents how they feel and how they perceive the situation.

4. The decision to redirect care away from supporting life to comfort measures must be accompanied by a discussion describing how intensive care support will be withdrawn. Be specific and involve parents in the plan.

D. Withdrawing life support

1. Once a decision has been made to withdraw life support, the family should be provided an environment that is quiet, private, and will accommodate everyone the family wishes to include.

2. Staffing should be arranged so that one nurse and one physician will be readily available to the family at all times.
3. Allow parents ample time to create memories and become a family. Allow them to hold, take pictures, bathe, and dress their infant before, during, or after withdrawing mechanical ventilation or other life support.
4. Discuss the entire process with parents, including endotracheal tube removal and pain control. Gently describe how the infant will look and measures that the staff will take to provide the infant with a comfortable, pain-free death. Let them know that death will not always occur immediately.
5. Arrange for baptism and spiritual support if desired.
6. Anticipate medications that may be required, leaving IV access in place. Discontinue muscle relaxation before extubation. The goal of medication use should be to ensure that the infant is as comfortable as possible.
7. When the infant is extubated, discontinue all unnecessary intravenous catheters and equipment.
8. Allow parents to hold their infant for as long as they desire after withdrawing life support. The nurse and attending physician should be nearby to assist the family and assess heart rate and comfort of the infant.
9. When the family has a surviving multiple, it is important that the care team acknowledge the difficulty that this will present both at the time of death and during the grieving process.
10. Autopsy should be discussed before or after death at the discretion of the attending physician.
11. Create a memory box including crib cards, photographs, clothing, a lock of hair, footprints, handprints, and any other mementos accumulated during the infant's life. Keep them in a designated place if the family does not desire to see or keep them at the time of death. They often change their mind later.
12. Be sure that the photographs of the infant have been taken. Parents of multiples will often want a photograph of both twins together or a family picture. It is helpful for the newborn intensive care unit (NICU) to have a digital camera and printer available.

III. BEREAVEMENT FOLLOW-UP

A. General principles. Each NICU should have a bereavement follow-up program in place that will provide continuing support to families as they begin the grieving process, assess their progress, and provide community referrals if necessary.

B. Hospital care
1. Before the family leaves the hospital they should understand that the staff will continue to support them through phone calls and follow-up meetings. They should understand the normal grieving process and what to expect in the following days and weeks. Obtain preferred contact information from family before discharge.
2. Continue to offer grief counseling and spiritual support.
3. Lactation support should be offered if appropriate and a plan made for lactation suppression and follow-up.
4. Provide assistance in making burial or cremation arrangements.
5. The family's obstetrician, pediatrician, and other community supports should be notified of the infant's death.
6. A packet of written grief materials and contact information should be provided before discharge.
7. A representative from the primary team or appropriately trained designee should assume responsibility for coordinating bereavement follow-up. This person will be responsible for arranging and documenting the follow-up process.
8. Provide assistance to the family as they leave the hospital without their child. If possible, arrange for prepaid valet parking or an escort to the door.

C. Follow-up after discharge
1. A phone call within the first few days after the infant's death.
2. A sympathy card, signed by members of the primary team sent to the family at home.

3. A follow-up meeting with the family approximately 4 to 6 weeks after the infant's death. Timing will depend on availability of autopsy results and the parents' preference. In some cases, the family will not want to return to the hospital or continue contact. The coordinator will be sure this is documented and arrange for the family to be followed through a primary-care provider or other community agency. Follow-up calls can still be made if the family consents.
4. Meetings should include a review of events surrounding the infant's death, results of the autopsy or other studies and implications for future pregnancies.
5. Assessment should be made to determine the coping ability of the family as they continue with the grieving process and referrals made to appropriate professionals or agencies including bereavement support groups if needed.
6. Card and phone call at 1-year anniversary.
7. Plan for future meetings if the family desires.

IV. STAFF EDUCATION AND SUPPORT
A. General principles
1. Caring for infants and families around the time of death is challenging and requires compassion and knowledge of the normal grieving process. Each NICU should create its own guidelines including orientation for all new staff, ongoing continuing education and conferences, designated staff members willing to mentor new staff, and a forum for discussing ethical issues.
2. Debriefing sessions with team members should be arranged following each death to provide support to team members and create a forum for discussion and education
3. A yearly memorial service for families and staff supported by the hospital provides a meaningful way to remember losses that have occurred each year.

Suggested Readings

Abe N, Catlin A, Mihara D. End of life in the NICU: A study of ventilator withdrawal. *Am J Matern Child Nurs* 2001;26(3):141–146.

Catlin A, Carter B. Creation of a neonatal end-of life palliative care protocol. *Neonatal Netw* 2002;21(4):37–49.

Chiswick M. Parents and end of life decisions in neonatal practice. *Arch Dis Child Fetal Neonatal Ed* 2001;85(1):F1–F3.

Gale G, Brooks A. Implementing a palliative care protocol in a newborn intensive care unit. *Adv Neonatal Care* 2006;6(1):37–53–e2.

Hutti MH. Social and professional support needs of families after perinatal loss. *J Obstet Gynecol Neonatal Nurs* 2005;34(5):630–638.

McHaffie HE, Laing IA, Lloyd DJ. Follow-up care of bereaved parents after treatment withdrawal from newborns. *Arch Dis Child Fetal Neonatal Ed* 2001;84(2):F125–F128.

McHaffie HE, Lyon AJ, Fowlie PW. Lingering death after treatment withdrawal in the neonatal intensive care unit. *Arch Dis Child Fetal Neonatal Ed* 2001;85(1):F4–F7.

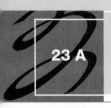

23 A

VIRAL INFECTIONS
Sandra K. Burchett and Nazan Dalgic

I. **INTRODUCTION.** Vertically transmitted (mother-to-child) viral infections of the fetus and newborn can generally be divided into two major categories. The first is **congenital infections,** which are transmitted to the fetus *in utero*. The second is **perinatal infections,** which are acquired intrapartum or in the postpartum period. Infections acquired through breastfeeding are in the latter category. Classifying these infections into congenital and perinatal categories highlights aspects of their pathogenesis in the fetus and newborn infant. Generally, when these infections occur in children or adults, they are benign; however, if the host is immunocompromised or if the immune system is not yet developed, such as in the neonate, clinical symptoms may be quite severe or even fatal. Congenital infections can have clinical manifestations that are apparent antenatally by ultrasonography or when the infant is born, whereas perinatal infections may not become clinically apparent until after the first few days or weeks of life. Although classically the congenital infections have gone by the acronym TORCH (T = toxoplasmosis, O = other, R = rubella, C = cytomegalovirus, H = herpes simplex virus), this term is now archaic and should be avoided. When congenital or perinatal infections are suspected, the diagnosis of each of the possible infectious agents should be considered separately and the most appropriate and rapid diagnostic test requested in order to implement therapy as quickly as possible. Useless information is often obtained when the diagnosis is attempted by drawing a single serum sample to be sent for measurement of TORCH titers. These antibodies are acquired by passive transmission to the fetus and merely reflect the maternal serostatus. The following discussion is divided by pathogen as to the usual timing of acquisition of infection (congenital or perinatal) and in approximate order of prevalence.

II. **CYTOMEGALOVIRUS (CMV) (CONGENITAL AND PERINATAL).** Disease manifestations are most commonly seen in neonates with congenital infection. CMV is a double-stranded and enveloped DNA virus; therefore infection is lifelong. It is a member of the herpesvirus family, is found only in humans, and derives its name from the histopathologic appearance of infected cells, which have abundant cytoplasm and both intranuclear and cytoplasmic inclusions, and does not result in rapid cell death. It is present in saliva, urine, genital secretions, breast milk, and blood/blood products of infected persons, and can be transmitted by exposure to any of these sources. Primary infection (acute infection) is usually asymptomatic in older infants, children, and adults, but may manifest with mononucleosis-like symptoms, including a prolonged fever and a mild hepatitis. Latent infection is asymptomatic unless the host becomes immunocompromised. CMV infection is very common, with seroprevalence in the United States between 50% and 85% by age 40. Forty percent or more of pregnant women in the United States are infected, with the lowest infection prevalence in young primigravidas. Vertical transmission can occur at any time in gestation or in the perinatal period and is usually asymptomatic, especially for women seropositive before pregnancy. However, there are reports that as many as 17% of all infants with symptomatic CMV are born to women with prior seropositivity.

    A. **Epidemiology.** Congenital CMV occurs in at least 1% of all live births in the United States and is the leading infectious cause of sensorineural hearing loss and developmental delay. Annually, of these 40,000 CMV-infected infants, 10% will have symptomatic disease. Additionally, 10% of the asymptomatic neonates will have significant sequelae. Therefore, at least 8,000 infants are severely affected by or die from CMV infection in the United States each year. Primary CMV infection occurs in 1% to 3% of pregnant women. It is estimated that 30% to 40% of fetuses of women with primary infection will become infected with CMV, and approximately 15% of these fetuses will develop significant disease. The risk of transmission to the fetus as a function of gestational age is uncertain, but infection during early gestation likely carries a higher risk of severe fetal disease.

B. Clinical manifestations. Symptomatic CMV infection of the fetus has two presentations.

1. Early manifestations can include a pattern consistent with an acute fulminant infection involving multiple organ systems and carries a high risk of mortality (as much as 30%). Findings with this presentation include petechiae or purpura (79%), hepatosplenomegaly (74%), jaundice (63%), prematurity and "blue-berry muffin spots" consistent with extramedullary hematopoiesis. **Laboratory abnormalities** include elevated hepatic transaminase and bilirubin levels (as much as half is conjugated), anemia, and thrombocytopenia. Hyperbilirubinemia may be present at birth or develop over time. It usually persists beyond the period of physiologic jaundice. Approximately one-third of these infants are preterm, and one-third have intrauterine growth restriction (IUGR).

2. A second early presentation includes those infants who are symptomatic but without life-threatening complications. These babies may have IUGR or disproportionate microcephaly (48%) with or without intracranial calcifications. The calcifications may occur anywhere in the brain, but are classically found in the periventricular area. Other neuroimaging and central nervous system (CNS) manifestations can include ventricular dilatation, cortical atrophy, migrational disorders such as lissencephaly and pachygyria and demyelination as well as chorioretinitis in approximately 10% to 15% of infants. Babies with CNS abnormalities almost always have developmental abnormalities and neurologic dysfunction, ranging from intelligence quotient (IQ) scores below 50, motor abnormalities, deafness, and visual problems to mild learning and language disability or mild hearing loss. Because sensorineural hearing loss is the most common sequela of CMV infection (60% in symptomatic and 5% in asymptomatic infants), any infant failing the newborn hearing screen should be quickly assessed for CMV infection. Infants with CMV infection should have hearing tested as neonates and young infants.

In contrast to symptomatic newborn infants, those with **asymptomatic infection** have no mortality, but 5% to 15% may have developmental abnormalities. These include hearing loss, mental retardation, motor spasticity, and microcephaly. Other problems that can be detected later in life include inguinal hernia and dental defects characterized by abnormal enamel production.

CMV infection is more common among HIV-1 infected infants, and coinfected infants may have more rapid progression of HIV-1 disease. Therefore, screening for CMV in HIV-exposed infants is important.

III. PERINATAL INFECTION. Perinatally acquired CMV infection may occur (i) from intrapartum exposure to the virus with in the maternal genital tract, (ii) from postnatal exposure to infected breast milk, (iii) from exposure to infected blood or blood products, or (iv) nosocomially through urine or saliva. The incubation period varies from 4 to 12 weeks. Almost all term infants who acquire infection perinatally from infected mothers remain asymptomatic. Many of these infections arise from mothers with reactivated viral excretion. In these cases, long-term developmental and neurologic abnormalities are infrequently seen. However, symptomatic perinatally acquired infections may occur at a higher frequency in preterm infants. Hearing abnormalities may also be detected in infants with perinatal CMV infection; therefore, hearing should be assessed in infants documented to have acquired CMV.

IV. CMV PNEUMONITIS. CMV has been associated with pneumonitis occurring in infants <4 months old. Symptoms and radiographic findings in CMV pneumonia are similar to those seen in afebrile pneumonia of other causes in neonates and young infants, including *Chlamydia trachomatis, Ureaplasma urealyticum,* and respiratory syncytial virus (RSV). Symptoms include tachypnea, cough, coryza, and nasal congestion.

Intercostal retractions and hypoxemia may be present, and apnea may occur. Radiographically, there is hyperinflation, diffuse increased pulmonary markings, thickened bronchial walls, and focal atelectasis. A small number of infants may have symptoms that are severe enough to require mechanical ventilation, and approximately 3% of infants die. Laboratory findings in CMV pneumonitis are nonspecific. Long-term sequelae include recurrent pulmonary problems, including wheezing, and, in some cases, repeated hospitalizations for respiratory distress. Whether this reflects congenital or perinatal CMV infection is unclear, but it does pose a risk, especially to the preterm infants. Conversely, merely finding CMV present in respiratory secretions of a preterm infant does not prove causality of symptomatology because CMV is present in saliva.

V. TRANSFUSION-ACQUIRED CMV INFECTION. In the past, significant morbidity and mortality could occur in newborn infants receiving CMV-infected blood or blood products. Those most severely affected were preterm, low birth-weight infants born to CMV-seronegative women. Symptoms typically developed 4 to 12 weeks after transfusion, lasted for 2 to 3 weeks, and consisted of respiratory distress, pallor, and hepatosplenomegaly. Hematologic abnormalities were also seen, including hemolysis, thrombocytopenia, and atypical lymphocytosis. Mortality was estimated to be 20% in very low birth weight infants. This is now rare, prevented by using blood/blood products from CMV-seronegative donors or filtered, leukoreduced products (see Chap. 26E).

VI. DIAGNOSIS. Congenital CMV infection should be suspected in any infant having typical symptoms of infection or if there is a maternal history of seroconversion or a mononucleosis-like illness in pregnancy. The diagnosis is made if CMV is identified in urine, saliva, blood, or respiratory secretions and defined as *congenital* infection if found within the first 2 weeks of life and as *perinatal* infection if after 4 weeks of life. There are three rapid diagnostic techniques:

A. Spin-enhanced culture or "shell vial." Virus can be isolated from urine or saliva, but CMV is concentrated in high titers in urine. For this technique, urine should be maintained at 4°C (ice or refrigerator) for transport and storage. The urine is then placed in viral tissue culture medium containing a coverslip on which tissue culture cells have been grown. If CMV is present, it infects the cells which are lysed and stained with antibody to CMV antigens. Virus can be detected with high sensitivity and specificity within 24 to 72 hours of inoculation. It is much more rapid than the standard tissue culture, which may take from 2 to 6 weeks for replication and identification.

B. CMV antigen. Peripheral blood can be centrifuged and the buffy coat spread on a slide. The neutrophils are then lysed and stained with an antibody to CMV pp65 antigen. Positive results confirm CMV infection and viremia; however, negative results do not rule out CMV infection. This test is usually used to follow efficacy of therapy.

C. CMV polymerase chain reaction (PCR). Commercial laboratories offer PCR to detect CMV in blood. The sensitivity of using this test as a diagnostic modality is unknown in neonatal CMV disease.

D. CMV IgG and IgM. The determination of serum antibody titers to CMV has limited usefulness for the neonate, although negative immunoglobulin G (IgG) titers in both maternal and infant sera are sufficient to exclude congenital CMV infection. The interpretation of a positive IgG titer in the newborn is complicated by the presence of transplacentally derived maternal IgG. Uninfected infants usually show a decline in IgG within 1 month and have no detectable titer by 4 to 9 months. Infected infants continue to produce IgG throughout the same time period. Tests for CMV-specific IgM have limitations but can help to elucidate infant infection.

If the diagnosis of congenital CMV infection is made, the infant should have a thorough physical and neurologic examination, a computed tomography (CT) scan of the brain (or magnetic resonance imaging [MRI]), an ophthalmologic examination, and a hearing test. Laboratory tests include a complete blood count, liver function tests, and cerebrospinal fluid (CSF) examination (if the CSF PCR is positive for CMV, the infant should be classified as having CNS disease). There are data from 56 CMV-infected infants with symptomatic disease that suggest that 90% of CMV-infected infants with an abnormal CT scan will have CNS sequelae; however, 29% of infants with a normal CT scan will also have sequelae.

VII. TREATMENT. Ganciclovir (9-[(13-dihydroxy-2-propoxy)methyl]guanine) and more recently valganciclovir have been effective in the treatment of and prophylaxis against dissemination of CMV in adult immunocompromised patients. In the earliest studies of ganciclovir treatment of infants with symptomatic CMV disease, most had thrombocytopenia and neutropenia during the course of therapy. Early ganciclovir studies showed a trend toward efficacy as assessed by stabilization or improvement of sensorineural hearing loss. Broader study is warranted because the most congenitally infected, symptomatic infants have poor neurodevelopmental outcome. Studies are planned using oral valganciclovir treatment for these infants. Questions remain as to the potential for future reproductive system effects because ganciclovir has been found to cause testicular atrophy in animal studies. Additionally, although there have been no controlled trials, hyperimmune CMV immunoglobulin might conceivably benefit infants with congenital CMV, especially those with a fulminant presentation.

VIII. PREVENTION

A. Screening. Because only 1% to 3% of women acquire primary CMV infection during pregnancy, with the overall risk of symptomatic fetal infection only 0.2%, many do not recommend screening for women at risk of seroconversion. Isolation of virus from the cervix or urine of pregnant women cannot be used to predict fetal infection. In cases of documented primary maternal infection or seroconversion, quantative PCR testing of amniotic fluid can determine whether the fetus acquired infection. However, counseling about a positive finding of fetal infection is difficult because 85% of infected fetuses will have mild or asymptomatic disease. Some investigators have found that higher CMV viral loads from the amniotic fluid correlated with abnormal neurodevelopmental outcome, but this is not proved. Presently, there is not enough information about fetal transmission and outcome to provide guidelines for obstetric management, such as recommendations for therapeutic abortion, even if primary maternal CMV infection is documented. The Centers for Disease Control and Prevention recommends that (i) pregnant women practise hand-washing with soap and water after contact with diapers or oral secretions; (ii) pregnant women who develop a mononucleosis-like illness during pregnancy should be evaluated for CMV infection and counseled about risks to the unborn child; (iii) antibody testing can confirm prior CMV infection; (iv) recovery of CMV from the cervix or urine of women near delivery does not warrant a cesarean section; (v) the benefits of breastfeeding outweigh the minimal risk of acquiring CMV; (vi) there is no need to screen for CMV or exclude CMV-excreting children from schools or institutions.

B. Immunization. Passive immunization with hyperimmune anti-CMV immuno-globulin and active immunization with a live attenuated CMV vaccine represent attractive therapies for prophylaxis against congenital CMV infections. However, data from clinical trials are lacking. Immune globulin might be considered as prophylaxis of susceptible women against primary CMV infection in pregnancy. Two live attenuated CMV vaccines have been developed, but their efficacy has not been clearly established. The possibility of reactivation of vaccine-strain CMV in pregnancy with subsequent infection of the fetus must be considered carefully before adequate field trials can be completed in women of child-bearing age.

C. Breast-milk restriction. Although breast milk is a common source for perinatal CMV infection in the newborn, symptomatic infection is rare, especially in term infants. In this setting, protection against disseminated disease may be provided by transplacentally derived maternal IgG or antibody in breast milk. However, there may be insufficient transplacental IgG to provide adequate protection in preterm infants. It remains unclear whether preterm infants should be screened for CMV seropositivity. In women of extremely premature infants known to be CMV positive, pasteurizing breast milk at 220°C or freezing breast milk, will reduce the titer of CMV although it will not eliminate active virus. At present there is no recommended method of minimizing the risk of exposure to CMV in infected breast milk.

D. Environmental restrictions. Day care centers and hospitals are potential high-risk environments for acquiring CMV infection. Not surprisingly, a number of studies confirmed an increased risk for infection in day care workers. However, there does not appear to be an increased risk for infection in hospital personnel. These studies demonstrated that good hand-washing and infection-control measures practiced in hospital settings may be sufficient to control the spread of CMV to workers. Unfortunately, such control may be difficult to achieve in day care centers. Good hand-washing technique should be suggested to pregnant women with children in day care, especially if they are known to be seronegative. The determination of the CMV susceptibility of these women by serology may be useful for counseling.

E. Transfusion product restrictions. The risk of transfusion-acquired CMV infection in the neonate has been almost eliminated by the use of CMV antibody-negative donors, by freezing packed red blood cells (PRBCs) in glycerol, or by removing the white blood cells. It is particularly important to use blood from one of these sources in preterm, low birth-weight infants (see Chap. 26E).

IX. HERPES SIMPLEX VIRUS (HSV: PERINATAL). HSV is a double-stranded, enveloped DNA virus with two virologically distinct types: types 1 and 2. HSV-2 is the predominant cause of neonatal disease (75%–80%), but both types produce clinically indistinguishable neonatal syndromes. At least 80% of the U.S population is infected with HSV type 1, the cause of recurrent orolabial disease, and 40% are infected with HSV-2, the predominant cause of recurrent genital disease, by young adulthood. Infection in the newborn occurs as a result of direct exposure, most commonly in the perinatal period from maternal genital disease. The virus can cause localized disease of the skin, eye, or mouth, or may disseminate by cell-to-cell contiguous spread or viremia. After adsorption and penetration into host cells, viral replication proceeds, resulting in cellular swelling, hemorrhagic necrosis, formation of intranuclear inclusions, cytolysis, and cell death.

A. Epidemiology. Because HSV-2 is more likely to recur in the genital tract and therefore accounts for most neonatal HSV infections, it is important to understand the potential for neonatal exposure to virus. The seroprevalence of HSV-2 varies according to locale in the United States, but is likely to be at least 30%. In a study of 779 women attending a sexually transmitted disease clinic, 47% had serologic evidence of HSV-2 infection, but only 22% had symptoms. The characteristic ulcerations of the genitalia were present only in two-thirds of the genital tracts from which HSV could be isolated, and the others had asymptomatic shedding or atypical lesions. It is estimated that 0.01% to 0.39% of all women shed virus at delivery, and approximately 1% of all women with a history of recurrent HSV infection asymptomatically shed HSV at delivery. However, when the birth canal is carefully visualized and those with asymptomatic lesions excluded, this rate of shedding may be nearer 0.5%. **It is critical to recognize that most mothers of infants with neonatal HSV do not have a history of HSV.** Infants at greatest risk of acquisition of infection are those born to mothers with newly acquired HSV during pregnancy (primary infection), in whom the rate of transmission of HSV is estimated to be 50%. Additionally, one-third of infants born to mothers with newly acquired HSV-2, although already infected with HSV-1 (nonprimary, first episode), may acquire HSV infection. Infants born to HSV-2–seropositive mothers (recurrent) have an approximate 3% risk of acquiring infection. This may well be due to protective maternal type-specific antibodies in the infant's serum or the birth canal. The overall incidence of newborn infection with HSV is estimated to be 1 in 3,000 to 1 in 20,000, or 200 to 1,333 infants, per year.

B. Intrapartum transmission. This is the most common cause of neonatal HSV and is primarily associated with active shedding of virus from the cervix or vulva at the time of delivery. As many as 95% of newborn infections occur as a result of intrapartum transmission. Several factors have been identified that relate to intrapartum transmission. The amount and duration of maternal virus shedding is likely to be a major determinate of fetal transmission. These are greatest with primary maternal infections. Maternal antibody to HSV is also important and is associated with a decreased risk of fetal transmission. In fact, when maternal antibody is present, the risk of acquisition of HSV, even for the newborn exposed to HSV in the birth canal, is very low. The exact mechanism of action of maternal antibody in preventing perinatal infection is not known, but transplacentally acquired antibody has been shown to reduce the risk of severe newborn disease following postnatal HSV exposure. The risk of intrapartum infection increases with ruptured membranes, especially when ruptured longer than 4 hours. Finally, direct methods for fetal monitoring, such as with scalp electrodes, increase the risk of fetal transmission in the setting of active shedding. It is best to avoid these techniques in women with a history of recurrent infection or suspected primary HSV disease.

C. Antenatal transmission. *In utero* infection has been documented but is uncommon. Spontaneous abortion has occurred with primary maternal infection before 20 weeks' gestation, but the true risk to the fetus of early-trimester primary infection is not known. Fetal infections may occur by either transplacental or ascending routes and have been documented in the setting of both primary and recurrent maternal disease. There may be a wide range of clinical manifestations, from localized skin or eye involvement to multiorgan disease and congenital malformations. Chorioretinitis, microcephaly, and hydranencephaly may be found in a small number of patients.

D. Postnatal transmission. There is evidence that a percentage of neonatal HSV infections result from postnatal exposure. Potential sources include symptomatic and asymptomatic oropharyngeal shedding by either parent, hospital personnel, or other contacts; maternal breast lesions; and nosocomial spread. Measures to minimize exposure from these sources are discussed in the subsequent text.

E. Clinical manifestations. Data from the National Institute of Allergy and Infectious Diseases (NIAID) Collaborative Antiviral Study Group (CASG) indicate that morbidity and mortality of neonatal HSV best correlates with three categories of disease. These are infection localized to the skin, eye, and/or mouth; encephalitis with or without localized mucocutaneous disease; and disseminated infection with multiple organ involvement. The NIAID CASG reported on the outcome of 210 infants with HSV infection who were randomized to receive either acyclovir or vidarabine antiviral therapy. Eight babies had congenital infection with signs (chorioretinitis, skin lesions, hydrocephalus) at birth. The highest mortality (>50%) was seen in infants having disseminated disease; hemorrhagic shock and pneumonitis were the principal causes of death. Of the survivors for whom follow-up was available, significant neurologic sequelae were seen in a high percentage of the infants with encephalitis and disseminated disease.

1. Skin, eye, and mouth infection. Approximately 50% of infants with HSV have disease localized to the skin, eye, or mucocutaneous membranes. Vesicles typically appear on the sixth to ninth day of neonatal life. A cluster of vesicles often develops on the presenting part of the body, where extended direct contact with virus may occur. Vesicles occur in 90% of infants with localized mucocutaneous infection, and recurrent disease is common. Furthermore, significant morbidity can occur in these infants despite the absence of signs of disseminated disease at the time of diagnosis; up to 10% of infants later show neurologic impairment, and infants with keratoconjunctivitis can develop chorioretinitis, cataracts, and retinopathy. Ophthalmologic and neurologic follow-up is important in all infants with mucocutaneous HSV. Infants with three or more recurrences of vesicles have an increased risk of neurologic complications.

2. CNS infection. Approximately one-third of neonates with HSV present with encephalitis in the absence of disseminated disease, and from 40% to 60% of these infants do not have mucocutaneous vesicles. These infants usually become symptomatic at 10 to 14 days of life with lethargy, seizures, temperature instability, and hypotonia. In the setting of disseminated disease, HSV is thought to invade the CNS from hematogenous spread. However, CNS infection in the absence of disseminated disease probably results from retrograde axonal spread. The latter condition most often occurs in infants having transplacentally derived viral-neutralizing antibodies, which may protect against widespread dissemination but not influence intraneuronal viral replication. Mortality is high without treatment and is approximately 15% with treatment, and approximately two-thirds of surviving infants have impaired neurodevelopment. Long-term sequelae from acute HSV encephalitis include microcephaly, hydranencephaly, porencephalic cysts, spasticity, blindness, chorioretinitis, and learning disabilities.

3. **Disseminated infection.** This is the most severe form of neonatal HSV infection. It accounts for approximately 22% of all infants with neonatal HSV infection and ends in mortality for 57% of the infants with this presentation. Pneumonitis is associated with greatest mortality. Symptoms usually begin within the first week of neonatal life. The liver, adrenals, and multiple other visceral organs are usually involved. Approximately two-thirds of infants also have encephalitis. Clinical findings include seizures, shock, respiratory distress, disseminated intravascular coagulation (DIC), and pneumonitis. A typical vesicular rash may be absent in as many as 20% of infants. Forty percent of the infants who survive have morbidity.

F. **Diagnosis.** HSV infection should be considered in the differential diagnosis of ill neonates with a variety of clinical presentations. These include CNS abnormalities, fever, shock, DIC, and/or hepatitis. HSV also should be considered in infants with respiratory distress without an obvious bacterial cause or a clinical course and findings consistent with prematurity. The possibility of concomitant HSV infection with other commonly encountered problems of the preterm infant should be considered. Viral isolation or fluorescent antibody detection in the appropriate clinical setting remains critical to the diagnosis. Combined HSV 1 and 2 serology is of little value, because many women are infected with HSV 1 and because these tests usually have a relatively slow turnaround time; however, obtaining type-specific antibody from the mother or the infant may help determine whether there was maternal exposure to either and prognosis. Additionally, specific IgM may not be detected for up to 3 weeks in neonates. However, the number of different viral antigen-specific antibodies produced seems to correlate with the extent of disseminated disease, and the presence of certain antigen-specific antibodies may have long-term prognostic value. For the infant with mucocutaneous lesions, tissue should be scraped from vesicles, placed in the appropriate viral transport medium, and promptly processed for culture by a diagnostic virology laboratory. Alternatively, virus can be detected directly when tissue samples are swabbed onto a glass slide and evaluated by direct fluorescent antibody (DFA) technique. Virus also can be isolated from the oropharynx and nasopharynx, conjunctivae, stool, and urine. In the absence of a vesicular rash, viral isolation from these sites may aid in the diagnosis of disseminated HSV or HSV encephalitis. With encephalitis, an elevated CSF protein level and pleocytosis are often seen, but initial values may be within normal limits. Therefore, serial CSF examinations may be very important. Electroencephalography and CT/MRI are also useful in the diagnosis of HSV encephalitis. Viral isolation from CSF is reported to be successful in as many as 40% of cases, and rates of detection in CSF by PCR may reach close to 100%. Laboratory abnormalities seen with disseminated disease include elevated hepatic transaminase levels, direct hyperbilirubinemia, neutropenia, thrombocytopenia, and coagulopathy. A diffuse interstitial pattern is usually observed on x-ray films of infants with HSV pneumonitis.

G. **Treatment.** Effective antiviral therapy (acyclovir, a nucleoside analog that selectively inhibits HSV replication) exists, but the timing of therapy is critical. Treatment is indicated for all forms of neonatal HSV disease. Initially NIAID CASG studies were carried out with vidarabine, which reduced the morbidity and mortality for all forms of neonatal HSV. Mortality with encephalitis was reduced from 50% to 15% and with disseminated disease from 90% to 70%. Later, studies from the CASG found that acyclovir is as efficacious as vidarabine for the treatment of neonatal HSV. Furthermore, acyclovir is a selective inhibitor of viral replication with minimal side effects on the host, and can be administered in relatively small volumes over short infusion times. Recommendations include treating infants with disease limited to the skin, eye, and mouth disease with 20 mg acyclovir/kg every 8 hours for 14 days, and those with CNS or disseminated disease for at least 21 days, or longer if the CSF PCR remains positive. Infants with ocular involvement should have an ophthalmologic evaluation and consider topical ophthalmic agents (1% trifluridine, 0.1% iododeoxyruidine, or 3% vidarabine) in addition to parenteral therapy. Oral therapy such as with valacyclovir is not recommended at this time for initial treatment. Some experts recommend acyclovir suppressive therapy at 300 mg/m^2/dose three times a day after the initial treatment period until 6 months of life with careful monitoring for neutropenia and anemia.

H. Prevention. Several trials have shown efficacy and safety of treating pregnant women with clinically symptomatic primary HSV infection with a 10-day course of acyclovir. Additionally, there is a suggestion that if a woman asymptomatically seroconverts during pregnancy that a course of acyclovir therapy beginning at 38 weeks' gestation might be helpful in prevention of active lesions at the time of delivery.

I. Management of the newborn at risk for HSV (see Table 23A.1). The principal problem in developing strategies for the prevention of HSV transmission is the inability to identify maternal shedding of virus at the time of delivery. Viral identification requires isolation in tissue culture, so any attempt to identify women who may be shedding HSV at delivery would require antenatal cervical cultures. Unfortunately, such screening cultures taken before labor fail to predict active excretion at delivery.

Until more rapid techniques such as a screening PCR are made available for the identification of HSV, the only clear recommendation that can be made is to deliver infants by cesarean section if genital lesions are present at the start of labor. The efficacy of this approach may diminish when membranes are ruptured beyond 4 hours. Nevertheless, it is generally recommended that cesarean section be considered even with membrane rupture of longer durations, although data showing efficacy beyond 4 hours are lacking. The upper time limit for membrane rupture has been suggested to be 12 hours to 24 hours. For women

TABLE 23A.1   Management of the Child Born to a Woman with Active Genital Herpes Simplex Virus (HSV) Infection

Maternal primary or first-episode infection:
- Consider offering an elective cesarean section, regardless of lesion status at delivery, or if membranes ruptured >4 h
- Swab infant's conjunctive and nasopharynx, and possibly collect urine for DFA and culture to determine exposure to HSV
- Treat with acyclovir if DFA or culture positive or signs of neonatal HSV

If cesarean section performed after 24 h of ruptured membranes or if vaginal delivery unavoidable:
- Swab infant's conjunctive and nasopharynx, and collect urine for DFA and culture to determine exposure to HSV
- Consider initiation of acyclovir while pending culture and DFA results or if signs of neonatal HSV

Recurrent infection, active at delivery:
- Cesarean section after 4 h of ruptured membranes or unavoidable vaginal delivery
- Swab infant's conjunctivae and nasopharynx, and possibly collect urine for DFA and culture to determine exposure to HSV
- Treat with acyclovir if culture positive or signs of HSV infection

DFA = direct fluorescent antibody.

with a history of prior genital herpes, careful examination should be performed to determine whether lesions are present when labor commences. If lesions are observed, cesarean section should be carried out. If no lesions are identified, vaginal delivery is appropriate, but a cervical swab should be obtained for culture. At this time, there are no data to support the prophylactic use of antiviral agents or immunoglobulin to prevent transmission to the newborn infant.

Infants inadvertently delivered vaginally in the setting of cervical lesions should be isolated from other infants in the nursery, and cultures should be obtained from the oropharynx/nasopharynx and conjunctivae. If the mother can be identified as having recurrent infection, the resultant neonatal infection rate is low, and parents should be instructed to consult their pediatrician when a rash or other clinical changes (lethargy, tachypnea, poor feeding) develop. Weekly pediatric follow-up during the first month is recommended. Infants with a positive culture from any site or the evolution of clinical symptomatology should immediately have cultures repeated and antiviral therapy started.

Before starting acyclovir therapy, the infant should have conjunctival, nasopharyngeal swabs for DFA and culture, urine for culture, and a CSF evaluation for pleocytosis and HSV DNA PCR. These infants should be evaluated for possible disseminated HSV, as well by liver function tests and possibly a chest radiograph.

J. Prevention. Infants and mothers with HSV lesions should be in contact isolation. Careful hand washing and preventing the infant from having direct contact with lesions should be emphasized. Breastfeeding should be avoided if there are breast lesions, and women with oral HSV should wear a mask while breastfeeding. Hospital personnel with orolabial HSV infection represent a low risk to the newborn, although the use of face masks should be recommended if active lesions are present. Of course, hand washing or use of gloves should again be emphasized. The exception to these guidelines is nursery personnel with herpetic whitlows. Because they have a high risk of viral shedding, and as transmission can occur despite the use of gloves, these individuals should not care for newborns.

X. PARVOVIRUS (CONGENITAL). Parvoviruses are small, unenveloped single-stranded DNA viruses that range in size from 18 to 26 mm. Humans are the only known host.

A. Epidemiology. Parvovirus transmission results after contact with respiratory secretions, blood/blood products, or by vertical transmission. Cases can occur sporadically or in outbreak settings (especially in schools in late winter and early spring). Secondary spread occurs to at least half of susceptible household contacts. Infection is very common, such that 90% of elderly persons are seropositive. The prevalence of infection increases throughout childhood, such that approximately one-half of women of childbearing age are immune and the other half are susceptible to primary infection. The annual seroconversion rate in these women is 1.5%; however, because assessment of parvovirus infection status is not part of routine prenatal testing and because clinical infection is often asymptomatic, the rate of fetal infection in women who seroconvert during pregnancy is unknown. Women who are parents of young children, elementary school teachers, or child-care workers may be at greatest risk for exposure. Unfortunately, the time of greatest transmissibility is before the onset of symptoms or rash. Additionally, 50% of contagious contacts may not have a rash, and 20% may be asymptomatic. The incubation period is usually 4 to 14 days but can be as long as 21 days. Rash and joint symptoms occur 2 to 3 weeks after infection. The virus is probably spread by means of respiratory secretions, which clear in patients with typical erythema infectiosum at or shortly after the onset of rash. The overall rate of vertical transmission of parvovirus from the mother with primary infection to her fetus is approximately one-third. The overall risk of fetal loss is greatest when maternal infection occurs in the first half of pregnancy and is approximately 3% to 6%. Fetal death usually occurs within 6 weeks of maternal infection. The risk of fetal hydrops is approximately 1%. Therefore, parvovirus B19 could be causal of as many as 1,400 cases of fetal death or hydrops fetalis each year in the United States.

B. Pathogenesis. The cellular receptor for parvovirus B19 is the P blood group antigen, which is found on erythrocytes, erythroblasts, megakaryocytes, endothelial cells, placenta, and fetal liver and heart cells. This tissue specificity correlates with sites of clinical abnormalities (which are usually anemia with or without thrombocytopenia and sometimes fetal myocarditis). Lack of the P antigen is extremely rare, but these persons are resistant to infection with parvovirus.

C. Clinical manifestations

1. **Disease in children.** Parvovirus B19 has been associated with a variety of rashes, including the typical "slapped cheek" rash of erythema infectiosum (fifth disease). In approximately 60% of school-age children with erythema infectiosum, fever occurs 1 to 4 days before the facial rash appears. Associated symptoms include myalgias, upper respiratory or gastrointestinal symptoms, and malaise, but these symptoms generally resolve with the appearance of the rash. The rash is usually macular, progresses to the extremities and trunk, and may involve the palms and soles. The rash may be pruritic and may recur. These children are likely most infectious before the onset of fever or rash. In group settings such as classrooms, the appearance of one clinically symptomatic child could reinforce the need for good hand-washing practices among potentially seronegative pregnant women.

2. **Disease in adults.** The typical school-age presentation of erythema infectiosum can occur in adults, but arthralgias and arthritis are more common. As many as 60% of adults with parvovirus B19 infection may have acute joint swelling, most commonly involving peripheral joints (symmetrically). Rash and joint symptoms occur 2 to 3 weeks after infection. Arthritis may persist for years and may be associated with the development of rheumatoid arthritis.

3. **Less common manifestations of parvovirus B19 infection**

   a. **Infection in patients with severe anemia or immunosuppression.** Parvovirus B19 has been clearly identified as a cause of persistent and profound anemia in patients with rapid red blood cell turnover such as in those with sickle cell disease, hemoglobin SC disease, thalassemia, hereditary spherocytosis, and cellular enzyme deficits, such as pyruvate kinase deficiency. Parvovirus B19 has also been associated with acute and chronic red blood cell aplasia in immunosuppressed patients.

   b. **Fetal infection.** Although parvovirus B19 has genotypic variation, no antigenic variation between isolates has been demonstrated. Parvoviruses tend to infect rapidly dividing cells and can be transmitted across the placenta, posing a potential threat to the fetus. Based primarily on the demonstration of viral DNA in fetal tissue samples, parvovirus B19 has been implicated in approximately 10% of cases of fetal nonimmune hydrops. The presumed pathogenic sequence is as follows:

   Maternal primary infection → Transplacental transfer of B19 virus → Infection of red blood cell precursors → Arrested red blood cell production → Severe anemia (Hb <8 g/dL) → Congestive heart failure → Edema.

   Furthermore, B19 DNA has been detected in cardiac tissues from aborted fetuses. It has been suggested that B19 may cause fetal myocarditis and that this may contribute to the development of hydrops. Finally, fetal hepatitis with severe liver disease has been documented. Although there have been rare case reports of infants with fetal anomalies and parvovirus infection, it is unlikely that parvovirus causes fetal anomalies; hence, therapeutic abortion should not be recommended, but rather the pregnancy should be followed carefully by frequent examination and ultrasonography.

D. Diagnosis. Parvovirus B19 will not grow in standard tissue cultures because humans are the only host. Determination of serum IgG and IgM levels is the most practical test. Serum B19 IgG is absent in susceptible hosts, and IgM appears by day 3 of an acute infection. Serum IgM may be detected in as many as 90% of patients with acute B19 infection, and serum levels begin to fall by the second to third month after infection. Serum IgG appears a few days after IgM and may persist for years. Serum or plasma can also be assessed for viral DNA by PCR and defines recent infection. Viral antigens may be directly detected in tissues by radioimmunoassay, enzyme-linked immunosorbent assay (ELISA), immunofluorescence, *in situ* nucleic acid hybridization, or PCR. These techniques may be valuable for certain clinical settings, such as the examination of tissues from fetuses with nonimmune hydrops or determination of infection (PCR).

E. Treatment. Treatment is generally supportive. Intravenous immunoglobulin (IVIG) has been used with reported success in a limited number of patients with severe hematologic disorders related to persistent parvovirus infection. The rationale for this therapy stems from the observations that (i) the primary immune response to B19 infection is the production of specific IgM and IgG, (ii) the appearance of systemic antibody coincides with the resolution of clinical symptoms, and (iii) specific antibody prevents infection. However, no controlled studies have been undertaken to establish the efficacy of IVIG prophylaxis or therapy for B19 infections. There are no recommendations for use of IVIG in pregnancy.

In the carefully followed pregnancy in which hydrops fetalis is worsening, intrauterine blood transfusions may be considered, especially if the fetal hemoglobin is <8g/dL. The risk/benefit of this procedure to the mother and fetus will need to be assessed because some hydrops will improve without intervention, there is some tangible percentage of fetal demise associated with the procedure, and in some cases, if there is also fetal myocardiopathy secondary to parvovirus infection, the cardiac function may be inadequate to handle transfusion. Attempts to identify other causes of fetal hydrops are obviously important. The possible contribution of cardiac dysfunction that may not respond to blood transfusions also should be considered.

F. Prevention. Three groups of pregnant women of interest when considering the potential risk of fetal parvovirus disease are those exposed to an infected household contact, schoolteachers, and health care providers. In each, the measurement of serum IgG and IgM levels may be useful to determine who is at risk or acutely infected after B19 exposure. The risk of fetal B19 disease is apparently very small for asymptomatic pregnant women in communities where outbreaks of erythema infectiosum occur. In this setting, no special diagnostic tests or precautions may be indicated. However, household contacts with erythema infectiosum place pregnant women at increased risk for acute B19 infection. The estimated risk of B19 infection in a susceptible adult with a household contact is approximately 50%. Considering an estimated risk of 5% for severe fetal disease with acute maternal B19 infection, the risk of hydrops fetalis is approximately 2.5% for susceptible pregnant women exposed to an infected household contact during the first 18 weeks of gestation. Management of these women may include the following:

1. **Determination of susceptibility of acute infection** by serum IgG and IgM and PCR.
2. For susceptible or acutely infected women, **serial fetal ultrasonography** to monitor fetal growth and the possible evolution of hydrops.
3. Serial determinations of **maternal serum α-fetoprotein (AFP)** (AFP may rise up to 4 weeks before ultrasonography evidence of fetal hydrops), although this use is questioned.
4. Determination of **fetal IgM or DNA PCR** by percutaneous umbilical blood sampling (PUBS). The utility of this is questionable given the relatively high-risk–benefit ratio at present, especially because it is unclear that obstetric management will be altered by results. It may be useful to confirm B19 etiology when hydrops fetalis is present.

The epidemiology of community outbreaks of erythema infectiosum suggests that the risk of infection to susceptible schoolteachers is approximately 19% (compared with 50% for household contacts). This would lower the risk of B19 fetal disease in pregnant schoolteachers to <1%. It is not obvious that special precautions are necessary in this setting. In fact, there is likely to be widespread inapparent infection in both adults and children, providing a constant background exposure rate that cannot be altered. Considering the high prevalence of B19, the low risk of severe fetal disease, and the fact that attempts to avoid potential high-risk settings only reduce but do not eliminate exposure, exclusion of pregnant schoolteachers from the workplace is not recommended.

A similar approach may be taken for pregnant health care providers where the principal exposure will be from infected children presenting to the emergency room or physician's office. However, in many cases, the typical rash of erythema infectiosum may already be present, at which time infectivity is low. Furthermore, precautions directed at minimizing exposure to respiratory secretions may be taken to decrease the risk of transmission. Particular care should be exercised on pediatric wards where there are immunocompromised patients or patients with hemolytic anemias in whom B19 disease is suspected. These patients may shed virus well beyond the period of initial clinical symptoms, particularly when presenting with aplastic crisis. In this setting, there may be a significant risk for the spread of B19 to susceptible health care workers or other patients at risk for B19-induced aplastic crisis. To minimize this risk, patients with aplastic crises from B19 infections should be maintained on contact precautions, masks should be worn for close contact, and pregnant health care providers should not care for these patients.

XI. **HUMAN IMMUNODEFICIENCY VIRUS (HIV: CONGENITAL AND PERINATAL).** HIV is a cytopathic RNA retrovirus. HIV-1 is the principal cause of HIV infection in the United States and throughout the world. The virus binds to the host $CD4^+$ cell. This virus/receptor complex then binds to a coreceptor, and the viral core enters the host cell cytoplasm. The virus uses reverse transcriptase to synthesize DNA from its viral RNA, and this viral DNA integrates into the host genome. On cell activation, the viral DNA is transcribed to RNA, and viral proteins are synthesized. The virion acquires its outer envelope coat on budding from the host cell surface and is then infectious for other $CD4^+$ cells. HIV contains genomic RNA within a core that is surrounded by an inner protein shell and an outer lipid envelope. The genome consists of the three genes found in all retroviruses *(gag, pol, env)*, along with at least six additional genes, including gp120, which is necessary for the binding of virus to target cells, and p24, which is the major core protein.

A. **Epidemiology.** As of the end of 2005, the Centers for Disease Control and Prevention reported that 956,666 cases of the acquired immunodeficiency syndrome (AIDS) had been reported, 530,756 deaths from AIDS had occurred, and that 425,910 people were living with AIDS. Approximately 80,000 people died yearly from AIDS from 1993 to 1997, and approximately 15,000 to 20,000 died yearly since 1997. The decreased death rate is in large part attributed to access to more potent antiretroviral therapies since 1996. Additional estimates include that approximately 1,200,000 people are living with HIV of whom 25% are aware of their infection, and that 40,000 persons in the United States become infected with HIV each year. These estimates are difficult because only AIDS is mandatorily reported in all states. Additionally, many persons who are HIV infected will not have been tested and therefore do not know their infection status. Approximately 20% of persons living with AIDS are women, most of childbearing age. One percent of cases are in children younger than 13 years (n = 9,348 as of the end of 2003), with approximately 175 to 200 infants and children reported each year with AIDS, predominantly through perinatal transmission. In women of childbearing age, the leading risk behavior is heterosexual contact with a known HIV-infected person or unknown risk behavior (presumably heterosexual contact with a person of unknown positive status). Previously, injection drug use accounted for the major risk behavior, but this is no longer the case.

The number of cases occurring in infants and children younger than 13 years rose rapidly until 1994. In that year, data from the Pediatric AIDS Clinical Trials Group Study 076 of the effectiveness of zidovudine (AZT) use antenatally, intrapartum, and for the neonate for the first 6 weeks of life became available. Currently, most states emphasize the importance of antenatal testing for HIV and offering zidovudine as part of the antiretroviral regimen for maternal health and to reduce vertical transmission. At present, approximately 90% of HIV-infected pregnant women receive antiretroviral therapy, including zidovudine at or before delivery. The epidemic in the United States has largely been curtailed in pediatrics; however, sub-Saharan Africa, Central and Southeast Asia, and Russia continue to have uncontrolled epidemics. In some countries, 40% of women of childbearing age are seropositive for HIV. World Health Organization statistics estimated that by the end of 2006, there would be 39.5 million persons living with AIDS (18 million women, 2.3 million children younger than 15 years). New HIV infections were estimated in 2006 to be 4.3 million (65% in sub-Saharan Africa) with 530,000 in children. Deaths in 2006 were 2.9 million (380,000 in children). Unquestionably, HIV poses one of the most serious and challenging health problems of the late 20th and early 21st centuries.

B. Pathogenesis. When HIV-infected lymphocytes are activated, such as in intercurrent illnesses, many virions may be transcribed, and the cell can be lysed or apoptosis is enhanced, each resulting in host cell death. Because $CD4^+$ lymphocytes are central to developing an appropriate immune response to almost all pathogens, the host with $CD4^+$ counts below $200/mm^3$ is susceptible to opportunistic infections and malignancies. In initial HIV infection, virus may first infect dendritic cells, viremia is present, and the lymphoid tissue is seeded. The host immune response is triggered, viremia is cleared, and 80% of patients become asymptomatic; for 20%, a rapidly progressive course ensues. In untreated patients, $CD4^+$ cell loss progresses, with the median duration of the asymptomatic phase being approximately 10 years in adults. After this phase, the patient becomes symptomatic, generally with opportunistic infections, and death occurs within 5 years.

At present, prevention of horizontal transmission relies on barrier protection for known HIV-infected persons and on reduction of viral load in genital fluids with antiretroviral therapy. Many developing countries have access to only limited antiretroviral therapy; however, over the last few years, many governments and nongovernmental organizations are offering HIV counseling and testing to pregnant women and offer antenatal and intrapartum prophylactic therapy to positive women. Breastfeeding has been found to increase the rate of perinatal transmission by approximately 14%; however, infant mortality is approximately equal to that in nonbreastfed infants in developing countries. Trials of continued maternal and/or infant prophylaxis with antiretroviral therapy as well as with early weaning and alternatives to breastfeeding are continuing. Additionally, some countries are able to offer antiretroviral therapy to HIV-infected women postpartum and the fathers of these babies, recognizing that even if the infant escapes HIV infection, he or she may become orphaned and therefore have a lower life expectancy unless the parents are treated. Contributions from wealthy foundations and governments in developed countries such as the United States have helped to put these treatment programs in place. Expansion of the monies needed for antiretroviral therapy has been seen by using generically manufactured drugs.

Infants with HIV infection have an initially high viral load, which declines over the first 5 years of life as the immune system develops. Current U.S. guidelines suggest treating all infants diagnosed with HIV infection in the first year of life so that the immune system can develop normally. After 1 year of age, suggestions for initiation of therapy based on $CD4^+$ cell count and HIV viral load are less specific, but include treating children with symptomatic infection and for those with the lowest $CD4^+$ cell percentages, regardless of age. Issues of when to initiate antiretroviral therapy must be individualized, and willingness of the care provider to assure the infant or child receives every dose every day is a critical component of success.

C. Transmission. There are three principal routes for HIV transmission: sexual contact, parenteral inoculation, and maternal–fetal or maternal–newborn transfer.

    1. Sexual contact. This remains the principal mode of transmission of HIV in the United States and worldwide. Both semen and vaginal secretions have been found to contain HIV. The principal risk behavior for mothers of children reported with AIDS is heterosexual contact.

    2. Parenteral transmission. Parenteral transmission of HIV results from the direct inoculation of infected blood or blood products. The groups affected have been intravenous drug users and patients receiving transfusions or factor concentrates. Careful screening of blood donors for risk factors for infection, universal HIV antibody and viral testing of donated blood, and the special preparation of clotting factor to eliminate the risk of viral contamination have greatly reduced the incidence of transfusion-acquired HIV. The most likely reason for false-negative HIV serology is the seronegative window that occurs between the time of initial infection and the production of antiviral antibody. The odds of transfusion-acquired HIV infection from the transfusion of a single unit of tested blood have been estimated to be from 1:250,000 to 1:150,000 (see Chap. 26E).

3. **Congenital and perinatal transmission.** More than 90% of pediatric AIDS cases have resulted from maternal transmission hematogenously throughout gestation, at birth, or postnatally through breast milk. The rate of transmission of HIV from untreated infected mothers to their fetuses and newborn infants has been estimated to be between 15% and 40%. HIV has been isolated from cord blood specimens, and products of conception have demonstrated HIV infection as early as 14 to 20 weeks' gestation; however, it is believed that most of the infection is transmitted in late third trimester or at delivery. The mechanism of transplacental transfer of HIV is not known, but HIV can infect trophoblast and placental macrophage (Hofbauer) cell lines. Neither infection nor quantity of virus present in the placenta correlate with congenital infection. This may suggest that the placenta in general acts as a protective barrier to transmission or conversely as a focus of potential transmission.

In a study of 100 sets of twins delivered to HIV-infected mothers, twin A was infected in 50% delivered vaginally and 38% delivered by cesarean. Twin B was infected in 19% of both vaginal and cesarean deliveries. This study—as well as the Women and Infants Transmission study and a meta-analysis of transmission studies—suggest that intrapartum infection occurs as a correlate of duration of ruptured membranes and that elective (without onset of labor) cesarean section deliveries may be preventive, especially if the HIV viral load is not controlled by antiretrovirals at delivery. Infants who are culture or DNA PCR or high-level RNA PCR positive in the first 3 days of life are considered to have been infected *in utero*; infants who test negative in the first 3 days and positive for HIV thereafter are considered to have peripartum-acquired HIV. This differentiation is relevant because offering potent antiretroviral therapy at the time of delivery, even in undiagnosed and/or untreated mothers, may be highly effective in reducing vertical transmission. Rapid diagnostic testing for HIV in previously untested women at presentation for delivery with institution of prophylactic therapy has been shown to reduce transmission. On the basis of this kind of information, investigators are targeting the intrapartum interval to offer potent, rapidly active preventive treatments such as antiretroviral therapy (especially using nevirapine). Intrapartum transmission is likely to account for at least 50% of HIV infections in infants.

Any instrumentation, including fetal scalp electrodes and pH sampling, during the intrapartum period that would expose the fetus to maternal blood and secretions should be avoided in HIV-positive women. Postpartum, the mother should be advised to avoid allowing her infant to contact her blood or secretions.

Studies have also suggested that in countries where breastfeeding is almost exclusively practiced, the transmission rate may be as much as 14% over the presumed rate seen that is due to *in utero* or intrapartum transmission. In studies of women in endemic areas who were not HIV infected at the time of delivery but who seroconverted postpartum, some infants seroconverted almost simultaneously with their mothers. Several investigators reported on infants born to women who were not HIV infected, but who were breastfed by an HIV-infected wet nurse and subsequently acquired HIV infection. It may be that infants who do not have maternally derived, passively transferred antibody to HIV or those infants whose mothers acquire primary HIV infection during lactation are at a higher risk of acquisition of HIV exposure through breast milk than are those who are probably exposed to virions and antibody together. Therefore, breastfeeding is contraindicated in countries in which formula preparations are safe and nutritionally replete; however, recent data have shown that the next best practice is exclusive breastfeeding rather than mixed and bottle feeding.

D. **HIV in pregnancy.** The HIV-infected pregnant woman should be counseled that completion of pregnancy probably does not worsen her prognosis. HIV-infected women should be carefully screened for other sexually transmitted diseases (gonorrhea, herpes, chlamydia, hepatitis B and C, and syphilis), as well as being tested for infection with CMV and toxoplasmosis. The mother should also have a tuberculin skin test and, when appropriate, be offered hepatitis B, pneumococcal, and influenza vaccines. If the $CD4^+$ count is below 350 per μL, she should be offered antiretroviral therapy, including zidovudine, for her own health care. Additionally, guidelines suggest that pregnant women should be treated with the same antiretroviral combinations and with the same goal of suppression of HIV viral load and maintenance or increase of $CD4^+$ lymphocytes as nonpregnant women. Exceptions to these recommendations include efavirenz which has shown teratogenic effects in animal studies, the combination of didanosine and stavudine which has been associated with rare cases of maternal hepatic steatosis and death, and nevirapine which has resulted in fulminant hepatitis in women with higher $CD4^+$ lymphocyte counts. Therefore, these agents should be used cautiously in pregnancy. All HIV-infected pregnant women should be offered at least zidovudine throughout pregnancy, even if the HIV viral load and $CD4^+$ cell count would not warrant initiation of therapy for their own health care. Currently in the United States, the rate of vertical transmission is <2% in women who are diagnosed and take antiretroviral therapy before delivery. This rate is <1% when the HIV viral load is suppressed at delivery. This essentially makes perinatal transmission of HIV a preventable disease when women have antenatal counseling and testing and receive antiretroviral therapy for themselves and their infants. HIV testing is not mandatory component of antenatal care; hence every obstetric provider and pediatrician should offer testing and counseling to all pregnant women so they may consider therapeutic options for themselves and prophylactic options for their fetuses. Infants born to untested women in New York and Connecticut are assessed for HIV exposure immediately after birth. Because this policy has been instituted, New York has seen an increase in antenatal testing and a decrease in vertical transmission. Data have shown that instituting zidovudine as a component of antiretroviral therapy antenatally, intrapartum, or even neonatally reduces transmission compared with that seen (~25%) when no antiretroviral therapy is received by the mother or the infant.

Pneumocystis carinii and possibly *Mycobacterium avium* intracellulare prophylaxis should be considered. Currently, prospective studies on HIV in pregnancy, such as through the Pediatric AIDS Clinical Trials Group (PACTG) or the Women and Infants Transmission Study, which are multicenter National Institutes of Health–sponsored investigations, are under way.

E. **HIV infection in children.** Most pediatric AIDS cases occurs in infants and young children, reflecting the preponderance of congenital and perinatally acquired infections. Where HIV infection is undiagnosed, 50% of pediatric AIDS cases are reported in the first year of life, and approximately 80% are reported by the age of 3. Of these patients, HIV-related symptoms occur in >80% in the first year of life (median age at onset of symptoms is 9 months). It is estimated that 20% of untreated infants with congenital/perinatal HIV infection will die within the first year of life, and 60% will have severe symptomatic disease by the age of 18 months. These patients are defined as "rapid progressors." These statistics reflect only pediatric AIDS cases reported to the Centers for Disease Control and Prevention and may reflect only the part of the spectrum of disease that is identified. Statistics are also heavily influenced by the natural disease progression in untreated children. It is possible that many infected children are undiagnosed and remain asymptomatic for years. Children should be prescribed antiretroviral regimens based on the goal of maintaining a CD4$^+$ lymphocyte percentage >15% and many experts would suggest 25%, along with a moderately low HIV viral load. As of this writing, in developed countries, pediatric HIV infection should be considered a chronic illness, not a disease with a limited lifespan or poor quality of life.

F. **Clinical manifestations.** The clinical presentation differs in children compared with adults. The HIV-infected newborn is usually asymptomatic, but may present with lymphadenopathy and/or hepatosplenomegaly. Generally the infant-infected peripartum does not develop signs or symptoms until after the first 2 weeks of life. These include lymphadenopathy and hepatosplenomegaly (as in adults), poor weight gain as might be found in chronic viral infection, and occasionally neuromotor abnormalities or encephalopathy. Before antiretroviral therapy was available to children, 50% to 90% of HIV-infected children had CNS involvement characterized by an encephalopathy that was often clinically devastating. Although the clinical presentation may vary, developmental delay or loss of developmental milestones and diminished cognitive function are common features. All too often an infant is diagnosed with AIDS between the ages of 2 and 6 months when he or she presents with *Pneumocystis jiroveciii* pneumonia. This is an interstitial pneumonia often without auscultatory findings. Patients present with low-grade fever, tachypnea, and often, tachycardia. Progressive hypoxia ensues and may result in mortality as high as 90%. This is the AIDS-defining illness at presentation in 37% of pediatric patients, with a peak incidence at the age of 4 months. Treatment is intravenous trimethoprim-sulfamethoxazole and steroids. Prophylaxis to prevent such life-threatening possibilities is of course preferable to acquisition of disease. On the basis of adult studies, early on the Centers for Disease Control and Prevention recommended offering prophylaxis to HIV-infected infants based on CD4$^+$ lymphocyte number and percent by age. Most infants with *Pneumocystis* pneumonia in the first year of life had CD4$^+$ cell counts lower than 1,500 per μL. It was recognized that fully 50% of these infants had either no CD4$^+$ cell assessment available or the count was above the 1,500/μL guideline. It is now recommended by the Public Health Service that all infants born to HIV-infected mothers be started on phencyclidine (PCP) prophylaxis at the age of 1 month until the infection and immune status of that infant is known.

A second condition, possibly unique to pediatric AIDS, is the development of chronic interstitial lung disease, referred to as *lymphoid interstitial pneumonitis* (LIP). LIP is characterized by a diffuse lymphocytic and plasma cell infiltrate. The clinical course of LIP is quite variable but may be progressive, resulting in marked respiratory distress (tachypnea, retractions, wheezing, hypoxemia). There is an association with Epstein-Barr virus infection, but the significance of this is uncertain. After the initial presentation, the prognosis appears to be more favorable for children with symptomatic HIV infection when the AIDS-defining illness is LIP. In addition to LIP, recurrent bacterial infections are a frequent feature of pediatric AIDS, owing in part to the early occurrence of B-cell dysfunction with dysfunctional hypergammaglobulinemia. Both focal and disseminated infections are encountered, with sepsis being most common. The organism usually isolated from the bloodstream is *Streptococcus pneumoniae*, but a variety of other bacteria have been recovered, especially from hospitalized patients. It will be interesting to see if this epidemiology holds true now that conjugated pneumococcal vaccines are standard of care for infants in the first 6 months of life. Other manifestations of HIV infection that may be more common in children are parotitis and cardiac dysfunction. Older children present with the more typical AIDS-defining opportunistic infections, as do adults when the CD4$^+$ count wanes.

G. **Diagnosis.** The diagnosis of HIV infection in adults is made by the detection of specific antibody by an ELISA with confirmation by Western blot analysis. Testing should be offered to anyone engaging in risk behaviors for HIV transmission and for all pregnant women. Testing requires counseling and informed consent.

Serology is of limited value in diagnosing vertically transmitted HIV infection in infants <15 months old, because maternal IgG crosses the placenta and can persist in infants throughout the first year or more of life. In the presence of an AIDS-defining illness and a positive antibody test, the diagnosis is made even if the infant is <15 months of age. However, the picture is less clear in infants with minimal or no symptomatology. Therefore, viral detection tests must be used to identify infected infants born to HIV-seropositive mothers. These include the following:

1. PCR to detect viral DNA in peripheral blood cells.

2. PCR for viral RNA in plasma (must be >10,000 copies/mL to be diagnostic).

3. *In vitro* cell culture of mononuclear cells.

The blood samples for these tests should be collected in anticoagulant, but not heparin. Sometimes the diagnosis is made with a positive p24 antigen detection in peripheral blood or *in situ* hybridization to detect HIV-specific DNA in infected cells.

Culture is sensitive and specific but is expensive, is technically difficult, and may require weeks before results are obtained. PCR generally correlates with cell culture and may be more quickly obtained. The mainstay of early viral diagnostic testing of the infant born to an HIV-infected mother remains HIV PCR to detect both viral RNA and DNA. The p24 antigen assay suffers from a lack of sensitivity, particularly in infants, and can be replaced by acid-dissociated p24 antigen detection, which has a much greater sensitivity. The importance of obtaining an early diagnosis is clear: to provide even very young infants the benefit of antiretroviral therapy, which is hoped to reduce viral load and possibly prevent or reduce the viral burden at sites such as the CNS, as well as to maintain normal numbers of CD4+ cells.

H. Treatment. The major part of the management of HIV infection is antiretroviral therapy. This should be offered to all symptomatic patients regardless of CD4$^+$ cell count. At present, there is no cure for HIV infection, but the goal of antiretroviral therapy is to suppress the HIV viral load to nondetectable and to maintain or reconstitute CD4$^+$ cell numbers to >25%. Generally, these agents are of three classes:

1. Nucleoside or nucleotide analog reverse transcriptase inhibitors (NRTIs) (e.g., zidovudine/AZT). These agents prevent viral RNA from being reverse-transcribed to DNA; therefore, infection of cells can be aborted.

2. Non-nucleoside analog reverse transcriptase inhibitors (NNRTIs) (e.g., nevirapine). These agents also act to prevent reverse transcription, but at a slightly different site on the enzyme. They are generally more potent than the NRTIs, but resistance can develop rapidly if the viral load is not controlled.

3. Protease inhibitors (PIs) act to prevent processing of viral proteins. These agents are quite potent, but are highly protein bound and therefore little crosses the placenta, making these excellent agents to treat maternal viral load but limit exposure of the fetus.

Generally, initial therapy is with two NRTIs and either a Pi or an NNRTI. Other possible therapies being investigated include other sites of action in the retroviral life cycle such as fusion and integrase inhibitors as well as immune-based therapies.

Optimization of nutrition, immunizations, prophylaxis against opportunistic infections (most notably Pneumocystis), and the prompt recognition and treatment of HIV-related complications (e.g., opportunistic infections, cardiac dysfunction) are paramount to the improvement in the longevity and the quality of life for HIV-infected patients. In the newborn, special attention should be given to the possibility of congenitally and perinatally transmitted pathogens, such as tuberculosis, toxoplasmosis, and sexually transmitted diseases, which may have a relatively high prevalence in HIV-infected adults.

I. Prevention. Trials to prevent mother-to-child transmission of HIV, have been highly successful in the United States. In February 1994, a large clinical trial conducted by the AIDS Clinical Trials Group was closed early owing to astonishing results. HIV-infected pregnant women with >200 CD4+ T cells were randomized to receive zidovudine or placebo, beginning at 14 weeks' gestation. The mothers randomized to receive zidovudine also received intrapartum zidovudine intravenously at 2 mg/kg for the first hour of labor followed by 1 mg/kg/hour until delivery, and their infants orally received zidovudine syrup at 2 mg/kg every 6 hours for the first 6 weeks of life. This trial (PACTG 076) closed when approximately 183 babies had been born to each cohort and had been assessed for HIV infection. Only 13 babies (8.3%) in the ziduovudine-receiving group were infected, whereas 40 babies (25.5%) in the placebo group were infected. As of February 1994, it has been the standard of care to offer zidovudine as part of the antiretroviral regimen to pregnant HIV-infected women with >200 CD4+ T cells following the 076 algorithm. The infection rate of babies born to mothers with <200 CD4+ T cells was also decreased with zidovudine use, as shown in PACTG 185. It has also been shown that an elective cesarean section (before onset of labor), can further reduce transmission if the HIV viral load remains >1,000 copies/mL, but that there is no added benefit if the HIV viral load is suppressed. Several studies have shown that higher maternal viral load, along with lower CD4+ T cell counts, is a strong correlate of vertical transmission; therefore, it is imperative to treat with an optimized antiretroviral regimen to suppress viral load. Resistance testing should also be considered because it is estimated that as many as 15% of previously untreated persons will have an HIV isolate that has resistance to one or more antiretrovirals. It is advised that care of HIV-infected pregnant women be offered in concert with skilled HIV obstetricians, internists, and pediatricians for optimal outcome. Current standard of care in the United States is to suppress maternal viral load to nondetectable during pregnancy (and after pregnancy to optimize the maternal health care) using combinations of the approved agents to treat HIV infection, except efavirenz, combination didanosine and stavudine, or nevirapine in women with better CD4+ cell numbers. The rate of transmission is <1% for women with a nondetectable viral load. Clearly these data challenge all health care providers to participate in offering testing and counseling to all pregnant women. Frequently, mothers may learn for the first time that they are HIV infected during their pregnancy. The appropriate social, nonjudgmental support network must be effectively in place to achieve the best pregnancy outcome possible. The mother's health, both medical and emotional, should not be subjugated to that of the fetus; rather, optimization of the mother–baby pair is key in effecting the best possible outcome.

J. Internationally, an exciting trial in Uganda (HIVNET 012) offered a single dose of nevirapine to HIV-infected women in labor and followed this with a single dose of nevirapine at 3 days of life to the infants. Approximately 10% of these infants were already HIV infected *in utero*; however, the rate of perinatal transmission was markedly reduced in the nevirapine arm. Nevirapine was found to readily cross the placenta, and with the two-dose regimen for the mother–infant pair, the nevirapine level in the infant's blood is above the level needed to reduce HIV viral load for at least a week. By 18 months of age, the infant mortality in the nevirapine-treated group equaled that in the other group, most likely because of HIV transmission from breast-milk feeding, which was essentially universal. Implementation of the two-dose nevirapine regimen is ongoing in developing countries, as are studies designed to prevent breast-milk transmission of HIV. Data from Thailand has shown a transmission rate of 2% using a combination of zidovudine as per 076 and nevirapine as per HIVNET 012 along with exclusive bottle feeding. Birth canal washes with a virostatic agent have been disappointing to date. Recent studies include active immunity with vaccines to the surface glycoprotein of HIV (gp120), much along the hepatitis B model. It is hoped that combinations of these approaches or newer ones will be able to reduce mother-to-child transmission of HIV to infants throughout the world born to women with any CD4+ count, regardless of antiretroviral availability or mandate to breast-feed.

Education plays an important role in the prevention of the spread of HIV infection. Informing the public about high-risk behaviors, such as intravenous drug use and unprotected sexual contact, is critical in curtailing this epidemic. The health care provider should take advantage of every patient contact to provide preventive education. Eliminating unwarranted fears about casual contact with HIV-infected individuals is also within the purview of the provider.

K. HIV and the health care worker. The transmission of HIV from patients to health care providers is very uncommon, as is transmission from care providers to patients. The greatest risk for transmission is from parenteral inoculation of infected blood by inadvertent needle sticks or cuts with contaminated sharp instruments. To minimize the risk of transmission of HIV, universal precautions have been recommended for all hospital environments. Particular emphasis in perinatal/neonatal medicine should be placed on the avoidance of blood and bloody secretions in the delivery room by the wearing of gowns, gloves, and eye protection (preferably goggles with side shields). Meconium and gastric aspirates should never be suctioned by mouth; special meconium suction adapters and catheters that can be attached to wall suction are generally available. Of special concern in the nursery is the recapping of needles after drawing blood from umbilical lines. If recapping is required, it is best to use cap-holding devices to avoid needle sticks. Also, syringes should not be tapped or "flicked" to remove air when obtaining arterial blood gas samples. Specific guidelines have been suggested for the recognition and management of occupational exposures to HIV. Types of exposures include percutaneous injury (needle sticks, cuts with sharp instruments), mucous membrane contact, and skin contact (particularly from skin with cuts, abrasions, or dermatitis, or for prolonged exposure or over a large area) with potentially infectious tissues or body fluids. The guidelines recommend procedures for serologic testing in the worker and the patient contact. The use of zidovudine for postexposure prophylaxis is also discussed. Review of these guidelines is recommended for all individuals at risk for occupational exposure to HIV. The average risk of contracting HIV per episode of percutaneous exposure to HIV-infected blood is estimated to be approximately 0.3%. It is unknown if postexposure zidovudine will further reduce this risk.

XII. HEPATITIS. Acute viral hepatitis is defined by the following clinical criteria: (i) symptoms consistent with viral hepatitis, (ii) elevation of serum aminotransaminase levels to >2.5 times the upper limit of normal, and (iii) the absence of other causes of liver disease. At least five agents have been identified as causes of viral hepatitis: hepatitis A virus (HAV) has no vertical transmission and will not be discussed; hepatitis B virus (HBV); hepatitis D virus (HDV); hepatitis C virus (HCV) (post-transfusion non-A, non-B hepatitis virus [NANB]); and hepatitis E virus (HEV) (enteric, epidemic NANB hepatitis virus). HDV, also referred to as the *delta agent*, is a defective virus that requires coinfection or superinfection with HBV. HDV is coated with hepatitis B surface antigen (HBsAg). Specific antibodies to HDV can be detected in infected individuals, but there is no known therapy to prevent infection in exposed HBsAg-positive patients. For the newborn, therapy directed at the prevention of HBV infection should also prevent HDV infection, because coinfection is required.

A. HBV (Perinatal and Congenital). This DNA virus is one of the most common causes of acute and chronic hepatitis worldwide. In endemic populations, the carrier state is high, and perinatal transmission is a common event. The risk of chronic infection is inversely proportional to age, with a 90% carriage rate following infection in neonates. The overall incidence of HBV infections in the United States is relatively low but still substantial. There are estimates of approximately 300,000 infections yearly, with 250 deaths from fulminate disease. As many as 1 million individuals are chronic carriers, approximately 25% of whom develop chronic active hepatitis. Patients with chronic active hepatitis are at increased risk for developing cirrhosis and hepatocellular carcinoma, and approximately 5,000 of these patients die each year from HBV-related hepatic complications (primarily cirrhosis). The incubation period for HBV infection is approximately 120 days (range 45–160 days). Transmission occurs by percutaneous or permucosal routes from infected blood or body fluids. Symptoms include anorexia, malaise, nausea, vomiting, abdominal pain, and jaundice.

1. **High-risk groups for HBV infection** in the United States include the following:
    a. **Persons born in endemic areas.** Alaskan natives and Pacific Islanders and natives of China, Southeast Asia, most of Africa, parts of the Middle East, and the Amazon basin; descendants of individuals from endemic areas.
    b. **Persons with high-risk behavior.** Men who have sex with men, intravenous drug use, and multiple sex partners.
    c. **Close contacts with HBV-infected persons** (sex partners, family members).
    d. **Selected patient populations,** particularly those receiving multiple blood or blood product transfusions.
    e. **Selected occupational groups,** including health care providers.
2. **Diagnosis.** The diagnosis is made by specific serology and by the detection of viral antigens. The specific tests are as follows:
    a. **HBsAg determination.** Usually found 1 to 2 months after exposure and lasts a variable period of time.
    b. **Anti-HB surface antigen (anti-HBs).** Appears after resolution of infection or immunization and provides long-term immunity.
    c. **Anti-HB core antigen (anti-HBc).** Present with all HBV infections and lasts for an indefinite period of time.
    d. **Anti-HBc IgM.** Appears early in infection, is detectable for 4 to 6 months after infection, and is a good marker for acute or recent infection.
    e. **HB e antigen (HbeAg).** Present in both acute and chronic infections and correlates with viral replication and high infectivity.
    f. **Anti-HB e antigen (anti-HBe).** Develops with resolution of viral replication and correlates with reduction in infectivity.
        Infectivity correlates best with HBeAg positivity, but any patient positive for HBsAg is potentially infectious. Acute infection can be diagnosed by the presence of clinical symptoms and a positive HBsAg or anti-HBc IgM. The chronic carrier state is defined as the presence of HBsAg on two occasions, 6 months apart, or the presence of HBsAg without anti-HBc IgM.
3. **Prevention.** The transmission of HBV from infected mothers to their newborns is thought to result primarily from exposure to maternal blood at the time of delivery. Transplacental transfer appears to occur in Taiwan, but this has not been found in other parts of the world, including the United States. In Taiwan there is a high chronic carrier rate that may be related to the transplacental transfer observed in that country. When acute maternal HBV infection occurs during the first and second trimesters of pregnancy, there is generally little risk to the newborns, because antigenemia is usually cleared by term and anti-HBs is present. Acute maternal HBV infection during late pregnancy or near the time of delivery, however, may result in a 50% to 75% transmission rate. Women with higher HBV viral loads are potentially also more likely to transmit HBV to their infants. Treatments such as lamivudine, tenofovir or adefovir, or etanercept may be suggested by infectious disease specialists to further reduce the possibility of transmission.

    The principal strategy for the prevention of neonatal HBV disease has been to use immunoprophylaxis for newborns at high risk for infection. Vaccination of these infants is also an important part of perinatal prevention and safeguards against postnatal exposure as well. Immunization of infants effectively reduced the risk of chronic HBV infection in Taiwan. Universal immunization of infants promises to be one of the best options for disease control in the United States and is now recommended for all infants born to HBsAg-negative mothers. Three doses before the age of 18 months should be given. High-risk populations, such as Alaskan natives, Pacific Islanders, and infants of immigrant mothers from areas where HBV is endemic, should receive the three-dose series by the age of 6 to 9 months. The recommended schedule is begun during the newborn period; the second dose is given 1 to 2 months later; and the third dose is given at the age of 6 months for infants of mothers with HBsAG positive or unknown status and between 6 and 18 months for infants of mothers with negative

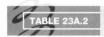

TABLE 23A.2	Doses of Hepatitis B Vaccines in Neonates*		
	Active immunization: either		
	Recombivax HB merck	**Engerix-B smithkline beecham**	**Passive immunization HBIg**
Infants of HBsAg-negative mothers	5 μg (0.5 mL)	10 μg (0.5 mL)	—
Infants of HBsAg-positive mothers	5 μg (0.5 mL)	10 μg (0.5 mL)	0.5 mL

HBIg = hepatitis B immunoglobulin; HBsAg = hepatitis B surface antigen.
*Both vaccine regimens use a three-dose schedule.

HBsAg status. The preterm infant born to an HBSAg-positive mother should be started on the immunization series and given treatment with hepatitis B immune globulin (HBIG) immediately (see Table 23A.2). Please consult the Red Book, Report of the Committee on Infectious Diseases, American Academy of Pediatrics for dosing based on gestational age and birth weight. Other methods of disease control have been considered and include delivery by cesarean section. In one study in Taiwan, cesarean delivery in conjunction with maternal immunization dramatically reduced the incidence of perinatally acquired HBV from highly infective mothers. These results are promising and may offer a potential adjunctive therapy for very high-risk situations (e.g., HBsAg/HBe-positive women). Currently, no specific recommendations can be made regarding mode of delivery.

It is recommended that all pregnant women be screened for HBsAg. Screening should be done early in gestation. If the test result is negative, no further evaluation is recommended unless there is a potential exposure history. When there is any concern about a possible infectious contact, development of acute hepatitis, or high-risk behavior in a nonimmunized woman, testing should be repeated. All infants born to mothers confirmed to be positive for HBsAg should receive HBIG in addition to recombinant hepatitis B vaccine. The first immunization and HBIG are given within the first 12 hours of life, and the vaccine is repeated at the ages of 1 and 6 months. If the mother has immigrated from an endemic area, HBIG also should be given unless the mother is found to be HBsAg-negative.

Postnatal transmission of HBV by the fecal-oral route probably occurs, but the risk appears to be small. Nevertheless, this possibility adds further support to the need for the immunization of infants born to HBsAg-positive women. Another potential route of infection is by means of breast milk. This mode of transmission appears to be very uncommon in developed countries; there has been no documented increase in the risk of HBV transmission by breastfeeding mothers who are HBsAg-positive. This is true although HBsAg can be detected in breast milk. Recommendations regarding breastfeeding in developed countries should be individualized, depending on how strongly breastfeeding is desired by the mother. The risk is certain to be negligible in infants who have received HBIG and hepatitis vaccine.

4. **Prevention of nosocomial spread.** HBsAg-positive infants pose a definite risk for nosocomial spread in the nursery. To minimize this risk, nursery personnel are advised to wear gloves and gowns when caring for infected infants. Of course, current universal precautions should be in effect in all nurseries, so the risk of exposure to blood and body secretions already should be minimized.

Immunization of health care workers is also strongly recommended, but if exposure should occur in a nonimmunized person, blood samples should be sent for hepatitis serology and HBIG administered as soon as possible unless the individual is known to be anti-HBs–positive. This should apply to personnel having close contact without appropriate precautions, as well as those exposed parenterally (e.g., from a contaminated needle).

B. HCV (Perinatal and Congenital). Hepatitis C is the agent responsible for most NANB hepatitis in transfusion or organ transplant recipients and is a single-strand RNA virus related to the Flavivirus family.

1. Epidemiology. At least five HCV subtypes have been characterized based on sequence heterogeneity of the viral genome. HCV is found worldwide, and different subtypes have been identified from the same area. Subtype 1 is the most common in the United States and has a poorer prognosis than other subtypes.

  a. Horizontal transmission. Injection drug use is now the most common risk behavior for infection. In addition to injection drug users and transfusion recipients, dialysis patients and sexual partners of HCV-infected persons may also be infected, but 50% of identified persons are unable to define a risk factor.

  b. Vertical transmission. Overall rate of transmission is approximately 5% from known hepatitis C–infected women to their infants. The transmission rate may well be much higher and may approach 70% when the pregnant mother has a high viral load as assessed by semiquantitative PCR. HCV is transmitted at a higher frequency if the mother is also HIV infected, but this has not been assessed in women with a controlled HIV viral load and lower semiquantitative HCV viral load. The mode of transmission is also unknown. Detection of HCV by RNA PCR in cord blood would suggest that at least in some cases, *in utero* transmission occurs. There is also a case report of one infant having been infected with an HCV strain different from all maternal strains at the time of delivery, suggesting *in utero* transmission. Conversely, PCR-negative infants at birth may develop PCR positivity later in infancy, suggesting perinatal infection. One study found 50% of vaginal samples collected at 30 weeks' gestation from HCV-positive mothers to contain HCV, suggesting the possibility of infection by passage through the birth canal. The potential risk of breastfeeding is not well defined. HCV has been detected in breast milk by PCR, but vertical transmission rates in breastfed and bottle-fed infants are similar. The Centers for Disease Control and Prevention currently states that maternal HCV infection is not a contraindication to breastfeeding. The decision to breast-feed should be discussed with the mother on an individual basis.

2. Clinical manifestations. HCV accounts for 20% to 40% of viral hepatitis in the United States. The incubation period is 40 to 90 days after exposure, and manifestations often present insidiously. Serum transaminase levels may fluctuate or remain chronically elevated for as long as 1 year. Chronic disease may result in as many as 60% of community-acquired HCV infections. Cirrhosis may result in as many as 20% of chronic disease cases, but may be less likely in pediatric patients.

3. Diagnosis. ELISA detects antibodies to three proteins (c100–3, c22–3, and c33c) that are components of HCV. This test may be able to detect infection as early as 2 weeks after exposure. Another serologic assay with even greater sensitivity is the radioimmunoblot assay, which detects antibodies to the three antigens detected by the ELISA and a fourth antigen, 5–5-1. Infants born to HCV-infected mothers will show evidence of passively acquired maternal antibody; therefore, to determine infection in the infant, RNA PCR, which detects the viral genome itself, must be performed. This assay can detect viremia within 1 week of infection in adults. In adults, approximately 70% of samples with detectable antibody will also be positive by PCR. This is a curious finding in that a serologic response does not provide adequate protection.

Persons who have had an acute infection that resolves will become antibody negative. Infants born to known seropositive women should be tested for HCV antibody and HCV RNA by PCR at the age of 1, and possibly by RNA PCR earlier to determine which infants to follow more closely. If both are negative, the infant is likely uninfected; if the PCR is negative, but the antibody positive, the infant should be retested at 18 months.

4. **Treatment.** Clinical trials suggest that symptomatic persons with chronic HCV infection may benefit from treatment with α-interferon and ribavirin, given for as long as a year. Side effects of this therapy include fever and myalgias, and the risk–benefit ratio must be carefully weighed.

5. **Prevention.** Blood products are screened for antibody to HCV. Presence of the antibody likely also indicates presence of virus, and the unit is discarded if antibody positive. Before blood products were screened and before the recognition that viremia often accompanied antibody positivity, some had recommended the use of immune globulin for prophylaxis for individuals exposed to HCV. This concept had transcended to the infant of the HCV-infected mother. There is *no* benefit to immune globulin given to the exposed infant or to the needle-stick recipient, as products containing antibody are excluded from the lot.

C. **HEV.** Enterically transmitted NANB viral hepatitis (HEV) is a single-stranded RNA virus that is similar to a calcivirus. It is primarily spread by fecal-contaminated water supplies. Epidemics have been documented in parts of Asia, Africa, and Mexico, and shellfish have been implicated as sources of infection. Incubation is 15 to 60 days. The clinical picture in infected individuals is similar to that of HAV infection, with fever, malaise, jaundice, abdominal pain, and arthralgia. HEV infection has an unusually high incidence of mortality in pregnant women. Treatment is supportive. The efficacy of immunoglobulin prophylaxis against this form of hepatitis is unknown, but because the infection is not endemic in the United States, commercial preparations in the United States would not be expected to be helpful.

D. **Hepatitis G virus (HGV).** HGV is a single-stranded RNA virus in the Flaviviridae family that shares 27% homology with HCV. HGV can be found worldwide and is found in approximately 1.5% of blood donors in the United States. Coinfection with HBV or HCV may be as much as 20%, suggesting common routes of transmission, such as transfusion or organ transplantation. Transplacental transmission is probably rare and may be associated with higher maternal viral loads. HGV is diagnosed by RNA PCR in research settings, and there is no current treatment or prophylactic therapy.

XIII. **VARICELLA-ZOSTER VIRUS ([V-ZV]: CONGENITAL OR PERINATAL).** The causative agent of varicella (chickenpox) is a DNA virus member of the herpesvirus family. The same agent is responsible for herpes zoster (shingles); hence, this virus is referred to as V-ZV. Chickenpox results from primary V-ZV infection, following which the virus may remain latent in sensory nerve ganglia. Zoster results from reactivation of latent virus later in life or if the host becomes immunosuppressed.

A. **Epidemiology.** Before the use of varicella vaccine, there were approximately 3 million cases of varicella yearly in the United States, primarily occurring in school-age children. Most adults have antibodies to V-ZV, indicating prior infection, even when there is thought to be no history of chickenpox. It follows that varicella is an uncommon occurrence in pregnancy. The precise incidence of gestational varicella is uncertain, but is certainly less than it was before widespread use of varicella vaccine. There are recommendations to immunize nonimmune adults who are at high risk of infection unless they are pregnant. Alternatively, zoster is primarily a disease of adults. The incidence of zoster in pregnancy is also unknown, but the disease is likely to be uncommon as well. The overall risk of the congenital varicella syndrome following maternal infection in the first trimester is 2%, 0.4% in the first 12 weeks of pregnancy, and 2% from 13 to 20 weeks' gestation. It is primarily seen with gestational varicella but may occur with maternal zoster. It appears that the primary mode of transmission of V-ZV is through respiratory droplets from patients with chickenpox. Spread through contact with vesicular lesions also can occur. Typically, individuals with chickenpox are contagious from 1 to 2 days before and 5 days after the onset of rash. Conventionally, a patient is no longer considered contagious when all vesicular lesions have dried and crusted over. The incubation period for primary disease extends from 10 to 21 days, with most infections occurring between 13 and 17 days. Transplacental transfer of V-ZV may take place, presumably secondary to maternal viremia, but the frequency of this event is unknown.

Varicella occurs in approximately 25% of newborns whose mothers developed varicella within the peripartum period. The onset of disease usually occurs 13 to 15 days after the onset of maternal rash. When the rash develops in the newborn within 10 days, it is presumed to result from *in utero* transmission. The greatest risk for severe disease is seen when maternal varicella occurs in the 5 days before or 2 days after delivery. In these cases, there is insufficient time for the fetus to acquire transplacentally derived V-ZV–specific antibodies. Symptoms generally begin 5 to 10 days after delivery, and the expected mortality is approximately 30%.

When *in utero* transmission of V-ZV occurs before the peripartum period, there is no obvious clinical impact in most fetuses; however, congenital varicella syndrome can occur.

B. Clinical manifestations

    1. Congenital varicella syndrome. There is a strong association between gestational varicella and a spectrum of congenital defects comprising a unique syndrome. Characteristic findings include cicatricial skin lesions, ocular defects, CNS abnormalities, IUGR, and early death. The syndrome most commonly occurs with maternal V-ZV infection in weeks 7 to 20 of gestation.

    2. Zoster. Zoster is uncommon in young infants but may occur as a consequence of *in utero* fetal infection with V-ZV. Similarly, children who develop zoster but have no history of varicella most likely acquired V-ZV *in utero*. Zoster in childhood is usually self-limiting, with only symptomatic therapy indicated in otherwise healthy children.

    3. Postnatal varicella. Varicella acquired in the newborn period as a result of postnatal exposure is generally a mild disease. Rarely, severe disseminated disease occurs in newborns exposed shortly after birth. In these instances, treatment with acyclovir may be beneficial. Varicella has been detected in breast milk by PCR; therefore, it may be prudent to defer breastfeeding at least during the period of time in which the mother is likely to be viremic and/or infectious.

C. Diagnosis. Infants with congenital varicella resulting from *in utero* infection occurring before the peripartum period do not shed virus, and the determination of V-ZV-specific antibodies is often confusing. Therefore, the diagnosis is made on the basis of clinical findings and maternal history. With neonatal disease, the presence of a typical vesicular rash and a maternal history of peripartum varicella or postpartum exposure are all that is required to make the diagnosis. Laboratory confirmation can be made by (i) culture of vesicular fluid, although the sensitivity of this method is not optimal because the virus is quite labile; (ii) demonstration of a fourfold rise in V-ZV antibody titer by the fluorescent antibody to membrane antigen (FAMA) assay or by ELISA. Antigen can also be detected from cells at the base of a vesicle by immunofluorescent antibody detection. The latter is sensitive, specific, and rapid and should be the preferred method of diagnosis when vesicles are present.

D. Treatment. Infants with congenital infection, resulting from *in utero* transmission before the peripartum period, are unlikely to have active viral disease, so antiviral therapy is not indicated. However, infants with perinatal varicella acquired from maternal infection near the time of delivery are at risk for severe disease. In this setting, therapy with acyclovir is generally recommended. Data are not available on the most efficacious and safe dose of acyclovir for the treatment of neonatal varicella, but minimal toxicity has been shown with the administration of 60 mg/kg divided every 8 hours for the treatment of neonatal HSV infection.

At the present time, there is no established immunotherapy for the treatment of V-ZV infections, but varicella-zoster immune globulin (VZIG) may be of prophylactic value. When administered within 72 hours of exposure, VZIG is effective in preventing or attenuating V-ZV infection. The dose for newborns is 125 units intramuscularly.

E. Prevention

1. **Vaccination** of women who are not immune to varicella should decrease the incidence of congenital and perinatal varicella. Women should not receive the vaccine if they are pregnant or in the 3 months before pregnancy. If this inadvertently occurs, the women should be enrolled in the National Registry. Additionally, acyclovir should also be considered for seronegative women exposed to varicella during pregnancy beginning 7 to 9 days postexposure and continuing 7 days. Women who acquire primary varicella during pregnancy should be treated with acyclovir for their own health as well as to prevent fetal infection.

2. **Management of varicella in the nursery.** The risk of horizontal spread of varicella following exposure in the nursery appears to be low, possibly because of a combination of factors, including (i) passive protection resulting from transplacentally derived antibody in infants born to varicella-immune mothers; (ii) brief exposure with a lack of intimate contact. Nevertheless, nursery outbreaks do occur, so steps should be taken to minimize the risk of nosocomial spread. The infected infant should be isolated in a separate room, and visitors and caregivers should be limited to individuals with a history of varicella. A new gown should be worn on entering the room, and good hand-washing technique should be used. Bedding and other materials should be bagged and sterilized. VZIG can be given to all other exposed neonates, but this can be withheld from full-term infants whose mothers have a history of varicella. Neonates at <28 weeks' gestation should be given VZIG postexposure regardless of maternal status. Exposed personnel without a history of varicella should be tested for V-ZV antibodies, and patient care by these individuals should be restricted as outlined below.

   In the regular nursery, all exposed infants will ordinarily be discharged home before they could become infectious. Occasionally, an exposed infant needs to remain in the nursery for >8 days, and in this circumstance, isolation may be required. In the neonatal intensive care unit, exposed neonates are generally cohorted and isolated from new admissions within 8 days of exposure. If there is antepartum exposure within 21 days of hospital admission for a mother without a history of varicella, the mother and infant should be discharged as soon as possible from the hospital. If the exposure was from a household contact with current disease, VZIG should be administered to both mother and infant before discharge. Alternatively, arrangements to isolate the infectious household contact from the mother and infant may be done before discharge. If the exposure occurred 6 days or less before admission and the mother is discharged within 48 hours, no further action is required. Otherwise, mothers hospitalized between 8 and 21 days after exposure should be kept isolated from the nursery and other patients.

   Personnel without a history of varicella should be kept from contact with a potentially infectious mother. If such an individual is inadvertently exposed, serologic testing (FAMA or ELISA) should be performed to determine susceptibility, and further contact should be avoided until immunity is proved. If the mother at risk for infection has not developed varicella 48 hours after the staff member was exposed, no further action is required. Alternatively, if a susceptible staff member is exposed to any individual with active varicella lesions or in whom a varicella rash erupts within 48 hours of the exposure, contact with any patients should be restricted for that staff member from day 8 through day 21 after exposure. Personnel without a history of varicella should have serologic testing, and if not immune, they should be vaccinated.

For mothers in whom varicella has occurred in the 21 days before delivery, if there were resolution of the infectious stage before hospitalization, maternal isolation is not required. The newborn should be isolated from other infants (room in with mother). If the mother has active varicella lesions on admission to the hospital, isolate the mother and administer VZIG (125 units intramuscularly) to the newborn if maternal disease began <5 days before delivery or within 2 days postpartum (not 100% effective, and may consider acyclovir in addition). The infant should be isolated from the mother until she is no longer infectious. If other neonates were exposed, VZIG may be administered; these infants may require isolation if they are still hospitalized by day 8 after exposure.

XIV. **ENTEROVIRUSES (CONGENITAL).** The enteroviruses are RNA viruses belonging to the Picornaviridae family. They are classified into four major groups: coxsackieviruses group A, coxsackieviruses group B, echoviruses, and polioviruses. All four groups cause disease in the neonate. Infections occur throughout the year, with a peak incidence between July and November. The viruses are shed from the upper respiratory and gastrointestinal tracts. In most children and adults, infections are asymptomatic or produce a nonspecific febrile illness.

A. **Epidemiology.** Most infections in newborns are caused by coxsackieviruses B and echoviruses. The mode of transmission appears to be primarily transplacental, although this is less well understood for echoviruses. Clinical manifestations are most commonly seen with transmission in the perinatal period.

B. **Clinical manifestations.** Symptoms in the newborn often appear within the first week postpartum. Clinical presentations vary from a mild nonspecific febrile illness to severe life-threatening disease. There are three major clinical presentations in neonates with enterovirus infections. Approximately 50% have meningoencephalitis, 25% have myocarditis, and 25% have a sepsis-like illness. The mortality (approximately 10%) is lowest for the group with meningoencephalitis. With myocarditis, there is a mortality of approximately 50%. The mortality from the sepsis-like illness is essentially 100%. Most (70%) of severe enteroviral infections in neonates are caused by echovirus 11.

C. **Diagnosis.** The primary task in symptomatic enterovirus infections is differentiating between viral and bacterial sepsis and meningitis. In almost all cases, presumptive therapy for possible bacterial disease must be initiated. Obtaining a careful history of a recent maternal viral illness, as well as that of other family members, particularly young siblings, and especially during the summer and fall months, may be helpful. The principal diagnostic laboratory aid generally available at this time is viral culture or PCR. Material for cultures should be obtained from the nose, throat, stool, blood, urine, and CSF and from blood, urine, stool, or CSF for PCR. Usually, evidence of viral growth can be detected within 1 week, although a longer time is required in some cases.

D. **Treatment.** In general, treatment of symptomatic enteroviral disease in the newborn is supportive only. There are no approved specific antiviral agents known to be effective against enteroviruses. However, protection against severe neonatal disease appears to correlate with the presence of specific transplacentally derived antibody. Furthermore, the administration of immune serum globulin appears to be beneficial in patients with a gammaglobulinemia who have chronic enteroviral infection. Given these observations, it has been recommended that high-dose immune serum globulin be given to infants with severe, life-threatening enterovirus infections. It may also be beneficial to delay the time of delivery if acute maternal enteroviral infection is suspected, provided there are no maternal or fetal contraindications. The clinical presentation in infants with a sepsis-like syndrome frequently evolves into shock, fulminant hepatitis with hepatocellular necrosis, and DIC. This expectation dictates close monitoring with early interventions for any signs of cardiovascular instability and coagulopathy. In the initial stages of treatment, broad-spectrum antibiotic therapy is indicated for possible bacterial sepsis. Later, with the recognition of progressive viral disease, some form of antibiotic prophylaxis to suppress intestinal flora may be helpful. Neomycin (25 mg/kg every 6 hours) has been recommended. Drugs designed to prevent attachment of enterovirus to the host cell (e.g., pleconaril) were under study, but are not currently available.

XV. RUBELLA (CONGENITAL). This human-specific RNA virus is a member of the Togavirus family. It causes a mild self-limiting infection in susceptible children and adults, but its effects on the fetus can be devastating.

A. Epidemiology. Before widespread immunization beginning in 1969, rubella was a common childhood illness: 85% of the population was immune by late adolescence and approximately 100% by ages 35 to 40 years. Epidemics occurred every 6 to 9 years, with pandemics arising with a greater and more variable cycle. During pandemics, susceptible women were at significant risk of exposure to rubella, resulting in a high number of fetal infections. A worldwide epidemic from 1963 to 1965 accounted for an estimated 11,000 fetal deaths and 20,000 cases of congenital rubella syndrome (CRS). Childhood immunization has dramatically reduced the number of cases of rubella in the United States. In fact, some states have omitted rubella serologic screening from standard antenatal diagnostic recommendations because the very few cases of CRS in recent years have been reported from unimmunized immigrants. The relative risk of fetal transmission and the development of CRS as a function of gestational age have been studied. With maternal infection in the first 12 weeks of gestation, the rate of fetal infection was 81%. The rate dropped to 54% for weeks 13 to 16, 36% for weeks 17 to 22, and 30% for weeks 23 to 30. During the last 10 weeks of gestation, the rate of fetal infection again rose: 60% for weeks 31 to 36 and 100% for weeks 36 and beyond. Fetal infection can occur at any time during pregnancy, but early-gestation infection may result in multiple organ anomalies. When maternofetal transmission occurred during the first 10 weeks of gestation, 100% of the infected fetuses had cardiac defects and deafness. Deafness was found in one-third of fetuses infected at 13 to 16 weeks, but no abnormalities were found when fetal infection occurred beyond the 20th week of gestation. There are also case reports of vertical transmission with maternal reinfection.

B. Clinical manifestations. Classically, CRS is characterized by the constellation of cataracts, sensorineural hearing loss, and congenital heart disease. The most common cardiac defects are patent ductus arteriosus and pulmonary artery stenosis. Common early features of CRS are IUGR, retinopathy, microphthalmia, meningoencephalitis, electroencephalographic abnormalities, hypotonia, dermatoglyphic abnormalities, hepatosplenomegaly, thrombocytopenic purpura, radiographic bone lucencies, and diabetes mellitus. The onset of some of the abnormalities of CRS may be delayed months to years. Many additional rare complications have been described, including myocarditis, glaucoma, microcephaly, chronic progressive panencephalitis, hepatitis, anemia, hypogammaglobulinemia, thymic hypoplasia, thyroid abnormalities, cryptorchidism, and polycystic kidney disease. A 20-year follow-up study of 125 patients with congenital rubella from the 1960s epidemic found ocular disease to be the most common disorder (78%), followed by sensorineural hearing deficits (66%), psychomotor retardation (62%), cardiac abnormalities (58%), and mental retardation (42%).

C. Diagnosis

1. Maternal infection. The diagnosis of acute rubella in pregnancy requires serologic testing. This is necessary because the clinical symptoms of rubella are nonspecific and can be seen with infection by other viral agents (e.g., enteroviruses, measles, human parvovirus). Furthermore, a large number of individuals may have subclinical infection. Several sensitive and specific assays exist for the detection of rubella-specific antibody. Viral isolation from the nose, throat, and/or urine is possible, but this is costly and not practical in most instances. **Symptoms** typically begin 2 to 3 weeks after exposure and include malaise, low-grade fever, headache, mild coryza, and conjunctivitis occurring 1 to 5 days before the onset of rash. The rash is a salmon-pink macular or maculopapular exanthem that begins on the face and behind the ears and spreads downward over 1 to 2 days. The rash disappears in the

5 to 7 days from onset, and posterior cervical lymphadenopathy is common. Approximately one-third of women may have arthralgias without arthritis. In women suspected of having acute rubella infection, confirmation can be made by demonstrating a fourfold or higher rise in serum IgG titers when measured at the time of symptoms and approximately 2 weeks later. The results of some assays may not directly correlate with a fourfold rise in titer, so other criteria for a significant increase in antibody may be required. When there is uncertainty about the interpretation of assay results, advice should be obtained from the laboratory running the test and an infectious diseases consultation.

2. **Recognized or suspected maternal exposure.** Any individual known to have been immunized with rubella vaccine after his or her first birthday is generally considered immune. However, it is best to determine immunity by measuring rubella-specific IgG, which has become a standard of practice in obstetric care. If a woman exposed to rubella is known to be seropositive, she is immune, and the fetus is considered not to be at risk for infection. Reinfections in previously immune women have been rarely documented, but the risk of fetal damage appears to be very small. If the exposed woman is known to be seronegative, a serum sample should be obtained 3 to 4 weeks after exposure for determination of titer. A negative titer indicates that no infection has occurred, whereas a positive titer indicates infection. Women with an uncertain immune status and a known exposure to rubella should have serum samples obtained as soon as possible after exposure. If this is done within 7 to 10 days of exposure, and the titer is positive, the patient is rubella immune and no further testing is required. If the first titer is negative or was determined on serum taken more than 7 to 10 days after exposure, repeat testing (~3 weeks later) and careful clinical follow-up are necessary. When both the immune status and the time of exposure are uncertain, serum samples for titer determination should be obtained 3 weeks apart. If both titers are negative, no infection has occurred. Alternatively, infection is confirmed if seroconversion or a fourfold increase in titer is observed. Further testing and close clinical follow-up are required if titer results are inconclusive. In this situation, specific IgM determination may be helpful. It should be emphasized that all serum samples should be tested simultaneously by the same laboratory when one is determining changes in titers with time. This can be accomplished by saving a portion of each serum sample before sending it for titer determination. The saved portion can be frozen until convalescent serum samples have been obtained.

3. **Congenital rubella infection.**
   a. **Antenatal diagnosis.** The risk of severe fetal anomalies is highest with acute maternal rubella infection during the first 16 weeks of gestation. However, not all early-gestation infections result in adverse pregnancy outcomes. Approximately 20% of fetuses may not be infected when maternal rubella occurs in the first 12 weeks of gestation, and as many as 45% of fetuses may not be infected when maternal rubella occurs closer to 16 weeks of gestation. Unfortunately, there is no foolproof method of determining infected from uninfected fetuses early in pregnancy, but *in utero* diagnosis is being investigated. One method that has been used with some success is the determination of specific IgM in fetal blood obtained by PUBS. Direct detection of rubella antigen and RNA in a chorionic villous biopsy specimen also has been used successfully. Although these techniques offer promise, their use may be limited by sensitivity and specificity or the lack of widespread availability.
   b. **Postnatal diagnosis.** Guidelines for the establishment of congenital rubella infection or CRS in neonates have been summarized by the Centers for Disease Control and Prevention. The diagnosis of congenital infection is made by one of the following:
      i. **Isolation of rubella virus** (oropharynx, urine). Notify the laboratory in advance as special culture medium needs to be prepared.
      ii. **Detection of rubella-specific IgM** in cord or neonatal blood.

        iii. Persistent rubella-specific titers over time (i.e., no decline in titer as expected for transplacentally derived maternal IgG). If, in addition, there are congenital defects, the diagnosis of CRS is made.

D. Treatment. There is no specific therapy for either maternal or congenital rubella infection. Maternal disease is almost always mild and self-limiting. If primary maternal infection occurs during the first 5 months of pregnancy, termination options should be discussed with the mother. More than one-half of newborns with congenital rubella may be asymptomatic at birth. If infection is known to have occurred beyond the 20th week of gestation, it is unlikely that any abnormalities will develop, and parents should be reassured. Nevertheless, hearing evaluations should be repeated during childhood. Closer follow-up is required if early-gestation infection is suspected or the timing of infection is unknown. This is true for asymptomatic infants as well as those with obvious CRS. The principal reason for close follow-up is to identify delayed-onset abnormalities or progressive disorders. In some cases, early interventions, such as therapy for glaucoma, may be critical. Unfortunately, there is no specific therapy to halt the progression of most of the complications of CRS.

E. Prevention. The primary means of prevention of CRS is by immunization of all susceptible persons. Immunization is recommended for all nonimmune individuals 12 months or older. Documentation of maternal immunity is an important aspect of good obstetric management. When a susceptible woman is identified, she should be reassured of the low risk of contracting rubella, but she should also be counseled to avoid contact with anyone known to have acute or recent rubella infection. Individuals with postnatal infection typically shed virus for 1 week before and 1 week after the onset of rash. On the other hand, infants with congenital infection may shed virus for many months, and contact should be avoided during the first year. Unfortunately, once exposure has occurred, little can be done to alter the chances of maternal and subsequently fetal disease. Although hyperimmune globulin has not been shown to diminish the risk of maternal rubella following exposure or the rate of fetal transmission, it should be given in large doses to any woman who is exposed to rubella and who does not wish to interrupt her pregnancy. The lack of proven efficacy must be emphasized in these cases.

    Susceptible women who do not become infected should be immunized soon after pregnancy. There have been reports of acute arthritis occurring in women immunized in the immediate postpartum period, and a small percentage of these women developed chronic joint or neurologic abnormalities or viremia. Vaccine-strain virus also may be shed in breast milk and transmitted to breast-fed infants, some of whom may develop chronic viremia. Therefore, it may be best to avoid breastfeeding in women receiving rubella vaccine. Conception also should be avoided for 3 months following immunization. Immunization during pregnancy is not recommended because of the theoretical risk to the fetus. Inadvertent immunizations during pregnancy have occurred, and fetal infection has been documented in a small percentage of these pregnancies. However, no cases of CRS have been identified. In fact, the rubella registry at the Centers for Disease Control and Prevention has been closed, with the following conclusions: The number of inadvertent immunizations during pregnancy is too small to be able to state with certainty that no adverse pregnancy outcomes will occur, but these would appear to be very uncommon. Therefore, it is still recommended that immunization not be carried out during pregnancy, but when this has occurred, reassurance of little risk to the fetus can be given.

XVI. RSV (NEONATAL). RSV is an enveloped RNA paramyxovirus that is the leading cause of bronchiolitis and can cause severe or even fatal lower respiratory tract disease, especially in preterm infants. Conditions that increase the risk of severe disease include cyanotic or complicated congenital heart disease, pulmonary hypertension, chronic lung disease, and immune-compromised states.

    A. Epidemiology. Humans are the only source of infection, spread by respiratory secretions as droplets or fomites, which can survive on environmental surfaces for hours. Spread by hospital workers to infants occurs, especially in the winter and early spring months in temperate climates. Viral shedding is 3 to 8 days, but in very young infants may take weeks. The incubation period is 2 to 8 days.

B. Diagnosis. Rapid diagnosis is made by immunofluorescent antigen testing of respiratory secretions. This test can have up to 95% sensitivity and is quite specific. Viral culture usually requires 3 to 5 days.

C. Treatment. Treatment is largely supportive, with hydration, supplemental oxygen, and mechanical ventilation as needed. Controversy exists as to whether albuterol nebulized therapy is beneficial. Ribavirin has been marketed for treatment of infants with RSV infection because it does have *in vitro* activity; however, efficacy has never been repeatedly proven in randomized trials. This makes the risk of ribavirin (aerosol route, potentially toxic side effects to health care personnel, and high cost) important to consider on a case-by-case basis. The use of palivizumab may be considered along with your infectious disease consultant for the most severely affected infants.

D. Prevention. Palivizumab (Synagis), a humanized mouse monoclonal antibody given intramuscularly, have been approved by the U.S. Food and Drug Administration (FDA) for prevention of RSV disease in children younger than 2 years of age with chronic lung disease or who were <35 weeks' gestation. Palivizumab is easy to administer, has a low volume and is given (15 mg/kg intramuscularly) just before and monthly throughout the RSV season (typically mid-November to March/April). Because the drug supply is limited, its protection incomplete, and is costly, the American Academy of Pediatrics has made the following recommendations regarding which high-risk infants should receive palivizumab:

  1. Infants who have required therapy for chronic lung disease within 6 months of the RSV season.
  2. Infants who are born at <32 weeks' gestation without chronic lung disease: up to 12 months of age if born at 28 weeks' gestation or less; up to 6 months of age if born at 29 to 32 weeks' gestation.
  3. Preterm infants 32 to 35 weeks <6 months of age who have two or more of the following risk factors: attending day care, with school-aged siblings in household, exposure to environmental pollutants, congenital abnormalities of the airways, or severe neuromuscular disease.
      If an RSV outbreak is documented in a high-risk unit (e.g., pediatric intensive care unit), primary emphasis should be placed on proper infection-control practices. The need for and efficacy of antibody prophylaxis in these situations has not been documented. Each unit should evaluate the risk to its exposed infants and decide on the need for treatment. If the patient stays hospitalized, this may only require one dose.
  4. Children who are 24 months of age or younger with hemodynamically significant cyanotic or acyanotic congenital heart disease.

E. Antibody preparations are not recommended for the following
  1. Healthy preterm babies greater than 32 weeks' gestation without other risk factors.
  2. Patients with hemodynamically insignificant heart disease.
  3. Infants with lesions adequately corrected by surgery; unless they continue to require medication for congestive heart failure.
      Palivizumab does not interfere with the routine immunization schedule.

Suggested Readings

American Academy of Pediatrics, Committee on Infectious Diseases. *2006 Red Book: Report of the committee on infectious diseases*, 27th ed. Elk Grove Village: American Academy of Pediatrics, 2006.

Bopanna SB, Rivera LB, Fowler KB, et al. Intrauterine transmission of cytomegalovirus to infants of women with preconceptual immunity. *N Engl J Med* 2001;344(18):1366–1371.

Cooper ER, Charurat M, Mofenson L, et al. Combination antiretroviral strategies for the treatment of pregnant HIV-1-infected women and prevention of perinatal HIV-1 transmission. *J Acquir Immune Defic Syndr* 2002;29(5):484–494.

Kimberlin DW, Lin C-Y, Jacobs RF, et al. Natural history of neonatal herpes simplex virus infections in the acyclovir era. *Pediatrics* 2001;108:223–229.

Mofenson LM, Lambert JS, Steihm ER, et al. Risk factors for perinatal transmission of human immunodeficiency virus type 1 in women treated with zidovudine. *N Engl J Med* 1999;341:385–393.

Perinatal HIV Guidelines Working Group. Public Health Service Task Force Recommendations for Use of Antiretroviral Drugs in Pregnant HIV-1 Infected Women for Maternal Health and Interventions to Reduce Perinatal HIV-1 Transmission in the United States. October 12, 2006 1–65. Available at http://aidsinfo.nih.gov/ContentFiles/PerinatalGL.pdf.

Working Group on Antiretroviral Therapy and Medical Management of HIV-Infected Children. *Guidelines for the use of antiretroviral agents in pediatric HIV infection.*October 26, Available at: http://aidsinfo.nih.gov/ContentFiles/PediatricGuidelines.pdf, 2006: 1–126.

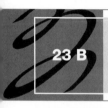

BACTERIAL AND FUNGAL INFECTIONS

23 B

Karen M. Puopolo

I. BACTERIAL SEPSIS AND MENINGITIS

A. Introduction. Bacterial sepsis and meningitis continue to be major causes of morbidity and mortality in newborns, particularly in low-birth-weight infants. In the 1990s, improvements in neonatal intensive care decreased the morbidity and mortality from early-onset sepsis (EOS) in term infants. Preterm infants, however, remain at high risk for both EOS and its sequelae. They are also at risk for hospital-acquired sepsis. Neonatal survivors of sepsis can have severe neurologic sequelae due to central nervous system (CNS) infection, as well as from secondary hypoxemia resulting from septic shock, persistent pulmonary hypertension, and severe parenchymal lung disease.

B. Epidemiology of EOS. Several studies report the incidence of EOS to vary from 1 to 4 cases per 1,000 live births. Recent data from the Centers for Disease Control (CDC) shows that the incidence of Group B Streptococcus (GBS) EOS has decreased with the implementation of recommendations for intrapartum antibiotic prophylaxis (IAP) against GBS. Multiple studies assessing the impact of GBS IAP policies have demonstated that the incidence of non-GBS EOS is unchanged or decreasing among term births; however, the incidence of non-GBS EOS is increasing among very-low-birth weight (VLBW) (<1,500 g, VLBW) infants.

C. Risk factors for EOS. Maternal and infant characteristics associated with the development of EOS have been most rigorously studied with respect to GBS EOS. Maternal factors predictive of GBS disease include intrapartum fever (>37.5°C), chorioamnionitis, and prolonged rupture of membranes (ROM) (>18 hours). Neonatal risk factors include prematurity (<37 weeks' gestation) and low birth weight (BW) (<2,500 g). The incidence of EOS is nearly ten times higher in infants with a BW <1,500 g than that for infants with normal BW.

D. Clinical presentation of EOS. Early-onset disease can manifest as asymptomatic bacteremia, generalized sepsis, pneumonia, and/or meningitis. The clinical signs of

EOS are usually apparent in the first hours of life; 90% of infants are symptomatic by 24 hours of age. Respiratory distress is the most common presenting symptom. Respiratory symptoms can range in severity from mild tachypnea and grunting, with or without a supplemental oxygen requirement, to respiratory failure. Persistent pulmonary hypertension of the newborn (PPHN) can also accompany sepsis. Other less specific signs of sepsis include irritability, lethargy, temperature instability, poor perfusion, and hypotension. Disseminated intravascular coagulation (DIC) with purpura and petechiae can occur in more severe septic shock. Gastrointestinal symptoms can include poor feeding, vomiting, and ileus. Meningitis may present with seizure activity, apnea, and depressed sensorium, but may complicate sepsis without specific neurologic symptoms, underscoring the importance of the lumbar puncture (LP) in the evaluation of sepsis.

Other diagnoses to be considered in the immediate newborn period in the infant with signs of sepsis include transient tachypnea of the newborn, meconium aspiration syndrome, intracranial hemorrhage, congenital viral disease, and congenital cyanotic heart disease. In infants presenting at more than 24 hours of age, closure of the ductus arteriosus in the setting of a ductal-dependent cardiac anomaly (such as critical coarctation of the aorta or hypoplastic left heart syndrome) can mimic sepsis. Other diagnoses that should be considered in the infant presenting beyond the first few hours of life with a sepsislike picture include bowel obstruction, necrotizing enterocolitis (NEC), and inborn errors of metabolism.

E. **Evaluation of the symptomatic infant for EOS. Laboratory evaluation** of the symptomatic infant suspected of EOS includes at minimum a complete blood count (CBC) with differential and blood culture. An elevated white blood cell (WBC) count with a predominance of immature granulocytes polymorphonuclear cells (PMN), a depressed total WBC ($<5,000$) and absolute neutropenia (PMN $<1,500$) are commonly found. However, a normal WBC and differential can be initially seen; a second WBC performed at 12 to 24 hours of age can be helpful in making a clinical diagnosis of infection. Other laboratory abnormalities can include hyperglycemia and metabolic acidosis. Thrombocytopenia as well as evidence of DIC (elevated prothrombin time [PT], partial thromboplastin time [PTT], and international normalized ratio [INR]; decreased fibrinogen) can be found in more severely ill infants. For infants with a strong clinical suspicion of sepsis, **a LP for cerebrospinal fluid (CSF) cell count, protein and glucose concentration, gram stain, and culture** should be performed before the administration of antibiotics if the infant is clinically stable. The LP may be deferred until after the institution of antibiotic therapy if the infant is clinically unstable, or if later culture results or clinical course demonstrate that sepsis was present.

Infants with respiratory symptoms should have a **chest radiograph** as well as other indicated evaluation such as arterial blood gas measurement. Radiographic abnormalities caused by retained fetal lung fluid or atelectasis, usually resolve within 48 hours. **Neonatal pneumonia** will present with persistent focal or diffuse radiographic abnormalities and variable degrees of respiratory distress. Neonatal pneumonia (particularly that caused by GBS) can be accompanied by primary or secondary surfactant deficiency.

F. **Treatment of EOS.** Empiric **antibiotic therapy** includes broad coverage for organisms known to cause EOS, usually a β-lactam antibiotic and an aminoglycoside. In our institutions, we use ampicillin (150 mg/kg/dose q12 hours) and gentamicin (3–4 mg/kg/dose q24 hours). We add a third-generation cephalosporin (cefotaxime or ceftazidime) to the empiric treatment of critically ill infants for whom there is a strong clinical suspicion for sepsis because of a recent increase the proportion of EOS caused by ampicillin-resistant enteric gram-negative organisms, primarily ampicillin-resistant *Escherichia coli*. (See Tables 23B.1 and 23B.2 for treatment recommendations). **Supportive treatments for sepsis** include the use of mechanical ventilation; exogenous surfactant therapy for pneumonia and respiratory distress syndrome (RDS); volume and pressor support for hypotension and poor perfusion; sodium bicarbonate for metabolic acidosis; and anticonvulsants for seizures. **Echocardiography** may be of benefit in the severely ill, cyanotic infant to determine

Organism	Antibiotic	Bacteremia	Meningitis
GBS	Ampicillin or penicillin G	10–14 d	21 d
E. coli	Cefotaxime or ampicillin and gentamicin	14 d	21 d
CONS	Vancomycin	7 d	14 d
Klebsiella, Serratia[†]	Cefotaxime or meropenem and gentamicin	14 d	21 d
Enterobacter, Citrobacter[‡]	Cefepime or meropenem and gentamicin	14 d	21 d
Enterococcus[§]	Ampicillin or vancomycin and gentamicin	10 d	21 d
Listeria	Ampicillin and gentamicin	10–14 d	21 d
Pseudomonas	Ceftazidime or piperacillin/tazobactam and gentamicin or tobramycin	14 d	21 d
S. aureus[¶]	Nafcillin	10–14 d	21 d
MRSA	Vancomycin	10–14 d	21 d

TABLE 23B.1 Suggested Antibiotic Regimens for Sepsis and Meningitis*

GBS = Group B Streptococcus; CONS = coagulase-negative staphylococci; MRSA = Methicillin-resistant *Staphylococcus aureus*.

* All treatment courses are counted from the first documented negative blood culture and assume that antibiotic sensitivity data are available for the organisms. In late-onset infections, all treatment courses assume central catheters have been removed. With CONS infections, the clinician may choose to retain the catheter during antibiotic treatment, but if repeated cultures remain positive, the catheters must be removed. Many infectious disease specialists recommend repeat lumbar punctures at the completion of therapy for meningitis to ensure eradication of the infection.
† The spread of plasmid-borne extended-spectrum beta-lactamases (ESBL) among enteric pathogens such as *E. coli*, *Klebsiella*, and *Serratia* is an increasing clinical problem. Recent literature suggests that ESBL-containing organisms can be effectively treated with cefepime or meropenem.
‡ *Enterobacter* and *Citrobacter* species have inducible, chromosomally-encoded cephalosporinases. Cephalosporins other than the fourth generation cefepime should not be used to treat infections with these organisms **even if** initial *in vitro* antibiotic sensitivity data suggest sensitivity to third-generation cephalosporins such as cefotaxime. There are some reports in the literature of cefepime-resistant *Enterobacter*.
§ Enterococci are resistant to all cephalosporins. Ampicillin-resistant strains of enterococci are common in hospitals, and require treatment with vancomycin. Treatment of vancomycin resistant strains (VRE) requires consultation with an infectious disease specialist.
¶ Uncomplicated methicillin-sensitive *S. aureus* and MRSA bacteremias may be treated for only 10 days if central catheters have been removed. Persistent bacteremias can require treatment for 3–4 weeks. Bacteremias complicated by deep infections such as osteomyelitis or infectious arthritis often require surgical drainage and treatment for up to 6 weeks. The use of additional agents such as daptomycin and rifampin to eradicate persistent *S. aureus* infection requires consultation with an infectious disease specialist.

if significant pulmonary hypertension or cardiac failure is present. Infants born at ≥34 weeks with symptomatic pulmonary hypertension may benefit from treatment with inhaled nitric oxide (**iNO**). A recent trial of the use of iNO in severely ill VLBW infants demonstrated no benefit of this therapy in the first 5 days of life. Extra-corporeal membrane oxygenation (**ECMO**) can be offered to infants ≥34 weeks if respiratory and/circulatory failure occurs despite all conventional measures of intensive care. ECMO is not generally available to infants less than 34 weeks gestation.

A variety of **adjunctive immunotherapies** for sepsis have been trialed since the 1980s to address deficits in immunoglobulin and neutrophil number and function.

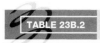

TABLE 23B.2 Neonatal Dosing of Common Intravenous Antibiotics

Antibiotic	Dosing regimen	
Ampicillin*	≤7 d	150 mg/kg/dose q12 h
	>7 d and <1.2 kg	100 mg/kg/dose q12 h
	>7 d and 1.2 kg–2.0 kg	50 mg/kg/dose q8 h
	>7 d and >2.0 kg	50 mg/kg/dose q6 h

In the case of **meningitis,** total daily ampicillin dose should be 300 mg/kg/day, divided by the age- and BW-appropriate interval.

Cefotaxime	≤7 d: 50 mg/kg/dose q12 h	
	>7 d: 50 mg/kg/dose q8 h	
Cefepime	50 mg/kg/dose q8 h	
Ceftazidime[†]	≤7 d: 50 mg/kg/dose q12 h	
	>7 d: 50 mg/kg/dose q8 h	
Clindamycin	≤29 wk: 7.5 mg/kg/dose q12 h	
	>29 wk: 7.5 mg/kg/dose q8 h	
Gentamicin[‡]	<35 wk: 3 mg/kg/dose q24 h	
	≥35 wk: 4 mg/kg/dose q24 h	
Meropenem	Sepsis: 20 mg/kg/dose q12 h	
	Meningitis: 40 mg/kg/dose q8 h	
Nafcillin	≤7 d and <2.0 kg	25 mg/kg/dose q12 h
	≤7 d and ≥2.0 kg	25 mg/kg/dose q8 h
	>7 d and <1.2 kg	25 mg/kg/dose q12 h
	>7 d and 1.2–2.0 kg	25 mg/kg/dose q8 h
	>7 d and >2.0 kg	25 mg/kg/dose q6 h
Penicillin G	GBS sepsis: 200,000 U/kg/day ÷ q8 h	
	GBS meningitis: 400,000 U/kg/day ÷ q8 h	
Vancomycin[§]	≤7 d and <1.2 kg	15 mg/kg/dose q24 h
	≤7 d and 1.2–2.0 kg	10 mg/kg/dose q12 h
	≤7 d and >2.0 kg	15 mg/kg/dose q12 h
	>7 d and <1.2 kg	15 mg/kg/dose q24
	>7 d and 1.2 – 2.0 kg	15 mg/kg/dose q12 h
	>7 d and >2 kg	10 mg/kg/dose q8 h

GBS = Group B Streptococcus.
* At our institution, we use ampicillin 150 mg/kg/dose q12 hours and gentamicin as empiric therapy for EOS.
[†] For meningitis, ceftazidime should be given at 50 mg/kg/dose q8 hours regardless of age.
[‡] Gentamicin levels: Trough <1.5 μg/mL Peak 6–15 μg/mL.
[§] Vancomycin levels: Trough 5–15 μg/mL We no longer monitor vancomycin peak levels at our institution.
See Appendix A for administrative guidelines.

Double-volume exchange transfusions, granulocyte infusions, the administration of intravenous immunoglobulin (IVIG), and treatment with granulocyte-colony stimulating factor (G-CSF) and granulocyte macrophage-colony stimulating factor (GM-CSF) have all been investigated with variable results.

1. **Double-volume exchange transfusion and granulocyte infusion.** Several experimental approaches have been taken replete neutrophils in neutropenic septic infants: (1) double-volume exchange transfusion with fresh whole blood, (2) infusion of fresh buffy-coat preparations, or (3) infusion of granulocytes collected by leukopheresis. Double-volume exchange with whole blood also provides platelets and removes bacteria, bacterial toxins, and circulating inflammatory

molecules. Two small, randomized, controlled trials of exchange transfusion with whole blood in infants with (largely gram-negative) sepsis were published in the 1990s. Both reported a 50% reduction in mortality in the infants undergoing exchange, and demonstrated increases in neutrophil number, improvement in neutrophil function and increases in immunoglobin concentration in the exchanged infants. A recent Cochrane review of four small trials of granulocyte transfusion in neutropenic neonates with sepsis concluded that there is insufficient evidence of survival benefit with this therapy. Both whole blood exchange transfusion and granulocyte infusion do present significant risks, including graft-versus-host disease; blood-group sensitization; and transmission of infections such as Cytomegalovirus (CMV), human immunodeficiency virus (HIV), and viral hepatitis. In addition, the emergent availability of these blood products (especially leukopheresed granulocytes) is limited in most centers. We do not currently use either of these treatments in the treatment of early- or late-onset sepsis.

2. **IVIG.** The use of IVIG in the acute treatment of neonatal sepsis is controversial. It is likely that any efficacy of IVIG would be highest in EOS, which in the United States is largely due to the encapsulated organisms GBS and *E. coli* K1, and in premature infants, who are most likely to have inadequate immunoglobulin reserves. A 2004 meta-analysis of 13 randomized trials of the use of IVIG in the acute treatment of suspected or proven neonatal sepsis showed a decrease in mortality of borderline significance. These trials were conducted in seven different countries, using different dosing regimens and/or immunoglobulin preparations. IVIG is expensive and has potential infectious risks, and most authorities have not endorsed the routine use of IVIG in the treatment of neonatal sepsis. However, in light of this meta-analysis, a single dose of IVIG at 750 mg/kg/dose for preterm infants (1 g/kg for term infants) with overwhelming sepsis is a reasonable adjunctive therapy in the seriously ill infant.

3. **Cytokines.** Recombinant G-CSF and GM-CSF have been shown to restore neutrophil levels in small studies of neutropenic growth-restricted infants, ventilator-dependent neutropenic infants born to mothers with preeclampsia, and in neutropenic infants with sepsis. A rise in the absolute neutrophil count (ANC) above $1,500/\text{mm}^3$ occurred in 24 to 48 hours. To date seven randomized, controlled trials of recombinant colony-stimulating factors have been reported, all enrolling small numbers of infants. Assessment of these trials is complicated by the use of different preparations, dosages, and durations of therapy, as well as variable enrollment criteria (differing gestational age ranges, presumed and culture-proven sepsis, neutropenic and nonneutropenic infants, early and late-onset of infection). None of the trials included neurodevelopmental follow-up. These studies suggest that G-CSF may result in lower mortality among neutropenic, septic VLBW infants, but overall there is currently insufficient evidence to support the routine use of these preparations in the acute treatment of neonatal sepsis.

G. **Evaluation of the asymptomatic infant at risk for EOS.** There are a number of clinical factors that place infants at risk for EOS. These factors also identify a group of asymptomatic infants who may have colonization or bacteremia that places them at risk for the development of symptomatic EOS. These infants include those born to mothers who have received inadequate IAP for GBS (see subsequent text) and those born to mothers with suspected chorioamnionitis. Blood cultures are the definitive determination of bacteremia. A number of laboratory tests have been evaluated for their ability to predict which of the at-risk infants will go on to develop symptomatic or culture-proven sepsis, but no single test has adequate sensitivity and specificity.

1. **Blood culture.** With advances in the development of computer-assisted, continuous-read culture systems, most blood cultures will be positive within 24 to 36 hours of incubation if organisms are present. Most institutions, including ours, empirically treat infants for sepsis for a minimum of 48 hours with the assumption that true positive cultures will turn positive within that period. At least 0.5 mL (and preferably 1 mL) of blood should be placed in most pediatric blood culture bottles. We use two culture bottles, one aerobic and one anaerobic.

Certain organisms causing EOS (such as *Bacteroides fragilis* [*B. fragilis*]) will only grow under anaerobic conditions. GBS, *Staphylococcus* species, and many gram-negative organisms grow in a facultative fashion, and the use of two culture bottles increases the likelihood of detecting low-level bacteremia with these organisms.

2. **WBC.** A total WBC <5,000; an ANC <1,000; and an immature to total neutrophil count (I:T ratio) >0.2 have all been correlated with the presence of bacterial infection. An elevated WBC (>20,000) is not predictive in newborn infants. The overall positive predictive value of WBC values is poor, as there are a number of neonatal conditions that result in neutrophilia and an elevated I:T ratio including maternal fever, neonatal asphyxia, meconium aspiration syndrome, pneumothorax, and hemolytic disease. Maternal pregnancy-induced hypertension and preeclampsia are associated with neonatal neutropenia as well as thrombocytopenia. WBC values can be useful, however, when placed in the clinical context and used as part of an algorithm to evaluate infants for sepsis risk. In addition, a repeat WBC obtained at 12 to 24 hours of age is more predictive of infection than a single determination at birth. Some centers use a "sepsis screen" (e.g., the use of an algorithm incorporating total WBC, I:T ratio, total band count, with or without C-reactive protein (CRP) values) to guide treatment decisions.

3. **C-reactive protein.** CRP is a nonspecific marker of inflammation or tissue necrosis. Elevations in CRP are found in bacterial sepsis and meningitis. A single determination of CRP at birth lacks both sensitivity and specificity for infection, but serial CRP determinations at birth, and at 12 hours and beyond have been used to manage infants at risk for sepsis. We do not use CRP measurements in the evaluation of infants at risk for sepsis.

4. **Cytokine measurements.** Advances in the understanding of the immune responses to infection and in the measurement of small peptide molecules have allowed investigation into the utility of these inflammatory molecules in predicting infection in neonates at risk. Serum levels of interleukin-6, interleukin-8, interleukin-10, interleukin-1 β, G-CSF, TNF-alpha, and procalcitonin, as well as measurements of inflammatory cell-surface markers such as CD64 have been variably correlated with culture-proven, clinical and viral sepsis. The need for serial measurements and the availability of the specific assays so far limit the use of cytokine markers in diagnosing neonatal infection. In addition, most studies have been performed on infants who are symptomatic and being evaluated for sepsis. None of these has yet proven useful in predicting infection in initially well-appearing infants. A combination of these measurements with more traditional markers of infection (WBC, CRP) may prove useful in making judgments about empiric treatment of sepsis in the absence of a positive blood culture.

5. **Other strategies. Gram stain of gastric aspirate contents** for bacteria and PMNs was once used to predict the presence of early onset infection but has fallen out of use due to poor specificity and sampling error. **Urine latex particle agglutination testing for GBS** remains available at some institutions; we have given up use of this test due to very poor predictive value. Latex particle testing of CSF for both GBS and *E. coli* K1 can be of use in evaluating CSF after the institution of antibiotic treatment.

6. **LP.** The use of routine LP in the evaluation of **asymptomatic neonates** at risk for EOS remains controversial. A recent retrospective review of 9,111 infants born at ≥34 weeks gestation from 150 neonatal intensive care unit (NICU)'s on whom a LP was performed found 95 cases of culture-proven meningitis. In 38% of these cases, the accompanying blood culture was sterile. Another retrospective study of CSF taken from a population of 169,849 infants identified 8 infants with culture-positive CSF, but with negative blood cultures and no CNS symptoms. In both studies the authors concluded that the selective use of LP in the evaluation of EOS may lead to missed diagnoses of meningitis. However, in both studies infants were not all evaluated for sepsis in the absence of symptoms, and the subjects were drawn from large numbers of hospitals with likely disparate

culture systems. Another study reviewed the results of sepsis evaluations in a population of 24,452 infants from a single institution. This study found 11 cases of meningitis, all in symptomatic infants; 10 of 11 corresponding blood cultures were positive for the same organism. No cases of meningitis were found in 3423 asymptomatic infants evaluated with LP.

Beginning in 1994, we stopped the routine use of LP for the evaluation of **asymptomatic term infants** at risk for EOS. A review of our own data from 1996–2003, a period during which IAP for GBS was implemented using a screening-based approach, revealed 20 cases of culture-positive meningitis from a population of over 70,000 deliveries. Only two cases occurred in term infants; both infants grew GBS from both blood and CSF cultures and both infants were symptomatic.

It is our current policy to perform LPs only on (1) infants with positive blood cultures and (2) symptomatic infants with negative blood cultures who are treated empirically for the clinical diagnosis of sepsis. Whenever clinically feasible, LPs are performed on symptomatic infants with a high suspicion for sepsis before administering antibiotics. When LPs are performed after the administration of antibiotics, a clinical evaluation of the presence of meningitis is made, taking into account the blood culture results, the CSF cell count, protein, and glucose levels as well as the clinical scenario. Whenever the CSF is being examined after the administration of antibiotics, we recommend sending two separate CSF samples for cell count from the same LP, to account for the role of possible fluctuation in CSF cell count measurements.

Normal CSF WBC counts in term, noninfected infants are variable, with most studies reporting a mean of <20 cells/mm^3, with ranges of up to 90 cells, and widely varying levels of polymorphonuclear cells on the differential. One recent study defined "noninfected" infants by negative bacterial blood, CSF and urine cultures, and negative viral CSF culture as well as negative enteroviral CSF polymerase chain reaction (PCR). This study reported a mean CSF WBC 7.3 $(+/-14)$/mm^3 with a range of 0 to 130 cells. The presence of blood in the CSF, due to subarachnoid or intraventricular hemorrhage, or to blood contamination of CSF samples by "traumatic" LPs, can yield abnormal cell counts that may be due to the presence of blood in the CSF rather than true infection. All these considerations emphasize the need for clinical judgment in the diagnosis of blood and CSF culture-negative meningitis.

H. Algorithm for the evaluation of the infant born at ≥35 weeks' gestation at risk for EOS. At the Brigham and Women's Hospital (BWH), an algorithm is used for the evaluation of asymptomatic, ≥35-week-gestation infants who are at risk for developing EOS. This algorithm incorporates both the evaluation of infants based on maternal GBS colonization, and an evaluation of infants at risk of EOS due to maternal intrapartum risk factors (see Fig. 23B.1). A total WBC <5,000 or an immature to total neutrophil ratio (I/T ratio) >0.2 is used to guide treatment decisions in the evaluation of the well-appearing infant at risk for sepsis. A single WBC determination is used in most cases to avoid multiple blood draws from otherwise asymptomatic infants (although significantly abnormal values are usually confirmed within 12 to 24 hours). We also take into account the impact of a clustering of risk factors for sepsis to guide treatment decisions. These guidelines are based on a delivery service for which a screening-based approach to GBS prophylaxis has been in place since 1996, and for which the vast majority of vaginal deliveries involve epidural placement (which alone can cause low-grade intrapartum fever). We use a fever threshold of 100.4°F (38°C) for evaluation in accordance with CDC and other published recommendations.

I. Specific organisms causing EOS. The bacterial species responsible for EOS vary by locality and time period. In the United States since the 1980s, GBS has been the leading cause of neonatal EOS. Despite the implementation of IAP against GBS, it remains the leading cause of EOS in term infants. However, coincident with the increased use of intrapartum IAP for GBS, gram-negative enteric bacteria have become the leading cause of EOS in preterm infants. Enteric bacilli causing EOS

Guidelines for the Management of Asymptomatic Infants Born
at ≥ 35 Weeks Gestation with Risk Factors for Early-Onset Sepsis

Maternal Fever ≥ 101° — **Yes** → CBC, Blood Culture. Treat with Antibiotics Regardless of GBS Status or IAP

↓ No

Proceed with Following Algorithm Depending on Maternal GBS Status

GBS +

Routine Care ← **Yes** — IAP ≥ 4 hrs PTD — **No** → Fever 100.4°F–100.9°F

↑ Yes ↓ No ↓ Yes

Csxn Intact Membranes — IAP ≥ 4 hrs PTD — **Yes**

↓ No ↓ No

CBC, Blood Culture Treat if WBC Abnormal

GBS –

Fever 100.4°F–100.9°F — **No** → Routine Care

↓ Yes

Any of the Following Present:
- FHR > 160's
- Chorioamnionitis
- ROM > 24 hrs
- < 37 wks Gestation

↓ Yes ↓ No

CBC, Blood Culture Treat with Antibiotics

CBC, Blood Culture Treat if WBC Abnormal

GBS Unknown

Fever 100.4°F–100.9°F

Routine Care ← **No**

↓ Yes (→ Any of the Following Present)

IAP ≥ 4 hrs PTD — **Yes** →

↓ No

CBC, Blood Culture Treat With Antibiotics

Abnormal WBC:

Total WBC < 5000 or
I:T ratio > 0.2

I:T - number immature PMN's divided by total number of all PMN's

IV Antibiotic therapy:

Ampicillin 150 mg/kg/dose q12 h
Gentamicin 4 mg/kg/dose q24 h

<u>Notes:</u> (1) Mother with previous child with GBS disease: the infant should have a CBC and blood culture drawn and antibiotics given IF there is IAP<4 hours prior to delivery, or if there is maternal fever ≥100.4° F

(2) Maternal fever that occurs within one hour of delivery should be treated like intrapartum fever, and the infant should be evaluated as outlined above.

THESE ARE GUIDELINES ONLY AND SHOULD NOT SUBSTITUTE
FOR CLINICAL JUDGEMENT.

Figure 23B.1. Guidelines for the evaluation of asymptomatic infants at risk for EOS. EOS = early-onset sepsis.

include *E. coli*, other enterobactericiae (*Klebsiella, Pseudomonas, Hemophilus,* and *Enterobacter* species) and the anaerobe *B. fragilis*. Less common organisms that can cause serious early-onset disease include *Listeria monocytogenes* and *Citrobacter diversus*. Staphylococci and enterococci can be found in EOS but are more commonly causes of nosocomial sepsis and are discussed under that heading in the subsequent text. Fungal species can cause EOS primarily in preterm infants; this is also discussed separately in the subsequent text.

1. GBS. GBS (*Streptococcus agalactiae*) frequently colonizes the human genital and gastrointestinal tracts, and the upper respiratory tract in young infants. In addition to causing neonatal disease, GBS is a frequent cause of urinary-tract infection (UTI), chorioamnionitis, postpartum endometritis, and bacteremia in pregnant women. There is some evidence suggesting that vaginal colonization with a high inoculum of GBS during pregnancy contributes to premature birth.

a. **Microbiology.** GBS are facultative diplococci that are easily cultivated in selective laboratory media. GBS are primarily identified by the Lancefield group B carbohydrate antigen, and are further subtyped into nine distinct serotypes (types Ia, Ib, II–VIII) by analysis of capsular polysaccharide composition. Most neonatal disease in the United States is currently caused by types Ia, Ib, II, III and type V GBS. Type III GBS are associated with the development of meningitis and are commonly a cause of late-onset GBS disease.

b. **Pathogenesis.** Neonatal GBS infection is acquired *in utero* or during passage through the birth canal. Because not all women are colonized with GBS, documented colonization with GBS is the strongest predictor of GBS EOS. Approximately 20% to 30% of American women are colonized with GBS at any given time. A longitudinal study of GBS colonization in a cohort of primarily young, sexually active women demonstrated that 45% of initially GBS-negative women acquired colonization at some time over a 12-month period. In the absence of IAP, approximately 50% of infants born to mothers colonized with GBS are found to be colonized with this organism at birth, and 1% to 2% of colonized infants develop invasive GBS disease. Lack of maternally derived, protective capsular polysaccharide-specific antibody is associated with the development of invasive GBS disease. Other factors predisposing the newborn to GBS disease are less well understood, but relative deficiencies in complement, neutrophil function and innate immunity may be important.

c. **Clinical risk factors for GBS EOS.** GBS bacteriuria during pregnancy is associated with heavy colonization of the rectovaginal tract, and is considered a significant risk factor for EOS. Black race and maternal age <20 years are associated with higher rates of GBS EOS, although it is not entirely clear whether this reflects only higher rates of GBS colonization in these populations. Multiple gestation is **not** an independent risk factor for GBS EOS. The odds ratios for the development of GBS EOS by specific risk factor are shown in Table 23B.3.

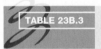

| TABLE 23B.3 | Risk Factors for Early-Onset Group B Streptococcus (GBS) Sepsis in the Absence of Intrapartum Antibiotic Prophylaxis |

Risk factor	Odds ratio (95% CI)
Maternal GBS colonization	204 (100–419)
BW <1,000 g	24.8 (12.2–50.2)
BW <2,500 g	7.37 (4.48–12.1)
Prolonged ROM >18 h	7.28 (4.42–12.0)
Chorioamnionitis	6.42 (2.32–17.8)
Intrapartum fever >37.5°C	4.05 (2.17–7.56)

CI = confidence interval; BW = birth weight; ROM = rupture of membranes.
Data from Benitz WE, Gould JB, Druzin MML. Risk factors for early-onset group B streptococcal sepsis: Estimation of odds ratios by critical literature review. *Pediatrics* 1999;103(6):e77.

d. Prevention of GBS infection. Multiple trials have demonstrated that the use of intrapartum penicillin or ampicillin significantly reduces the rate of neonatal colonization with GBS and the incidence of early-onset GBS disease. IAP for the prevention of GBS EOS can be administered to pregnant women during labor based on (1) specific risk factors for early-onset GBS infection or on (2) the results of antepartum screening of pregnant women for GBS colonization. In 1996, the CDC published consensus guidelines for the prevention of neonatal GBS disease that endorsed the use of **either** a risk factor-based or screening-based approach. The CDC later conducted a large retrospective cohort study of over 600,000 births that demonstrated the superiority of the screening-based approach to the prevention of neonatal GBS disease. The CDC issued revised guidelines for the prevention of early-onset GBS disease in 2002. "Prevention of Perinatal Group B Streptococcal Disease," (*MMWR* 1 Vol. 51, No. RR11:1–22, 08/16/2002) can be accessed on the Internet at http://www.cdc.gov/mmwr/preview/mmwrhtml/rr5111a1.htm or in PDF form at http://www.cdc.gov/mmwr/PDF/RR/RR5111.pdf. The highlight of the revised guidelines is the recommendation of **universal screening of pregnant women for GBS by rectovaginal culture are 35 to 37 weeks' gestation and management of IAP based on screening results** (see Fig. 23B.2). Pregnant women with documented GBS bacteriuria during pregnancy or who previously delivered an infant who developed invasive GBS disease need not be screened as these women should be given IAP **regardless of current GBS colonization status.** Recommendations were also made for the use of GBS prophylaxis in women experiencing threatened preterm labor (see Fig. 23B.3).

The revised guidelines address concerns over the documented emergence of GBS resistance to erythromycin and clindamycin, antibiotics frequently used for IAP in the penicillin-allergic woman. The CDC continues to recommend penicillin or ampicillin for IAP. In the penicillin-allergic woman, it is now recommended that any GBS isolates identified on screening be tested

---

Vaginal and rectal GBS screening cultures at 35–37 weeks' gestation for **ALL** pregnant women (unless patient had GBS bacteriuria during the current pregnancy or a previous infant with invasive GBS disease)

Intrapartum prophylaxis indicated	**Intrapartum prophylaxis not indicated**
• Previous infant with invasive GBS disease • GBS bacteriuria during current pregnancy • Positive GBS screening culture during current pregnancy (unless a planned cesarean delivery, in the absence of labor or amniotic membrane rupture, is performed) • Unknown GBS status (culture not done, incomplete, or results unknown) and any of the following: • Delivery at <37 weeks' gestation* • Amniotic membrane rupture 18 hours • Intrapartum temperature 100.4° F (38.0° C)†	• Previous pregnancy with a positive GBS screening culture (unless a culture was also positive during the current pregnancy) • Planned cesarean delivery performed in the absence of labor or membrane rupture (regardless of maternal GBS culture status) • Negative vaginal and rectal GBS screening culture in late gestation during the current pregnancy, regardless of intrapartum risk factors

*If onset of labor or rupture of amniotic membranes occurs at <37 weeks' gestation and there is a significant risk for preterm delivery (as assessed by the clinician), a suggested algorithm for GBS prophylaxis management is provided (Figure 3).

†If amnionitis is suspected, broad-spectrum antibiotic therapy that includes an agent known to be active against GBS should replace GBS prophylaxis.

Figure 23B.2. *2002 CDC Revised Guidelines for the Prevention of Early Onset GBS Disease.* Indications for intrapartum antibiotic prophylaxis to prevent perinatal GBS disease under a universal prenatal screening strategy based on combined vaginal and rectal cultures collected at 35 to 37 weeks' gestation from all pregnant women. CDC = Centers for Disease Control; GBS = Group B Streptococcus.

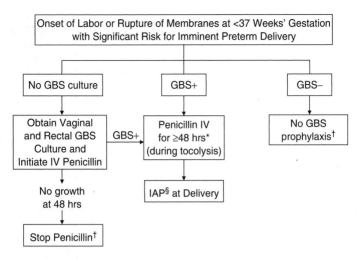

*Penicillin should be continued for a total of at least 48 hours, unless delivery occurs sooner. At the physician's discretion, antibiotic prophylaxis may be continued beyond 48 hours in a GBS culture-positive woman if delivery has not yet occurred. For women who are GBS culture positive, antibiotic prophylaxis should be reinitiated when labor likely to proceed to delivery occurs or recurs.

†If delivery has not occurred within 4 weeks, a vaginal and rectal GBS screening culture should be repeated and the patient should be managed as described, based on the result of the repeat culture.

§Intrapartum antibiotic prophylaxis.

Figure 23B.3. *2002 CDC Revised Guidelines for the Prevention of Early Onset GBS Disease.* Sample algorithm for GBS prophylaxis for women with threatened preterm delivery. This algorithm is not an exclusive course of management. Variations that incorporate individual circumstances or institutional preferences may be appropriate. CDC = Centers for Disease Control; GBS = Group B Streptococcus.

for antibiotic susceptibility. For the woman deemed to be **not at high risk** for penicillin anaphylaxis, cefazolin is recommended for IAP; for the woman deemed to be at high risk for anaphylaxis, clindamycin or erythromycin are recommended for sensitive strains; vancomycin is recommended if resistance is documented or susceptibility data is unavailable.

The development of a **vaccine for GBS** could eliminate the need for most IAP. Capsular polysaccharide-based vaccines alone and polysaccharide-tetanus toxoid vaccines have been developed and tested in phase I and II trials. For greatest efficacy, the development of a multivalent vaccine (serotypes Ia, Ib, II, III, and V) or inclusion of a GBS protein common to most serotypes will be needed.

e. **Current status of GBS EOS.** CDC active surveillance data for the United States in 2004 demonstrates that the incidence of GBS EOS has fallen to 0.34 cases per 1,000 live births (compared to 1.7 cases per 1,000 live births in 1993.) We recently evaluated the reasons for persistent GBS EOS despite the use of a screening-based approach to IAP at the BWH. We found that most GBS EOS in term infants now occurs in infants born to women with **negative** antepartum screens for GBS colonzation. Many of the mothers in this study had other intrapartum risk factors for sepsis, underscoring the importance of continued evaluation of infants at risk for EOS in the era GBS prophylaxis.

Bacterial culture remains the CDC-recommended standard for detection of maternal GBS colonization. In 2002, the FDA approved the first **PCR-based rapid diagnostic test** (IDI-Strep B test) for use in detection of maternal GBS colonization. The test can be completed in one hour and potentially allows for screening of pregnant women on presentation for delivery. A recent comparison of the IDI-Strep B test with antenatal culture and intrapartum culture demonstrated that the PCR-based diagnostic was more sensitive than antenatal culture in predicting intrapartum GBS status. Due to the costs and technicalities of providing continuous support for a real-time PCR-based diagnostic, most obstetric services continue to rely on antenatal culture-based screening programs.

   f. Evaluation of infants after maternal GBS IAP. The revised CDC guidelines include a recommended algorithm for the evaluation of infants born to mothers exposed to IAP. **We have incorporated these guidelines into our policy for the evaluation of the asymptomatic ($\geq$35-week) infant at risk for EOS** (see Fig. 23B.1).

   g. Treatment of infants with invasive GBS disease. When GBS is identified as the sole causative organism in EOS, empiric antibiotic treatment should be narrowed to ampicillin (200 to 300 mg/kg/day) or penicillin G (250,000 to 450,000 U/kg/day) alone, with the higher dosing reserved for cases complicated by meningitis. The total duration of therapy should be at least 10 days for sepsis without a focus, 14–21 days for meningitis, and 28 days for osteomyelitis. Bone and joint infections that involve the hip or shoulder require surgical drainage in addition to antibiotic therapy.

   h. Recurrent GBS infection. Recurrent GBS infections are infrequent, with reported incidences ranging from 1% to 6%. Infants usually fail to have a specific antibody response after infection with GBS, and GBS can be isolated from mucosal surfaces of infants even after appropriate antibiotic treatment for invasive disease. Occasionally reinfection with a new strain of GBS occurs. Treatment of recurrent GBS infections is the same as for primary infection except that susceptibility testing of the GBS strain to penicillin is recommended if not routinely performed. Rifampin, which eliminates colonization in other infections such as meningococcal disease, does not reliably eradicate mucous membrane colonization with GBS.

2. _E. coli_ and other enteric gram-negative bacilli. With the implementation of IAP against GBS, an **increasing proportion** of EOS cases are caused by gram-negative organisms. Whether GBS IAP policies are contributing to an absolute increase in the **incidence** of EOS caused by gram-negative organisms, and in particular, of ampicillin-resistant gram-negative organisms, is a matter of ongoing controversy. In 2003, CDC researchers published a review of 23 reports of EOS in the era of GBS prophylaxis. This review concluded that there is no evidence of an increase in non-GBS EOS among term infants. **However, worrisome increases in non-GBS EOS and ampicillin-resistant EOS are reported in preterm, and particularly in VLBW, infants.** We have analyzed EOS at the BWH from 1990–2006, comparing the period 1990–92 (no GBS IAP policy) to 1997–2006 (screening-based GBS IAP policy). We found an **absolute decrease in the incidence** of all-cause EOS in both term and VLBW infants, and no increases in non-GBS EOS, _E. coli_ EOS or ampicillin-resistant EOS in term or VLBW infants. Trends in the microbiology of EOS likely vary to some extent by institution, and may be influenced by local obstetrical practices as well as by local variation in indigenous bacterial flora.

   a. Microbiology and pathogenesis. _E. coli_ are aerobic gram-negative rods found universally in the human intestinal tract and commonly in the human vagina and urinary tract. There are hundreds of different lipopolysaccharide (LPS), flagellar, and capsular antigenic types of _E. coli_, but EOS _E. coli_ infections, particularly those complicated by meningitis, are primarily due to strains with the K1-type polysaccharide capsule. _E. coli_ with the K1 antigen are resistant to the bacteriocidal effect of normal human serum; strains that possess both a complete LPS and K1 capsule have been shown to specifically evade both complement-mediated bacteriolysis and neutrophil-mediated killing. The K1 antigen has been shown to be a primary factor in the development of meningitis in a rat model of *E. coli* infection. The K1 capsule is a poor immunogen, however, and despite widespread carriage of this strain in the population, there is usually little protective maternal antibody available to the infant. In addition to the K1 antigen, surface fimbriae, or pili are have been associated with adherence to vaginal and uroepithelial surfaces and may also function as a virulence mechanism in EOS.

b. Treatment. As noted in the preceding text, when there is a strong clinical suspicion for sepsis in a critically ill infant, the possibility of ampicillin-resistant *E. coli* must be considered. The addition of a third-generation cephalosporin such as cefotaxime or ceftazidime is recommended in this setting. *E. coli* bacteremia should be treated with a total of 14 days of antibiotic according to the identified sensitivities. *E. coli* meningitis is treated with a 21-day course of cefotaxime (see Tables 23B.1 and 23B.2).

3. Listeria monocytogenes. Although uncommon, *L. monocytogenes* deserves special note due to its unique role in pregnancy. *L. monocytogenes* are gram-positive, β-hemolytic, motile bacteria that frequently cause disease in animals, and most commonly infect humans through the ingestion of contaminated food. These bacteria do not cause significant disease in immunocompetent adults, but can cause severe illness in the immunocompromised (i.e., renal transplant patients), in pregnant women and their fetuses, and in newborns. There is human epidemiologic evidence and evidence in animal models of listeriosis that indicate that *L. monocytogenes* is particularly virulent in pregnancy. The bacteria readily invades the placenta and can infect the developing fetus either by ascending infection, direct tissue invasion or hematogenous spread, causing spontaneous abortion or preterm labor and delivery, and often fulminant early-onset disease. Like GBS, *L. monocytogenes* can also cause late-onset neonatal infection, the pathogenesis of which is not fully understood. Over 90% of late-onset infections are complicated by meningitis.

The true incidence of listeriosis in pregnancy is difficult to determine because many cases are undiagnosed when they result in spontaneous abortion of the previable fetus. The incidence of EOS due to *L. monocytogenes* is often quoted as 13 cases per 100,000 live births; the incidence in the recent CDC active surveillance effort in Atlanta and San Francisco was 2.4 cases per 100,000 live births. Listeriosis can result from ingestion of contaminated food such as soft cheeses, deli meat, and hot dogs. Infection in pregnant woman may not be recognized, or may cause a mild febrile illness with or without gastrointestinal symptoms before resulting in pregnancy loss or preterm labor. Epidemic outbreaks of listerosis affecting both pregnant and nonpregnant adults are reported. Epidemic outbreaks in the United States in 2000 and 2002 were linked to turkey deli meat; an outbreak in 2001 linked to homemade, unpasteurized Mexican-style cheese resulted in five stillbirths, three premature deliveries, and two infected newborns among ten infected pregnant women.

a. Microbiology and pathogenesis. *L. monocytogenes* are distinguished from other gram-positive rods by tumbling motility that is most prominent at room temperature. The organisms can be gram-variable and depending on growth stage, can also appear coccilike, and can therefore be initially misdiagnosed on gram stain. *L. monocytogenes* is an intracellular pathogen that can invade cells as well as persist in phagocytic cells (monocytes, macrophages.) *Listeria* possess a variety of virulence factors, including surface proteins that promote cellular invasion, and enzymes (listeriolysin O, phospholipase) that enhance the ability of the organism to persist intracellularly. On pathologic examination of tissues infected with *Listeria*, miliary granulomas, and areas of necrosis and suppuration are seen. The liver is prominently involved. Both T-cell-mediated killing as well as immunoglobulin M (IgM)-complement-mediated killing are involved in host response to listeriosis. Deficiencies in both of these arms of the newborn immune system may contribute to the virulence of *L. monocytogenes* in the neonate; similarly, it is hypothesized that local downregulation of the immune response in the pregnant uterus may account for proliferation of the bacteria in the placenta.

b. Treatment. EOS due to *L. monocytogenes* is treated with ampicillin and gentamicin for 14 days; meningitis is treated for 21 days. *L. monocytogenes* is resistant to cephalosporins. In the case of meningitis, it is recommended that LPs be repeated daily until sterilization of the CSF is achieved. Additional therapy with rifampin or trimethoprim-sulfamethoxazole, as well as cerebral imaging is recommended if the organism persists in the CSF for longer than 2 days. We have noted that *L. monocytogenes* can persist in the stool of preterm infants even after adequate systemic treatment of the infection. Proper infection control measures must be observed to prevent nosocomial spread of the organism.

4. Other organisms responsible for EOS. Bacteria causing EOS vary with time and locality. Beyond GBS and *E. coli*, there are a number of pathogens that cause EOS in the United States in the era of IAP for GBS. Viridans streptococci (species such as *Streptococcus mitis, Streptococcus oralis, and Streptococcus sanguis*, which are part of the oral flora), Enterococci and *Staphylococcus aureus* are next in frequency. *Listeria*, a variety of gram-negative organisms (*Klebsiella, Hemophilus, Enterobacter, Pseudomonas* species) and the anaerobe *B. fragilis* cause most of the remaining infections. Gram-negative organisms, especially *Hemophilus influenzae* and *Klebsiella*, predominate in some Asian and South American countries.

J. LOS. Late-onset neonatal sepsis is defined as occurring from 8 to 90 days of life. Late-onset sepsis (LOS) can be divided into two distinct entities: disease occurring in otherwise healthy term infants in the community, and disease affecting premature infants in the NICU. The latter is often referred to as hospital-acquired sepsis, as the risk factors for LOS in premature infants are related to the necessities of their care (i.e., the presence of central lines) and the bacteria that cause LOS are often acquired in the NICU. For epidemiologic purposes, LOS infections occurring in VLBW infants in the NICU are defined as those occuring at >72 hours of life.

This section is primarily devoted to LOS in the NICU population, but disease in otherwise **healthy term and near-term infants** deserves mention. In these infants, LOS is largely caused by GBS and gram-negative species such as *E. coli* and *Klebsiella* species. Causes of bacteremia in older infants (such as *Streptococcus pneumoniae*, and *Neisseria meningititis*) occur less frequently. The **risk factors for late-onset GBS disease** are not as well defined as for early-onset disease, but like early-onset disease are related to colonization of the infant from maternal (or less commonly, hospital) sources and lack of maternally derived protective antibody. The use of IAP for GBS has had no significant impact on the rate of GBS LOS, remaining at approximately 0.3–0.5 cases per 1,000 live births from 1990–2004. The rate of GBS LOS actually exceeded that of EOS GBS for the first time in 2003. Preterm infants account for a disproportionate number of GBS late-onset infections; active surveillance by the CDC for 2004 revealed that 55% of late-onset GBS cases occurred in infants born at <37 weeks gestation. GBS LOS is more often complicated by meningitis that early-onset disease, and is predominantly caused by polysaccharide serotype III strains. Although mortality from GBS LOS is low (0%–9% in term and preterm infants, respectively), sequelae in survivors of GBS meningitis can be severe, ranging from hearing loss to severe global brain damage.

Gram-negative bacteremia is often associated with UTI. Different series report 20% to 30% of UTIs in infants under 1 month are complicated by bacteremia. Mortality is low if promptly treated, and sequelae are few unless meningitis occurs. *L. monocytogenes* can also cause late-onset disease, with onset commonly by 30 days of life, and can account for up to 20% of LOS in some centers. Late-onset listeriosis is frequently complicated by meningitis, but unlike late-onset GBS meningitis, the morbidity and long-term sequelae are infrequent if the disease is diagnosed and treated in timely fashion.

Term infants with LOS generally present with fever and/or poor feeding and lethargy to the private pediatrician or emergency department. Evaluation in the

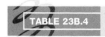

TABLE 23B.4	Risk Factors for Late-onset Sepsis in Infants with Birth Weight Less Than 1,500 g

Birth weight <750 g
Presence of central venous catheters (umbilical, percutaneous, and tunneled)
Delayed enteral feeding
Prolonged hyperalimentation
Mechanical ventilation
Complications of prematurity
Patent ductus arteriosus
Bronchopulmonary dysplasia
Necrotizing enterocolitis

Data from Stoll BJ, Hanson N, Fanaroff AA, et al. Late onset sepsis in very low birth weight neonates: The experience of the NICHD Neonatal Research Network. *Pediatrics* 2002;110(2): 285–291 and Makhoul IR, Sujov P, Smolkin T, et al. Epidemiologic, clinicial and microbiologic characteristics of late-onset sepsis among very low birth weight infants in Israel: A national survey. *Pediatrics* 2002;109(1): 34–39.

infant younger than 3 months old in most centers includes at minimium a CBC, urinalysis, CSF cell count, glucose and protein and cultures of blood, urine, and CSF. Infants under 1 month are generally hospitalized for empiric IV therapy that includes coverage for GBS, *Listeria*, and gram-negative organisms (commonly ampicillin and cefotaxime); over 1 month, management varies in different centers.

K. Epidemiology of LOS in premature infants. Most LOS occurs in the NICU among low-birth-weight infants. The National Institute of Child Health and Human Development (NICHD) Neonatal Research Network data from 1998–2000 revealed that 21% of their VLBW cohort had at least one episode of blood-culture-proven sepsis beyond 3 days of life. Overall mortality was 18% of infected infants versus 7% of uninfected infants. The mortality among infants with gram-negative infections was about 40%, and 30% with fungal infections.

L. Risk factors for LOS. A number of clinical factors are associated with an increased risk of LOS (Table 23B.4). The incidence of LOS is inversely related to BW. The risk of developing LOS associated with central catheters, hyperalimentation, and mechanical ventilation are all increased with longer duration of these therapies.

M. Microbiology of LOS. Nearly half of cases of LOS are caused by coagulase-negative staphylococci (CONS). In the NICHD study, 22% of cases of LOS were caused by other gram-positive organisms (*Staphylococcus aureus*, Enterococcus, GBS); 18% by gram-negative organisms (*E. coli, Klebsiella, Pseudomonas, Enterobacter, Serratia*), and 12% by fungal species (*Candida albicans* and *Candida parapsilosis*). The distribution of organisms causing LOS may vary significantly at individual centers. We reviewed cases of LOS occurring in the BWH's NICU from 1995–2004. Although the overall incidence of LOS among VLBW infants did not differ between the BWH and the NICHD network centers, the **distribution of pathogens** causing LOS in our population differs from that reported by the NICHD Network. These differences are primarily due to a higher incidence of *S. aureus* infections, and a lower incidence of fungal infections. Awareness of local variation in the microbiology of LOS is important in choosing empiric antibiotic therapy for the acutely infant in whom LOS is suspected.

  1. CONS. CONS are a heterogeneous group of gram-positive organisms with a structure similar to *S. aureus*, but these organisms lack protein A and have different cell wall components. *Staphylococcus epidermidis* is the primary cause of NICU disease. CONS universally colonize the skin of NICU patients. They are believed to cause bacteremia by first colonizing the surfaces of central catheters. A polysaccharide surface adhesin (PSA), as well as several other surface components have been implicated in adherence to and colonization of the catheter surface; subsequent biofilm and slime production inhibit the ability of the host to eliminate the organism. Most CONS are resistant to penicillin, semisynthetic penicillins, and gentamicin, and empiric treatment for LOS in the NICU usually includes vancomycin. CONS disease is rarely fatal even to the VLBW infant, and rarely if ever causes meningitis or site-specific disease. However, CONS disease can cause systemic instability resulting in temporary cessation of enteral feeding and/or escalation of ventilatory support, and is associated with prolonged hospitalization and poorer overall outcome.

2. **Staphylococcus aureus.** S. aureus is an encapsulated gram-positive organism that elaborates multiple adhesins, virulence-associated enzymes, and toxins to cause a wide range of serious disease, including bacteremia, meningitis, cellulitis, omphalitis, osteomyelitis, and arthritis. S. aureus is distinguished from CONS by the production of coagulase, and by the presence of protein A, a component of the cell wall that contributes to virulence by binding to the Fc portion of immunoglobulin G (IgG) antibody and blocking opsonization. LOS caused by S. aureus can be result in significant morbidity. Disease is frequently complicated by focal site infections (soft tissue, bone, and joint infections are commonly observed in neonates) and marked by persistent bacteremia despite antibiotic administration. Joint infections often require open surgical drainage and can lead to joint destruction and permanent disability. The treatment of methicillin-sensitive S. aureus (MSSA) requires the use of semisynthetic penicillins such as nafcillin or oxacillin.

Methicillin-resistant Staphylococcus aureus (MRSA) is an increasingly recognized pathogen in NICUs. Resistance to semi-synthetic penicillins is mediated by chromosomal acquisition of the mecA gene, found on different types of staphylococcal chromosomal cassette mec (SCCmec) elements. The mecA gene encodes a modified penicillin-binding protein (PBP) with a low affinity for methicillin. Once acquired, the modified PBP replaces similar proteins on the bacterial cell membrane and results in resistance to all β-lactam antibiotics. The recent emergence of MRSA infections in NICU's appears to track the increase in these infections in both general hospital settings and in the community. MRSA isolates can be grouped as hospital-acquired or community-acquired in origin. Uniform resistance to all common antibiotics except for vancomycin characterizes hospital-acquired isolates. Community-acquired isolates are usually resistant only to β-lactam antibiotics and erythromycin. Community-acquired isolates also differ in that they often carry distinct types of SCCmec elements and distinct virulence elements such as the Panton-Valentine leukocidin. Distinguishing between the two types of organisms can be important for determining the source of epidemic outbreaks of MRSA disease within individual units as well as for developing effective infection control measures. Whatever the source of the organism, however, it can be rapidly spread within the NICU by nosocomial transmission on the hands of caregivers. Infection control measures including identification of colonized infants by routine surveillance and cohorting and isolation of colonized infants may be required to prevent spread and persistence of the organism. MRSA infections usually require treatment with **vancomycin.** As with MSSA infections, MRSA infections can be complicated by deep-tissue involvement and persistent bacteremia that may require surgical debridement for resolution. Although it cannot be used as a single agent, rifampin can be a helpful adjunctive therapy for persistent MRSA infection. Consultation with an infectious diseases specialist is recommended regarding the utility of adding newer gram-positive antibiotics (the oxazolidinone antibiotic linezolid or the lipopeptide antibiotic daptomycin) to eradicate persistent MRSA bacteremia.

3. **Enterococci.** Formerly categorized as members of Group D Streptococci, both Enterococcus faecalis and Enterococcus faecium cause LOS in premature infants. These organisms are associated with indwelling catheters; they are encapsulated organisms that produce both biofilm and slime and can adhere to and persist on catheter surfaces as described in the preceding text for CONS. Although disease

can be complicated by meningitis and is sometimes associated with NEC, enterococcal LOS is associated with low overall mortality. Enterococci are resistant to cephalosporins and often resistant to penicillin G and ampicillin; treatment requires the synergistic effect of an aminoglycoside with ampicillin or vancomycin. Vancomycin-resistant enterococci (VRE) present a significant problem in adult intensive-care settings, and outbreaks have occurred in NICUs as well. VRE of *faecium* origin can be treated with Synercid (quinupristin/dalfopristin) but this combination is not effective against *E. faecalis*. VRE outbreaks may also require the institution of infection control measures (surveillance to identify colonized infants, isolation and cohorting of those colonized) to control spread and persistence of the organism.

4. **Gram negative organisms:** LOS caused by gram-negative organisms is complicated by a 40% mortality rate in the NICHD cohort. *E. coli* were discussed under EOS (see I.I.2).

   a. ***Pseuodomonas aeruginosa.*** Mortality associated with *P. aeruginosa* sepsis in low-birth-weight infants is high (76% in the NICHD cohort). A number of bacterial factors, including LPS, mucoid capsule, adhesins, invasins, and toxins (notably exotoxin A) contribute to its extreme virulence in premature infants as well as in debilitated adults and burn victims. Both LPS and the mucoid capsule help the organism avoid opsonization and secreted proteases inactivate complement, cytokines, and immunoglobulin. The lipid A moiety of LPS (endotoxin) causes the typical aspects of gram-negative septicemia (i.e., hypotension, DIC). Exotoxin A is antigenically distinct from diptheria toxin, but acts by the same mechanism: adenovirus death protein (ADP)-ribosylation of eukaryotic elongation factor 2 results in inhibition of protein synthesis and cell death. *P. aeruginosa* is present in the intestinal tract of approximately 5% of healthy adults, but colonizes premature infants at much higher rates due to nosocomial acquisition of the bacteria. Selection of the bacteria, likely due to the resistance of *Pseudomonas* to most common antibiotics, also plays a role in colonization; prolonged exposure to intravenous antibiotics is an identified risk factor for LOS with *Pseudomonas*. *Pseudomonas* can be found in environmental reservoirs in ICUs (i.e., sinks, respiratory equipment), and outbreaks of nosocomial disease have been linked to both environmental sources and spread by the hands of healthcare workers.

   Treatment requires a combination of two agents active against *Pseudomonas*, such as ceftazidime, piperacillin/tazobactam, gentamicin, or tobramycin. Generally a β-lactam–based antibiotic combined with an aminoglycoside is preferred; however, both extended-spectrum beta-lactamases (ESBL) and constitutive AmpC-type β-lactamases are emerging in Pseudomonal species (see subsequent text) and treatment must be guided by isolate antibiotic sensitivity testing. A survey of neonatologists' practices in the treatment of LOS reveals that the most common antibiotics empirically used are vancomycin and gentamicin. When an infant presents as severely ill, or when the infant becomes acutely sicker during or after standard antibiotic treatment, consideration should be given to empiric coverage for *Pseudomonas* until blood culture results are available.

   b. ***Enterobacter species:*** Like *E. coli*, *Enterobacter* species are LPS-containing, gram-negative rods that are normal constituents of colonic flora that can cause overwhelming sepsis in low-birth-weight infants. The most common isolates are *Enterobacter cloacae* and *Enterobacter aerogenes*. *Enterobacter sakazakii* has received publicity due to outbreaks of disease caused by contamination of powdered infant formulas with this organism. Since 1990, there have been multiple reports of increases in the proportion of LOS attributable to *Enterobacter*, and as well as epidemic outbreaks of cephalosporin-resistant *Enterobacter* in NICUs. *Enterobacter* species contain chromosomally encoded, inducible β-lactamases (AmpC-encoded cephalosporinases) and treatment with third-generation cephalosporins, even if the initial isolate appears to be sensitive, can result in the emergence of cephalosporin-resistant organisms. In addition, stably derepressed, high-level constitutive AmpC-producing strains of *Enterobacter, Citrobacter* and *Serratia* have been reported. The fourth-generation cephalosporin cefepime is relatively stable against AmpC-type β-lactamases. ESBL's, (discussed in the subsequent text) have also been reported in *Enterobacter* species. Given the increasing concern about cephalosporin resistance among infectious disease experts, cefepime or meropenem and gentamicin is usually recommended for treatment of infections caused by *Enterobacter* species. Infection control measures and restriction of cephalosporin use can be effective in controlling outbreaks of resistant organisms.

N. Symptoms and evaluation of LOS. The spectrum of symptoms in LOS ranges from a mild increase in apnea to fulminant sepsis. Lethargy, an increase in the number or severity of apneic spells, feeding intolerance, temperature instability, and/or an increase in ventilatory support all may be early signs of LOS—or may be part of the variability in the course of the VLBW infant. The difficulty in distinguishing between these two in part explains the frequency of evaluation for LOS; in the NICHD study, 62% of VLBW infants had at least one blood culture drawn after day of life 3. With mild symptoms and a low suspicion for the presence of sepsis, it is reasonable to draw a CBC with differential and a blood culture and wait for the results of the CBC (while monitoring the infant's symptoms closely) before beginning empiric antibiotic therapy. If the CBC is abnormal or the infant's status worsens, empiric antibiotic therapy should be started. If the suspicion for sepsis is still low, and/or the clinical impression is that a CONS infection is likely, it is not unreasonable to obtain a blood culture only. Ideally cultures of urine and CSF should also be obtained before antibiotic therapy, both to guide empiric therapy and to ensure proper follow-up (such as renal imaging if a UTI is present.) A recent study of late-onset infection in VLBW infants underscores the importance of **performing a LP in the evaluation of LOS** in this population. Two-thirds of a cohort of over 9,000 infants had one or more blood cultures drawn after 72 hours of life; one-third had a LP. Culture-proven meningitis was diagnosed in 134 infants (5% of those on whom a LP was performed) and in 45/134 cases, the coincident blood culture was negative.

If a previously well, convalescing premature infant presents primarily with increased apnea with or without UTI symptoms, consideration should be given to a viral source of infection as well. Tracheal or nasal aspirate should be sent for rapid analysis and culture to rule out respiratory syncytial virus (RSV), parainfluenze, and influenzae A and B if seasonally appropriate.

O. Treatment of LOS. Tables 23B.1 and 23B.2 list suggested antibiotic regimens for selected organisms. Note that for many antibiotics dosing is dependent on gestational and postnatal age (see also Appendix A). A recent study addressed the issue of **central line removal** in culture-proven LOS. This study demonstrated that bacteremic infants experience fewer complications of infection if central lines are removed promptly upon identification of a positive culture. This was particularly true for infections caused by *S. aureus* and gram-negative organisms.

ESBL's are plasmid-encoded bacterial enzymes that confer resistance to a variety of penicillins and cephalosporins. ESBL's are distinguished from the generally chromosomally encoded AmpC-type enzymes by sensitivity to clavulanate. Nosocomial gram-negative pathogens that commonly colonize and cause disease in VLBW infants (such as *E. coli, Enterobacter, Klebsiella, Pseudomonas and Serratia*) are increasingly found to harbor these resistance enzymes. ESBL organisms have become a significant problem in adult ICU's and since 2000, there have been multiple reports of outbreaks of ESBL-producing organisms in NICU's, primarily with ESBL-containing *Klebsiella* species. Risk factors for acquiring ESBL organisms include low gestational age and use of third-generation cephalosporins. Current recommendations to control outbreaks of these organisms include restriction of third-generation cephalosporin use and the same infection control measures (routine surveillance for colonization, cohorting and isolation of colonized infants) as are needed for control of MRSA. Treatment of ESBL infections should ideally include consultation with infectious diseases specialists; carbapenems, cefepime and piperacillin/tazobactam are currently most effective, with increasing rates of co-resistance reported for aminoglycosides and fluoroquinolones.

P. Prevention of LOS. In addition to significant mortality, LOS is associated with prolonged hospitalization and overall poorer outcome in VLBW infants compared to those that remain uninfected. A number of strategies to lower rates of LOS have been studied.

1. **IVIG.** Multiple studies have been conducted using prophylactic administration of IVIG to address the relative deficiency of immunoglobulin in low-birth-weight infants and prevent LOS. A meta-analysis of these 19 trials revealed that although the use of IVIG to prevent LOS resulted in a 3% to 4% decrease in LOS, IVIG was not associated with a decrease in mortality or other serious outcomes and is generally not recommended.

2. **GCSF.** GCSF has been shown to resolve preeclampsia–associated neutropenia, and may thereby decrease the rate of LOS in this population of infants. One trial of GM-CSF in premature neonates with the clinical diagnosis of early-onset disease did not improve mortality but was associated with acquiring fewer nosocomial infections over the subsequent 2 weeks.

3. **Antibiotic restriction.** Limitation of the use of broad-spectrum antibiotics in neonatal, pediatric and adult ICUs has been inconsistently associated with decreases rates of patient colonization with antibiotic-resistant organisms. This practice is reported to be successful in case reports of outbreaks of specific antibiotic-resistant organisms, but has failed in other reports to reduce overall acquisition of antibiotic-resistant organisms. **However, the widespread emergence of ESBL and AmpC-type β-lactamase resistance in nosocomial gram-negative pathogens has led to an increased awareness of the risk of empiric use of third-generation cephalosporins among infectious diseases experts.** Cycling of antibiotics used for empiric treatment has not been successful in preventing LOS. Some studies suggest that substitution of oxacillin for vancomycin in the empiric treatment of LOS is not likely to cause significant morbidity in VLBW infants because of the low virulence of the organism, and may decrease the acquisition and spread of VRE and other antibiotic-resistant organisms.

4. **Hygiene practices.** Reinforcement of hand-washing policies, use of waterless hand disinfectants, restriction of artificial fingernails and nail polish, and cohorting and isolation of patients colonized with resistant organisms, have all been reported to decrease the risk of LOS.

5. **Prophylactic vancomycin.** A meta-analysis of several trials of low-dose vancomycin administration to VLBW infants demonstrated that the administration of prophylactic vancomycin reduced the incidence of both total LOS and CONS-associated infections, but did not improve mortality or length of hospitalization. Prophylactic vancomycin IV lock solution has been studied with some success in decreasing CONS infection. Antibiotic-impregnated catheters are not currently available for VLBW infants. There is concern that widespread use of vancomycin in these ways will lead to the increased emergence of vancomycin-resistant organisms.

6. **Establishment of early enteral feedings** in VLBW infants may have the greatest effect on reducing LOS by reducing exposure to hyperalimentation and allowing for decreased use of central catheters. **Breast-milk** feeding may also help decrease nosocomial infection rates among VLBW infants, both by its numerous infection-protective properties (i.e., secretory immunoglobulin A [IgA], lactoferrin, lysozyme) and by aiding in the establishment of enteral feeds. A retrospective cohort study of 212 VLBW infants from a single center revealed lower rates of LOS in infants receiving breast milk (29%) versus infants receiving formula (47%).

7. Revised "**Guidelines for the Prevention of Intravascular Catheter-Related Infections**" were issued in 2002 and are available on the Internet at http:// pediatrics.aappublications.org/cgi/reprint/110/5/e51. These guidelines were

developed by an interdisciplinary working group including the American Academy of Pediatrics (AAP) and the CDC, and include specific recommendations for neonates. Topics addressed include: catheter insertion techniques; catheter and catheter site care; type and duration of use of IV administration sets and parenteral fluids; duration of use of umbilical catheters; indications for central catheter removal; use of prophylactic antiseptic and antimicrobial agents.

II. ANAEROBIC BACTERIAL INFECTIONS. Anaerobic bacteria comprise a significant portion of the oral, vaginal, and gastrointestinal flora. Although many anaerobes are of low virulence, a few anaerobic organisms can cause both EOS and LOS. These organisms include *B. fragilis, Peptostreptococcus,* and *Clostridia perfringens.* Necrotizing enterolitis and/or bowel perforation can be complicated by anaerobic sepsis alone or in a polymicrobial infection. In addition to bacteremia, *B. fragilis* can cause abdominal abscesses, meningitis, omphalitis, cellulitis at the site of fetal scalp monitors, endocarditis, osteomyelitis, and arthritis in the neonate.

A. Treatment of anaerobic infections. Bacteremia and/or meningitis are treated with intravenous antibiotics; abscesses and other focal infections often require surgical drainage. *B. fragilis* is a gram-negative rod, and although oral *Bacteroides* species are sensitive to penicillin, *B. fragilis* usually requires treatment with drugs such as metronidazole, chloramphenicol, clindamycin, cefoxitin, or imipenem. Occasional strains of *B. fragilis* are also resistant to clindamycin, cefoxitin and/or imipenem. Most other cephalosporins and vancomycin are ineffective against *B. fragilis.* *Peptostreptococcus* and *Clostridia* are gram-positive organisms that are sensitive to penicillin G. NEC and intestinal perforations are treated with ampicillin, gentamicin, and clindamycin to provide coverage for the spectrum of organisms that can complicate these illnesses.

B. Neonatal tetanus. This syndrome is caused by the effect of a neurotoxin produced by the anaerobic bacterium *Clostridium tetani.* Infection can occur by invasion of the umbilical cord due to unsanitary childbirth or cord care practices. It has historically been a significant cause of neonatal mortality in developing countries. An estimated 215,000 deaths due to neonatal tetanus occurred worldwide in 1998. The World Health Organization (WHO) set a 2005 neonatal tetanus worldwide elimination target. This has been achieved in many developing countries, but neonatal tetanus persists in remote and poverty-ridden regions, associated with lack of adequate maternal tetanus toxoid immunization and unsanitary delivery settings. This disease is virtually nonexistent in the United States. The last reported case of neonatal tetanus in the United States is from 1998, and was caused by the application of cosmetic clay to the umbilical stump of an infant born to an unvaccinated mother. Infected infants develop hypertonia and muscle spasms including trismus and consequent inability to feed. Treatment consists of the administration of tetanus toxoid (500 U IM) and penicillin G (100 to 300,000 U/kg/day for 10 to 14 days) as well as supportive care with mechanical ventilation, sedatives, and muscle relaxants. Neonatal tetanus does not result in immunity to tetanus and infants require standard tetanus immunizations after recovery.

III. FUNGAL INFECTIONS

A. Mucocutaneous candidiasis. Fungal infections in the well term infant are generally limited to mucocutaneous disease involving *C. albicans.* *Candida* species are normal commensal flora beyond the neonatal period and rarely cause serious disease in the immunocompetent host. Immaturity of host defenses and colonization with *Candida* before complete establishment of normal intestinal flora probably contribute to the pathogenicity of *Candida* in the neonate. Oral and gastrointestinal colonization with *Candida* occurs before the development of oral candidiasis (thrush) or diaper dermatitis. *Candida* can be acquired through the birth canal, or through the hands or breast of caretakers. Nosocomial transmission in the nursery setting has been documented, as has transmission from feeding bottles and pacifiers.

Oral candidiasis in the young infant is treated with a nonabsorbable oral antifungal medication, which has the advantages of little systemic toxicity and concomitant treatment of the intestinal tract. **Nystatin** oral suspension (100,000 U/mL) is standard treatment (1 mL is applied to each side of the mouth every 6 hours, for a minimum of 10 to 14 days). Ideally treatment is continued for several days after lesions resolve. **Gentian violet** (1%, applied once or twice) remains an approved and effective treatment for thrush, but it does not eliminate intestinal fungal colonization. This topical dye has fallen out of favor in the United States; it stains skin and clothing, can irritate the mucosa with prolonged use, and has been shown to be mutagenic *in vitro*. **Miconazole** oral gel (20 mg/g) is more effective than nystatin, but is not available in the United States. Systemic **fluconazole** is highly effective in treating chronic mucocutaneous candidiasis in the immunocompromised host. A 2002 pilot study demonstrated the superiority of oral fluconazole over nystatin suspension in curing thrush in otherwise healthy infants, but fluconazole is not currently approved for this use. Infants with chronic, severe thrush refractory to treatment should be evaluated for an underlying congenital or acquired immunodeficiency.

Oral candidiasis in the **breastfed infant** is often associated with superficial or ductal candidiasis in the mother's breast. Concurrent treatment of both the mother and infant is necessary to eliminate continual cross-infection. Breastfeeding of term infants can continue during treatment. Mothers with breast ductal candidiasis who are providing expressed breast milk for VLBW infants should be advised to withhold expressed milk until treatment has been instituted. Freezing does not eliminate *Candida* from expressed breast milk.

Candidal diaper dermatitis is effectively treated with topical agents such as 2% nystatin ointment, 2% miconazole ointment, or 1% clotrimazole cream. Concomitant treatment with oral nystatin to eliminate intestinal colonization is often recommended, but not well studied. It is reasonable to use simultaneous oral and topical therapy for refractory candidal diaper dermatitis.

B. Systemic candidiasis. Systemic candidiasis is a serious form of nosocomial infection in VLBW infants. Recent data on late-onset candidal sepsis from the NICHD Neonatal Research Network showed that 7% of a cohort of 4,579 infants with BW <1,000 g developed candidal sepsis or meningitis, primarily caused by *C. albicans* and *C. parapsilosis*. One-third of these infants died. Invasive candidiasis is associated with overall poorer neurodevelopmental outcomes and higher rates of threshold retinopathy of prematurity, compared to matched VLBW control infants. Gastrointestinal tract colonization of the low-birth-weight infants often precedes invasive infection, and **risk factors for colonization and invasive disease** are similar. The most significant epidemiologic factors specific to candidal LOS in the NICHD cohort were BW <1,000 g, delay in enteral feeding and exposure to third-generation cephalosporins. Other clinical factors include markers of illness severity such as 5-minute Apgar <5, shock, DIC and prolonged intubation, as well as the presence of central venous catheters and the need for parenteral nutrition and intralipid infusions. The use of H2-blockers or systemic steroids have also been identified as independent risk factors for the development of invasive fungal infection.

1. Microbiology. Disseminated candidiasis is primarily caused by *C. albicans* and *C. parapsilosis* in preterm infants, but infection with *Candida tropicalis, Candida lusitaniae*, and *Candida glabrata* and *Candida krusei* are reported in recent CDC surveillance data. The pathogenicity of *C. albicans* is associated with the variable production of a number of toxins, including an endotoxin. *C. albicans* can be acquired perinatally as well as postnatally. *C. parapsilosis* has emerged as the second most common cause of disseminated neonatal candidiasis in recent years. Studies suggest that *C. parapsilosis* is primarily a nosocomial pathogen, in that it is acquired at a later age than *C. albicans*, and is associated with colonization of healthcare workers' hands. In the recent NICHD study, fungal species (primarily *C. albicans* versus *C. parapsilosis*) did not independently predict death or later neurodevelopmental impairment, and a delay in removal of central catheters was associated with higher mortality rates from *Candida* LOS regardless of species.

2. Clinical manifestations. Candidiasis due to *in utero* infection can occur. Congenital cutaneous candidiasis can present with severe, widespread, and desquamating skin involvement. Pulmonary candidiasis can occur in isolation or with disseminated infection and presents as a severe pneumonia. Most cases of systemic candidiasis, however, present as LOS in VLBW infants, most often after the third week of life. The initial clinical features of **late-onset invasive candidiasis** are often nonspecific, and can include lethargy, increased apnea or need for increased ventilatory support, poor perfusion, feeding intolerance, and hyperglycemia. Hyperthermia can be present, an otherwise unusual sign of sepsis in the low-birth-weight infant. Both the total WBC and the differential can be normal early in the course of infection, and although thrombocytopenia is a consistent feature, it is not universally found at presentation. The clinical picture is initially difficult to distinguish from sepsis caused by CONS infection, and contrasts with the abrupt onset of septic shock that often accompanies LOS caused by gram-negative organisms. Candidemia can be complicated by meningitis and brain abscess, as well as end-organ involvement of the kidneys, heart, joints, and eyes (endopthalmitis). The fatality rate of disseminated candidiasis is high relative to that found in CONS infections, and increases in the presence of CNS involvement.

3. **Diagnosis.** *Candida* can be cultured from standard pediatric blood culture systems; the time to identification of a positive culture is usually by 48 hours, although late identification (beyond 72 hours) does occur more frequently than with bacterial species. Specialized fungal isolator tubes can aid in the identification of fungal infection if it is suspected by allowing for direct culture on selective media. Both fungal culture and fungal staining (KOH preparation) of urine obtained by suprapubic aspiration (SPA) can be helpful in making the diagnosis of systemic candidiasis. Specimens obtained by bag urine collection or bladder catheterization are difficult to interpret as they can be readily contaminated with colonizing species. We have obtained urine by SPA from VLBW infants under bedside ultrasound guidance for maximal safety. Before the initiation of antifungal therapy, CSF should be obtained for cell count and fungal culture.

4. **Treatment.** Systemic candidiasis is treated with **amphotericin B**, 0.5 to 1 mg/kg/day for durations of 7 to 14 days after a documented negative blood culture and for longer periods if specific end organ infection is present. All common strains of Candida other than *C. lusitaniae* are sensitive to amphotericin. This medication is associated with a variety of dose-dependent immediate and delayed toxicities in older children and adults and can cause phlebitis at the site of infusion. Febrile reactions to the infusion do not usually occur in the low-birth-weight infant (although renal and electrolyte disturbances can occur) and we start infants at the higher 1 mg/kg dose from the beginning of treatment. The medication is given slowly (over 4–6 hours) to minimize the risk of seizures and arrhythmias during the infusion. There is increased experience in VLBW babies with **liposomal preparations of amphotericin B** and we now use this formulation routinely for invasive candidiasis. Doses of 5 mg/kg/day can be used without toxicity, and the medication can be given over 2 hours with less irritation at the site of infusion. There are concerns that liposomal amphotericin is not effective in renal candidiasis. It is recommended that CNS disease be treated with an additional second agent, commonly **5'-fluorocytosine (flucytosine 5-FC) (100 to 150 mg/kg/day) or fluconazole (6 mg/kg/day).** Flucytosine achieves good CNS penetration, and appears to be safe in infants, but is only available for enteral administration, limiting its utility in sick VLBW infants. Bone marrow and liver toxicity has occurred in adults and correlates with elevated serum levels of the medication. Serum levels can be monitored (<100 μg/mL is desirable.) Fluconazole is safe for use in infants, and can be successfully used for primary treatment of candidemia. It should not be used as until candidal speciation is completed, because *C. krusei* and *C. glabrata* are frequently resistant to fluconazole.

   Removal of central catheters in place when candidemia is identified is essential to the eradication of the infection. Delayed catheter removal is associated with persistent candidemia and increased mortality.

Further evaluation of the infant with invasive candidiasis should include renal and brain ultrasonography to rule out fungal abscess formation and opthalmologic examination to rule out enopthalmitis. In infants who are persistently fungemic despite catheter removal and appropriate therapy, an echocardiogram to rule out endocarditis or vegetation formation is warranted.

5. **Prevention.** Minimizing use of broad-spectrum antibiotics (particularly cephalosporins) and H2-blockers may be helpful in preventing disseminated candidiasis. The CDC recommends changing infusions of lipid suspensions every 12 hours to minimize microbial contamination; solutions of parenteral nutrition and lipid mixtures should be changed every 24 hours. Three randomized trials and three retrospective cohort studies of prophylactic fluconazole administration to prevent invasive fungal infection in VLBW infants have been published since 2001. All the trials demonstrated decreased rates of colonization with fungal species, and most also demonstrated decreased rates of invasive fungal infection. The largest randomized trial of infants with BW <1,000 g demonstrated a 63% decrease in colonization and statistically significant decrease in invasive fungal disease (from 20% in placebo group to 0% in treatment group), with no adverse effects. A meta-analysis of the three randomized trials also revealed a reduced risk of death before hospital discharge in the fluconazole-treated group. Two other studies have attempted to achieve these same goals with more limited use of fluconazole. One study used compared twice-weekly use of fluconazole to a more frequent regimen, and another used fluconazole in VLBW infants only when they were treated with broad-spectrum antibiotic therapy for longer than three days. Both studies demonstrated decreased rates of fungal colonization and invasive fungal disease with these regimens. The widespread implementation of any fluconazole prophylaxis regimen, however, has been limited by concerns regarding the emergence of azole-resistant fungal species. It has been noted that when infants receiving prophylaxis do become colonized or develop invasive fungal disease, the isolates are more likely to be non-*albicans*, less fluconazole-sensitive *Candida* species. These risks must be balanced with the potentially severe consequences of invasive fungal infection (in the NICHD cohort, 73% of infants with LOS fungal sepsis died or survived with significant neurodevelopmental impairment) as well as the frequency of LOS fungal infection in an individual NICU in making a decision to implement a fluconazole prophylaxis policy.

C. **Malassezia furfur.** This organism is a lipophilic dermatophyte that readily colonizes infants in neonatal units, and is found in 30% to 60% of neonates over time. *M. furfur* requires exogenous long-chain fatty acids for growth and readily contaminates and proliferates in intravenous lipid preparations as well as the catheters used for administration of lipids. It causes a nonspecific sepsis syndrome. *M. furfur* grows poorly in standard pediatric blood culture bottles, but isolation is optimized by the addition of a lipid source to the bottles, or by the use of fungal isolator systems and the addition of sterile olive oil to the selective media. In most reported cases, removal of the contaminated central catheter results in cure; amphotericin B is effective when catheter removal alone does not resolve the fungemia.

IV. **FOCAL BACTERIAL INFECTIONS**

A. **Skin Infections.** The newborn may develop a variety of rashes associated with both systemic and focal bacterial disease. Responsible organisms include all of the usual causes of EOS (GBS, enteric gram-negative rods, and anaerobes) as well as gram-positive organisms that specifically colonize the skin—staphylococci and other streptococci. Colonization of the newborn skin occurs with organisms acquired from vaginal flora as well as from the environment. **Sepsis** can be accompanied by skin manifestations such as maculopapular rashes, erythema multiforme, and petechiae or purpura. **Localized infections** can arise in any site of traumatized skin: in the scalp at lesions caused by intrapartum fetal monitors or blood gas samples; in the penis and surrounding tissues due to circumcision; in the extremities at sites of venipuncture or IV placement; in the umbilical stump (omphalitis.) Generalized pustular skin infections can occur due to *S. aureus*, occasionally in epidemic fashion.

1. **Cellulitis** usually occurs at traumatized skin sites as noted in the preceding text. Localized erythema and/or drainage in a term infant (e.g., at a scalp electrode site) can be treated with careful washing and local antisepsis with antibiotic ointment (bacitracin or mupirocin ointment) and close monitoring. Cellulitis at sites of intravenous access or venipuncture in premature infants must be addressed in a more aggressive fashion due to the risk of local and systemic spread, particularly in the VLBW infant. If the premature infant with a localized cellulitis is well appearing, a CBC and blood culture should be obtained and intravenous antibiotics administered to provide coverage primarily for skin flora (i.e., oxacillin or nafcillin and gentamicin). If MRSA is a concern in a particular setting, vancomycin should be substituted for nafcillin. If blood cultures are negative, the infant can be treated for a total of 5 to 7 days with resolution of the cellulitis. If an organism grows from the blood culture, a LP should be performed to rule out meningitis and careful physical examination should be performed to rule out accompanying osteomyelitis or septic arthritis. Therapy is guided by the organism identified (see Tables 23B.1 and 23B.2).

2. **Pustulosis.** Infectious pustulosis is usually caused by *S. aureus* and must be distinguished from the benign neonatal rash erythema toxicum and transient pustular melanosis (see Chapter 34). The pustules are most commonly found in the axillae, groin, and periumbilical area; both erythema toxicum and transient pustular melanosis have a more generalized distribution. Lesions can be unroofed after cleansing in sterile fashion with betadine or 4% chlorhexidine, and contents aspirated and analyzed by gram stain and culture. Gram stain of infectious pustules will reveal neutrophils and gram-positive cocci, whereas Wright stain of erythema toxicum lesions will reveal predominantly eosinophils and no (or a few contaminating) organisms. Gram stain of transient pustular melanosis lesions will reveal neutrophils but no organisms. Cultures of the benign rashes will be sterile or grow contaminating organisms such as *S. epidermidis*. Treatment of pustulosis caused by *S. aureus* is tailored to the degree of involvement and condition of the infant. A few lesions in a healthy term infant may be treated with topical mupirocin and oral therapy with medications such as amoxicillin/clavulonate, dicloxacillin, or cephalexin. More extensive lesions, systemic illness, or pustulosis occuring in the premature infant requires intravenous therapy with nafcillin or oxacillin.

    Some strains of *S. aureus* produce toxins that can cause **bullous lesions or scalded skin syndrome.** The cutaneous changes are due to local and systemic spread of toxin. Although blood cultures may be negative, intravenous antibiotics should be given (nafcillin or oxacillin) until the progression of disease stops and skin lesions are healing.

    Pediatricians who diagnose infectious pustulosis in an infant under 2 weeks of age should report the case to the birth hospital; **epidemic outbreaks due to nosocomial acquistion in newborn nurseries** are often recognized in this way because the rash may not occur until after hospital discharge. When such outbreaks are recognized in the nursery or NICU, hospital infection control experts should be consulted. Appropriate steps may include surveillance cultures of staff members and newborns and cohorting of colonized infants.

3. **Omphalitis.** Omphalitis is characterized by erythema and/or induration of the periumbilical area with purulent discharge from the umbilical stump. The infection can progress to widespread abdominal wall cellulitis or necrotizing fasciitis; complications such as peritonitis, umbilical arteritis or phlebitis, hepatic vein thrombosis, and hepatic abscess have all been described. Responsible organisms include both gram-positive and gram-negative species. Treatment consists of a full sepsis evaluation (CBC, blood culture, LP) and empiric intravenous therapy with oxacillin or nafcillin and gentamicin. With serious disease progression, broader-spectrum gram-negative coverage with a cephalosporin or piperacillin/tazobactam should be considered. As noted in II.A, Treatment of Anaerobic Infections, invasion of the umbilical stump by *Clostridia tetani* under

conditions of poor sanitation can result in neonatal tetanus in the infant of an unimmunized mother.

B. Conjunctivitis (ophthalmia neonatorum). This condition refers to inflammation of the conjunctiva within the first month of life. Causative agents include topical medications (chemical conjunctivitis), bacteria, and herpes simplex viruses. Chemical conjunctivitis is most commonly seen with silver nitrate prophylaxis, requires no specific treatment, and usually resolves within 48 hours. Bacterial causes include *Neisseria gonorrhoeae*, and *Chlamydia trachomatis*, as well as staphylococci, streptococci, and gram-negative organisms. In the United States where routine birth prophylaxis against opthalmia neonatorum is practiced, the incidence of this disease is reported to be approximately 1.6%. In developing countries in the absence of prophylaxis, the incidence is 20% to 25% and remains a major cause of blindness.

1. **Prophylaxis against infectious conjunctivitis.** One percent silver nitrate solution (1 to 2 drops to each eye), 0.5% erythromycin opthlamic ointment (1-cm strip to each eye), and 2.5% povidone-iodine solution (1 drop to each eye) administered within 1 hour of birth are all effective in the prevention of opthalmia neonatorum. In a trial comparing the use of these three agents conducted in Kenya, povidone-iodine was shown to be slightly more effective against both *C. trachomatis* and other causes of infectious conjunctivitis, and equally effective against *N. gonorrhoeae* and *Staphylococcus aureus*. Povidone-iodine was associated with less noninfectious conjunctivitis and is less costly than the other two agents; in addition, this agent is not associated with the development of bacterial resistance. In our institution, where most mothers receive prenatal care and the incidences of chlamydia and gonorrhea are low, we use erythromycin ointment, primarily because the medication does not stain. Silver nitrate or povidone-iodine are the preferred agents in areas where the incidence of penicillinase-producing *N. gonorrhoeae* is high.

2. ***N. gonorrhoeae.*** Pregnant women should be screened for *N. gonorrhoeae* as part of routine prenatal care. High-risk women or women without prenatal care should be screened at delivery. If a mother is known to have untreated *N. gonorrhoeae* infection, the infant should receive **ceftriaxone 25 to 50 mg/kg IV or IM (not to exceed 125 mg) at birth.**

   Gonococcal conjunctivitis presents with chemosis, lid edema, and purulent exudate beginning 1 to 4 days after birth. Clouding of the cornea or panophthalmitis can occur. Gram stain and culture of conjunctival scrapings will confirm the diagnosis. The treatment of infants with uncomplicated gonococcal conjunctivitis requires only a single dose of ceftriaxone (25 to 50 mg/kg IV or IM, not to exceed 125 mg). Additional topical treatment is unnecessary. However, infants with gonococcal conjunctivitis should be hospitalized and screened for invasive disease (i.e., sepsis, meningitis, arthritis). Scalp abscesses can result from internal fetal monitoring. Treatment of these complications is ceftriaxone (25 to 50 mg/kg/day IV or IM q24 hours) or cefotaxime (25 mg/kg IV or IM q12 hour) for 7 to 14 days (10 to 14 days for meningitis). The infant and mother should be screened for coincident chlamydial infection.

3. ***C. trachomatis.*** Pregnant women should be screened for ***C. trachomatis*** as part of routine prenatal care. Prophylaxis for infants born to mothers with untreated chlamydial infection is not indicated. Chlamydial conjunctivitis is the most common identified cause of infectious conjunctivitis in the United States. It presents with variable degrees of inflammation, yellow discharge, and eyelid swelling 5 to 14 days after birth. Conjunctival scarring can occur, although the cornea is usually not involved. Examination of conjunctival scrapings for chlamydia by DNA probe testing is currently used for diagnosis of chlamydia at our institution. Direct fluorescent-antibody and enzyme-linked immunoassay (ELISA)-based detection methods are also available, but culture-based detection is technically involved and takes several days to complete. Chlamydial conjunctivitis is treated with oral **erythromycin base or ethylsuccinate 40 mg/kg/day divided into 4 doses for 14 days.** Topical treatment alone is not adequate, and is unnecessary when systemic therapy is given. An association of oral erythromycin therapy and

infantile hypertrophic pyloric stenosis has been reported in infants younger than 6 weeks. Infants should be monitored for this condition. The efficacy of treatment is approximately 80%, and infants must be evaluated for treatment failure and the need for a second course of treatment. Infants should also be evaluated for the concomitant presence of chlamydial pneumonia. The treatment for pneumonia is the same as for conjunctivitis, in addition to necessary supportive respiratory care.

4. Other bacterial conjunctivitis. Other causes are generally diagnosed by culture of eye exudate. *S. aureus, E. coli,* and *H. influenzae* can cause conjunctivitis that is usually easily treated with local ophthalmic ointments (erythromycin or gentamicin) without complication. Very severe cases caused by *H. influenzae* may require parenteral treatment and evaluation for sepsis and meningitis. *P. aeruginosa* can cause a rare and devastating form of conjunctivitis that requires parenteral treatment.

C. Pneumonia. The diagnosis of **neonatal pneumonia** is challenging. It is difficult to distinguish primary (occurring from birth) neonatal bacterial pneumonia clinically from sepsis with respiratory compromise, or radiographically from other causes of respiratory distress (hyaline membrane disease, retained fetal lung fluid, meconium aspiration, amniotic fluid aspiration). Persistent focal opacifications on chest radiograph due to neonatal pneumonia are uncommon and their presence should prompt some consideration of noninfectious causes of focal lung opacification (such as congenital cystic lesions or pulmonary sequestration). The causes of neonatal bacterial pneumonia are the same as for EOS, and antibiotic treatment is generally the same as for sepsis. The infant's baseline risk for infection, radiographic and laboratory studies, and most important, the clinical progression must all be taken into account when making the diagnosis of neonatal pneumonia.

The diagnosis of **nosocomial, or ventilator-associated pneumonia** in neonates who are ventilator-dependent due to chronic lung disease or other illness, is equally challenging. Culture of tracheal secretions in infants who are chronically ventilated can yield a variety of organisms, including all the causes of EOS and LOS as well as (often antibiotic-resistant) gram-negative organisms that are endemic within a particular NICU. A distinction must be made between colonization of the airway and true tracheitis or pneumonia. Culture results must be taken together with the infant's respiratory and systemic condition, as well as radiographic and laboratory studies when making the diagnosis of nosocomial pneumonia.

Ureaplasma urealyticum deserves mention with respect to chronically ventilated infants. This mycoplasmal organism frequently colonizes the vagina of pregnant women, and has been associated with chorioamnionitis, spontaneous abortion and premature delivery, and infection of the premature infant. Infection with *Ureaplasma* has been studied as a contributing factor to the development of chronic lung disease, but the role of the organism and the value of diagnosis and treatment is unclear. *Ureaplasma* requires special culture conditions and will grow within 2 to 5 days. It will not be identified on routine bacterial culture. It is sensitive to erythromycin, but is difficult to eradicate, and few data are available on the dosing, treatment duration, and efficacy of treatment when this organism is found in tracheal secretions. Only two small randomized trials of erythromycin treatment to prevent chronic lung disease have been published and neither demonstrated a change in the incidence or severity of bronchopulmonary dysplasia (BPD).

D. UTI. The incidence of UTIs in the first month of life is reported to range from 0.1% to 1%, but is perhaps higher in preterm infants. UTIs may occur secondary to bacteremia, or bacteremia may occur secondary to primary UTI. The incidence is higher in male infants than female infants. The most common causative organisms are gram-negative, such as *E. coli,* but enterococci can also cause UTI. Culture of urine is not routinely recommended as part of the evaluation for EOS, but is an essential part of the evaluation for LOS (see section I.N). The most common presenting symptoms in term and older preterm infants are fever, lethargy, and poor feeding; younger preterm infants will present as for LOS. Diagnosis is made by urinalysis and urine culture. Culture of urine obtained from a bag collection or diaper is of little value as it will commonly be contaminated with skin and fecal flora. Specimens should be obtained by bladder catheterization or SPA with sterile technique. Ultrasound guidance can be useful in performing SPA in the VLBW infant. Empiric treatment in term and preterm infants is as for LOS (see I.J); antibiotic choice and treatment duration is guided by blood, urine, and CSF culture results. If the urine culture **alone** is positive in a term infant, treatment is completed with oral therapy once the infant is afebrile. Treatment duration in the absence of a positive blood or CSF culture is 10 to 14 days. It is recommended that infants with UTI undergo renal ultrasound and vesicourethrocytogram (VCUG) imaging to identify any underlying anatomic or functional abnormalities (i.e., reflux) that may have contributed to the development of the UTI. Infants should receive UTI prophylaxis with amoxicillin (10 to 20 mg/kg once per day) after completing UTI treatment until imaging studies are performed.

E. Osteomyelitis and septic arthritis. These focal infections are rare in newborns, and may result from hematogenous seeding in the setting of bacteremia, or direct extension from a skin source of infection. The most common organisms are *S. aureus*, GBS, and gram-negative organisms including *Neisseria gonorrhoeae*. Symptoms include localized erythema, swelling, and apparent pain or lack of spontaneous movement of the involved extremity. The hip, knee, and wrist are commonly involved in septic arthritis, and the femur, humerus, tibia, radius, and maxilla are the most common bone sites of infection. The evaluation should be as for sepsis, including blood, urine, and CSF culture, and culture of any purulent skin lesions. Needle aspiration of an infected joint is sometimes possible, and plain film and ultrasound can aid in diagnosis. Empiric treatment is with nafcillin or oxacillin and gentamicin, and/or vancomycin if MRSA is a concern, and is later tailored to any identified organisms. Joint infections commonly require surgical drainage; material can be sent for gram stain and culture at surgery. Duration of therapy is 3 to 4 weeks. Significant disability can result from joint or growth plate damage.

Suggested Readings

Benjamin DK, Stoll BJ, Fanaroff AA, et al. Neonatal candidiasis among extremely low birth weight infants: Risk factors, mortality rates, and neurodevelopmental outcomes at 18 to 22 months. *Pediatrics* 2006;117(1):84–92.

Hyde TB, Hilger TM, Reingold A, et al. Trends in incidence and antimicrobial resistance of early-onset sepsis: Population-based surveillance in San Francisco and Atlanta. *Pediatrics* 2002;110(4):690–695.

Isenberg SJ, Apt L, Wood M. A controlled trial of povidone-iodine as prophylaxis against ophthalmia neonatorum. *N Engl J Med* 1995;332(9):562–566.

Kaufman D, Boyle R, Hazen KC, et al. Fluconazole prophylaxis against fungal colonization and infection in preterm infants. *N Engl J Med* 2001;345(23):1660–1666.

Moore MR, Schrag SJ, Schuchat A. Effects of intrapartum antimicrobial prophylaxis for prevention of group-B-streptococcal disease on the incidence and ecology of early-onset neonatal sepsis. *Lancet Infect Dis* 2003;3:201–213.

O'Grady NP, Alexander M, Dellinger EP, et al. Guidelines for the prevention of intravascular catheter-related infections. *Pediatrics* 2002;110(5):e51.

Stoll BJ, Hanson N, Fanaroff AA, et al. Late-onset sepsis in very low birth weight neonates: The experience of the NICHD Neonatal Research Network. *Pediatrics* 2002;110 (2 Pt 1):285–291.

TUBERCULOSIS

Jennifer L. Anderson, John P. Cloherty, and
Dara Brodsky

23 C

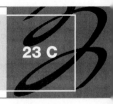

I. **INCIDENCE.** The World Health Organization (WHO) estimates that one-third of the world's population is infected by the acid-fast bacillus (AFB) *Mycobacterium tuberculosis* with 8 million new cases each year and 2 million deaths per year (1,2). Between 1985 and 1992, there was a 20% increase in the reported cases of **tuberculosis (TB)** in the United States (1). This increase was greatest in young adults and children and has been attributed to five factors: the human immunodeficiency virus (HIV) epidemic; recent immigration to the United States from areas with a high prevalence of TB; increased transmission in high-risk facilities (prisons, hospitals, nursing homes, and homeless shelters); development of multidrug-resistant TB; and the decrease in public health TB services (3).

Intensified strategic measures initiated in 1989 have steadily reduced the incidence of TB in the United States. Indeed, there were only 14,093 cases reported in the United States in 2005, the lowest recorded since reporting was initiated in 1953 (4). However, the Centers for Disease Control's (CDC) goal of eliminating TB from the United States by 2010 remains a challenge because of a deceleration in the decline of TB from 7.1% per year in 1993 to 2000 to 3.8% per year in 2001 to 2005 (4). In addition, the number of multidrug-resistant TB cases in the United States has increased to 13.3%, and there continues to be an increase in the number of TB cases among foreign-born persons (4–6). The increase in TB among foreign-born persons is due to increased immigration to the United States and emigration from countries with higher rates of TB (7).

The rate of decline of TB in the pediatric population has not been as significant as in adults (5). Indeed, foreign-born children younger than 5 years had the highest rate of TB between 1993 and 1998 among different age groups (5). Because the highest risk group for mortality from TB is patients <5 years of age, and untreated TB in the newborn is fatal in approximately 40% to 50% of cases, pediatricians and neonatologists should maintain a high index of suspicion for this disease.

II. **TRANSMISSION AND PATHOGENESIS.** TB is transmitted by respiratory droplet nuclei, which can remain suspended in the air for several hours. Under normal conditions, *M. tuberculosis* organisms are only transmissible from disease sites in the respiratory system: larynx, bronchi, and pulmonary interstitium. The risk of infectivity from pulmonary TB increases if the sputum smear is positive for AFB in addition to a positive culture; the chest radiograph shows pulmonary cavities; or there is a prolonged period of symptoms without treatment (8). Extrapulmonary TB can act as a source of transmission only rarely, which is related to medical/surgical procedures that create aerosols from infected tissue. One rare but critical exception is congenital transmission, which can arise from maternal bloodborne or occult genitourinary TB.

The **incubation stage** occurs after a person has become infected after exposure to a person with contagious pulmonary TB (3). Usually exposure has to be close (e.g., in an enclosed room) for an extended period (e.g., 1 day or more of cumulative exposure). After being inspired by a new host, the smaller respiratory droplets may travel to the alveoli, where they are ingested by alveolar macrophages; most bacilli are destroyed while the remaining bacilli multiply. Following cellular death, the organisms are released and can spread to the regional lymph nodes and the bloodstream. During this incubation stage, the tuberculin skin test with purified protein derivative (PPD) remains negative (if the person had not been previously sensitized), and the chest x-ray (CXR) is normal. As immunologic sensitivity to the mycobacteria builds, the skin test result is more likely to be positive, and within 8 weeks, sensitivity can be detected with the skin test in most newly infected individuals. Sensitivity to tuberculin may take longer to evolve in neonates and children (3). In all age groups, after the infection is established, the CXR may be normal or minimally abnormal, because of enlarged lymph nodes or focal infiltrates (3).

The initial infection can then progress directly to TB **disease**. The likelihood of direct progression to disease is increased by weakened cellular immunity (HIV infection, neonatal period, chronic high-dose steroid therapy, treatment with tumor necrosis α–inhibiting drugs, immunosuppression for preventing organ-transplant rejection). In any individual who has been recently infected, TB disease can emerge after a quiescent (latent) period. In approximately half of cases, this occurs within 2 years. Therefore, the treatment of latent infection is urged for those with infection within the prior 2 years, as demonstrated by diagnosis of infection after recent known exposure or by a skin test conversion. The disease can take decades to emerge, presumably after intercurrent declines in immunity (6). The reactivation of latent infection is more likely in individuals with specific underlying illnesses, for example, pneumosilicosis and diabetes. Although TB disease involves only the lungs in two-thirds of cases, it also can affect any organ system. Extrapulmonary manifestations of TB are more common in immunosuppressed patients and occur in 25% to 35% of infants and young children with disease (7).

III. **MATERNAL TUBERCULOSIS.** Clear distinctions must be made between latent tuberculosis infection (LTBI) and TB disease. The diagnosis, treatment, and health implications are different. LTBI is common in populations that are at risk of exposure, and it is not an immediate threat to the mother, the fetus or newborn, or the wider community. Diagnosing LTBI creates opportunities for preventing future TB disease, but this requires health care systems that can supervise treatment for LTBI. Public health departments can take this role, or they can provide consultation. In contrast with LTBI, TB disease is rare, but it is an immediate threat to the mother and the fetus or newborn, and it creates an infection-control hazard in the health care setting and the wider community.

A. **Latent tuberculosis infection**
  1. **Diagnosis (PPD).** There should be a low threshold for obtaining a PPD in pregnant women. Skin testing should be done on all pregnant women who are exposed to a person with TB; are immigrants from areas with a high incidence of TB; have increased susceptibility to TB because of HIV infection, diabetes, gastrectomy; live in a high prevalence area; or work in a profession with a high probability of exposure (9). Pregnancy does not alter the response to a tuberculin skin test, and there have been no adverse effects on women or their infants from tuberculin testing (3).

     A positive PPD reaction in an asymptomatic woman is the most common method of diagnosing TB infection during pregnancy in the United States. Forty-eight to 72 hours after placement of a PPD (5 units), a positive result is defined as follows:

     a. Induration ≥5 mm if the person is immunosuppressed (e.g., HIV seropositive), has close contact with person(s) who have infectious TB disease, or has radiographic fibrotic pulmonary lesions.

     b. Induration ≥10 mm if the person is an intravenous drug user, has an underlying medical disorder (including chronic renal failure, diabetes mellitus, malnutrition, leukemia, gastrectomy), is foreign-born from high TB prevalence area, resident of long-term facility or shelter, lives in a medically underserved region, or is a health care worker in high-risk areas.

     c. Induration ≥15 mm without risk factors (3,9).

     Whenever there is a positive reaction to PPD, it is essential to determine if it is due to a LTBI or TB disease. A complete history should be taken to assess for presence of clinical manifestations of TB disease. In addition, a CXR should be obtained (see III.B).

  2. **Treatment** (6,10,11). There is some debate about whether to treat **asymptomatic pregnant women who have a positive PPD, negative sputum, and normal CXR**. Because treatment with isoniazid (INH) is associated with hepatitis during pregnancy, some feel that therapy should be delayed until after delivery if the woman is immunocompetent, does not have a known TB exposure, and

is otherwise healthy. On the other hand, a pregnant woman who is a recent converter (within the last 2 years), has had recent contact with an infectious person, or is immunosuppressed (e.g., HIV seropositive) should receive INH and pyridoxine for 9 months beginning in the second trimester. TB disease must be excluded before undertaking treatment.

B. Tuberculosis disease

1. Diagnosis

   a. Chest radiography. If the tuberculin skin test is positive or there is clinical evidence of TB, a CXR should be obtained to determine if there is active disease. An abdominal shield is required to protect the fetus from the x-ray. Radiographic findings consistent with active disease include adenopathy, focal or multinodular infiltrates, cavitation, and decreased expansion of the upper lobes of the lung (9). Because radiographic findings may be normal despite TB disease, further evaluation (e.g., sputum cultures) is necessary if symptoms are present.

   b. Maternal signs and symptoms. The clinical manifestations of TB during pregnancy are identical to those in nonpregnant women. Although many women may be asymptomatic, possible symptoms include cough (74%), weight loss (41%), fever (30%), malaise and fatigue (30%), or hemoptysis (20%) (12). Malaise, fatigue, and vomiting can often be mistaken for other pregnancy-associated conditions. Extrapulmonary involvement can lead to mastitis, miliary TB, TB meningitis, and more commonly, involvement of the lymph nodes, bones, or kidneys.

   c. Culture. Any pregnant woman suspected of having TB (positive PPD reaction, suspicious or positive CXR and/or clinical manifestations), should have three early morning sputum samples obtained for acid-fast staining, culture (isolation can take up to 6 weeks), and susceptibility testing (7,12). Because 5% to 10% of pregnant women with TB exhibit extrapulmonary disease, a complete evaluation is essential, and if indicated, lymph node or liver biopsies should be obtained for staining and culture. A peritoneal fibrinous exudate at cesarean section or an infected placenta may assist in the diagnosis of TB in the mother and/or neonate. If there is evidence of active TB, close contacts should be tested for the disease.

2. Treatment (6,10,11) (see Fig. 23C.1).
If active TB is diagnosed during pregnancy (positive culture, clinical or radiographic evidence), prompt initial therapy with INH, rifampin (RIF), and ethambutol (EMB) is recommended. Pyridoxine (50 mg daily) is added to this regimen because of the increased requirement of this vitamin (B_6) during pregnancy and because it might help prevent INH-related neuropathy. The length of therapy of each drug is dependent upon the sensitivity results of the organism. If the bacilli are sensitive to INH and RIF, EMB should be discontinued and INH and RIF continued for 9 months. If the bacilli are sensitive to only one medication (INH or RIF), that drug and EMB are required for 12 to 18 months. If extrapulmonary manifestations are present, prolonged therapy may be warranted. All patients with active TB should be isolated in a room with an independent air-handling system and negative air pressure (13). Notify the local health department so that a contact investigation can be done.

    INH, RIF, and EMB appear to be relatively safe for the fetus, and the benefit of treatment outweighs the potential risk to the fetus. Although streptomycin (STREP) is often used to treat TB, it is contraindicated in pregnant women because it can cause ototoxicity in the fetus. There are no data on the effects of pyrazinamide (PZA) in pregnancy, so it should be avoided if possible. Consult an expert if a pregnant woman has multidrug-resistant TB and therefore requires treatment with medications that are usually contraindicated in pregnancy or have unknown fetal effects. Although anti-TB medications pass through breast milk, the amount transmitted is low and there is little effect on the neonate. For all patients with TB disease, supervision of treatment by the health department or direct observation of doses (DOT) is indicated.

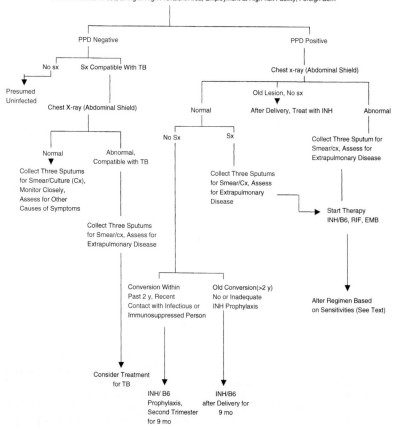

Figure 23C.1. Diagnosis and treatment of tuberculosis in the pregnant woman. PPD = purified protein derivative; TB = tuberculosis; HIV = human immunodeficiency virus; INH = isoniazid; RIF = rifampin; EMB = ethambutol. Data from refs. (3,8,9).

IV. TUBERCULOSIS OF THE FETUS OR NEWBORN

A. Pathogenesis (7,9,10,14). Although **congenital TB** is rare (~300 reported cases), it can be acquired in the following ways:

1. Hematogenous spread through the umbilical vein from an infected placenta to the fetal liver and lungs (can also involve the gastrointestinal tract, bone marrow, skin, or mesenteric nodes).

2. Aspiration or ingestion of infected amniotic fluid, *in utero* or at the time of birth, leading to primary infection in the lungs or gastrointestinal tract. Congenital TB is most often diagnosed in a neonate born to a mother with tuberculous endometritis or miliary TB.

The diagnosis of congenital TB requires the presence of TB lesions in the first week of life, primary hepatic lesions, maternal placental or genital TB, or exclusion of postnatal transmission after an extensive investigation. If none of these findings are present, the infection was probably acquired **postnatally** in the following ways:

a. Inhalation (most common) or ingestion of infected respiratory droplets.

b. Contamination of traumatized skin or mucous membranes.

B. Neonatal signs and symptoms (3). The clinical manifestations of TB in the neonate vary in relation to the duration, mechanism, and location of the infection in the infant. Although symptoms may be present at birth, they are more commonly observed in the second or third week of life. Clinical manifestations are often nonspecific and include hepatic and splenic enlargement (76%); respiratory distress (72%); fever (48%); lymphadenopathy (38%); abdominal distension (24%); lethargy and irritability (21%); ear discharge (17%); and skin papules (14%). In addition, apnea, failure to thrive, jaundice, and central nervous system signs can occur. Infection is more likely to disseminate in neonates compared with older children and adults.

Most infected infants will have an abnormal CXR (infiltrates or miliary pattern in 50%), and almost all infected infants will have an initial negative PPD. The PPD (5 units, 0.1 cc) is more likely to be positive (defined in children <4 years of age as ≥ 10 mm) if infection has been present for 4 to 6 months. Stains for AFB and cultures should be performed on blood, urine, three early morning gastric aspirates, tracheal aspirates, and cerebrospinal fluid (CSF). Abnormal liver function tests suggest disseminated disease. Tissue from lymph nodes, liver, lung, bone marrow, skin lesions, and the placenta may reveal organisms on pathologic examination and culture. Drug sensitivities should be performed on any organism grown from these cultures as well as organisms grown from maternal isolates. If all direct smears are negative and the infant is ill, antituberculosis therapy should be started until the diagnosis of TB is excluded. HIV testing should be done on all neonates with TB because the treatment regimen is longer for coinfection.

C. Management

1. Congenital TB (7,11) (see Table 23C.1). Neonates with suspected TB should have a tuberculin skin test, CXR, lumbar puncture, and cultures obtained as part of the initial management. In addition, the placenta should be cultured and examined histologically. Initiate treatment of the neonate with INH, RIF, PZA, and an aminoglycoside such as amikacin. This initial regimen provides broad coverage, because neonates are at greater risk of developing extrapulmonary TB (e.g., meningitis, miliary TB, bone and joint disease). If extrapulmonary TB is diagnosed, the infant should receive 2 months of this broad therapy followed by 7 to 10 months of INH and RIF. Corticosteroids should be added if TB meningitis is confirmed. If the infant has multidrug-resistant TB, a prolonged (12–18 months) four-drug regimen is often recommended in consultation with a TB specialist. Because the yield of culturing bacilli in the neonate is low, the clinician may need to rely on the mother's susceptibilities to determine treatment. In contrast with older children who have adequate pyridoxine levels, infants who are breast-feeding and receiving INH should be supplemented with pyridoxine owing to relatively low levels of this vitamin in breast milk. Consider isolating infants with congenital TB because they typically have a high inoculum of organisms in their tracheal aspirates (13). Consult a TB specialist during neonatal therapy.

2. Asymptomatic neonate, active infection in the mother (7,15). Assess the infant for clinical evidence of TB, place a PPD, obtain a CXR, send three gastric aspirates for smear and culture, perform a lumbar puncture, and examine the placenta for organisms. If there is evidence of neonatal disease, treat as in congenital TB (see IV.C.1); if there is no evidence of neonatal disease, the infant is at high risk and should receive INH daily. If the bacillus is INH resistant, give RIF for 6 months. If the bacilli is INH and RIF resistant, consult a specialist.

Continue INH therapy in the infant until the mother is culture negative for 3 to 4 months. At that time, if the neonate has a positive PPD without evidence of clinical or radiographic TB, continue INH for a total of 9 months (12 months if infant is HIV seropositive). In contrast, if the neonate has a negative PPD,

TABLE 23C.1 Commonly Used Medications for Treatment of TB Infection in Neonates and Children (11)

Drug	Activity	Dosage (mg/kg/d)	Side effects
Isoniazid (INH) Tablets (100 or 300 mg) (syrup unstable), also IM	Bactericidal	10–15 (or 20–30 mg/kg twice weekly)	Peripheral neuropathy, hepatotoxic, allergic reactivity
Rifampin (RIF) Capsules (150 or 300 mg) (syrup unstable), also IV	Bactericidal	10–20 (or 10–20 mg/kg twice weekly)	Orange discoloration of body fluids, hepatotoxic, vomiting, thrombocytopenia
Pyrazinamide (PZA) Tablets (500 mg)	Bactericidal	20–40 (or 50 mg/kg twice weekly)	Hepatotoxic, hyperuricemia
Streptomycin (STREP) 400 mg/mL in 2.5-mL vials	Bactericidal	20–40 IM (12 wk maximal use)	Ototoxic, nephrotoxic, rash Monitor renal function and hearing screens
Ethambutol (EMB) Tablets (100 or 400 mg)	Bacteriostatic, bactericidal (higher doses)	15–25 (or 50 mg/kg twice weekly)	Optic neuritis, allergic reactivity, gastrointestinal symptoms Monitor visual fields, acuity, and color discrimination.

INH can be discontinued if the mother is adherent and there is adequate clinical response to therapy. Repeat skin testing at 3 months and, if positive, reevaluate the infant for disease. In all scenarios, close clinical monitoring of the neonate is necessary.

As soon as a mother is diagnosed with active TB, notify the local health department, so that a contact investigation can be performed, and separate the infant from the mother. Once the infant is receiving chemotherapy, further isolation is not required unless the mother is severely ill, noncompliant, or has multidrug-resistant TB. When the infant and mother are reunited, breast-fed infants should receive pyridoxine.

3. **Asymptomatic neonate, mother with positive PPD and abnormal CXR** (11,15). Separate the infant and mother until the mother has been evaluated. If the mother has active TB, follow protocol as in IV.C.2. If the mother has inactive pulmonary disease, the infant is at low risk of infection and does not require therapy. If the mother has not been treated in the past, however, she requires therapy to prevent reactivation. Evaluate household members for TB. Closely monitor neonate with PPD (testing every 3 months for 1 year, yearly thereafter) and frequent clinical evaluations.

4. **Asymptomatic neonate, mother with positive PPD, negative sputum and normal CXR** (7,15). In this situation, the infant is not separated from the mother. Although the mother requires INH postpartum, the infant does not need therapy. Evaluate household members for TB. If disease cannot be excluded in household members, or if disease is found in the family, further skin testing is required in the neonate.

5. **Neonate with TB exposure in the nursery** (7). Although neonates exposed to TB in the nursery have a low risk for acquiring disease, infection can occur. If the exposure is considered to be significant, the infant should be skin tested and, even if negative, treated with INH for 3 months. The skin test should then be repeated; if it is still negative, therapy can be stopped. If the skin test is positive, the infant should be treated with INH for 9 months with close clinical monitoring. To prevent transmission of TB in the nursery, personnel should be skin tested yearly.

V. **BACILLUS CALMETTE-GUERIN (BCG)** (11,16). BCG is a live, attenuated vaccine prepared from *Mycobacterium bovis*. Although BCG vaccination has recently been shown to prevent serious forms of TB in children, its efficacy in the prevention of pulmonary disease in adolescents and adults remains uncertain. Although vaccination is currently used in more than 100 countries, the indications in the United States are limited to select groups that meet defined criteria: (i) infants and children (PPD-negative and HIV seronegative) with prolonged exposure to untreated, ineffectively treated contagious persons, or multidrug-resistant contagious persons if removal from the source is not possible; or (ii) nontuberculin reactors working in homeless shelters or health care facilities in high-risk multidrug-resistant TB areas (provided infection-control precautions have not been successful).

Before administering the BCG vaccine, consult a local TB specialist. When BCG is given, closely follow the instructions on the insert. Infants of age <2 months do not need tuberculin testing (unless congenital infection is suspected), whereas older children typically require a negative PPD before receiving BCG. Infants <30 days of age should receive one-half the recommended dose. If the indications for vaccination persist after 1 year of age, they should receive a full vaccine dose if their PPD is <5 mm. Preliminary data suggest that BCG may have minimal effectiveness in premature infants. Patients with burns or generalized skin infection should not receive BCG. In the United States, BCG is also contraindicated in HIV-infected persons, infants of HIV-infected mothers and persons receiving high-dose corticosteroids. Outside the United States, the WHO recommends that asymptomatic HIV-infected children living in areas with a high incidence of TB should receive BCG. Owing to the unknown effects of BCG on the fetus, the vaccine is not recommended during pregnancy.

Following BCG vaccination, pustular formation often occurs at the injection site within 3 weeks and often leads to a permanent scar. Other complications are infrequent but may include ulceration at the injection site, lymphadenitis, and possible osteitis; disseminated BCG may occur in severely immunodeficient patients. Adverse reactions can be treated with anti-TB medications in consultation with a TB expert. Report all adverse reactions to the manufacturer.

It is recommended that tuberculin reactivity following BCG vaccination should be documented. Initial testing should be performed 3 months after injection and induration size should be documented. In the future, if the PPD induration increases ($\geq$10 mm if <35 years of age; $\geq$15 mm if $\geq$35 years of age), newly acquired TB infection should be suspected. Although BCG administration may limit the future diagnostic utility of the PPD, studies have shown that most children who receive BCG in infancy have a negative PPD at 5 years of age.

 ## ACKNOWLEDGMENTS

The authors would like to thank John A. Jereb, MD, FAAP (Division of Tuberculosis Elimination, Centers for Disease Control and Prevention) for his critical review of this manuscript.

References

1. Small PM, Fujwara PI. Management of TB in the US. *N Engl J Med* 2001;345(3):189.
2. Dye C, Scheele S, Dolin P, et al. Global burden of tuberculosis. *JAMA* 1999;282:677.
3. Starke JR. Tuberculosis. *Clin Perinatol* 1997;24(1):107.
4. Centers for Disease Control and Prevention. Trends in tuberculosis—united states, 2005. *Morb Mortal Wkly Rep*, 2006;55(11):305–308.
5. Talbot ET, Moore M, McCray E, et al. Tuberculosis among foreign-born persons in the US, 1993–1998. *JAMA* 2000;284(22):2894.
6. Centers for Disease Control and Prevention. Core curriculum on TB. Available at: http://www.cdc.gov/nchstp/tb/pubs/corecurr/. Accessed 2006.
7. Starke JR, Smith MD. Tuberculosis. In: Remington JS, Klein JO, eds. *Infectious diseases of the fetus and newborn infant*, 5th ed. Philadelphia: WB Saunders, 2001.
8. Abernathy RS. Tuberculosis: An update. *Pediatr Rev* 1997;18(2):50.
9. Riley L. Pneumonia and TB in pregnancy. *Infect Dis Clin North Am* 1997;11(1):119.
10. Laibl VR, Sheffield JS. Tuberculosis in pregnancy. *Clin Perinatol* 2005;32:739–747.
11. American Academy of Pediatrics. Tuberculosis. In: Pickering LK, ed. *2006 Red book: Report of the committee on infectious diseases*, 27th ed. Elk Grove Village: American Academy of Pediatrics, 2006:678.
12. Jacobs RF, Abernathy RS. Management of TB in pregnancy and the newborn. *Clin Perinatol* 1988;15(2):305.
13. Guidelines for preventing the transmission of mycobacterium tuberculosis in heath-care settings, 2005 (www.cdc.gov/nchstp/tb/Federal_Register/New_Guidelines/TBICGuidelines.pdf). Accessed 2005.
14. Cantwell MF, Shehab ZM, Costello AM, et al. Congenital tuberculosis. *N Engl J Med* 1994;330(15):1051.
15. Mallory MD, Jacobs RF, Congenital tuberculosis. *Semin Pediatr Infect Dis* 1999;10(3):177.
16. Centers for Disease Control and Prevention. The role of BCG vaccine in the prevention and control of TB in the US. *Morb Mortal Wkly Rep* 1996;45(RR-4):1–18.

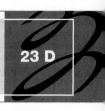

SYPHILIS
Louis Vernacchio

23 D

I. PATHOPHYSIOLOGY

A. Acquired syphilis is a sexually transmitted infection caused by the spirochete *Treponema pallidum*. The incubation period is typically about 3 weeks but could range from 9 to 90 days. The disease has three clinically recognizable stages.

1. **Primary syphilis** is manifest by one or more chancres (painless indurated ulcers) at the site of inoculation, typically the genitalia, anus, or mouth. It is often accompanied by regional lymphadenopathy.

2. **Secondary syphilis** occurs 3 to 6 weeks after the appearance of the chancre, often after the chancre has resolved. The secondary stage is characterized by a polymorphic rash, most commonly maculopapular, generalized, and involving the palms and soles. Sore throat, fever, headache, diffuse lymphadenopathy, myalgias, arthralgias, alopecia, condylomata lata, and mucous membrane plaques may also be present. The symptoms resolve without treatment. Some patients develop recurrences of the manifestations of secondary syphilis.

3. **Latent syphilis** is defined as those periods of time with no clinical symptoms but positive serologic evidence of infection. A variable latent period usually follows the manifestations of secondary syphilis, sometimes interrupted by recurrences of the secondary symptoms.

4. **Tertiary syphilis** usually occurs 4 to 12 years after the secondary stage and is characterized by gummata—nonprogressive, localized lesions that may occur in the skin, bones, or viscera. These lesions are thought to be due to a pronounced immunologic reaction. The tertiary stage can also be marked by cardiovascular syphilis, especially inflammation of the great vessels.

5. **Neurosyphilis** may occur at any stage of the disease. Early manifestations include meningitis and neurovascular disease. Late manifestations include dementia, posterior column disease (tabes dorsalis), and seizures, among others.

B. Congenital syphilis results from transplacental passage of *T. pallidum*. The risk of transmission to the fetus correlates largely with the duration of maternal infection—the more recent the maternal infection, the more likely transmission to the fetus will occur. During the primary and secondary stages of syphilis, the likelihood of transmission from an untreated women to her fetus is extremely high, approaching 100%. After the secondary stage, the likelihood of transmission to the fetus declines steadily until it reaches approximately 10% to 30% in late latency. Transplacental transmission of *T. pallidum* can occur throughout pregnancy.

Congenital infection may result in stillbirth, hydrops fetalis, or premature delivery. Most affected infants will be asymptomatic at birth, but clinical signs usually develop within the first 3 months of life. The most common signs of early congenital syphilis include hepatomegaly, skeletal abnormalities (osteochondritis, periostitis, pseudoparalysis), skin and mucocutaneous lesions, jaundice, pneumonia, splenomegaly, anemia, and watery nasal discharge (snuffles). If untreated, late manifestations appear after 2 years of age and may include neurosyphilis, bony changes (frontal bossing, short maxilla, high palatal arch, Hutchinson teeth, saddle nose), interstitial keratitis, and eighth nerve deafness, among others.

II. EPIDEMIOLOGY.

The incidence of primary and secondary syphilis in the United States, which had increased significantly throughout the 1980s and early 1990s, underwent a dramatic decline to a historic low of 2.1 cases per 100,000 population in 2000. Since then, the infection rate has risen somewhat to 2.7/100,000, although this rise has been largely due to an increase among men who have sex with men. The syphilis rate among women has continued to decline, to a rate of 0.8/100,000 in 2004. The incidence of syphilis is significantly higher in African Americans (9.0/100,000 in 2004), in urban areas, and in the Southern United States.

Along with the decreasing incidence of primary and secondary syphilis among women, the number of cases of congenital syphilis in the United States has declined from a recent high of 4,410 cases reported to the Centers for Disease Control and Prevention (CDC) in 1991 to 353 cases in 2004 (8.8 cases per 100,000 live births).

The most important risk factors for congenital syphilis are lack of prenatal health care and maternal illicit drug use, particularly cocaine use. Clinical scenarios that contribute to the occurrence of congenital syphilis include lack of prenatal care; no serologic test for syphilis (STS) performed during pregnancy; a negative STS in the first trimester, without repeat test later in pregnancy; a negative maternal STS around the time of delivery in a woman who was recently infected with syphilis but had not converted her STS yet; laboratory error in reporting STS results; delay in treatment of a pregnant woman identified as having syphilis; and failure of treatment in an infected pregnant woman.

III. DIAGNOSIS OF SYPHILIS

A. Serologic tests for syphilis

1. **Nontreponemal tests** include the rapid plasma reagin (RPR) test, the venereal disease research laboratory (VDRL) test, and the automated reagin test (ART). These tests measure antibodies directed against a cardiolipin-lecithin-cholesterol antigen from *T. pallidum* and/or its interaction with host tissues. These antibodies give quantitative results, are helpful indicators of disease activity, and are useful for follow-up after treatment. Titers usually rise with each new infection and fall after effective treatment. A sustained fourfold decrease in titer of the nontreponemal test with treatment demonstrates adequate therapy; a similar increase after treatment suggests reinfection.

   Nontreponemal tests will be positive in approximately 75% of cases of primary syphilis, nearly 100% of cases of secondary syphilis, and 75% of cases of latent and tertiary syphilis. In secondary syphilis, the RPR or VDRL test result is usually positive in a titer >1:16. In the first attack of primary syphilis, the RPR or VDRL test will usually become nonreactive 1 year after treatment whereas in secondary syphilis the test will usually become nonreactive approximately 2 years after treatment. In latent or tertiary syphilis, the RPR or VDRL test may become nonreactive 4 or 5 years after treatment, or may never turn completely nonreactive. A notable cause of false-negative nontreponemal tests is the prozone phenomenon, a negative or weakly positive reaction that occurs with very high antibody concentrations. In this case, dilution of the serum will result in a positive test.

   In 1% of cases, a positive RPR or VDRL result is not caused by syphilis. This has been called a *biologic false-positive (BFP) reaction* and is probably related to tissue damage from various causes. Acute BFPs, which usually resolve in approximately 6 months, may be caused by certain viral infections (particularly infectious mononucleosis, hepatitis, measles, and varicella), endocarditis, intravenous drug abuse, and mycoplasma or protozoa infections. Rarely, BFPs are seen as a result of pregnancy alone. Patients with BFPs usually have low titers (1:8 or less) and nonreactive treponemal tests. Chronic BFPs may be seen in chronic hepatitis, cirrhosis, tuberculosis, extreme old age, malignancy (if associated with excess gamma globulin), connective tissue disease, or autoimmune disease. Patients with systemic lupus erythematosus may have a positive RPR or VDRL test result. The titer is usually 1:8 or less.

2. **Treponemal tests** include the fluorescent treponemal antibody absorption test (FTA-ABS) and the *Treponema pallidum* particle agglutination (TP-PA) test. Although these tests are more specific than nontreponemal tests, they are also more expensive and labor-intensive and are therefore not used for screening. Rather, they are used to confirm positive nontreponemal tests. The treponemal tests correlate poorly with disease activity and usually remain positive for life, even after successful therapy, and therefore should not be used to assess treatment response.

False-positive treponemal tests occur occasionally, particularly in other spirochetal diseases such as Lyme disease, yaws, pinta, leptospirosis, and rat-bite fever; nontreponemal tests should be negative in these situations. Also, in some cases where antibodies to DNA are present, such as in systemic lupus erythematosus, rheumatoid arthritis, polyarteritis, and other autoimmune diseases, a false-positive FTA-ABS test result may occur. Rarely, pregnancy itself will cause a false-positive treponemal test.

B. Cerebrospinal fluid (CSF) testing for neurosyphilis should be done using VDRL test. A cell count and protein concentration should also be performed. A positive CSF VDRL test result is diagnostic of neurosyphilis, but a negative CSF VDRL test result does not exclude neurosyphilis. The FTA-ABS test is recommended by some experts for CSF testing because it is more sensitive than the VDRL test; however, contamination with blood during the lumbar puncture may result in a false-positive CSF FTA-ABS test result. A negative CSF FTA-ABS test result is good evidence against neurosyphilis. The RPR test should not be used for CSF testing.

C. New tests under investigation for the diagnosis of syphilis include the following:

1. FTA-ABS 19S Immunoglobulin M (IgM) test. This test detects antitreponemal IgM antibodies. Because IgM does not cross the placenta, a positive test in newborn serum should indicate congenital syphilis. This test represents an advance over previous antitreponemal IgM tests that were very nonspecific; however, because of continued problems with diagnostic accuracy, it is not currently recommended for clinical use.

2. Polymerase chain reaction (PCR). PCR can detect the presence of the *T. pallidum* genome in a clinical specimen, and therefore should be helpful in diagnosing congenital syphilis and neurosyphilis. PCR is not yet widely available for clinical use but may become more so in the near future.

IV. SCREENING AND TREATMENT OF PREGNANT WOMEN FOR SYPHILIS

A. All pregnant women should be screened for syphilis with a nontreponemal STS. Testing should be performed at the first prenatal visit and, in high-risk populations, should also be repeated at 28 to 32 weeks' gestation and at delivery. When a woman presents in labor with no history of prenatal care or if results of previous testing are unkown, an STS should be performed at delivery and the infant should not be discharged from the hospital until the test results are known. In women at very high risk, consideration should be given to a repeat STS 1 month postpartum to capture the rare patient who was infected just before delivery but had not yet seroconverted. All positive nontreponemal STS in pregnant women should be confirmed with a treponemal test.

B. Pregnant women with a reactive nontreponemal STS confirmed by a reactive treponemal STS should be treated unless previous adequate treatment is clearly documented and follow-up nontreponemal titers have declined at least fourfold. Treatment depends on the stage of infection:

1. Primary and secondary syphilis. Benzathine penicillin G 2.4 million units IM in a single dose. Some experts recommend a second dose of 2.4 million units IM 1 week after the first dose.

2. Early latent syphilis (without neurosyphilis). Treatment is the same as in primary and secondary syphilis.

3. Late latent syphilis over 1-year duration or syphilis of unknown duration (without neurosyphilis). Benzathine penicillin G in a total dose of 7.2 million units given as 2.4 million units IM weekly for 3 weeks.

4. Tertiary syphilis (without neurosyphilis). Benzathine penicillin G in a total dose of 7.2 million units given as 2.4 million units IM weekly for 3 weeks.

5. Neurosyphilis. Aqueous crystalline penicillin G 18 to 24 million units daily administered as 3 to 4 million units IV every 4 hours for 10 to 14 days. If compliance can be assured, an alternative regimen of procaine penicillin 2.4 million units IM daily plus probenecid 500 mg orally 4 times a day for 10 to 14 days may be used. At the end of these therapies, some experts recommend benzathine penicillin G 2.4 million units IM weekly for up to 3 weeks.

6. Penicillin-allergic patients. There are no proven alternatives to penicillin for the prevention of congenital syphilis. If an infected pregnant woman has a history of penicillin allergy, she should be skin-tested against the major and minor penicillin determinants. If these test results are negative, penicillin may be given under medical supervision. If the test results are positive, the patient should be desensitized and then given penicillin. Desensitization should be done in consultation with an expert and in a facility where emergency treatment is available.

7. **Human immunodeficiency virus (HIV)-infected pregnant women** receive the same treatment as HIV-negative pregnant women, except that treatment for primary and secondary syphilis and early latent syphilis may be extended to three weekly doses of benzathine penicillin G 2.4 million units IM per week.

8. **The Jarisch-Herxheimer reaction**—the occurrence of fever, chills, headache, myalgias, and exacerbation of cutaneous lesions—may occur after treatment of pregnant women for syphilis. Fetal distress, premature labor, and stillbirth are rare but possible. Patients should be made aware of the possibility of such reactions, but concern about such complications should not delay treatment.

9. If a mother is treated for syphilis in pregnancy, **monthly follow-up should be provided.** A sustained fourfold decrease in nontreponemal titer should be seen with successful treatment. All patients with syphilis should be evaluated for other sexually transmitted diseases, such as chlamydia, gonorrhea, hepatitis B, and HIV.

V. EVALUATION AND TREATMENT OF INFANTS FOR CONGENITAL SYPHILIS. No newborn should be discharged from the hospital until the mother's serologic syphilis status is known. Screening of newborn serum or cord blood in place of screening maternal blood is not recommended because of potential false-negative results.

A. Any infant born to a mother with a reactive nontreponemal test confirmed by a treponemal test should be evaluated with the following:

1. **Complete physical examination** looking for evidence of congenital syphilis (see I.B).

2. **Quantitative nontreponemal test (RPR or VDRL).** This test should be performed on infant serum, not on cord blood because of potential false-negatives and false-positives. Because immunoglobulin G (IgG) is readily transported across the placenta, the infant's serum RPR or VDRL test result will be positive even if the infection was not transmitted. The infant's titer should begin to fall by 3 months and become nonreactive by 6 months if the antibody is passively acquired. If the baby was infected, the titer will not fall and may rise. The tests may be negative at birth if the infection was acquired late in pregnancy. In this case, repeating the test later will confirm the diagnosis.

3. **Pathologic examination** of the placenta or umbilical cord using specific fluorescent antitreponemal antibody staining, if available.

4. **Darkfield microscopic examination** of direct fluorescent antibody staining of any suspicious lesions or body fluids (e.g., nasal discharge).

B. The CDC recommends classifying infants evaluated for congenital syphilis into one of the following four scenarios:

1. **Scenario one**

a. **Any** of the following is evidence of **proven or highly probable disease:**

i. **Abnormal physical examination** consistent with congenital syphilis.

ii. **Nontreponemal titer** that is **fourfold higher** than the mother's titer (**note** that the absence of a fourfold or greater titer does not exclude congenital syphilis).

iii. **Positive darkfield** or **fluorescent antibody test** of body fluid(s).

b. Further evaluation of infants with proven or highly probable disease should include the following:

i. **CSF analysis for VDRL, cell count, and protein concentration.** Note that, in the neonatal period, interpretation of CSF values may be difficult. Normal values of protein and white blood cells (WBC) are higher in preterm infants. Values up to 25 WBC/mm^3 and 150 mg protein/dL may be normal (Table 36.1).

ii. **Complete blood count (CBC)** with differential and platelet count.

      iii. Other tests as clinically indicated, including long-bone radiographs, chest radiograph, liver function tests, cranial ultrasonography, ophthalmologic examination, and auditory brainstem responses.

  c. Treatment for infants with proven or highly probable disease should consist of either of the following:

      i. Aqueous crystalline penicillin G 100,000 to 150,000 units/kg/day IV, administered as 50,000 units/kg/dose IV every 12 hours during the first 7 days of life and every 8 hours thereafter for a toal of 10 days.

      ii. Procaine penicillin G 50,000 units/kg/dose IM daily in a single dose for 10 days.

2. Scenario two

  a. Infants who have a normal physical examination and a serum quantitative nontreponemal titer the same or less than fourfold the maternal titer and **any of** the following:

      i. Maternal treatment not given, inadequate, or not documented.

      ii. Maternal treatment with erythromycin or any other **nonpenicillin** regimen.

      iii. Maternal treatment administered **<4 weeks before delivery.**

  b. Such infants should be evaluated with the following:

      i. CSF analysis for VDRL, cell count, and protein concentration.

      ii. CBC with differential and platelet count.

      iii. Long-bone radiographs.

  c. Treatment of such infants should consist of one of the following:

      i. Aqueous crystalline penicillin G 100,000 to 150,000 units/kg/day IV, administered as 50,000 units/kg/dose IV every 12 hours during the first 7 days of life and every 8 hours thereafter for a total of 10 days.

      ii. Procaine penicillin G 50,000 units/kg/dose IM daily in a single dose for 10 days.

      iii. If the complete evaluation is normal (CBC with differential and platelets, CSF analysis with VDRL, cell count, and protein concentration, and long-bone radiographs) and follow-up is certain, **a single dose of benzathine penicillin G** 50,000 units/kg IM **may be substituted for the full 10-day course.** If any part of the evaluation is abnormal or not interpretable (e.g., CSF sample contaminated with blood), or if follow-up is not certain, then the full 10-day course of parenteral therapy should be given.

3. Scenario three

  a. Infants who have a normal physical examination and a serum quantitative nontreponemal titer the same as or less than fourfold the maternal titer and **all of** the following:

      i. Maternal treatment during pregnancy with a penicillin regimen appropriate for the stage of infection, and >4 weeks before delivery.

      ii. No evidence of maternal reinfection or relapse

  b. Such infants require no further evaluation

  c. Such infants should be treated with a **single dose of benzathine penicillin G** 50,000 units/kg IM.

4. Scenario four

  a. Infants who have a normal physical examination and a serum quantitative nontreponemal titer the same as or less than fourfold the maternal titer and **both of** the following:

      i. Adequate maternal treatment before pregnancy

      ii. Maternal nontreponemal titer remained low and stable before and during pregnancy and at delivery (VDRL ≤1:2 or RPR ≤1:4).

  b. Such infants require no further evaluation

  c. No treatment is required; however some experts recommend a single dose of benzathine penicillin G 50,000 units/kg IM, particularly if follow-up is uncertain.

C. Evaluation and treatment of infants and children **older than 1 month**.

Children identified as having a reactive STS after the neonatal period should have maternal serology and treatment records reviewed to determine if the child has congenital or acquired syphilis.

1. If the child is at risk for congenital syphilis, **evaluation should include the following:**
   a. **CSF analysis for VDRL,** cell count, and protein concentration.
   b. **CBC with differential and platelet count**
   c. **Other tests as clinically indicated,** including long-bone radiographs, chest radiograph, liver function tests, cranial ultrasonography, ophthalmologic examination, and auditory brainstem responses.
2. **Treatment should consist of aqueous crystalline penicillin G** 200,000 to 300,000 units/kg/day IV divided every 4 to 6 hours for 10 days. Some experts also suggest administering a single dose of benzathine penicillin G 50,000 units/kg IM following the 10-day course of IV therapy.

D. Some experts would treat all newborns with a positive STS because it may be difficult to document that the mother had adequate treatment and falling serologic titers, a low titer may be present in latent maternal syphilis, infected newborns may have no clinical signs at birth, and follow-up/compliance may be difficult in populations at risk for congenital syphilis. If the mother has received an appropriate penicillin regimen >1 month before delivery, the infant's clinical and laboratory examination are normal, and follow-up is assured, some would follow up the infant without treatment.

VI. FOLLOW-UP OF INFANTS TREATED FOR CONGENITAL SYPHILIS. All seroreactive infants should have a physical examination and nontreponemal titer every 2 to 3 months until the test becomes nonreactive or the titer decreases fourfold. If the titer is found to increase or remain reactive at 6 to 12 months, the infant should undergo reevaluation for signs of active syphilis and retreatment should be seriously considered. Infants with possible neurosyphilis (abnormal or uninterpretable CSF results at the time of initial diagnosis) should undergo repeat CSF examination at 6-month intervals until the CSF is normal. If the CSF VDRL test result remains positive at any 6-month interval, retreatment is recommended. If the CSF VDRL test result is negative, but the CSF cell count and/or protein concentration are not declining or remain abnormal at 2 years, retreatment is recommended.

VII. INFECTION CONTROL. Nasal secretions and open syphilitic lesions are highly infectious. Strict bodily fluid precautions should be taken. Health care personnel as well as family members and other visitors should wear gloves when handling infants with congenital syphilis until therapy has been administered for at least 24 hours. Those who have had close contact with an infected infant or mother before precautions were taken should be examined and tested for infection and treatment should be considered.

A. Infants and their mothers at risk for syphilis or are infected with syphilis should be evaluated for other sexually transmitted diseases such as hepatitis B, gonorrhea, chlamydia, and HIV.

B. Assistance and guidance in syphilis testing and treatment are available from the CDC, Atlanta, Georgia, and state health departments.

Suggested Readings

American Academy of Pediatrics. Syphilis. In: Pickering LK, Baker CJ, Long SS, eds. *Red book: 2006 report of the committee on infectious diseases*, 27th ed. Elk Grove Village: American Academy of Pediatrics, 2006:631–644.

Ingall D, Sanchez P, Baker CJ. Syphilis. In: Remington J, Klein J, eds. *Infectious diseases of the fetus and newborn infant*. Philadelphia: Elsevier Saunders, 2006.

Lago EG, Rodrigues LC, Fiori RM, et al. Congenital syphilis: Identification of two distinct profiles of maternal characteristics associated with risk. *Sex Transm Dis* 2004;31:33–37.

Workowski KA, Berman SM. Sexually transmitted diseases treatment guidelines, 2006. *MMWR Recomm Rep* 2006;55:22–34.

LYME DISEASE
John A. F. Zupancic and John P. Cloherty

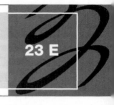

I. LYME DISEASE (Lyme borreliosis) is the most common vector-borne disease in the United States. The causative organism is the spirochete *Borrelia burgdorferi,* which is transmitted to humans through the bite of tick species including the deer tick, Ixodes scapularis. White-footed mice and deer are important in the life cycle of the tick. Distribution of Lyme disease correlates with the distribution of these hosts. Most cases in the United States are clustered in the northeast from Massachusetts to Maryland, in the midwest in Wisconsin and Minnesota, or in California. There have been cases reported from all states and also Canada, Europe, China, Japan, and Russia. Humans are the most likely to be infected in June, July, and August.

The clinical manifestations of Lyme disease may be divided into three stages. In the **early localized** stage, an annular, erythematous, nonpruritic rash known as *erythema chronicum migrans* presents at site of a tick bite, usually within 1 to 2 weeks. The early localized stage may also present with multiple erythema migrans lesions, fever, myalgia and arthralgia. Patients with **early disseminated** disease may present with multiple erythema migrans lesions, neurologic involvement (meningitis, cranial nerve palsy, and peripheral radiculopathy) and carditis (atrioventricular block and myocardial dysfunction). **Late** disease manifests as recurrent pauciarticular arthritis, peripheral neuropathy, and cognitive impairment.

Early case reports and case series confirmed that transplacental transmission of *B. burgdorferi* was possible and raised concerns about a congenital Lyme disease syndrome analogous to that seen with other spirochetal infections such as syphilis. A wide variety of clinical manifestations were noted, with most initial concerns being focused on congenital cardiac malformations and fetal death. However, epidemiologic studies have not supported an association between congenital infection and adverse fetal or neonatal outcomes. A prospective study of 2,014 pregnant women showed no association between seropositivity or history of tick bite and congenital malformations, low birth weight, or fetal death. A report by the same authors compared 2504 infants born in an endemic region to 2,507 delivered in a nonendemic region. This study showed a significant increase in the rate of congenital cardiac malformations in the endemic compared with the nonendemic region, but notably no association within the endemic region between seropositivity and cardiac malformation. Similarly, in a retrospective case–control study of 796 patients with congenital heart disease and 704 control infants, there was no association between cardiac anomalies and clinical evidence of Lyme disease during pregnancy. Although these studies were limited by the low prevalence of Lyme disease, it appears from available evidence that any increased risk for adverse neonatal effects of prenatal Lyme borreliosis are likely to be small. There is no evidence that *B. burgdorferi* is transmitted in human milk.

II. DIAGNOSIS. Lyme disease may be diagnosed by the appearance of a typical rash (erythema migrans) in women living in or visiting an area where cases of Lyme disease have been previously reported. However, the spectrum of clinical symptoms may be quite variable. As discussed, there is no accepted syndrome of congenital Lyme borreliosis. Serologic testing begins with acute and convalescent enzyme immunoassay (EIA) or immunofluorescence assay (IFA) to detect immunoglobulin M (IgM) antibodies against *B. burgdorferi*. The IgM titer peaks at 3 to 6 weeks after infection, and may be negative for patients with isolated erythema migrans, those who are pregnant, or those who have been treated early. In addition, false-positive EIA and IFA results occur secondary to cross-reaction with other spirochetal and viral infections and autoimmune disease. Therefore, positive or equivocal EIA or IFA test results should be confirmed with Western immunoblot. If central nervous system involvement is suspected, spinal fluid serology should also be obtained. Polymerase chain reaction for detection of *B. burgdorferi* is currently investigational.

III. **TREATMENT OF MOTHERS AND THE NEWBORN.** Patients known to have Lyme disease or who are suspected of having Lyme disease during pregnancy should be treated. The treatment is the same as for nonpregnant persons except that doxycycline is contraindicated.

    A. **Tick bite.** Prophylactic treatment of tick bites in endemic areas is not generally recommended, although this is sometimes prescribed in nonpregnant individuals, particularly those with prolonged duration of attachment (>72 hours).

    B. **Localized early Lyme disease.** Amoxicillin 500 mg PO TID for 14 to 21 days or cefuroxime axetil 500 mg PO BID for 14 to 21 days. For penicillin-allergic patients, erythromycin 500 mg PO QID for 14 to 21 days is an alternative; however, macrolides appear to be less effective, and these patients should therefore be closely followed up.

    C. **Disseminated early Lyme disease or any manifestations of late disease.** Ceftriaxone 2 g IV once daily for 14 to 28 days or penicillin G 18 to 24 million units IV every day divided q4h. Patients with isolated cranial nerve palsy, first- or second-degree heart block, or arthritis without neurologic manifestations may be treated with oral therapy as for localized early Lyme disease.

    D. **Newborn of mother with confirmed Lyme disease in pregnancy.** The relative risk of fetal transmission as a function of severity of maternal disease, chronicity of maternal disease, or choice of antibiotic and route of administration is not known. Similarly, data are lacking on the optimal therapy for the newborn infant with symptoms of acute Lyme disease. In one report, a 38-week fetus born to a mother who developed acute Lyme disease 1 week before delivery developed petechiae and a vesicular rash that resolved with the intravenous administration of penicillin G for 10 days. If an infant is thought to have Lyme disease, treatment with penicillin or ceftriaxone intravenously should be given for 14 to 21 days after studies are taken from blood and spinal fluid. If a mother was treated for Lyme disease with erythromycin during pregnancy, consideration should be given to treatment of the infant with penicillin or ceftriaxone.

    E. **Prevention of Lyme disease.** A recombinant vaccine against the outer surface protein of *B. burgdorferi* was licensed by the Food and Drug Administration (FDA) in 1998 for individuals between 15 and 70 years of age. It was not recommended for use in pregnant women. The vaccine was withdrawn from the market in 2002 by the manufacturer owing to lack of demand. In the absence of a vaccine, prevention rests on avoidance of heavily tick-infested areas, use of appropriate tick and insect repellents, and careful examination for and removal of ticks as soon as possible after attachment.

Suggested Readings

American Academy of Pediatrics. Committee on infectious diseases. Prevention of Lyme disease. *Pediatrics* 2000;105:142.

American Academy of Pediatrics. Lyme disease. In: Pickering LK, Baker CJ, Long SS, et al. eds. *Red book: 2006 report of the committee of infectious disease*, 27th ed. Elk Grove Village: American Academy of Pediatrics, 2006:428–433.

Silver HM. Lyme disease during pregnancy. *Infect Dis Clin North Am* 1997;11:93.

Strobino B, Abid S, Gewitz M. Maternal Lyme disease and congenital heart disease: A case-control study in an endemic area. *Am J Obstet Gynecol* 1999;180:711.

Strobino BA, Williams CL, Abid S, et al. Lyme disease and pregnancy outcome: A prospective study of two thousand prenatal patients. *Am J Obstet Gynecol* 1993;169:367.

Wormser GP, Nadelman RB, Dattwyler RJ, et al. Practice guidelines for the treatment of Lyme disease. *Clin Infect Dis* 2000;31(Suppl 1):1.

CONGENITAL TOXOPLASMOSIS
Regine M. Fortunov

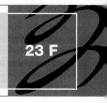

I. **TOXOPLASMA GONDII,** an obligate, intracellular protozoan parasite, is an important human pathogen, especially for the fetus, newborn, and immunocompromised patient.

II. **EPIDEMIOLOGY.** *T. gondii* is ubiquitous and commonly causes human infection worldwide.

    A. The prevalence of *TOXOPLASMA* antibody increases with age and varies by geographic location and population. Data from one area or population may not accurately be generalized to other areas or populations. The reported prevalence of *T. gondii* antibodies in women of childbearing age ranges from 3% to 40% (average 15%) in the United States and 4% to 80% worldwide. Women without antibiodies are at risk for acute toxoplasmosis during pregnancy.

    B. Seroconversion during pregancy also varies by geographic location. Rates range from 1.5% in France, a high prevalance country, to 0.17% in Norway, a low prevalence country. The National Collaborative Perinatal Project (National Institutes of Health) estimated the rate at 1.1 in 1,000 in the United States.

    C. The reported incidence of congenital toxoplamsosis in the United States has decreased during the last 20 years from a high of 2 in 1,000 to 1 in 10,000.

III. **PATHOPHYSIOLOGY**

    A. The cat, the only definitive host, is usually asymptomatic. During acute infection, millions of oocysts are shed daily in the stool for 2 weeks or longer. Oocysts may remain viable in the soil for >1 year in some climates.

    B. Other animals become infected by ingesting the oocysts resulting in tissue cysts containing viable organisms predominately in muscle and brain.

    C. Normal children and adults are susceptible to acute infection if they lack specific antibody to the organism. Both humoral and cell-mediated immunity are important in the control of infection. Transmission usually occurs by direct ingestion of oocysts or ingestion of the cysts in undercooked meat. After acute parasitemia, the organism forms tissue cysts in multiple organs, including muscle and brain, which probably persist for life. Usually these are of little consequence to the normal host, but progressive, localized, or reactivated disease may occur.

    D. Human congenital infection

        1. Placental pathology suggests that parasites from the maternal circulation invade and multiply within placental cells before reaching the fetal circulation. This delay in transmission from the placenta to the fetus ranges from <4 weeks to >16 weeks.

        2. The congenital infection risk increases when acute maternal infection occurs later in pregnancy. The average transmission rate is 15% for the first trimester, 60% for the third trimester, and may approach 90% at term. The fetal disease severity, however, is inversely proportional to gestational age. Without prenatal therapy, most fetuses infected in the first trimester die in utero or in the neonatal period, or have severe central nervous system (CNS) and ophthalmologic disease. Conversely, most fetuses infected in the second trimester, and all infants infected in the third trimester, have mild or subclinical disease in the newborn period.

        3. Congenital infections after chronic maternal infection are associated with serologic relapse are extremely rare. Maternal immune dysfunction, including human immunodeficiency virus (HIV), should be suspected.

IV. **DIAGNOSIS.** All neonates suspected to have congenital toxoplasmosis based on symptoms, maternal acute *Toxoplasma* infection during pregnancy, or maternal HIV with a history of chronic *Toxoplasma* infection should be evaluated.

A. **Clinical presentation.** There are four recognized patterns of presentation for congenital toxoplasmosis.
   1. **Neonatal symptomatic disease** is usually severe and neurologic signs predominate.
   2. **Symptomatic disease in the first 3 months of age** is most often seen with premature infants but can also be found in full-term neonates and can be severe.
   3. **Sequelae or relapse in infancy through adolescence of a previously undiagnosed infection** may be ocular (chorioretinitis) or neurologic (seizures, late cerebrospinal fluid (CSF) obstruction).
   4. **Subclinical infection.** At present, the outcome of a newborn that is asymptomatic cannot be predicted. Most infants with congenital toxoplasmosis (80%–90%) do not have overt signs of infection at birth but may have retinal and CNS abnormalities when further testing is performed. The New England Regional Newborn Screening program (1986–1992) identified 52 cases of congenital toxoplasmosis of 635,000 infants screened for IgM antibody to *T. gondii*. Fifty infants were full term, asymptomatic and had normal physical examinations. After confirming congenital infection, CNS or retina abnormalities were identified in 19 of 48 infants.
B. **Specific symptoms.** Hydrocephalus, chorioretinitis, and intracranial calcifications are the classic triad, but disease is usually a clinical spectrum.
   1. **Neurologic.** These can include microcephaly or bulging fontanelle with increased head circumference, seizures, opisthotonos, paralysis, swallowing difficulties, respiratory distress, and deafness. Encephalitis may be present with CSF abnormalities or calcifications (discussed in the subsequent text). The neonate may have evidence of endocrine dysfunction or difficulties with temperature regulation depending on the areas of brain affected. Active encephalitis and obstructive hydrocephalus from edema and inflammation may respond well to treatment.
   2. **Ophthalmologic.** Toxoplasmosis is one of the most common causes of chorioretinitis and can lead to visual impairment. Lesions not seen in the newborn period may develop during the first several years of life if congenital infection is not treated. External findings can include strabismus, nystagmus, cataracts, and microcornea. **Focal necrotizing retinitis,** yellow–white cotton-like patches, is usually bilateral. Macular lesions are more common than peripheral. Inflammatory exudates may prevent visualization of the fundus. Retinal edema is common. In the National Collaborative Congenital Toxoplasmosis (NCCT) study of patients with eye disease, 22% of patients had active lesions if not treated in the first year compared to 8% of treated patients. **Chorioretinal scars** were seen in 100% of untreated patients versus 74% of treated patients. Other manifestations include phthisis (destruction of the globe), retinal detachment, optic atrophy, iritis, scleritis, uveitis, and vitreitis. Patients may have both retinopathy of prematurity and toxoplasmic chorioretinitis.
   3. **Other common symptoms** include hepatosplenomegaly, persistent conjugated hyperbilirubinemia (from liver damage or hemolysis), and thrombocytopenia. Some patients have lymphadenopathy, anemia, hypogammaglobulinemia, or nephrotic syndrome.
   4. **Rare** presentations include erythroblastosis and hydrops fetalis, myocarditis, vomiting, diarrhea, feeding problems, and respiratory distress (from interstitial pneumonitis, superinfection, or lesions affecting respiratory control centers).
   5. **Special cases.** Infected infants are commonly born premature (25%–50%). Monozygotic twins often have similar patterns of infection in contrast to dizygotic twins. Neonates born to HIV-infected mothers are often asymptomatic only to develop severe disseminated infection during the first weeks or months of age.
C. **Laboratory studies.** Diagnosis may be made by serology, polymerase chain reaction (PCR), histology, or isolation of the parasite. Currently, only Massachusetts and New Hampshire screen all neonates.
   1. **Postnatal *Toxoplasma*-specific immunoglobulin (Ig) pattern after acute infection**

a. **IgG** appears within 1 to 2 weeks, peaks at 1 to 2 months, and persists throughout life. Transplacental IgG antibody disappears by 6 to 12 months of age. For patients with seroconversion or a fourfold rise in IgG antibody titer, perform IgM testing.

b. **IgM** appears within 2 weeks, peaks at 1 month, and declines to undetectable within 6 to 9 months (uncommonly years). Because IgM does not cross the placenta, this test may be very useful in determining congenital infection. If maternal blood contamination is possible, repeat the IgM, IgA, and IgE testing in a few days.

c. **IgA** rises rapidly, and it usually disappears by 7 months (uncommonly >1 year). IgA may have greater sensitivity for neonates compared to IgM assays.

d. **IgE** rises rapidly and does not persist as long as IgM and IgA (<4 months).

e. **In congenital toxoplasmosis,** antibody production varies significantly and is affected by treatment.

2. **Serologic laboratory tests**

   a. **The Sabin-Feldman dye test (IgG)** uses the uptake of methylene blue by *Toxoplasma* tachyzoites (organisms appear swollen and blue). The tachyzoite membranes lyse in the presence of complement and IgG-specific antibody (organisms appear thin and unstained). There is extensive experience with this test particularly as an antenatal screen for maternal seroconversion in pregnancy.

   b. **Indirect fluorescent antibody (IFA) (IgG, IgM)** uses fluorescein-tagged antiserum against Ig to detect antibody binding to *Toxoplasma* slide preparations. In general, IgG IFA and the dye test qualitatively agree. IgM IFA will detect only 25% to 50% of congenital infections.

   c. **Double–sandwich enzyme-linked immunosorbant assay (ELISA) (IgM, IgA, IgE)** uses wells coated with specific antibody to IgM to detect IgM in serum. A second antibody to IgM linked to an enzyme is added. The enzyme converts substrate into a fluorescent signal.

   d. **The immunosorbent agglutination assay (ISAGA) (IgM, IgA, IgE)** measures *Toxoplasma*-specific antibody captured from sera by the agglutination of a particulate antigen preparation. Sensitivity is 75% to 80%. IgM ISAGA is more sensitive and specific than IgM IFA or IgM ELISA for congenitial toxoplasmosis.

   e. **Differential agglutination test (AC/HS) (IgG)** compares agglutination titers for sera against formalin-fixed tachyzoites (HS antigen) with those against acetone- or methanol-fixed tachyzoites (AC antigen). The different test preparations display antigens present at different times in infection so the relative titers with each preparation may be indicative of acute versus remote infection.

   f. **Avidity testing (IgG)** may differentiate acute versus remote infection. IgG antibodies produced early in infection have low avidity, but avidity increases over time. High-avidity IgG antibodies against *Toxoplasma* exclude infection occuring within the preceding 3 months and is useful in early pregnancy.

   g. We strongly recommend that a *Toxoplasma* reference laboratory perform all PCR testing and confirm all positive IgM test results. PCR and the recommended serologic tests discussed here are available as panels and are performed by the *Toxoplasma* Serology Laboratory Palo Alto, CA.

3. **Recommended serum serology.** *Toxoplasma* specific IgG, IgM, IgA, and IgE testing should be performed in neonates suspected to have congenital toxoplasmosis and their mothers.

   a. **Recommended neonatal tests.** Sabin-Feldman dye test (IgG), IgM ISAGA, IgA ELISA, IgE ISAGA or ELISA.

   b. **Recommended maternal tests.** Sabin-Feldman dye test (IgG), IgM ELISA, IgA ELISA, IgE ISAGA or ELISA, AC/HS.

4. **PCR** can detect *T. gondii* in the peripheral blood buffy coat, CSF cell pellet, or amniotic fluid. **Amniotic fluid PCR** is recommended to diagnose fetal infection. Higher parasite DNA levels can be found in cases where infection occurred

earlier in gestation or were more severe. A negative amniotic fluid PCR does not rule out fetal infection as the accuracy range is wide and parasite transmission from the mother to the fetus may be delayed. PCR sensitivity for the B1 gene is high between 17 to 21 weeks' gestation (>90%), and is lower after 21 weeks (50%–60%). Antenatal maternal therapy to prevent or treat fetal infection should extend until delivery even with a negative result.

D. Other diagnostic testing

1. **Peripheral blood count** often demonstrates leukocytosis or leukopenia. Early manifestations include lymphocytopenia, or monocytosis. Eosinophilia may be seen (may be >30%), as well as thrombocytopenia.

2. **Liver function tests**

3. Serum **glucose-6-phosphate dehydrogenase screen** (before starting sulfadiazine)

4. **Creatinine and urine analysis**

5. **Quantitative Igs** are recommended to determine a baseline.

6. **CSF** findings include xanthochromia, mononuclear pleocytosis and elevated protein content (may be very high). Persistence of *Toxoplasma*-specific immunoglobulin (IgM) may indicate active infection. *Toxoplasma*-specific IgG has been seen and quantitative IgG levels should be determined as a baseline. Treatment may decrease these findings. PCR is the preferred method to detect parasite from CSF.

7. **Auditory brain stem response to 20 dB**

E. Head computed tomography (CT) scan without contrast is the preferred study. One study reported a clear relationship between the lesions on CT scan, neurologic signs, and the date of maternal infection.

1. CT scan may detect **calcifications** not seen by ultrasonography. They may be single or multiple and are usually limited to intracranial structures. Common locations include periventricular, scattered in the white matter, and the basal ganglia (often caudate). The pattern may be indistinguishable from that seen with cytomegalovirus infection. Lesions can decrease or resolve with treatment.

2. **Hydrocephalus** is usually due to periaqueductal obstruction. Massive hydrocephalus may develop in as quickly as 1 week.

3. **Cortical atrophy** can be seen as well as porencephalic cysts.

F. Pathologic findings

1. **Histology** may demonstrate tachyzoites (acute toxoplasmosis) or cysts (acute or chronic toxoplasmosis) in tissue or body fluids.

2. **Tissue or mouse culture** to isolate the parasite from peripheral blood buffy coat or the placenta may require 1 or 6 weeks, respectively.

G. Differential diagnosis

1. The clinical and laboratory findings are common to congenital infections by **rubella, cytomegalovirus, syphilis, and neonatal herpes simplex virus.**

2. Other disorders to be considered include hepatitis B, varicella, bacterial sepsis, hemolytic diseases, metabolic disorders, immune thrombocytopenia, histiocytosis, congenital leukemia and congenital lymphocytic choriomeningitis virus syndrome.

V. TREATMENT OF MATERNAL/FETAL INFECTION

A. Toxoplasmosis symptoms in the adult may be transient and nonspecific (usually lymphadenopathy and fatigue). Ninety percent of women infected during pregnancy report no clinical illness and most cases are undiagnosed without universal antibody screening.

1. **Antenatal screening** allows early diagnosis of acute maternal, fetal, and neonatal infection, and improves outcomes. Routine screening throughout pregnancy is performed in other countries, such as France, but not currently in the United States. Positive Sabin-Feldman dye tests (or equivalent assay) should be confirmed by IgM double–sandwich ELISA. IgG avidity can help establish the timing of infection. **It is strongly recommended that a *Toxoplasma* reference laboratory confirm all serology suggesting infection before treatment, fetal testing, or abortion.**

B. Medications. Prompt treatment may prevent irreversible in utero retinal and brain damage.

1. **Spiramycin** is recommended before 18 weeks' gestation and until term if the fetus is uninfected by 18 week amniotic fluid PCR. This macrolide antibiotic reduces or delays vertical transmision to the fetus through high placental levels (3–5 times maternal serum levels). However, if transmission occurs, disease severity may be unaltered. This drug lacks U.S. Food and Drug Administation (FDA) approval in the United States.

2. **Pyrimethamine, sulfadiazine, and folinic acid** are recommended for confirmed fetal infections after 18 weeks' gestation (or when unable to perform amniocentesis) and all acute maternal infections after 24 weeks (amniotic fluid PCR sensitivity is poor after 24 weeks). Fetal infections diagnosed before 17 weeks should be treated with sulfadiazine alone until after the first trimester as pyrimethamine may affect organogenesis. Treatment of infections acquired between 21 and 24 weeks with negative amniotic fluid PCR should be individualized.

3. **Prenatal diagnosis** by amniotic fluid PCR should be performed, if possible, in every case of acute infection during pregnancy. After maternal treatment with primethamine and sulfadiazine, diagnosis during infancy may be difficult as infants may lack typical clinical or serologic features. **Ultrasonographic monitoring** is also important as ventricular dilation is an indirect sign of fetal infection and may develop rapidly.

4. **Therapeutic abortion** is considered by some families. When infection occurs before 16 weeks' gestation, prognosis can be severe with brain necrosis despite lack of ventricular dilation by ultrasonography.

C. Patient education. The best way to prevent congenital toxoplasmosis is to prevent acute maternal infection during pregnancy through education of women of childbearing age.

1. **Cats.** Keep indoors. Only feed dry, canned, or cooked food. Change litter daily and disinfect the litter box for 5 minutes with nearly boiling water. If possible avoid the litter if pregnant or wear gloves.

2. **Food.** Cook meat till well done. Do not eat raw eggs. Wash fruits and vegetables well before eating. Wash hands, cutting boards and utensils well after contact with raw meat, eggs or vegetables.

3. **Gardening.** Wear gloves.

VI. TREATMENT OF NEONATAL INFECTION

A. Medications. Therapy is recommended, regardless of symptoms, to prevent the high incidence of sequelae, resolve acute symptoms, and improve outcomes. As current medications do not eradicate *T. gondii* and primarily act against the tachyzoite form not tissue cysts (especially from neural tissue and the eye), extended therapy until 1 year of age is recommended.

1. **Pyrimethamine** (1 mg/kg every 12 hours for 2 days, then daily for until 2 to 6 months of age, then 3 times weekly until 1 year of age), and **sulfadiazine** (50 mg/kg every 12 hours until 1 year of age) act synergistically and can result in symptom resolution within the first few weeks of therapy.

2. **Side effects** of sulfadiazine include crystalluria, hematuria, hypersensitivity, and bone marrow suppression. Alternative medications for atopy or severe intolerance of sulfadiazine include clindamycin, azithromycin, and atovaquone. Pyrimethamine (a dihydrofolate reductase inhibitor) can induce bone marrow suppression; patients should be monitored by a complete blood count, differential, and platelet count twice weekly. Neutropenia is more frequent than megaloblastic anemia or thrombocytopenia. Other less frequent side effects include gastrointestinal distress, convulsions, and tremor. **Folinic acid** (10 mg 3 times weekly until 1 week after pyrimethamine stopped) helps prevent bone marrow suppression, but temporary therapy cessation or dose modification may be required.

3. **Prednisone** (0.5 mg/kg every 12 hours) is recommended for active CNS disease (CSF protein exceeding 1 g/dL) or active chorioretinitis, which threatens vision. The dose can be tapered and discontinued when symptoms improve.

4. The same treatment is recommended for infants born to mothers infected with **HIV** and *T. gondii*. Combination with antiretrovirals such as zidovudine, however, may increase bone marrow toxicity. Treatment may be discontinued after 1 year if the infant CD^{4+} count is >200 cells/mm^3.

B. **Ventricular shunting** for ventricular dilation is recommended although systematic outcome data is unavailable. A perioperative head CT scan to assess adequacy of drainage and subdural bleeding (after pressure reduction) may help with prognosis. After treatment with ventricular shunt and medications, some patients experience significant improvement in hydrocephalus with brain cortical expansion and growth. Intelligence quotient (IQ) may be within normal range.

C. **Multidisciplinary consultation** is usually helpful for patient management. Specialty consultation is typically required for.

  1. **Infectious diseases.** Congenital infection is frequently subclinical, has symptoms similar to other infections and diseases, and serologic diagnosis may be difficult.

  2. **Ophthalmology.** Retinal evaluation is recommended.

  3. **Neurosurgery.** Recommended for ventricular dilation.

  4. **Neurodevelopmental pediatrics.** Follow-up is suggested every 3 to 6 months for 1 year then as needed.

D. The **NCCT** Study has reported outcomes in a series of children with congenital infection. Treatment improved early outcomes for many congenitally infected children. All children who died had severe infection at birth.

  1. With treatment, **chorioretinitis** usually resolved within 1 to 2 weeks and did not relapse during therapy. Relapse after treatment may occur, often during adolescence, and risk factors are unknown. **Visual impairment** is a prominent sequela even with treatment in 85% of the patients at 5 years with severe disease at birth and 15% of neonates with none or mild disease. Most retinal disease causing impairment was present at birth. Acuity may be adequate for reading and daily activities even with large macular scars. Poor acuity has affected school performance and cognitive development for some patients. Retinal scaring can cause retinal detachment. Owing to the risk of new lesions and poor visual acuity, **ophthalmoscopic examinations are recommend every 3 months until 18-months-old and then yearly.**

  2. With treatment, 80% of patients with severe disease at birth had normal motor function and 73% had an IQ >70 at follow-up compared to >80% of untreated childern who had IQ scores <70 at 4 years. All patients with none to moderate disease at birth had normal motor and cognitive function. Despite the good **cognitive outcomes**, patients' IQ scores often are 15 points lower than their closest sibling ($p < 0.05$). Children asymptomatic at birth may have varying degress of impairment. No **hearing impairment** was observed compared to previous reports. With treatment, the **head CT findings** improved. After encephalitis resolution with treatment, antiepiletic medications could be discontinued in some patients.

  3. With treatment, other signs of infection including thrombocytopenia, hepatitis, and rashes resolved within 1 month.

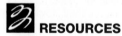

RESOURCES

Congenital toxoplasmosis study group (US) 773-834-4152

Toxoplasma Serology Laboratory at the Palo Alto Medical Foundation Research Institute, Ames Bldg, 795 El Camino Real, Palo Alto, CA 94301-2302 (Tel: (650) 853-4828, Fax (650) 614-3292, Email: toxolab@pamf.org,Web: http://www.pamf.org/serology/

Suggested Readings

McLeod R, Boyer K, Karrison T, et al. Outcome of treatment for congenital toxoplasmosis, 1981–2004: The National Collaborative Chicago-based, Congenital Toxoplasmosis Study. *Clin Infect Dis* 2006;42:1383–1394.

RESPIRATORY DISTRESS SYNDROME
Kushal Y. Bhakta

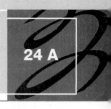

$\mathcal{T}$he primary cause of respiratory distress syndrome (RDS), also known as hyaline membrane disease, is inadequate pulmonary surfactant due to preterm birth. The manifestations of the disease are caused by the resultant diffuse alveolar atelectasis, edema, and cell injury. Subsequently, serum proteins that inhibit surfactant function leak into the alveoli. The increased water content, immature mechanisms for clearance of lung liquid, lack of alveolar-capillary apposition, and low surface area for gas exchange typical of the immature lung also contribute to the disease. Significant advances made in the management of RDS include the development of prenatal diagnosis to identify infants at risk, prevention of the disease by antenatal administration of glucocorticoids, improvements in perinatal and neonatal care, advances in respiratory support, and surfactant replacement therapy. As a result, the mortality from RDS has decreased. However, the survival of increasing numbers of extremely immature infants has provided new challenges, and RDS remains an important contributing cause of neonatal mortality and morbidity.

I. IDENTIFICATION
A. Perinatal risk factors
1. **Factors** that affect the state of lung development at birth include prematurity, maternal diabetes, and genetic factors (white race, history of RDS in siblings, male sex). Thoracic malformations that cause lung hypoplasia, such as diaphragmatic hernia, may also increase the risk for surfactant deficiency. Genetic disorders of surfactant production and metabolism include surfactant protein B and surfactant protein C gene mutations, and mutations of the ABCA3 gene, whose product is an adenosine triphosphate (ATP)-binding cassette transporter localized to the lamellar bodies of alveolar type II cells. These rare disorders cause a severe RDS-like picture, often in term infants, and are usually fatal without lung transplantation.
2. **Factors** that may acutely impair surfactant production, release, or function include perinatal asphyxia in premature infants and cesarean section without labor. Infants delivered before labor starts do not benefit from the adrenergic and steroid hormones released during labor, which increase surfactant production and release. As a result, RDS may be seen in late preterm or early term infants delivered by elective cesarean section.

B. Prenatal prediction
1. **Assessment** of fetal lung maturity (FLM). Prenatal prediction of lung maturity can be made by testing amniotic fluid obtained by amniocentesis.
   a. **The lecithin-sphingomyelin** (L/S) ratio is performed by thin-layer chromatography. Specific techniques vary among laboratories and may affect the results. In general, the risk of RDS is very low if the L/S ratio is >2. Exceptions to the prediction of pulmonary maturity with an L/S ratio >2 are infants of diabetic mothers (IDMs), intrapartum asphyxia, and erythroblastosis fetalis. Possible exceptions are intrauterine growth restriction (IUGR), abruptio placentae, preeclampsia, and hydrops fetalis. Contaminants, such as blood and meconium, affect the interpretation of results. Blood and meconium tend to elevate an immature L/S ratio and depress a mature L/S ratio. As a result, an L/S ratio over 2 in a contaminated specimen is probably mature, and a ratio under 2 is probably immature.

      b. The TDx-FLM II measures the surfactant-albumin ratio using fluorescent polarization technology. It appears to predict clinically significant RDS when a cutoff of >45 mg/g is used for mature results. Contamination with blood or meconium may interfere with interpretation of this test, although the extent and direction are uncertain.

      c. Lamellar body counts in the amniotic fluid have also been used as a rapid and inexpensive test to determine FLM. Lamellar bodies are "packages" of phospholipids produced by type II alveolar cells, and are present in amniotic fluid in increasing numbers with advancing gestational age. In one study, a count of >50,000 lamellar bodies/microliter predicted lung maturity.

  2. Antenatal corticosteroid therapy should be given to pregnant women 24 to 34 weeks' gestation with intact membranes or with preterm rupture of the membranes (ROM) without chorioamnionitis, who are at high risk for preterm delivery within the next 7 days. Treatment at gestational ages <24 weeks is of questionable efficacy. This strategy induces sufactant production and accelerates maturation of the lungs and other fetal tissues, resulting in a substantial reduction of RDS, intraventricular hemorrhage (IVH), necrotizing enterocolitis, and perinatal mortality. A full course consists of two doses of betamethasone (12 mg IM) separated by a 24-hour interval, or four doses of dexamethasone (6 mg IM) at 12-hour intervals, although incomplete courses may improve outcome. Contraindications to treatment include chorioamnionitis or other indications for immediate delivery. Betamethasone may be preferable; a higher risk of periventricular white matter injury was observed in infants whose mothers received dexamethasone compared with those exposed to betamethasone. In a study by the NICHD Neonatal Research Network, antenatal treatment with betamethasone showed a statistically significant decease in neonatal mortality, and a trend toward less IVH and severe retinopathy of prematurity compared to antenatal treatment with dexamethasone.

C. Postnatal diagnosis. A premature infant with RDS has clinical signs shortly after birth. These include tachypnea, retractions, flaring of the nasal alae, grunting, and cyanosis. The classic radiographic appearance is of low-volume lungs with a diffuse reticulogranular pattern and air bronchograms.

II. MANAGEMENT. The keys to the management of infants with RDS are (i) to prevent hypoxemia and acidosis (this allows normal tissue metabolism, optimizes surfactant production, and prevents right-to-left shunting); (ii) to optimize fluid management (avoiding hypovolemia and shock, on the one hand, and edema, particularly pulmonary edema, on the other); (iii) to reduce metabolic demands; (iv) to prevent worsening atelectasis and pulmonary edema; (v) to minimize oxidant lung injury; and (vi) to minimize lung injury caused by mechanical ventilation.

A. Surfactant replacement therapy is one of the best-studied therapies in neonates. It has been shown in numerous clinical trials to be successful in ameliorating RDS. These trials have examined the effects of surfactant preparations delivered through the endotracheal tube either within minutes of birth (prophylactic treatment) or after the symptoms and signs of RDS are present (selective or "rescue" treatment). Surfactants of human, bovine, or porcine origin and synthetic preparations have been studied. In general, these studies have shown improvement in oxygenation and decreased need for ventilator support lasting hours to days after treatment and, in many of the larger studies, decreased incidence of air leaks and death. Survanta (a bovine lung extract), Infasurf (a calf lung extract), and Curosurf (a porcine lung extract) are currently available in the United States.

  1. Timing. Prophylactic treatment of surfactant deficiency, before lung injury occurs, results in better distribution and less lung injury than supplementation once respiratory failure is severe. "Early rescue" (before 2 hours of age) is preferable to delayed treatment, although whether prophylactic treatment is better than early treatment is uncertain. In a meta-analysis of eight randomized controlled trials comparing the effects of prophylactic surfactant administration to surfactant treatment of established RDS, prophylactic treatment decreased the risk of air leak and neonatal mortality, with a trend toward a decreased risk of IVH. In general, we administer early rescue surfactant as soon as the diagnosis of RDS is made and after adequate oxygenation, ventilation, perfusion, and monitoring have been established, usually within the first hour of age. Prophylactic therapy is justifiable in very premature infants (27 weeks or less) who have a high incidence of RDS, in centers that have several skilled staff available to attend each delivery, so that resuscitation is not delayed by surfactant administration. Local conditions such as equipment to provide warmed, humidified, blended air/oxygen, and full monitoring facilities in the delivery room will also influence the decision.

2. **The response to surfactant therapy** varies from baby to baby. The causes of this variability include timing of treatment and patient factors such as other concurrent illnesses and degree of lung immaturity. Delayed resuscitation, insufficient lung inflation, improper ventilator strategies, and excessive fluid administration may negate the benefits of surfactant therapy. The combined use of antenatal corticosteroids and postnatal surfactant when indicated improves neonatal outcome more than postnatal surfactant therapy alone.

   In infants with established RDS, repeated surfactant treatment results in greater improvement in oxygenation and ventilation, a decreased risk of pneumothorax, and a trend toward improved survival when compared to single-dose therapy. However, there is no clear benefit to more than four doses of Survanta or Infasurf or three doses of Curosurf. Whether all infants should be retreated, or only those who meet certain criteria for severity of illness at the recommended intervals for retreatment is unresolved. We generally retreat infants who still require mechanical ventilation with mean airway pressures above 7 cm H_2O and fractional concentration of inspired oxygen (Fio_2) over 0.30 up to the maximum number of doses, although most infants require only one or two doses.

3. **Administration.** The Survanta dose is 4 mL (100 mg phospholipid)/kg of body weight. It is administered during brief disconnection from the ventilator, in quarter doses through a feeding tube that is cut to a length just slightly longer than that of the endotracheal tube. The baby is ventilated for at least 30 seconds, or until stable between quarter doses. Changes in positioning of the infant during administration are routine and intended to facilitate distribution. However, studies suggest that other strategies of administration, such as omitting the position changes, do not result in loss of efficacy, although delivery that is too slow does. Careful observation is necessary during treatment. Desaturation, bradycardia, and apnea are frequent adverse effects. Administration should be adjusted according to the infant's tolerance. Apnea commonly occurs at slow ventilation rates, so the rate should be at least 30 breaths per minute during administration. In addition, some infants respond rapidly and need careful adjustment of ventilator settings to prevent hypotension or pneumothorax secondary to sudden improvement in compliance. Others become transiently hypoxic during treatment and require additional oxygen. Subsequent doses of Survanta, if needed, are given at 6-hour intervals.

   The initial dose of Infasurf is 3 mL/kg (105 mg/kg phospholipid), divided into two aliquots; subsequent doses are given at 12-hour intervals, if needed. · The initial dose of Curosurf is 2.5 mL/kg (200 mg/kg phospholipid); subsequent doses of 1.25 mL/kg are given at 12-hour intervals, if needed. Specific instructions about administration of these preparations are available on the package insert.

4. **Complications.** Pulmonary hemorrhage is an infrequent adverse event after surfactant therapy. It most commonly occurs in extremely low birth weight (ELBW) infants, in males, and in infants who have clinical evidence of patent ductus arteriosus (PDA). The risk is decreased by antenatal glucocorticoid therapy and by early postnatal treatment of PDA with indomethacin.

   Surfactant treatment has not consistently reduced the incidence of intraventricular hemorrhage, necrotizing enterocolitis (NEC), and retinopathy of prematurity. Although these disorders tend to be associated with severe RDS, they are primarily caused by immaturity of other organs. Likewise, most studies have not demonstrated a reduced incidence of bronchopulmonary dysplasia (BPD) particularly in the smallest infants, who are at the highest risk. However, the reduction in mortality attributable to surfactant therapy has not typically been associated with a large increase in rates of BPD, suggesting that surfactant therapy prevents BPD in some infants. No significant difference has been shown in infants treated with surfactant versus placebo with regard to both neurodevelopmental outcomes and physical growth.

B. Oxygen

1. **Delivery of oxygen** should be sufficient to maintain oxygen saturations in the 88% to 95% range, a range generally sufficient to meet metabolic demands. In the smallest infants (<1,250 g birth weight), lower oxygen saturation targets (85%–92%) may be preferable. Higher than necessary Fio_2 levels should be avoided because of the danger of potentiating the development of lung injury and retinopathy of prematurity. The oxygen is warmed, humidified, and delivered through an air-oxygen blender that allows precise control over the oxygen concentration. For infants with acute RDS, oxygen is ordered by concentration to be delivered to the infant's airway, not by flow, and oxygen concentration is checked at least hourly. It should be titrated to the targeted oxygen saturation, which should be monitored continuously. When ventilation with an anesthesia bag is required during suctioning of the airway, during insertion of an endotracheal tube, or for an apneic spell, the oxygen concentration should be similar to that before bagging to avoid hyperoxia and should be adjusted in response to continuous monitoring.

2. **Blood gas monitoring** (see Chap. 24C). During the acute stages of illness, frequent sampling may be required to maintain arterial blood gases within appropriate ranges. Arterial blood gases (arterial oxygen tension [Pao_2], arterial carbon dioxide tension [$Paco_2$], and pH) should be measured 30 minutes after changes in respiratory therapy, such as alteration in the Fio_2, ventilator pressures, or rate. We use indwelling arterial catheters for this purpose. To monitor trends in oxygenation continuously, we use pulse oximeters. In more stable infants, capillary blood from warmed heels may be adequate for monitoring $Paco_2$ and pH.

C. Continuous positive airway pressure

1. **Indications.** We begin continuous positive airway pressure (CPAP) therapy as soon as possible after birth in infants (see Chap. 24B) with RDS who have mild respiratory distress, require an Fio_2 below 0.4 to maintain the targeted oxygen saturation, and have $Paco_2$ <55 to 60 mm Hg. Early CPAP therapy may reduce the need for mechanical ventilation and the incidence of long-term pulmonary morbidity. In infants with RDS, CPAP appears to help prevent atelectasis, thereby minimizing lung injury and preserving the functional properties of surfactant, and allowing reduction of oxygen concentration as the Pao_2 rises. In each infant, however, the relative benefits of endotracheal intubation and mechanical ventilation in order to administer artificial surfactant should be weighed. It is uncertain whether brief intubation and administration of surfactant followed by extubation to CPAP is comparable to surfactant treatment with continued mechanical ventilation and extubation from low levels of support. We use the latter strategy for surfactant administration.

   If CPAP enables the infant to inspire on a more compliant portion of the pressure–volume curve, $Paco_2$ may fall. However, minute ventilation may decrease on CPAP, particularly if the distending pressure is too great. We obtain a chest radiograph before or soon after starting CPAP to confirm the diagnosis of RDS and to exclude disorders in which this type of therapy should be approached with caution, such as air leak.

2. **Methods of administering CPAP.** We usually begin CPAP through nasal prongs or nasopharyngeal tube using a continuous-flow ventilator. We generally start at 5 to 7 cm H_2O pressure, using a flow high enough to avoid rebreathing (5–10 L/minute), then adjust the pressure in increments of 1 to 2 cm H_2O to a maximum of 8 cm H_2O, observing the baby's respiratory rate and effort and monitoring oxygen saturation. A nasogastric tube is always placed to decompress swallowed air. Simpler CPAP delivery utilizing tubing submerged in sterile

water to deliver the desired CPAP pressure ("bubble" CPAP) is also used, and may have some benefits over use of a continuous-flow ventilator. Variable flow CPAP devices, which reduce the work of breathing, especially during expiration, are available, although significant clinical benefits have not been observed with their use.

3. Problems encountered with CPAP

   a. CPAP may interfere with venous return to the heart and thereby decrease cardiac output. Positive pressure may be transmitted to the pulmonary vascular bed, raising pulmonary vascular resistance and thereby promoting right-to-left shunting. The risk of these phenomena increases as lung compliance increases as RDS resolves. In this circumstance, reduction of the CPAP may improve oxygenation.

   b. Hypercarbia may indicate that CPAP is too high and tidal volume is thereby reduced.

   c. The use of nasal prongs or nasopharyngeal tubes may be unsuccessful if crying or mouth opening prevents adequate transmission of pressure or if the infant's abdomen becomes distended despite insertion of a nasogastric tube. In these situations, endotracheal intubation is often necessary.

4. Weaning. As the infant improves, we begin by reducing the Fio_2 in decrements of 0.05 to maintain the targeted oxygen saturation. Generally, when Fio_2 is <0.30, CPAP can be reduced to 5 cm H_2O, following oxygen saturation. Physical examination will provide evidence of respiratory effort during weaning, and chest radiographs may help estimate lung volume. Lowering of the distending pressure should be attempted with caution if the lung volumes appear low and alveolar atelectasis persists. We generally discontinue CPAP if there is no distress and the Fio_2 remains <0.3.

D. Mechanical ventilation (see Chap. 24B)

1. The initiation of ventilator therapy is influenced by the decision to administer surfactant (see II. A). The goals, once mechanical ventilation is initiated, are to limit tidal volume without losing lung volume or promoting atelectasis and to wean to extubation as soon as possible. Indications to start ventilation are a respiratory acidosis with a $Paco_2$ >55 mm Hg or rapidly rising, a Pao_2 <50 mm Hg or oxygen saturation <90% with an Fio_2 above 0.50, or severe apnea. The actual levels of Pao_2 and $Paco_2$ necessitating intervention depend on the course of the disease and the size of the infant. For example, a high $Paco_2$ early in the course of RDS will generally indicate the need for ventilator support, while the same $Paco_2$ when the infant is recovering might be managed, after careful evaluation, by observation and repeated sampling before any intervention is made.

2. Ventilators. A continuous-flow, pressure-limited, time-cycled ventilator is useful for ventilating newborns because pressure waveforms, inspiratory and expiratory duration, and pressure can be varied independently and because the flow of gas permits unobstructed spontaneous breathing. Synchronized intermittent mechanical ventilation (SIMV), which synchronizes with the infant's own respiratory effort, is preferred (see Chap. 24B). Other modes of pressure-limited ventilation, including assist-control, pressure support, and volume-guarantee are used as well, although clinical benefits have not been shown with these newer modes of mechanical ventilation.

High-frequency oscillatory ventilation (HFOV) may be useful to minimize lung injury in very small and/or sick infants who require very high peak inspiratory pressures and oxygen concentration to maintain adequate gas exchange and to manage infants in whom air leak syndromes complicate RDS.

   a. Initial settings. We generally start mechanical ventilation with a peak inspiratory pressure of 20 to 25 cm H_2O, positive end-expiratory pressure (PEEP) of 4 to 6 cm H_2O, frequency of 25 to 30 breaths per minute, inspiratory duration of 0.3 to 0.4 seconds, and the previously required Fio_2 (usually 0.50–1). Because of the short lung time constant in early RDS, faster rates (40–60 breaths per minute) with a shorter inspiratory time (0.2 seconds) may also be used. It is useful to ventilate the infant first by hand, using an anesthesia bag and manometer to determine the actual pressures required. The infant should be observed for color, chest motion, and respiratory effort, and the examiner should listen for breath sounds and observe changes in oxygen saturation. Adjustments in ventilator settings may be required on the basis of these observations or arterial blood gas results.

   b. Adjustments (see Chap. 24B). $Paco_2$ should be maintained in the range of 45 to 55 mm Hg. Acidosis may exacerbate RDS. Therefore, if relative hypercapnia is accepted to minimize lung injury, meticulous control of any metabolic acidosis is necessary. Rising $Paco_2$ levels may indicate the onset of complications, including atelectasis, air leak, or symptomatic PDA. Pao_2 usually rises in response to increases in Fio_2 or mean airway pressure. Some infants have pulmonary hypertension resulting in right-to-left shunting through fetal pathways; in these infants, interventions to reduce pulmonary vascular resistance may improve oxygenation (see 24F). More commonly, premature infants remain hypoxemic because of shunting through atelectatic lung and respond to measures that improve lung recruitment, including HFOV.

3. **Care of the infant receiving ventilator therapy** includes scrupulous attention to vital signs and clinical condition. Fio_2 and ventilator settings must be checked frequently. Oxygen saturation should be monitored continuously. Blood gas levels should be checked at least every 4 to 6 hours during the acute illness, or more frequently if the infant's condition is changing rapidly, and 30 minutes following changes in ventilator settings. Airway secretions may require periodic suctioning using closed (in-line) suction devices.

4. **Danger signs**
   a. If an infant receiving CPAP or mechanical ventilation deteriorates, the following should be suspected:
      i. Blocked or dislodged endotracheal tube.
      ii. Malfunctioning ventilator.
      iii. Air leak.
   b. Remedial action. The infant should be removed from the ventilator and ventilated with an anesthesia bag, which should be immediately available at the bedside. An appropriate suction catheter is passed to determine patency of the tube, and the tube position is checked by auscultation of breath sounds or by laryngoscopy. If there is any doubt, the tube should be removed and the infant should be ventilated by bag and mask pending replacement of the tube. The ventilator should be checked to ensure that Fio_2 settings are appropriate. The baby's chest is auscultated and transilluminated to check for pneumothorax (see Chap.24E). If pneumothorax is suspected, chest radiographs should be obtained, but if the infant's condition is critical, immediate aspiration by needle is both diagnostic and therapeutic. Hypotension secondary to hemorrhage, capillary leak, or myocardial dysfunction also can complicate RDS and should be treated by blood volume expansion or pressors or both. Pneumopericardium and pulmonary or intraventricular hemorrhage can also cause a sudden deterioration. Immediate attention to treatable conditions is appropriate.

5. **Weaning.** As the infant shows signs of improvement, weaning from the ventilator should be attempted. Specific steps to reduce inspiratory pressure, PEEP rate, and Fio_2 depend on the infant's blood gases, physical examination, and responses.
   a. The settings at which mechanical ventilation can be successfully discontinued will vary with the size, condition, respiratory drive, and individual pulmonary mechanics of the infant. Infants weighing <2 kg are usually best weaned to ventilator rates of approximately 20 breaths per minute and then extubated if they are stable on Fio_2 <0.30 and peak inspiratory pressure <18 cm H_2O. Larger infants may tolerate extubation from higher settings. We frequently use CPAP through nasal prongs or nasopharyngeal tubes to stabilize lung volumes after extubation, especially in smaller infants.
   b. Failure to wean may result from a number of causes, of which the following is a partial list.

i. Pulmonary edema may be present owing to capillary leak during acute stages of the illness or may develop secondary to patency of the ductus arteriosus. However, diuretic treatment in the acute phase of RDS is not helpful.

ii. Recovery of the lung from RDS is not uniform, and segmental or lobar atelectasis, edema, or interstitial emphysema may delay weaning.

iii. As the infant's lungs become more compliant, the inspiratory and expiratory times may have to be increased to allow optimal inflation and deflation of the lungs.

iv. Other reasons include onset of BPD or of apnea of prematurity. We frequently begin caffeine therapy before extubation in infants <30 weeks' gestation to improve respiratory drive and prevent apnea (see Chap. 24I). Glottic or subglottic edema resulting in obstruction may respond to inhaled racemic epinephrine; a brief course of systemic glucocorticoids may rarely be needed.

E. Supportive therapy

1. Temperature (see Chap. 12). Temperature control is crucial in all low birth weight infants, especially in those with respiratory disease. If the infant's temperature is too high or low, metabolic demands increase considerably. If oxygen uptake is limited by RDS, the increased demand cannot be met. An incubator or a radiant warmer must be used to maintain a neutral thermal environment for the infant.

2. Fluids and nutrition (see Chaps. 9 and 10)

a. **Infants with RDS** initially require intravascular administration of fluids. We generally start fluid therapy at 60 to 80 mL/kg/day, using dextrose 10% in water. Very low birth weight (VLBW) infants in whom poor glucose tolerance and large transcutaneous losses are expected are usually started at 100 to 120 mL/kg/day. ELBW infants may be started as high as 120 to 140 mL/kg/day, although use of humidified incubators will dramatically decrease insensible losses and resultant fluid requirements. Phototherapy, skin trauma, and radiant warmers increase insensible losses. Excessive fluid administration may cause pulmonary edema and increases the risk for a symptomatic PDA. The key to fluid management is careful monitoring of serum electrolytes and body weight, and frequent adjustments in fluids as indicated. Fluid retention is common in infants with RDS. However, extremely immature infants often lack renal concentration efficiency and have enormous evaporative losses if not placed in humidified incubators.

b. **By the second day,** we usually add sodium (2 mEq/kg/day), potassium (1 mEq/kg/day), and calcium (100 to 200 mg/kg/day) to the fluids. If it seems unlikely that adequate enteral nutrition will be achieved within several days, total parenteral nutrition should be started by the first day after birth.

c. **In most infants with RDS,** spontaneous diuresis occurs on the second to fourth day, preceding improvement in pulmonary function. Diuresis and improvement in pulmonary compliance occurs much sooner in surfactant treated infants, often within hours. If diuresis and improvement in lung disease do not occur by 1 to 2 weeks of age, this may indicate the onset of BPD (see Chap. 24J).

3. Circulation is assessed by monitoring the heart rate, blood pressure, and peripheral perfusion. Judicious use of blood or a volume expander (normal saline) may be necessary, and pressors may be used to support the circulation. In general, we attempt to limit crystalloid administration (attempting to avoid both capillary leak of fluid into inflamed lung parenchyma and the excessive administration of sodium from repeated boluses of saline). We often use dopamine (starting at 5 μg/kg/minute) to maintain adequate blood pressure and cardiac output and ensure improved tissue perfusion and urine output, and avoid metabolic acidosis. After the first 12 to 24 hours, hypotension and poor perfusion can also result from a large left-to-right shunt through a PDA, so careful assessment is warranted. The volume of blood drawn should be monitored and, in very low birth weight infants who are sick with RDS, generally should be replaced by packed red blood cell (PRBCs) transfusion when the hematocrit falls below 35% to 40%.

4. **Possible infection.** Because pneumonia or sepsis (classically with group B Streptococcus) can duplicate the clinical signs and radiographic appearance of RDS, we obtain blood cultures and complete blood counts with differential from all infants with RDS and treat with broad-spectrum antibiotics (ampicillin and gentamicin) for at least 48 hours.

F. **Acute complications**

1. **Air leak** (see Chap. 24E). Pneumothorax, pneumomediastinum, pneumoperi-cardium, or interstitial emphysema should be suspected when an infant with RDS deteriorates, typically with hypotension, apnea, bradycardia, or persistent acidosis.

2. **Infection** (see Chap. 23) may accompany RDS and may present in a variety of ways. Also, instrumentation, such as catheters or respiratory equipment, provides access for organisms to invade the immunologically immature preterm infant. Whenever there is suspicion of infection, appropriate cultures should be obtained and antibiotics administered promptly.

3. **Intracranial hemorrhage** (see Chap. 27B). Infants with severe RDS are at increased risk for intracranial hemorrhage and should be monitored with cranial ultrasound examinations.

4. **PDA** (see Chap. 25 frequently complicates RDS. PDA typically presents as pulmonary vascular pressures begin to fall. If untreated, it may result in increasing left-to-right shunt and ultimately cause heart failure, manifested by respiratory decompensation and cardiomegaly. The systemic consequences of the shunt may include low mean blood pressure, metabolic acidosis, decreased urine output, and worsening jaundice due to impaired organ perfusion. We generally treat infants, especially those weighing <1,500 g, with intravenous indomethacin if they develop any signs of a symptomatic PDA, such as a systolic or continuous murmur, hyperdynamic precordium, bounding pulses, or widened pulse pressure. In infants who weigh <1,000 g, we treat with indomethacin when a PDA first becomes clinically apparent (i.e., presence of ductal murmur without the signs or symptoms of a large left-to-right shunt). We reserve surgical ligation for infants in whom indomethacin is contraindicated (e.g., those with renal failure or necrotizing enterocolitis) or those in whom two courses of indomethacin have failed. In larger infants who are improving steadily despite PDA and who have no evidence of heart failure, mild fluid restriction and time may result in closure. Intravenous ibuprofen is also available for pharmacologic closure of the PDA, and may have fewer renal side effects compared with indomethacin.

G. **Long-term complications** include BPD (see Chap. 24J), and other complications of prematurity, including neurodevelopmental impairment and retinopathy of pre-maturity. The risk of these complications increases with decreasing birth weight and gestational age.

Suggested Readings

Halliday HL. Recent clinical trials of surfactant treatment for neonate. *Biol Neonate* 2006;89(4):323–329.

Hamvas A. Inherited surfactant protein-B deficiency and surfactant protein-C associated disease: Clinical features and evaluation. *Semin Perinatol* 2006;30(6):316–326.

Ramanathan R. Surfactant therapy in preterm infants with respiratory distress syn-drome and in near-term or term newborns with acute RDS. *J Perinatol* 2006;26 (Suppl 1):S51–S56.

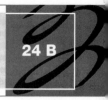

MECHANICAL VENTILATION
Eric C. Eichenwald

24 B

I. **GENERAL PRINCIPLES.** Mechanical ventilation is an invasive life support procedure with many effects on the cardiopulmonary system. The goal is to optimize both gas exchange and clinical status at minimum Fio$_2$ (fractional concentration of inspired oxygen) and ventilator pressures/tidal volume. The ventilator strategy employed to accomplish this goal depends, in part, on the infant's disease process. In addition, recent advances in technology have brought more options for ventilatory therapy of newborns.

II. **TYPES OF VENTILATORY SUPPORT**
A. **Continuous positive airway pressure (CPAP)**
1. **CPAP is usually administered by means of a ventilator.** Any system used to deliver CPAP should allow continuous monitoring of the delivered pressure, and be equipped with safety alarms to indicate when the pressure is above or below the desired level. Alternatively, CPAP may be delivered by a simplified system providing blended oxygen flowing past the infant's airway with the end of the tubing submerged in 0.25% acetic acid in sterile water solution to the desired depth to generate pressure ("bubble CPAP").
2. **General characteristics.** A continuous flow of heated, humidified gas is circulated past the infant's airway typically at a set pressure of 3 to 8 cm H$_2$O, maintaining an elevated end-expiratory lung volume while the infant breathes spontaneously. The air–oxygen mixture and airway pressure can be adjusted. CPAP is usually delivered by means of nasal prongs or a nasopharyngeal tube. Prolonged endotracheal CPAP should not be used because the high resistance of the endotracheal tube increases the work of breathing, especially in small infants. Positive-pressure hoods and continuous-mask CPAP are not recommended.
3. **Advantages**
   a. CPAP is less invasive than mechanical ventilation and causes less barotrauma.
   b. When used early in infants with respiratory distress syndrome (RDS), it can help prevent alveolar and airway collapse, which might result in deterioration of Pao$_2$, and thereby reduce the need for mechanical ventilation.
   c. CPAP decreases the frequency of obstructive and mixed apneic spells in some infants.
4. **Disadvantages**
   a. CPAP does not improve ventilation and may worsen it.
   b. CPAP provides inadequate respiratory support in the face of severe changes in pulmonary compliance and resistance.
   c. Maintaining nasal or nasopharyngeal CPAP in large, active infants may be technically difficult.
   d. Swallowed air can elevate the diaphragm and must be removed by a gastric tube.
5. **Indications**
   a. Early treatment of premature infants with minimal respiratory distress and minimal need for supplemental oxygen (mild RDS) to prevent atelectasis.
   b. Moderately frequent apneic spells.
   c. After recent extubation.
   d. Weaning chronically ventilator-dependent infants.
B. **Pressure-limited, time-cycled, continuous-flow** ventilators are used most frequently in newborns with respiratory failure.
1. **General characteristics.** A continuous flow of heated and humidified gas is circulated past the infant's airway; the gas is a selected mixture of air with

oxygen. Maximum inspiratory pressure (P_I), positive end-expiratory pressure (PEEP), and respiratory timing (rate and duration of inspiration and expiration) are selected.

2. Advantages

   a. The continuous flow of fresh gas allows the infant to make spontaneous respiratory efforts between ventilator breaths (intermittent mandatory ventilation, IMV).

   b. Good control is maintained over respiratory pressures.

   c. Inspiratory and expiratory time can be independently controlled.

   d. The system is relatively simple and inexpensive.

3. Disadvantages

   a. Tidal volume is poorly controlled.

   b. The system does not respond to changes in respiratory system compliance.

   c. Spontaneously breathing infants who breathe out of phase with too many IMV breaths ("bucking" or "fighting" the ventilator) may receive inadequate ventilation and are at increased risk for air leak.

4. Indications. Useful in any form of lung disease in infants.

C. Synchronized and patient-triggered (assist/control, or pressure support) ventilators are adaptations of conventional pressure-limited ventilators used for newborns.

1. General characteristics. These ventilators combine the features of pressure-limited, time-cycled, continuous-flow ventilators with an airway pressure, air flow, or respiratory movement sensor. By measuring inspiratory flow or movement, these ventilators deliver intermittent positive-pressure breaths at a fixed rate in synchrony with the baby's inspiratory efforts ("synchronized IMV," or synchronized intermittent mandatory ventilation [SIMV]). During apnea, SIMV ventilators continue to deliver the set IMV rate. In patient-triggered ventilation, a positive pressure breath is delivered with every inspiratory effort. As a result, the ventilator delivers more frequent positive pressure breaths, usually allowing a decrease in the peak inspiratory pressure (PIP) needed for adequate gas exchange. During apnea, the ventilator in patient-triggered mode delivers an operator-selected IMV ("control") rate. In some ventilators, synchronized IMV breaths can be supplemented by pressure-supported breaths in the spontaneously breathing infant. Ventilators equipped with a flow sensor can also be used to monitor delivered tidal volume continuously by integration of the flow signal.

2. Advantages

   a. Synchronizing the delivery of positive pressure breaths with the infant's inspiratory effort reduces the phenomenon of breathing out of phase with IMV breaths ("fighting" the ventilator). This may decrease the need for sedative medications and aid in weaning mechanically ventilated infants.

   b. Pronounced asynchrony with ventilator breaths during conventional IMV has been associated with the development of air leak and intraventricular hemorrhage. Whether the use of SIMV or assist/control ventilation reduces these complications is not known.

3. Disadvantages

   a. Under certain conditions, the ventilators may inappropriately trigger a breath because of artifactual signals, or fail to trigger because of problems with the sensor.

   b. Few data are available on the effects of patient-triggered ventilation in newborns. Pressure support ventilation may not be appropriate for small premature infants with irregular respiratory patterns and frequent apnea because of the potential for significant variability in ventilation.

   c. It is more expensive and complicated to use than a conventional pressure-limited device.

4. Indications. SIMV can be used when a conventional pressure-limited ventilator is indicated. If available, it may be the preferable mode of ventilator therapy in infants who are breathing spontaneously while on IMV. The indications for assist/control and pressure support ventilation have not been established, although are under active investigation.

D. Volume-cycled ventilators are rarely used in newborn infants, although recent advances in technology have renewed interest in this mode of ventilation in selected situations. Only volume-cycled ventilators specifically designed for newborns should be used.

    1. General characteristics. Volume-cycled ventilators are similar to pressure-limited ventilators except that the operator selects the volume delivered, rather than the PIP. "Volume guarantee" is a mode of SIMV in which the ventilator targets an operator-chosen tidal volume during mechanically delivered breaths.

    2. Advantages. The pressure automatically varies with respiratory system compliance to deliver the selected tidal volume, theoretically minimizing variability in minute ventilation.

    3. Disadvantages

        a. The system is complicated and requires more skill to operate.

        b. Because tidal volumes in infants are small, most of the tidal volume selected is lost in the ventilator circuit or from air leaks around uncuffed endotracheal tubes. A separate in-line tidal volume monitor may be helpful.

        c. It is more expensive than a pressure-limited device.

    4. Indications. May be useful if lung compliance is rapidly changing.

E. The high frequency ventilator (HFV) is an important adjunct to conventional mechanical ventilation in newborns. The recommended uses and the ventilatory strategies employed with HFVs continue to evolve with clinical experience. Three types of HFVs are approved for use in newborns: a high-frequency oscillator (HFO), a high-frequency flow interrupter (HFFI), and a high-frequency jet (HFJ) ventilator.

    1. General characteristics. Available HFVs are similar despite considerable differences in design. All HFVs are capable of delivering extremely rapid rates (300–1,500 breaths/minute, 5–25 Hz; 1 Hz = 60 breaths/minute) with tidal volumes equal to or smaller than anatomic dead space. These ventilators apply continuous distending pressure to maintain an elevated lung volume; small tidal volumes are superimposed at a rapid rate. HFJ ventilators are paired with a conventional pressure-limited device, which is used to deliver intermittent "sigh" breaths to help prevent atelectasis. "Sigh" breaths are not used with HFO ventilation. Expiration is passive (i.e., dependent on chest wall and lung recoil) with HFFI and HFJ machines, while it is active with HFO. The mechanisms of gas exchange with HFV are incompletely understood.

    2. Advantages

        a. HFVs can achieve adequate ventilation while avoiding the large swings in lung volume required by conventional ventilators and associated with lung injury. Because of this, they may be useful in pulmonary air leak syndromes (pulmonary interstitial emphysema (PIE), pneumothorax), or in infants failing conventional mechanical ventilation.

        b. HFV allows the use of a high mean airway pressure (MAP) for alveolar recruitment and resultant improvement in ventilation-perfusion ($\dot{V}/\dot{Q}$) matching. This may be advantageous in infants with severe respiratory failure requiring high MAP to maintain adequate oxygenation on a conventional mechanical ventilator.

    3. Disadvantages. Despite theoretic advantages of HFV, no significant benefit of this method has been demonstrated in routine clinical use over more conventional ventilators. Only one rigorously controlled study found a small reduction in bronchopulmonary dysplasia (BPD) in infants at high risk treated with high-frequency oscillatory ventilation (HFOV) as the primary mode of ventilation. This experience is likely not generalizable, however, as other studies have shown no difference. These ventilators are more complex and expensive, and there is less long-term clinical experience. The initial studies with HFO suggested an increased risk of significant intraventricular hemorrhage, although this complication has not been observed in recent clinical trials. Studies comparing the different types of HFVs are unavailable; therefore, the relative advantages or disadvantages of HFO, HFFI, and HFJ, if any, are not characterized.

4. **Indications.** HFVs are primarily used as a rescue therapy for infants failing conventional ventilation. Both HFJ and HFO ventilators have been shown to be superior to conventional ventilation in infants with air leak syndromes, especially PIE. Because of the potential for complications, we do not use high-frequency ventilation as the primary mode of ventilatory support in infants.

F. **Negative pressure.** These infant versions of the adult "iron lung" are rarely used because nursing access is limited by the negative-pressure cylinder and because the neck seal makes them feasible only for large babies. Their use is restricted to older infants with neuromuscular problems who can therefore be ventilated without an endotracheal tube.

III. INDICATIONS FOR RESPIRATORY SUPPORT. See Chapter 36 for intubation procedures and proper selection of endotracheal tube sizes.

A. **Indications** for CPAP in the preterm infant with RDS include the following:

1. Recently delivered premature infant with minimal respiratory distress and low supplemental oxygen requirement (to prevent atelectasis).
2. Respiratory distress and requirement of Fio_2 above 0.30 by hood.
3. Fio_2 above 0.40 by hood.
4. Clinically significant retractions and/or distress after recent extubation.
5. In general, infants with RDS who require Fio_2 above 0.35 to 0.40 on CPAP should be intubated, ventilated, and given surfactant replacement therapy. In some neonatal intensive care units (NICUs), intubation for surfactant therapy in infants with RDS is followed by immediate extubation to CPAP. This method of surfactant delivery requires more investigation before it is routinely recommended. We use mechanical ventilation for all infants who are given surfactant.

B. Relative indications for mechanical ventilation in any infant include the following:

1. Frequent intermittent apnea unresponsive to drug therapy.
2. Early treatment when use of mechanical ventilation is anticipated because of deteriorating gas exchange.
3. Relieving "work of breathing" in an infant with signs of respiratory difficulty.
4. Administration of surfactant therapy in infants with RDS.

C. **Absolute indications for mechanical ventilation**

1. Prolonged apnea.
2. Pao_2 below 50 mm Hg or Fio_2 above 0.80. This indication may not apply to the infant with cyanotic congenital heart disease.
3. $Paco_2$ above 60 mm Hg with persistent acidemia.
4. General anesthesia.

IV. HOW VENTILATOR CHANGES AFFECT BLOOD GASES

A. **Oxygenation (see Table 24B.1)**

1. **Fio_2.** The goal is to maintain adequate tissue oxygen delivery. Generally, this can be accomplished by achieving a Pao_2 of 50 to 70 mm Hg. This results in a hemoglobin saturation of 88% to 95% (see Fig. 24B.1). Increasing inspired oxygen is the simplest and most direct means of improving oxygenation. In premature infants, the risk of retinopathy and pulmonary oxygen toxicity argue for minimizing Pao_2. For infants with other conditions, the optimum Pao_2 may be higher. Direct pulmonary oxygen toxicity begins to occur at Fio_2 values greater than 0.60 to 0.70.

2. **MAP**

a. MAP is the average area under the curve of the pressure waveform. Many ventilators now display MAP or can be equipped with a device to do so; it may also be calculated using the following equation: MAP = $([PIP - PEEP][T_I]/T_I + T_E) + PEEP$. MAP is increased by increases in PEEP, inspiratory pressure (P_I), inspiratory time (T_I), rate, and flow rate. All these changes lead to higher Pao_2, but each has different effects on $Paco_2$. For a given rise in MAP, increasing PEEP gives the greatest improvement in Pao_2. Other ways to raise MAP are to increase P_I and prolong T_I.

b. Optimum MAP results from a balance between optimizing Pao_2, minimizing direct oxygen toxicity, minimizing barotrauma, achieving adequate

TABLE 24B.1   Ventilator Manipulations to Increase Oxygenation

Parameter	Advantage	Disadvantage
↑ Fio_2	Minimizes barotrauma Easily administered	Fails to affect $\dot{V}/\dot{Q}$ matching Direct toxicity, especially >0.06
↑ P_I	Critical opening pressure Improves $\dot{V}/\dot{Q}$	Barotrauma: air leak, BPD
↑ PEEP	Maintains FRC/prevents collapse Splints obstructed airways Regularizes respiration	Shifts to stiffer compliance Curve Obstructs venous return Increases expiratory work and CO_2 Increases dead space
↑ T_I	Increases MAP without increases P_I "Critical opening time"	Necessitates slower rates, higher P_I Lower minute ventilation for given P_I — PEEP combination
↑ Flow	Square wave — maximizes MAP	Greater shear force, more barotrauma Greater resistance at greater flows
↑ Rate	Increases MAP while using lower P_I	Inadvertent PEEP with high rates or long-term constant

↑ = increase; BPD = bronchopulmonary dysplasia; Fio_2 = fractional concentration of inspired oxygen; FRC = functional residual capacity; P_I = inspiratory pressure; T_I = inspiratory time; MAP = mean airway pressure; PEEP = positive end-expiratory pressure; $\dot{V}/\dot{Q}$ = ventilation-perfusion ratio. All manipulations (except Fio_2) result in higher mean airway pressure (MAP).

ventilation, and minimizing adverse cardiovascular effects. Ventilator-induced lung injury is probably most closely related to peak-to-peak swings in lung volume, although changes in airway pressure are also implicated.

    c. MAP as low as 5 cm H_2O may be sufficient in infants with normal lungs, whereas 20 cm H_2O or more may be necessary in severe RDS. Excessive MAP may impede venous return and adversely affect cardiac output.

3. Ventilation (see Table 24B.2)

    a. CO_2 elimination depends on minute ventilation. Since minute ventilation is the product of respiratory rate and tidal volume, increases in ventilator rate will lowerPaco_2. Increases in tidal volume can be achieved by increasing the P_I on pressure-cycled ventilators or by increasing volume on volume-limited machines. Because tidal volume is a function of the difference between P_I and PEEP, a reduction in PEEP also improves ventilation. At very low tidal volumes, the volume of dead space becomes important and may lead to CO_2 retention.

    b. Optimal Paco_2 varies according to disease state. For very immature infants or infants with air leak, a Paco_2 of 50 to 60 mm Hg may be tolerated to minimize ventilator-induced lung injury, provided pH is >7.25.

V. DISEASE STATES

  A. Effects of diseases. Respiratory failure can result from numerous illnesses through a variety of pathophysiologic mechanisms. Optimal ventilatory strategy must take into account the pathophysiology, expected time course, and particular vulnerabilities of the patient.

  B. Pulmonary mechanics influence the ventilator strategy selected.

    1. Compliance is the stiffness or distensibility of the lung and chest wall, that is, the change in volume (ΔV) produced by a change in pressure (ΔP), or $\Delta V/\Delta P$. It is decreased with surfactant deficiency, excess lung water, and lung fibrosis. It is also decreased when the lungs are hyperexpanded.

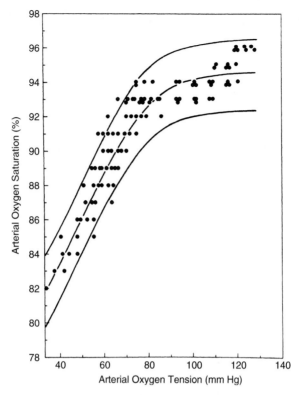

Figure 24B.1. Comparison of paired measurements of oxygen saturation by pulse oximetry and of oxygen tension by indwelling umbilical artery oxygen electrode. The lines represent ±2 standard deviations. (Modified from Wasunna A, Whitelaw AG. Pulse osimetry in preterm infants. *Arch Dis Child* 1987;62:957.)

2. **Resistance is the impediment** to airflow due to friction between gas and airways (airway resistance) and between tissues of the lungs and chest wall (viscous tissue resistance). Almost half of airway resistance is in the upper airways, including the endotracheal tube when in use. Resistance is high in diseases characterized by airway obstruction, such as meconium aspiration and BPD. Resistance can change rapidly if, for example, secretions partially occlude the endotracheal tube.

3. **Time constant** is the product of compliance and resistance. This is a measure of the time it takes to equilibrate pressure between the proximal airway and the alveoli. Expiratory time constants are somewhat longer than inspiratory ones. When time constants are long, as in meconium aspiration, care must be taken to set ventilator inspiratory times and rates that permit adequate inspiration to deliver the required tidal volume and adequate expiration to avoid inadvertent PEEP.

4. **Functional residual capacity (FRC)** is a measure of the volume of the lungs at end-expiration. FRC is decreased in diseases that permit alveolar collapse, particularly surfactant deficiency.

5. **$\dot{V}/\dot{Q}$ matching.** Diseases that reduce alveolar surface area (through atelectasis, inflammatory exudates, or obstruction) permit intrapulmonary shunting of desaturated blood. The opposite occurs in persistent pulmonary hypertension,

TABLE 24B.2   Ventilator Manipulations to Increase Ventilation and Decrease $Paco_2$

Parameter	Advantage	Disadvantage
↑ Rate	Easy to titrate Minimizes barotrauma	Maintains same dead space/tidal volume May lead to inadvertent PEEP
↑ P_I	Better bulk flow (improved dead space/tidal volume)	More barotrauma Shifts to stiffer compliance curve
↓ PEEP	Widens compression Pressure Decreases dead space Decreases expiratory load Shifts to steeper compliance curve	Decreases MAP Decreases oxygenation/alveolar collapse Stops splinting obstructed/closed airways
↑ Flow	Permits shorter T_I, longer T_E	More barotrauma
↑ T_E	Allows longer time for passive expiration in face of prolonged time Constant	Shortens T_I Decreases MAP Decreases oxygenation

↓ = decrease; T_E = expiratory time; Fio_2 = fractional concentration of inspired oxygen; ↑ = increase; T_I = inspiratory time; MAP = mean airway pressure; $Paco_2$ = partial pressure of carbon dioxide, arterial; P_I = peak inspiratory pressure; PEEP = positive end-expiratory pressure.

when extrapulmonary shunting diverts blood flow away from the ventilated lung. Both mechanisms result in systemic recirculation of desaturated blood.

6. **Work of breathing** is especially important in the smallest infants and those with chronic lung disease, whose high airway resistance, decreased lung compliance, compliant chest wall, and weak musculature may overwhelm their metabolic energy requirements and impede growth.

C. **Specific disease states.** Several of the more common neonatal disease processes are described in the subsequent text and are presented in Table 24B.3 along with the optimal ventilatory strategies. Before initiating ventilatory support, however, clinicians must evaluate for mechanical causes of distress, including pneumothorax or airway obstruction.

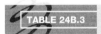

TABLE 24B.3   Neonatal Pulmonary Physiology by Disease State

Disease	Compliance mL/cm H_2O	Resistance cm H_2O/mL/s	Time constant (s)	FRC (mL/kg)	$\dot{V}/\dot{Q}$ matching	Work
Normal term	4–6	20–40	0.25	30	—	—
RDS	↓↓	—	↓↓	↓	↓/↓↓	↑
Meconium aspiration	—/↓	↑/↑↑	↑	↑/↑↑	↓↓	↑
BPD	↑/↓	↑↑	↑	↑↑	↓↓/↓	↑↑
Air leak	↓↓	—/↑	—/↑	↑↑	↓/↓↓	↑↑
VLBW apnea	↓	—	↓↓	—/↓	↓/—	—/↑

BPD = bronchopulmonary dysplasia; ↓ = decrease; /, either/or; FRC = functional residual capacity; ↑ = increase; — = little or no change; RDS = respiratory distress syndrome; $\dot{V}/\dot{Q}$ = ventilation-perfusion ratio; VLBW = very low birth weight.

1. **RDS** (see Chap. 24A)

   a. **Pathophysiology.** RDS is caused by surfactant deficiency, which results in a severe decrease in compliance (stiff lung). This causes diffuse alveolar collapse with $\dot{V}/\dot{Q}$ mismatching and increased work of breathing.

   b. **Surfactant replacement.** We recommend intubation and initiation of mechanical ventilation early in the course of RDS in order to provide surfactant therapy promptly. The distinctive time course of escalation, plateau, and weaning in classic RDS has changed with the use of surfactant therapy. Ventilatory strategy should anticipate the increased risk of pneumothorax as compliance increases and time constants lengthen, especially with the rapid improvements that can be seen after surfactant administration. In all approaches, a $Paco_2$ value higher than the physiologic value is acceptable to minimize ventilator-induced lung injury.

   c. **Ventilator strategy**

      i. **CPAP.** In mildly affected infants who may not require intubation and surfactant administration, CPAP is used early in the disease course to prevent further atelectasis. CPAP is initiated at 5 to 6 cm H_2O, and increased to a maximum of 7 to 8 cm H_2O, although occasionally higher pressures may be used. CPAP is titrated by clinical assessment of retractions and respiratory rate and by observation of O_2 saturation. Alternatively, in infants with slightly more severe RDS, consideration may be given to intubation for surfactant administration, a short period of mechanical ventilation, followed by CPAP as gas exchange improves.

      ii. Mechanical ventilation is used when $\dot{V}/\dot{Q}$ mismatching is so severe that increased Fio_2 and CPAP are inadequate, or in infants who tire from the increased work of breathing. Recent data suggest that a ventilator strategy that avoids large changes in tidal volume (V_T) may reduce ventilator-induced lung injury. The objective of all strategies of assisted ventilation in the infant with RDS should be to provide the lowest level of ventilatory support possible to support adequate oxygenation and ventilation while attempting to reduce acute and chronic lung injury secondary to barotrauma/volutrauma and oxygen toxicity. Our preferred approach is to maintain the appropriate MAP with a T_I initially set at 0.3 second and rate of approximately 20 to 40 breaths/minute. Rarely, a longer T_I is required to provide adequate oxygenation. This ventilatory approach requires a moderate P_I to provide adequate minute ventilation and to maintain alveolar recruitment.

      iii. **P_I and PEEP.** P_I, applied to recruit alveoli, is initially estimated by good chest excursion and is usually 20 to 25 cm H_2O. PEEP is set at 4 to 5 cm H_2O and may go up to 6 cm H_2O. Higher PEEP may interfere with cardiac output and should be avoided in acute RDS.

      iv. **Flow.** Flow rates of 7 to 12 L/minute are needed to provide a relatively square pressure waveform. Higher flows may be required at very high P_I (>35 cm H_2O).

      v. Rates are generally set initially at 20 to 40 breaths/minute, and adjusted by blood gas results.

      vi. **Weaning.** When the patient becomes stable, Fio_2 and P_I are weaned first, alternating with rate, in response to assessment of chest excursion, oxygen saturation, and blood gas results. Extubation is usually successful when ventilator rates are <20 to 25 breaths/minute. Caffeine citrate may be used to facilitate spontaneous breathing before extubation and may increase the success rate of extubation in very low birth weight infants.

      vii. **Advantages and disadvantages.** This ventilatory strategy maximizes alveolar recruitment, but with a potential for greater barotrauma secondary to the higher P_I and volutrauma secondary to higher V_T.

      viii. **Alternative ventilator strategies.** An alternative approach to mechanical ventilation in RDS relies on high rates to maintain MAP while reducing P_I and V_T to minimize barotrauma/volutrauma. Rates of 60 to

80 breaths/minute are used, with T_I as low as 0.2 second. Inadvertent PEEP is not encountered because the time constant in RDS may be as short as 0.05 second. P_I is set as low as 12 to 18 cm H_2O, with PEEP of 4 to 5 cm H_2O. Initial settings are based on auscultation of good breath sounds and are increased as needed to maintain adequate minute ventilation and oxygenation. In general, pressure is weaned first, although the rate remains high, or by 10% drops in rate alternating with pressure, as tolerated. This ventilator strategy may minimize barotrauma due to P_I and utilizes lower V_T, with the disadvantage of less alveolar recruitment and consequent need for higher Fio_2 to maintain adequate oxygen saturation.

High-frequency ventilation may be initiated if conventional ventilation fails to maintain adequate gas exchange. High-frequency ventilation should be used only by clinicians familiar with its use. We consider the use of HFV when the MAP required for adequate gas exchange exceeds 10 to 11 cm H_2O in small infants and 12 cm H_2O in larger infants, or if air leak occurs. Strategies differ depending on whether HFJ, HFO, or HFFI is used. We prefer HFOV over other available HFV because of its ease of use and applicability in a wide range of pulmonary diseases and infant weights.

a) **HFJ ventilation.** HFJ requires a special adapter for a standard endotracheal tube to allow connection to the jet port of the ventilator.

1) **P_I and PEEP.** Peak pressures on the jet ventilator are initially set approximately 20% lower than on those being used with conventional ventilation, and adjusted to provide adequate chest vibration assessed clinically and by blood gas determinations. P_I, PEEP, and Fio_2 are adjusted as needed to maintain oxygenation. CO_2 elimination is dependent on the pressure difference (P_I–PEEP). Because of the lower peak pressures required to ventilate, PEEP may be increased to 8 to 10 cm H_2O if needed to improve oxygenation.

2) **Rate.** The frequency is usually set at 420 breaths/minute, with an inspiratory jet valve on-time of 0.02 second.

3) **Conventional ventilator settings.** Once the HFJ is properly adjusted, the conventional ventilator rate is decreased to 2 to 10 breaths/minute to help maintain alveolar recruitment, with P_I set at 2 to 3 cm H_2O lower than the jet P_I. In air leak syndromes, it may be advantageous to provide no sigh breaths from the conventional ventilator as long as the PEEP is set high enough to maintain lung volume.

4) **Weaning** from HFJ ventilation is accomplished by decreasing the jet P_I in response to blood gas determinations and the Fio_2. PEEP is weaned as tolerated if pressures higher than 4 to 5 cm H_2O are used. Frequency and jet valve on-time are generally not adjusted.

5) **Similar strategies** outlined for the HFJ apply in use of the HFFI.

b) **HFOV.** With HFO, operator-selected parameters include MAP, frequency, and piston amplitude.

1) **MAP.** In RDS, the initial MAP selected is usually 2 to 5 cm H_2O higher than that being used on the conventional ventilator to enhance alveolar recruitment. MAP used with HFO is titrated to O_2 requirement and to provide adequate lung expansion on chest x-ray. Care must be exercised to avoid lung hyperinflation, which might adversely affect oxygen delivery by reducing cardiac output.

2) **Frequency is usually set at 10 to 15 Hz.** Inspiratory time is set at 33%.

3) **Amplitude.** Changes in piston amplitude primarily affect ventilation. It is set to provide adequate chest vibration, assessed clinically and by blood gas determinations.

4) **Flow rates** of 8 to 15 L/minute are usually adequate.

5) **Weaning.** In general, FiO_2 is weaned first, followed by MAP in decrements of 1 to 2 cm H_2O once the FiO_2 falls below 0.6. Piston amplitude is adjusted by frequent assessment of chest vibration and blood gas determinations. Frequency is usually not adjusted. In both HFJ and HFO, we usually wean to extubation after transfer back to conventional ventilation, although infants can be extubated directly from HFV.

2. Meconium aspiration syndrome (MAS) (see Chap. 24K)

a. **Pathophysiology.** MAS results from aspiration of meconium-stained amniotic fluid. The severity of the syndrome is related to the associated asphyxial insult and the amount aspirated. The aspirated meconium causes acute airway obstruction, marked airway resistance, scattered atelectasis with $\dot{V}/\dot{Q}$ mismatching, and hyperexpansion due to obstructive ball–valve effects. The obstructive phase is followed by an inflammatory phase 12 to 24 hours later that results in further alveolar involvement. Aspiration of other fluids (such as blood or amniotic fluid) has similar but milder effects.

b. **Ventilator strategy.** Because of the ball–valve effects, the application of positive pressure may result in pneumothorax or another air leak, so initiating mechanical ventilation requires careful consideration of the risks and benefits. Low levels of PEEP (4–5 cm H_2O) are helpful in splinting open partially obstructed airways and equalizing $\dot{V}/\dot{Q}$ matching. Higher levels may lead to hyperinflation. If airway resistance is high and compliance is normal, a slow-rate, moderate-pressure strategy is needed. If pneumonitis is more prominent, more rapid rates can be used. Sedation or muscle relaxation may be used to minimize the risks of air leak in severe MAS because of the high transpulmonary pressures these large infants can generate when "fighting" the ventilator and the ball–valve hyperexpansion caused by their disease. Use of synchronized IMV may be helpful. Weaning may be rapid if the illness is primarily related to airway obstruction or prolonged if complicated by barotrauma and severe inflammation. The use of surfactant therapy in more severe cases of MAS may improve lung compliance and oxygenation, and should be considered.

High-frequency ventilation has also been successfully used in infants with MAS who are failing conventional ventilation or who have suffered air leak. The strategies are similar to those described in the preceding text. During HFO, slower frequencies (8–10 Hz) may be useful to improve oxygenation in severe cases.

3. BPD (see VII.A.1)

a. **Pathophysiology.** BPD results from injury to the alveoli and airways. Bleb formation may lead to poor recoil. Fibrosis and excess lung water may cause stiffer compliance. Airways may be narrowed and fibrotic or hyperreactive. The upper airways may be overdistended and conduct airflow poorly. BPD is marked by shifting focal atelectasis, hyperinflation with $\dot{V}/\dot{Q}$ mismatching, chronic and acute increases in airway resistance, and a significant increase in the work of breathing.

b. **Ventilator strategy.** The optimal strategy is to wean infants off the ventilator as soon as possible to prevent further barotrauma and oxygen toxicity. If this is not feasible, ventilator settings should be minimized to permit tissue repair and long-term growth. Rates as low as 10 to 15 breaths/minute should generally be avoided to prevent increased work of breathing, but longer TI (0.4–0.5 second) may be used to maintain FRC. Higher pressures are sometimes required (20–30 cm H_2O) because of the stiff lungs, although the high resistance prevents transfer of most of this to the alveoli. Oxygenation should be maintained (saturations of 90%–92%), but higher $PaCO_2$ values can be permitted (55–65 mm Hg), provided the pH is normal. Acute decompensations can result from bronchospasm and interstitial fluid accumulation. These must be treated with adjustment of P_I, bronchodilators, and diuretics. Acute BPD "spells" in which oxygenation and airway resistance worsen rapidly are due to larger airway collapse, and may be treated successfully with higher PEEP (7–8 cm H_2O). Frequent rapid desaturations secondary to acute decreases in FRC with crying or infant movement respond to changes in Fio_2, but may also be partially ameliorated by using higher PEEP. Weaning is a slow and difficult process, decreasing rate by 1 to 2 breaths/minute or 1-cm H_2O decrements in P_I every day when tolerated. Fortunately, with improved medical and ventilatory care of these infants, it is rare for infants with BPD to require tracheostomy for chronic ventilation.

4. **Air leak (see Chap. 24E)**
   a. **Pathophysiology.** Pneumothorax and PIE are the two most common air leak syndromes. Pneumothorax results when air ruptures into the pleural space. In PIE, the interstitial air substantially reduces tissue compliance as well as recoil. In addition, peribronchial and perivascular air may compress the airways and vascular supply, causing "air block."
   b. **Ventilator strategy.** Since air is driven into the interstitium throughout the ventilatory cycle, the primary goal is to reduce MAP through any of its components (P_I, T_I, PEEP) and to rely on increased Fio_2 to provide oxygenation. This strategy holds for all air leak syndromes. If dropping the MAP is not tolerated, other techniques may be tried. Because the time constants for interstitial air are much longer than those for the alveoli, we sometimes use very rapid conventional rates (up to 60 breaths/minute), which may preferentially ventilate the alveoli.

      High-frequency ventilation is an important alternative therapy for severe air leak and, if available, may be the ventilatory treatment of choice. HFV strategies for air leak differ from those used in diffuse alveolar disease. As described for conventional ventilation, the ventilatory goal in air leak syndromes is to decrease MAP, relying on Fio_2 to provide oxygenation. With HFJ and HFFI, PEEP is maintained at lower levels (4–6 cm H_2O), and few to no sigh breaths provided. With HFO, the MAP initially used is the same as that being used on the conventional ventilator, and the frequency set at 15 Hz. While weaning, MAP is decreased progressively, tolerating higher Fio_2 in the attempt to limit the MAP exposure.

5. **Apnea (see Chap. 24I)**
   a. **Pathophysiology.** Occasionally, apnea is severe enough to warrant ventilator support, even in the absence of pulmonary disease. This may result from apnea of prematurity, during or following general anesthesia, or from neuromuscular paralysis.
   b. **Ventilator strategy.** For infants completely dependent on the ventilator, the goal should be to provide "physiologic" ventilation using moderate PEEP (3–4 cm H_2O), low gas flow, and normal rates (30–40 breaths/minute), with P_I adjusted to prevent hyperventilation (10–18 cm H_2O). Prolonged T_I is unnecessary. For infants requiring a ventilator because of intermittent but prolonged apnea, low rates (12–15 breaths/minute) may be sufficient.

VI. ADJUNCTS TO MECHANICAL VENTILATION

A. **Sedation** can be used when agitation or distress is associated with excessive liability of oxygenation and hypoxemia. Although this problem is more common in the neonate receiving long-term ventilation, acutely ill newborns may occasionally benefit from sedation. Morphine (0.05–0.1 mg/kg) or fentanyl (1–3μg/kg) can be used but may lead to dependence. Lorazepam (0.05–0.1 mg/kg/dose given every 4–6 hours) or midazolam (0.05–0.1 mg/kg/dose given every 2–4 hours) has been used in more mature infants and in more chronic situations because of its long duration of action. In preterm infants, nonpharmacologic methods, such as limiting environmental light and noise and providing behavioral supports, may help decrease agitation and limit the need for sedative medications. As discussed, synchronized IMV or ventilation may also help diminish agitation and ventilatory liability.

B. Muscle relaxation with pancuronium bromide (0.1 mg/kg/dose, repeated as needed) is rarely used, but may be indicated in some infants who continue to breathe out of phase with the ventilator after attempts at finding appropriate settings and sedation have failed. High Fio_2 requirement (>0.75) or PIP (>30 cm H_2O) are also relative indications for muscle relaxation. Although unequivocal data are not available, gas exchange may be improved in some infants following muscle relaxation, and the occurrence of chronic lung disease may be reduced. Prolonged muscle relaxation leads to fluid retention and may result in deterioration in compliance. Sedation is routinely administered to infants receiving muscle relaxants.

C. Blood gas monitoring (see Chap. 24C). All infants receiving mechanical ventilation require continuous monitoring of oxygen saturation and intermittent blood gas measurements.

VII. COMPLICATIONS AND SEQUELAE. As a complex and invasive technology, mechanical ventilation can result in numerous adverse outcomes, both iatrogenic and unavoidable.

A. Barotrauma/volutrauma and oxygen toxicity

1. **Bronchopulmonary dysplasia** (BPD) is related to increased airway pressure and changes in lung volume, although oxygen toxicity, anatomic and physiologic immaturity, and individual susceptibility also contribute.

2. **Air leak** is directly related to increased airway pressure. Risk is increased at MAPs in excess of 14 cm H_2O.

B. Mechanical

1. Obstruction of endotracheal tubes may result in hypoxemia and respiratory acidosis.

2. Equipment malfunction, particularly disconnection, is not uncommon and requires functioning alarm systems and vigilance.

C. Complications of invasive monitoring

1. Peripheral arterial occlusion with infarction (see Chap. 26F).

2. Aortic thrombosis from umbilical arterial catheters, occasionally leading to renal impairment and hypertension.

3. Emboli from flushed catheters, particularly to the lower extremities, the splanchnic bed, or even the brain.

D. Anatomic

1. Subglottic stenosis.

2. Palatal grooves from prolonged orotracheal intubation.

3. Vocal cord damage.

Suggested Reading

Carlo W. Assisted ventilation. In: Klaus M.H, Fanaroff A.A, eds. *Care of the high risk neonate*, 5th ed. Philadelphia: WB Saunders, 2001.

BLOOD GAS AND PULMONARY FUNCTION MONITORING
James M. Adams

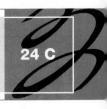

24 C

I. **GENERAL PRINCIPLES.** Blood gas monitoring in neonatal critical care units provides for (i) assessment of pulmonary gas exchange; (ii) determination of hemoglobin-oxygen saturation and arterial oxygen content; and (iii) evaluation, although limited, of adequacy of tissue oxygen delivery. Both invasive and noninvasive techniques are used in the clinical setting. Most pulmonary function monitoring in neonatal intensive care currently is focused on parameters of oxygenation.

II. **OXYGEN USE AND MONITORING.** In emergency situations sufficient oxygen to abolish cyanosis should be administered. Oxygen monitoring should be initiated as soon as possible. Monitoring of acute and chronic oxygen use is necessary to reduce risk of injury to the lungs or the immature retina of the premature infant.

   A. **Arterial blood gas measurements.** Arterial Po_2 and Pco_2 are direct indicators of efficiency of pulmonary gas exchange in babies with acute lung disease. Arterial oxygen tension (Pao_2), measured under steady state conditions from an indwelling catheter, is presently the "gold standard" for oxygen monitoring.

   1. **Usual values.** Most sources consider 50 to 80 mm Hg to be an acceptable target range for newborn Pao_2. Premature infants receiving mechanical ventilation often exhibit wide swings in Pao_2 values. In such circumstances, a random single blood gas value may not accurately reflect the overall trend of oxygenation.

   2. **Sampling.** To minimize sampling and dilutional artifacts, arterial blood gas samples should be collected in dry heparin syringes that are commercially available for this purpose. Most modern blood gas analyzers allow determination of blood gas values, as well as other whole blood parameters, on 0.2 to 0.3 mL samples. Samples should be analyzed within 15 minutes or preserved on ice if sent to a remote laboratory site. Blood gas sampling by percutaneous puncture is utilized when the need for measurement is infrequent or an indwelling catheter is not available. However, the discomfort of the puncture may result in agitation and a fall in Pao_2, such that the value obtained underestimates the true steady state value.

   B. **Capillary blood gas determination.** This technique requires extensive warming of the extremity, free-flowing puncture, and strictly anaerobic collection. Under these conditions, capillary sampling may be useful for determination of pH and Pco_2. Proper collection techniques are often difficult to guarantee in the clinical setting, however, and capillary sampling should not be used for determination of Pao_2.

   C. **Continuous blood gas analysis** through an indwelling catheter has been advocated to provide rapid, real-time data and reduce the volume of blood required for repeated blood gas measurements. Recent technology has utilized fiber optic systems with optical sensors inserted into vascular catheters already in place. These devices have been used for circuit monitoring during neonatal extracorporeal membrane oxygenation (ECMO) and for monitoring of premature infants through umbilical artery catheters. Reported correlation with measured Pao_2 values is good in some studies but bias and precision of measurements deteriorate for Pao_2 values above 70 mm Hg. The sensors cannot be threaded into some brands of umbilical catheters smaller than 5 Fr. Little data exist regarding the accuracy of arterial blood pressure recordings using these systems. Optical sensor technology has also been employed in the form of small in-line blood gas analyzers contained in a closed infusion system connected to an umbilical or peripheral artery catheter. With these systems blood is withdrawn into the sensor chamber periodically for blood gas analysis then infused back into the catheter. Most studies involving these devices are small and data are lacking regarding complications, cost effectiveness, and impact on need for subsequent transfusion. At the moment they are best viewed as trend monitoring devices and a specific role in neonatal intensive care has not been established.

D. Noninvasive oxygen monitoring provides real-time trend data that is particularly useful in babies exhibiting frequent swings in PaO_2 and oxygen saturation. Noninvasive devices also may reduce the frequency of blood gas sampling in some patients.

1. **Pulse oximetry** has become the primary tool for noninvasive oxygen monitoring in neonates. This technique is less complex than transcutaneous monitoring and does not require calibration or the level of user sophistication necessary with transcutaneous O_2 monitors. Major brands of pulse oximeters provide continuous measurement of hemoglobin–oxygen saturation (SpO_2) with a high level of accuracy ($\pm 3\%$) when compared to control values measured by co-oximetry.

   a. **General characteristics.** Oximeters depend on different absorption characteristics of oxygenated versus reduced hemoglobin for various wavelengths of light. Differences in transmission of two (usually red and near infrared) or more wavelengths through tissues with pulsatile blood flow are measured. Using the measured values, the proportion of oxygenated and reduced hemoglobin is calculated and displayed as percent saturation.

   b. **Disadvantages.** Patient movement and the low amplitude pulse wave of premature infants may introduce artifacts that result in false episodes of desaturation. At least two manufacturers have introduced recent software upgrades that significantly reduce these sources of false low saturation values in neonates. Other potential sources of artifact include inappropriate sensor placement, presence of high-intensity light (some phototherapy devices), fetal hemoglobin values $>50\%$ and presence of carboxyhemoglobin or methemoglobin. Pulse oximetry does not measure the PaO_2; therefore, it is insensitive in detecting hyperoxemia. Due to the shape of the oxyhemoglobin dissociation curve, if SpO_2 is $>95\%$, PaO_2 is unpredictable. Under such conditions PaO_2 may well be >100 mm Hg.

   c. **Targeted saturation values.** Recent studies suggest a strategy of targeted SpO_2 values in preterm infants is associated with less need for supplemental oxygen and a reduction in adverse pulmonary events. Oxygen supplemented preterm infants maintained at SpO_2 values of 89% to 94% have fewer exacerbations of chronic lung disease and are less likely to need supplemental oxygen at 36 weeks' postmenstrual age than those maintained at higher values. We Maintain SpO_2 at 85% to 95% (85% to 92% if <29 wk gestation) range, where arterial PO_2 rarely will exceed 90 mm Hg and avoid persistent saturation values above 95% in premature infants receiving oxygen. Some pulse oximeters provide a histogram that allows the user to determine proportion of total saturation values falling within specific ranges.

2. **Transcutaneous oxygen monitoring** ($P_{tc}O_2$). In trained hands transcutaneous oxygen monitoring can be useful in management of acute cardiopulmonary disease during the first 2 weeks of life or if arterial catheterization is not possible. This technique has been largely supplanted by pulse oximetry.

   a. **General characteristics.** Transcutaneous oxygen monitors use a heated sensor similar to a miniature blood gas electrode applied to the skin with an occlusive dressing that protects the sensor site from contamination by room air. The skin surface is heated to $43.5°C$ to $44°C$ to maximize skin surface blood flow and oxygen diffusion to the sensor site.

   b. **Potential artifacts.** Under proper conditions, skin surface PO_2 will correlate closely with true arterial PO_2. However, the device requires frequent calibration and change of electrode site and is highly dependent upon user training and expertise. Correlation with PaO_2 is poor in presence of circulatory insufficiency, during use of some vasodilator medications, and if operated at low sensor temperature. Increasing skin maturation after 3 to 4 weeks of age also limits reliability. All of these artifacts produce underestimation of true PaO_2, especially in the presence of hyperoxemia. If the transcutaneous monitor is used, $PtCO_2$ should be correlated periodically with arterial blood gas values.

    c. Target values. Target $PtCO_2$ range is usually 40 to 80 mm Hg.

III. ASSESSMENT OF PULMONARY VENTILATION. Assessment of alveolar ventilation by direct or noninvasive measurement of PCO_2 is receiving renewed emphasis because of potential association of low values and brain or lung injury in preterm infants. Also, ventilator strategies to prevent lung injury by avoiding excessive volume distension of the immature lung emphasize "permissive hypercarbia" and tolerate PCO_2 values in the range of 50 to 65 mm Hg.

    A. Blood gas determination. As is the case with oxygen monitoring, a $PaCO_2$ value obtained at steady state from an indwelling arterial catheter provides the most accurate indicator of alveolar ventilation. Lack of a catheter, however, limits the availability of this sampling for many patients. Blood obtained by percutaneous arterial puncture is an alternative but may not reflect steady state values because of artifacts introduced by pain and agitation.

        1. Venous blood from a central catheter may also be useful in certain circumstances. If alveolar ventilation and circulatory function are normal, venous PCO_2 usually exceeds arterial values by 5 to 6 mm Hg. However, if significant hypoventilation or circulatory dysfunction is present, this relationship is unpredictable.

        2. Capillary blood gases. PCO_2 and pH values obtained from properly collected capillary blood can closely reflect arterial values. The extremity must be warmed and a free-flowing blood sample collected under strictly anaerobic conditions without squeezing the extremity. In smaller premature infants these conditions are difficult to achieve.

    B. Transcutaneous CO_2 monitoring. Most current transcutaneous oxygen monitor sensors also include a transcutaneous CO_2 electrode. Accurate $PtCCO_2$ values, however, are more difficult to obtain than values for transcutaneous oxygen tension. Tissue diffusion rates and temperature coefficients for carbon dioxide are different than those for oxygen. Gas calibration of the electrode is required and a calibration factor must be built into the algorithm. Transcutaneous carbon dioxide tension exceeds that of arterial blood by a mean of 4 mm Hg but this gradient may more than double in the presence of hypercapnia. The need for a high level of user attention and expertise has limited applicability of this technique in routine clinical practice.

    C. Capnography. The utility of end-tidal carbon dioxide measurements in neonates is limited by several factors. Mechanical ventilation typically occurs at relatively rapid rates compared to adult strategies and most ventilator circuits deliver a continuous fresh flow of gas throughout the respiratory cycle. This limits the ability to obtain a true end-expiratory plateau. Also, arterial–alveolar CO_2 gradients are high in babies with primary lung disease because of maldistribution of ventilation (mean 6–10 mm Hg). Resulting end-tidal measurements tend to significantly underestimate arterial PCO_2 values in patients with hypoventilation. However, the technique may be useful for trend monitoring in babies with more uniform distribution of ventilation, such as those in the routine postoperative setting.

IV. PULMONARY GRAPHICS MONITORING. Several devices have been marketed in recent years for bedside pulmonary function testing in infants and young children. Likewise, most newer generation ventilators have software algorithms and flat panel screens to display a variety of measured or calculated parameters graphically. Despite the added cost and increasing availability of these modalities, evidence of beneficial effect on neonatal outcomes is lacking. Several techniques have been advocated in limited studies.

    A. Measurement of tidal volume. Tidal volume measurements may be used to assist in manual adjustment of ventilator settings. Alternatively, such measurements may form the basis for software-automated ventilator adjustments designed to maintain a defined range of delivered tidal volume ("volume guarantee") or consistent tidal volume delivery employing minimal peak airway pressure ("pressure-regulated volume control"). However, several technical issues may limit efficacy of these modalities. Marked variations in measured tidal volume exist among devices from different manufacturers. Although newer modes of ventilation may improve consistency of delivered tidal volume, a significant proportion of values still remain outside the target range. Reasons for these discrepancies include differences in the site of measurements in ventilator systems, variations in tubing system compliance and use of differing strategies to compensate for endotracheal tube leaks. In addition, some software algorithms average adjustments in tidal volume over several breaths. Despite these shortcomings, tidal volume measurements employing the same device consistently over time may provide clinically useful information during chronic mechanical ventilation and may be helpful with weaning following surfactant treatment where rapid changes in lung compliance and delivered tidal volume are of significant concern.

B. Flow volume loops. The use of positive end-expiratory pressure (PEEP) is an important tool in management of infants with congenital or acquired bronchomalacia (a common complication of severe bronchopulmonary dysplasia [BPD]). Limited case studies have reported use of real-time flow volume loop tracings to guide in determination of optimal PEEP to oppose airway collapse. However, indices that quantitate the flow volume relationship have not been validated in young infants. Because of rapid breathing, onset of inspiration often occurs before end-expiratory closure of the loop is achieved. As a result "normal" tracings are difficult to obtain and clinical application of this technique in small infants is limited.

Suggested Reading
Askie L, Henderson-Smart D, Irwig L, et al. Oxygen-saturation targets and outcomes in extremely preterm infants. *N Engl J Med* 2003;349:959–967.

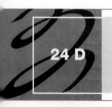

EXTRACORPOREAL MEMBRANE OXYGENATION
24 D

Gerhard K. Wolf and John H. Arnold

I. BACKGROUND. Extracorporeal membrane oxygenation (ECMO) is a technique of life support for neonates in cardiac or respiratory failure not responding to conventional therapy.

ECMO has been offered to >20,000 neonates worldwide to date (see Tables 24D.1 and 24D.2). The use of ECMO for neonatal respiratory failure has been declining since the early 1990s, whereas the use of ECMO for cardiac failure is increasing. This trend is associated with improved ventilator management and the institution of surfactant and nitric oxide for neonatal respiratory failure.

II. INDICATIONS AND CONTRAINDICATIONS

A. Respiratory failure. The indications for neonatal ECMO are (i) reversible respiratory failure and (ii) a predicted mortality with conventional therapy great enough to warrant the risks of ECMO. ECMO is also considered in patients with life-threatening air leaks not manageable with optimal ventilatory support and chest drainage. **Oxygenation index (OI)** is a measure of the severity of respiratory failure and is calculated as: $OI = $ mean arterial blood pressure$(MAP) \times Fio_2/Pao_2 \times 100$. It is essential to document OIs from serial blood gases over time, as the OI may vary. ECMO indications vary among different centers. Commonly used criteria include two OIs of >40 within 1 hour, one OI of 60 on high frequency ventilation, or one OI of 40 combined with cardiovascular instability.

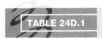

Neonatal	Total patients	Survived ECLS	Survival to discharge or transfer
TABLE 24D.1 Overall Outcomes for Neonatal ECMO by Indication, Extracorporeal Life Support Organization (ELSO) 2006			
Respiratory	20,258	17,273 (85%)	15,482 (76%)
Cardiac	2,599	1,505 (58%)	954 (38%)
ECMO-CPR	233	144 (65%)	88 (39%)

CPR = cardiopulmonary resuscitation; ECLS = extracoporeal life support; ECMO = extracorporeal membrane oxygenation.
ECLS, January 2006, Published by the Extracorporeal Life Support Organization, Ann Arbor, Michigan. "Total Patients"-refers to all neonatal ECMO therapies reported in the ELSO registry. "ECMO-CPR" refers to neonatal patients placed emergently on ECMO during cardiopulmonary resuscitation.

B. Cardiac failure. ECMO provides biventricular support for neonates with cardiac failure. ECMO for congenital heart defects (hypoplastic left heart syndrome, coarctation of the aorta, pulmonary atresia, total anomalous venous return) is offered as a bridge to definitive treatment until the neonate's condition has stabilized. Other cardiac indications are failure to wean from cardiopulmonary bypass, cardiomyopathy, and pulmonary hypertension.

C. Rapid-response ECMO (ECMO-cardiopulmonary resuscitation [CPR]). ECMO in the setting of a witnessed cardiorespiratory arrest is offered in centers with a rapid response team. Response times from the arrest to cannulation are ideally 15 to 30 minutes. A readily primed circuit and an ECMO team must be available 24 hours/day. Effective CPR before cannulation is essential for a favorable outcome during rapid-response ECMO.

D. *Ex utero* intrapartum treatment (EXIT) procedure. The vessels are cannulated during a cesarean section while the neonate remains on placental support. Indications include severe congenital diaphragmatic hernia, lung tumors, and airway obstructing lesions such as large neck masses and mediastinal tumors.

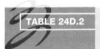

Neonatal categories	Total runs	Percentage survived
TABLE 24D.2 Neonatal Respiratory Runs by Diagnosis, Extracorporeal Life Support Organization (ELSO) 2006		
MAS	6,866	94
CDH	4,881	52
PPHN/PFC	3,153	78
Sepsis	2,444	75
RDS	1,403	84
Pneumonia	277	58
Air leak syndrome	101	71
Other	1,385	63

CDH = congenital diaphragmatic hernia; MAS = meconium aspiration syndrome; PFC = persistent fetal circulation; PPHN = persistent pulmonary hypertension of the newborn; RDS = respiratory distress syndrome.

E. **Contraindications.** ECMO should only be offered for reversible conditions. Absolute contraindications in our institution are significant intraventricular or intraparenchymal hemorrhage, weight <1,500 g, gestational age <34 weeks, lethal congenital abnormality, and continuous CPR for more than an hour before ECMO support.

III. **PHYSIOLOGY**

A. **Flow.** Venous drainage is always passive from the patient to the ECMO circuit. The cessation of venous drainage (hypovolemia, cardiac tamponade, pneumothorax) causes an automatic shutdown of the circuit, as any negative pressure could introduce air into the circuit. Flow is determined by venous return and the ECMO pump.

B. **Venoarterial (V-A) ECMO.** V-A ECMO supports the cardiac and the respiratory systems, and is indicated for primary cardiac failure or respiratory failure combined with secondary cardiac failure. In V-A ECMO, the blood is drained from a vein (internal jugular vein, femoral vein) and returned into the arterial system (internal carotid artery). The patient's total cardiac output (CO) is the sum of the native CO and the pump flow generated by the circuit: $CO_{total} = CO_{native} + CO_{circuit}$

C. **Venovenous (V-V) ECMO.** V-V ECMO supports only the respiratory system and is indicated for isolated respiratory failure. V-V ECMO spares accessing the carotid artery. In V-V ECMO, the blood is drained as well as returned to the jugular vein through a double-lumen cannula. Some of the blood is immediately recirculated into the ECMO circuit. The rest of the oxygenated blood goes to the right side of the heart, into the pulmonary vascular bed, into the left side of the heart and into the systemic circulation. As a requirement for V-V ECMO, the internal jugular vein has to be large enough for a 14-French double-lumen cannula. Converting to V-A ECMO is considered in the presence of additional hypotension, cardiac failure, or metabolic acidosis. Technical difficulties related to large recirculation in the venous cannula can also lead to the need to convert to V-A ECMO. In our institution, the carotid artery is already identified at the time of V-V cannulation. For conversion to V-A ECMO, the venous cannula is left in place and an additional arterial cannula is inserted into the internal carotid artery.

D. **Oxygen delivery.** Oxygen delivery is the product of CO and arterial oxygen content. During ECMO, many factors contribute to oxygen delivery. Arterial oxygen content is determined by the gas exchange in the membrane oxygenator and the gas exchange from the neonate's lung. CO is only altered during V-A ECMO and is determined by the ECMO flow and the infant's native CO.

E. **Carbon dioxide removal.** Carbon dioxide (CO_2) removal is achieved by the membrane and the patient's lung. The amount of CO_2 removed is dependent on the $Paco_2$ of blood circulating through the membrane, the surface area of the membrane, and the gas flow through the membrane lung ("sweep gas flow"). As physiologic pulmonary function and tidal volume improve, the $Paco_2$ decreases. CO_2 removal is extremely efficient during ECMO, to the point that additional CO_2 has to be added into the circuit in order to prevent hypocarbia and respiratory alkalosis.

F. **Cerebral perfusion.** Cerebral perfusion during shock is rapidly restored after initiation of V-A ECMO. On the other hand, venous drainage and arterial perfusion to the brain are impaired by large bore cannulas during ECMO. Collateral circulation to the brain during V-A-ECMO is maintained through the circle of Willis. The carotid artery is frequently ligated after decannulation from ECMO, although reconstruction of the carotid artery has been successfully performed. Impairments to arterial reconstructions are an intimal flap, arterial thrombosis, infections, or excessive tension on attempt of reconstruction. In our institution, the carotid artery was successfully reconstructed in 25% of patients. It is unclear whether carotid arterial reconstruction improves neurologic outcome.

G. **Renal perfusion.** During V-A ECMO, the arterial pulse-pressure wave may become dampened as the roller pump contributes significantly to the patient's CO. Recent animal models have suggested that renal perfusion is not different during V-A as compared to V-V ECMO. Unclamping the bridge during V-A ECMO directs flow away from the patient and may be associated with a decrease in blood pressure and renal perfusion.

IV. MANAGEMENT

A. Pre-ECMO. In preparation for cannulation, the following should be available: central venous access to the patient, postductal arterial catheter, cross-matched blood in the blood bank, complete blood count, coagulation profile, head ultrasonographic examination. Platelets should be transfused for a platelet count <50,000/mL. An echocardiogram should be done before ECMO in order to rule out structural abnormalities. During V-A ECMO, it may be difficult to identify pulmonary hypertension or certain congenital lesions such as total anomalous venous return, as the right atrium is decompressed and blood flow through the lung is decreased.

B. Membrane. The appropriate membrane for a neonate is a 0.8 m^2 or 1.5 m^2 membrane oxygenator. The resulting total volume of a neonatal ECMO circuit is 600 mL.

C. Saline priming. Patients who are placed on ECMO emergently can be started on a saline-primed circuit. Instead of blood products, the circuit is primed with normal saline. In centers with rapid-response ECMO, a saline-primed, sterile circuit is always available, minimizing the time to initiate ECMO therapy. The neonate's own blood volume is initially diluted with the normal saline from the ECMO circuit. This causes a drop in hematocrit and a transient decrease in oxygen carrying capacity. The hematocrit is later restored by using ultrafiltration and transfusing packed red blood cells (PRBCs).

D. Blood priming. Patients who are placed on ECMO nonemergently are started on a blood-primed circuit. Orders for the initial prime of a neonatal circuit are as follows: 500 mL of PRBC (cytomegalovirus [CMV] negative, <7 days old), 200 mL of fresh frozen plasma, 2 units of cryoprecipitate, 2 units of platelets (not concentrated). Heparin and Tham (Tris-hydroxymethyl-aminomethane, also "Tris") buffer, and calcium gluconate are added to the circuit. Circuit pH, ionized calcium and potassium levels are checked before going on to ECMO. Hyperkalemia of the circuit is treated with calcium and bicarbonate.

E. Cannulation. The ECMO cannulation is performed by cardiac or pediatric surgeons at the bedside, in the cardiac catheterization laboratory or in the operating room. A surgical cutdown- -approach is preferred over transcutaneous cannulation. The neonate is sedated and paralyzed with fentanyl, midazolam, and pancuronium. Heparin 30 units/kg is administered 3 minutes before cannulation. The vein is cannulated first. The catheter is introduced aproximately 6.5 cm to the right atrium and sutured in place. In V-A ECMO, the artery is cannulated in a similar manner. In full term neonates, the arterial cannula is introduced 3.5 cm into the aortic arch. Once the patient is on ECMO, 2 units of platelets and 2 units of cryoprecipitate are administered. On initiation of ECMO, vasopressors can be rapidly weaned. The neonate may become markedly hypertensive on initiation of ECMO therapy. Hydralazine 0.1 to 0.4 mg/kg/dose is administered to treat hypertension.

F. ECMO therapy. ECMO pump flow rate is generally 100 to 120 mL/kg. Sweep gas flow rate is 1 to 2.5 L/minute for a 0.8 m^2 membrane. A safety check is conducted every 4 hours. This safety check includes searching for blood clots and circuit inspection for leaks. The bridge is unclamped every 15 minutes to prevent clot formation. Elective circuit changes are made only if one of the following indications is met: (i) excessive clotting in the circuit; (ii) elevation of the premembrane pressure (>350 mm Hg), indicating membrane clotting and failure; (iii) membrane failure proved by inadequate change from pre- to postmembrane PaO_2 and $PaCO_2$; (iv) excessive platelet consumption; (v) 120 hours of therapy with Amicar and (vi) an uncorrectable coagulopathy that is thought to be caused by the circuit/membrane. If a circuit needs to be changed, a new circuit is primed, the patient is cycled off ECMO, the old circuit is cut away, and the new circuit is connected, with care being taken to keep air out of the system.

G. Anticoagulation. Heparin is used in all patients to prevent clot formation. The whole blood–activated clotting time (ACT) is used to monitor heparin infusion and avoid hemorrhagic complications. ACT is kept at 180 to 200 seconds.

H. **Blood products.** Prothrombin time is maintained at <17 seconds using fresh frozen plasma, fibrinogen is kept above 150 mg/dL using cryoprecipitate, and the platelet count is maintained above 150,000 using concentrated platelets. The hematocrit is kept above 35% to facilitate oxygen delivery.

I. **Amicar.** ε-Aminocaproic acid lowers the incidence of hemorrhagic complications associated with ECMO, including intracranial and postoperative hemorrhage. Negative effects are increased clot formation in the circuit. Patients who are considered to be at high risk for bleeding complications are given Amicar. They include infants who (i) are <37 weeks' gestational age, (ii) have sepsis, (iii) have prolonged hypoxia or acidosis (pH 7.1) before ECMO, or (iv) have grade I or II intraventricular hemorrhage. A loading dose of Amicar (100 mg/kg) is given followed by a 30 mg/kg/hour infusion. After 72 hours of Amicar, the patient is assessed for further risks of bleeding complications. If these risks still exist, Amicar is continued and the circuit is changed at 120 hours. Otherwise, the Amicar infusion is discontinued.

J. **Antibiotics.** Broad-spectrum antibiotics are routinely administered to lower the risk of infection while on ECMO therapy.

K. **Analgesia and sedation.** Patients are sedated with an opioid/benzodiazepine combination. Drugs of choice are morphine 0.05 mg/kg/hour and lorazepam 0.05 to 0.1 mg/kg/dose every 4 to 6 hours. Note that fentanyl is absorbed in large quantities by the ECMO membrane, leading to suboptimal analgesia. Fentanyl can be used during ECMO cannulation, but should not be used during ECMO.

L. **Fluids and nutrition.** Nutrition is administered through the parenteral route. Gastric feeding during ECMO is avoided, as it may increase the rate of necrotizing enterocolitis. Lipid administration should not exceed 1 g/kg/day, to prevent lipid accumulation and embolism in the circuit. Lipids should be administered directly to the patient and not to the circuit. Dextrose and amino acid solution (parenteral nutrition) can be administered through the circuit.

M. **Ultrafiltration.** An ultrafilter is placed in line with the ECMO circuit. The goal is to normalize fluid balance in patients who have excessive positive fluid balance. Indications are urine output of <0.5 mL/kg/hour, positive fluid balance >500 mL/24 hours, failed diuretic therapy.

N. **Neurologic assessment.** Head ultrasonographic examinations are performed within 24 hours of cannulation, and every other day while the patient is receiving ECMO support. Electroencephalograms are performed when seizure activity is suspected.

O. **Ventilator strategy.** The goal of the ventilator strategy on ECMO is to let the lung "rest," yet not to allow total lung collapse. Typical settings are peak inspiratory pressure (PIP) = 25 cm H_2O, positive end-expiratory pressure (PEEP) = 5 cm H_2O, rate = 10, inspiratory time 1 seconds, and Fio_2 = 0.4. With a patient on V-A ECMO for pneumothorax and air leak, apneic oxygenation with Fio_2 = 1 should be considered starting at continuous positive airway pressure (CPAP) settings of 12 cm H_2O and decreasing until no further air leaks are present. Endotracheal suctioning is performed every 4 hours. During ECMO, lung function is assessed as follows: (i) as lung function improves, CO_2 removal increases and oxygenation by the lung improves, resulting in better gas exchange. Sweep gases can be adjusted accordingly; (ii) chest radiographs show gradual resolution of pulmonary edema; (iii) as pulmonary edema resolves, lung mechanics improve and expired tidal volumes increase.

P. **Conditioning and cycling.** "Conditioning" means challenging the patient by reducing the ECMO support to evaluate the gas exchange accomplished by the lungs. Sweep gas flow is reduced; Fio_2 is increased to 1 and the respiratory rate is increased to 25/minute; the flow of the ECMO pump is weaned to 100 mL/minute in 50 mL increments; and serial arterial blood gases are obtained. If the postductal saturation falls below 95%, the ECMO settings are resumed. "Cycling" means transiently removing the patient from the ECMO circuit. In V-A ECMO, the venous and arterial cannulae are clamped, the bridge is opened, and the ECMO blood flow "cycles" from the arterial to the venous side through the bridge, without perfusing the patient. In V-V ECMO, the sweep gas flow is interrupted ("capped"), while the circuit continues to flow.

Q. Decannulation. The patient's lung disease has to be improved enough to tolerate moderate ventilator settings. Our criteria for decannulation are as follows: PIP = 30 cm H_2O; PEEP = 5 cm H_2O; rate = 25 breaths/minute; and Fio_2 = 0.35; Pao_2 over 60 mm Hg; $Paco_2$ = 40 to 50 mm Hg; pH <7.5. When these criteria are used, patients rarely require recannulation. At the time of decannulation from V-A ECMO, we attempt to reconstruct the common carotid artery. The jugular vein is routinely ligated. Two units of concentrated platelets are given following decannulation.

Discontinuation of ECMO support is also considered in the following situations: when the disease process becomes irreversible, failure to wean successfully, neurologic events (devastating neurologic examination, significant intracranial hemorrhage), or multiorgan failure.

V. COMPLICATIONS

A. Neurologic. Sequelae resulting in neurologic damage often originate from acidosis and hypoxia before commencement of ECMO. According to the extracorporeal life support (ECLS) registry, intracranial hemorrhage has occurred in 6% and infarction of the central nervous system (CNS) in 8.4% of neonates during ECMO therapy. Small intracranial hemorrhages are managed by optimizing clotting factors and using Amicar. Larger intracranial hemorrhages may force discontinuation of ECMO.

B. Mechanical. Poor venous return to the circuit causes the pump to shut down in order to avoid air entrainment. Causes for poor venous return from the patient to the ECMO circuit include hypovolemia, pneumothorax, or tamponade physiology. Mechanical reasons for poor venous return related to the ECMO circuit are poor catheter position, small venous catheter diameter, excessive catheter length, kinked tubing, and insufficient hydrostatic column length (height of patient above pump head). Initially, fluids are administered while other reasons for poor return are ruled out.

C. Cardiovascular. Hemodynamic instability during ECMO may be a result of hypovolemia, vasodilation during septic inflammatory response, arrhythmias, and pulmonary embolism. Volume overload, especially in the setting of capillary leak, may worsen chest wall compliance and further compromise gas exchange.

VI. OUTCOME

A. Survival. The ECLS database reports the outcomes of ECMOtherapies worldwide since 1985. A total of 20,258 neonatal ECMO runs in neonates were reported for respiratory disorders through January 2006. The most common indication was meconium aspiration syndrome (MAS), followed by congenital diaphragmatic hernia, persistent pulmonary hypertension of the newborn, sepsis, neonatal respiratory distress syndrome, and air leak. Seventy-six percent of patients survived the ECMO therapy to hospital discharge or transfer. For cardiac ECMO in neonates, a total of 2,599 cases were reported, with 38% surviving to hospital discharge. For ECMO-CPR in neonates (total 223 cases), the survival to hospital discharge was 39% (Tables 24D.1, 24D.2). Mortality at 7 years of age after completion of the UK-collaborative ECMO trial was 33% in the ECMO group and 59% in the conventional group (see Table 24D.3).

B. Neurodevelopment. Neurologic follow-up was assessed 7 years after completion of the UK-collaborative ECMO trial (Table 24D.3). Both the ECMO and conventional therapy groups had problems and impaired neurologic outcome, but the ECMO group performed better in each task. Both groups had notable difficulties with learning and processing tasks. Progressive sensorineural hearing loss was observed in both groups. There was no difference in cognitive skills, 76% of the children in each group recorded a cognitive level within the normal range. Comparing the survivors in both groups, 55% in the ECMO group versus 50% in the conventional group survived without disabilities. This study suggests that the underlying disease is the major influence on morbidity, and that the beneficial effect of ECMO is still present after 7 years.

| TABLE 24D.3 | Overall Status by 7 Yr of Age | |

Overall status by 7 yr of age	ECMO (n = 93) (%)	Conventional (n = 92) (%)
Deaths	31 (33)	54 (59)
Lost to follow-up	6 (6)	4 (4)
Children with:		
Severe disability	3 (3)	0
Moderate disability	9 (10)	6 (7)
Mild disability	13 (14)	11 (12)
Children with:		
Impairment only	21 (23)	15 (16)
No abnormal signs or disability	10 (11)	2 (2)
Assessed survivors with no disability	31/56 (55)	17/34 (50)

ECMO = extracorporeal membrane oxygenation.
Follow-up after completion of the McNally H, Bennett CC, Elbourne D, et al. UK Collaborative ECMO Trial Group. United Kingdom collaborative randomized trial of neonatal extracorporeal membrane oxygenation: Follow-up to age 7 years. *Pediatrics* 2006;117(5):e845–e854.

Suggested Readings

Bartlett RH. Extracorporeal life support: History and new directions. *ASAIO J* 2005;51(5): 487–489.

McNally H, Bennett CC, Elbourne D, et al. UK Collaborative ECMO Trial Group. United Kingdom collaborative randomized trial of neonatal extracorporeal membrane oxygenation: Follow-up to age 7 years. *Pediatrics* 2006;117(5):e845–e854.

Van Meurs Krisa, Zwischenberger JB, eds. *ECMO: Extracorporeal cardiopulmonary support in critical care*, 3rd ed. Ann Arbor: ELSO, (This book can be ordered online at http://www.elso.med.umich.edu/publications.htm. 2006.)

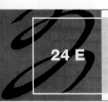

24 E

PULMONARY AIR LEAK*
Mohan Pammi Venkatesh

I. BACKGROUND

   A. Incidence and risk factors. Risk factors for air leak in premature infants include respiratory distress syndrome (RDS), mechanical ventilation, sepsis, and pneumonia. Surfactant therapy for RDS has markedly decreased the incidence of pneumothorax. Risk factors in term infants are aspiration of meconium, blood, or amniotic fluid; pneumonia; congenital malformations; and mechanical ventilation.*

---

*This is a Revision of Chapter 24E by Dr. Mark T. Ogino in the 5th edition of *Manual Of Neonatal Care*.

B. **Pathogenesis.** Air leak syndromes arise through a common mechanism. Transpulmonary pressures that exceed the tensile strength of the noncartilagenous terminal airways and alveolar saccules can damage the respiratory epithelium. Loss of epithelial integrity permits air to enter the interstitium, causing **pulmonary interstitial emphysema**. Persistent elevation in transpulmonary pressure facilitates the dissection of air toward the visceral pleura and/or the hilum through the peribronchial and perivascular spaces. In rare circumstances, air can enter the pulmonary veins and result in an **air embolus**. Rupture of the pleural surface allows the adventitial air to decompress into the pleural space, causing **pneumothorax**. Following a path of least resistance, air can dissect from the hilum and into the mediastinum, resulting in **pneumomediastinum**, or into the pericardium, resulting in **pneumopericardium**. Air in the mediastinum can decompress into the pleural space, the fascial planes of the neck and skin (**subcutaneous emphysema**), or the retroperitoneum. In turn, retroperitoneal air can rupture into the peritoneum (**pneumoperitoneum**) or dissect into the scrotum or labial folds.

1. Elevations in transpulmonary pressure can occur during the infant's first breaths when negative inspiratory pressure can increase to as much as 100 cm H_2O. Uneven ventilation due to atelectasis, surfactant deficiency, pulmonary hemorrhage, or retained fetal lung fluid can increase transpulmonary pressure. In turn, this leads to alveolar overdistention and rupture. Similarly, aspiration of blood, amniotic fluid, or meconium can facilitate alveolar overdistention by a ball-valve mechanism.

2. In the presence of pulmonary disease, positive pressure ventilation increases the risk of air leak. The high airway pressure required to achieve adequate oxygenation and ventilation in infants with poor pulmonary compliance (e.g., pulmonary hypoplasia, RDS, inflammation, pulmonary edema) further increases this risk. Excessive transpulmonary pressures can occur when ventilator pressures are not decreased as pulmonary compliance improves. This situation sometimes occurs in infants with RDS who improve rapidly after surfactant treatment. Mechanically ventilated preterm infants who make expiratory efforts against ventilator breaths are also at increased risk for pneumothorax.

3. Direct trauma to the airways can also cause air leak. Laryngoscopes, endotracheal tubes, suction catheters, and malpositioned feeding tubes can damage the lining of the airways and provide a portal for air entry.

II. TYPES OF AIR LEAKS

A. **Pneumothorax.** Spontaneous pneumothorax occurs in 0.07% of otherwise healthy-appearing neonates. One in ten of these infants is symptomatic. The high inspiratory pressures and uneven ventilation that occur in the initial stages of lung inflation may contribute to this phenomenon. Pneumothorax is more common in newborns treated with mechanical ventilation for underlying pulmonary disease. Clinical signs of pneumothorax range from insidious changes in vital signs to the complete cardiovascular collapse that frequently accompanies a tension pneumothorax. As intrathoracic pressure rises, there is decreased lung volume, mediastinal shift, compression of the large intrathoracic veins, and increased pulmonary vascular resistance. The net effect is an increase in central venous pressure, a decrease in preload, and, ultimately, diminished cardiac output. A pneumothorax must be considered in mechanically ventilated infants who develop unexplained alterations in hemodynamics, pulmonary compliance, or oxygenation and ventilation.

1. **Diagnosis**
   a. **Physical examination**
      i. Signs of respiratory distress include tachypnea, grunting, flaring, and retractions.
      ii. Cyanosis.
      iii. Chest asymmetry with expansion of the affected side.
      iv. Episodes of apnea and bradycardia.
      v. Shift in the point of maximum cardiac impulse.
      vi. Diminished or distant breath sounds on the affected side.
      vii. Abdominal distension from displacement of the diaphragm.

viii. Alterations in vital signs. With smaller collections of extrapulmonary air, compensatory increases may occur in heart rate and blood pressure. As the amount of air in the pleural space increases, central venous pressure rises and severe hypotension, bradycardia, apnea, hypoxia, and hypercapnia may occur.

b. Arterial blood gases. Changes in arterial blood gas measurements are nonspecific and demonstrate a decreased Po_2 and increased Pco_2 (and decreased pH).

c. Chest radiograph. Anteroposterior (AP) views may show a hyperlucent hemithorax, a separation of the visceral from the parietal pleura, flattening of the diaphragm, and mediastinal shift. Smaller collections of intrapleural air can be detected beneath the anterior chest wall by obtaining a cross-table lateral view; however, an AP view is needed to identify the affected side. The lateral decubitus view, with the side of suspected pneumothorax up, may be helpful in detecting a small pneumothorax and may help differentiate skin folds, congenital lobar emphysema, cystic adenomatoid malformations, and surface blebs that occasionally give the appearance of intrapleural air.

d. Transillumination. A high-intensity fiberoptic light source may demonstrate a pneumothorax. This technique is less sensitive in infants with chest-wall edema or severe pulmonary interstitial edema (PIE), in extremely small infants with thin chest walls, or in full-term infants with thick chest walls or dark skin. We often obtain a baseline transillumination in infants at high risk for air leak.

e. Needle aspiration. In a rapidly deteriorating clinical situation, thoracentesis may confirm the diagnosis and be therapeutic (see II.2.b).

2. Treatment

a. Conservative therapy. Close observation may be adequate for infants who have no underlying lung disease or complicating therapy (such as mechanical ventilation), are in no significant respiratory distress, and have no continuous air leak. The extrapulmonary air will usually resolve in 24 to 48 hours. Although some of these infants may require an increase in their ambient O_2 concentration, we do not routinely administer 100% oxygen.

b. Needle aspiration. Thoracentesis with a "butterfly" needle or intravenous catheter with an inner needle can be used to treat a symptomatic pneumothorax. Needle aspiration may be curative in infants not receiving mechanical ventilation and is frequently a temporizing measure in mechanically ventilated infants. In infants with severe hemodynamic compromise, thoracentesis may be a life-saving procedure.

i. Attach a 23- or 25-gauge butterfly needle or 22- or 24-guage intravenous catheter to 10- to 20-cc syringe previously fitted with a three-way stopcock.

ii. Identify the second or third intercostal space in the midclavicular line, and prepare the overlying skin with an antibacterial solution.

iii. Insert the needle firmly into the intercostal space and pass it just above the top of the third rib. This will minimize the chance of lacerating an intercostal artery, as these vessels are located on the inferior surface of the ribs. As the needle is inserted, have an assistant apply continuous suction with the syringe. A rapid flow of air into the syringe occurs when the needle enters the pleural space. Once the pleural space has been entered, stop advancing the needle. This will reduce the risk of puncturing the lung while the remaining air is evacuated.

iv. A continuous air leak can be aspirated while a chest tube is being inserted (see II.2.c). The "butterfly" needle can be left in place and if an intravenous catheter is used, the needle can be removed and the plastic catheter left in place for further aspiration. A short piece of IV extension tubing, for example, a "T" connector, attached to the intravenous catheter hub will allow flexibility during repeated aspirations. Otherwise, withdraw the needle after the air flow has ceased.

c. Chest tube drainage. Chest tube drainage is generally needed to evacuate pneumothoraces that develop in infants receiving positive pressure ventilation.

Frequently, these air leaks are continuous and will result in severe hemodynamic compromise if left untreated.

i. Insertion of a chest tube

a) Select a chest tube of the appropriate size; French size 10 (smaller) and 12 (larger) catheters are adequate for most infants.

b) Prepare the chest area with an antiseptic solution. Infiltrate the subcutaneous tissues overlying the fourth to sixth rib at the midaxillary line with a 1% lidocaine solution. We administer an appropriate dose of narcotic for pain management.

c) In the midaxillary line in the sixth intercostal space (ICS), parallel to the rib, make a small incision (1–1.5 cm) through the skin. Incisions of breast tissue should be avoided by locating the position of the nipple and surrounding tissue. An alternative site is in the anterior-superior portion of the chest wall; however, due to the possible complications of injury to the internal mammary artery and other regional vessels, we do not routinuely use this approach.

d) With a small curved hemostat, dissect the subcutaneous tissue overlying the rib. Make a subcutaneous track to the fourth ICS. Care should be taken to avoid the nipple area, the pectoralis muscle, and the axillary artery.

e) Enter the pleural space in the fourth ICS at the intersection of the nipple line just anterior to the midaxillary line with the closed hemostat. Guide the tip over the top of the rib to avoid trauma to the intercostal artery. Push the hemostat through the intercostal muscles and parietal pleura. Listen for a rush of air to indicate pleural penetration. Spread the tips to widen the opening and leave the hemostat in place. We use trochars cautiously because their use may increase the risk of lung perforation.

f) Grasp the end of the chest tube with the tips of the mosquito hemostat. The chest tube and the hemostat should be in a parallel orientation. Direct the chest tube through the skin incision, into the pleural opening, and between the opened tips. After the pleural space has been entered, direct the chest tube anteriorly and cephalad by rotating the curved points of the hemostat. Release the hemostat and advance the chest tube a few centimeters. Be certain that the side ports of the chest tube are in the pleural space.

g) The chest tube will "steam up" once it has been placed into the pleural space.

h) Direct the chest tube to the location of the pleural air. Placement in the anterior pleural space is generally most effective for infants in the supine position.

i) Palpate the chest wall around the entry site to confirm that the chest tube is not in the subcutaneous tissues.

j) Attach the chest tube to a Heimlich valve (for transport) or an underwater drainage system such as a Pleur-evac. Apply negative pressure (10–20 cm H_2O) to the underwater drainage system.

k) Using 3-0 or 4-0 silk, close the skin incision. We place a purse-string suture around the tube or a single interrupted suture on either side of the tube. Secure the chest tube by wrapping and then tying the skin suture tails around the tube. A second loop may be placed around the chest tube at a position 2 to 4 cm from the skin surface.

l) Cover the insertion site with petrolatum gauze and a small, clear, plastic, adhesive surgical dressing. We avoid extensive taping or large dressings, as they interfere with chest examination and may delay the discovery of a displaced chest tube.

m) AP and lateral chest radiographs are obtained to confirm tube position and ascertain drainage of the pleural air.

n) Radiographs may reveal chest tubes that are ineffective in evacuating extrapulmonary air. The most common cause of failure is tube placement in the posterior pleural space or the subcutaneous tissue. Other causes for ineffective drainage are tubes that perforate the lung, diaphragm, or mediastinum. Extrapulmonary air not in the pleural space, such as a pneumomediastinum or a subpleural pulmonary pseudocyst, will not be drained by a chest tube. Complications of chest tube insertion include hemorrhage, lung perforation, cardiac tamponade, and phrenic nerve injury.

ii. **Removal of a chest tube.** When the infant's lung disease has improved and the chest tube has not drained air for 24 to 48 hours, we discontinue suction and leave the tube under water seal. If radiographic examination shows no reaccumulation of extrapulmonary air in the next 12 to 24 hours, the chest tube is removed. A narcotic is given for pain control before the chest tube removal. To reduce the chance of introducing air into the pleural space, cover the chest wound with a small occlusive dressing while removing the tube. Remove the chest tube during expiration in spontaneously breathing infants and during inspiration in mechanically ventilated infants. A manual mechanical or bagged breath can insure removing the chest tube during the inspiratory phase.

   a) Persistent pneumothorax refractory to routine measures may improve with high-frequency oscillation ventilation (HFOV); some infants require extracorporeal membrane oxygenation (ECMO) (see Chap. 24D). We sometimes place catheters under ultrasonography or fluoroscopic guidance to drain air collections that are inaccessible by standard techniques. We often initiate HFOV to minimize mean airway pressure and resolve airleaks in mechanically ventilated infants. In patients with severe air leaks, oxygen supplementation is often increased so that mean airway pressure can be minimized.

iii. **Complications**

   a) Profound ventilatory and circulatory compromise can occur and, if untreated, result in death.

   b) Intraventricular hemorrhage may result, possibly secondary to a combination of fluctuating cerebrovascular pressures, impaired venous return, hypercapnia, hypoxia, and acidosis.

   c) Inappropriate antidiuretic hormone secretion may occur.

B. **Pulmonary interstitial emphysema (PIE)** occurs most often in mechanically ventilated, extremely preterm infants with RDS or sepsis. Interstitial air can be localized or can spread to involve significant portions of one or both lungs. Interstitial air can dissect toward the hilum and the pleural surface through the adventitial connective tissue surrounding the lymphatics and pulmonary vessels. This can compromise lymphatic drainage and pulmonary blood flow. PIE alters pulmonary mechanics by decreasing compliance, increasing residual volume and dead space, and enhancing ventilation/perfusion mismatch. Rupture of interstitial air into the pleural space and mediastinum can result in pneumothorax and pneumomediastinum, respectively.

1. **Diagnosis**

   a. PIE frequently develops in the first 48 hours of life.

   b. PIE may be accompanied by hypotension, bradycardia, hypercarbia, hypoxia, and acidosis.

   c. PIE has two radiographic patterns: cystlike and linear. Linear lucencies radiate from the lung hilum. Occasionally, large cystlike blebs give the appearance of a pneumothorax.

2. **Treatment**

   a. If possible, attempt to decrease mean airway pressure by lowering peak inspiratory pressure, positive end expiratory pressure (PEEP), and inspiratory time. We often use high-frequency oscillatory ventilation in infants with PIE to avoid large swings in lung volume.

   b. Unilateral PIE may improve if the infant is positioned with the affected lung dependent.

    c. Endotracheal suctioning and manual positive pressure ventilation should be minimized.

    d. Severe localized PIE that has failed to improve with conservative management may require collapse of the affected lung by selective bronchial intubation or occlusion or, rarely, surgical resection.

  3. Complications. PIE may precede more severe complications such as pneumothorax, pneumopericardium, or an air embolus.

C. Pneumomediastinum. Mediastinal air can develop when pulmonary interstitial air dissects into the mediastinum or when direct trauma occurs to the airways or the posterior pharynx.

  1. Diagnosis

    a. Physical examination. Heart sounds may appear distant.

    b. Chest radiograph. Air collections are central and usually elevate or surround the thymus. This results in the characteristic "spinnaker sail" sign. A pneumomediastinum is best seen on a lateral view.

  2. Treatment

    a. Pneumomediastinum is of little clinical importance, and specific drainage procedures are usually unnecessary.

    b. Rarely, cardiorespiratory compromise may develop if the air is under tension and does not decompress into the pleural space, the retroperitoneum, or the soft tissues of the neck. This situation may require mediastinostomy drainage.

    c. If the infant is mechanically ventilated, reduce mean airway pressure if possible.

  3. Complications. Pneumomediastinum may be associated with other air leaks.

D. Pneumopericardium. Pneumopericardium is the least common form of air leak in newborns but the most common cause of cardiac tamponade. Asymptomatic pneumopericardium is occasionally detected as an incidental finding on a chest radiograph. Most cases occur in preterm infants with RDS treated with mechanical ventilation, preceded by PIE and pneumomediastinum. The mortality rate for critically ill infants who develop pneumopericardium is 70% to 80%.

  1. Diagnosis. Pneumopericardium should be considered in mechanically ventilated newborn infants who develop acute or subacute hemodynamic compromise.

    a. Physical examination. Although infants may initially have tachycardia and decreased pulse pressure, hypotension, bradycardia, and cyanosis may ensue rapidly. auscultation reveals muffled or distant heart sounds. A pericardial knock (Hamman sign) or a characteristic millwheel-like murmur (bruit de moulin) may be present.

    b. Chest radiograph. Anteroposterior views show air surrounding the heart. Air under the inferior surface of the heart is diagnostic.

    c. Transillumination. A high-intensity fiberoptic light source may illuminate the substernal region. Flickering of the light with the heart rate may help differentiate pneumopericardium from pneumomediastinum or a medial pneumothorax.

    d. Electrocardiogram (ECG). Decreased voltages, manifest by a shrinking QRS complex, are consistent with pneumopericardium.

  2. Treatment

    a. Conservative management. Asymptomatic infants not receiving positive pressure ventilation can be managed expectantly. Vital signs are closely monitored (especially changes in pulse pressure). Frequent chest radiographs are obtained until the pneumopericardium resolves.

    b. Needle aspiration. Cardiac tamponade is a life-threatening event that requires immediate pericardiocentesis.

      i. Prepare the subxiphoid area with antiseptic solution.

      ii. Attach a 20- to 22-gauge intravenous catheter with an inner needle to a short piece of IV extension tubing that, in turn, is connected to a three-way stopcock and a 20-mL syringe.

      iii. In the subxiphoid space, insert the catheter at a 30- to 45-degree angle and toward the infant's left shoulder.

    iv. Have an assistant aspirate with the syringe as the catheter is advanced. Once air is aspirated, stop advancing the catheter.

    v. Slide the plastic catheter over the needle and into the pericardial space.

    vi. Remove the needle, reattach the IV tubing to the hub of the plastic catheter, evacuate the remaining air, and withdraw the catheter. If air leak persists, prepare for pericardial tube placement.

    vii. If blood is aspirated, immediately withdraw the catheter to avoid lacerating the ventricular wall. The complications of pericardiocentesis include hemopericardium and laceration of the right ventricle or left anterior descending coronary artery.

  c. Continuous pericardial drainage. Pneumopericardium often progresses to cardiac tamponade and may recur. A pericardial tube may be needed for continuous drainage. We manage the pericardial tube like a chest tube, although less negative pressure (5–10 cm H_2O) is used for suction.

  3. Complications. Ventilated infants who have a pneumopericardium drained by needle aspiration frequently (80%) have a recurrence. Recurrent pneumopericardium can occur days after apparent resolution of the initial event.

E. Other types of air leaks

  1. Pneumoperitoneum. Intraperitoneal air may result from extrapulmonary air that decompresses into the abdominal cavity. Usually the pneumoperitoneum is of little clinical importance, but it must be differentiated from intraperitoneal air resulting from a perforated viscus. Rarely, pneumoperitoneum can impair diaphragmatic excursion and compromise ventilation. In these cases, continuous drainage may be necessary.

  2. Subcutaneous emphysema. Subcutaneous air can be detected by palpation of crepitus in the face, neck, or supraclavicular region. Large collections of air in the neck, although usually of no clinical significance, can partially occlude or obstruct the compressible, cartilaginous trachea of the premature infant.

  3. Systemic air embolism. An air embolism is a rare but usually fatal complication of pulmonary air leak. Air may enter the vasculature either by disruption of the pulmonary venous system or by inadvertent injection through an intravascular catheter. The presence of air bubbles in blood withdrawn from an umbilical artery catheter can be diagnostic.

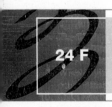

PERSISTENT PULMONARY HYPERTENSION OF THE NEWBORN
24 F
Linda J. Van Marter

I. DEFINITION. Persistent pulmonary hypertension of the newborn (PPHN) is the result of disruption in the normal perinatal fetal-neonatal circulatory transition. The disorder is characterized by sustained elevation in pulmonary vascular resistance (PVR) at birth. Survivors of PPHN are at risk of adverse sequelae including chronic pulmonary disease, neurodevelopmental disabilities, hearing impairment, and brain injury. Improved ventilator management, treatment with inhaled nitric oxide (iNO), and extracorporeal membrane oxygenation (ECMO) have led to improved survival among infants with PPHN.

  A. Perinatal circulatory transition. The normal perinatal circulatory transition is characterized by a rapid fall in PVR accompanying the first breath and a marked increase in systemic vascular resistance (SVR) following the clamping of the umbilical cord. Humoral mediators released in response to the rise in arterial oxygen content and pH cause vasorelaxation of the pulmonary circulation and constriction of the ductus arteriosus. These events raise SVR relative to PVR and cause functional closure of the foramen ovale and signal the change in the pulmonary and systemic circulations from parallel to series circuits. PPHN physiology mimics the fetal circulation in which PVR exceeds SVR and right-to-left hemodynamic shunting occurs through the foramen ovale and/or ductus arteriosus. Before birth, this circulatory configuration results in systemic delivery of oxygenated blood from the placental circulation; in postnatal life it causes diminished pulmonary perfusion and systemic hypoxemia.

II. EPIDEMIOLOGIC ASSOCIATIONS. PPHN occurs at a rate of 1 to 2 per 1,000 live births and is most common among full-term and post-term infants. Perinatal risk factors reported in association with PPHN include meconium-stained amniotic fluid and maternal conditions such as fever, anemia, and pulmonary disease. Case-control studies of risk factors for PPHN have shown associations between PPHN and a number of antenatal factors, including maternal diabetes mellitus, urinary tract infection during pregnancy, selective serotonin reuptake inhibitors (SSRIs), aspirin, and nonsteroidal anti-inflammatory drug consumption during pregnancy. Although mechanisms of antenatal pathogenesis remain uncertain, there are a number of perinatal and neonatal conditions with established links with PPHN.

A. Intrauterine or perinatal asphyxia is the most common associated diagnosis. Prolonged fetal stress and hypoxemia might result in remodeling and abnormal muscularization of the smallest pulmonary arteries. Acute birth asphyxia also causes release of vasoconstricting humoral factors and suppression of pulmonary vasodilators, probably contributing to pulmonary vasospasm.

B. Pulmonary parenchymal disease, including surfactant deficiency, pneumonia, and aspiration syndromes, such as meconium aspiration, cause hypoxia-induced pulmonary hypertension. In most such cases, the pulmonary hypertension eventually resolves, suggesting a vasospastic contribution; however, even in reversible PPHN, the characteristic pulmonary vascular remodeling cannot be excluded. The risk of hypertension appears to be greater when the fetus is of more advanced gestational age, although PPHN has been reported among late preterm or more immature infants especially those who have experienced intrauterine growth restriction.

C. Abnormalities of pulmonary development are associated with a different structural form of PPHN including alveolar capillary dysplasia, congenital diaphragmatic hernia, and various other forms of pulmonary parenchymal hypoplasia.

D. Myocardial dysfunction, myocarditis, intrauterine constriction of the ductus arteriosus, and several forms of congenital heart disease, including left- and right-sided obstructive lesions, lead to pulmonary hypertension.

E. Pneumonia and/or sepsis of bacterial or viral origin can initiate PPHN. Underlying pathophysiologic mechanisms that contribute to pulmonary hypertension in this clinical setting include suppression of nitric oxide (NO) production, endotoxin-mediated myocardial depression, and pulmonary vasoconstriction associated with release of thromboxanes and leukotrienes.

F. Although familial recurrence of PPHN is uncommon, genetic predisposition might influence PPHN risk. Infants with PPHN have low plasma levels of arginine and NO metabolites and have a greater likelihood of specific polymorphisms at position 1,405 of the carbamoyl-phosphate synthetase gene. Although no specific polymorphisms of NO synthase genes have been reported in association, diminished endothelial nitric oxide synthase (eNOS) expression has been demonstrated among infants with PPHN.

III. PATHOLOGY AND PATHOPHYSIOLOGY

A. Pulmonary vascular remodeling is pathognomonic of idiopathic PPHN and has been reported among infants with fatal PPHN. Abnormal muscularization of the normally nonmuscular intracinar arteries, with increased medial thickness of the larger muscular arteries, results in a decreased cross-sectional area of the pulmonary vascular bed and elevated PVR. Mechanisms leading to such vascular remodeling are under investigation. One possible stimulus to pulmonary vascular remodeling is fetal hypoxemia. Humoral growth factors released by hypoxia-damaged endothelial cells promote vasoconstriction and overgrowth of muscular media. Laboratory and limited clinical data suggest that vascular changes might also occur following fetal exposure to nonsteroidal anti-inflammatory agents, that cause constriction of the fetal ductus arteriosus and associated fetal pulmonary overcirculation.

B. Pulmonary hypoplasia affects both alveolar and pulmonary arteriolar development. It may be seen as an isolated anomaly or with congenital diaphragmatic hernia, oligohydramnios syndrome, renal agenesis (i.e., Potter syndrome), or remodeling or vasoconstriction of impaired fetal breathing.

C. Reversible pulmonary vasospasm is the likely pathophysiologic mechanism among infants with nonfatal PPHN. The underlying disease process, the associated conditions, and the maturity of the host each appear to modulate the pathophysiologic response. Hypoxia induces profound pulmonary vasoconstriction and this response is exaggerated by acidemia. Neural and humoral vasoactive substances each might contribute to the pathogenesis of PPHN, the response to hypoxemia, or both. These include factors associated with platelet activation and production of arachidonic acid metabolites. Suppression of endogenous NO, prostacyclin, or bradykinin production and release of thromboxanes (A_2 and its metabolite, B_2), and leukotrienes (C_4 and D_4), appear to mediate the increased PVR seen with sepsis and/or hypoxemia.

D. Myocardial dysfunction with elevated PVR

1. Right ventricular (RV) dysfunction can be caused by intrauterine closure of the ductus arteriosus, which results in altered fetal hemodynamics, postnatal pulmonary hypertension, RV failure, and a right-to-left shunt at the atrial level. RV failure resulting in altered diastolic compliance can cause right-to-left atrial shunting even in the absence of elevated PVR.

2. Left ventricular (LV) dysfunction causes pulmonary venous hypertension and secondary pulmonary arterial hypertension, often to suprasystemic levels, contributing to right-to-left hemodynamic shunting through the ductus arteriosus. Treating this form of pulmonary hypertension requires an approach that improves LV function, rather than simply lowering PVR.

E. Mechanical factors that influence PVR include cardiac output and blood viscosity. Low cardiac output recruits fewer pulmonary arteriolar channels and raises PVR by this mechanism as well as by its primary effect of lowering mixed venous oxygen content. Hyperviscosity, associated with polycythemia, reduces pulmonary microvasculature perfusion.

IV. DIAGNOSIS. PPHN should be routinely considered in evaluating the cyanotic newborn.

A. Among cases of suspected PPHN, the most common **alternative diagnoses** are uncomplicated severe pulmonary parenchymal disease, sepsis, and congenital heart disease.

B. The **physical examination** of the infant with PPHN is generally most remarkable for evidence of cyanosis and severe illness along with signs of any associated diagnoses. Among infants with PPHN, the cardiac examination might be notable for a prominent precordial impulse, a single or narrowly split and accentuated second heart sound, and/or a systolic murmur consistent with tricuspid regurgitation.

C. A **gradient in oxygenation** between simultaneous preductal (right upper extremity or head) and postductal (lower extremity or abdomen) arterial blood gas (ABG) values or transcutaneous oxygen saturation measures documents the presence of a ductus arteriosus right-to-left hemodynamic shunt. A 10% or greater pre-/postductal difference in oxygen saturation in the absence of structural heart disease suggests PPHN. A subset of infants with PPHN have hemodynamic shunting only at the level of the foramen ovale. The absence of a significant ductal shunt, however, does not exclude pulmonary hypertension associated with an isolated atrial right-to-left hemodynamic shunt, as a subset of infants with PPHN have hemodynamic shunting only at the level of the foramen ovale.

D. The **chest radiograph** usually appears normal or shows associated pulmonary parenchymal disease. The cardiothymic silhouette usually is normal; pulmonary blood flow is normal or diminished.

E. The **electrocardiogram (ECG)** most commonly shows RV predominance that is within the range considered normal for age. Less commonly, the ECG might reveal signs of myocardial ischemia or infarction.

F. An **echocardiographic study** should be performed in all infants with suspected PPHN to evaluate hemodynamic shunting and ventricular function as well as to exclude cyanotic congenital heart disease. Color Doppler examination is a technology that is useful to assess the presence of intracardiac or ductal shunting. Additional echocardiographic markers, such as flattened or septum bowed to the left, suggest pulmonary hypertension. Pulmonary artery pressure can be estimated using continuous-wave Doppler sampling of the velocity of the tricuspid regurgitation jet, if present.

G. Other diagnostic considerations. A number of disorders, some of which are associated with secondary pulmonary hypertension, are misdiagnosed as PPHN. Therefore, an important aspect of the evaluation of the infant with presumed PPHN is the effort to rule out competing conditions, including the following:

1. Structural cardiovascular abnormalities associated with right-to-left ductal or atrial shunting include the following:

a. Obstruction to pulmonary venous return: infradiaphragmatic total anomalous pulmonary venous return, hypoplastic left heart, cor triatriatum, congenital mitral stenosis.

b. Myopathic LV disease: endocardial fibroelastosis, Pompe disease

c. Obstruction to LV outflow: critical aortic stenosis, supravalvar aortic stenosis, interrupted aortic arch, coarctation of the aorta.

d. Obligatory left-to-right shunt: endocardial cushion defect, arteriovenous malformation, hemitruncus, coronary arteriovenous fistula.

e. Miscellaneous disorders: Ebstein anomaly, transposition of the great arteries.

2. LV or RV dysfunction associated with right-to-left hemodynamic shunting. LV dysfunction, due to ischemia or obstruction caused by myopathic LV disease or obstruction to LV outflow, might present with a right-to-left ductus arteriosis shunt. RV dysfunction may be associated with right-to-left atrial shunting as a result of decreased diastolic compliance and elevated end-diastolic pressure. These diagnoses must be differentiated from idiopathic PPHN caused by pulmonary vascular remodeling or vasoconstriction.

H. Signs favoring cyanotic congenital cardiac disease over PPHN include cardiomegaly, weak pulses, active precordium, pulse differential between upper and lower extremities, pulmonary edema, grade 3+ murmur, and persistent pre- and postductal arterial oxygen tension (Pao$_2$) at or <40 mmHg.

V. MANAGEMENT. The infant with PPHN constitutes a medical emergency in which immediate, appropriate intervention is critical to reverse hypoxemia, improve pulmonary and systemic perfusion, and minimize hypoxic-ischemic end-organ injury. Adequate respiratory support yields normoxemia and neutral or slightly alkalotic acid–base balance that facilitate the normal perinatal circulatory transition. Once stability is achieved, weaning should be accomplished conservatively with careful attention to the infant's tolerance of each step in tapering cardiorespiratory support.

A. Supplemental oxygen. Hypoxia is a powerful pulmonary vasoconstrictor. Therefore, the use of supplemental oxygen to achieve normoxia or hyperoxia is the most important therapy used to reduce abnormally elevated PVR. In the presence of hypoxemia, sufficient supplemental oxygen should be administered to any near-term or full-term newborn to maintain postductal oxygen saturations >95% and he/she should undergo continuous noninvasive pre- and postductal monitoring of oxygenation. The effects of oxygen therapy also should be evaluated with a postductal ABG analysis. Arterial access will be needed for blood gas and blood pressure monitoring if the baby does not demonstrate immediate improvement.

B. Intubation and mechanical ventilation. Mechanical respiratory support is instituted when hypoxemia persists despite maximal administration of supplemental oxygen, the Pao$_2$ is borderline despite supplementation with 100% oxygen and/or respiratory failure is demonstrated by marked hypercarbia and acidemia. Specific approaches to respiratory support and mechanical ventilation vary among medical centers. We recommend an approach that maintains adequate oxygenation and mild hyperventilation, until stability is achieved for 12–24 hours' after initially attempting to keep the oxygen saturation above 95%, arterial carbon dioxide tension (Paco₂) at 35 to 45 mm Hg, and pH at 7.35–7.45.

1. The nature of the underlying pulmonary parenchymal abnormality, if any, and the infant's clinical lability or stability are important factors to consider when choosing the specific respiratory management strategy.

    a. In the absence of pulmonary alveolar disease, high intrathoracic pressure may impede cardiac output and elevate PVR. In providing respiratory support to this group of infants, we recommend a strategy of rapid, low-pressure, short inspiratory time mechanical ventilation in an effort to minimize effects of ventilation on pulmonary venous return and cardiac output.

    b. When PPHN complicates parenchymal pulmonary disease, ventilator strategies should be address the optimal approach for the primary pulmonary disease. High-frequency oscillatory ventilation (HFOV) is often useful in treating infants whose PPHN is associated with severe pulmonary parenchymal disease. HFOV also has proved to be the most effective means of delivering iNO to infants whose PPHN is complicated by parenchymal disease.

C. **iNO.** NO is a naturally occurring substance produced by endothelial cells. Whether produced by pulmonary endothelium or delivered through the ventilator circuit, NO diffuses into smooth muscle cells, increases intracellular cyclic guanosine monophosphate (cGMP), relaxes the vascular smooth muscle, and causes pulmonary vasodilation. In the circulation, NO is bound by hemoglobin and biologically inactivated and, therefore, iNO causes little or no systemic vasodilation or hypotension. iNO administered by conventional or high-frequency ventilation in doses of 5 to 20 parts permillion (ppm) causes pulmonary but not systemic vasodilation and, thus, selectively decreases PVR. In a systematic review conducted by the Cochrane Collaboration, iNO was deemed useful in reducing the need for ECMO among term infants with severe respiratory failure. Methemoglobinemia is a serious potential toxicity of iNO treatment and, therefore, methemoglobin levels must be monitored daily in infants being treated with iNO. Another potential complication is rebound hypoxemia that occurs when iNO is tapered too rapidly. For this reason, iNO must be tapered very gradually and not discontinued entirely until adequate oxygenation can be maintained at an iNO dose of 1 ppm. Because not all infants with PPHN respond to iNO and some may deteriorate rapidly, we recommend treatment of critically ill infants with PPHN at a center where both iNO and ECMO are readily accessible.

    1. iNO is most effective when administered after adequate alveolar recruitment. This can be accomplished among infants PPHN with diffuse pulmonary disease by the concomitant use of HFOV and/or surfactant treatment.

D. **ECMO.** ECMO often is lifesaving therapy for infants with PPHN who fail conventional management and/or iNO treatment. Among term or near-term infants meeting ECMO criteria (Alveolar-arterial oxygen difference [AaDo₂] >600 or oxygenation index [OI] >30 on two ABGs ≥30 minutes apart), both iNO and HFOV appear to reduce the need for ECMO treatment. Therefore, if the infant's clinical status permits, a brief trial of HFOV and/or iNO might prove useful before commencing ECMO.

E. **Sedation and analgesia.** Because catecholamine release activates pulmonary α-adrenergic receptors, thereby potentially raising PVR, a narcotic analgesic that blocks the stress response, such as fentanyl infusion (2 to 5 μg/kg/hour), is a useful adjunct therapy. In rare instances, we use neuromuscular blockade with pancuronium (0.1 mg/kg/dose; every 1–4 hours PRN) to accomplish muscle relaxation and fully synchronize the infant's breathing with mechanical ventilation.

F. **Metabolic alkalosis.** Correction of acidosis is second in importance only to oxygenation in the treatment of PPHN. Alkalosis, rather than hypocarbia, is the physiologic stimulus that reduces PVR. Alkalosis can be achieved by gentle hyperventilation, and/or conservative use of metabolic therapy with sodium bicarbonate with careful attention to the associated sodium load. Among infants with PPHN, we recommend maintaining the pH at 7.35 to 7.45. Because of past reports of serious neonatal complications associated with the use of Tromethamine (THAM) we do not recommend its use for treatment of infants with PPHN.

G. **Hemodynamic support.** Optimal cardiac output is necessary to maximize tissue oxygenation and mixed venous oxygen content. In the short term, this is accomplished by optimizing systemic blood pressure to override the elevated PVR, effectively reducing or eliminating the right-to-left hemodynamic shunt. Because many infants with PPHN have PVR that is at or near normal systemic blood pressures, it is reasonable to set initial treatment goals of raising systemic blood pressure to levels of 50 to 75 mm Hg (systolic) and 45 to 55 mm Hg (mean).

   1. **Volume expansion.** Intravascular volume support with normal saline (0.9% NS) or packed red blood cells may be important adjunctive therapies for infants with pathophysiologic conditions associated with intravascular volume depletion (e.g., hemorrhage, hydrops, capillary leak) or decreased SVR (e.g., septic shock) or systemic hypotension. In treating infants with evidence of marked capillary leak, we minimize the use of 5% albumin because it also leaks from capillaries and worsens interstitial edema.

   2. **Pharmacologic treatment.** In the clinical setting of PPHN, vasopressors, such as dopamine, dobutamine, and/or epinephrine, often are necessary to achieve adequate cardiac output. When cardiac function is very poor, cardiotonic medications such as milrinone, that both enhance cardiac output and lower PVR, might prove useful.

H. **Correction of metabolic abnormalities.** Biochemical abnormalities might contribute to right-to-left shunting by impairing cardiac function. Correction of hypoglycemia and hypocalcemia is important in treating infants with PPHN in order to provide adequate substrates for myocardial function and appropriate responses to inotropic agents.

I. **Correction of polycythemia.** Hyperviscosity, associated with polycythemia, increases PVR and is associated with release of vasoactive substances through platelet activation. Partial exchange transfusion to reduce the hematocrit to 50% to 55% should be considered in the infant with PPHN whose central hematocrit exceeds 65%.

J. **Additional pharmacologic agents.** Pharmacologic therapy is directed at the simultaneous goals of optimizing cardiac output, enhancing systemic blood pressure, and reducing PVR. Consideration of associated and differential diagnoses and the known or hypothetical pathogenesis of the right-to-left shunt may prove helpful in selecting the best agent or combination of agents for a particular infant.

   1. Dopamine is often used in moderate (3 to 5 μg/kg/minute) to high (6 to 30 μg/kg/minute) doses for support of systemic blood pressure and improved cardiac output by means of α- and β-adrenergic receptor stimulation. Dopamine in low doses (1 to 2 μg/kg/minute) also offers the benefit of enhanced mesenteric and renal blood flow. Dobutamine, a synthetic catecholamine with a chemical structure similar to that of isoproterenol, has an inotropic more than a chronotropic effect on the heart through β1-adrenergic stimulation. Dopamine may increase PVR, through α-adrenergic effects, especially at higher infusion rates (>10 μg /kg/minute).

   2. Epinephrine (0.03 to 0.10 μg/kg/minute) stimulates both α- and β-adrenergic receptors; therefore, it is primarily useful in raising systemic blood pressure through enhanced cardiac output and marked peripheral vasoconstriction. Caution is advised in using epinephrine infusion because pulmonary α-adrenergic receptor stimulation might result in pulmonary vasoconstriction and elevated PVR and other oxygen perfusion (e.g., renal and mesenteric) might be reduced.

   3. At the present time, data are insufficient to support the use of other proposed medical therapies for PPHN, including sildenafil, adenosine, magnesium sulfate, calcium channel blockers, inhaled prostacyclin, inhaled ethyl nitrite, and inhaled or intravenous tolazoline.

K. Treatment controversies. There is substantial inter-institutional variation in approaches to diagnosis and management of PPHN. A few centers have reported successful treatment of PPHN without the use of mechanical ventilation, iNO, or ECMO.

VI. **POSTNEONATAL OUTCOMES AMONG INFANTS WITH PPHN.** The combined availability of iNO and ECMO led to reductions in PPHN-associated mortality from 25% to 50% to 10% to 15%. Survivors of PPHN remain at substantial risk of medical and neurodevelopmental sequelae. Controlled clinical trials suggest that the risk of morbid sequelae is not affected by specific PPHN treatment(s). Infants who develop PPHN are at approximately 20% risk of rehospitalization within 1 year of discharge, and have a 20% to 46% risk of audiologic, neurodevelopmental, or cognitive impairments.

Suggested Readings

Dakshinamurti S. Pathophysiologic mechanisms of persistent pulmonary hypertension of the newborn. *Pediatr Pulmonol* 2005;39:492–503.

Hernandez-Diaz S, Van Marter LJ, Werler M, et al. Risk factors for persistent pulmonary hypertension of the newborn. *Pediatrics* 2007; in press.

Ichinose F, Roberts JD, Zapol WM. Inhaled nitric oxide: A selective pulmonary vasodilator: Current uses and therapeutic potential. *Circulation* 2004;109:3106–3111.

Konduri GG. New approaches for persistent pulmonary hypertension of newborn. *Clin Perinatol* 2004;31:591–611.

Ostrea EM, Villanueva-Uy ET, Natarajan G, et al. Persistent pulmonary hypertension of the newborn. *Pediatr Drugs* 2006;8:179–188.

Sokol GM, Ehrenkranz RA. Inhaled nitric oxide therapy in neonatal hypoxic respiratory failure: Insights beyond primary outcomes. *Semin Perinatol* 2003;27:311–319.

Travadi JN, Patole SK. Phosphdiesterase inhibitors for persistent pulmonary hypertension of the newborn: A review. *Pediatr Pulmonol* 2003;36:529–535.

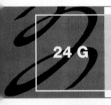

TRANSIENT TACHYPNEA OF THE NEWBORN

24 G

Nancy A. Louis

I. **DEFINITION.** Transient tachypnea of the newborn (TTN), otherwise known as *wet lung*, is observed clinically as a relatively mild, self-limited disorder most commonly affecting infants who are born at or near term gestation. The disorder is characterized by tachypnea with signs of mild respiratory distress including retractions and cyanosis; decreased oxygen saturation is usually alleviated by supplemental oxygen with Fio_2 <0.40.

II. **PATHOPHYSIOLOGY.** The transition to air breathing requires rapid clearance of fetal lung fluid, which is mediated primarily by transepithelial sodium reabsorption through amiloride-sensitive sodium channels in the alveolar epithelial cells. This is likely facilitated by the changes in the maternal–fetal hormonal milieu that normally accompany the onset of spontaneous labor at term. Disruption or delay in clearance of fetal lung liquid from a number of conditions results in the transient pulmonary edema that characterizes TTN. Retained fluid accumulates in the peribronchiolar lymphatics and bronchovascular spaces, causing compression and bronchiolar collapse with areas of air trapping and hyperinflation. These changes result in a net decrease in lung compliance accounting for the clinical manifestations of the condition.

III. **RISK FACTORS.** Premature birth, precipitous birth, and operative birth without labor have all been associated with an increased risk of TTN. This has been attributed to altered sodium transport and associated abnormal fluid clearance possibly due to the absence of hormonal changes that normally accompany the onset of spontaneous labor. Delayed cord clamping or cord milking, promoting placental–fetal transfusion, leads to an elevation in the infant's central venous pressure, disrupting clearance of fluid by the thoracic duct or pulmonary lymphatics, is also associated with TTN. Additional risk factors include male gender and birth to an asthmatic mother. The mechanism underlying the gender-associated risk and the increased associated with maternal asthma is unclear although there is speculation that these infants have an altered sensitivity to catecholamines that may play a role in delayed clearance of lung fluid. Macrosomia and multiple gestations also increase the risk of TTN. The associations between TTN and other obstetric factors such as excessive maternal sedation, prolonged labor, and complications resulting in administration of large amounts of intravenous fluids to the mother have been less consistent.

IV. CLINICAL PRESENTATION. Affected term or late preterm infants present within the first 6 hours of birth with tachypnea; respiratory rates are typically >80 breaths/minute.

   A. The tachypnea is accompanied by mild to moderate respiratory distress with cyanosis, subcostal retractions, and increased anteroposterior diameter of the chest secondary to air trapping. These signs are accompanied by nasal flaring and expiratory grunting, reflecting the effort to compensate for decreased lung compliance.

   B. Auscultation usually reveals good air entry, and crackles may or may not be appreciated. TTN usually occurs in the absence of cardiac, central nervous system (CNS), hematologic, or metabolic sources of respiratory distress. As the care of the infant of TTN is primarily supportive, it is important to rule out these other sources of respiratory distress that require more targeted and aggressive intervention.

   C. Signs of TTN usually persist for 12 to 24 hours in cases of mild disease, but can last up to 48 to 72 hours in more severe cases.

   D. In premature infants, TTN may accompany respiratory distress syndrome (RDS) caused by surfactant deficiency. Retained fetal lung liquid may complicate surfactant administration due to heterogeneous lung expansion leading to further decreases in lung compliance and areas of air trapping. These factors may combine to result in increased requirements for ventilatory support and supplemental oxygen.

V. DIFFERENTIAL DIAGNOSIS AND EVALUATION. Determination of the diagnosis of TTN requires the exclusion of other potential etiologies for mild to moderate respiratory distress presenting in the first 6 hours of age. The differential diagnosis includes pneumonia/sepsis, cyanotic congenital heart disease, RDS, pulmonary hypertension, meconium aspiration, CNS insults accompanied by central hyperventilation as seen in term infants with hypoxic-ischemic encephalopathy (HIE), and polycythemia.

   A. Careful **history** of factors such as prematurity, meconium, risk factors for sepsis, or perinatal depression events can help narrow the potential diagnosis.

   B. A **sepsis evaluation**, including complete blood count (CBC) and appropriate cultures can provide information concerning possible pneumonia or sepsis. If risk factors or laboratory data suggest sepsis, or if respiratory distress does not improve within 4 hours, we initiate broad-spectrum antibiotics.

   C. **Arterial blood gas measurement** provides more specific determination of the extent of hypoxemia and adequacy of ventilation. An infant with TTN breathing room air may demonstrate mild hypoxemia and a mild respiratory acidosis that usually resolves over 24 hours. In contrast, the presence of respiratory alkalosis is consistent with tachypnea due to central hyperventilation accompanying CNS pathology. With persistent or extreme hypoxemia, cardiac evaluation including four extremity blood pressures, electrocardiogram (EKG), and a hyperoxia test should be considered.

   D. The **chest radiograph** of the infant with TTN demonstrates prominent perihilar streaking due to engorgement of periarterial lymphatics with accumulation of interstitial fluid along the bronchovascular spaces. Mild to moderate cardiomegaly is usually present. Additionally, coarse, fluffy densities are seen due to liquid-filled alveoli. Fluid in the minor fissure, pleural effusions, and widening of the interlobar fissures may be observed. Hyperinflation due to air trapping secondary to bronchiolar collapse may be accompanied by flattening of the diaphragms. The radiograph usually shows evidence of clearing by 12 to 18 hours with complete resolution by 48 to 72 hours. The rapid resolution of these findings helps distinguish the process from bacterial pneumonia and meconium aspiration. The presence of increased pulmonary vascularity in the absence of cardiomegaly may represent total anomalous pulmonary venous return in a term infant or a patent ductus arteriosus (PDA) in a preterm infant.

VI. TREATMENT. Treatment is mainly supportive with provision of supplemental oxygen, as needed. In some infants, lung recruitment and expansion can be improved through use of continuous positive airway pressure (CPAP). Despite the apparent role for fluid retention in the pathogenesis of TTN, diuretic therapy has been shown to have no significant effect on the clinical course. Infants with sustained respiratory rates >60 breaths/minute should not be fed orally; therefore, these infants should be maintained either with gavage feedings for respiratory rates between 60 and 80 or NPO with intravenous fluids for more severe tachypnea.

VII. COMPLICATIONS. Although TTN is a self-limited process, supportive therapy may be accompanied by complications. The use of CPAP is associated with an increased risk of air leak. Delayed initiation of oral feeds may interfere with parental bonding and establishment of breastfeeding, and prolong hospital stay.

VIII. PROGNOSIS. The prognosis for these infants is excellent. There are no significant long-term residual effects. TTN is not associated with any increased risk of reactive airways disease.

Suggested Readings

Jain L, Dudell G. Respiratory transition in infants delivered by cesarean section. *Semin Perinatol* 2006;30:296–304.

Jain L, Eaton DC. Physiology of fetal lung fluid clearance and the effect of labor. *Semin Perinatol* 2006;30:34–43.

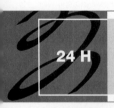

24 H PULMONARY HEMORRHAGE
Nancy A. Louis

I. DEFINITION. Pulmonary hemorrhage is defined on **pathologic** examination as the presence of erythrocytes in the alveoli, interstitium, or both, with those infants surviving longer than 24 hours showing a predominance of interstitial hemorrhage. Confluent hemorrhage involving at least two lobes of the lungs is termed *massive pulmonary hemorrhage*. There is less agreement about the **clinical** definition. We define pulmonary hemorrhage as the presence of hemorrhagic fluid in the trachea accompanied by respiratory decompensation requiring increased respiratory support or intubation within 60 minutes of the appearance of the fluid.

II. EPIDEMIOLOGY. Clinically apparent pulmonary hemorrhage occurs at a rate of 1 to 12 per 1,000 live births. Accurate incidence rates are difficult to ascertain as the clinical definition is not uniform and definitive diagnosis requires pathologic examination, which may be unavailable either because the event is not fatal or because permission for pathologic examination is not obtained. In high-risk groups such as premature and growth-restricted infants, the incidence increases to as many as 50 per 1,000 live births. In autopsy studies, pulmonary hemorrhage of any degree is much more prevalent. Some studies report hemorrhage in up to 68% of autopsied neonates, with severe pulmonary hemorrhage occurring in 19% of infants dying in the first week after birth. In most cases, death occurred 2 to 4 days after birth. Massive pulmonary hemorrhage was observed in 1.7% to 28% of infants in large autopsy studies. It was only infrequently suspected before death.

III. **PATHOGENESIS.** The underlying mechanisms of pulmonary hemorrhage remain uncertain.

   A. Studies of tracheal aspirates and fluid obtained from these infants reveal a relatively low erythrocyte concentration relative to whole blood suggesting that the clinical condition results from hemorrhagic pulmonary edema rather than direct hemorrhage into the lung.

   B. Acute left ventricular failure, often caused by hypoxia and acidosis, may lead to increased pulmonary capillary pressure with rupture of some blood vessels and transudation from others. This may be the final common pathway of many of the conditions associated with pulmonary hemorrhage.

   C. Factors that alter the integrity of the epithelial–endothelial barrier in the alveolus or that change the filtration pressure across these membranes may predispose infants to pulmonary hemorrhage.

IV. **PREDISPOSING FACTORS**

   A. Risk factors include conditions predisposing the infant to increased left ventricular filling pressures, increased pulmonary blood volume, compromised pulmonary venous drainage, or poor cardiac contractility.

   B. Retrospective autopsy surveys have correlated pulmonary hemorrhage with several conditions including respiratory distress syndrome (RDS), intrauterine growth restriction, intrauterine and intrapartum asphyxia, infection, congenital heart disease, oxygen toxicity, maternal blood aspiration, diffuse pulmonary emboli, and urea cycle defects accompanied by hyperammonemia.

   C. Patent ductus arteriosus (PDA). Increased pulmonary blood flow and compromised ventricular function accompanying dropping pulmonary resistance in the setting of a PDA is a significant risk factor.

   D. Thrombocytopenia and vascular leak accompanying conditions such as sepsis appear to increase the risk for pulmonary hemorrhage. Coagulopathy is also associated with the occurrence of pulmonary hemorrhage, although it remains unclear whether it is an inciting factor or a result of the hemorrhage.

   E. Exogenous surfactant. There has been considerable debate as to whether exogenous surfactant therapy increases the risk of pulmonary hemorrhage. *In vitro* studies have demonstrated an increased risk of erythrocyte lysis on exposure to artificial surfactant. A meta-analysis of 11 surfactant trials that prospectively reported the clinical occurrence of pulmonary hemorrhage showed an increased risk of pulmonary hemorrhage of approximately 50% in infants treated with exogenous surfactant. This finding was mainly the result of a significant increase in pulmonary hemorrhage in infants treated with synthetic surfactant preparations as a preventative strategy. The risk of pulmonary hemorrhage was not significantly increased in infants treated with either natural or synthetic surfactant using a rescue strategy. Additionally, autopsy data from five synthetic surfactant studies demonstrated no difference in the incidence of pulmonary hemorrhage at autopsy for infants treated with synthetic surfactant versus those receiving an air placebo. The reported increase in pulmonary hemorrhage may result from surfactant-associated changes in hemodynamics and lung compliance with increased pulmonary perfusion occurring in the setting of compromised left ventricular function rather than an effect of surfactant on the integrity of the pulmonary endothelial barrier.

V. **DIAGNOSIS.** The clinical diagnosis of pulmonary hemorrhage is made when sudden cardiorespiratory decompensation occurs in the setting of hemorrhagic fluid in the respiratory tract. Only a small percentage of pulmonary hemorrhages observed at autopsy are evident clinically. This is most likely due to the difficulty in diagnosing hemorrhage confined to the interstitial space without spread to the airways. In the absence of hemorrhagic secretions, respiratory deterioration is usually attributed to other causes.

A. Clinical diagnosis of pulmonary hemorrhage can sometimes be facilitated by the radiographic changes that accompany it. These nonspecific changes include diffuse opacification of one or both lungs accompanied by air bronchograms.

B. Laboratory studies mainly reflect the accompanying cardiorespiratory decompensation with metabolic or mixed acidosis, a drop in hematocrit, and sometimes evidence of coagulopathy. In most cases, the coagulopathy is probably a result of the hemorrhage rather than a precipitating factor.

VI. TREATMENT. Because the underlying pathogenesis is unclear, treatment remains supportive. The general approach involves clearing the airways of hemorrhagic fluid and restoring adequate ventilation. Better understanding of pathogenesis is required in order to allow further refinement of therapeutic approaches.

A. Use of elevated positive end-expiratory pressure (PEEP) of 6 to 8 cm H_2O helps to decrease the efflux of interstitial fluid into the alveolar space.

B. Hemodynamic instability should be corrected with volume resuscitation including packed red blood cell (PRBC) replacement, with the addition of pressor support, as needed.

C. Acidosis should be corrected through restoration of adequate ventilation and blood pressure followed by bicarbonate administration, as needed.

D. Echocardiographic evaluation may assist in evaluation of ventricular function, need for pressor support, and the possible contribution of a PDA. If hemodynamically significant, a PDA should be closed either pharmacologically or surgically.

E. Additional potential contributing factors such as coagulopathy and sepsis must be addressed.

F. It is uncertain whether using high-frequency ventilation to provide high mean airway pressure while limiting tidal volume excursions is more effective than conventional ventilation to minimize further interstitial and alveolar fluid accumulation.

G. A role for surfactant therapy following pulmonary hemorrhage has been considered either for continued treatment of primary surfactant deficiency in RDS or for treatment of secondary surfactant deficiency resulting from hemorrhagic airway edema. Experimental studies indicate that surfactant activity may be inhibited by hemoglobin and plasma components in the airspace and this inhibition may be reversed in the presence of sufficient surfactant. Additionally, a retrospective case review revealed a decrease in the oxygenation index (OI) of infants given surfactant following pulmonary hemorrhage although the OI remains significantly elevated above that seen before the hemorrhage. Decreased lung compliance following a hemorrhage may prevent or attenuate further surfactant-associated changes in pulmonary perfusion that conferred an increased risk of pulmonary edema before the hemorrhage. The potential benefits of surfactant therapy in these cases require further investigation and treatment should be decided on a case-by-case basis.

VII. PROGNOSIS. The prognosis is difficult to establish in part due to the difficulty in establishing a clinical diagnosis of this condition. Pulmonary hemorrhage was thought to be uniformly fatal before mechanical ventilation, although this was based on pathologic diagnosis and therefore excluded infants with milder hemorrhages who survived. A small retrospective case study of very low birth weight infants with pulmonary hemorrhage suggests that although mortality remains high, the occurrence of pulmonary hemorrhage does not significantly increase the risk of later pulmonary or neurodevelopmental disabilities among survivors.

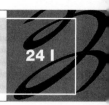

APNEA
Ann R. Stark
24 I

I. BACKGROUND

A. Definition. Apnea is defined as the cessation of airflow. Apnea is pathologic (an apneic spell) when absent airflow is prolonged (usually 20 seconds or more) or accompanied by bradycardia (heart rate <100 beats/minute) or cyanosis. Bradycardia and cyanosis are usually present after 20 seconds of apnea, although they can occur more rapidly in the small premature infant. After 30 to 45 seconds, pallor and hypotonia are seen, and infants may be unresponsive to tactile stimulation.

B. Classification of apnea is based on whether absent air flow is accompanied by continued inspiratory efforts and upper airway obstruction. Most spells are central or mixed apnea.

1. Central apnea occurs when inspiratory efforts are absent.

2. Obstructive apnea occurs when inspiratory efforts persist. Airway obstruction is present.

3. Mixed apnea occurs when airway obstruction with inspiratory efforts precedes or follows central apnea.

C. Incidence. Apneic spells occur frequently in premature infants. The incidence of apnea increases with decreasing gestational age. As many as 25% of all premature infants who weigh <1,800 g (~34 weeks' gestational age) have at least one apneic episode. Essentially all infants <28 weeks' gestational age have apnea.

1. Onset. Apneic spells generally begin at 1 or 2 days after birth; if they do not occur during the first 7 days, they are unlikely to occur later.

2. Duration. Apneic spells persist for variable periods postnatally and usually cease by 37 weeks' gestational age. In infants born before 28 weeks' gestation, however, spells often persist beyond term gestational age. In a study in which infants were monitored at home, significant apnea and/or bradycardia were recorded up to 43 weeks' gestational age in 20% of preterm infants who were free of spells for at least 5 days before discharge and in 33% of those who had spells observed during that period. The clinical significance of these events is uncertain.

3. Term infants. Apneic spells occurring in infants at or near term are always abnormal and are nearly always associated with serious, identifiable causes, such as birth asphyxia, intracranial hemorrhage, seizures, or depression from medication. Failure to breathe at birth in the absence of drug depression or asphyxia is generally caused by irreversible structural abnormalities of the central nervous system (CNS).

II. PATHOGENESIS.

Several mechanisms have been proposed to explain apnea in premature infants. Many clinical conditions have also been associated with apneic spells, and some may be causative.

A. Developmental immaturity of central respiratory drive is a likely contributing factor, because apneic spells occur more frequently in immature infants.

1. The occurrence of apnea may correlate with brainstem neural function. The frequency of apnea decreases over a period in which brainstem conduction time of the auditory evoked response shortens as gestational age increases.

2. Breathing in infants is strongly influenced by sleep state. Active or rapid eye movement (REM) sleep is marked by irregularity of tidal volume and respiratory frequency. REM sleep predominates in preterm infants, and apneic spells occur more frequently in this state than in quiet sleep.

B. Chemoreceptor response

1. In preterm infants, hypoxia results in transient hyperventilation, followed by hypoventilation and sometimes apnea, in contrast to the response in adults. In addition, hypoxia makes the premature infant less responsive to increased levels of carbon dioxide. Therefore, hypoxemia may be involved in the pathogenesis of some apneic spells.

2. The ventilatory response to increased carbon dioxide is decreased in preterm infants with apnea compared with a matched group without apnea, which suggests that abnormal respiratory control may contribute to the pathogenesis of apnea.

C. Reflexes. Active reflexes invoked by stimulation of the posterior pharynx, lung inflation, fluid in the larynx, or chest wall distortion can precipitate apnea in infants. These reflexes may be involved in the apnea that is sometimes associated, for example, with vigorous use of suction catheters in the pharynx or with fluid in the upper airway during feeding.

D. Respiratory muscles. Ineffective ventilation may result from impaired coordination of the inspiratory muscles (diaphragm and intercostal muscles) and the muscles of the upper airway (larynx and pharynx).

1. Airway obstruction contributes to mixed and obstructive apneic spells. The site of this obstruction is usually the upper pharynx, which is vulnerable because of poor muscle tone, especially in REM sleep. Passive neck flexion, pressure on the lower rim of a face mask, and submental pressure (all encountered during nursery procedures) can obstruct the airway in infants and lead to apnea, especially in a small premature infant. Spontaneously occurring airway obstruction is seen more frequently when preterm infants assume a position of neck flexion.

2. Nasal obstruction can lead to apnea, especially in preterm infants, who usually do not switch to oral breathing after nasal occlusion.

E. Gastroesophageal reflux is common in preterm infants. However, no association has been demonstrated between apnea of prematurity and gastroesophageal reflux.

III. MONITORING AND EVALUATION. All infants <35 weeks' gestational age should be monitored for apneic spells for at least the first week after birth because of the risk of apneic spells in this group. Monitoring should continue until no significant apneic episode has been detected for at least 5 days. Because impedance apnea monitors may not distinguish respiratory efforts during airway obstruction from normal breaths, heart rate should be monitored in addition to, or instead of, respiration. Even with careful monitoring, some prolonged spells of apnea and bradycardia may not be recognized.

A. When a monitor alarm sounds, one should remember to respond to the infant, not the monitor, checking for bradycardia, cyanosis, and airway obstruction.

B. Most apneic spells in premature infants respond to tactile stimulation. Infants who fail to respond to stimulation should be ventilated during the spell with bag and mask, generally with a fractional concentration of inspired oxygen (Fio_2) of under 0.40 or equal to the Fio_2 before the spell to avoid marked elevations in arterial oxygen tension (Po_2).

C. After the first apneic spell, the infant should be evaluated for a possible underlying cause (see Table 24I.1); if a cause is identified, specific treatment can then be initiated. One should be particularly alert to the possibility of a precipitating cause in infants who are more than 34 weeks' gestational age. Evaluation should include a history and physical examination, arterial blood gas measurement with continuous oxygen saturation monitoring, complete blood count, and measurement of blood glucose, calcium, and electrolyte levels.

IV. TREATMENT. When apneic spells are repeated and prolonged (i.e., more than two to three times/hour) or when they require frequent bag and mask ventilation, treatment should be initiated in order of increasing invasiveness and risk.

A. General measures

1. **Specific therapy** should be directed at an underlying cause, if one is identified.

2. **In general,** oxygen saturation should be maintained between 85% and 95%, with supplemental oxygen provided if needed.

3. **Care should be taken** to avoid reflexes that may trigger apnea. Suctioning of the pharynx should be done carefully, and oral feedings should be avoided.

4. **Positions of extreme flexion** or extension of the neck should be avoided, to reduce the likelihood of airway obstruction.

TABLE 24I.1	Evaluation of an Infant with Apena	
Potential cause	**Associated history of signs**	**Evaluation**
Infection	Feeding intolerance, lethargy, temperature instability	Complete blood count, cultures, if appropriate
Impaired oxygenation	Cyanosis, tachypnea, respiratory distress	Continuous oxygen monitoring, arterial blood gas measurement, chest x-ray examination
Metabolic disorders	Jitteriness, poor feeding, lethargy, CNS depression, irritability	Glucose, calcium, electrolytes
Drugs	CNS depression, hypotonia, maternal history	Magnesium, screen for toxic substances in urine
Temperature instability	Lethargy	Monitor temperature of patient and environment
Intracranial pathology	Abnormal neurologic examination, seizures	Cranial ultrasonographic examination

CNS = central nervous system.

5. **Decreasing the environmental temperature** to the low end of the neutral thermal environment range may lessen the number of spells. Avoiding swings in environmental temperature may prevent apnea.
6. **Whether blood transfusion reduces the frequency of apneic spells** in some infants is controversial. We consider a transfusion of packed red blood cells (PRBCs) if the hematocrit is <25% and the infant has episodes of apnea and bradycardia that are frequent or severe while methylxanthine levels are therapeutic (see Chap. 26).

B. **Nasal continuous positive airway pressure** (CPAP) at moderate levels (4–6 cm H_2O) can reduce the number of mixed and obstructive apneic spells. It is especially useful in infants <32 to 34 weeks' gestational age and those with residual lung disease.

C. **Methylxanthine therapy** markedly reduces the number of apneic spells and the need for mechanical ventilation. Mechanisms by which methylxanthines may decrease apnea include (i) respiratory center stimulation; (ii) antagonism of adenosine, a neurotransmitter that can cause respiratory depression; and (iii) improvement of diaphragmatic contractility.

1. We treat frequent and/or severe apnea with caffeine citrate. We use a loading dose of 20 mg/kg of caffeine citrate (10 mg/kg caffeine base) orally or intravenously over 30 minutes, followed by maintenance doses of 5 to 8 mg/kg (2.5 to 5 mg/kg caffeine base) in one daily dose beginning 24 hours after the loading dose.

   a. If apnea continues, we give an additional dose of 10 mg/kg caffeine citrate, and increase the maintenance dose by 20%.

   b. Caffeine serum levels of 5 to 20 μg/mL are considered therapeutic. We do not routinely measure serum drug concentration because of the wide therapeutic index and the lack of an established dose–response relationship. However, we measure drug concentration in infants with signs of toxicity or liver dysfunction, and sometimes in those with persistent apnea.

   c. Caffeine is generally discontinued at 34 to 36 weeks' gestational age if no apneic spells have occurred for 5 to 7 days. The effect of caffeine likely remains for approximately 1 week after it has been discontinued. We continue monitoring until no apnea has been detected for at least 5 days after that period.

2. Additional short-term or long-term benefits of caffeine therapy and risks are uncertain. In a report of short-term outcomes from a large multicenter ongoing trial in infants 500 to 1,250 g birth weight, the frequency of bronchopulmonary dysplasia (BPD) and of treatment of patent ductus arteriosus (PDA) with drug or surgery was less in infants treated with caffeine compared to placebo. Weight gain was less during the first 3 weeks after randomization in infants treated with caffeine, but not at 4 and 6 weeks. In a preliminary report, caffeine reduced the rate of survival without neurodevelopmental disability at 18 to 21 months corrected age.

3. Most reports of side effects of methylxanthines in newborns are based on experience with theophylline. These included tachycardia; signs of gastrointestinal dysfunction, including abdominal distention, feeding intolerance, or vomiting; or jitteriness and irritability. Caffeine appears to be less toxic than theophylline and is well tolerated. There may be no change in heart rate in infants treated with caffeine, in contrast to the tachycardia often associated with theophylline therapy. Diuresis and urinary calcium excretion occur with both drugs. Metabolic changes, including increased glucose and insulin levels, occur following a theophylline loading dose in some infants.

4. We do not use doxapram, a respiratory stimulant that may reduce apnea if methylxanthine therapy has failed. Side effects of doxapram include hyperactivity, jitteriness, seizures, hyperglycemia, mild liver dysfunction, and hypertension. In addition, benzyl alcohol is used as a preservative.

D. Mechanical ventilation may be required if the other interventions are unsuccessful.

V. PERSISTENT APNEA. In some infants, especially those born at <28 weeks' gestation, apneic spells may persist at 37 to 40 weeks' postmenstrual age, when the infant may be otherwise ready for discharge home from the nursery. There is no consensus yet on the appropriate management of these infants, but efforts are directed at reducing the risk of apneic spells so that the child can be cared for at home.

A. Recordings of impedance pneumography and electrocardiogram (ECGs) for 12 to 24 hours ("pneumograms") can be used to document the occurrence of apnea and bradycardia during that time period, but they do not predict the risk of sudden infant death syndrome (SIDS).

B. Continued use of caffeine may be helpful in infants whose spells recur when the drug is discontinued. Attempts to withdraw the drug can be made at intervals of approximately 2 months while the child is closely monitored.

C. Some infants are cared for with cardiorespiratory monitoring at home, although few data are available on its effectiveness. Extensive psychosocial support must be provided for the parents, who should be skilled in cardiopulmonary resuscitation (CPR) and in the use of the monitor. Routine home monitoring of asymptomatic preterm infants is not indicated.

VI. STRATEGIES TO PREVENT SIDS. Although the peak incidence of SIDS occurs after the newborn period, parents frequently express concern about their child's risk. Although SIDS occurs more frequently in premature or low birth weight infants, a history of apnea of prematurity does not increase this risk.

We encourage strategies that may reduce the risk of SIDS.

A. Sleeping position. Prone sleeping position increases the risk of SIDS, and sleeping on the back reduces the risk. In general, babies should be placed on their back to sleep on a firm surface. The exceptions include preterm infants with respiratory disease, infants with symptomatic gastroesophageal reflux, and infants with craniofacial abnormalities or evidence of upper airway obstruction. For these infants, soft bedding should be avoided. The American Academy of Pediatrics (AAP) recommends a sleeping environment that is separate from but near the mother. Use of a pacifier during sleep also appears to reduce the risk of SIDS.

B. Smoking. Infants exposed to maternal smoking during pregnancy and postnatally have a higher risk of SIDS. Smoking should be avoided by parents, and infants should not be exposed to smoke.

C. **Overheating.** Infants exposed to excessively high room temperatures or overheating from excess wrapping have an increased risk of SIDS. Caregivers should avoid practices that result in overheating.

D. **Breastfeeding.** Infants who were never breastfed have a higher risk of SIDS than do breastfed infants. We encourage breastfeeding for many reasons (see Chap. 11).

Suggested Readings

American Academy of Pediatrics Task Force on SIDS. The changing concept of Sudden Infant Death Syndrome: Diagnostic coding shifts, controversies regarding the sleeping environment, and new variables to consider in reducing risk. *Pediatrics* 2005;116:1245–1255.

Ramanathan R, Corwin MJ, Hunt CE, et al. Cardiorespiratory events recorded on home monitors. *JAMA* 2001;285:2199.

Schmidt B, Roberts RS, Davis P, et al. Caffeine therapy for apnea of prematurity. *N Engl J Med* 2006;354:2112–2121.

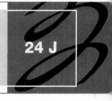

BRONCHOPULMONARY DYSPLASIA/CHRONIC LUNG DISEASE

24 J

Richard B. Parad

I. **DEFINITION.** A National Institutes of Health (NIH) conference proposed definitions for bronchopulmonary dysplasia (BPD), also known as *chronic lung disease* (CLD), of prematurity, which is a more general term. For infants born at <32 weeks' gestation who remain in oxygen for the first 28 days, at 36 weeks postmenstrual age (PMA) mild BPD is defined as no supplemental oxygen requirement, moderate BPD is requirement of supplemental O_2 <30% and severe BPD is requirement of $\geq$30% O_2 and/or continuous positive airway pressure (CPAP) or ventilator support. For infants born at $\geq$32 weeks, BPD is defined as a supplemental O_2 requirement for first 28 days with severity level based on oxygen requirement at 56 days. A physiologic definition of BPD has been proposed based on SaO_2 during a room air challenge performed at 36 weeks (or 56 days for infants >32 weeks), or before hospital discharge, with SaO_2 <90% the cutoff at which supplemental O_2 is required. Lung parenchyma usually appears abnormal on chest radiographs.This definition can include term babies with meconium aspiration syndrome, pneumonia, and certain cardiac and gastrointestinal (GI) anomalies who require chronic ventilatory support. BPD is associated with the development of chronic respiratory morbidity.

II. **EPIDEMIOLOGY.** Approximately 3,000 to 7,000 cases of BPD are estimated to occur in the United States each year. Infants <1,250 g birth weight are most susceptible to developing this condition. Differences in populations (race/ethnicity/socioeconomic status), clinical practices, and definitions account for a wide variation in the rate reported among centers. The risk is decreased in African-Americans and girls. In spite of attempts to clarify the clinical definition, only 40% of those infants requiring O_2 at 36 weeks go on to develop chronic respiratory morbidity, and infants without O_2 requirement at 36 weeks are still at increased risk for chronic respiratory morbidity.

III. **PATHOGENESIS**

A. **Acute lung injury** is caused by the combination of oxygen toxicity, barotrauma, and volutrauma from mechanical ventilation. Cellular and interstitial injury results in the release of proinflammatory cytokines (interleukin 1β [IL-1β],

IL-6, IL-8, tumor necrosis factor-α [TNF-α]) that cause secondary changes in alveolar permeability and recruit inflammatory cells into interstitial and alveolar spaces; further injury from proteases, oxidants, and additional chemokines and chemoattractants cause ongoing inflammatory cell recruitment and leakage of water and protein. Airway and vascular tone may be altered. Alveolar development is interrupted and parenchyma is destroyed, leading to emphysematous changes. Sloughed cells and accumulated secretions not cleared adequately by the damaged mucociliary transport system cause inhomogeneous peripheral airway obstruction that leads to alternating areas of collapse and hyperinflation and proximal airway dilation. Bombesin-like protein, a proinflammatory peptide produced by neuroendocrine cells, has been shown to be elevated in the urine of infants who subsequently develop BPD.

B. In the chronic phase of lung injury, the interstitium may be altered by fibrosis and cellular hyperplasia that results from excessive release of growth factors and cytokines, leading to insufficient repair. Interstitial fluid clearance is disrupted, resulting in pulmonary fluid retention. Airways develop increased muscularization and hyperreactivity. The physiologic effects are decreased lung compliance, increased airway resistance, and impaired gas exchange with resulting ventilation-perfusion mismatching and air trapping.

C. Factors that may contribute to the development of BPD include the following:

1. **Immature lung substrate.** The lung is most susceptible before alveolar formation begins. Injury at this stage may cause an arrest of alveolarization.

2. **Inadequate activity** of the antioxidant enzymes superoxide dismutase, catalase, glutathione peroxidase, and/or deficiency of free radical sinks such as vitamin E, glutathione, and ceruloplasmin may predispose the lung to oxygen toxicity. Similarly, inadequate antiprotease protection may predispose the lung to injury from the unchecked proteases released by recruited inflammatory cells.

3. **Excessive early intravenous fluid administration** and persistent left-to-right shunt through the patent ductus arteriosus (PDA). Although prophylactic PDA ligation does not prevent BPD, persistent left-to-right shunt may still be a contributing factor.

4. **Intrauterine or perinatal infection** may contribute to the etiology of BPD or modify its course. Ureaplasma urealyticum has been associated with BPD in premature infants, although it remains unclear whether this relationship is causal. Chlamydia trachomatis and cytomegalovirus can cause gradually developing pneumonitis.

5. **Familial airway hyperreactivity.**

6. **Increased inositol clearance,** leading to diminished plasma inositol levels and decreased surfactant synthesis or impaired surfactant metabolism.

7. **An increase in vasopressin** and a decrease in atrial natriuretic peptide release may alter pulmonary and systemic fluid balance in the setting of obstructive lung disease.

IV. CLINICAL PRESENTATION

A. Physical examination typically reveals tachypnea, retractions, and rales on auscultation.

B. Arterial blood gas (ABG) analysis shows hypoxemia and hypercarbia with eventual metabolic compensation for the respiratory acidosis.

C. The chest radiograph appearance changes as the disease progresses. In early descriptions of BPD, stage I had the same appearance as respiratory distress syndrome (RDS), stage II showed diffuse haziness with increased density and normal to low lung volumes, stage III demonstrated streaky densities with bubbly lucencies and early hyperinflation, and stage IV showed hyperinflation with larger hyperlucent areas interspersed with thicker, streaky densities. Not all infants progressed to stage IV, and some transitioned directly from stage I to stage III. Radiographic abnormalities often persisted into childhood. *New BPD*, a term coined to distinguish the different histology and radiographic findings of the most immature very low birth weight (VLBW) infants, is often associated with stage II changes.

D. Cardiac evaluation. Nonpulmonary causes of respiratory failure should be excluded. Electrocardiogram (ECG) can show persistent or progressive right ventricular hypertrophy if *cor pulmonale* develops. Left ventricular hypertrophy may develop with systemic hypertension. Two-dimensional echocardiography may be useful in excluding left-to-right shunts (see Chap. 25). Biventricular failure is unusual when good oxygenation is maintained and the development of pulmonary hypertension is avoided.

E. Pulmonary function testing, if done, will show increased respiratory system resistance (Rrs) and decreased dynamic compliance (Crs).

F. Pathologic changes are detectable in severe cases by the first few days after birth. By the end of the first week, necrotizing bronchiolitis, obstruction of small airway lumens by debris and edema, and areas of peribronchial and interstitial fibrosis are present. Emphysematous changes and significant impairment in alveolar development result in diminished surface area for gas exchange. Changes in both large airways (glandular hyperplasia) and small airways (smooth muscle hyperplasia) likely form the histologic basis for reactive airway disease. Pulmonary vascular changes associated with pulmonary hypertension may be seen. Arrest of alveolariztion is more significant at lower gestational ages.

V. INPATIENT TREATMENT. The goals of treatment during the neonatal intensive care unit (NICU) course are to minimize further lung injury (baro- and volutrauma, oxygen toxicity, inflammation), maximize nutrition, and diminish oxygen consumption.

A. Mechanical ventilation

1. Acute phase. Ventilator adjustments are made to minimize airway pressures and tidal volumes although providing adequate gas exchange (see Chap. 24B).

In most circumstances, we avoid hyperventilation (keeping arterial carbon dioxide tension [$Paco_2$] at >55 mm Hg, with pH >7.25) and maintain oxygen saturation (Sao_2) at 90% to 95% or lower and arterial oxygen tension (Pao_2) 60 to 80 mm Hg. We do not routinely use high-frequency oscillatory ventilation because most available evidence suggests that this technique does not prevent BPD in high-risk infants. Early CPAP with avoidance of mechanical ventilation, and earlier transition from IMV to CPAP are management strategies that may be associated with decreased BPD risk.

2. Chronic phase. Once baseline ventilator settings are established with an arterial carbon dioxide tension ($Paco_2$) not higher than 65 mm Hg, we maintain the ventilator rate without weaning until a pattern of steady weight gain is established.

B. Supplemental oxygen is supplied to maintain the Pao_2 >55 mm Hg. The Sao_2 should be correlated with Pao_2 in each infant. A trial designed to lower retinopathy of prematurity (ROP) incidence showed that lower target Sao_2 led to a decreased risk of developing BPD by setting oximeter alarm limits at 85% to 93% for infants <32 weeks' gestation and then relaxing the range to 87% to 97% at 32 weeks.

When <30% oxygen concentration is required by hood, we supply oxygen by nasal cannula. If adequate Sao_2 cannot be maintained on <1 L/min of flow, hood oxygen should be restored. We use a flowmeter that is accurate at low rates, and gradually decrease the flow of 100% oxygen although maintaining the appropriate Sao_2. Alternatively, flow can be decreased to the lowest marking on the flowmeter, as tolerated, and then oxygen concentration can be decreased. Hypopharyngeal Fio_2 can be estimated from that delivered by nasal cannula (see Fig. 24J.1). Sao_2 should remain >90% during sleep, feedings, and active periods before supplemental oxygen is discontinued.

C. Surfactant replacement therapy decreases the combined outcome of CLD or death at 28 days of age, although it has made little or no impact on the overall incidence of CLD. Meta-analyses suggest the incidence is decreased in larger premature infants, but is higher in smaller premature infants who would have died without surfactant therapy.

D. Aggressive early management of a hemodynamically significant PDA is recommended (see Chap. 25).

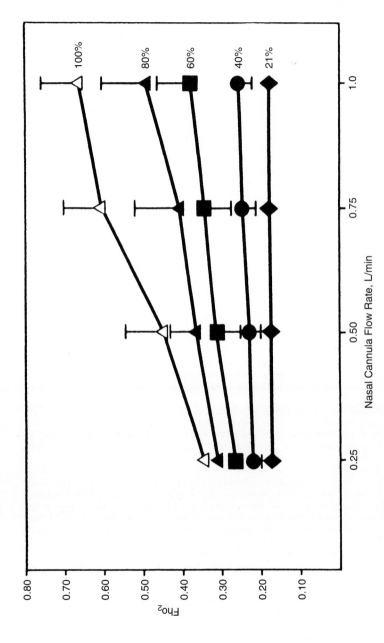

Figure 24J.1. Approximate conversion from nasal cannula flow Fio_2 to hypopharyngeal Fio_2 (Fho_2). Fio_2 = fraction of inspired oxygen. (From Vain NE, Prudent LM, Stevens DP, et al. Regulation of oxygen concentration delivered to infants through nasal cannulas. *Am J Dis Child* 1989;143:1459. By Permission.)

E. Monitoring (see Chap. 24C)

1. **ABG analysis** is used to monitor gas exchange and confirm noninvasive monitoring values.

2. **We use continuous pulse oximetry** for long-term monitoring of infants with CLD, set oximeter alarm limits at 85% to 93% for infants <32 weeks' gestation and relax the range to 87% to 97% at 32 weeks. The long-term goal is to keep the Pao_2 >55 mm Hg.

3. **Capillary blood gas** (CBG) values are useful to monitor pH and Pco_2. Because pH and Pco_2 sometimes vary from central values, we compare them with ABG values. If CBG and ABG values are similar, we monitor stable ventilator-dependent infants with pulse oximetry and one or two CBG analyses per day; less frequent CBG tests are obtained for patients receiving oxygen by nasal cannula.

4. **Pulmonary function testing** is used in some centers to document functional responses to trials of bronchodilators, and diuretics (see V.G.1–4).

F. Fluid management. Fluid intake is limited to the minimum required. Initially, we provide intake adequate to maintain urine output at least 1 mL/kg/hour and serum sodium concentration of 140 to 145 mEq/L. Subsequently, we provide 130 to 150 mL/kg/day to supply sufficient calories for growth. We regularly recalculate fluid intake for weight gain, once it is above birth weight. Later, when respiratory status is stable, fluid restriction is gradually released.

G. Drugs. When the infant remains ventilator dependent on restricted fluid intake in the absence of PDA or intercurrent infection, additional pharmacotherapeutic trials (usually >24 hours) should be considered.

1. **Prevention.** In multicenter randomized clinical trials:

   a. **Vitamin A** (5,000 U IM, three times weekly for the first 28 days of age) reduced the incidence of CLD in extremely low birth weight (ELBW) infants by 10%. Although we routinely treat ELBW infants with vitamin A using this protocol, the impact on long-term outcomes is uncertain.

   b. **In <27-week infants,** intratracheal recombinant human Cu/Zn superoxide dismutase administered intratracheally every 48 hours while intubated resulted in an approximately 50% reduction in use of asthma medications, emergency room visits, and hospitalizations in the first year of life. This treatment remains investigational.

   c. Caffeine citrate (20 mg/kg loading dose and 5 mg/kg daily maintenance) started during the first 10 days of life in infants 500 to 1250 g birth weight reduced the rate of BPD from 47% to 36%. In a preliminary report, caffeine treatment also improved the rate of survival without neurodevelopmental disability at 18 to 21 months corrected age.

2. **Pulmonary fluid retention** is treated with diuretics. Diuretics indirectly attenuate symptoms of respiratory distress and result in decreased Rrs and increased Crs; gas exchange is variably affected. An acute clinical response may be seen within 1 hour, although maximal effect may not be achieved until 1 week of therapy. The clinical improvement is likely due to decreased lung water content, with decreased interstitial and peribronchial fluid resulting in less resistance and better compliance. The mechanisms of action may be due to either diuresis or nondiuretic effects. Diuretics have not been shown to improve clinical outcomes such as duration of ventilator dependence, hospital length of stay, or long-term outcome.

   a. **Furosemide is used initially** at a dose of 0.5 to 1.0 mg/kg intravenously one to two times daily. The dose may be given at the time of blood transfusions if these have been associated with increased pulmonary fluid and respiratory distress. Immature infants are at increased risk of toxicity from larger or more frequent doses because of the prolonged drug half-life. Side effects include hypercalciuria, nephrocalcinosis, ototoxicity, electrolyte imbalance, and nephrolithiasis. We use lower doses or combine furosemide with other diuretics to avoid the need for compensation with electrolyte supplementation (see G.8). Alternate-day furosemide therapy may be effective in the chronic stage of the disease with fewer side effects.

b. Chlorothiazide. We prefer treatment with chlorothiazide (20 to 40 mg/kg/day orally, divided BID). Chlorothiazide decreases calcium excretion and, if used in combination with furosemide, may minimize calcium loss and reverse nephrocalcinosis due to furosemide. The combination also allows the use of a lower furosemide dose.

3. Bronchodilators. Acute obstructive episodes or chronically increased resistance may be related to increased airway tone or bronchospasm and may respond to bronchodilator therapy. Infants with developing CLD may benefit as early as the second week of age.

a. Administration of nebulized β-adrenergic agonists (BAAs) results in decreased Rrs and increased Crs. Tachycardia is the major limiting side effect. Newer agents have increased β2 specificity with less β1 toxicity. We use an albuterol metered-dose inhaler (MDI) with a spacer device (1 puff) or nebulized 0.5% solution (5 mg/mL) 0.02 to 0.04 mL/kg (up to 0.1 mL total in 2 mL of normal saline solution) every 6 to 8 hours. In ventilated infants, for efficiency, our preference is an MDI with a spacer device placed in line with the ventilator near the endotracheal tube

b. Muscarinic agents. MDI (1 puff) or nebulized (25 mg/kg/dose) ipratropium bromide increases Crs and decreases Rrs. Combination MDI containing both BAAs and muscarinic agents may provide a synergistic effect, but this has not been studied in preterm infants.

c. Theophylline is infrequently used as a bronchodilator because most infants with BPD are treated with caffeine citrate for apnea. Although not well studied, infants treated with caffeine for apnea may have improved Crs.

4. Postnatal corticosteroids. In early trials, treatment with glucocorticoids (usually dexamethasone) in infants who remained ventilator-dependent for 2 to 3 weeks resulted in increased Crs, decreased Rrs, diminished oxygen requirement, and earlier extubation. However, treatment with glucocorticoids does not appear to have a substantial impact on long-term pulmonary outcomes, such as duration of supplemental oxygen requirement, length of hospital stay, or mortality. Subsequent trials of earlier treatment, recurrent pulses, and lower doses have yielded inconsistent results as either a prophylactic or attenuating agent. Randomized trials of inhaled glucocorticoids also did not demonstrate improved pulmonary outcome. In addition to short-term side effects, including hypertension, hyperglycemia, and spontaneous GI performation, long-term follow-up of infants treated with postnatal corticosteroids, primarily dexamethasone, has raised concerns about delays in neurodevelopment and growth. Because of this potential harm and lack of well-established long-term benefit, routine use of corticosteroids is discouraged, and reserved only for infants with progressive respiratory failure that is refractory to all other therapies. If treatment with glucocorticoids is undertaken, we discuss the potential neurodevelopmental harm with parents before use. Although this regimen has not been tested in clinical trials, we use a short course and relatively low dose of dexamethasone to reduce ventilator settings and facilitate extubation (see Table 24J.1). Treatment with hydrocortisone may provide similar short-term benefit without adverse neurologic consequences, but further studies are needed.

a. Common acute complications of dexamethasone include glucose intolerance, systemic hypertension, and transient catabolic state. Total neutrophil counts, band counts, and platelet counts increase during steroid treatment. Hypertrophic cardiomyopathy sometimes occurs, but is transient and does not appear to affect cardiac function. GI perforation and gastric ulcerations can occur. Adrenal suppression is transient.

b. Postextubation airway edema, with stridorous obstruction (see VI.A) leading to respiratory failure, may be attenuated with dexamethasone, 0.25 mg/kg/dose every 12 hours starting 8 to 12 hours before the next extubation. Edema also may be acutely diminished with nebulized racemic epinephrine.

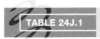

TABLE 24J.1	Suggested Course of Dexamethasone Treatment for Severe BPD	
Length of Course	**Day**	**Dose**
Short	1	0.1 mg/kg q12h
	2	0.075 mg/kg q12h
	3	0.05 mg/kg q12h
	May repeat weekly, if necessary	
Long	1 and 2	0.1 mg/kg q12h
If no response after 48–72 h of this dosing, stop.		
If response:		
	3 and 4	0.075 mg/kg q12h
	5 6, and 7	0.05 mg/kg q12h
	8	OFF
	9	0.05 mg/kg q12h
	10	END

5. **Cromolyn** acts on both airway and pulmonary vascular tone. Prophylactic treatment of reactive airways attenuates symptoms in infants with CLD who develop asthma during the first year of life. Use in the NICU setting has not been well evaluated. Dosing can be either with MDI and spacer, or nebulized (10 to 20 mg q6–8h).

6. **Inhaled nitric oxide** (iNO). In animal models of BPD, iNO may act to relax airway and pulmonary vascular tone, and diminish lung inflammation. Two recent multicenter clinical trials assessed the potential efficacy of iNO in attenuating or preventing BPD using different treatment regimens. One trial found BPD was reduced in infants >1,000 g although not for the overall group; the other found overall benefit that was limited to those treated at 7 to 14 days. Because benefit is unclear, and both safety and long-term impact have not yet been established on follow-up, therapy is not considered standard of care. Additional trial data are pending.

7. **Pain management.** Pain management and sedation are used for physical or autonomic signs of pain or discomfort. These responses may interfere with the ability to ventilate and oxygenate. Oral sucrose, morphine sulfate or fentanyl, phenobarbital, short-acting benzodiazepines, or chloral hydrate are used (see Chap. 37).

8. **Electrolyte supplements.** Hyponatremia, hypokalemia, and hypochloremia with secondary hypercarbia are common side effects of chronic diuretic therapy that are corrected by lowering the diuretic dose or adding NaCl and KCl supplements. Adequate sodium intake should be provided. Serum sodium level can fall below 130 mEq/L before intervention is required. Although hypochloremia may occur with compensated respiratory acidosis, low serum chloride concentration from diuretic-induced loss and inadequate intake can cause metabolic alkalosis and $Paco_2$ elevation. Hypochloremia may also contribute to poor growth. Chloride deficit can be corrected with potassium chloride. Monitoring should be carried out at regular intervals until equilibrium is reached.

H. Nutrition (see Chap. 10)

1. **Metabolic rate** and energy expenditure are elevated in BPD although caloric intake is poor. Providing more calories by the administration of lipids instead of carbohydrates lowers the respiratory quotient, thereby diminishing CO_2 production. To optimize growth, wasteful energy expenditure should be minimized

and caloric intake maximized. Prolonged parenteral nutrition is often required. As enteral feeding is started, we feed by orogastric or nasogastric tube and limit oral feeding to avoid tiring the infant. We generally advance to 30 cal/oz formula.

2. **Vitamin, trace element, and other dietary supplementation.** Vitamin E and antioxidant enzymes diminish oxidant toxicity, although vitamin E supplementation does not prevent BPD. Vitamin A may promote epithelial repair and minimize fibrosis. Selenium, zinc, and copper are trace elements vital to antioxidant enzyme function, and inadequate intake may interfere with protection.

I. Blood transfusions. We generally maintain hematocrit approximately 30% to 35% (hemoglobin 8–10 g/dL) as long as supplemental oxygen is needed. Fluid-sensitive patients may benefit from furosemide given immediately following the transfusion. Improved oxygen delivery may allow better reserves for growth in the infant with increased metabolic demands.

J. Behavioral factors. As with all sick infants, care is best provided with individualized attention to behavioral and environmental factors (see Chap. 14).

VI. ASSOCIATED COMPLICATIONS

A. Upper airway obstruction. Trauma to the nasal septum, larynx, trachea, or bronchi is common after prolonged or repeated intubation and suctioning. Abnormalities include laryngotracheobronchomalacia, granulomas, vocal cord paresis, edema, ulceration with pseudomembranes, subglottic stenosis, and congenital structural anomalies. Stridor may develop when postextubation edema is superimposed on underlying stenosis. Abnormalities are not excluded by the absence of stridor and may be asymptomatic, becoming symptomatic at the time of a viral upper respiratory tract infection. Flexible fiberoptic bronchoscopy should be used to evaluate stridor, hoarseness, persistent wheezing, recurrent obstruction, or repeated extubation failure.

B. Cor pulmonale. Pulmonary hypertension may have reversible and fixed components. Chronic hypoxemia leads to hypoxic vasoconstriction, pulmonary hypertension, and eventual right ventricular hypertrophy and failure. Decrease in cross-sectional perfusion area and abnormal peripheral muscularization of more peripheral vessels have been documented. Left ventricular function also can be affected. The ECG should be followed up. Supplemental oxygen is used to maintain the PaO_2 >55 mm Hg. Further studies may be required to define the dysfunction and evaluate therapy. Pulmonary vasodilators including hydralazine and nifedipine have variable efficacy and should only be tried during pulmonary artery pressure and PaO_2 monitoring. Echocardiographic studies can exclude structural heart disease, assess left ventricular function, and estimate pulmonary vascular resistance and right ventricular function.

C. Systemic hypertension, sometimes with left ventricular hypertrophy, may develop in BPD infants receiving prolonged O_2 therapy.

D. Systemic-to-pulmonary shunting. Left-to-right shunt through collateral vessels (e.g., bronchial arteries) can occur in BPD. The risk factors include chest tube placement, thoracic surgery, and pleural inflammation. When left-to-right shunt is suspected and echocardiography fails to show intracardiac or PDA shunting, collaterals may be demonstrated by angiography. Occlusion of large vessels has been associated with clinical improvement.

E. Metabolic imbalance secondary to diuretics (see V.G.2 and 8)

F. Infection. Because these chronically ill and malnourished infants are at increased risk, episodes of pulmonary and systemic decompensation should be evaluated for infection. Monitoring by Gram stain of tracheal aspirates may help distinguish endotracheal tube colonization from tracheobronchitis or pneumonia (presence of organisms and neutrophils). Viral and fungal infections should be considered when fevers or pneumonia develop. In infants with more severe clinical courses, we frequently culture tracheal aspirates for possible infection with *Ureaplasma* sp. and *Mycoplasma hominis* and may treat with erythromycin if these organisms are identified.

G. Central nervous system (CNS) dysfunction Dysfunction. A neurologic syndrome presenting with extrapyramidal signs has been described in infants with CLD.

H. Hearing loss. Ototoxic drugs (furosemide, gentamicin) and ischemic or hypoxemic CNS injury increase the risk for sensorineural hearing loss. Screening with auditory brainstem responses should be performed at discharge (see Chap. 35B).

I. ROP (see Chap. 35A). ELBW infants with BPD are at highest risk for developing ROP. The use of phenylephrine-containing eyedrops before eye examinations can cause an increase in airway resistance in some infants with CLD.

J. Nephrocalcinosis is frequently documented on ultrasonographic examination and has been linked to the use of furosemide and possibly steroids. Hematuria and passage of stones may occur. Most infants are asymptomatic, with eventual spontaneous resolution, but renal function should be followed (see Chap. 31).

K. Prematurity, inadequate calcium and phosphorus retention, and prolonged immobilization can lead to osteoporosis. Calcium loss due to furosemide and corticosteroids may also contribute. Supplementation with vitamin D, calcium, and phosphorus should be optimized (see Chap. 25B).

L. Gastroesophageal reflux (GER). We try to document and treat GER when reflux or aspiration may contribute to pulmonary decompensation, apnea, or feeding intolerance with poor growth.

M. The incidence of inguinal hernia is increased by the presence of the patent processus vaginalis in VLBW infants, particularly boys, with CLD. If the hernia is reducible, surgical correction should be delayed until respiratory status is improved. Spinal rather than general anesthesia avoids reintubation and postoperative apnea.

N. Early growth failure may result from inadequate intake and excessive energy expenditure and may persist after clinical resolution of pulmonary disease. Premature withdrawal of supplemental oxygen should be avoided because it may contribute to slowing of growth.

VII. DISCHARGE PLANNING. The timing of discharge depends on the availability of home-care support systems and parental readiness (see Chap. 16).

A. Weight gain and oxygen therapy. Supplemental oxygen should be weaned when the SaO_2 is maintained >92% to 94%, no significant periods of desaturations occur during feedings and/or sleep, good weight gain has been established, and respiratory status is stable (see V.B and VI.N). We prefer to delay discharge until oxygen has been discontinued. However, if long-term oxygen supplementation seems likely in an infant who is stable, growing, and has capable caretakers, we offer the option of home oxygen therapy.

B. Teaching. The involvement of parents in caregiving is vital to the smooth transition from hospital to home care. Parents should be taught cardiopulmonary resuscitation (CPR) and early signs of decompensation. Teaching about equipment use, medication administration, and nutritional guidelines should begin when discharge planning is initiated.

C. Baseline values. Baseline values of vital signs, daily weight gain, discharge weight and head circumference, blood gases, SaO_2, hematocrit, electrolytes, and the baseline appearance of the chest radiograph and ECG must be documented at discharge. This information is useful to evaluate subsequent changes in clinical status. An eye examination and hearing screening should be performed before discharge.

VIII. OUTPATIENT THERAPY

A. Oxygen. Supplemental oxygen can be delivered by tanks or oxygen concentrator. Portable tanks allow mobility. Weaning is based on periodic assessment of SaO_2.

B. Medications. Infants receiving diuretics require monitoring of electrolytes. When the infant is stable, we allow him or her to outgrow the diuretic dose by 50% before discontinuing the drug. Bronchodilators are tapered when respiratory status is stable in room air. Nebulized medications are tapered last. Discontinued medications should remain available for early use when symptoms recur.

C. Immunizations. In addition to standard immunizations, infants with CLD should receive pneumococcal and influenza vaccines and palizumab (Synagis) (see Chap. 23A).

D. **Nutrition.** Weight gain is a sensitive indicator of well-being and should be closely monitored. Caloric supplementation is often required to maintain good growth after discharge. At discharge, we supplement calories in a transitional formula.

E. **Passive smoke exposure.** Because smoking in the home increases respiratory tract illness in children, parents of CLD infants should be discouraged from smoking and should minimize the child's exposure to smoke-containing environments.

IX. OUTCOME

A. **Mortality.** Mortality is estimated at 10% to 20% during the first year of life. The risk increases with duration of oxygen exposure and level of ventilatory support. Death is frequently caused by infection. The risk of sudden unexpected death may be increased, but the cause is unclear.

B. **Long-term morbidity**

1. **Pulmonary.** Tachypnea, retractions, dyspnea, cough, and wheezing can be seen for months to years in seriously affected children. Although complete clinical recovery can occur, underlying pulmonary function, gas exchange, and radiographic abnormalities may persist beyond adolescence. The impact of persistent minor abnormalities of function and growth on long-term morbidity and mortality is not known. Reactive airway disease occurs more frequently, and infants with CLD are at increased risk for bronchiolitis and pneumonia. The rehospitalization rate for respiratory illness during the first 2 years of life is approximately twice that of matched control infants.

2. **Neurodevelopmental** delay/neurologic deficits. BPD is not clearly an independent predictor of adverse neurologic outcome. Early behavioral differences do exist, however, between VLBW infants with CLD and RDS controls. Later outcome varies widely; one-third to two-thirds of infants with BPD are normal by 2 years, and subsequent improvement may occur in some of the remaining infants. Our experience suggests specific motor coordination delays and visual-perceptual impairment may occur, rather than overall lower IQ, with resulting mean Bayley scores 1 standard deviation below the normal mean by ages 4 to 6 years.

3. **Growth failure.** The degree of long-term growth delay is inversely proportional to birth weight and probably is influenced by the severity and duration of CLD. Weight is most affected, and head circumference is least affected. Delayed growth occurs in one-third to two-thirds of these infants at 2 years. One-third of our school-age population is 3 standard deviations below the mean for height and weight.

Suggested Readings

Aly H. Is there a strategy for preventing bronchopulmonary dysplasia? Absence of evidence is not evidence of absence. *Pediatrics* 2007;119(4):818–820.

Bancalari E. Bronchopulmonary dysplasia. *Semin Neonatol* 2003;8(1):1–91.

D'Alton M, Gross I, Bhandari V, Guest eds. BPD: State of the Art. *Semin Perinatol* 2006;30(4):163–232.

Ehrenkranz RA, Walsh MC, Vohr BR, et al. Validation of the national institutes of health consensus definition of bronchopulmonary dysplasia. *Pediatrics* 2005;116(6):1353–1360.

Jobe AH, Bancalari E. Bronchopulmonary dysplasia. *Am J Respir Crit Care Med* 2001;163:1723–1729.

Kinsella JP, Greenough A, Abman SH, Bronchopulmonary dysplasia. *Lancet* 2006;367:1421–1431, www.thelancet.com.

Walsh MC, Szefler S, Davis J, et al. Summary proceedings from the bronchopulmonary dysplasia group. *Pediatrics* 2006;117;S52–S56.

MECONIUM ASPIRATION
Leslie L. Harris and Ann R. Stark

24 K

I. BACKGROUND

A. **Cause.** Acute or chronic hypoxia and/or infection can result in the passage of meconium *in utero*. In this setting, gasping by the fetus or newly born infant can cause aspiration of amniotic fluid contaminated by meconium. Meconium aspiration before or during birth can obstruct airways, interfere with gas exchange, and cause severe respiratory distress (see Fig. 24K.1).

B. **Incidence.** Meconium-stained amniotic fluid (MSAF) complicates delivery in approximately 8% to 15% of live births. The incidence of MSAF in preterm infants is very low. Most babies with MSAF are 37 weeks or older, and most meconium-stained infants are postmature and small for gestational age. Approximately 5% of neonates born through MSAF develop meconium aspiration syndrome (MAS). MSAF is associated with an increased risk of respiratory disorders, and approximately 50% of these infants require mechanical ventilation.

II. PATHOPHYSIOLOGY.
Meconium is a sterile, thick, black–green odorless material that results from the accumulation of debris in the fetal intestine during the third month of gestation. The componetns of meconium include: water (72%–80%), desquamated cells from the intestine and skin, gastrointestinal mucin, lanugo hair, fatty material from the vernix caseosa, amniotic fluid and intestinal secretions, blood-group specific glycoproteins and bile.

A. **Passage of meconium in utero.** MSAF may result from a post-term fetus with rising motilin levels and normal gastrointestinal function, vagal stimulation produced by cord or head compression, or *in utero* fetal stress. Amniotic fluid that is thinly stained is described as *watery*. Moderately stained fluid is opaque without particles and fluid with thick meconium with particles is sometimes called *pea soup*.

B. **Aspiration of meconium.** In the presence of fetal stress, gasping by the fetus can result in aspiration of meconium before, during or immediately following delivery. Severe MAS appears to be caused by pathologic intrauterine processes, primarily chronic hypoxia, acidosis, and infection. Meconium has been found in the lungs of stillborn infants and infants who died soon after birth without a history of aspiration at delivery.

C. **Effects of meconium aspiration.** When aspirated into the lung, meconium may stimulate the release of cytokines and vasoactive substances that result in cardiovascular and inflammatory responses in the fetus and newborn. Meconium itself, or the resultant chemical pneumonitis, mechanically obstructs the small airways, causes atelectasis and a "ball-valve" effect with resultant air trapping and possible air leak. Aspirated meconium leads to vasospasm, hypertrophy of the pulmonary arterial musculature, and pulmonary hypertension that lead to extrapulmonary right-to-left shunting through the ductus arteriosus or the foramen ovale and results in worsened ventilation–perfusion ($\dot{V}/\dot{Q}$) mismatch, leading to severe arterial hypoxemia. Approximately one third of infants with MAS develop persistent pulmonary hypertension of the newborn (PPHN), which contributes to the mortality associated with this syndrome (see Chapter 24F). Aspirated meconium also inhibits surfactant function.

D. **Classification of respiratory disease.** Mild MAS is a disease requiring <40% oxygen for <48 hours. Moderate MAS is a disease requiring >40% oxygen for >48 hours without air leak. Severe MAS is a disease requiring assisted ventilation for >48 hours, often associated with PPHN.

E. **Sequelae.** *In utero* passage of meconium in term infants has been associated with and increased risk of perinatal and neonatal mortality, severe acidemia, need for

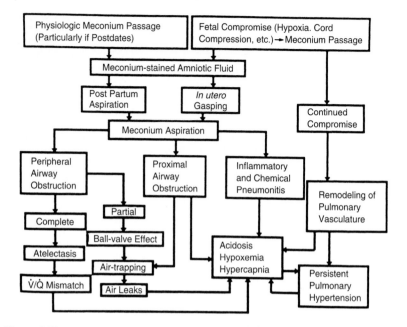

Figure 24K.1. Pathophysiology of meconium aspiration. V̇/Q̇, ventilation-perfusion ratio. (From Wiswell T, Bent RC. Meconium staining and the meconium aspiration syndrome: Unresolved issues. *Pediatr Clin North Am* 1993;40:955. Used with permission.)

caesarean section delivery, need for intensive care and oxygen administration, and adverse neurologic outcome. Preterm infants who pass meconium before delivery have similar adverse effects, as well as an increased incidence of grade 3 to 4 intraventricular hemorrhage, cystic periventricular leukomalacia, and cerebral palsy.

III. PREVENTION OF MAS

A. Prevention of passage of meconium *in utero.* Mothers at risk for uteroplacental insufficiency include those with preeclampsia or increased blood pressure, chronic respiratory or cardiovascular disease, poor uterine growth, post-term pregnancy, and heavy smokers. These women should be carefully monitored during pregnancy. During labor the fetal heart rate should be monitored, with fetal scalp blood samples obtained for pH determination when indicated.

B. Amnioinfusion. The use of amnioinfusion in women whose labor is complicated by MSAF does not reduce neonatal morbidity related to meconium aspiration, although the technique effectively treats repetitive variable fetal heart rate decelerations by relieving umbilical cord compression in labor. A large randomized trial of amnioinfusion for women with thick meconium-stained fluid with or without variable fetal heart rate decelerations showed no reduction of the risk of moderate or severe MAS, perinatal death, or caesarean delivery. However, the study did not have adequate power to determine definitively if amnioinfusion may benefit the group with variable decelerations.

C. Timing and mode of delivery. In pregnancies that continue past the due date, induction as early as 41 weeks may help prevent MAS by avoiding passage of meconium. Delivery mode does not appear to significantly impact the risk of aspiration.

IV. MANAGEMENT OF INFANTS DELIVERED THROUGH MECONIUM-STAINED FLUID.

Oropharyngeal and nasopharyngeal suctioning on the perineum and routine tracheal intubation and aspiration of meconium in vigorous infants are not effective in preventing

MAS. Infants should be assessed and intervention reserved for infants who are depressed or have respiratory distress.

A. Initial assessment. At a delivery complicated by MSAF, the clinician should determine whether the infant is vigorous, demonstrated by heart rate >100 beats per minute, spontaneous respirations, and good tone (spontaneous movement or some degree of flexion). The infant will be depressed approximately 20% to 30% of the time.

1. If the infant appears vigorous, routine care should be provided, regardless of the consistency of the meconium.

2. If respiratory distress develops or the infant becomes depressed, the trachea should be intubated under direct laryngoscopy and intratracheal suctioning performed. Visualization of the cords without suctioning is not adequate because significant meconium may be present below the cords.

3. In questionable cases, it is safer to intubate and suction, as MAS can occur in infants delivered through thinly stained amniotic fluid.

B. Suctioning technique

1. The infant should be placed on a radiant warmer and given free-flow oxygen.

2. Delay drying and stimulation, and postpone emptying of any gastric contents until the infant has stabilized.

3. A clinician (e.g., pediatrician, anesthesiologist, advanced practice nurse) should intubate the trachea under direct laryngoscopy, preferably before inspiratory efforts have been initiated. A 3.0 mm or 3.5 mm internal-diameter endotracheal tube is used in term infants.

4. After intubation, the tube is attached to wall suction at a pressure of 80 to 100 mm Hg by means of a plastic adapter (Neotech Meconium Aspirator, Neotech Products, Chatsworth, CA). Continuous suction is applied as the tube is being withdrawn; the procedure is repeated until the trachea is cleared or resuscitation needs to be initiated.

5. Avoid positive pressure ventilation, if possible, until tracheal suctioning is accomplished.

C. Complications of intubation include bleeding, laryngospasm, stridor, apnea, and cyanosis. This procedure should be accomplished rapidly, and ventilation with oxygen should be initiated before significant bradycardia occurs. The infant's general condition must not be ignored in persistent attempts to clear the trachea. Because a few inspiratory efforts by the infant will move the meconium from the trachea to the smaller airways, exhaustive attempts to remove it are unwise.

V. MANAGEMENT OF MAS

A. Observation. Infants who are depressed at birth and have had meconium suctioned from the trachea are at risk for meconium aspiration pneumonia and should be observed closely for respiratory distress.

1. A chest radiograph may help determine those infants who are most likely to develop respiratory distress, although a significant number of asymptomatic infants will have an abnormal-appearing chest film. The classic roentgenographic findings are diffuse, assymmetric patchy infiltrates, areas of consolidation, and hyperinflation.

2. Monitoring of oxygen saturation during this period aids assessment of the severity of the infant's condition and avoids hypoxemia.

B. Routine care

1. The infant should be maintained in a neutral thermal environment and tactile stimulation should be minimized.

2. Blood glucose and calcium levels should be assessed and corrected if necessary. Severely depressed infants may have severe metabolic acidosis that may need to be corrected.

3. Fluids should be restricted as much as possible to prevent cerebral and pulmonary edema.

4. Infants may also require specific therapy for hypotension and poor cardiac output, including cardiotonic medications such as dopamine.

5. Circulatory support with normal saline or packed red blood cells should be provided in patients with marginal oxygenation. In infants with substantial oxygen and ventilator requirements, we usually maintain a hemoglobin concentration above 15 g (hematocrit above 40%).

6. Renal function should be continuously monitored (see Chapter 27C).

C. Oxygen therapy. Management of hypoxemia should be accomplished by increasing the inspired oxygen concentration and by monitoring blood gases and pH. An indwelling arterial catheter is usually required for blood sampling. It is crucial to provide sufficient oxygen, because repeated hypoxic insults may result in ongoing pulmonary vasoconstriction and contribute to the development of PPHN.

D. Assisted ventilation

1. Continuous positive airway pressure (CPAP). If Fio_2 requirements exceed 0.40, a trial of CPAP may be considered. CPAP is often helpful, and the appropriate pressures must be individualized for each infant. However, CPAP may sometimes aggravate air trapping and should be instituted with caution if hyperinflation is apparent clinically or radiographically.

2. Mechanical ventilation. Infants with very severe disease may have severe gas exchange abnormalities. Mechanical ventilation is indicated for excessive carbon dioxide retention ($Paco_2$ >60 mm Hg) or for persistent hypoxemia (Pao_2 <50 mm Hg).

a. In these infants, higher inspiratory pressures (approximately 30–35 cm H_2O) are more often required than in infants with respiratory distress syndrome; the positive end-expiratory pressure (PEEP) selected (usually 3–6 cm H_2O) should depend on the individual's response. Adequate expiratory time should be permitted to prevent air trapping behind partly obstructed airways.

b. Useful starting points are an inspiratory time of 0.4 to 0.5 seconds at a rate of 20 to 25 breaths per minute. Some infants may respond better to conventional ventilation at more rapid rates with inspiratory times as short as 0.2 seconds.

c. High-frequency ventilation with jet or oscillatory ventilators may be successful in infants with severe MAS who fail to improve with conventional ventilation, and in those who develop air-leak syndromes. There are no prospective, randomized controlled trials comparing the efficacy of the various ventilator modes in MAS.

d. The use of sedation and muscle relaxation may be warranted in some infants who require mechanical ventilation.

E. Medications

1. Antibiotics. Differentiating between bacterial pneumonia and meconium aspiration by clinical course and chest x-ray findings may be difficult. Although few infants with MAS have documented infections, the use of broad-spectrum antibiotics (e.g., ampicillin and gentamicin) is usually indicated in infants when an infiltrate is seen on chest radiograph. Blood cultures should be obtained to identify bacterial disease, if present, and to determine length of antibiotic course.

2. Surfactant. Endogenous surfactant activity may be inhibited by meconium. Surfactant treatment of MAS may improve oxygenation and reduce pulmonary complications and the need for extracorporeal membrane oxygenation (ECMO). We do not routinely use surfactant to treat infants with MAS. However, in infants whose clinical status continues to deteriorate and who require escalating support, surfactant adminsitration may be helpful. We do not recommend washing meconium from the lungs with bronchioalveolar surfactant lavage.

3. Corticosteroids. We do not recommend the use of corticosteroids in MAS, although this approach has been proposed to reduce inflammation induced by meconium and minimize prostaglandin-mediated pulmonary vasoconstriction.

F. Complications

1. Air leak. Peumothorax or pneumomediastium occurs in approximately 15% to 33% of patients with MAS. Air leaks occur more frequently with mechanical ventilation, especially in the setting of air trapping. A high index of suspicion for air leak is necessary. Equipment should be available to evacuate a pneumothorax promptly (see Chapter 24E).

2. **PPHN** is associated with MAS in approximately one third of cases and contributes to the mortality associated with this syndrome (see Chapter 24F). Depending on the extent of hypoxemia, echocardiography should be performed to ascertain the degree to which the right-to-left shunting is contributing to the infant's overall hypoxemia and to exclude congenital heart disease as the etiology. In severely ill infants with MAS and PPHN, inhaled nitric oxide (iNO) reduces the need for ECMO.

3. **Pulmonary sequelae.** Approximately 5% of survivors require supplemental oxygen at 1 month, and a substantial proportion may have abnormal pulmonary function, including increased functional residual capacity, airway reactivity, and higher incidence of pneumonia.

Suggested Readings

Ahanya SN, Lakshmanan J, Morgan B, et al. Meconium passage in utero: Mechanisms, consequences, and management. *Obstet Gynecol Surv* 2005;60:45–56.

Fraser WD, Hofmeyr J, Lede R, The Amnioinfusion Trial Group. Amnioinfusion for the prevention of the meconium aspiration syndrome. *N Engl J Med* 2005;353:909–917.

Velaphi S, Vidyasagar D. Intrapartum and postdelivery management of infants born to mothers with meconium-stained amniotic fluid: Evidence-based recommendations. *Clin Perinatol* 2006;33:29–42.

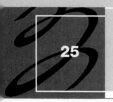

25 CARDIAC DISORDERS
Stephanie Burns Wechsler and Gil Wernovsky

I. **INTRODUCTION.** At the beginning of the twentieth century, Dr. William Osler wrote in his textbook of medicine that congenital heart disease was of "limited clinical interest as in a large proportion of cases the anomaly is not compatible with life, and in others, nothing can be done to remedy the defect or even relieve the symptoms." In the years since 1938, when Dr. Robert Gross first successfully ligated a patent ductus arteriosus (PDA) in a 7-year-old girl at Children's Hospital, Boston (with a 17-day postoperative stay, 12 of which were for "general interest in the case") the outlook for children with congenital heart disease has improved dramatically. This remarkable progress is due to synergistic advances in pediatric and fetal cardiology, cardiac surgery, neonatology, cardiac anesthesia, intensive care, and nursing.

In critical lesions, the ultimate prognosis for the patient depends in part on (i) a timely and accurate assessment of the structural anomaly and (ii) the evaluation and resuscitation of secondary organ damage. It is therefore crucial that pediatricians and neonatologists be able to rapidly evaluate and participate in the initial medical management of neonates with congenital heart disease. A multidisciplinary approach involving several subspecialty services is frequently required, especially because one-fifth of patients with severe congenital heart disease may be premature and/or weigh <2,500 g at birth. Although neonates (as a group) may have a slightly higher surgical mortality than term infants, the secondary effects of the unoperated lesion on the heart, lung, and brain may be quite severe. These secondary changes may include chronic congestive heart failure (CHF), failure to thrive, frequent infections, irreversible pulmonary vascular changes, delayed cognitive development, or focal neurologic deficits. For these reasons, at Children's Hospital in Boston primary surgical correction is carried out early in life, often in the neonatal period. This chapter is intended as a practical guide for the initial evaluation and management, by pediatricians and neonatologists, of neonates and infants suspected of having congenital heart disease. For a detailed discussion of the individual lesions, the clinician should consult current textbooks of pediatric cardiology and cardiac surgery.

II. **INCIDENCE AND SURVIVAL.** The incidence of moderate to severe structural congenital heart disease in live born infants is 6 to 8 per 1,000 live births. This incidence has been relatively constant over the years and in different areas around the world. More recent higher incidence figures appear to be due to the inclusion of more trivial forms of congenital heart disease, such as tiny ventricular septal defects that are detected more frequently by highly sensitive echocardiography. Data from the New England Regional Infant Cardiac Program suggest that approximately 3 per 1,000 live births have heart disease that results in death or requires cardiac catheterization or surgery during the first year of life. Most of these infants with congenital heart disease are identified by the end of the neonatal period. The most common congenital heart lesions presenting in the first weeks of life are summarized in Table 25.1. Recent advances in diagnostic imaging, cardiac surgery, and intensive care have reduced the operative risks for many complex lesions; the hospital mortality following all forms of neonatal cardiac surgery has significantly decreased in the past decade.

III. **CLINICAL PRESENTATIONS OF CONGENITAL HEART DISEASE IN THE NEONATE.** The timing of presentation and accompanying symptomatology depends on (i) the nature and severity of the anatomic defect, (ii) the *in utero* effects (if any) of the structural lesion, and (iii) the alterations in cardiovascular physiology secondary to the effects of the transitional circulation: **closure of the ductus arteriosus**

TABLE 25.1	Top Five Diagnoses Presenting at Different Ages[*]

Diagnosis	Percentage of patients
Age on admission: 0–6 d (n = 537)	
D-Transposition of great arteries	19
Hypoplastic left ventricle	14
Tetralogy of Fallot	8
Coarctation of aorta	7
Ventricular-septal defect	3
Others	49
Age on admission: 7–13 d (n = 195)	
Coarctation of aorta	16
Ventricular septal defect	14
Hypoplastic left ventricle	8
D-Transposition of great arteries	7
Tetralogy of Fallot	7
Others	48
Age on admission: 14–28 d (n = 177)	
Ventricular septal defect	16
Coarctation of aorta	12
Tetralogy of Fallot	7
D-Transposition of great arteries	7
Patent ductus arteriosus	5
Others	53

[*]Reprinted with permission from Flanagan MF, Yeager SB, Weindling SN. Cardiac disease. In: MacDonald MG, Mullett MD, Seshia MMK, eds. *Avery's neonatology: Pathophysiology and management of the newborn,* 6th ed. Philadelphia: Lippincott Williams & Wilkins, 2005.

and the **fall in pulmonary vascular resistance.** This chapter focuses primarily on cardiovascular abnormalities with critical effects in the neonatal period.

In the first few weeks of life, the many heterogeneous forms of heart disease present in a surprisingly limited number of ways (in no particular order nor mutually exclusive): (i) cyanosis; (ii) CHF (with the most extreme presentation being cardiovascular collapse or shock); (iii) an asymptomatic heart murmur; and (iv) arrhythmia. With increasing frequency, neonates with congenital heart disease have been diagnosed before delivery by fetal echocardiography and are therefore born with a presumptive diagnosis into an expectant team of physicians and nurses. In many neonates, however, congenital heart disease is not suspected until after birth. The clinician may be diverted away from a diagnosis of heart disease because of the report of a "normal" prenatal ultrasonography performed for screening purposes. Finally, the diagnosis of "heart disease" should never divert the clinician from a complete noncardiac evaluation with a thorough search for additional or secondary medical problems—occasionally the neonate with complex congenital heart disease and hypoxemia has inadequate attention paid to an initial and continued assessment of an adequate airway and ventilation.

A. Cyanosis

1. **Clinical findings.** Cyanosis (bluish tinge of the skin and mucous membranes) is one of the most common presenting signs of congenital heart disease in the neonate. Although cyanosis usually indicates underlying hypoxemia (diminished

level of arterial oxygen saturation), there are a few instances when cyanosis is associated with a normal arterial oxygen saturation. Depending on the underlying skin complexion, clinically apparent cyanosis is usually not visible until there is >3 g/dL of **desaturated** hemoglobin in the arterial system. Therefore, the degree of visible cyanosis depends on both the severity of hypoxemia (which determines the percent of oxygen saturation) as well as the hemoglobin concentration. For example, consider two infants with similar degrees of hypoxemia—each having an arterial oxygen saturation of 85%. The polycythemic newborn (hemoglobin of 22 g/dL) will have 3.3 g/dL (15% of 22) desaturated hemoglobin and be more easily appreciated to be cyanotic than the anemic infant (hemoglobin of 10 g/dL) who will only have 1.5 g/dL (15% of 10) desaturated hemoglobin. An additional note, true central cyanosis should be a generalized finding (i.e., not acrocyanosis, blueness of the hands and feet only, which is a normal finding in a neonate).

Because determining cyanosis by visual inspection can be challenging for the reasons mentioned, there has been recent interest in adding routine lower extremity pulse oximetry measurement as a screening test for otherwise asymptomatic congenital heart disease. There is conflicting data on the efficacy and cost-effectiveness of this screening method, but it would appear that it is most effective when the pulse oximetry reading is done in a lower extremity in infants >24 hours old with further evaluation by echocardiogram for readings <95% in room air.

2. **Differential diagnosis.** Differentiation of cardiac from respiratory causes of cyanosis in the neonatal intensive care unit (NICU) is a common problem. Pulmonary disorders are frequently the cause of cyanosis in the newborn due to intrapulmonary right-to-left shunting. Primary lung disease (pneumonia, hyaline membrane disease, pulmonary arteriovenous malformations, etc.); pneumothorax; airway obstruction; extrinsic compression of the lungs (congenital diaphragmatic hernia, pleural effusions, etc.); and central nervous system abnormalities may produce varying degrees of hypoxemia manifesting as cyanosis in the neonate. For a more complete differential diagnosis of pulmonary causes of cyanosis in the neonate, see Chapter 24. Finally, clinical cyanosis may occur in an infant without hypoxemia in the setting of methemoglobinemia or pronounced polycythemia. Table 25.2 summarizes the differential diagnosis of cyanosis in the neonate.

Cyanosis due to congenital heart disease can be broadly grouped into those lesions with (i) decreased pulmonary blood flow and intracardiac right-to-left shunting and (ii) normal to increased pulmonary blood flow with intracardiac mixing (complete or incomplete) of the systemic and pulmonary venous return. Specific lesions and lesion specific management are covered in more detail in section V.

B. **CHF**

1. **Clinical findings.** CHF in the neonate (or in a patient of any age) is a **clinical** diagnosis made on the basis of the existence of certain signs and symptoms rather than on radiographic or laboratory findings (although these may be supportive evidence for the diagnosis). Signs and symptoms of CHF occur when the heart is unable to meet the metabolic demands of the tissues. Clinical findings are frequently due to homeostatic mechanisms attempting to compensate for this imbalance. In early stages, the neonate may be tachypneic and tachycardic with an increased respiratory effort, rales, hepatomegaly, and delayed capillary refill. In contrast to adults, edema is rarely seen. Diaphoresis, feeding difficulties, and growth failure may be present. Finally, CHF may present acutely with cardiorespiratory collapse, particularly in "left-sided" lesions (see V.A). *Hydrops fetalis* is an extreme form of intrauterine CHF.

2. **Differential diagnosis.** The age when CHF develops depends on the hemodynamics of the responsible lesion. When heart failure develops in the first weeks of life, the differential diagnosis includes (i) a structural lesion causing severe pressure and/or volume overload, (ii) a primary myocardial lesion

TABLE 25.2	**Differential Diagnosis of Cyanosis in the Neonate**

Primary cardiac lesions

Decreased pulmonary blood flow, intracardiac right-to-left shunt

    Critical pulmonary stenosis

    Tricuspid atresia

    Pulmonary atresia/intact ventricular septum

    Tetralogy of Fallot

    Ebstein anomaly

    Total anomalous pulmonary venous connection with obstruction

Normal or increased pulmonary blood flow, intracardiac mixing

    Hypoplastic left heart syndrome

    Transposition of the great arteries

    Truncus arteriosus

    Tetralogy of Fallot/pulmonary atresia

    Complete common atrioventricular canal

    Total anomalous pulmonary venous connection without obstruction

    Other single-ventricle complexes

Pulmonary lesions (intrapulmonary right-to-left shunt) (see Chap. 24)

Primary parenchymal lung disease

    Aspiration syndromes (e.g., meconium and blood)

    Respiratory distress syndrome

    Pneumonia

Airway obstruction

    Choanal stenosis or atresia

    Pierre Robin syndrome

    Tracheal stenosis

    Pulmonary sling

    Absent pulmonary valve syndrome

Extrinsic compression of the lungs

    Pneumothorax

    Pulmonary interstitial or lobar emphysema

    Chylothorax or other pleural effusions

    Congenital diaphragmatic hernia

    Thoracic dystrophies or dysplasia

Hypoventilation

    Central nervous system lesions

    Neuromuscular diseases

    Sedation

    Sepsis

Pulmonary arteriovenous malformations

Persistent pulmonary hypertension (see Chap. 24F)

Cyanosis with normal P_{O_2}

    Methemoglobinemia

    Polycythemia*

*In the case of polycythemia, these infants have plethora and venous congestion in the distal extremities, which gives the appearance of distal cyanosis; these infants actually are not hypoxemic (see text).

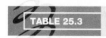

TABLE 25.3 Differential Diagnosis of Congestive Heart Failure in the Neonate

Pressure overload
Aortic stenosis
Coarctation of the aorta

Volume overload
Left-to-right shunt at level of great vessels
Patent ductus arteriosus
Aorticopulmonary window
Truncus arteriosus
Tetralogy of Fallot, pulmonary atresia with multiple aorticopulmonary collaterals
Left-to-right shunt at level of ventricles
Ventricular septal defect
Common atrioventricular canal
Single ventricle without pulmonary stenosis (includes hypoplastic left heart syndrome)
Arteriovenous malformations

Combined pressure and volume overload
Interrupted aortic arch
Coarctation of the aorta with ventricular septal defect
Aortic stenosis with ventricular septal defect

Myocardial dysfunction
Primary
Cardiomyopathies
Inborn errors of metabolism
Genetic
Myocarditis
Secondary
Sustained tachyarrhythmias
Perinatal asphyxia
Sepsis
Severe intrauterine valvar obstruction (e.g., aortic stenosis)
Premature closure of the ductus arteriosus

causing myocardial dysfunction, or (iii) arrhythmia. Table 25.3 summarizes the differential diagnoses of CHF in the neonate.

C. Heart murmur. Heart murmurs are not uncommonly heard when examining neonates. Estimates of the prevalence of heart murmurs in neonates vary widely from <1% to >50% depending on the study. Murmurs heard in newborns in the first days of life are often associated with structural heart disease of some type, and therefore may need further evaluation, particularly if there are any other associated clinical symptoms.

Pathologic murmurs tend to appear at characteristic ages. Semilunar valve stenosis (systolic ejection murmurs) and atrioventricular valvar insufficiency (systolic regurgitant murmurs) tend to be noted very shortly after birth, on the first day of life. In contrast, murmurs due to left-to-right shunt lesions (systolic regurgitant ventricular septal defect murmur or continuous PDA murmur) may not be heard until the second to fourth week of life, when the pulmonary vascular resistance has decreased and the left-to-right shunt increases. Therefore, the **age**

of the patient when the murmur is first noted and the **character of the murmur** provide important clues to the nature of the malformation.

D. Arrhythmias. See VIII, Arrhythmias of this chapter for a detailed description of identification and management of the neonate with an arrhythmia.

E. Fetal echocardiography. It is increasingly common for infants to be born with a diagnosis of probable congenital heart disease due to the widespread use of obstetric ultrasonography and fetal echocardiography. This may be quite valuable to the team of physicians caring for mother and baby, guiding plans for prenatal care, site and timing of delivery, as well as immediate perinatal care of the infant. The recommended timing for fetal echocardiography is 18 to 20 weeks gestation although reasonable images can be obtained as early as 16 weeks, and transvaginal ultrasonography may be used for diagnostic purposes in fetuses in the first trimester. Indications for fetal echocardiography are summarized in Table 25.4.

TABLE 25.4	**Indications for Fetal Echocardiography**

Fetus-related indications
  Suspected congenital heart disease on screening ultrasonography
  Fetal chromosomal anomaly
  Fetal extracardiac anatomic anomaly
  Fetal cardiac arrhythmia
    Persistent bradycardia
    Persistent tachycardia
    Irregular rhythm
  Nonimmune hydrops fetalis
Mother-related indications
  Congenital heart disease
  Maternal metabolic disease
    Diabetes mellitus
    Phenylketonuria
  Maternal rheumatic disease (such as systemic lupus erythematosus)
  Maternal environmental exposures
    Alcohol
    Cardiac teratogenic medications
      Amphetamines
      Anticonvulsants
        Phenytoin
        Trimethadione
        Carbamazepine
        Valproate
      Isotretinoin
      Lithium carbonate
  Maternal viral infection
    Rubella
Family related Indications
  Previous child or parent with congenital heart disease
  Previous child or parent with genetic disease associated with congenital heart disease

It is important to note, however, that most cases of prenatally diagnosed congenital heart disease occur in pregnancies without known risk factors. Most severe forms of congenital heart disease can be accurately diagnosed by fetal echocardiography. Coarctation of the aorta, small ventricular and atrial septal defects, total anomalous pulmonary venous return, and mild aortic or pulmonary stenosis are abnormalities that may be missed by fetal echocardiography. In general, in complex congenital heart disease, the main abnormality is noted; however, the full extent of cardiac malformation may be better determined on postnatal examinations.

Fetal tachy- or bradyarrhythmias (intermittent or persistent) may be detected on routine obstetric screening ultrasonographic examinations; this should prompt more complete fetal echocardiography to rule out associated structural heart disease, assess fetal ventricular function, and further define the arrhythmia.

Fetal echocardiography has allowed for improved understanding of the *in utero* evolution of some forms of congenital heart disease. This, in turn, has opened up the possibility of fetal cardiac intervention. Recent successes in limited, selected cases of fetal cardiac intervention suggests that this is a promising new method of treatment for congenital heart disease.

IV. EVALUATION OF THE NEONATE WITH SUSPECTED CONGENITAL HEART DISEASE. As noted, the suspicion of congenital heart disease in the neonate typically follows one of a few clinical scenarios. Circulatory collapse is, unfortunately, not an uncommon means of presentation for the neonate with congenital heart disease. It must be emphasized that **emergency treatment of shock precedes definitive anatomic diagnosis.** Although sepsis may be suspected and treated, the signs of low cardiac output should always alert the examining physician to the likely possibility of congenital heart disease.

A. Initial evaluation

    1. Physical examination. A complete physical examination provides important clues to the anatomic diagnosis. Inexperienced examiners frequently focus solely on the presence or absence of cardiac murmurs, but much more additional information should be obtained during a complete examination. A great deal may be learned from simple visual inspection of the infant. Cyanosis may first be apparent on inspection of the mucous membranes and/or nailbeds (see III. A.1). Mottling of the skin and/or an ashen, gray color are important clues to severe cardiovascular compromise and incipient shock. While observing the infant, particular attention should be paid to the pattern of respiration including the work of breathing and use of accessory muscles.

    Before auscultation, palpation of the distal extremities with attention to temperature and capillary refill is imperative. The cool neonate with delayed capillary refill should always be evaluated for the possibility of severe congenital heart disease. While palpating the distal extremities, note the presence and character of the distal pulses. Diminished or absent distal pulses are highly suggestive of obstruction of the aortic arch. Palpation of the precordium may provide an important clue to the presence of congenital heart disease. The presence of a precordial thrill usually indicates at least moderate pulmonary or aortic outflow obstruction, although a restrictive ventricular septal defect with low right ventricular pressure may present with a similar finding. A hyperdynamic precordium suggests a sizeable left-to-right shunt.

    During auscultation, the examiner should first pay particular attention to the heart rate, noting its regularity and/or variability. The heart sounds, particularly the second heart sound, can be helpful clues to the ultimate diagnosis as well. A split second heart sound is a particularly important marker of the existence of two semilunar valves, although it is often difficult to be sure of S2 splitting with the rapid heart rate of a neonate. Differentiating an S3 from an S4 heart sound is challenging in a tachycardic newborn; however, a gallop rhythm of either type is unusual and suggests the possibility of a significant left-to-right shunt or myocardial dysfunction. Ejection clicks suggest pulmonary or aortic valvar stenosis.

The presence and intensity of systolic murmurs can be very helpful in suggesting the type and severity of the underlying anatomic diagnosis; systolic murmurs are usually due to (i) semilunar valve or outflow tract stenosis, (ii) atrioventricular valve regurgitation, or (iii) shunting through a septal defect. Diastolic murmurs are **always** indicative of cardiovascular pathology. For a more complete description of auscultation of the heart, refer to one of the cardiology texts listed at the end of the chapter.

A careful search for other anomalies is essential, because congenital heart disease is accompanied by at least one extracardiac malformation 25% of the time. Table 25.5 summarizes malformation and chromosomal syndromes commonly associated with congenital heart disease.

2. **Four-extremity blood pressure.** Measurement of blood pressure should be taken in both arms and both legs. Usually an automated Dynamapp is used, but in a small neonate with pulses that are difficult to palpate, manual blood pressure measurement with Doppler amplification may be necessary for an accurate measurement. A systolic pressure that is >10 mm Hg higher in the upper body compared to the lower body is abnormal and suggests coarctation of the aorta, aortic arch hypoplasia, or interrupted aortic arch. It should be noted that a systolic blood pressure gradient is quite specific for an arch abnormality but not sensitive; a systolic blood pressure gradient will not be present in the neonate with an arch abnormality in whom the ductus arteriosus is patent and nonrestrictive. Therefore, the lack of a systolic blood pressure gradient in newborn does **not** conclusively rule out coarctation or other arch abnormalities, but the presence of a systolic pressure gradient is diagnostic of an aortic arch abnormality.

3. **Chest x-ray.** A frontal and lateral view (if possible) of the chest should be obtained. In infants, particularly newborns, the size of the heart may be difficult to determine due to overlying thymus. Nevertheless, useful information can be gained from the chest x-ray. In addition to heart size, notation should be made of visceral and cardiac situs (dextrocardia and *situs inversus* are frequently accompanied by congenital heart disease.) The aortic arch side (right or left) can frequently be determined; a right-sided aortic arch is associated with congenital heart disease in >90% of patients. Dark or poorly perfused lung fields suggests decreased pulmonary blood flow, whereas diffusely opaque lung fields may represent increased pulmonary blood flow or significant left atrial hypertension.

4. **Electrocardiogram (ECG).** The neonatal ECG reflects the hemodynamic relations that existed *in utero*; therefore, the normal ECG is notable for right ventricular predominance. As many forms of congenital heart disease have minimal prenatal hemodynamic effects, the ECG is frequently "normal for age" despite significant structural pathology (e.g., transposition of the great arteries, tetralogy of Fallot, etc.). Throughout the neonatal period, infancy, and childhood, the ECG will evolve due to the expected changes in physiology and the resulting changes in chamber size and thickness that occur. Because most findings on a neonate's ECG would be abnormal in an older child or adult, it is essential to refer to age-specific charts of normal values for most ECG parameters. Refer to Tables 25.6 and 25.7 for normal ECG values in term and premature neonates.

When interpreting an ECG, the following determinations should be made: (i) rate and rhythm; (ii) P, QRS, and T axes; (iii) intracardiac conduction intervals; (iv) evidence for chamber enlargement or hypertrophy; (v) evidence for pericardial disease, ischemia, infarction, or electrolyte abnormalities; and (vi) if the ECG pattern fits with the clinical picture. When the ECG is abnormal, one should also consider incorrect lead placement; a simple confirmation of lead placement may be done by comparing QRS complexes in limb lead I and precordial lead V_6—each should have a similar morphology if the limb leads have been properly placed. The ECG of the premature infant is somewhat different from that of the term infant (Table 25.7).

TABLE 25.5 Chromosomal Anomalies, Syndromes, and Associations Commonly Associated with Congenital Heart Disease

	Approximate incidence or mode of inheritance	Extracardiac features	Cardiac features
CHROMOSOMAL ANOMALIES			
Trisomy 13 (Patau syndrome)	1/5,000	SGA, facies (midfacial hypoplasia, cleft lip and palate, microphthalmia coloboma, low-set ears); brain anomalies (microcephaly holoprosencephaly); aplasia cutis congenita of scalp; polydactyly	$\geq$80% have cardiac defects, VSD most common
Trisomy 18 (Edward syndrome)	1/3,000 (female-male = 3:1)	SGA; facies (dolicocephaly, prominent occiput, short palpebral fissures, low-set posteriorly rotated ears, small mandible); short sternum; rocker-bottom feet; overlapping fingers with "clenched fists"	>95% have cardiac defects, VSD most common (sometimes multiple); redundant valvar tissue with regurgitation often affecting more than one valve (polyvalvar disease)
Trisomy 21 (Down syndrome)	1/660	Facies (brachycephaly, flattened occiput, midfacial hypoplasia, mandibular prognathism, upslanting palpebral fissures, epicanthal folds, Brushfield spots, large tongue); simian creases, clinodactyly with short fifth finger; pronounced hypotonia	40%–50% have cardiac defects, CAVC, VSD most, common, also TOF, ASD, PDA; complex congenital heart disease is very rare
45,X (Turner syndrome)	1/2,500	Lymphedema of hands, feet; short stature; short webbed neck; facies (triangular with downslanting palpebral fissures, low-set ears); shield chest	25%–45% have cardiac defects, coarctation, bicuspid aortic valve most common
SINGLE-GENE DEFECTS			
Noonan syndrome	AD	Facies (hypertelorism, epicanthal folds, downslanting palpebral fissures, ptosis); low-set ears; short-webbed neck with low hairline; shield chest, cryptorchidism in men	50% have cardiac detect, usually valvar pulmonary stenosis, also ASD, hypertrophic CM

Syndrome		Features	Cardiac Findings
Holt-Oram syndrome	AD	Spectrum of upper limb and shoulder girdle anomalies	≥50% have cardiac defect, usually ASD or VSD
Alagille syndrome	AD	Cholestasis; facies (micrognathism, broad forehead, deep-set eyes); vertebral anomalies, ophthalmologic abnormalities	Cardiac findings in 90%. Peripheral pulmonic stenosis most common
GENE DELETION SYNDROMES			
Williams syndrome (Deletion 7q11)	1/7,500	SGA, FIT; facies ("elfin" with short palpebral fissures, periorbital fullness or puffiness, flat nasal bridge, stellate iris, long philtrum, prominent lips); fussy infants with poor feeding, friendly personality later in childhood; characteristic mental deficiency (motor more reduced than verbal performance)	50%–70% have cardiac defect, most commonly supravalvar aortic stenosis; other arterial stenoses also occur, including PPS, COA, renal artery and coronary artery stenoses
DiGeorge syndrome (Deletion 22q11)	1/6,000	Thymic hypoplasia/aplasia; parathyroid hypoplasia/aplasia; cleft palate or velopharyngeal incompetence	IAA and conotruncal malformations including truncus, TOF
ASSOCIATIONS			
VACTERL		Vertebral defects; anal atresia; TE fistula; radial and renal anomalies; limb defects	Approximately 50% have cardiac defect, most commonly VSD
CHARGE		Coloboma; choanal atresia; growth and mental deficiency; genital hypoplasia (in men); ear anomalies and/or deafness	50%–70% have cardiac defect, most commonly conotruncal anomalies (TOF, DORV, truncus arteriosus)

AD = autosomal dominant; AR = autosomal recessive; CM = cardiomyopathy; CoA = coarctation of the aorta; CAVC = complete atrioventricular canal; DORV = double outlet right ventricle; FIT = failure to thrive; IAA = interrupted aortic arch; PDA = patent ductus arteriosus; PPS = peripheral pulmonary stenosis; SGA = small for gestational age; TOF = tetralogy of Fallot; TEF = tracheoesophageal fistula; VSD = ventricular septal defect.

TABLE 25.6 ECG Standards in Newborns

Measure	Age (D)			
	0–1	**1–3**	**3–7**	**7–30**
Term infants				
Heart rate (beats/mm)	122(99–147)	123(97–148)	128(100–160)	148 (114–177)
QRS axis (degrees)	135(91–185)	134(93–188)	133(92–185)	108(78–152)
PR interval, II (s)	0.11 (0.08–0.14)	0.11 (0.09–0.13)	0.10 (0.08–0.13)	0.10 (0.08–0.13)
QRS duration (s)	0.05 (0.03–0.07)	0.05 (0.03–0.06)	0.05 (0.03–0.06)	0.05 (0.03–0.08)
V1, R amplitude (mm)	13.5 (6.5–23.7)	14.8 (7.0–24.2)	12.8 (5.5–21.5)	10.5 (4.5–18.1)
V1, S amplitude (mm)	8.5 (1.0–18.5)	9.5 (1.5–19.0)	6.8 (1.0–15.0)	4.0 (0.5–9.7)
V6, R amplitude (mm)	4.5 (0.5–9.5)	4.8 (0.5–9.5)	5.1 (1.0–10.5)	7.6 (2.6–13.5)
V6, S amplitude (mm)	3.5 (0.2–7.9)	3.2 (0.2–7.6)	3.7 (0.2–8.0)	3.2 (0.2–3.2)
Preterm infants				
Heart rate (beats/mm)	141(109–173)	150(127–182)	164(134–200)	170(133–200)
QRS axis (degrees)	127(75–194)	121 (75–195)	117(75–165)	80(17–171)
PR interval (s)	0.10 (0.09–0.10)	0.10 (0.09–1.10)	0.10 (0.09–0.10)	0.10 (0.09–0.10)
QRS duration (s)	0.04	0.04	0.04	0.04
V1, R amplitude (mm)	6.5 (2.0–12.6)	7.4 (2.6–14.9)	8.7 (3.8–16.9)	13.0 (6.2–21.6)
V1 S amplitude (mm)	6.8 (0.6–17.6)	6.5 (1–0–16.0)	6.8 (0.0–15.0)	6.2 (1.2–14.0)
V6, R amplitude (mm)	11.4 (3.5–21.3)	11.9 (5.0–20.8)	12.3 (4.0–20.5)	15.0 (8.3–21.0)
V6, S amplitude (mm)	15.0 (2.5–26.5)	13.5 (2.6–26.0)	14.0 (3.0–25.0)	14.0 (3.1–26.3)

Sources: Davignon A, Rautaharja P, Boiselle E, et al. Normal ECG Standards for Infants and Children. *Pediatr Cardiol* 1980;1(2):123–131.
Sreenivasan VV, Fisher BJ, Liebman J, et al. Longitudinal Study of the Standard Electrocardiogram in the Healthy Premature Infant During the First Year of Life. *Am J Cardiol* 1973;31(1):57–63.

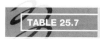

TABLE 25.7	ECG Findings in Premature Infants (Compared to Term Infants)

Rate

Slightly higher resting rate with greater activity-related and circadian variation (sinus bradycardia to 70, with sleep not uncommon)

Intracardiac conduction

PR and QRS duration slightly shorter

Maximum QT_C <0.44 s (longer than for term infants, QT_C <0.40 s)

QRS complex

QRS axis in frontal plane more leftward with decreasing gestational age

QRS amplitude lower (possibly due to less ventricular mass)

Less right ventricular predominance in precordial chest leads

Source: Reproduced with permission from Thomaidis C, Varlamis G, Karemperis S. Comparative Study of the Electrocardiograms of Healthy Full Term and Premature Infants. *Acta Paediatr Scand* 1988;77(5):653–657.

5. **Hyperoxia test.** In **all** neonates with suspected critical congenital heart disease (not just those who are cyanotic), a hyperoxia test should be considered. **This single test is perhaps the most sensitive and specific tool in the initial evaluation of the neonate with suspected recent disease.** In sites with timely access to echocardiography, a complete hyperoxia test may not be performed; however, it is important to realize what a valuable test this can be when echo is not easily and quickly available.

To investigate the possibility of a fixed, intracardiac right-to-left shunt, the arterial oxygen tension should be measured in room air (if tolerated) followed by repeat measurements with the patient receiving 100% inspired oxygen (the "hyperoxia test"). If possible, the arterial partial pressure of oxygen (PO_2) should be measured directly through arterial puncture, although properly applied transcutaneous oxygen monitor (TCOM) values for PO_2 are also acceptable. **Pulse oximetry cannot be used** for documentation; in a neonate given 100% inspired oxygen, a value of 100% oxygen saturation may be obtained with an arterial PO_2 ranging from 80 torr (abnormal) to 680 torr (normal, see III.A.1).

Measurements should be made (by arterial blood gas or TCOM) at both "preductal" and "postductal" sites and the exact site of PO_2 measurement must be recorded, because some congenital malformations with desaturated blood flow entering the descending aorta through the ductus arteriosus may result in "differential cyanosis" (as seen in persistent pulmonary hypertension of the newborn). A markedly higher oxygen content in the upper versus the lower part of the body can be an important diagnostic clue to such lesions, including all forms of critical aortic arch obstruction or left ventricular outflow obstruction. There are also the rare cases of "reverse differential cyanosis" with elevated lower-body saturation and lower upper-body saturation. This occurs only in children with transposition of the great arteries with an abnormal pulmonary artery to aortic shunt due to coarctation, interruption of the aortic arch, or suprasystemic pulmonary vascular resistance ("persistent fetal circulation").

When a patient breathes 100% oxygen, an arterial PO_2 of >250 torr in both upper and lower extremities virtually eliminates critical structural cyanotic heart disease (a "passed" hyperoxia test.) An arterial PO_2 of <100 in the absence of clear-cut lung disease (a "failed" hyperoxia test) is most likely due to intracardiac right-to-left shunting and is virtually diagnostic of cyanotic congenital heart disease. Patients who have an arterial PO_2 between 100 and 250

may have structural heart disease with complete intracardiac mixing and greatly increased pulmonary blood flow, as is occasionally seen with single-ventricle complexes such as hypoplastic left heart syndrome. **The neonate who "fails" a hyperoxia test is very likely to have congenital heart disease involving ductal-dependent systemic or pulmonary blood flow, and should receive prostaglandin E1 (PGE$_1$) until anatomic definition can be accomplished** (see IV.B.2).

B. Stabilization and transport. On the basis of the initial evaluation, if an infant has been identified as likely to have congenital heart disease, further medical management must be planned as well as arrangements made for a definitive anatomic diagnosis. This may involve transport of the neonate to another medical center where a pediatric cardiologist is available.

1. Initial resuscitation. For the neonate who presents with evidence of decreased cardiac output or shock, initial attention is devoted to the basics of advanced life support. A stable airway must be established and maintained as well as adequate ventilation. Reliable vascular access is essential, usually including an arterial line. In the neonate, this can most reliably be accomplished through the umbilical vessels. Volume resuscitation, inotropic support, and correction of metabolic acidosis are required with the goal of improving cardiac output and tissue perfusion (see Chap. 17).

2. PGE$_1$. The neonate who "fails" a hyperoxia test (or has an equivocal result in addition to other signs or symptoms of congenital heart disease) as well as the neonate who presents in shock within the first 3 weeks of life is highly likely to have congenital heart disease. These neonates are very likely to have congenital lesions that include anatomic features with ductal-dependent systemic or pulmonary blood flow, or in whom a PDA will aid in intercirculatory mixing.

PGE$_1$, administered as a continuous intravenous infusion, has important side effects that must be anticipated. PGE$_1$ causes apnea in 10% to 12% of neonates, usually within the first 6 hours of administration. Therefore, the infant who will be transferred to another institution while receiving PGE$_1$ should be intubated for maintenance of a stable airway before leaving the referring hospital. In infants who will not require transport, intubation may not be required but continuous cardiorespiratory monitoring is essential. In addition, PGE$_1$ typically causes peripheral vasodilation and subsequent hypotension in many infants. A separate intravenous line should be secured for volume administration in any infant receiving PGE$_1$, especially those who require transport.

Specific information regarding other adverse reactions, dose, and administration of PGE$_1$ is in section VII.A.

The authors cannot overemphasize the need to begin PGE$_1$ in **any** neonate in whom congenital heart disease is strongly suspected (i.e., a failed hyperoxia test and/or severe, acute CHF). In the neonate with ductal-dependent pulmonary blood flow, oxygen saturation will typically improve and the pulmonary blood flow remain secure until an anatomic diagnosis and plans for surgery are made. In neonates with transposition of the great arteries, maintenance of a patent ductus improves intercirculatory mixing. Most important, **neonates who present in shock in the first few weeks of life have duct-dependent systemic blood flow until proved otherwise;** resuscitation will not be successful unless the ductus in opened. In these cases, it is appropriate to begin an infusion of PGE$_1$ even **before** a precise anatomic diagnosis can be made by echocardiography.

It is prudent to remeasure arterial blood gases and reassess perfusion, vital signs, and acid–base status within 15 to 30 minutes of starting a PGE$_1$ infusion. Rarely, patients may become more unstable after beginning PGE$_1$. This is usually due to lesions with left atrial hypertension (hypoplastic left heart syndrome with restrictive patent foramen ovale, subdiaphragmatic total anomalous pulmonary venous return, mitral atresia with restrictive patent foramen ovale, transposition of the great arteries with intact ventricular septum with restrictive patent foramen ovale). In these lesions, deterioration on PGE_1 is often a helpful diagnostic finding, and **urgent** plans for echocardiography and possible interventional catheterization or surgery should be made.

3. **Inotropic agents.** Continuous infusions of inotropic agents, usually the sympathomimetic amines, can improve myocardial performance as well as perfusion of vital organs and the periphery. Care should be taken to replete intravascular volume before institution of vasoactive agents. **Dopamine** is a precursor of norepinephrine and stimulates β-1, dopaminergic, and α-adrenergic receptors in a dose-dependent manner. Dopamine can be expected to increase mean arterial pressure, improve ventricular function, and improve urine output with a low incidence of side effects at doses <10 μg/kg/minute. **Dobutamine** is an analog of dopamine, with predominantly β-1 effects and relatively weak β-2 and α-receptor stimulating activity. In comparison with dopamine, dobutamine lacks renal vasodilating properties, has less chronotropic effect (in adult patients), and does not depend on norepinephrine release from peripheral nerves for its effect. There are few published data available concerning the use of dobutamine in neonates, although clinical experience has been favorable. A combination of low-dose dopamine (up to 5 μg/kg/minute) and dobutamine may be used to minimize the potential peripheral vasoconstriction induced by high doses of dopamine while maximizing the dopaminergic effects on the renal circulation. See VII.B for details of administration of inotropic agents, and additional pharmacologic agents (see Chap. 17).

4. **Transport.** After initial stabilization, the neonate with suspected congenital heart disease often needs to be transferred to an institution that provides subspecialty care in pediatric cardiology and cardiac surgery. A successful transport actually involves two transitions of care for the neonate: (i) from the referring hospital staff to the transport team; (ii) from the transport team to the accepting hospital staff. The need for accurate, detailed, and complete communication of information between all these teams cannot be overemphasized. If possible, the pediatric cardiologist who will be caring for the patient should be included in the discussions of care while the neonate is still at the referring hospital.

Reliable **vascular access** should be secured for the neonate receiving continuous infusions of PGE_1 or inotropic agents. Umbilical lines placed for resuscitation and stabilization should be left in place for transport; the neonate with congenital heart disease may potentially require cardiac catheterization through this route.

Particular attention should be paid to the patient's airway and respiratory effort before transport. In general, all neonates receiving a PGE_1 infusion should be **intubated for transport** (see IV.B.2). Neonates with probable or definite congenital heart disease will most likely require surgical or interventional catheterization management during the hospitalization; therefore, it is likely that they will be intubated at some point. Because there is real risk in not intubating these infants, as a general rule, all should be intubated for transport unless there is a compelling reason not to do so. All intubated patients should have gastric decompression by nasogastric or orogastric tube.

Acid–base status and oxygen delivery should be checked with an arterial blood gas before transport. Although most noncardiac patients are transported receiving supplemental oxygen at or near 100%, this is often **not** the inspired oxygen concentration of choice for the neonate with congenital heart disease (see V for details of lesion-specific care). This management decision for transport is particularly important for those infants with duct-dependent systemic blood flow and complete intracardiac mixing with single ventricle physiology, and emphasizes the need to consult with a pediatric cardiologist before transport to achieve optimal intratransport patient care.

Finally, it is important to remember in neonates that **hypotension** is a late finding in shock. Therefore, other signs of incipient decompensation, such as persistent tachycardia and poor tissue perfusion, are important to note and treat before transport. Before leaving the referring hospital, the patient's current hemodynamic status (distal perfusion, heart rate, systemic blood pressure, acid–base status, etc.) should be reassessed and relayed to the receiving hospital team.

C. Confirmation of the diagnosis

1. **Echocardiography.** Two-dimensional echocardiography, supplemented with Doppler and color Doppler has become the primary diagnostic tool for anatomic definition in pediatric cardiology. Echocardiography provides information about the structure and function of the heart and great vessels in a timely fashion. Though not an invasive test *per se*, a complete echocardiogram on a newborn suspected of having congenital heart disease may take an hour or more to perform, and may therefore not be well tolerated by a sick and/or premature newborn. Temperature instability due to exposure during this extended time of examination may be a problem in the neonate. Extension of the neck for suprasternal notch views of the aortic arch may be problematic, particularly in the neonate with respiratory distress or with a tenuous airway. Therefore, in sick neonates, **close monitoring by a medical staff person other** than the one performing the echocardiogram is recommended, with attention to vital signs, respiratory status, temperature, etc.

2. **Cardiac catheterization**

   a. **Indications** (see Table 25.8). Neonatal cardiac catheterization has changed a great deal in its focus. In the current era, cardiac catheterization is rarely necessary for anatomic definition of intracardiac structures (although catheterization is still necessary for definition of the distal pulmonary arteries, aortic–pulmonary collaterals, and certain types of coronary artery anomalies) or for physiologic assessment as Doppler technology has assumed

---

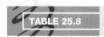 **TABLE 25.8**   **Indications for Neonatal Catheterization**

Interventions

Therapeutic

    Balloon atrial septostomy

    Balloon pulmonary valvuloplasty*

    Balloon aortic valvuloplasty*

    Balloon angioplasty of native coarctation of the aorta*

    Coil embolization of abnormal vascular communications

Diagnostic

    Endomyocardial biopsy

Anatomic definition (not visualized by echocardiography)

Coronary arteries

    Pulmonary atresia/intact ventricular septum

    Transposition of the great arteries

    Tetralogy of Fallot

Aortic to pulmonary artery collateral vessels

    Tetralogy of Fallot

Distal pulmonary artery anatomy

Hemodynamic measurements

*These interventions have alternative surgical options and are controversial based on institutional experience (see text).

Normal Newborn

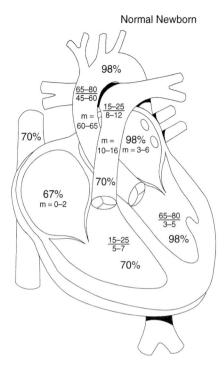

Figure 25.1. Typical hemodynamic measurements obtained at cardiac catheterization in a newborn, term infant without congenital or acquired heart disease. In this (and subsequent diagrams), oxygen saturations are shown as percentages, and typical hemodynamic pressure measurements in mm Hg are shown. In this example, the transition from fetal to infant physiology is complete; the pulmonary vascular resistance has fallen, the ductus arteriosus has closed, and there is no significant shunt at the foramen ovale. m = mean value.

an increasingly important role in this regard. Increasingly, catheterization is performed for catheter-directed therapy of congenital lesions. See Fig. 25.1 for normal newborn oxygen saturation and pressure measurements obtained during cardiac catheterization.

- **b. Interventional catheterization.** Since the first balloon dilation of the pulmonary artery reported by Kan in 1982, balloon valvuloplasty has become the procedure of choice in many types of valvar lesions, even extending to critical lesions in the neonate. At Children's Hospital, balloon valvuloplasty is considered the initial treatment of choice for both pulmonary and aortic stenosis, with a >90% immediate success rate in the neonate. The application of balloon dilation of native coarctation of the aorta is controversial (see the subsequent text).
- **c. Preparation for catheterization.** Catheterization in the neonate is not without its attendant risks; young age, small size, and interventional procedures are risk factors for complications. With appropriate anticipatory care, complications can be minimized. In addition to basic medical stabilization (see IV.B), specific attention to airway management is crucial. Sedation and analgesia are necessary, but will depress the respiratory drive in the neonate. When catheterizing a neonate, intubation and mechanical ventilation should be strongly considered, especially if an intervention is contemplated. In our institution, a **separate staff person not performing the catheterization** is present during the study, dedicated to the supervision of the infant's overall hemodynamic and respiratory status.

  Supervision of the neonate undergoing catheterization should also include periodic evaluation of the patient's body temperature, acid–base status, serum glucose, and monitoring of blood loss. All infants undergoing interventional catheterization such as balloon procedures should have 10 to 25 mL/kg packed red blood cells (PRBCs) typed and crossmatched **in the cathertization laboratory** during the procedure. Intravenous lines are recommended in the upper extremities or head (because the lower body will be draped and inaccessible during the case) in order to provide unobstructed access for medications, volume infusions, etc. Finally, the neonate may have the catheterization performed through umbilical vessels that were previously used for the administration of fluid, glucose, PGE_1, inotropic agents, or blood administration. Therefore, a peripheral line should be started and medications changed to that site before transfer of the neonate to the cardiac catheterization laboratory.

Consultation with the pediatric cardiologist who will be performing the case beforehand will help clarify these issues and allow the infant to be well prepared and monitored during the case.

V. "LESION-SPECIFIC" CARE FOLLOWING ANATOMIC DIAGNOSIS

A. **Duct-dependent systemic blood flow.** Commonly referred to as **left-sided obstructive lesions,** this group of lesions includes a spectrum of hypoplasia of left-sided structures of the heart ranging from isolated coarctation of the aorta to hypoplastic left heart syndrome. These infants typically present in cardiovascular collapse as the ductus arteriosus closes, with resultant systemic hypoperfusion; they may also present more insidiously with symptoms of CHF (see III.B). Although all infants with significant left-sided lesions and duct-dependent systemic blood flow require prostaglandin-induced patency of the ductus arteriosus as part of the initial management, additional care varies somewhat with each lesion.

1. **Aortic stenosis** (see Fig. 25.2). Morphologic abnormalities of the aortic valve may range from a bicuspid, nonobstructive, functionally normal valve to a unicuspid, markedly deformed and severely obstructive valve, which greatly

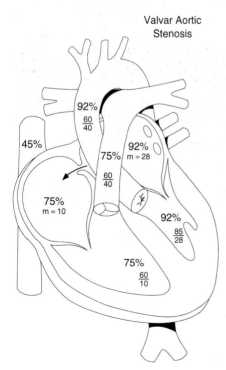

Valvar Aortic
Stenosis

Figure 25.2. Critical valvar aortic stenosis with a closed ductus arteriosus. Typical anatomic and hemodynamic findings include (i) a morphologically abnormal, stenotic valve; (ii) poststenotic dilatation of the ascending aorta; (iii) elevated left ventricular end diastolic pressure and left atrial pressures contributing to pulmonary edema (mild pulmonary venous and arterial desaturation); (iv) a left-to-right shunt at the atrial level (note increase in oxygen saturation from superior vena cava to right atrium); (v) pulmonary artery hypertension (also secondary to the elevated left atrial pressure); (vi) only a modest (25 mm Hg) gradient across valve. The low measured gradient (despite severe anatomic obstruction) across the aortic valve is due to a severely limited cardiac output, as evidenced by the low mixed venous oxygen saturation (45%) in the superior vena cava.

limits systemic cardiac output from the left ventricle. By convention, "severe" aortic stenosis is defined as a peak systolic gradient from left ventricle to ascending aorta of at least 60 mm Hg. "Critical" aortic stenosis results from severe anatomic obstruction with accompanying left ventricular failure and/or shock, regardless of the measured gradient. Patients with critical aortic stenosis have severe obstruction present *in utero* (usually due to a unicuspid, "plate-like" valve), with resultant left ventricular hypertrophy and, frequently, endocardial fibroelastosis. Associated left-sided abnormalities such as mitral valve disease and coarctation are not uncommon. Following closure of the ductus, the left ventricle must supply all of the systemic cardiac output. In cases of severe myocardial dysfunction, clinical CHF or shock will become apparent.

Initial management of the severely affected infant includes treatment of shock, stable vascular access, airway management and mechanical ventilation, sedation and muscle paralysis, inotropic support and institution of PGE_1. Positive end-expiratory pressure (PEEP) is helpful to overcome pulmonary venous desaturation from pulmonary edema secondary to left atrial hypertension. For a patient with critical aortic stenosis to benefit from a PGE_1 infusion, there must be a small patent foramen ovale to allow effective systemic blood flow (pulmonary venous return) to cross the atrial septum and ultimately enter the systemic vascular bed through the ductus. Inspired oxygen should be limited to a fractional concentration of inspired oxygen (FiO_2) of 0.5 to 0.6 unless severe hypoxemia is present.

Following anatomic definition of left ventricular size, mitral valve and aortic arch anatomy by echocardiography, cardiac catheterization or surgery should be performed as soon as possible to perform aortic valvotomy. With either type of therapy, patient outcome will depend largely on (i) the degree of relief of the obstruction, (ii) the degree of aortic regurgitation, (iii) associated cardiac lesions (especially left ventricular size), and (iv) the severity of end-organ dysfunction secondary to the initial presentation (e.g., necrotizing enterocolitis or renal failure). All patients with aortic stenosis will require life-long follow-up, as stenosis frequently recurs. Multiple procedures in childhood are common.

2. **Coarctation of the aorta** (see Fig. 25.3) is an anatomic narrowing of the descending aorta, most commonly at the site of insertion of the ductus arteriosus (i.e.,"juxtaductal"). Additional cardiac abnormalities are common, including bicuspid aortic valve (which occurs in 80% of patients) and ventricular septal defect (which occurs in 40% of patients). In addition, hypoplasia or obstruction of other left-sided structures including the mitral valve, the left ventricle, and the aortic valve are not uncommon and must be evaluated during the initial echocardiographic evaluation.

In utero, systemic blood flow to the lower body is through the PDA. Following ductal closure in the newborn with a critical coarctation, the left ventricle must suddenly generate adequate pressure and volume to pump the entire cardiac output past a significant point of obstruction. This sudden pressure load may be poorly tolerated by the neonatal myocardium and the neonate may become rapidly and critically ill because of lower body hypoperfusion.

As in critical aortic stenosis, initial management of the severely affected infant includes treatment of shock, stable vascular access, airway management and mechanical ventilation, moderate supplemental oxygen, sedation and muscle paralysis, inotropic support, and institution of PGE_1. PEEP is helpful to overcome pulmonary venous desaturation from pulmonary edema secondary to left atrial hypertension. In some infants, PGE_1 is unsuccessful in opening the ductus.

In infants with symptomatic coarctation, surgical repair is performed as soon as the infant has been resuscitated and medically stabilized. Usually the procedure is performed through a left lateral thoracotomy incision. In infants with symptomatic coarctation and a large, coexisting ventricular septal defect, consideration should be given to repair both defects in the initial procedure

Coarctation
of the Aorta

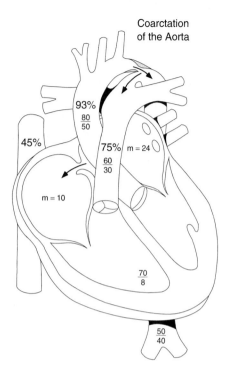

Figure 25.3. Coarctation of the aorta in a critically ill neonate with a nearly closed ductus arteriosus. Typical anatomic and hemodynamic findings include (i) "juxtaductal" site of the coarctation; (ii) a bicommissural aortic valve (seen in 80% of patients with coarctation); (iii) narrow pulse pressure in the descending aorta and lower body; (iv) a bidirectional shunt at the ductus arteriosus. As in critical aortic stenosis (see Fig. 25.2) there is an elevated left atrial pressure, pulmonary edema, a left-to-right shunt at the atrial level, pulmonary artery hypertension, and only a moderate (30 mm Hg) gradient across the arch obstruction. The low measured gradient (despite severe anatomic obstruction) across the aortic arch is due to low cardiac output.

through a median sternotomy. Balloon dilation of native coarctation is not routinely done at our institution because of the high incidence of restenosis and aneurysm formation, especially given the safe and effective surgical alternative.

3. **Interrupted aortic arch** (see Fig. 25.4) consists of complete atresia of a segment of the aortic arch. There are three anatomic subtypes of interrupted aortic arch based on the location of the interruption: distal to the left subclavian artery (type A); between the left subclavian artery and the left carotid artery (type B); and between the innominate artery and the left carotid artery (type C). Type B is the most common variety. More than 99% of these patients have a ventricular septal defect; abnormalities of the aortic valve and narrowed subaortic regions are associated anomalies.

Infants with interrupted aortic arch are completely dependent on a PDA for lower body blood flow therefore become critically ill when the ductus closes. Immediate management is similar to that described for coarctation (see V.A.2); PGE_1 infusion is essential. All other resuscitative measures will be ineffective if blood flow to the lower body is not restored. Oxygen saturations should be measured in the upper body; pulse oximetry readings in the lower body are reflective of the pulmonary artery oxygen saturation, and are typically lower than that distributed to the central nervous system and coronary arteries. High concentrations of inspired oxygen may result in low pulmonary vascular resistance, a large left-to-right shunt, and a "run-off" during diastole from the lower body into the pulmonary circulation. Inspired oxygen levels should therefore be minimized, aiming for normal (95%) oxygen saturations in the **upper** body.

Surgical reconstruction should be performed as soon as metabolic acidosis (if present) has resolved, end-organ dysfunction is improving, and the patient is hemodynamically stable. The repair typically entails a corrective approach

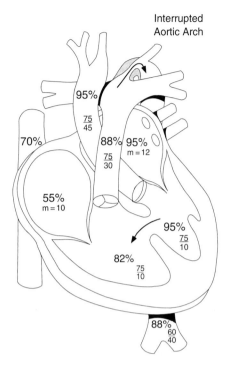

Interrupted
Aortic Arch

Figure 25.4. Interrupted aortic arch with restrictive patent ductus arteriosus. Typical anatomic and hemodynamic findings include (i) atresia of a segment of the aortic arch between the left subclavian artery and the left common carotid (the most common type of interrupted aortic arch—"type B"); (ii) a posterior malalignment of the conal septum resulting in a large ventricular septal defect and a narrow subaortic area; (iii) a bicuspid aortic valve occurs in 60% of patients; (iv) systemic pressure in the right ventricle and pulmonary artery (due to the large, nonrestrictive ventricular septal defect); (v) increased oxygen saturation in the pulmonary artery due to left-to-right shunting at the ventricular level; (vi) "differential cyanosis" with a lower oxygen saturation in the descending aorta due to a right-to-left shunt at the patent ductus. Note the lower blood pressure in the descending aorta due to constriction of the ductus; opening the ductus with PGE$_1$ results in equal upper and lower extremity blood pressures, but continued "differential cyanosis." PGE$_1$ = prostaglandin E1.

through a median sternotomy, with arch reconstruction (usually an end-to-end anastomosis) and closure of the ventricular septal defect. Arch reconstruction and a pulmonary artery band (through a lateral thoracotomy) are generally not recommended, typically reserved for patients with multiple ventricular septal defects.

4. **Hypoplastic left heart syndrome** (see Fig. 25.5A and 25.5B) represents a heterogeneous group of anatomic abnormalities in which there is a small to absent left ventricle with hypoplastic to atretic mitral and aortic valves. Before surgery, the right ventricle supplies both the pulmonary and systemic blood flows (through the PDA) with the proportion of cardiac output going to either circuit dependent on the relative resistances of these vascular beds.

At this point the continued fall in pulmonary vascular resistance results
As the pulmonary vascular resistance begins to fall (Fig. 25.5A), blood flow is preferentially directed to the pulmonary circulation at the expense of the systemic circulation. As systemic blood flow decreases, stroke volume and heart rate increase as a mechanism to preserve systemic cardiac output. The right ventricle becomes progressively volume overloaded with mildly elevated end-diastolic and left atrial pressures. The infant may be tachypneic or in respiratory distress, hepatomegaly may be present. The greater proportion of pulmonary venous return in the mixed ventricular blood results in a mildly decreased systemic arterial oxygen saturation (80%), and visible cyanosis may be mild or absent. Not infrequently, these infants are discharged from the nursery as normal newborns.

At this point the continued fall in pulmonary vascular resistance results in a progressive increase in pulmonary blood flow and relative decrease in systemic cardiac output. As the total right ventricular output is limited by heart rate and stroke volume, there is the onset of clinically apparent CHF, right ventricular dilation and dysfunction, progressive tricuspid regurgitation,

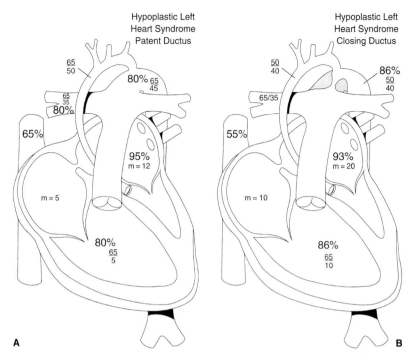

Figure 25.5. A: Hypoplastic left heart syndrome in a 24-hour-old patient with falling pulmonary vascular resistance and a nonrestrictive ductus arteriosus. Typical anatomic and hemodynamic findings include (i) atresia or hypoplasia of the left ventricle, mitral, and aortic valves; (ii) a diminutive ascending aorta and transverse aortic arch, usually with an associated coarctation; (iii) coronary blood flow is usually **retrograde** from the ductus arteriosus through the tiny ascending aorta; (iv) systemic arterial oxygen saturation (in Fio_2 of 0.21) of 80%, reflecting relatively balanced systemic and pulmonary blood flows—the pulmonary artery and aortic saturations are equal (see text); (v) pulmonary hypertension secondary to the nonrestrictive ductus arteriosus; (vi) minimal left atrial hypertension; (vii) normal systemic cardiac output (note superior vena cava oxygen saturation of 65%) and blood pressure (65/45). **B:** Acute circulatory collapse following constriction of the ductus arteriosus in hypoplastic left heart syndrome. These neonates are typically in shock with poor perfusion, tachycardia, acidosis, and in respiratory distress. The anatomic features are similar to those in Fig.25.5A, with the exception of the narrowed ductus arteriosus. Note (i) the low cardiac output (as evidenced by the low mixed venous oxygen saturation in the superior vena cava of 55%); (ii) narrow pulse pressure; (iii) elevated atrial and ventricular end-diastolic pressure—elevated left atrial pressure may cause pulmonary edema (note left atrial saturation of 93%); (iv) significantly increased pulmonary blood flow, as reflected in an arterial oxygen saturation (in Fio_2 of 0.21) of 86%.

poor peripheral perfusion with metabolic acidosis, decreased urine output, and pulmonary edema. Arterial oxygen saturation approaches 90%.

Alternatively, a sudden deterioration takes place with rapidly progressive CHF and shock as the ductus arteriosus constricts (Fig. 25.5B). There is decreased systemic perfusion and increased pulmonary blood flow, which is largely independent of the pulmonary vascular resistance. The peripheral pulses are weak to absent. Renal, hepatic, coronary, and central nervous system perfusion is compromised, possibly resulting in acute tubular necrosis, necrotizing enterocolitis, or cerebral infarction or hemorrhage. A vicious cycle may also result from inadequate retrograde perfusion of the ascending aorta (coronary blood supply), with further myocardial dysfunction and continued compromise of coronary blood flow. The pulmonary to systemic flow ratio approaches infinity as systemic blood flow nears zero. Therefore, one has the paradoxical presentation of profound metabolic acidosis in the face of a relatively high PO_2 (70–100 mm Hg).

The arterial blood gas may represent the single best indicator of hemodynamic stability. Low arterial saturation (75%–80%) with normal pH indicates an acceptable balance of systemic and pulmonary blood flow with adequate peripheral perfusion, whereas elevated oxygen saturation (>90%) with acidosis represents significantly increased pulmonary and decreased systemic flow with probable myocardial dysfunction and secondary effects on other organ systems.

Resuscitation of these neonates involves pharmacologic maintenance of ductal patency with PGE_1 and ventilatory maneuvers to **increase** pulmonary resistance. In our experience, a mild respiratory acidosis (e.g., pH 7.35) is appropriate for most of these infants. It is important to note that **hyperventilation and/or supplemental oxygen is usually of no significant benefit and may be harmful** by causing excessive pulmonary vasodilation and pulmonary blood flow at the expense of the systemic blood flow.

Hypotension in these infants is more frequently caused by increased pulmonary blood flow (at the expense of systemic flow) rather that due to intrinsic myocardial dysfunction. Although small to moderate doses of inotropic agents are frequently beneficial, **large doses of inotropic agents may have a deleterious effect,** depending on the relative effects on the systemic and pulmonary vascular beds. Preferential selective elevations of systemic vascular tone will secondarily increase pulmonary blood flow, and careful monitoring of mean arterial blood pressure and arterial oxygen saturation is warranted.

Similar to the patient with critical aortic stenosis, in order for the neonate with hypoplastic left heart syndrome to benefit from a PGE_1 infusion, there must be at least a small patent foramen ovale to allow for effective systemic blood flow (pulmonary venous return) to cross the atrial septum and ultimately enter the systemic vascular bed through the ductus. An infant with hypoplastic left heart syndrome and a severely restrictive or absent patent foramen ovale will be critically ill with profound cyanosis (oxygen saturation <60%–65%), and will not improve after the institution of PGE_1. **In these neonates, emergent balloon dilation of the atrial septum may be necessary.**

Medical therapy may be briefly palliative; however, surgical therapy is necessary for survival of infants with hypoplastic left heart syndrome. After a period of medical stabilization and support to allow for recovery of ischemic organ system injury (particularly of the kidneys, liver, central nervous system, and the heart itself), surgical relief of left-sided obstruction is required. Surgical intervention involves either staged reconstruction (with a neonatal Norwood procedure followed by a Fontan operation later in childhood) or neonatal cardiac transplantation. Recent results from both reconstructive surgery and transplantation have vastly improved the outlook for infants born with this previously 100% fatal condition.

B. Duct-dependent pulmonary blood flow. This underlying physiology is shared by a diverse group of lesions with the common finding of restricted pulmonary blood flow due to severe pulmonary stenosis or complete pulmonary atresia. Closure of the ductus arteriosus results in marked cyanosis.

  1. Pulmonary stenosis (see Fig. 25.6) with obstruction to pulmonary blood flow may occur at several levels: (i) within the body of the right ventricle; (ii) at the pulmonary valve (as pictured in Fig. 25.6); (iii) in the peripheral pulmonary arteries. Valvar pulmonary stenosis with an intact ventricular septum is the second most common form of congenital heart disease; "critical" obstruction occurs more rarely. Grading of the degree of pulmonary stenosis is similar to that of aortic stenosis (see V.A.1) with severe pulmonary stenosis defined as a peak systolic gradient from right ventricle to pulmonary artery of 60 mm Hg or more. By convention, "critical" pulmonary stenosis is defined as severe valvar obstruction with associated hypoxemia due to a right-to-left shunt

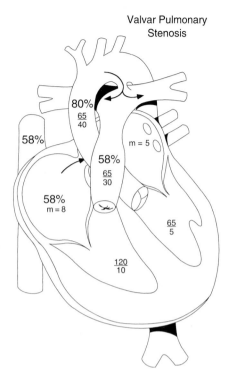

Valvar Pulmonary
Stenosis

Figure 25.6. Critical valvar pulmonary stenosis in a neonate with a nonrestrictive patent ductus arteriosus while receiving PGE_1. Typical anatomic and hemodynamic findings include (i) thickened, stenotic pulmonary valve; (ii) poststenotic dilatation of the main pulmonary artery with normal-sized branch pulmonary arteries; (iii) right ventricular hypertrophy with suprasystemic pressure; (iv) a right-to-left shunt at the atrial level through the patent foramen ovale with systemic desaturation (80%); (v) suprasystemic right ventricular (RV) pressure with a 55 mm Hg peak systolic ejection gradient; (vi) systemic pulmonary artery pressure (due to the nonrestrictive patent ductus); (vii) pulmonary blood flow through the patent ductus arteriosus. PGE_1 = prostaglandin E1.

at the foramen ovale. Critical pulmonary stenosis may be associated with hypoplasia of the right ventricle and/or tricuspid valve and significant right ventricular hypertrophy. The pressure in the right ventricle is often higher than the left ventricular pressure (i.e., suprasystemic) in order to eject blood past the severe narrowing. Due to the longstanding (*in utero*) increased right ventricular pressure, there is typically a hypertrophied, noncompliant right ventricle with a resultant increase in right atrial filling pressure. When right atrial pressure exceeds left atrial pressure, a right-to-left shunt at the foramen ovale results in cyanosis and hypoxemia. There may be associated right ventricular dysfunction and/or tricuspid regurgitation.

After initial stabilization of the patient and definitive diagnosis by echocardiography, transcatheter balloon valvotomy is the treatment of choice for this lesion, although surgical valvotomy may be used in specific cases. Despite successful relief of the obstruction during catheterization, cyanosis is usually not completely relieved, but rather resolves gradually over the first weeks of life as the right ventricle becomes more compliant, tricuspid regurgitation lessens, and there is less right to left shunting at the atrial level. Successful balloon valvuloplasty is associated with excellent clinical results among patients; the need for repeat procedures is quite low.

2. **Pulmonary atresia with intact ventricular septum ("hypoplastic right heart syndrome,"** see Fig. 25.7) is comparable to hypoplastic left heart syndrome in that there is atresia of the pulmonary valve with varying degrees of right ventricular and tricuspid valve hypoplasia. Perhaps the most important associated anomaly is the presence of coronary artery–myocardial–right ventricular sinusoidal connections. The coronary arteries may be quite abnormal, including areas of stenoses or complete atresia. Myocardial perfusion

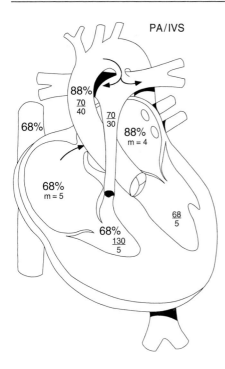

PA/IVS

88%
70/40

70/30

68%

88%
m = 4

68%
m = 5

68
5

68%
130/5

Figure 25.7. Pulmonary atresia (PA) with intact ventricular septum (IVS) in a neonate with a nonrestrictive patent ductus arteriosus while receiving PGE_1. Typical anatomic and hemodynamic findings include (i) hypertrophied, hypoplastic right ventricle; (ii) hypoplastic tricuspid valve and pulmonary annulus; (iii) atresia of the pulmonary valve with no antegrade flow; (iv) suprasystemic right ventricular pressure; (v) pulmonary blood flow through the patent ductus; (vi) right-to-left shunt at the atrial level with systemic desaturation. Many patients have significant coronary abnormalities with sinusoidal or fistulous connections to the hypertensive right ventricle or significant coronary stenoses (not shown). PGE_1 = prostaglandin E1.

may therefore be dependent on a hypertensive right ventricle to supply the distal coronary arteries; surgical relief of the pulmonary atresia (with a right ventricular-to-pulmonary artery connection) may lead to myocardial infarction and death. The presence of sinusoidal connections between the right ventricle and the coronary arteries is associated with poorer long-term survival. Because there is no outlet of the right ventricle, there is typically suprasystemic pressure in the right ventricle and some tricuspid regurgitation. There is an obligatory right-to-left shunt at the atrial level and pulmonary blood flow is entirely dependent on a PDA.

Although the cornerstone of initial management is PGE_1 infusion to maintain ductal patency, a more permanent and reliable form of pulmonary blood flow must be surgically created for the infant to survive. Surgical management is often preceded by catheterization to define the coronary artery anatomy. In patients without significant coronary abnormalities, pulmonary blood flow is established by creating an outflow for the right ventricle by pulmonary valvotomy and/or right ventricular outflow tract augmentation. Usually at the time of this procedure, a systemic-to-pulmonary artery shunt (most often a Blalock-Taussig shunt) is constructed to also augment pulmonary blood flow. In patients with "right ventricular dependent" coronary arteries, a systemic-to-pulmonary artery shunt is the typical procedure performed in the neonate.

3. **Tricuspid atresia** (see Fig. 25.8) involves complete absence of the tricuspid valve and therefore no direct communication from right atrium to right ventricle. The right ventricle may be severely hypoplastic or completely absent. More than 90% of patients have an associated ventricular septal defect, allowing blood to pass from the left ventricle to the right ventricular outflow and pulmonary arteries. Most patients have some form of additional pulmonary stenosis. In 70% of cases, the great arteries are normally aligned with the

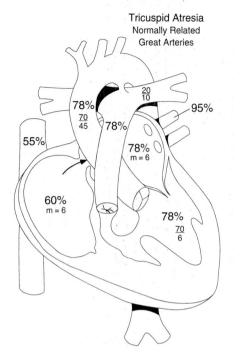

Tricuspid Atresia
Normally Related
Great Arteries

Figure 25.8. Tricuspid atresia with normally related great arteries and a small patent ductus arteriosus. Typical anatomic and hemodynamic findings include (i) atresia of the tricuspid valve; (ii) hypoplasia of the right ventricle; (iii) restriction to pulmonary blood flow at two levels: a (usually) small ventricular septal defect and a stenotic pulmonary valve; (iv) all systemic venous return must pass through the patent foramen ovale to reach the left ventricle; (v) complete mixing at the left atrial level, with systemic oxygen saturation of 78% (in Fio_2 of 0.21), suggesting balanced systemic and pulmonary blood flow ("single ventricle physiology" — see text.)

ventricles; however, in the remaining 30% the great arteries are transposed. An atrial level communication is necessary for blood to exit the right atrium; there is an obligatory right-to-left shunt at this level. In patients with normally related great arteries, pulmonary blood flow is derived from the right ventricle; if the right ventricle (or its connection with the left ventricle through a ventricular septal defect) is severely diminutive, the pulmonary blood flow may be duct-dependent; closure of the ductus leads to profound hypoxemia and acidosis.

Immediate medical management is primarily aimed at maintenance of adequate pulmonary blood flow. In the usual case of severe pulmonary stenosis and limited pulmonary blood flow, PGE_1 infusion maintains pulmonary blood flow through the ductus arteriosus. Surgical creation of a more permanent source of pulmonary blood flow (usually a Blalock-Taussig shunt) is undertaken as soon as possible. More complex cases (e.g., with transposition) may require more extensive palliative procedures.

4. **Tetralogy of fallot** (see Fig. 25.9) consists of right ventricular outflow obstruction, a ventricular septal defect (of the anterior malalignment variety), "overriding" of the aorta over the ventricular septum, and hypertrophy of the right ventricle. There is a wide spectrum of anatomic variation encompassing these findings, depending particularly on the site and severity of the right ventricular outflow obstruction. The severely cyanotic neonate with tetralogy most likely has severe right ventricular outflow tract obstruction and a large right-to-left shunt at the ventricular level through the large ventricular septal defect. Pulmonary blood flow may be duct-dependent.

Immediate medical management involves establishing adequate pulmonary blood flow usually with PGE_1 infusion, although some have attempted balloon dilation of the right ventricular outflow tract. Detailed anatomic definition particularly regarding coronary artery anatomy, the presence of additional

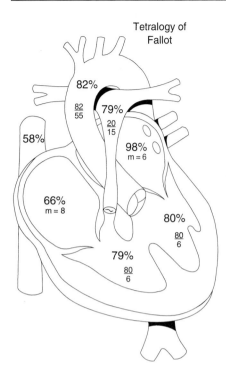

Tetralogy of
Fallot

82%

82
55

79%

20
15

58%

98%
m = 6

66%
m = 8

80%

80
6

79%

80
6

Figure 25.9. Tetralogy of Fallot. Typical anatomic and hemodynamic findings include (i) an anteriorly displaced infundibular septum, resulting in subpulmonary stenosis, a large ventricular septal defect, and overriding of the aorta over the muscular septum; (ii) hypoplasia of the pulmonary valve, main, and branch pulmonary arteries; (iii) equal right and left ventricular pressures; (iv) a right-to-left shunt at ventricular level, with a systemic oxygen saturation of 82%.

ventricular septal defects, and the sources of pulmonary blood flow (systemic to pulmonary collateral vessels) is necessary before surgical intervention. If echocardiography is not able to fully show these details, then diagnostic catheterization is performed. Surgical repair of the **asymptomatic** child with tetralogy of Fallot is usually recommended within the first 6 months of life. The **symptomatic** (i.e., severely cyanotic) neonate should have operative intervention. Complete repair is generally performed at our institution, although a systemic-to-pulmonary artery shunt is sometimes employed in unusual cases such as multiple ventricular septal defects or coronary anomalies.

5. **Ebstein anomaly** (see Fig. 25.10A and 25.10B) is an uncommon but grave anatomic lesion when it presents in the neonatal period. Anatomically there is "downward displacement" of the tricuspid valve into the body of the right ventricle. The tricuspid valve is frequently regurgitant resulting in marked right atrial enlargement and a large right-to-left shunt at the atrial level; there is little forward flow out the right ventricular outflow tract into the pulmonary circulation. The prognosis for neonates presenting with profound cyanosis due to Ebstein anomaly is quite grave. Surgical options are controversial and generally reserved for the severely symptomatic child. Further complicating the medical condition, Ebstein anomaly is often associated with Wolff-Parkinson-White (WPW) syndrome and supraventricular tachycardia (SVT).

Medical management is aimed at supporting the neonate through the initial period of transitional circulation. Because of elevated pulmonary vascular resistance, pulmonary blood flow may be quite severely limited with profound hypoxemia and acidosis as a result. PGE_1 is used to maintain a PDA; other measures to decrease pulmonary vascular resistance and promote antegrade pulmonary blood flow (such as a high level of supplemental oxygen and maintaining a mild respiratory alkalosis) are helpful. Recently, nitric oxide has

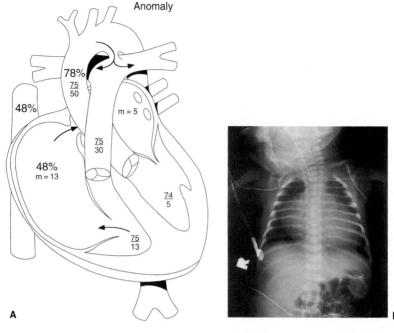

Figure 25.10. A: Ebstein anomaly (with large nonrestrictive ductus arteriosus). Typical anatomic and hemodynamic findings include (i) inferior displacement of the tricuspid valve into the right ventricle, which may also cause subpulmonary obstruction; (ii) diminutive muscular right ventricle; (iii) marked enlargement of the right atrium due to "atrialized" portion of right ventricle as well as tricuspid regurgitation; (iv) right-to-left shunting at the atrial level (note arterial oxygen saturation of 78%); (v) a left-to-right shunt and pulmonary hypertension secondary to a large patent ductus arteriosus supplying the pulmonary blood flow; (vi) low cardiac output (note low mixed venous oxygen saturation in the superior vena cava). **B:** Chest radiograph in a neonate with severe Ebstein anomaly and no significant pulmonary blood flow from the ductus arteriosus. The cardiomegaly is due to marked dilation of the right atrium. The pulmonary vascular markings are diminished due to the decreased pulmonary blood flow. Hypoplasia of the lungs is common due to the large heart causing a "space-occupying lesion."

been used with limited success. An important contributor to the high mortality rate in the neonate with severe Ebstein anomaly is the associated pulmonary hypoplasia that is present (due to the massively enlarged right heart *in utero*, Fig. 25.10B).

C. Parallel circulation/transposition of the great arteries (see Fig. 25.11). Transposition of the great arteries is defined as an aorta arising from the morphologically right ventricle and the pulmonary artery from the morphologically left ventricle. Approximately one-half of all patients with transposition have an associated ventricular septal defect.

In the usual arrangement, this creates a situation of "parallel circulations" with systemic venous return being pumped through the aorta back to the systemic circulation, and pulmonary venous return being pumped through the pulmonary artery to the pulmonary circulation. Following separation from the placenta, neonates with transposition are dependent on mixing between the parallel systemic and pulmonary circulations in order for them to survive. In patients with an intact ventricular septum, this communication exists through the PDA and the patent

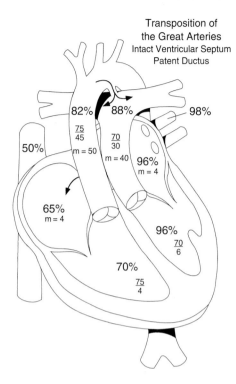

Transposition of
the Great Arteries
Intact Ventricular Septum
Patent Ductus

82%   88%   98%

$\frac{75}{45}$ $\frac{70}{30}$

50%   m = 50   m = 40   96%

m = 4

65%
m = 4

96%

$\frac{70}{6}$

70%

$\frac{75}{4}$

Figure 25.11. Transposition of the great arteries with an intact ventricular septum, a large patent ductus arteriosus (on PGE_1) and atrial septal defect (status post balloon atrial septostomy). Note the following: (i) the aorta arises from the anatomic right ventricle, and the pulmonary artery from the anatomic left ventricle; (ii) "transposition physiology," with a higher oxygen saturation in the pulmonary artery than in the aorta; (iii) "mixing" between the parallel circulations (see text) at the atrial (after balloon atrial septostomy) and ductal levels; (iv) shunting from the left atrium to the right atrium through the atrial septal defect (not shown) with equalization of atrial pressures; (v) shunting from the aorta to the pulmonary artery through the ductus arteriosus; (vi) pulmonary hypertension due to a large ductus arteriosus. PGE_1 = prostaglandin E_1.

foramen ovale. These patients are usually clinically cyanotic within the first hours of life leading to their early diagnosis. Those infants with an associated ventricular septal defect typically have somewhat improved mixing between the systemic and pulmonary circulations and may not be as severely cyanotic.

In neonates with transposition of the great arteries and an intact ventricular septum, a very low arterial Pao_2 (15–20 torr) with high $Paco_2$ (despite adequate chest motion and ventilation) and metabolic acidosis are markers for severely decreased effective pulmonary blood flow and need urgent attention. The initial management of the severely hypoxemic patient with transposition includes (i) **ensure adequate mixing** between the two parallel circuits and (ii) **maximize mixed venous oxygen saturation.**

In patients who do not respond with an increased arterial oxygen saturation to the opening of the ductus arteriosus with prostaglandin (usually these neonates have very restrictive atrial defects and/or pulmonary hypertension), **the foramen ovale should be emergently enlarged by balloon atrial septostomy.** Hyperventilation and treatment with sodium bicarbonate are important maneuvers to promote alkalosis, lower pulmonary vascular resistance, and increase pulmonary blood flow (which increases atrial mixing following septostomy).

In transposition of the great arteries, most of the systemic blood flow is recirculated systemic venous return. In the presence of poor mixing, much can be gained by increasing the mixed venous oxygen saturation, which is the **major determinant of systemic arterial oxygen saturation.** These maneuvers include (i) decreasing the whole body oxygen consumption (muscle relaxants, sedation, mechanical ventilation) and (ii) improving oxygen delivery (increase cardiac output with inotropic agents, increase oxygen-carrying capacity by treating anemia). Coexisting causes of pulmonary venous desaturation (e.g., pneumothorax) should

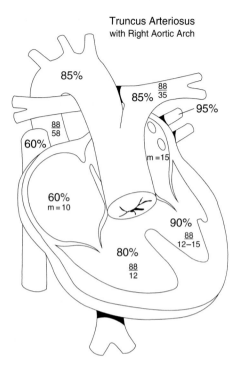

Truncus Arteriosus
with Right Aortic Arch

Figure 25.12. Truncus arteriosus (with right aortic arch). Typical anatomic and hemodynamic findings include (i) a single artery arises from the conotruncus giving rise to coronary arteries (not shown), pulmonary arteries, and brachiocephalic vessels; (ii) abnormal truncal valve (quadricuspid shown) with stenosis and/or regurgitation common; (iii) right-sided aortic arch (occurs in ~30% of cases); (iv) large conoventricular ventricular septal defect; (v) pulmonary artery hypertension with a large left-to-right shunt (note superior vena cava oxygen saturation of 60% and pulmonary artery oxygen saturation of 85%); (vi) complete mixing (of the systemic and pulmonary venous return) occurs at the great vessel level.

also be sought and treated. Increasing the Fio_2 to 100% will have little effect on the arterial PO_2, unless it serves to lower pulmonary vascular resistance and increase pulmonary blood flow.

In the current era, definitive management is surgical correction with an arterial switch operation in the early neonatal period. If severe hypoxemia persists despite medical management, mechanical support with extracorporeal membrane oxygenation (ECMO) or an urgent arterial switch operation may be indicated.

D. Lesions with complete intracardiac mixing

1. Truncus arteriosus (see Fig. 25.12) consists of a single great artery arising from the heart, which gives rise to (in order) the coronary arteries, the pulmonary arteries, and the brachiocephalic arteries. The truncal valve is often anatomically abnormal (only 50% are tricuspid), and is frequently thickened, stenotic, and/or regurgitant. A coexisting ventricular septal defect is present in >98% of cases. The aortic arch is right-sided in approximately one-third of cases; other arch anomalies such as hypoplasia, coarctation and interruption are seen in 10% of cases. Extracardiac anomalies are present in 20% to 40% of cases. Thirty five percent of patients with truncus arteriosus have a deletion of chromosome 22 at 22q11, detectable by fluorescence *in situ* hybridization (FISH) testing.

The overwhelming majority of infants with truncus arteriosus present with symptoms of CHF in the first weeks of life. The infants may be somewhat cyanotic, but CHF symptoms and signs are usually dominant. The pulmonary blood flow is increased, with significant pulmonary hypertension common. The natural history of truncus arteriosus is quite bleak. Left unrepaired, only 15% to 30% survive the first year of life. Furthermore, in survivors of the immediate neonatal period, the occurrence of accelerated irreversible pulmonary vascular disease is common, making surgical repair in the neonatal period (or as soon as the diagnosis is made) the treatment of choice. "Medical management" of heart failure would be considered only a temporizing measure until surgical correction can be accomplished.

2. **Total anomalous pulmonary venous connection** (see Fig. 25.13A and 25.13B) occurs when all pulmonary veins drain into the systemic venous system with complete mixing of pulmonary and systemic venous return usually in the right atrium. The systemic blood flow is therefore dependent on an obligate shunt through the patent foramen ovale into the left heart. The anomalous connections of the pulmonary veins may be (i) supracardiac (usually into the right superior vena cava or to the innominate vein through a persistent

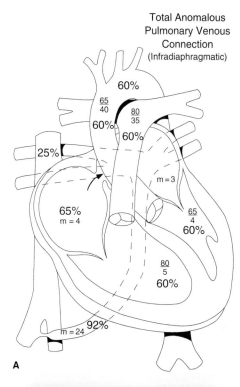

Total Anomalous
Pulmonary Venous
Connection
(Infradiaphragmatic)

A

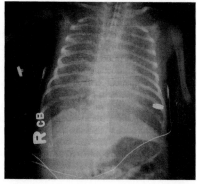

B

Figure 25.13. A: Infradiaphragmatic total anomalous pulmonary venous connection. Note the following: (i) pulmonary venous confluence does not connect with the left atrium, but descends to connect with the portal circulation below the diaphragm. This connection is frequently severely obstructed; (ii) obstruction to pulmonary venous return results in significantly elevated pulmonary venous pressures, decreased pulmonary blood flow, pulmonary edema, and pulmonary venous desaturation (92%); (iii) systemic to suprasystemic pressure in the pulmonary artery (in the absence of a patent ductus arteriosus, pulmonary artery pressures may exceed systemic pressures when severe pulmonary venous obstruction is present); (iv) all systemic blood flow must be derived through a right-to-left shunt at the foramen ovale; (v) nearly equal oxygen saturations in all chambers of the heart (i.e., complete mixing at right atrial level), with severe hypoxemia (systemic oxygen saturation 60%) and low cardiac output (mixed venous oxygen saturation 25%). **B:** Chest radiograph in a 16-hour-old neonate with severe infradiaphragmatic obstruction to pulmonary venous return. Note the pulmonary edema, small heart, and hyperinflated lungs (on mechanical ventilation). Despite high inflating and positive end-expiratory pressures and an FiO_2 of 1, the arterial blood gas revealed a pH of 7.02, arterial carbon dioxide tension ($PaCO_2$) of 84, and an arterial oxygen tension (PaO_2) of 23 torr. Emergent surgical management is indicated.

vertical vein); (ii) cardiac (usually to the right atrium or coronary sinus); (iii) subdiaphragmatic (usually into the portal system); or (iv) mixed drainage.

In patients with total connection below the diaphragm, the pathway is frequently obstructed with severely limited pulmonary blood flow, pulmonary hypertension, and profound cyanosis. This form of total anomalous pulmonary venous connection is a surgical emergency, with minimal beneficial effects from medical management. Although PGE_1 will maintain ductal patency, the limitation of pulmonary blood flow in these patients is **not** due to limited antegrade flow into the pulmonary circuit, but rather due to outflow obstruction at the pulmonary veins. In the current era of prostaglandin, ventilatory support, and advanced medical intensive care, obstructed total anomalous pulmonary venous connection represents one of the few remaining lesions that requires emergent, "middle of the night" surgical intervention. Early recognition of the problem (Fig. 25.13B) and prompt surgical intervention (surgical anastomosis of the pulmonary venous confluence to the left atrium) are necessary in order for the infant to survive. Patients with a mild degree of obstruction typically have minimal symptoms, with many neonates escaping recognition until later in infancy when they present with signs and symptoms of CHF.

3. **Complex single ventricles.** There are multiple complex anomalies that share the common physiology of complete mixing of the systemic and pulmonary venous return, frequently with anomalous connections of the systemic and/or pulmonary veins, and with obstruction to one of the great vessels (usually the pulmonary artery). In cases with associated polysplenia or asplenia and abnormalities of visceral situs, the term *heterotaxy syndrome* is frequently applied. Physiologically, systemic blood flow and pulmonary blood flow is determined by the balance of anatomic and/or vascular resistance in the systemic and pulmonary circulations. In the well-balanced single ventricle, the oxygen saturation in the pulmonary artery and the aorta will be essentially the same (usually in the high 70–low 80% range) with a normal pH on arterial blood gas ("single ventricle physiology.") It is beyond the scope of this chapter to define this heterogeneous group of patients further, although all will fail a hyperoxia test, most have significantly abnormal ECGs, and the diagnosis of complex congenital heart disease is rarely in doubt (even before anatomic confirmation with echocardiography). As there is complete mixing of venous return and essentially a single pumping chamber, initial management is similar to that described for hypoplastic left heart syndrome (see V.A.4).

E. **Left-to-right shunt lesions.** For the most part, infants with pure left-to-right shunt lesions are not diagnosed because of severe systemic illness, but rather due to the finding of a murmur or symptoms of CHF usually occurring in the late neonatal period or beyond. The lesion of this group most likely to require attention in the neonatal nursery is that of a PDA.

1. **PDA** is not particularly common in term newborns and rarely causes CHF. However, the frequency that a premature neonate will develop a hemodynamically significant left-to-right shunt through a PDA is inversely proportional to advancing gestational age and weight.

The typical presentation of a PDA begins with a harsh systolic ejection murmur heard over the entire precordium, but loudest at the left upper sternal border and left infraclavicular areas. As the pulmonary vascular resistance decreases, the intensity of the murmur increases and later becomes continuous (i.e., extends through the second heart sound). The peripheral pulses increase in amplitude ("bounding pulses"), the pulse pressure widens to >25 mm Hg, the precordial impulse becomes hyperdynamic, and the patient's respiratory status deteriorates (manifesting as tachypnea or apnea, carbon dioxide retention, and an increasing mechanical ventilation requirement). Serial chest x-rays show an increase in heart size and the lungs may appear more radiopaque.

It is important to remember that this typical progression of clinical signs is **not specific** only for a hemodynamically significant PDA. Other lesions may produce bounding pulses, a hyperdynamic precordium, and cardiac enlargement (e.g., an arteriovenous fistula or an aorticopulmonary window). Generally, however, the clinical assessment of a premature infant with the typical findings of a hemodynamically significant ductus is adequate to guide therapeutic decisions. If the diagnosis is in doubt, an echocardiogram will clarify the anatomic diagnosis.

Initial medical management includes increased ventilatory support, fluid restriction, and diuretic therapy. In symptomatic patients, indomethacin is initially used for nonsurgical closure of PDA in the premature neonate, and is effective in approximately 80% of cases. Birth weight does not affect the efficacy of indomethacin, and there is no increase in complications associated with surgery after unsuccessful indomethacin therapy. In asymptomatic patients, the efficacy of prophylactic administration of indomethacin is controversial. Adverse reactions to indomethacin include transient oliguria, electrolyte abnormalities, decreased platelet function, and hypoglycemia. Contraindications to use of indomethacin and dosing information is noted in Appendix A.

Indications for closure of a PDA vary from institution to institution. In general, we recommend medical treatment for mechanically ventilated premature infants weighing <1,000 g when a patent ductus first becomes apparent, regardless of the presence of signs or symptoms of a significant left-to-right shunt. For infants larger than 1,000 g, we recommend treatment with indomethacin only after cardiovascular or respiratory signs of a hemodynamically significant ductus develop. Some infants who fail to respond to the first course of treatment with indomethacin may respond to a second course.

Symptomatic patients who do not respond to a second treatment with indomethacin or cannot tolerate indomethacin therapy due to side effects should undergo surgical ligation following echocardiographic documentation of the patent ductus.

Ibuprofen has been recently approved for use in the newborn in the United States. It is as effective in closing a PDA as indomethacin but appears to have a better safety profile (more normal urine output, less elevation of blood urea nitrogen (BUN) and creatinine, less decrease in mesenteric blood flow, and improved autoregulation of cerebral blood flow). Rates of necrotizing enterocolitis, gastrointestinal bleeding, and intraventricular hemorrhage were not significantly diminished in the group treated with ibuprofen compared with those treated with indomethacin. Unlike indomethacin, early prophylactic use of ibuprofen has not been found to reduce the rate of intraventricular hemorrhage. The ibuprofen lysine has not been associated with an increased incidence of pulmonary hypertension and chronic lung disease reported with the use of the ibuprofen trishydroxy aminomethane (THAM) preparation. Pharmacokinetic studies have not shown that ibuprofen lysine displaces bilirubin from albumin. We are now using ibuprofen lysine (Neoprofen) as an option for PDA closure after the first day of life (see Appendix A).

2. **Complete atrioventricular canal** (see Fig. 25.14) consists of a combination of defects in the (i) endocardial portion of the atrial septum, (ii) the inlet portion of the ventricular septum, and (iii) a common, single atrioventricular valve. Because of the large net left-to-right shunt, which increases as the pulmonary vascular resistance falls, these infants typically present early in life with CHF. There may be some degree of cyanosis as well, particularly in the immediate neonatal period before the pulmonary vascular resistance has fallen. In the absence of associated right ventricular outflow tract obstruction, pulmonary artery pressures are at systemic levels; pulmonary vascular resistance is frequently elevated, particularly in patients with trisomy 21.

Approximately 70% of infants with complete atrioventricular canal have trisomy 21; notation of the phenotypic findings of Down syndrome often lead to evaluation of the patient for possible congenital heart disease (Table 25.5). In the immediate neonatal period, these infants may have an equivocal hyperoxia test because there may be some right-to-left shunting through the large intracardiac connections. Symptoms of congestive failure ensue during the first weeks of

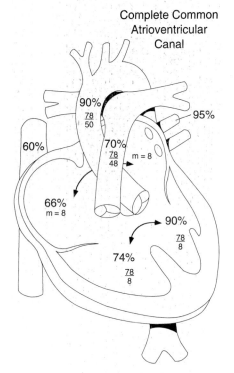

Complete Common
Atrioventricular
Canal

90%
78/50

95%

60%

70%
78/48   m = 8

66%
m = 8

90%
78/8

74%
78/8

Figure 25.14. Complete common atrioventricular canal. Typical anatomic and hemodynamic findings include (i) large atrial and ventricular septal defects of the endocardial cushion type; (ii) single, atrioventricular valve; (iii) pulmonary artery hypertension (due to large ventricular septal defect); (iv) bidirectional shunting (with mild hypoxemia) at atrial and ventricular level when pulmonary vascular resistance is elevated in the initial neonatal period. With subsequent fall in pulmonary vascular resistance, the shunt becomes predominantly left-to-right with symptoms of congestive heart failure.

life as the pulmonary vascular resistance falls and the patient develops a marked left-to-right shunt. These patients have a characteristic ECG finding of a "superior axis" (QRS axis from 0 to—180 degrees; see Fig. 25.15) which can be a useful clue for the presence of congenital heart disease in an infant with trisomy 21.

Most patients with complete atrioventricular canal will require medical treatment for symptomatic CHF, although prolonged medical therapy in patients with failure to thrive and symptomatic heart failure is not warranted. Complete surgical repair is undertaken electively approximately 4 to 6 months of age, with earlier repair in symptomatic patients. In our experience, corrective surgery for complete atrioventricular canal can be performed successfully in early infancy with good results.

3. **Ventricular septal defect** is the most common cause of CHF after the initial neonatal period. Moderate to large ventricular septal defects become hemodynamically significant as the pulmonary vascular resistance decreases and pulmonary blood flow increases due to a left-to-right shunt across the defect. As this usually takes 2 to 4 weeks to develop, term neonates with ventricular septal defect and symptoms of CHF should be investigated for coexisting anatomic abnormalities, such as left ventricular outflow tract obstruction, coarctation of the aorta, or PDA. Premature infants, who have a lower initial pulmonary vascular resistance, may develop clinical symptoms of heart failure earlier or require longer mechanical ventilation compared with term infants.

Ventricular septal defects may occur anywhere in the ventricular septum and are usually classified by their location (see Fig. 25.16). Defects in the membranous septum are the most common type. The diagnosis of ventricular septal defect is usually initially suspected on physical examination of the

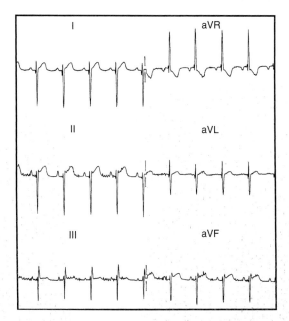

Figure 25.15. Superior ("northwest") axis as seen on the electrocardiogram (only frontal plane leads shown) in a newborn with complete atrioventricular canal. Note the initial upward deflection of the QRS complex (and subsequent predominantly negative deflection) in leads I and aVF. A superior axis (0–180 degrees) is present in 95% of patients with endocardial cushion defects.

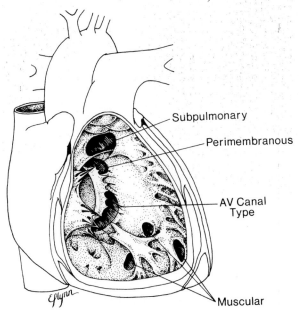

Figure 25.16. Diagram of types of ventricular septal defects as viewed from the right ventricle. AV = arteriovenous (Fyler DC, ed. Nadas' Pediatric Cardiology, first edition. Hanley & Belfus, Inc., Mosby-Year Book, Inc., 1992.)

infant; echocardiography confirms the diagnosis and localizes the defect in the ventricular septum. Because a large number (as many as 90% depending on the anatomic type and size) of ventricular septal defects may close spontaneously in the first few months of life, surgery is usually deferred beyond the neonatal period. In large series, only 15% of all patients with ventricular septal defects ever become clinically symptomatic. Medical management of CHF includes digoxin, diuretics, and caloric supplementation. Growth failure is the most common symptom of CHF not fully compensated by medical management. When it occurs, failure to thrive is an indication for surgical repair of the defect.

F. Cardiac surgery in the neonate. In the past, because of the perceived high risk of open-heart surgery early in life, critically ill neonates were mostly subjected to palliative procedures or prolonged medical management. The unrepaired circulation and residual hemodynamic abnormalities frequently resulted in secondary problems of the heart, lungs, brain, as well as more nonspecific problems of failure to thrive, frequent hospitalizations, and infections. In addition, there are difficult-to-quantitate psychologic burdens to the family of a chronically ill infant.

Low birth weight should not be considered an absolute contraindication for surgical repair. In one series, prolonged medical therapy in low birth weight infants to achieve further weight gain in the presence of a significant hemodynamic burden did not improve the survival rate, and prolonged intensive care management was associated with nosocomial complication. We feel that the symptomatic neonate with congenital heart disease should be repaired as early as possible, to prevent the secondary sequelae of the congenital lesion on the heart, lungs, and brain.

Recently, improvements in surgical techniques, cardiopulmonary bypass, and intensive care of the neonate and infant have resulted in significant improvements in surgical mortality and quality of life in the survivors. It is beyond the scope of this chapter to describe the multiple surgical procedures currently employed in the management of congenital heart disease; the reader is referred to Table 25.9 and general texts of cardiac surgery.

VI. ACQUIRED HEART DISEASE

A. Myocarditis may occur in the neonate as an isolated illness or as a component of a generalized illness with associated hepatitis and/or encephalitis. Myocarditis is usually the result of a viral infection (coxsackie, rubella, and varicella are most common), although other infectious agents such as bacteria and fungi as well as noninfectious conditions such as autoimmune diseases also may cause myocarditis. Although the clinical presentation (and in some cases endomyocardial biopsy) makes the diagnosis, specific identification of the etiologic agent is currently not made in most cases.

The infant with acute myocarditis presents with signs and symptoms of CHF (see III.B.1) and/or arrhythmia (see VIII). The course of the illness is frequently fulminant and fatal; however, full recovery of ventricular function may occur if the infant can be supported and survive the acute illness. Supportive care including supplemental oxygen, diuretics, inotropic agents, afterload reduction, and mechanical ventilation is frequently used. In severe cases, mechanical support of the myocardium with ECMO or ventricular assist devices can be considered. Care should be used when administering digoxin, due to the potential for the potentiation of arrhythmias or complete heart block (CHB).

B. Transient myocardial ischemia with myocardial dysfunction may occur in any neonate with a history of perinatal asphyxia. Myocardial dysfunction may be associated with maternal autoimmune disease such as systemic lupus erythematosus. A tricuspid or mitral regurgitant murmur is often heard. An elevated serum creatine kinase MB fraction or cardiac troponin level may be helpful in determining the presence of myocardial damage. Supportive treatment is dictated by the severity of myocardial dysfunction.

C. Hypertrophic and dilated cardiomyopathies represent a rare and multifactorial complex of diseases, complete discussion of which is beyond the scope of this chapter. The differential diagnoses includes primary diseases (e.g., genetic causes as well as metabolic, storage, and neuromuscular disorders) or secondary diseases

TABLE 25.9

Common Neonatal Operations and Their Early Sequelae

Lesion	Surgical repair (Eponym)	Early postoperative sequelae	
		Common	Rare
Corrective procedures			
TGA	Arterial switch procedure (Jatene) **1.** Division and reanastomosis of PA to RV and aorta to LV (anatomically correct ventricles) **2.** Translocation of coronary arteries **3.** Closure of septal defects if present	Transient decrease in cardiac output 6–12 h after surgery	Coronary ostial stenosis or occlusion/sudden death Hemidiaphragm paresis Chylothorax
	Atrial switch procedure (Senning or Mustard) **1.** Intra-atrial baffling of systemic venous return to LV (to PA) and pulmonary venous return to RV(to AO) **2.** Closure of septal defects if present	Supraventricular tachycardia Sick sinus syndrome Tricuspid regurgitation	Pulmonary or systemic venous obstruction
TOF	**1.** Patch closure of VSD through ventriculotomy or right atrium **2.** Enlargement of RVOT with infundibular patch or muscle bundle resection **3.** ±Pulmonary valvotomy **4.** ±Transannular RV to PA patch **5.** ±RVto PA conduit	Pulmonary regurgitation (if transannular patch, valvotomy, or nonvalved conduit) Transient RV dysfunction Right-to-left shunt through PFO, usually resolves post- operatively as RV function improves	Residual left-to-right shunt at VSD patch Residual RVOT obstruction Junctional ectopic tachycardia Complete heart block

(continued)

TABLE 25.9 *(Continued)*

Lesion	Surgical repair (Eponym)	Early postoperative sequelae	
		Common	**Rare**
COA	Resection with end-to-end anastomosis, or Subclavian flap (Waldhaussen), or Patch augmentation	Systemic hypertension Absent left-arm pulse (if Waldhaussen)	Ileus Hemidiaphragm paresis Vocal cord paresis Chylothorax
PDA	Ligation (±division) of PDA using open thoracotomy and direct visualization or video-assisted thoracoscopic visualization	—	Hemidiaphragm paresis Vocal cord paresis Chylothorax Interruption of left PA or descending aorta
TAPVC	1. Reanastomosis of pulmonary venous confluence to posterior aspect of left atrium 2. Division of connecting vein	Pulmonary hypertension Transient low cardiac output	Residual pulmonary venous obstruction
Truncus arteriosus	1. Closure of VSD; baffling LV to truncus (neoaorta) 2. Removal of PAs from truncus 3. Conduit placement from RV to PAs	Reactive pulmonary hypertension Transient RV dysfunction with right-to-left shunt through PFO Hypocalcemia (DiGeorge syndrome)	Truncal valve stenosis or regurgitation Residual VSD Complete heart block

Palliative procedure			
HLHS*	Stage I (Norwood) **1.** Connection of main PA to aorta with reconstruction of aortic arch **2.** Systemic-to-pulmonary shunt **3.** Atrial septectomy	Low systemic cardiac output due to excessive pulmonary blood flow	Aortic arch obstruction Restrictive atrial septal defect
Complex lesions with decreased pulmonary blood flow*	Systemic-to-pulmonary shunt (using prosthetic tube = modified Blalock-Taussig shunt; using subclavian artery = classic Blalock-Taussig shunt)	Excessive pulmonary blood flow and mild congestive heart failure	Hemidiaphragm paresis Vocal cord paralysis Chylothorax Seroma
Complex lesions with excessive pulmonary blood flow*	Ligation of main PA, creation of systemic-to-pulmonary shunt PA band (prosthetic or Silastic constriction of main PA)	—	PA distortion Aneurysm of main PA

TGA = transposition of the great arteries; PA = pulmonary artery; RV = right ventricle; LV = left ventricle; AO = aorta; TOF = tetralogy of Fallot; VSD = ventricular septal detect; RVOT = right ventricular outflow tract; PFO = patent foramen ovale; PDA = patent ductus arteriosus; COA = coarctation of the aorta; TAPVC = total anomalous pulmonary venous connection; HLHS = hypoplastic left heart syndrome.

*In patients with a single ventricle, the goal is to separate pulmonary and systemic venous return, rerouting systemic venous blood directly to pulmonary arteries (Fontan operation) though this is done in late infancy or early childhood.

Source: Adapted from Wernovsky G, Erickson LC, Weasel DL. Cardiac emergencies. In: May HL, ed. *Emergency medicine.*, Boston: Little, Brown and Company, **1992**.

(e.g., end-stage infection, ischemic, endocrine, nutritional, drugs, etc.) The reader is referred to texts of pediatric cardiology for more complete discussion.

The most common hypertrophic cardiomyopathy presenting in neonates is that type seen in **infants born to diabetic mothers.** Echocardiographically and hemodynamically, these infants are indistinguishable from patients with other types of hypertrophic cardiomyopathy. They are different in one important respect: their cardiomyopathy will completely resolve in 6 to 12 months. Noting a systolic ejection murmur, with or without CHF, in the infant of a diabetic mother should raise the question of congenital heart disease including hypertrophic cardiomyopathy. Treatment is supportive addressing the infant's particular symptoms of CHF. Propranolol has been used successfully in some patients with severe obstruction. Most patients require no specific care and no long-term cardiac follow-up. (See Chap. 1)

VII. PHARMACOLOGY

A. PGE$_1$. PGE$_1$ has been used since the late 1970s to pharmacologically maintain patency of the ductus arteriosus in patients with duct-dependent systemic or pulmonary blood flow. PGE$_1$ must be administered as a continuous parenteral infusion. The usual starting dose is 0.05 to 0.1 µg/kg/minute. Once a therapeutic effect has been achieved, the dose may often be decreased to as low as 0.025 µg/kg/minute without loss of therapeutic effect. The response to PGE$_1$ is often immediate if patency of the ductus is important for the hemodynamic state of the infant. Failure to respond to PGE$_1$ may mean that the initial diagnosis was incorrect, the ductus is unresponsive to PGE$_1$ (usually only in an older infant), or the ductus is absent. The infusion site has no significant effect on the ductal response to PGE$_1$. Adverse reactions to PGE$_1$ include apnea (10%–12%), fever (14%), cutaneous flushing (10%), bradycardia (7%), seizures (4%), tachycardia (3%), cardiac arrest (1%), and edema (1%). See Table 25.10 for recommended mixing and dosing protocol for PGE$_1$.

B. Sympathomimetic amine infusions are the mainstay of pharmacologic therapies aimed at improving cardiac output and are discussed in detail elsewhere in this book. Catecholamines, endogenous (dopamine, epinephrine), or synthetic (dobutamine, isoproterenol), achieve an effect by stimulating myocardial and vascular adrenergic receptors. These agents must be given as a continuous parenteral infusion. They may be given in combination to the critically ill neonate in an effort to maximize the positive effects of each agent while minimizing the negative effects. While receiving catecholamine infusions, patients should be closely monitored, usually with an electrocardiographic monitor and an arterial catheter. Before beginning sympathomimetic amine infusions, intravascular volume should be repleted if necessary, although this may further compromise a congenital lesion with coexisting volume overload. Adverse reactions to catecholamine infusions include tachycardia (which increases myocardial oxygen consumption), atrial and

TABLE 25.10	**Suggested Preparation of Prostaglandin E$_1$**	
Add 1 ampule (500 µg/1 mL) to:	Concentration (µg/mL)	ml/hr X weight (kg), needed to infuse 0.1 µg/kg/min
200 mL	2.5	2.4
100 mL*	5	1.2
50 mL	10	0.6

*Usually the most convenient dilution, provides one-fourth of maintenance fluid requirement. Usually mix in dextrose-containing solution for newborns.
Source: Adapted from Wernovsky G, Erickson LC, Wessel DL. Cardiac emergencies. In: May HL, ed. *Emergency medicine.*, Boston: Little, Brown and Company, 1992.

Drug	Usual dose (µg/kg/min)	Effect
Dopamine	1–5	↑ urine output, ↑ HR (slightly), ↑ contractility
	6–10	↑ HR, ↑ contractility, ↑ BP
	11–20	↑ HR, ↑ contractility, ↑ SVR, ↑ BP
Dobutamine	1–20	↑ HR (slightly), ↑ contractility, ↓ SVR
Epinephrine	0.05–0.50	↑ HR, ↑ contractility, ↑ SVR, ↑ BP
Isoproterenol	0.05–1.00	↑ HR, ↑ contractility, ↓ SVR, ↓ PVR

These infusions may be mixed in intravenous solutions containing dextrose and/or saline. For neonates, dextrose-containing solutions with or without salt should usually be chosen. Calculation for convenient preparation of IV infusions:

$$6 \times \frac{\text{desired dose (µg/kg/min)}}{\text{desired rate (mL/h)}} \times \text{weight (kg)} = \frac{\text{mg drug}}{100\ \text{mL fluid}}$$

(HR = heart rate; BP = blood pressure; SVR = systemic vascular resistance; PVR = pulmonary vascular resistance.)

ventricular arrhythmias, and increased afterload due to peripheral vasoconstriction (which may decrease cardiac output). See Table 25.11 for recommended mixing and dosing of the sympathomimetic amines.

C. Afterload reducing agents

1. **Phosphodiesterase inhibitors** such as **milrinone** are **bipyridine** compounds that selectively inhibit cyclic nucleotide phosphodiesterase. These nonglycosidic and nonsympathomimetic agents exert their effect on cardiac performance by increasing cyclic adenosine monophosphate (cAMP) in the myocardial and vascular muscle, but do so independently of β-receptors. Cyclic AMP promotes improved contraction through calcium regulation through two mechanisms: (i) activation of protein kinase (which catalyzes the transfer of phosphate groups from adenosine triphosphate [ATP]) leading to faster calcium entry through the calcium channels, and (ii) activation of calcium pumps in the sarcoplasmic reticulum resulting in release of calcium.

   There are three major effects of phosphodiesterase inhibitors: (i) increased inotropy, with increased contractility and cardiac output as a result of cAMP-mediated increase in trans-sarcolemmal calcium flux; (ii) vasodilatation, with increase in arteriolar and venous capacitance as a result of cAMP-mediated increase in uptake of calcium and decrease in calcium available for contraction; and (iii) increased lusitropy, or improved relaxation properties during diastole.

   Indications for use include low cardiac output with myocardial dysfunction and elevated systemic vascular resistance (SVR) not accompanied by severe hypotension. Side effects have been minimal and are typically the need for volume infusions (5–10 mL/kg) following loading dose administration. See Appendix A for dosing information.

   The use of phosphodiesterase inhibitors after cardiac surgery in the pediatric patient population has been shown to increase cardiac index and decrease SVR without a significant increase in heart rate. Phosphodiesterase inhibitors are the second-line drug (after dopamine) in the treatment of low cardiac output in neonates, infants, and children following cardiopulmonary bypass in our institution.

2. **Other vasodilators** improve low cardiac output principally by decreasing impedance to ventricular ejection; these effects are especially helpful after cardiac surgery in children and in adults when SVR is particularly elevated.

   Sodium nitroprusside is the most widely used afterload reducing agent. It acts as a nitric oxide donor, increasing intracellular cyclic guanosine monophosphate (cGMP), which effects relaxation of vascular smooth muscle in both arterioles and veins. The overall effect is a decrease in atrial filling pressure and SVR with a concomitant increase in cardiac output. The vasodilatory effects of nitroprusside occur within minutes with intravenous administration. The principal metabolites of sodium nitroprusside are thiocyanate and cyanide; thiocyanate toxicity is unusual in children with normal hepatic and renal function, and monitoring of cyanide and thiocyanate concentrations in children may not be correlated with clinical signs of toxicity.

In neonates with low cardiac output, there may be an increase in urine output and improvement in perfusion with institution of nitroprusside, but there can also be a significant drop in blood pressure necessitating care in its use.

Many other agents have been used as arterial and venous vasodilators to treat hypertension, reduce ventricular afterload and SVR, and improve cardiac output. A second nitrovasodilator, **nitroglycerine,** principally **a venous dilator,** also has rapid onset of action and a short half-life ($\sim$2 minutes). Tolerance may develop after several days of continuous infusion. Nitroglycerine is used extensively in adult cardiac units for patients with ischemic heart disease; experience in pediatric patients is more limited. **Hydralazine** is more typically used for acute hypertension; its relatively long half-life limits its use in postoperative patients with labile hemodynamics. The angiotensin converting enzyme inhibitor **enalapril** similarly has a relatively long half-life (2–4 hours) which limits its use in the acute setting. β**-blockers** (e.g., propranolol, esmolol, labetolol), although excellent in reducing blood pressure, may have deleterious effects on ventricular function. **Calcium channel blockers** (e.g., verapamil) may cause hypotension and severe bradycardia in the neonate and should **rarely be used.** All intravenous vasodilators must be used cautiously in patients with moderate to severe lung disease; their use has been associated with increased intrapulmonary shunting and acute reductions of Pao_2.

D. Digoxin (see Appendix A) remains important for the treatment of CHF and arrhythmia. A "digitalizing dose" (with a total dose of 30 µg/kg in 24 hours for term infants and 20 µg/kg in 24 hours in premature infants) is usually only used for treatment of arrhythmias or severe heart failure. One-half of this **total digitalizing dose (TDD)** may be given IV, IM, or PO, followed by one-fourth of the TDD every 8 to 12 hours for the remaining two doses. An initial maintenance dose of one-fourth to one-third of the TDD (range 5–10 µg/kg/day) may then be adjusted according to the patient's clinical response, renal function, and tolerance for the drug (see Appendix A for further details). Infants with mild symptoms, primary myocardial disease, renal dysfunction, or the potential for atrioventricular block may be digitalized using only the maintenance dose (omitting the loading dose). The maintenance dose is divided into equal twice daily doses, 12 hours apart.

Digoxin toxicity most commonly manifests with gastrointestinal upset, somnolence, and sinus bradycardia. More severe digoxin toxicity may cause high-grade atrioventricular block and ventricular ectopy. Infants suspected of having digoxin toxicity should have a digoxin level drawn and further doses withheld. The therapeutic level is <1.5 ng/mL with probable toxicity occurring at levels >4.0 ng/mL. In infants particularly, however, digoxin levels do not always correlate well with therapeutic efficacy nor with toxicity.

Digoxin toxicity in neonates is usually manageable by withholding further doses until the signs of toxicity resolve and by correcting electrolyte abnormalities (such as hypokalemia), which can potentiate toxic effects. Severe ventricular arrhythmias associated with digoxin toxicity may be managed with phenytoin, 2 to 4 mg/kg over 5 minutes, or lidocaine, 1 mg/kg loading dose, followed by an infusion at 1 to 2 mg/kg per hour. Atrioventricular block is usually unresponsive to atropine. Severe bradycardia may be refractory to these therapies and require temporary cardiac pacing.

The use of digoxin-specific antibody Fab (antigen-binding fragments) preparation (Digibind; Burroughs Wellcome) is reserved for those patient with evidence of severe digoxin intoxication and clinical symptoms of refractory arrhythmia and/or atrioventricular block; in these patients it is quite effective. Calculation of the Digibind dose in milligrams is as follows: (serum digoxin concentration in nanograms per milliliter × 5.6 × the body weight in kilograms/1,000) × 64. The dose is given as a one-time intravenous infusion. A second dose of Digibind may be given to those patients who continue to have clinical evidence of residual toxicity. Skin testing for hypersensitivity is recommended before the first dose.

E. Diuretics (see Appendix A) are frequently used in patients with CHF often in combination with digoxin. **Furosemide,** 1 to 2 mg/kg per dose, usually results in a brisk diuresis within an hour of administration. If no response is noted in an hour, a second dose (double the first dose) may be given. Chronic use of furosemide may produce urinary-tract stones as a result of its calciuric effects. A more potent diuretic effect may be achieved using a combination of a thiazide and a "loop" diuretic such as furosemide. Combination diuretic therapy may be complicated by hyponatremia and hypokalemia. Oral or intravenous potassium supplementation (3–4 mEq/kg/day) or an aldosterone antagonist usually should accompany the use of thiazide and/or "loop" diuretics to avoid excessive potassium wasting. It is important to carefully monitor serum potassium and sodium levels when beginning or changing the dose of diuretic medications. When changing from an effective parenteral to oral dose of furosemide, the dose should be increased by 50% to 80%. Furosemide may increase the nephro- and ototoxicity of concurrently used aminoglycoside antibiotics. Detailed discussion of alternative diuretics (e.g., chlorothiazide, spironolactone, etc.) is found elsewhere in the text (see Appendix A).

VIII. ARRHYTHMIAS

A. Initial evaluation. When evaluating any infant with an arrhythmia it is essential to simultaneously assess the electrophysiology and hemodynamic status. If the baby is poorly perfused and/or hypotensive, reliable intravenous access should be secured and a level of resuscitation employed appropriate for the degree of illness. As always, **emergency treatment of shock should precede definitive diagnosis.** It should be emphasized, however, there is **rarely** a situation in which it is justified to omit a 12-lead ECG from the evaluation of an infant with an arrhythmia, the exceptions being ventricular fibrillation or torsade de pointes with accompanying hemodynamic instability. These arrhythmias frequently require immediate defibrillation but are extremely rare arrhythmias in neonates and young infants.

In nearly all circumstances, appropriate therapy (short- and long-term) depends on an accurate electrophysiologic diagnosis. Determination of the mechanism of a rhythm disturbance is most often made from a 12-lead ECG in the abnormal rhythm compared to the patient's baseline 12-lead ECG in sinus rhythm. Although rhythm strips generated from a cardiac monitor can be helpful supportive evidence of the final diagnosis, they are typically **not** diagnostic and should **not** be the only documentation of arrhythmia if at all possible.

The three broad categories for arrhythmias in neonates are (i) tachyarrhythmias, (ii) bradyarrhythmias, and (iii) irregular rhythms. An algorithm for approaching the differential diagnosis of tachyarrhythmias can be consulted (see Fig. 25.17) in most cases. When analyzing the ECG for the mechanism of arrhythmia, a stepwise approach should be taken in three main areas: (i) **rate** (variable, too fast, or too slow); (ii) **rhythm** (regular or irregular, paroxysmal or gradual); and (iii) **QRS morphology.**

B. Differential diagnosis and initial management in the hemodynamically stable patient

1. Narrow QRS complex tachycardias

a. SVTs are the most common symptomatic arrhythmias in all children including neonates. SVTs usually have (i) a rate >200 beats/minute, frequently "fixed" with no beat-to-beat variation in rate; (ii) rapid onset and termination (in reentrant rhythms); and (iii) normal ventricular complexes on the surface ECG. The infant may initially be asymptomatic, but later may

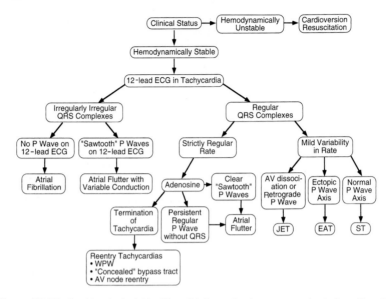

Figure 25.17. Algorithm for bedside differential diagnosis of narrow complex tachycardias, the most common type of arrhythmia in neonates. Note that, regardless of the mechanism of tachycardia, if the patient is hemodynamically unstable, immediate measures to resuscitate the infant including cardioversion are required. Also, treatment with adenosine is helpful therapeutically as well as diagnostically. In general, tachycardias that terminate (even briefly) after adenosine are of the reentry type. ECG = electrocardiogram; JET = junctional ectopic tachycardia; EAT = ectopic atrial tachycardia; ST = sinus tachycardia; WPW = Wolff-Parkinson-White syndrome.

become irritable, fussy, and refuse feedings. CHF usually does not develop before 24 hours of continuous SVT; however, heart failure is seen in 20% of patients after 36 hours and in 50% after 48 hours.

SVT in the neonate is almost always "reentrant," involving either an accessory atrioventricular pathway and the atrioventricular node, or due to atrial flutter. Approximately half the number of these patients will manifest preexcitation (delta wave) on the ECG when not in tachycardia (WPW syndrome, see Fig. 25.18). In rarer cases, the reentrant circuit may be within the atrium itself (atrial flutter) or within the atrial ventricular (AV) node

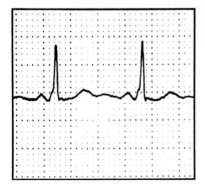

Figure 25.18. Wolff-Parkinson-White syndrome. Note the characteristic "slurred" initial QRS deflection and short PR interval that can occur in any lead; lead I only pictured here.

(AV node reentrant tachycardia). Patients with SVT may have associated structural heart disease; evaluation for structural heart disease should be considered in all neonates with SVT. Another rare cause of SVTs in a neonate is ectopic atrial tachycardia, in which the distinguishing features are an abnormal P wave axis, normal QRS axis, and significant variability in the overall rate.

Long-term medical therapy for SVT in the neonate is based on the underlying electrophysiologic diagnosis. For patients without demonstrable WPW syndrome, **digoxin** is the initial therapy in patients without CHF. Digitalization is described in section VII.D and Appendix A. Vagal maneuvers (facial/malar ice wrapped in a towel to elicit the "diving reflex") may be tried in stable neonates. Direct pressure over the eyes should be avoided. Parenteral digitalization usually abolishes the arrhythmia within 10 hours. If digoxin successfully maintains the patient in sinus rhythm, it typically is continued for 6 to 12 months. Although digoxin has long been the mainstay of treatment for SVT, reliance on this drug acutely has decreased, as more efficacious and faster-acting agents have become available such as β-blockers.

Digoxin is avoided in chronic management of WPW syndrome because of its potential for enhancing antegrade conduction across the accessory pathway. **Propranolol** is used as the initial and chronic drug therapy for patients with SVT due to the WPW syndrome, to avoid the potential facilitation of antegrade (atrioventricular) conduction through the accessory pathway. Treatment with propranolol may be associated with apnea and hypoglycemia; therefore neonates started on propranolol, especially premature infants, should be observed on a continuous cardiac monitor and have serial serum glucose checks for 1 to 2 days.

The addition or substitution of other antiarrhythmic drugs such as amiodarone alone or in combination may be necessary and should be done only in consultation with a pediatric cardiologist. In neonates, **verapamil should only rarely be used** because it has been associated with sudden death in babies.

In utero **SVT** may be suspected when a very rapid fetal heart rate is noted by the obstetrician during prenatal care. The diagnosis is confirmed by fetal echocardiography. At that time, an initial search for congenital heart disease and fetal hydrops may be made. *In utero* treatment of the immature fetus with SVT may be accomplished by treatment of the mother with antiarrhythmic drugs that cross the placenta. Digoxin, flecainide, and other anti-arrhythmic drugs have been successful therapies. Failure to control the fetal SVT in the presence of fetal hydrops is an indication for delivery. Cesarean delivery of an infant in persistent SVT may be necessary, as the fetal heart rate will not be a reliable indicator of fetal distress.

  b. **Sinus tachycardia** in the neonate is defined as persistent heart rate >2 standard deviations above the mean for age with normal ECG complexes including a normal P wave morphology and axis. Sinus tachycardia is common and occurs particularly in response to systemic events such as anemia, stress, fever, high levels of circulating catecholamines, hypovolemia, and xanthine (e.g., aminophylline) toxicity. An important clue to the existence of sinus tachycardia, in addition to its normal ECG morphology, is that the rate is not fixed but rather will vary by 10% to 20% over time. Medical management consists of identifying and treating the underlying cause.

2. **Wide-complex tachycardias**
  a. **Ventricular tachycardia** in the neonate is relatively rare and is usually associated with severe medical illnesses including hypoxemia, shock, electrolyte disturbances, digoxin toxicity, and catecholamine toxicity. It may rarely be due to an abnormality of the electrical conducting system of the heart such as prolonged QTc syndrome and intramyocardial tumors. Wide and frequently bizarre QRS complexes with a rapid rate are diagnostic;

this ECG pattern may be simulated by SVT in patients with WPW syndrome, in whom there is antegrade conduction through the anomalous pathway (SVT with "aberration"). Ventricular tachycardia is a potentially unstable rhythm commonly with hemodynamic consequences. The underlying cause should be rapidly sought and treated. The hemodynamically stable patient should be treated with a lidocaine bolus, 1 to 2 mg/kg, followed by a lidocaine infusion, 20–50 µg/kg/minute. Direct current cardioversion (starting dose to 1–2 J/kg) should be used if the patient is hemodynamically compromised, though will frequently be ineffective in the presence of acidosis. If a severe acidosis (pH <7.2) is present, it should be treated with hyperventilation and/or sodium bicarbonate before cardioversion. Phenytoin, 2 to 4 mg/kg, may be effective if the arrhythmia is due to digoxin toxicity (see VII.D).

b. Ventricular fibrillation in the neonate is almost always an agonal (preterminal) arrhythmia. There is a coarse irregular pattern on ECG with no identifiable QRS complexes. There are no peripheral pulses or heart sounds on examination. Cardiopulmonary resuscitation should be instituted and defibrillation (starting dose 1–2J/Kg) performed. A bolus of lidocaine, 1 mg/kg, followed by a lidocaine infusion should be started. Once the infant has been resuscitated, the underlying problems should be evaluated and treated.

3. Bradycardia

a. Sinus bradycardia in the neonate is not uncommon especially during sleep or during vagal maneuvers, such as bowel movements. If the infant's perfusion and blood pressure are normal, transient bradycardia is not of major concern. Persistent sinus bradycardia may be secondary to hypoxemia, acidosis, and elevated intracranial pressure. Finally, a stable sinus bradycardia may occur with digoxin toxicity, hypothyroidism, or sinus node dysfunction (usually a complication of cardiac surgery).

b. Heart block

i. First-degree atrioventricular block occurs when the PR interval is >0.15 seconds. In the neonate, first-degree atrioventricular block may be due to a nonspecific conduction disturbance; medications (e.g., digoxin); myocarditis; hypothyroidism; or associated with certain types of congenital heart disease (e.g., complete atrioventricular canal or ventricular inversion). No specific treatment is generally indicated.

ii. Second-degree atrioventricular block. Second-degree atrioventricular block refers to **intermittent** failure of conduction of the atrial impulse to the ventricles. Two types have been described: (i) Mobitz I (Wenckebach phenomenon) and (ii) Mobitz II (intermittent failure to conduct P waves, with a constant PR interval). Second-degree atrioventricular block may occur with SVT, digitalis toxicity, or a nonspecific conduction disturbance. No specific treatment is usually necessary other than diagnosis and treatment of the underlying cause.

iii. CHB refers to **complete** absence of conduction of any atrial activity to the ventricles. CHB typically has a slow, constant ventricular rate that is independent of the atrial rate. CHB is frequently detected *in utero* as fetal bradycardia. Although CHB may be secondary to surgical trauma, **congenital** CHB falls into two main categories. The most common causes include (i) anatomic defects (ventricular inversion and complete atrioventricular canal) and (ii) fetal exposure to maternal antibodies related to systemic rheumatologic disease such as lupus erythematosus. The presence of CHB without structural heart disease should alert the clinician to investigate the mother for rheumatologic disease. In cases of *in utero* CHB caused by maternal antibodies related to lupus erythematosus the prognosis may be poor. If there is a high risk of developing CHB (previous fetus with CHB, miscarriage, abnormal fetal echocardiography) treatment in pregnancy with dexamethasone, azathioprine, IV gamma globulin or plasmapheresis should be considered.

Symptoms related to CHB are related both to the severity of the associated cardiac malformation (when present) and the degree of bradycardia. Fortunately, the fetus with CHB adapts well by increasing stroke volume, and will usually come to term without difficulty. Infants with isolated congenital CHB usually have a heart rate >50 beats/minute, are asymptomatic, and grow normally.

   4. **Irregular rhythms**
      a. **Premature atrial contractions (PACs, see Fig. 25.19)** are common in neonates, are usually benign, and do not require specific therapy. Most PACs

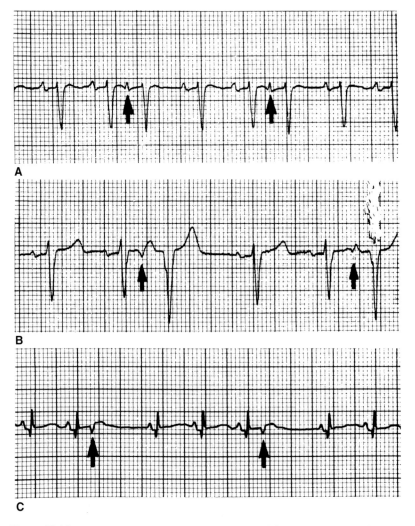

Figure 25.19. Premature atrial contractions (*arrows*) causing: **(A)** early ventricular depolarization with a normal QRS complex; **(B)** early ventricular depolarization with "aberration" of the QRS complex; **(C)** block at the atrioventricular node. (Fyler DC, ed. Nadas' Pediatric Cardiology, first edition. Hanley & Belfus, Inc., Mosby-Year Book, Inc., 1992.)

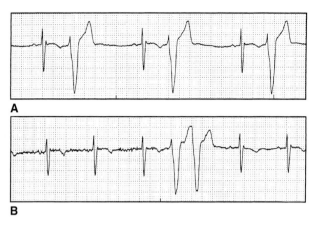

Figure 25.20. Premature ventricular contractions. **A:** PVCs alternating with normal sinus beats (ventricular bigeminy) are usually not indicative of significant pathology. **B:** Paired PVCs ("couplet") are a potentially more serious rhythm and require further investigation.

result in a normal QRS morphology (Fig. 25.19A), distinguishing them from premature ventricular contractions (PVCs). If the PAC occurs while the atrioventricular node is partially repolarized, an aberrantly conducted ventricular depolarization pattern may be observed on the surface ECG (Fig. 25.19B). If the premature beat occurs when the atrioventricular node is refractory (i.e., early in the cardiac cycle, occurring soon after the normal sinus beat), the impulse will not be conducted to the ventricle ("blocked") and may therefore give the appearance of a marked sinus bradycardia (Fig. 25.19C).

b. Premature ventricular contractions (PVCs, see Fig. 25.20) are "wide QRS complex" beats that occur when a ventricular focus stimulates a spontaneous beat before the normally conducted sinus beat. Isolated PVCs are not uncommon in the normal neonate and do not generally require treatment. Although PVCs frequently occur sporadically, they occasionally are grouped, such as every other beat (bigeminy, Fig. 25.20A), every third beat (trigeminy), etc. These more frequent PVCs are typically no more worrisome than isolated PVCs, though their greater frequency usually prompts a more extensive diagnostic workup. PVCs may be caused by digoxin toxicity, hypoxemia, electrolyte disturbances, catecholamine, or xanthine toxicity. PVCs occurring in groups of two or more (i.e., couplets, triplets, etc; Fig. 25.20B) are pathologic and "high grade"; they may be a marker for myocarditis or myocardial dysfunction and further evaluation should be strongly considered.

C. Emergency treatment in the hemodynamically compromised patient. With all therapies described in the following, it is important to have easily accessible resuscitation equipment available before proceeding with these antiarrhythmic interventions.

1. Tachycardias

a. Adenosine. Adenosine has become the drug of choice for acute management. Adenosine transiently blocks AV node conduction, allowing termination of rapid reentrant rhythms involving the AV node. It must be given by very rapid intravenous push because its half-life is 10 seconds or less. Due to this short half-life, adenosine is a relatively safe medication; however, it has been reported to cause transient AV block severe enough to require pacing (albeit briefly) so it should be used with caution and in consultation with a pediatric cardiologist. Adenosine, by virtue of its acute action on the AV node, is frequently **diagnostic** as well. Patients who respond with abrupt termination of the SVT have reentrant tachycardias involving the AV node; those with SVT due to atrial flutter will have acute AV block and easily visible flutter waves with reappearance of SVT in 10 to 15 seconds.

   b. **Cardioversion.** In the hemodynamically unstable patient, the **first** line of therapy is synchronized direct current cardioversion. The energy should start at 1 J/kg and be increased by a factor of 2 if unsuccessful. Care should be taken to avoid skin burns and arcing of the current outside the body by only using electrical transmission gel with the paddles. Paddle position should be anterior–posterior if possible.

   c. **Transesophageal pacing.** When available, esophageal overdrive pacing is a very effective maneuver for terminating tachyarrhythmias. The close proximity of the left atrium to the distal esophagus allows electrical impulses generated in the esophagus to be transmitted to atrial tissue; burst pacing may then terminate reentrant tachyarrhythmias.

2. **Bradycardias.** Therapeutic options for treating a symptomatic bradyarrhythmia are more limited. A transvenous pacemaker is a temporary measure in severely symptomatic neonates while preparing for placement of permanent epicardial pacemaker leads; however, transvenous pacing in a small neonate is technically difficult and frequently requires fluoroscopy. A number of transcutaneous pacemakers (Zoll) are available but long-term use must be avoided due to cutaneous burns. An isoproterenol infusion may temporarily increase the ventricular rate and cardiac output in an infant with CHF. The treatment of choice for sinus node dysfunction is transesophageal pacing at an appropriate rate, but this can only be accomplished with intact atrioventricular conduction and is not effective in patients with CHB. For the infant with transient bradycardia (due to increased vagal tone), intravenous atropine may be used.

Suggested Readings

Aranda JV, Thomas R. Systemic review: Intravenous ibuprofen in preterm newborns. *Semin Perinatol* 2006;30(3):114–120.

Allen HD, Gutgesell HP, Clark EB, et al. *Moss and Adams' heart disease in infants, children and adolescents including the fetus and young adult,* 6th ed. Philadelphia: Lippincott Williams & Wilkins, 2001.

Fyler DC. Report of the New England regional infant cardiac program. *Pediatrics* 1980;65(Suppl):377–461.

Hoffman JIE, Kaplan S. The incidence of congenital heart disease. *J Am Coll Cardiol* 2002; 39(12):1890–1900.

Jonas RA, DiNardo J, Laussen PC, et al. *Comprehensive surgical management of congenital heart disease.* Hodder Arnold, 2004.

Keane JF, Fyler DC, Lock JE. *Nadas' pediatric cardiology,* 2nd ed. WB Saunders, 2006.

Kovalchin JP, Silverman NH. The impact of fetal echocardiography. *Pediatr Cardiol* 2004;25(3):299–306.

Liske MR, Greeley CS, Law DJ, et al. Report of the tennessee task force on screening newborn infants for critical congenital heart disease. *Pediatrics* 2006;118(4):e1250–e1256.

Mavroudis C, Backer C. *Pediatric cardiac surgery,* 3rd ed. Mosby, 2003.

Rein AJ, Omokhodion SI, Nir A, et al. Significance of a cardiac murmur as the sole clinical sign in the newborn. *Clin Pediatr* 2000;39(9):511–520.

Saar P, Hermann W, Muller-Ladner U, et al. Connective tissue diseases and pregnancy. *Rheumatology* 2006;45:iii30–iii32.

Shah SS, Ohlsson A. Ibuprofen for the prevention of PDA in preterm and/or low birth weight infants. *Cochrane Database Syst Rev* 2006;(1):CD004213.

Tworetzky W, Wilkins-Haug L, Jennings RW, et al. Balloon dilation of severe aortic stenosis in the fetus; potential for prevention of hypoplastic left heart syndrome: Candidate selection, technique, and results of successful intervention. *Circulation* 2004;110(15):2125–2131.

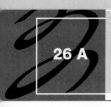

ANEMIA
Helen A. Christou, Kevin Shannon, and David H. Rowitch

26 A

I. HEMATOLOGIC PHYSIOLOGY OF THE NEWBORN (1–5). Significant changes occur in the red blood cell (RBC) mass of an infant during the neonatal period and ensuing months. The evaluation of anemia must take into account this developmental process, as well as the infant's physiologic needs.

A. Normal development: the physiologic anemia of infancy (1)

1. *In utero*, the fetal aortic oxygen saturation is 45%; erythropoietin levels are high, RBC production is rapid. The fetal liver is the major site of erythropoietin production.

2. After birth, the oxygen saturation is 95%, and erythropoietin is undetectable. RBC production by day 7 is <1/10th the level *in utero*. Reticulocyte counts are low, and the hemoglobin level falls (see Table 26A.1).

3. Despite dropping hemoglobin levels, the ratio of hemoglobin A to hemoglobin F increases, and the levels of 2,3-diphosphoglycerate (2,3-DPG) (which interacts with hemoglobin A to decrease its affinity for oxygen, thereby enhancing oxygen release to the tissues) are high. As a result, oxygen delivery to the tissues actually increases. This physiologic "anemia" is not a functional anemia in that oxygen delivery to the tissues is adequate. Iron from degraded RBCs is stored.

4. At 8 to 12 weeks, hemoglobin levels reach their nadir (see Table 26A.2), oxygen delivery to the tissues is impaired, renal erythropoietin production is stimulated, and RBC production increases.

5. Infants who have received transfusions in the neonatal period have lower nadirs than normal because of their higher percentage of hemoglobin A (1).

6. During this period of active erythropoiesis, iron stores are rapidly utilized. The reticuloendothelial system has adequate iron for 15 to 20 weeks in term infants. After this time, the hemoglobin level decreases if iron is not supplied.

B. Anemia of prematurity is an exaggeration of the normal physiologic anemia (Tables 26A.1 and 26A.2).

1. RBC mass and iron stores are decreased because of low birthweight; however, hemoglobin concentrations are similar in preterm and term infants.

2. The hemoglobin nadir is reached earlier than in the term infant because of the following:

   a. RBC survival is decreased in comparison with the term infant.

   b. There is a relatively more rapid rate of growth in premature babies than in term infants. For example, a premature infant gaining 150 g/week requires approximately a 12 mL/week increase in total blood volume.

   c. Many preterm infants have reduced red cell mass and iron stores because of iatrogenic phlebotomy for laboratory tests.

   d. Vitamin E deficiency is common in small premature infants, unless the vitamin is supplied exogenously.

3. The hemoglobin nadir in premature babies is lower than in term infants because erythropoietin is produced by the term infant at a hemoglobin level of 10 to 11 g/dL but is produced by the premature infant at a hemoglobin level of 7 to 9 g/dL. Many preterm infants have reduced red cell mass and iron stores because of iatrogenic phlebotomy for laboratory tests. This reflects the lower oxygen requirements in healthy preterm infants rather than a defect in erythropoietin production (1).

436

| TABLE 26A.1 | Hemoglobin Changes in Babies in the First Year of Life |

Week	Hemoglobin level		
	Term babies	Premature babies (1,200–2,500 g)	Small premature babies (<1,200 g)
0	17.0	16.4	16.0
1	18.8	16.0	14.8
3	15.9	13.5	13.4
6	12.7	10.7	9.7
10	11.4	9.8	8.5
20	12.0	10.4	9.0
50	12.0	11.5	11.0

Source: From Glader B, Naiman JL. Erythrocyte disorders in infancy. In: Taeusch HW, Ballard RA, Avery ME, eds. *Diseases of the newborn*, Philadelphia: WB Saunders, 1991.

4. Iron administration before the age of 10 to 14 weeks does not increase the nadir of the hemoglobin level or diminish its rate of reduction. However, this iron is stored for later use.

5. Once the nadir is reached, RBC production is stimulated, and iron stores are rapidly depleted because less iron is stored in the premature infant than in the term infant.

II. ETIOLOGY OF ANEMIA IN THE NEONATE (6)

A. Blood loss is manifested by a decreased or normal hematocrit (Hct), increased or normal reticulocyte count, and a normal bilirubin level (unless the hemorrhage is retained) (4,5). If blood loss is recent (e.g., at delivery), the Hct and reticulocyte count may be normal and the infant may be in shock. The Hct will fall later because of hemodilution. If the bleeding is chronic, the Hct will be low, the reticulocyte count up, and the baby normovolemic.

1. Obstetric causes of blood loss, including the following malformations of placenta and cord:
   a. Abruptio placentae.
   b. Placenta previa.
   c. Incision of placenta at cesarean section.

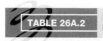

| TABLE 26A.2 | Hemoglobin Nadir in Babies in the First Year of Life |

Maturity of baby at birth	Hemoglobin level at nadir	Time of nadir (wk)
Term babies	9.5–11.0	6–12
Premature babies (1,200–2,500 g)	8.0–10.0	5–10
Small premature babies (<1,200 g)	6.5–9.0	4–8

Source: From Glader B, Naiman JL. Erythrocyte disorders in infancy. In: Taeusch HW, Ballard RA, Avery ME, eds. *Diseases of the newborn*. Philadelphia: WB Saunders, 1991.

    d. Rupture of anomalous vessels (e.g., vasa previa, velamentous insertion of cord, or rupture of communicating vessels in a multilobed placenta).

    e. Hematoma of cord caused by varices or aneurysm.

    f. Rupture of cord (more common in short cords and in dysmature cords).

  2. Occult blood loss

    a. Fetomaternal bleeding may be chronic or acute. It occurs in 8% of all pregnancies, and in 1% of pregnancies the volume may be as large as 40 mL. The diagnosis of this problem is by Kleihauer-Betke stain of maternal smear for fetal cells (2). Chronic fetal-to-maternal transfusion is suggested by a reticulocyte count >10%. Many conditions may predispose to this type of bleeding:

      i. Placental malformations—chorioangioma or choriocarcinoma.

      ii. Obstetric procedures—traumatic amniocentesis, external cephalic version, internal cephalic version, breech delivery.

      iii. Spontaneous fetomaternal bleeding.

    b. Fetoplacental bleeding

      i. Chorioangioma or choriocarcinoma with placental hematoma.

      ii. Cesarean section, with infant held above the placenta.

      iii. Tight nuchal cord or occult cord prolapse.

    c. Twin-to-twin transfusion

  3. Bleeding in the neonatal period may be due to the following causes:

    a. Intracranial bleeding associated with:

      i. Prematurity.

      ii. Second twin.

      iii. Breech delivery.

      iv. Rapid delivery.

      v. Hypoxia.

    b. Massive cephalhematoma, subgaleal hemorrhage, or hemorrhagic caput succedaneum.

    c. Retroperitoneal bleeding.

    d. Ruptured liver or spleen.

    e. Adrenal or renal hemorrhage.

    f. Gastrointestinal bleeding:

      i. Peptic ulcer.

      ii. Necrotizing enterocolitis.

      iii. Nasogastric catheter.

      iv. Maternal blood swallowed from delivery or breast should be ruled out by the Apt test (see Chap. 26B).

    g. Bleeding from umbilicus.

  4. Iatrogenic causes. Excessive blood loss may result from blood sampling with inadequate replacement.

B. Hemolysis is manifested by a decreased Hct, increased reticulocyte count, and an increased bilirubin level (1,2).

  1. Immune hemolysis (see Chap. 18)

    a. Rh incompatibility.

    b. ABO incompatibility.

    c. Minor blood group incompatibility (e.g., c, E, Kell, Duffy).

    d. Maternal disease (e.g., lupus), autoimmune hemolytic disease, rheumatoid arthritis (positive direct Coombs test in mother and newborn, no antibody to common red cell antigen Rh, AB, etc.), or drugs (e.g., penicillin antibodies in mother or infant, child on penicillin) (7).

  2. Hereditary RBC disorders

    a. RBC membrane defects such as spherocytosis, elliptocytosis, or stomatocytosis.

    b. Metabolic defects — glucose-6-phosphate dehydrogenase (G6PD) deficiency (significant neonatal hemolysis due to G6PD deficiency is usually seen only in Mediterranean or Asian G6PD-deficient men; blacks in the United States have a 10% incidence of G6PD deficiency but rarely have significant neonatal problems unless an infection or drug is operative), pyruvate-kinase deficiency, 5'-nucleotidase deficiency, and glucose-phosphate isomerase deficiency.

   c. Hemoglobinopathies

     i. α- and γ-Thalassemia syndromes.

     ii. α- and γ-Chain structural abnormalities.

  3. Acquired hemolysis

    a. Infection — bacterial or viral.

    b. Disseminated intravascular coagulation.

    c. Vitamin E deficiency and other nutritional anemias (1).

    d. Microangiopathic hemolytic anemia hemangioma, renal artery stenosis, and severe coarctation of the aorta.

 C. Diminished RBC production is manifested by a decreased Hct, decreased reticulocyte count, and normal bilirubin level.

  1. Diamond-Blackfan syndrome.

  2. Congenital leukemia or other tumor.

  3. Infections, especially rubella and parvovirus (see Chap. 23).

  4. Osteopetrosis, leading to inadequate erythropoiesis.

  5. Drug-induced suppression of RBC production.

  6. Physiologic anemia or anemia of prematurity (see I.A and I.B).

III. DIAGNOSTIC APPROACH TO ANEMIA IN THE NEWBORN (see Table 26A.3)

 A. The **family history** should include questions about anemia, jaundice, gallstones, and splenectomy.

 B. The **obstetric history** should be evaluated.

 C. The **physical examination** may reveal an associated abnormality and provide clues to the origin of the anemia.

  1. Acute blood loss leads to shock, with cyanosis, poor perfusion, and acidosis.

  2. Chronic blood loss produces pallor, but the infant may exhibit only mild symptoms of respiratory distress or irritability.

  3. Chronic hemolysis is associated with pallor, jaundice, and hepatosplenomegaly.

 D. Complete blood cell count. Capillary blood Hct is 3.7% to 2.7% higher than venous Hct. Warming the foot reduced the difference from 3.9% to 1.9% (1,2).

 E. Reticulocyte count (elevated with chronic blood loss and hemolysis, depressed with infection and production defect).

 F. Blood smear (Table 26A.3).

 G. Coombs test and bilirubin level.

 H. Apt test (see Chap. 26B) on gastrointestinal blood of uncertain origin.

 I. Kleihauer-Betke preparation of the mother's blood. A 50-mL loss of fetal blood into the maternal circulation will show up as 1% fetal cells in the maternal circulation (2).

 J. Ultrasound of abdomen and head.

 K. Parental testing — complete blood cell count, smear, and RBC indices are useful screening studies. Osmotic fragility testing and RBC enzyme levels (e.g., G6PD, pyruvate kinase) may be helpful in selected cases.

 L. Studies for infection (toxoplasmosis, rubella, cytomegalovirusand herpes simplex [TORCH]; see Chap. 23).

 M. Bone marrow (rarely used except in cases of bone marrow failure from hypoplasia or tumor).

IV. THERAPY

 A. Transfusion (see Chap. 26E)

  1. Indications for transfusion. The decision to transfuse must be made in consideration of the infant's condition and physiologic needs (8).

   a. Infants with significant respiratory disease or congenital heart disease (e.g., large left-to-right shunt) may need their Hct maintained above 40%. Transfusion with adult RBCs provides the added benefit of lowered oxygen affinity, which augments oxygen delivery to tissues. Blood should be fresh (3 to 7 days' old) to ensure adequate 2,3-DPG levels.

   b. Healthy, asymptomatic newborns will self-correct a mild anemia, provided that iron intake is adequate.

TABLE 26A.3 Classification of Anemia in the Newborn

Reticulocytes	Bilirubin	Coombs test	RBC morphology	Diagnostic possibilities
Normal or ↓	Normal	Negative	Normal	Physiologic anemia of infancy or prematurity; congenital hypoplastic anemia; other causes of decreased production
Normal or ↑	Normal	Negative	Normal	Acute hemorrhage (fetomaternal, placental, umbilical cord, or internal hemorrhage)
↑	↑	Positive	Hypochromic microcytes	Chronic fetomaternal hemorrhage
			Spherocytes	Immune hemolysis (blood group incompatibility or maternal autoantibody)
Normal or ↑	↑	Negative	Spherocytes	Hereditary spherocytosis
			Elliptocytes	Hereditary elliptocytosis
			Hypochromic microcytes	α- or γ-Thalassemia syndrome
			Spiculated RBCs	Pyruvate-kinase deficiency
			Schistocytes and RBC fragments	Disseminated intravascular coagulation; other microangiopathic processes
			Bite cells (Heinz bodies with supravital stain)	Glucose-6-phosphate dehydrogenase deficiency
			Normal	Infections; enclosed hemorrhage (cephalohematoma)

↓ = decreased; ↑ = increased; RBC = red blood cell.
Source: Adapted from the work of Dr. Glader B. Director of Division of hematology-oncology. California: Children's Hospital at Stanford 1991 (3).

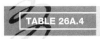

TABLE 26A.4	**Transfusion Guidelines for Premature Infants**

1. Asymptomatic infants with Hct <21% and reticulocytes <100, 000/UL (2%)

2. Infants with Hct <31% and hood O_2 <36% or mean airway pressure <6 cm H_2O by CPAP or IMV or >9 apneic and bradycardic episodes per 12 h or 2/24 h requiring bag and mask ventilation while on adequate methylxanthine therapy or HR >180/min or RR >80/min sustained for 24 h or weight gain of <10 g/d for 4 d on 100 Kcal/kg/d or having surgery

3. Infants with Hct <36% and requiring >35% O_2 or mean airway pressure 6–8 cm H_2O by CPAP or IMV

CPAP = continuous positive airway pressure by nasal or endotracheal route; HR = heart rate; Hct = hematocrit; IMV = intermittent mandatory ventilation; RR = respiratory rate.
From the multicenter trial of recombinant human erythropoietin for preterm infants.
Source: Data from Straus RG. Erythropoietin and neonatal anemia (Editorial). *N Engl J Med* 1994;330:1227.

    c. Infants with ABO incompatibility who do not have an exchange transfusion may have protracted hemolysis and may require a transfusion several weeks after birth. If they do not have enough hemolysis to require treatment with phototherapy, they will usually not become anemic enough to need a transfusion.

    d. Premature babies may be quite comfortable with hemoglobin levels of 6.5 to 7 mg/dL. The level itself is not an indication for transfusion. Sick infants (e.g., with sepsis, pneumonia, or bronchopulmonary dysplasia) may require increased oxygen-carrying capacities and therefore need transfusion. Growing premature infants may also manifest a need for transfusion by exhibiting poor weight gain, apnea, tachypnea, or poor feeding (8). Transfusion guidelines are shown in Table 26A.4. Despite efforts to adopt uniform transfusion critera, significant variation in transfusion practices among neonatal intensive care units (NICUs) has been reported (9). In our units when we instituted the practice of requiring parental permission for elective transfusion, the transfusion rate dropped markedly for premature infants. Similarly, a major reduction in blood exposure was observed in control infants that were enrolled on a clinical trial of recombinant erythropoietin that stipulated strict transfusion criteria (1,10).

  2. **Blood products and methods of transfusion** (see Chap. 26E and [2])

    a. **Packed RBCs.** The volume of transfusion may be calculated as follows:

$$\frac{\text{Weight in kilogram} \times \text{blood volume per kilogram} \times (\text{Hct desired} - \text{Hct observed})}{\text{Hct of blood to be given}} = \text{volume of transfusion}$$

      The average newborn blood volume is 80 mL/kg; the Hct of packed RBCs is 60% to 80% and should be checked before transfusion. We generally transfuse 15 to 20 mL/kg; larger volumes may need to be divided.

    b. **Whole blood** is indicated when there is acute blood loss.

    c. **Isovolemic transfusion** with high Hct-packed RBCs may be required for severely anemic infants, when routine transfusion of the volume of packed RBCs necessary to correct the anemia would result in circulatory overload (see Chap. 18).

    d. **Irradiated** RBCs are recommended in premature infants weighing <1,200 g. Premature infants may be unable to reject foreign lymphocytes in transfused blood. **We use irradiated blood for all neonatal transfusions.**

Leukocyte depletion with third-generation transfusion filters has substantially reduced the risk of exposure to foreign lymphocytes and cytomegalovirus (CMV) (4,11). However, blood from CMV-negative donors for neonatal transfusion may be preferable.

e. **Directed-donor transfusion** is requested by many families. Irradiation of directed-donor cells is especially important, given the human leukocyte antigen (HLA) compatibility among first-degree relatives and the enhanced potential for foreign lymphocyte engraftment.

f. Because of concern for multiple exposure risk associated with repeated transfusions in extremely low birth weight (ELBW) infants, **we recommend transfusing stored RBCs from a single unit reserved for an infant** (12).

B. Prophylaxis

1. **Term infants** should be sent home from the hospital on iron-fortified formula (2 mg/kg/day) if they are not breastfeeding (13).

2. **Premature infants** (preventing or ameliorating the anemia of prematurity). The following is a description of our usual nutritional management of premature infants from the point of view of providing RBC substrates and preventing additional destruction:

a. **Iron** supplementation in the preterm infant prevents late iron deficiency (14). We routinely supplement iron in premature infants at a dose of 2 to 4 mg of elemental iron/kg/day once full enteral feeding is achieved (see Chap. 10).

b. **Mother's milk** or formulas similar to mother's milk in that they are low in linoleic acid are used to maintain a low content of polyunsaturated fatty acids in the RBCs (3).

c. **Vitamin E** (15 to 25 IU of water-soluble form) is given daily until the baby is 38 to 40 weeks' postconceptional age (this is usually stopped at discharge from the hospital).

d. **These infants should be followed up carefully,** and additional iron supplementation may be required.

e. **Methods and hazards of transfusion** are described in Chap. 26E.

f. **Recombinant human erythropoietin (rh-EPO)** has been evaluated as a promising measure in ameliorating anemia of prematurity (10,15–19). Although studies in which we participated showed that rh-EPO stimulates red cell production and decreases the frequency and volume of RBC transfusions administered to premature infants, we do not recommend it as a routine procedure (10,16,17). Though many studies have shown that erythropoietin treatment is of limited benefit in reducing the number of transfusions once strict transfusion criteria are instituted, this therapy may have a role in selected cases. For infants in whom it is desirable to maintain a relatively high Hct, for example, babies with bronchopulmonary dysplasia or cyanotic congenital heart disease, initiation of erythropoietin may play a role in decreasing late transfusions.

Preterm infants require higher doses of erythropoietin on a per kilogram basis than children or adults because of a larger volume of distribution and the requirement for a brisk rate of red cell production to keep pace with rapid growth and to compensate for iatrogenic blood loss. A dose of 200 to 250 units/kg administered 3 days/week is sufficient to stimualte erythropoiesis and higher doses are not indicated as iron availability rapidly becomes limiting. For this reason, preterm babies who are receiving erythropoietin should receive at least 6 mg/kg/day of elemental iron in divided doses.

Complementary strategies to reduce phlebotomy losses and the use of conservative standardized transfusion criteria have contributed to significant reductions in transfusions. Therefore, any benefits of erythropoietin therapy are likely to depend upon careful targeting to the population that is most likely to benefit (18). Table 26A.5 provides a set of guidelines for rh-EPO administration in current use in the University of California, San Francisco (UCSF) Intesive Care Nursery.

TABLE 26A.5	Guidelines for Use of Erythropoietin

Introduction: these guidelines approximate the criteria from the large controlled trials of rh-EPO in preterm infants and are in current use in the UCSF Intensive Care Nursery; for other situations in which rh-EPO may be useful (e.g., bronchopulmonary dysplasia [BPD], late anemia after intrauterine transfusion), consultation with a pediatric hematologist is recommended

Eligibility criteria
1. Birth weight ≤1,250 g and gestation <31 wk with all of the following:
    a. Total caloric intake ≥50 kcal/kg/d, with >one-half enteral
    b. Hct <40% or 40%–50% but falling 2% per day
    c. Mean airway pressure <11 cm H_2O and Fio_2 <0.40
    d. Postnatal age >6 d and gestational age <33 wk
2. Any infant with birth weight 1,251–1,500 g and phlebotomy losses >5 mL/kg/wk who meet criteria (a–d) earlier
3. Exclusions: major anomalies, dysmorphic syndromes, hemolytic anemia, active major infection

Dose and duration: 750 units/kg/wk subcutaneously divided into three doses (e.g., 250 units/kg on Mon, Wed, Fri) discontinue rh-EPO when infant reaches 34-wk gestational age; (multiple patients can be treated using the same vial of rh-EPO)

Iron: Start oral iron at 2 mg/kg/d as soon as tolerated and increase to 4 mg/kg/d when feeds reach 100 mL/kg; when at full feeds, begin preterm vitamins; if not on iron after 2 wk of rh-EPO treatment consider:
1. Intravenous iron (1 mg/kg/d in intravenous alimentation fluid) or
2. Discontinue rh-EPO

Monitoring of rh-EPO therapy
1. **Measure Hct and reticulocyte count weekly.** Reticulocyte count should reach 200,000 after 1–2 wk of treatment with rh-EPO; if Hct reaches 45% without transfusion, discontinue rh-EPO, and consult with hematology before restarting
2. **Posttherapy.** Hct and reticulocyte count is expected to decline; endogenous EPO will be released only when the infant becomes anemic (usually with Hct in the mid-1920s); only then will reticulocytes rise again; if reticulocyte count has not started to rise at the time of the infant's discharge, alert the primary MD to the need to follow the Hct and reticulocyte count as an outpatient

Hct = hematocrit; rh-EPO = recombinant human erythropoietin.

References
1. Bifano EM, Ehrenkranz Z, eds. Perinatal hematology. *Clin Perinatol* 1995;23(3).
2. Blanchette V, Doyle J, Schmidt B, et al. Hematology. In: Avery GB, ed. *Neonatology*, 4th ed. Philadelphia: Lippincott–Raven Publishers, 1994:952.
3. Glader B, Naiman JL. Erythrocyte disorders in infancy. In: Taeusch HW, Ballard RA, Avery ME, eds. *Diseases of the newborn*. Philadelphia: WB Saunders, 1991.
4. Nathan DG, Oski FA. *Hematology of infancy and childhood*. Philadelphia: WB Saunders, 1992.
5. Oski FA, Naiman JL. *Hematologic problems in the newborn*, 3rd ed. Philadelphia: WB Saunders, 1982.
6. Molteni RA. Prenatal blood loss. *Pediatr Rev* 1990;12:47.
7. Clayton EM, Altshuler J, Bove JR, et al. Penicillin antibody as a cause of positive direct antiglobulin tests. *Am J Clin Pathol* 1965;44:648.
8. Ross MP, Christensen RD, Rothstein G, et al. A randomized trial to develop criteria for administering erythrocyte transfusions to anemic preterm infants 1 to 3 months of age. *J Perinatol* 1989;9:246.

9. Ringer SA, Richardson DK, Sacher RA, et al. Variations in transfusion practice in neonatal intensive care. *Pediatrics* 1998;101:194.
10. Shannon KM, Keith JF, Mentzer WC, et al. Recombinant human erythropoietin stimulates erythropoiesis and reduces erythrocyte transfusions in preterm infants. *Pediatrics* 1995;95:1.
11. Andreu G. Role of leucocyte depletion in the prevention of transfusion-induced cytomegalovirus infection. *Semin Hematol* 1991;28(Suppl 5):26.
12. Strauss RG. Blood banking issues pertaining to neonatal red blood cell transfusions. *Transfus Sci* 1999;21(1):7.
13. Committee on Nutrition AAP. Iron-fortified infant formulas. *Pediatrics* 1989;84:1114.
14. Hall RT, Wheeler RE, Benson J, et al. Feeding iron-fortified premature formula during initial hospitalization to infants less than 1800 grams birthweight. *Pediatrics* 1993;92:409.
15. Maier RF, Obladen M, Seigalla P, et al. European Multicentre Erythropoietin Study Group. The effect of epoietin beta (recombinant human erythropoietin) on the need for transfusion in very low-birth-weight infants. *N Engl J Med* 1994;330:1173.
16. Straus RG. Erythropoietin and neonatal anemia (Editorial). *N Engl J Med* 1994;330:1227.
17. Willmas JA. Erythropoietin—not yet a standard treatment for anemia of prematurity. *Pediatrics* 1995;95:9.
18. Soubasi V, Kremenopoulos G, Diamandi E, et al. In which neonates does early recombinant human erythropoietin treatment prevent anemia of prematurity? Results of a randomized, controlled study. *Pediatr Res* 1993;34(5):675.
19. http://www.uptodate.com: anemia/prematurity/epo. Accessed 2006.

AQ1

26 B BLEEDING
Allen M. Goorin and Ellis J. Neufeld

$\mathcal{T}$he hemostatic mechanism in the neonate differs from that in the older child. In neonates, there is decreased activity of several clotting factors, diminished platelet function, and suboptimal defense against clot formation. A detailed review of the subject is provided in reference (1).

I. ETIOLOGY
A. Deficient clotting factors
1. **Transitory deficiencies** of the procoagulant vitamin K–dependent factors II, VII, IX, and X; and anticoagulant proteins C and S are characteristic of the newborn period and may be accentuated by the following:
   a. **The administration of total parenteral alimentation or antibiotics or the lack of administration of vitamin K** to premature infants.
   b. **Term infants may develop vitamin K deficiency** by day 2 or 3 if they are not supplemented with vitamin K parenterally, because of negligible stores and inadequate intake.
   c. **The mother might have received certain drugs during pregnancy that can cause bleeding in the first 24 hours of the infant's life.**

i. Phenytoin (Dilantin), phenobarbital, and salicylates interfere with the vitamin K effect on synthesis of clotting factors.

ii. Coumadin compounds given to the mother interfere with the synthesis of vitamin K–dependent clotting factors by the livers of both the mother and the fetus, and the bleeding may not be immediately reversed by administration of vitamin K.

2. Disturbances of clotting may be related to associated diseases such as disseminated intravascular coagulation (DIC) due to infection, shock, anoxia, necrotizing enterocolitis (NEC), renal vein thrombosis (RVT), or the use of vascular catheters. Any significant liver disease may interfere with the production of clotting factors by the liver.

    a. Extracorporeal membrane oxygenation (ECMO) in neonates with critical cardiopulmonary disease is a special case of coagulopathy related to consumption of clotting factors in the bypass circuit plus therapeutic anticoagulation (2,3).

3. Inherited abnormalities of clotting factors

    a. X-linked recessive (expressed predominantly in men; affected women should raise concern of Turner syndrome, partial X deletions, or unbalanced X chromosome inactivation):

        i. Factor VIII levels are decreased in the newborn with hemophilia A (1 in 5,000 boys) (4).

        ii. Hemophilia B, or Christmas disease is due to an inherited deficiency of factor IX (1 in 25,000 boys) (4).

            One-third of patients with severe hemophilia express "new mutations", so family history alone cannot rule out the problem.

    b. Autosomal dominant (expressed in boys and girls with one parent affected):

        i. von Willebrand disease (VWD) is due to decreased levels and functional activity of von Willebrand factor (VWF), which acts as a carrier for factor VIII, and as a platelet-aggregation agent. VWD is the most common inherited coagulation defect (up to 1% of the population as assayed by factor levels) (4). Neonatal levels of VWF are elevated in normal subjects because of maternal estrogen.

        ii. Dysfibrinogenemia (very rare) is due to fibrinogen structural mutations.

    c. Autosomal recessive (occurs in both boys and girls; the parents are carriers). In order of frequency, deficiencies of factors XI, VII, V, X, II, fibrinogen, and factor XIII are all encoded by autosomal genes. Factor XII is a special case because deficiency causes long partial thromboplastin time (PTT), but never causes bleeding. Combined factor V and VIII deficiency is caused by defect in the common processing protein ERGIC-53 (5).

        i. Severe factor VII or factor XIII deficiency can present as intracranial hemorrhage in neonates.

        ii. Factor XI deficiency is incompletely recessive because heterozygotes may have unpredictable bleeding problems with surgery or trauma.

        iii. VWD Type III (rare, complete absence of VWF) (4).

B. Platelet problems (see Chap. 26D)

    1. Qualitative disorders include hereditary conditions (e.g., Storage pool defects, Glanzmann thrombasthenia, Bernard-Soulier syndrome, platelet-type VWD (6)) and transient disorders that result from the mother's use of antiplatelet agents.

    2. Quantitative disorders include the following:

        a. Immune thrombocytopenia (maternal idiopathic thrombocytopenic purpura [ITP] or neonatal alloimmune thrombocytopenia [NAIT]) (7).

        b. Maternal preeclampsia or HELPP syndrome (see Chap. 2C), or severe uteroplacental insufficiency.

        c. DIC due to infection or asphyxia,

        d. inherited marrow failure syndromes, including Fanconi anemia and congenital amegakaryocytic thrombocytopenia.

        e. Congenital leukemia.

        f. Inherited thrombocytopenia syndromes, including gray-platelet syndrome and the macrothrombocytopenias, such as May-Hegglin syndrome (6).

g. Consumption of platelets in clots or vascular lesions, without DIC. Examples include vascular malformations, notably Kasabach-Merritt phenomenon from Kaposiform hemangioendotheliomas; RVT; and NEC.

h. Heparin-induced thrombocytopenia (HIT) deserves special consideration for several reasons. First, this condition leads to platelet activation and risk of thrombosis more than bleeding. Second, it is probably rare in neonates, although the antibody can be detected by ELISA assays after cardiac surgery. Finally, in neonates, the antibody may be maternal, as with other antibodies passed across the placenta.

C. Other potential causes of bleeding are **vascular** in etiology, and may include central nervous system hemorrhage, pulmonary hemorrhage, arterial-venous (A-V) malformations, and hemangiomas.

D. Miscellaneous problems

1. Trauma (see Chap. 20):

a. Rupture of spleen or liver associated with breech delivery.

b. Retroperitoneal or intraperitoneal bleeding may present as scrotal ecchymosis.

c. Subdural hematoma, cephalhematoma, or subgaleal hemorrhage (the latter may be associated with vacuum extraction).

2. Liver dysfunction.

II. DIAGNOSTIC WORKUP OF THE BLEEDING INFANT

A. The **history** includes (a) family history of excessive bleeding or clotting; (b) maternal medications (e.g. aspirin, phenytoin); (c) pregnancy and birth history; (d) maternal history of a birth of an infant with a bleeding disorder; and (e) any illness, medication, anomalies, or procedures done to the infant.

B. Examination. The crucial decision in diagnosing and managing the bleeding infant is determining whether the infant is sick or well (see Table 26B.1).

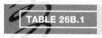

TABLE 26B.1   Differential Diagnosis of Bleeding in the Neonate

| Clinical evaluation | Laboratory studies | | | Likely diagnosis |
	Platelets	PT	PTT	
"Sick"	D−	I+	I+	DIC
	D−	N	N	Platelet consumption (infection, necrotizing enterocolitis, renal vein thrombosis)
	N	I+	I+	Liver disease
	N	N	N	Compromised vascular integrity (associated with hypoxia, prematurity, acidosis, hyperosmolality)
"Healthy"	D−	N	N	Immune thrombocytopenia, occult infection, thrombosis, bone marrow hypoplasia (rare), or bone marrow infiltrative disease
	N	I+	I+	Hemorrhagic disease of newborn (vitamin K deficiency)
	N	N	I+	Hereditary clotting factor deficiencies
	N	N	N	Bleeding due to local factors (trauma, anatomic abnormalities); qualitative platelet abnormalities (rare); factor XIII deficiency (rare)

PT = prothrombin time; PTT = partial thromboplastin time; D− = decreased; I+ = increased; DIC = disseminated intravascular coagulation; N = normal.
(Modified from Glader BE, Amylon MD. Bleeding disorders in the newborn infant. In: Taeusch HW, Ballard RA, Avery ME, Eds. *Diseases of the newborn*. Philadelphia: WB Saunders, 1991.)

1. **Sick infant.** Consider DIC, viral or bacterial infection, or liver disease (hypoxic/ ischemic injury may lead to DIC).
2. **Well infant.** Consider vitamin K deficiency, isolated clotting factor deficiencies, or immune thrombocytopenia. Maternal blood in the infant's gastrointestinal tract will not cause symptoms in the infant.
3. **Petechiae, small superficial ecchymosis, or mucosal bleeding** suggest a platelet problem.
4. **Large bruises** suggest deficiency of clotting factors, DIC, liver disease, or vitamin K deficiency.
5. **Enlarged spleen** suggests possible congenital infection or erythroblastosis.
6. **Jaundice** suggests infection, liver disease, or resorption of a large hematoma.
7. **Abnormal retinal findings** suggest infection (see Chap. 23).

C. **Laboratory tests** (see Table 26B.2)
   1. **The Apt test** is used to rule out maternal blood. If the child is well and only GI bleeding is noted, an Apt test is performed on gastric aspirate or stool to rule out the presence of maternal blood swallowed during labor or delivery or from a bleeding breast. A breast pump can be used to collect milk to confirm the presence of blood in the milk, or the infant's stomach can be aspirated before and after breast-feeding.
      a. **Procedure.** Mix one part bloody stool or vomitus with five parts water; centrifuge it and separate the clear pink supernatant (hemolysate); add 1 mL of sodium hydroxide 1% (0.25 M) to 4 mL of hemolysate.
      b. **Result.** Hemoglobin A (HbA) changes from pink to yellow brown (maternal blood); hemoglobin F (HbF) stays pink (fetal blood).
   2. **Peripheral blood smear** is used to determine the number, size, and kind of platelets and the presence of fragmented red blood cells (RBCs) as seen in DIC. Large platelets reflect either young platelets (implying an immune cause of thrombocytopenia) or congenital macrothrombocytopenias.

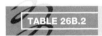

TABLE 26B.2	Normal Values for Laboratory Screening Tests in the Neonate		
Laboratory test	**Premature infant having received vitamin K**	**Term infant having received vitamin K**	**Child 1–2 mo of age**
Platelet count/μL	150,000–400,000	150,000–400,000	150,000–400,000
PT (s)*	14–22	13–20	12–14
PTT (s)*	35–55	30–45	25–35
Fibrinogen (mg/dL)	150–300	150–300	150–300

PT = prothrombin time; PTT = partial thromboplastin time.
*Normal values may vary from laboratory to laboratory, depending on the particular reagent employed. In full-term infants who have received vitamin K, the PT and PTT values generally fall within the normal "adult" range by several days (PT) to several weeks (PTT) of age. Small premature infants (under 1500 g) tend to have longer PT and PTT than larger babies. In infants with hematocrit levels >60%, the ratio of blood to anticoagulant (sodium citrate 3.8%) in tubes should be 19:1 rather than the usual ratio of 9:1; otherwise, spurious results will be obtained, because the amount of anticoagulant solution is calculated for a specific volume of plasma. Blood drawn from heparinized catheters should not be used. The best results are obtained when blood from a clean venipuncture is allowed to drip directly into the tube from the needle or scalp vein set. Factor levels II, VII, IX, and X are decreased. Three-day-old full-term baby not receiving vitamin K has levels similar to a premature baby. Factor XI and XII levels are lower in preterm infants than in term infants and account for prolonged PTT. Fibrinogen, factor V, and factor VII are normal in premature and term infants. Factor XIII is variable.
(Data from normal laboratory values at the Hematology Laboratory, The Children's Hospital, Boston; Alpers JB, Lafonet MT, eds. *Laboratory Handbook.* Boston: The Children's Hospital, 1984.)

3. **Significant bleeding** from thrombocytopenia **is usually associated with platelet counts under 20,000 to 30,000/mm³ or less,** except in alloimmune thrombocytopenia due to antibodies against the platelet alloantigen, HPA1 (also known as PLA1), which may cause bleeding in platelet counts up to 50,000 platelets/mm³ (see Chap. 26D) because the antibody interferes with platelet surface fibrinogen receptor, glycoprotein IIb–IIIa.

4. **Prothrombin time (PT)** is a test of the "extrinsic" clotting system. Factor VII and tissue factor activate factor X; Factor Xa activates prothrombin (II) to form thrombin, with factor Va as a cofactor. Thrombin cleaves fibrinogen to fibrin.

5. **PTT** is a test of the so-called intrinsic clotting system and of the activation of factor X by factors XII, XI, IX, and VIII, as well as the factors of the common coagulation pathway (factors V and II and fibrinogen).

6. **Fibrinogen** can be measured on the same sample as that used for PT. It may be decreased in liver disease and consumptive states.

7. **D-Dimer assays** measure degradation products of fibrin found in the plasma of patients with DIC and in patients with liver disease who have problems clearing fibrin split products (FSP). D-Dimers are formed from the action of plasmin on the fibrin clot, generating derivatives of cross-linked fibrin containing D-dimer. Normal levels depend on the type of assay used. Levels are higher in DIC, deep vein thrombosis, and pulmonary embolism. False-positive D-dimers are common in the intensive care unit (ICU) setting, because trivial clotting from catheter tips and other causes give positive results in this sensitive assay.

8. **Specific factor assays and Von Willebrand panels** for patients with positive family history **can be measured in cord blood, or by venipuncture after birth.** Age-specific norms must be consulted.

9. **Bleeding times are to be discouraged in all patients, but especially in neonates.** This test measures response to a standardized razor blade cut, and does not predict surgical bleeding. The apparatus is not well suited to infants, and should never be used.

10. Platelet function analysis using instruments such as the PFA100 may be useful as a screening test for VWD or platelet dysfunction in some settings, but confirmatory specific assays are required for positive tests.

III. **TREATMENT OF NEONATES WITH ABNORMAL BLEEDING PARAMETERS WHO HAVE NOT HAD CLINICAL BLEEDING.** In one study, preterm infants with respiratory distress syndrome (RDS) or term infants with asphyxia were treated for abnormal bleeding parameters (without DIC) to correct the hemostatic defect. Although the treatment was successful in correcting the defect, no change in mortality was seen in comparison with controls (8).

In general, we treat clinically ill infants or infants weighing <1,500 g with fresh-frozen plasma (FFP, 10 mL/kg) if the PT or PTT or both are more than two times normal for age or with platelets (1 unit) (see IV.C) if the platelet count is under 20,000/mm³ (see Chaps. 26D and 26E). This will vary with the clinical situations, trend of the laboratory values, impending surgery, and so forth. Some babies will receive platelets if their platelet count is <50,000/mm³, particularly in known NAIT with HPA1 (PLA1) sensitization.

IV. **TREATMENT OF BLEEDING**

A. **Vitamin K₁ (Aquamephyton).** An intravenous or intramuscular dose of 1 mg is administered in case the infant was not given vitamin K at birth. Infants receiving total parenteral nutrition and infants receiving antibiotics for more than 2 weeks should be given at least 0.5 mg of vitamin K₁ (IM or IV) weekly to prevent vitamin K depletion. Ideally, Vitamin K rather than FFP should be given for long PT and PTT due to vitamin K deficiency, rather than plasma, which should be reserved for bleeding or emergencies.

B. **FFP** (see Chap. 26E) (10 mL/kg) is given intravenously for active bleeding and is repeated every 8 to 12 hours as needed, or as a drip of 1 cc/kg/hour. This is used because it replaces the clotting factors immediately.

C. **Platelets** (see Chap. 26D). If there is no increased platelet destruction (as a result of DIC, immune platelet problem, or sepsis), 1 unit of platelets given to a 3-kg infant will raise the platelet count to 50,000 to 100,000/mm^3. If no new platelets are made or transfused, the platelet count will drop slowly over 3 to 5 days. If available, platelets from the mother or from a known platelet-compatible donor should be used if the infant has an alloimmune platelet disorder. The blood of the donor should be matched for Rh factor and type and washed, because RBCs will be mixed in the platelet concentrates. Platelets are irradiated before transfusion.

D. Fresh whole blood (see Chaps. 26A and 26E). The baby is given 10 mL/kg; more is given as needed.

E. Clotting factor concentrates (see Chap. 26E). When there is a known deficiency of factor VIII or IX, the plasma concentration should be raised to normal adult levels (50% to 100% of pooled normal control plasma, or 0.5 to 1 unit/mL) to stop serious bleeding. Recombinant-DNA derived factor VIII and IX should be used if the diagnosis is clear. If severe von Willebrand's disease is considered, a VWF-containing, plasma derived factor VIII concentrate should be used. For other factor deficiencies, 10 mL/kg of FFP will transiently raise the factor level approximately to 20% of adult control. Cryoprecipitate is the best concentrated source of fibrinogen or factor XIII.

F. Disorders due to problems other than hemostatic proteins. Diagnosis and treatment should be aimed at the underlying cause (e.g., infection, liver rupture, catheter, or NEC).

G. Treatment of specific disorders

1. DIC. The baby usually appears sick and may have petechiae, GI hemorrhage, oozing from venipunctures, infection, asphyxia, or hypoxia. The platelet count is decreased, and PT and PTT are increased. Fragmented RBCs are seen on the blood smear. Fibrinogen is decreased, and D-dimers are increased. Treatment involves the following steps:

a. The underlying cause should be treated (e.g., sepsis, NEC, herpes). This is **always** the most important factor in treatment of DIC, and determines success of overall treatment.

b. Confirm that Vitamin K$_1$ has been given.

c. Platelets and FFP are given as needed to keep the platelet count over 50,000/mL and to stop the bleeding. FFP contains anticoagulant proteins, which may slow down or stop ongoing consumption.

d. If the bleeding persists, one of the following steps should be taken, depending on the availability of blood, platelets, or FFP:

i. Exchange transfusion with fresh citrated whole blood or reconstituted whole blood (packed RBCs, platelets, FFP).

ii. Continued transfusion with platelets, packed red cells, and FFP as needed.

iii. Administration of cryoprecipitate (10 mL/kg) for hypofibrinogenemia.

e. If consumption coagulopathy is associated with thrombosis of large vessels and not with concurrent bleeding, **heparinization without a bolus may be considered** (e.g., 10–15 units/kg/hour as a continuous infusion). Platelets and plasma are continued to be given after the heparin has been started. Platelet counts should be kept at or above 50,000/mL. Heparin is best monitored by functional heparin levels, with a goal of 0.2 to 0.4 units/mL, aiming on the lower side in patients with mild concurrent bleeding. The plasma is essential to provide ATIII and other anticoagulant proteins. Heparinization is generally contraindicated in the presence of intracranial hemorrhage, and if bleeding accompanies DIC and thrombosis concurrently, heparinization is complicated. Consult an expert immediately (see Chap. 26F.)

2. Hemorrhagic disease of the newborn (HDN) occurs in 1 out of every 200 to 400 neonates not given vitamin K prophylaxis.

a. In the healthy infant, **HDN may occur when the infant is not given vitamin K.** The infant may have been born in a busy delivery room, at home, or transferred from elsewhere. Bleeding and bruising may occur after the infant is 48 hours old. The platelet level is normal, and PT and PTT are prolonged. If there is active bleeding, 10 mL/kg of FFP and an IV dose of 1 mg of vitamin K are given.

b. **If the mother has been treated with phenytoin (Dilantin), primidone (Mysoline), methsuximide (Celontin), or phenobarbital, the infant may be vitamin K deficient and bleed during the first 24 hours.** The mother should be given vitamin K, 24 hours before delivery (10 mg of vitamin K_1 IM). The newborn should have PT, PTT, and platelet counts monitored if any signs of bleeding occur. The usual dose of vitamin K_1 (1 mg) should be given to the baby postpartum and repeated in 24 hours. Repeated infusions of FFP are given if any bleeding occurs.

c. **Delayed hemorrhagic disease** of the newborn from vitamin K deficiency can occur at 4 to 12 weeks of age. This may happen in breast-fed infants who are not receiving supplementation. Infants who are undergoing treatment with broad-spectrum antibiotics or infants with malabsorption (liver disease, cystic fibrosis) are at greater risk of hemorrhagic disease. Vitamin K_1, 1 mg/week orally for the first 3 months of life, may prevent late hemologic disease of the newborn. An oral preparation as used in Europe has not yet been approved in the United States. Although blood tests show that breast-fed infants are at potential risk for HDN, HDN has not been reported in infants who received intramuscular vitamin K at birth (1,9).

References

1. Monagle P, Andrew M. Developmental hemostasis: Relevance to newborns and infants. In: Nathan DG, Orkin SH, Ginsburg D, eds. *Hematology of infancy and childhood.* Philadelphia: WB Saunders, 2003:121–168.
2. Plotz FB, van Oeveren W, Bartlett RH, et al. Blood activation during neonatal extracorporeal life support. *J Thorac Cardiovasc Surg* 1993;105:823–832.
3. Robinson TM, Kickler TS, Walker LK, et al. Effect of extracorporeal membrane oxygenation on platelets in newborns. *Crit Care Med* 1993;21:1029–1034.
4. Montgomery RR, Gill JC, Scott JP. Hemophilia and von Willebrand disease. In: Nathan DG, Orkin SH, Ginsburg D, eds. *Hematology of infancy and childhood.* Philadelphia: WB Saunders, 2003:1547–1576.
5. Bauer K. Rare hereditary coagulation factor abnormalities. In: Nathan DG, Orkin SH, Ginsburg D, eds. *Hematology of infancy and childhood.* Philadelphia: WB Saunders, 2003:1577–1596.
6. Poncz M. Inherited platelet disorders. In: Nathan DG, Orkin SH, Ginsburg D, eds. *Hematology of infancy and childhood.* Philadelphia: WB Saunders, 2003:1527–1546.
7. Wilson DB. Acquired platelet defects. In: Nathan DG, Orkin SH, Ginsburg D, eds. *Hematology of infancy and childhood.* Philadelphia: WB Saunders, 2003:1597–1630.
8. Turner T. Treatment of premature infants with abnormal clotting parameters. *Br J Hematol* 1981;47:65.
9. Committee on fetus and newborn, A. A. P. Controversies concerning vitamin K and the newborn. *Pediatrics* 2003;112:191–192.

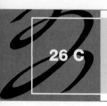

POLYCYTHEMIA
Allen M. Goorin

26 C

*A*s the central (venous) hematocrit rises, there is increased viscosity and decreased blood flow; when the hematocrit increases to >60%, there is a fall in oxygen transport (1) (see Fig. 26.1). Newborns have erythrocytes that are less deformable than the erythrocytes of adults. As viscosity increases, there is impairment of tissue oxygenation and decreased

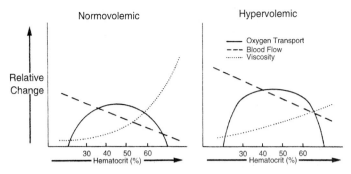

Figure 26.1. Effect of hematocrit on viscosity, blood flow, and oxygen transport. (Adapted from Glader B, Naiman JL. Erythrocyte disorders in infancy. In: Taeusch HW, Ballard RA, Avery ME, eds. *Diseases of the newborn*. Philadelphia: WB Saunders, 1991.)

glucose in plasma, and a tendency to form microthrombi. If these events occur in the cerebral cortex, kidneys, or adrenal glands, significant damage may result. Hypoxia and acidosis increase viscosity and deformity further. Poor perfusion increases the possibility of thrombosis.

I. DEFINITIONS

A. Polycythemia is defined as venous hematocrit of over 65% (2), a venous hematocrit of over 64% or more at 2 hours of age (3), and an umbilical venous or arterial hematocrit of over 63% or more (3). The mean venous hematocrit of term infants is 53% in cord blood, 60% at 2 hours of age, 57% at 6 hours of age, and 52% at 12 to 18 hours of age (3).

B. Hyperviscosity is defined as viscosity >14.6 cP at a shear rate of 11.5/s as measured by a viscometer (4). The relationship between hematocrit and viscosity is nearly linear below a hematocrit of 60%, but viscosity increases exponentially at a hematocrit of 70% or greater (Fig. 26.1) (1,5).

Other factors may alter viscosity. These include plasma proteins, especially fibrinogen, and local blood flow (3). The hyperviscosity syndrome is usually seen only in infants with venous hematocrits above 60%.

II. INCIDENCE.

The incidence of polycythemia in newborns is increased in babies who are small for gestational age (SGA) and in post-term babies; on average it is 0.4% to 5% (3,6,7).

III. CAUSES OF POLYCYTHEMIA (3)

A. Placental red cell transfusion

1. Delayed cord clamping may occur either intentionally or in unattended deliveries.

    a. When the cord is clamped within 1 minute after birth, the blood volume of the infant is 83.4 mL/kg.

    b. When the cord is clamped 2 minutes after delivery, the blood volume of the infant is 93 mL/kg.

    c. In newborns with polycythemia, blood volume per kilogram of body weight varies inversely in relation to birth weight (see Fig. 26.2).

2. Cord stripping (thereby pushing more blood into the infant).

3. Holding the baby below the mother at delivery.

4. Maternal-to-fetal transfusion is diagnosed with the Kleihauer-Betke stain technique of acid elution to detect maternal cells in the circulation of the newborn (see Chap. 26A).

5. Twin-to-twin transfusion (see Chap. 7).

6. Forceful uterine contractions before cord clamping.

B. Placental insufficiency (increased fetal erythropoiesis secondary to chronic intrauterine hypoxia)

1. SGA infants.

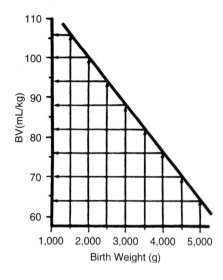

Figure 26.2. Nomogram designed for clinical use, correlating blood volume per kilogram with birth weight in polycythemic neonates. BV, blood volume. (From Rawlings JS, Pettett G, Wiswell T. et al. Estimated blood volumes in polycythemic neonates as a function of birth weight. *J Pediatr*, 1982;101:594.)

    2. Maternal hypertension syndromes (toxemia, renal disease, etc.).

    3. Postmature infants.

    4. Infants born to mothers with chronic hypoxia (heart disease, pulmonary disease).

    5. Pregnancy at high altitude.

    6. Maternal smoking.

C. Other conditions

    1. Infants of diabetic mothers (increased erythropoiesis).

    2. Some large-for-gestational-age (LGA) babies.

    3. Infants with congenital adrenal hyperplasia, Beckwith-Wiedemann syndrome, neonatal thyrotoxicosis, congenital hypothyroidism, trisomy 21, trisomy 13, trisomy 18.

    4. Drugs (maternal use of propranolol).

    5. Dehydration of infant.

IV. CLINICAL FINDINGS. Most infants with polycythemia are asymptomatic. Clinical symptoms, syndromes, and laboratory abnormalities that have been described in association with polycythemia include the following:

    A. Central nervous system (CNS). Poor feeding, lethargy, hypotonia, apnea, tremors, jitteriness, seizures, cerebral venous thrombosis.

    B. Cardiorespiratory. Cyanosis, tachypnea, heart murmurs, congestive heart failure, cardiomegaly, elevated pulmonary vascular resistance, prominent vascular markings on chest x-ray.

    C. Renal. Decreased glomerular filtration, decreased sodium excretion, renal vein thrombosis, hematuria, proteinuria.

    D. Other. Other thrombosis, thrombocytopenia, poor feeding, increased jaundice, persistent hypoglycemia, hypocalcemia, testicular infarcts, necrotizing enterocolitis (NEC), priapism, disseminated intravascular coagulation.

       All of these symptoms may be associated with polycythemia/hyperviscosity but may not be caused by it. They are common symptoms in many neonatal disorders.

V. SCREENING. The routine screening of all newborns for polycythemia/hyperviscosity is being advocated by some authors (8,9). The timing and site of blood sampling alter the hematocrit value (10,11). We do not routinely screen well term newborns for this syndrome, because there are few data showing that treatment of asymptomatic patients with partial exchange transfusion is beneficial in the long term (2,3,12).

VI. DIAGNOSIS. The capillary blood or peripheral venous hematocrit level should be determined in any baby who appears plethoric, who has any predisposing cause of polycythemia, who has any of the symptoms mentioned in IV, or who is not well for any reason.

   A. Depending on local perfusion, the **capillary blood hematocrit** will be 5% to 20% higher than the central hematocrit (3). Warming the heel before drawing blood for a capillary hematocrit determination will give a better correlation with the peripheral venous or central hematocrit. If the capillary blood hematocrit is above 65%, the peripheral venous hematocrit should be determined. The hematocrit should be measured with an automated hematology analyzer. Most of the old studies of hematocrits were done with spun hematocrits, which may give falsely high levels (3).

   B. Few hospitals are equipped to measure blood viscosity. If the equipment is available, the test should be done, because some infants with venous hematocrits under 65% will have hyperviscous blood (7).

VII. MANAGEMENT

   A. Any child with symptoms that could be due to hyperviscosity should have a **partial exchange transfusion if the peripheral venous hematocrit is >65%.**

   B. **Asymptomatic infants** with a peripheral venous hematocrit between 60% and 70% **can usually be managed by increasing fluid intake and repeating the hematocrit in 4 to 6 hours.**

   C. Most neonatologists perform an **exchange transfusion when the peripheral venous hematocrit is >70% in the absence of symptoms, but this is a controversial** issue (2,10–13).

   D. The following formula can be used to calculate the exchange with albumin 5% or normal saline that will bring the hematocrit to 50% to 60%. In infants with polycythemia, the blood volume varies inversely with the birth weight (Fig. 26.2). **Usually we take the blood from the umbilical vein and replace it with albumin 5% or normal saline in a peripheral vein.** Because randomized trials show no advantage with albumin, and there is less chance of infection, nonhuman products, such as saline, are preferred. There are many methods of exchange (see Chap. 18).

Volume of exchange in mL

$$= \frac{(\text{blood volume/kg} \times \text{weight in kg}) \times (\text{observed hematocrit} - \text{desired hematocrit})}{\text{observed hematicrit}}$$

Example: A 3-kg infant, hematocrit 75%, blood volume 80 mL/kg—to bring hematocrit to 50%:

$$\text{Volume of exchange(in mL)} = \frac{(80 \text{ mL} \times 3 \text{ kg}) \times (75 - 50)}{75}$$
$$= \frac{240 \text{ mL} \times 25}{75}$$
$$= 80\text{-mL exchange}$$

The total volume exchanged is usually 15 to 20 mL/kg of body weight. This will depend on the observed hematocrit. (Blood volume may be up to 100 mL/kg in polycythemic infants.)

VIII. OUTCOME

   A. **Infants with polycythemia and hyperviscosity who have decreased cerebral blood flow velocity and increased vascular resistance develop normal cerebral blood flow following partial exchange transfusion** (10). They also have improvement in systemic blood flow and oxygen transport (3,4,11,12).

   B. **The long-term neurologic outcome** in infants with asymptomatic polycythemia/hyperviscosity, whether treated or untreated, **remains controversial.**

   1. One trial with small numbers of randomized patients has shown decreased IQ scores in school-age children who had neonatal hyperviscosity syndrome, irrespective of whether the newborns were treated or not (2,14).

2. Another retrospective study, with small numbers of patients, showed no difference in the neurologic outcome of patients with asymptomatic neonatal polycythemia, irrespective of whether they were treated or not (15).
3. Some earlier preliminary prospective studies favored treatment (13,16).
4. A small prospective study showed no difference at follow-up between control infants and those with hyperviscosity, between those with symptomatic and asymptomatic hyperviscosity, and between asymptomatic infants treated with partial exchange transfusion and those who were observed. Analysis revealed that other perinatal risk factors and race, rather than polycythemia or partial exchange transfusion, significantly influenced the long-term outcome (3,12).
5. An increased incidence of NEC following partial exchange transfusions by umbilical vein has been reported (13,17). NEC was not seen in one retrospective analysis of 185 term polycythemic babies given partial exchange transfusions with removal of blood from the umbilical vein and reinfusion of a commercial plasma substitute through peripheral veins (18).
6. A large prospective, randomized clinical trial comparing partial exchange transfusion with symptomatic care (increased fluid intake, etc.) equally balanced for risk factors and the etiologies of the polycythemia will be necessary to give guidelines for treatment of the asymptomatic newborn with polycythemia/hyperviscosity.
7. Partial exchange transfusion will lower hematocrit, decrease viscosity, and reverse many of the physiologic abnormalities associated with polycythemia/hyperviscosity but has not been shown to significantly change the long-term outcome of these infants (3).

References

1. Glader B. Erythrocyte disorders in infancy. In: Taeusch HW, Ballard RA, Avery ME, eds. *Diseases of the newborn*, 6th ed. Philadelphia: WB Saunders, 1991.
2. Delaney-Black VD, et al. Neonatal hyperviscosity: Association with lower achievement and IQ scores at school age. *Pediatrics* 1989;83:662.
3. Wexner EJ. Neonatal polycythemia and hyperviscosity. *Clin Perinatol* 1995;22:693.
4. Swernam SM, et al. Hemodynamic consequences of neonatal polycythemia. *J Pediatr* 1987;110:443.
5. Ramamurthy RSJ, et al. Postnatal alteration in hematocrit and viscosity in normal and polycythemic infants. *J Pediatr* 1987;110:929.
6. Lindermann R, et al. Evaluation and treatment of polycythemia in the neonate. In: Christensen RD, ed. *Hematologic problems of the neonate*. Philadelphia: WB Saunders, 2000.
7. Wirth FH, et al. Neonatal hyperviscosity I. Incidence. *J Pediatr* 1979;63:833.
8. Drew JH, et al. Neonatal whole blood hyperviscosity: The important factor influencing later neurologic function is the viscosity, and not the polycythemia. *Clin Hemorheol Microcirc* 1997;17:67.
9. Wiswell TE, et al. Neonatal polycythemia: Frequency of clinical manifestations and other associated findings. *Pediatrics* 1986;78:26.
10. Oski FA, Naiman JL. *Hematologic problems in the newborn*, 3rd ed. Philadelphia: WB Saunders, 1982:87–96.
11. Phibbs RH, et al. Hematologic problems. In: Klaus MH, Fanaroff AA, eds. *Care of the high risk neonate*. Philadelphia: WB Saunders, 1993:421.
12. Bada H, Korones SB, Pourcyrous M, et al. Asymptomatic syndrome of polycythemic hyperviscosity: Effect of partial plasma transfusion. *J Pediatr* 1992;120:578.
13. Black VD, et al. Neonatal polycythemia and hyperviscosity. *Pediatr Clin North Am* 1982;5:1137.
14. Black VD, et al. Developmental and neurologic sequelae in neonatal hyperviscosity syndrome. *Pediatrics* 1982;69:426.
15. Host A, et al. Late prognosis in untreated neonatal polycythemia with minor or no symptoms. *Acta Paediatr Scand* 1982;71:629.

16. Goldberg K, et al. Neonatal hyperviscosity. II. Effect of partial plasma exchange transfusion. *Pediatrics* 1982;69:419.
17. Black VD, et al. Gastrointestinal injury in polycythemic term infants. *Pediatrics* 1985;76:225.
18. Hein HA, et al. Partial exchange transfusion in term, polycythemic neonates: Absence of association with severe gastrointestinal injury. *Pediatrics* 1987;80:75.

THROMBOCYTOPENIA

Allen M. Goorin and John P. Cloherty

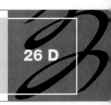

26 D

*N*eonatal thrombocytopenia is a platelet count of $<150,000/mm^3$. The causes include increased consumption or decreased production (rare). Consumption may be caused by antibodies, mechanical problems, or intravascular coagulation. The incidence in the general neonatal population is small ($\sim$0.1% of cord blood had counts $<50,000$), and most neonates with thrombocytopenia have only a modest reduction in platelet counts ($50,000-100,000$). These are generally self-resolved (1). More serious reductions, $<20,000$, or $50,000$ with bleeding, warrant evaluation and intervention.

In contrast, thrombocytopenia in the neonatal intensive care unit (NICU) is quite common. Indeed, in one prospective study, thrombocytopenia developed in 22% of 807 NICU admissions. The etiology in approximately 80% of cases is generally consumptive. This is particularly true for sick infants, in whom thrombocytopenia may represent just part of a spectrum of consumptive coagulopathy (2). The most severe sequelae of severe thrombocytopenia, such as intracranial hemorrhage, are associated with alloimmunization or are related to the degree of prematurity.

Thrombocytopenia may precede delivery. A recent retrospective review observed an incidence of approximately 5% of thrombocytopenia in fetal blood samplings. Congenital infections or chromosomal disorders accounted for almost half of these (reflecting the indications for the fetal blood sampling itself). Antibody-mediated causes included both maternal autoimmune and alloimmune conditions (3).

I. DIAGNOSIS (SEE FIG. 26D.1)
   A. Maternal history. There may be a history of thrombocytopenia, bleeding before or during pregnancy, a previous splenectomy, drug use, or infection. A history of pre- or postnatal bleeding in a previous pregnancy is important.
   B. Infant. The baby may seem healthy or may appear sick. There may be petechiae or large bruises, hepatosplenomegaly, jaundice, limb enlargement, hemangioma, or bruits (4).
   C. Laboratory studies
      1. Mother. Platelet count and platelet typing (if the maternal count is normal).
      2. Baby. Complete blood count (CBC), platelet count, prothrombin time (PT), and partial thromboplastin time (PTT).
II. THERAPY
   A. Platelet transfusion
      1. Indications
         a. When there is bleeding or platelets are $<20,000$: there have been few prospective controlled trials of the best time to transfuse platelets in neonates. One

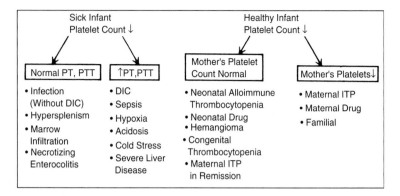

Figure 26D.1. Clinical status in neonatal thrombocytopenia with features that determine a quick differential diagnosis. PT = prothrombin time; PTT = partial thromboplastin time; DIC = disseminated intravascular coagulation; ITP = immune thrombocytopenic purpura; ↑ = increase; ↓ = decrease.

attempt randomized sick preterm infants to conventional therapy (typically keeping platelets >50,000) versus maintaining platelets >150,000 with one to three transfusions over the first week of life. There was no difference in the rate of intracranial hemorrhage in either group (5).

    b. This confirms that routine platelet transfusion does not help in severe prematurity, but it does not address the issue of minimum number to which platelet counts should be allowed to fall.

  2. Source. Use a random donor, except for the infant with alloimmune thrombocytopenia. In this case, use the mother's platelets after appropriate testing (washed to remove the alloantibody) or platelets from a platelet antigen–compatible donor.

  3. Quantity. One unit of platelets/3 kg raises the platelet count by 50,000 to 100,000/ mL, unless there is peripheral destruction of the platelets.

  4. Frequency. The normal half-life of platelets is 4 to 5 days; it is shorter if there is increased platelet consumption.

  5. Route. Give platelets intravenously through a peripheral vein. Never give platelets through an arterial line or into the liver (umbilical line) because thrombosis may occur.

  6. Irradiate all platelet transfusions for newborns.

 B. Steroid therapy in bleeding infants. Prednisone 2 mg/kg/day (prednisolone IV) may reduce bleeding.

 C. In an emergency, **whole blood may be used for exchange transfusion.**

III. THROMBOCYTOPENIA WITH DECREASED PLATELET SURVIVAL

 A. Immune. In immune thrombocytopenias (ITP), maternal antibody crosses the placenta, resulting in destruction of neonatal platelets. Considerable amounts of antibody may cross, resulting in thrombocytopenias that persist for several weeks. It is called an **autoantibody** when the antibody is directed against an antigen on the mother's own platelets shared in common with the baby's platelets. **Alloantibodies** are antibodies directed against antigens on the baby's platelets (and, perforce, paternal platelets) but not present on maternal platelets.

  1. Auto-maternal ITP. These include various autoimmune syndromes such as systemic lupus erythematosus (SLE).

    a. Clinical picture. The baby usually has mild to moderate thrombocytopenia (20,000 to 50,000) and is healthy, but has petechiae or bruising. There may be increased bruising at the vitamin K injection site or bleeding at circumcision or heel-stick sites. The mother usually has thrombocytopenia or a history of ITP.

b. **Pathophysiology.** Maternal autoantibodies cross the placenta and bind to neonatal platelets. A normal maternal platelet count does not rule out this cause, as the maternal count may reflect compensated increased destruction. Although it is rare, one center had 11 mothers with normal platelet counts, in whom alloimmune differences were excluded, who delivered 17 infants with severe thrombocytopenia. In 10 of these 11 mothers, the center was able to identify a maternal autoanti-GP1b antibody and subsequently demonstrate compensated maternal thrombocytolysis or hypersplenism (6). This may be more common if the mother has had a splenectomy. Elicit a **maternal history** of thrombocytopenia or symptoms of autoimmune syndromes. Maternal thrombocytopenia at delivery is common (at delivery ~7% of women have platelet counts <150,000). Almost all infants born to women with thrombocytopenia are either unaffected or have mild to moderate reductions that are self-resolving. Only 1 of 756 of infants born to women with incidental thrombocytopenia, 5 of 1,414 with hypertension, and 4 of 46 with ITP had cord blood platelet counts <50,000, and all of them were >20,000 and without sequelae (1). Identification of autoantibody on maternal platelets is not sufficient to diagnose an autoimmune cause. There was elevated platelet-associated immunoglobulin G(IgG) (not directed against Gp1b) in the serum of approximately one-third of mothers of infants with documented anti-HPA-1a alloimmune thrombocytopenia (7).

c. **Treatment of autoimmune thrombocytopenia**

i. **Prenatal management.** Even if the mother has true ITP, it appears that fetal hemorrhage *in utero* is very rare, compared with the small but definite risk of such hemorrhage in alloimmune thrombocytopenia (1,8). One uncontrolled study (3) showed a 3.6-fold increase in neonatal platelet counts following steroid administration to mothers with ITP and positive antiplatelet antibodies. Prednisone, 10 to 20 mg QD, was given for 10 to 14 days before delivery.

A small prospective randomized trial of low-dose betamethasone (1.5 mg/day orally from day 259 to day 273 and 1 mg until delivery) failed to prevent thrombocytopenia in newborns (9). These discrepant data need further study before steroid administration becomes routine practice. Intravenous gamma globulin (IGG) given prenatally to the mother with ITP has not been clearly shown to affect the fetal platelet count. Percutaneous umbilical blood sampling (PUBS) is beginning to be used as a safe, accurate, and direct method of obtaining the fetal platelet counts. In experienced hands, the mortality from this procedure is <1% (8). This may still be too great a risk for cases of maternal ITP (see Chap. 1). There may be little correlation between fetal and maternal platelet counts. Mothers who have had recent platelet counts <80,000, who are on steroids, or who have had a splenectomy are at increased risk of having a child with significant thrombocytopenia. Because a cesarean section reduces trauma to the infant, it would decrease the risk of bleeding in the occasional infant who is severely thrombocytopenic. The issue of when to do cesarean sections in mothers known to have ITP is controversial. The maternal mortality from cesarean sections in most centers is the same as from vaginal deliveries. Our usual management of these cases is to allow vaginal delivery to progress until a fetal scalp platelet count can be done. If the fetal scalp platelet count is >50,000 and labor is progressing normally, the infant is delivered vaginally. If these criteria are not met, then a cesarean section is done. One should remember that obstetricians would like a maternal platelet count of 50,000 to 100,000 before they are willing to operate, and anesthesiologists are often unwilling to give epidural anesthesia to mothers with platelet counts <100,000. The use of steroids, IgG, PUBS, or cesarean sections in the prenatal management of maternal ITP is controversial and requires cooperation between the obstetrician, neonatologist, hematologist, and family. These therapies are not usually required in maternal ITP (4,7).

ii. **Postnatal treatment** of infants affected by maternal ITP may include platelet transfusion, steroids, IgG, or exchange transfusion (treatment is as in Chap. 26B, III,IV).

2. **Alloimmune thrombocytopenia.** Maternal serum that shows antibodies that react against the father's but not against the mother's own platelets demonstrates an alloantibody. Of 19 fetuses known to be at risk for alloimmune thrombocytopenia (typically because of severely affected siblings from a prior delivery), 6 had platelet counts <20,000 and 3 suffered intracranial bleeding episodes, 2 of which were antenatal (1). Hence, alloimmune thrombocytopenia, although uncommon, when present, may result in severe hemorrhagic complications *in utero*. We have seen one mother who had recurrent episodes of severe fetal hemorrhage. Most cases are secondary to anti-HPA-1 (P1A-1) antibody; however, there are also numerous other antigens as targets (see Table 26D.1) (10).

a. **Clinical picture.** The baby appears healthy but has petechiae, bruising, bleeding, and a low platelet count (often <20,000). The mother has a normal platelet count; it may be her first pregnancy, or she may have a history of a previously affected pregnancy. There may be a history of alloimmune thrombocytopenia in children born to the mother's sisters.

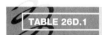

TABLE 26D.1   **Platelet-Specific Alloantigen Systems**

New HPA nomenclature	Original designations	White phenotype frequency	Clinical alloimmune syndromes described
HPA-1a	Zw^a, $P1^{A1}$	0.97	NAIT, PTP, PTR, PAT, TAT
HPA-1b	Zw^b, $P1^{A2}$	0.27	NAIT, PTP, PTR
HPA-2a	Ko^b	0.992	—
HPA-2b	Ko^a, Sib^a	0.169	NAIT, PTR
HPA-3a	Bak^a, Lek^a	0.85	NAIT, PTP
HPA-3b	Bak^b, Lek^b	0.66	NAIT, PTP, PTR
HPA-4a	Pen^a, Yuk^b	>0.999	NAIT, PTP
HPA-4b	Pen^b, Yuk^a	<0.0001	NAIT
HPA-5a	Br^b, Zav^b	0.99	NAIT
HPA-5b	Br^a, Zav^a, Hc^a	0.21	NAIT, PTP, PTR, PAT
HPA-6b	Tu^a, Ca	<0.007	NAIT
HPA-7b	Mo^a	<0.002	NAIT
HPA-8b	Sr^a	<0.01	NAIT
—	$P1^{E1}$	0.999	—
—	$P1^{E2}$	0.05	NAIT
—	Gov^a	0.81	NAIT, PTP
—	Gov^b	0.74	—
—	Va^a	<0.004	NAIT
—	Nak^a GPIV isoantibody	0.9966	PTR

HPA = human platelet antigen; NAIT = neonatal alloimmune thrombocytopenia; PAT = passive alloimmune thrombocytopenia; PTR = platelet transfusion refractoriness; PTP = post-transfusion purpura; TAT = transplant-associated thrombocytopenia.
Source: Adapted from Burrows RF, Kelton JG. Prenatal thrombocytopenia. *Clin Perinatol* 1995;22:779.

b. **Pathophysiology.** Approximately 97% of whites are HPA-1a positive and, hence approximately 3% of pregnancies involve an HPA-1a negative mother carrying an HPA-1a positive fetus. Roughly 1 in 1,000 to 5,000 deliveries is affected; therefore, 3% of pregnancies at risk are actually affected (1,11). There is a link between maternal production of alloantibodies and HLA type DR-3; there may be other factors that also regulate maternal antibody formation (12). Virtually all identified platelet antigens have been implicated in neonatal alloimmune thrombocytopenia (NAIT) (13). In one series of 295 patients with suspected NAIT referred to a platelet serology reference laboratory, only 36% were found to have platelet-specific antibody. Two-thirds of them were anti-HPA-1a directed, and 4% anti-HPA-3a (6). Twenty-four percent revealed only HLA antibodies, although the presence of an anti-HLA antibody does not prove that the antibody resulted in the thrombocytopenia.

c. **Diagnostic evaluation.** DNA techniques that define platelet-specific polymorphisms add to the diagnostic armamentarium but do not eliminate the usefulness of serologic techniques (14). The identification of numerous polymorphisms, including those in Table 26D.1, makes the role of a centralized platelet serology laboratory paramount (2). The Blood Center of Wisconsin (1–800-245-3117), Tom Kickler (Johns Hopkins, Baltimore, Maryland), and Scott Murphy (Temple University, Philadelphia, Pennsylvania) have excellent laboratories providing outside diagnostic services. Proper identification of the cause of the thrombocytopenia may be more important for the proper management of future pregnancies than for acute treatment of the thrombocytopenic infant. In cases of paternal heterozygosity, amniocentesis will identify the platelet antigen genotype of the fetus (10). Although controversial, the antenatal treatment of alloimmune thrombocytopenia with Percutaneous umbilical blood sampling (PUBS) and administration of IVIG to the mother may affect the natural history of a disorder associated with intracranial hemorrhage during the third trimester (7,10,11).

Infusion of maternal compatible platelets at the time of cordocentesis may decrease the incidence of hemorrhage during the procedure.

DNA testing is performed on 1 to 5 mL of the mother's and the infant's (or, alternatively, the father's) blood. Serologic testing typically requires testing of both maternal serum and paternal platelets, as testing of the affected infant's platelets generally proves impossible because of thrombocytopenia. Again, not all infants of HPA-1a (P1A1)-negative women with documented anti-HPA-1a (P1A1) Ab are thrombocytopenic; use caution when interpreting treatment results of such "high-risk" women (12).

d. **Treatment**

i. **Prenatal treatment.** Intravenous gamma globulin (IVGG), steroids, prenatal (by PUBS) platelet transfusion, fetal scalp platelet counts in labor, and elective cesarean section should be considered as management tools on a case-by-case basis with cooperation between the obstetrician, neonatologist, and hematologist. We may now many cases where the mother has had treatment with IVGG with good outcome. If the fetal platelet count is >50,000/ mL as measured by PUBS or fetal scalp platelet count, we allow **vaginal delivery** if presentation and labor are normal. If these criteria are not met, a **cesarean section** is done.

ii. **Postnatal treatment** (see II.)

a) **Platelet transfusion.** If the diagnosis is known to be alloimmune neonatal thrombocytopenia, the mother's platelets are collected 24 hours before delivery. If the baby has a platelet count of <20,000/mL, or if the baby shows any signs of bleeding, the mother's platelets (P1A1 negative) are transfused into the baby. The mother's serum will have P1A1-positive antibody, which potentially can react with the newborn's platelets. Using washed maternal platelets resuspended in plasma will avoid this complication. If there is an emergency secondary to bleeding in the newborn, and the mother's platelets have not been previously collected, either the mother's whole blood or platelets from a previously typed P1A1-negative platelet donor can be used. Random platelets should be used if there is serious bleeding and P1A1-negative platelets are not available. To avoid the possibility that the infant will develop **graft-versus-host disease (GVHD),** the blood products should be irradiated (see Chap. 26E).

Apheresis services are generally not necessary, as a single unit of antigen negative platelets should give a 50,000 to 100,000 boost. By collecting the platelet-rich plasma from the mother and reinfusing the red blood cells to the mother, there can be multiple collections over the ensuing several days. Although an apheresis unit could be obtained and aliquoted to achieve a platelet supply for up to 5 days of transfusions, it is unclear that this benefits the patient (15).

   b) **Gamma globulin (IgG).** There has been successful postnatal use of intravenous IgG 0.4 g/kg/day for 2 to 5 days (8,16). This is our routine treatment now. Other centers use 1 g/kg/day for 2 days.

   c) **Prednisone (Prednisolone IV).** Usually, 2 mg/kg/day is given to newborns with continued low platelet counts or continued bleeding (8).

 iii. **Treatment of additional children.** It is important to make the diagnosis for other children and to refer the family to a high-risk center for additional pregnancies. Sisters of P1A1-negative mothers should have platelet typing done to foresee problems. If they are P1A1-negative and their husbands are P1A1-positive, anticipatory planning is indicated. Three platelet serology laboratories are The Blood Center of Southeastern Wisconsin (1-800-245-3117), Tom Kickler (Johns Hopkins, Baltimore, Maryland), and Scott Murphy's lab (Temple University, Philadelphia, Pennsylvania).

 iv. **Outcome.** Roughly 20% of all infants with identified cases of NAIT have intracranial hemorrhages. As many as half of these occur antenatally. We have seen two fetal deaths with bleeding associated with fetal alloimmune thrombocytopenia. Obtain a cranial ultrasonographic study after delivery to document any intracranial bleeding, because intracranial hemorrhages are sometimes clinically silent.

3. **Drug-induced.** Although a long list of drugs is associated with neonatal thrombocytopenia, it is unclear how many of them are the true cause. If the mother has an antibody that results in thrombocytopenia by immune mechanisms, the infant may become thrombocytopenic if given the same medication. (Treatment is as in Chapter 26B.)

B. **Peripheral consumption of platelets**
 1. **Disseminated intravascular coagulation (DIC) (see Chap. 26B).**
    a. **Clinical picture.** The infant appears sick and has thrombocytopenia, a prolonged PT, and a prolonged PTT. There is a decrease in fibrinogen, and an increase in D-dimers.
    b. **Therapy**
      i. Treat the underlying disorder (e.g., sepsis, acidosis, hypoxia, or hypothermia). Give vitamin K and replace clotting factors and platelets.
     ii. Perform exchange transfusion with fresh whole blood for patients with active bleeding that does not respond to repeated plasma and platelet transfusions.
 2. **Giant hemangioma (Kasabach-Merritt syndrome)** (4)
    a. **Clinical picture.** The baby appears healthy, and has a large hemangioma and thrombocytopenia.
    b. **Therapy** involves platelet transfusion, clotting factors, and prednisone. Most hemangiomas involute by 1 to 2 years of age, so attempt medical management. We and others have had good results treating some of these hemangiomas with α-interferon but an increase in cerebral palsy in

children treated with α-interferon has stopped us from using this therapy. Embolization or surgery is sometimes necessary.

3. Necrotizing enterocolitis (see Chap. 32)
    a. Clinical picture. Thrombocytopenia with necrotizing enterocolitis.
    b. Therapy. Treat the underlying disorder and give platelet transfusions as necessary.

4. Type IIB von Willebrand disease may present as thrombocytopenia secondary to platelet aggregation in newborns (3).

C. Direct toxic injury to platelets
  1. Sepsis may be of bacterial or viral origin. Therapy involves treatment of the underlying disorder. Platelet transfusion is necessary if there is bleeding.
    a. Thrombocytopenia as an early sign of sepsis in newborns is nonspecific, although high mean platelet volume and high platelet distribution widths correlated with late sepsis.
    b. There is some evidence that an immune mechanism may be involved in the thrombocytopenia of neonatal sepsis.
  2. Drug injury. Thiazides, tolbutamide, hydralazine, and aspirin have been implicated. Therapy involves the removal of the offending drug, and giving platelet transfusion if there is bleeding. Maternal ingestion of **aspirin** during pregnancy should be avoided. If ingestion occurs within 1 week of delivery, 90% of newborns will have bleeding tendencies. Maternal use of aspirin has been associated with a reduced mean birth weight of the offspring, prolongation of gestation and labor, increased blood loss at delivery, and increased perinatal mortality (4).
  3. Neonatal cold injury. Massive pulmonary hemorrhage secondary to hyperaggregation of platelets has been associated with infants who die while being rewarmed.

D. Hypersplenism
  1. Clinical picture. The baby has an enlarged spleen and thrombocytopenia; there may or may not be hemolytic anemia. The condition is associated with congenital hepatitis, congenital viral infection, and portal vein thrombosis.
  2. Therapy. Treat the underlying disorder. Administer platelet transfusion if there is bleeding. Splenectomy is the last resort for uncontrollable bleeding.

E. Familial shortened platelet survival results from intrinsic problems with platelets. Production may also be abnormal.
  1. Wiskott-Aldrich syndrome is manifested by the presence of abnormal, small platelets.
  2. May-Hegglin anomaly is an autosomal dominant disorder in which the infant has giant, bizarre platelets with Döhle bodies, abnormal platelet survival, and impaired production of platelets.
  3. Bernard-Soulier syndrome is demonstrated by the presence of large platelets with granules clumped to appear as a nucleus.

IV. THROMBOCYTOPENIA WITH NORMAL PLATELET SURVIVAL AND DECREASED PLATELET PRODUCTION
  A. Toxic injury to megakaryocytes due to bacterial or viral infections or drug-induced injury.
  B. Congenital thrombocytopenias due to syndrome of thrombocytopenia with absent radii, Fanconi anemia, familial thrombocytopenias, or marrow aplasia, which may be isolated or general.
  C. Marrow infiltration due to neonatal leukemia, congenital neuroblastoma, or storage disease.

V. THROMBOCYTOPENIA ASSOCIATED WITH ERYTHROBLASTOSIS FETALIS. The mechanism may possibly involve platelet trapping in the liver and spleen, anoxia with secondary intravascular coagulation, or associated antiplatelet antibodies.

VI. THROMBOCYTOPENIA AFTER EXCHANGE OR OTHER TRANSFUSION. Blood more than 24 hours old has few viable platelets.

VII. THE MANAGEMENT OF A HIGH-RISK FETUS requires orchestration of interventional obstetricians, reference laboratory, and comprehensive blood bank services. A review of platelet problems in the newborn is found in reference (4).

References

1. Burrows RF. Fetal thrombocytopenia and its relation to maternal thrombocytopenia. *N Engl J Med* 1993;329:1463.
2. Pao M, Karlowicz M, Kickler T, et al. Importance of platelet serologic testing for defining the cause of neonatal thrombocytopenia. *Am J Pediatr Hematol Oncol* 1991; 13:71.
3. DeCarolis S, Noia G, DeSantis M, et al. Immune thrombocytopenic purpura and percutaneous umbilical blood sampling: An open question. *Fetal Diagn Ther* 1993;8:154.
4. Beardsley DS. Platelet abnormalities in infancy and childhood. In: Nathan DG, Oski FA, eds. *Hematology of infancy and childhood*, 5th ed. Philadelphia: WB Saunders, 1998.
5. Andrew M, Vegh P, Caco C, et al. A randomized, controlled trial of platelet transfusions in thrombocytopenic premature infants. *Pediatrics* 1993;123:285.
6. Schnell M, McFarland JG, Besa EC, et al. Serologic investigation of 295 cases of suspected neonatal alloimmune thrombocytopenia [Abstract]. *Transfusion* 1994;34 (Suppl 16):64.
7. Kaplan C, Morel-Kopp MC, Clemenceau S, et al. Fetal and neonatal alloimmune thrombocytopenia: Current trends in diagnosis and therapy. *Transfus Med* 1992;2:265.
8. Bussel JB, Kaplan C, McFarland J, et al. Recommendations for the evaluation and treatment of neonatal autoimmune and alloimmune thrombocytopenia. *Thromb Haemost* 1991;65:631.
9. Christiaens GC, Nieuwenhuis HK, Von dem Borne AEGK, et al. Idiopathic thrombocytopenic purpura in pregnancy: A randomized trial on the effect of antenatal low dose corticosteroids on neonatal platelet counts. *Br J Obstet Gynaecol* 1990;97:893.
10. Bussel JB, Zabusky MR, Berkowitz RL, et al. Fetal alloimmune thrombocytopenia. *N Engl J Med* 1997;337:23.
11. Burrows RF, Kelton JG. Prenatal thrombocytopenia. *Clin Perinatol* 1995;22:779.
12. Blanchette VS, Chen L, de Friedberg ZS, et al. Alloimmunization to the P1A1 platelet antigen: Results of a prospective study. *Br J Haematol* 1990;74:209.
13. Menell JS, Bussel JB, Gianopoulas JG, et al. Antenatal management of the thrombocytopenias. *Clin Perinatol* 1994;21:591.
14. McFarland JG, Aster RH, Bussel JB, et al. Prenatal diagnosis of neonatal alloimmune thrombocytopenia using allele-specific oligonucleotide probes. *Blood* 1991;78:2276.
15. Karpatkin M. Platelet counts in infants of women with autoimmune thrombocytopenia: Effect of steroid administration to the mother. *N Engl J Med* 1981;305:936.
16. Amato M, Pasquier S, Besa EC, et al. Treatment of neonatal thrombocytopenia. *J Pediatr* 1985;107:650.
17. Kickler TS. Elevated platelet-associated IgG in PLA1-negative mothers following sensitization to the PLA-1 antigen during pregnancy. *Vox Sang* 1992;63:210.
18. Cines DB, McKenzie SE, Siegel DL, et al. Immune thrombocytopenia Purpura. *N Engl J Med* 2002;13:995.
19. Schmidt BK. Coagulation screening in high risk neonates: A prospective cohort study. *Arch Dis Child* 1992;67:1196.
20. Hohlfeld P, Forestier F, Kaplan C, et al. Fetal thrombocytopenia: A retrospective survey of 5194 fetal blood samplings. *Blood* 1994;84:1851.
21. Tchernia G, Morel-Kopp MC, Yvart J, et al. Neonatal thrombocytopenia and hidden maternal autoimmunity. *Br J Haematol* 1993;84:457.
22. Warkentin TE, Keltan JG. Platelet lifecycle: Quantitative disorders. In: Handen RI, Lux SE, Stossel TP, eds. *Blood principles and practice of hematology*, 2nd ed. Lippincott Williams & Wilkins, 2003.

BLOOD PRODUCTS USED IN THE NEWBORN
Steven R. Sloan

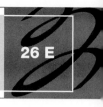

I. WHOLE BLOOD AND BLOOD COMPONENT TRANSFUSIONS

A. General principles. Blood components consist of packed red blood cells (PRBCs), platelets, frozen plasma, fresh frozen plasma (FFP), cryoprecipitate (CRYO), and granulocytes (1). In addition, intravenous immunoglobulin (IVIG) is purified from blood. In some special cases, whole blood, usually in the form of reconstituted whole blood, can be used. However, in most cases blood components are preferred because each component has specific optimal storage conditions and component therapy maximizes the use of blood donations.

B. Side effects

1. Infectious diseases. A variety of infectious diseases can be transmitted by blood transfusion. Human immunodeficiency virus (HIV), hepatitis B virus (HBV), hepatitis C virus (HCV), syphilis, human T-lymphotropic virus (HTLV) I/II and West Nile virus (WNV) are screened for using medical history questionnaires and laboratory tests, but new pathogens can enter the blood supply. The risk of acquiring a transfusion-transmitted infectious disease is too low to be accurately measured but the values have been calculated and are shown in Table 26E.1 (2–4).

Cytomegalovirus (CMV) can also be transmitted by blood but this is rare if the blood is leukoreduced and/or it tests negative for antibodies to CMV (5). Other diseases known to be capable of being transmitted by blood transfusions include malaria, babesiosis, and Chagas disease. Animal studies suggest that variant Creutzfeldt-Jakob disease (vCJD) can also be transmitted by blood transfusion and some probable cases of transfusion-transmitted vCJD in humans have been reported (6,7).

C. Special considerations. Whole blood, platelets, and RBCs can be leukoreduced by filtration or irradiated to reduce the incidence of specific complications.

1. Leukoreduction. Leukoreduction filters remove approximately 99.9% of the white blood cells from RBCs and platelets. In addition, most platelets collected by apheresis are leukoreduced even without additional filtration. Benefits of leukoreduction include the following (8):

a. Decreased immunization to antigens on leukocytes such as human leukocyte antigen (HLA) antigens.

b. Decreased rate of febrile transfusion reactions.

c. Minimization of a possible (and controversial) immunomodulatory effect of blood transfusions.

d. Decreased rate of CMV transmission.

Although the first three indications are not essential for neonates, neonates often receive leukoreduced blood components to decrease transmission of CMV.

2. Irradiation. Irradiation prevents transfusion-associated graft-versus-host disease (TA-GVHD) from transfused leukocytes in cellular blood components. Among those at risk are premature infants and children with certain congenital immunodeficiencies. To prevent this fatal consequence of transfusion, all PRBCs, platelets, and granulocytes are irradiated at Children's Hospital, Boston, unless blood is emergently needed.

Some people donate blood for specific patients, providing what is commonly known as *directed or designated blood*. Directed donations have a small increase in rate of infectious disease transmission. The difference is minimal and parents often want to donate for their children. Transfusion of paternal RBCs or platelets is contraindicated if the neonate's plasma contains antibodies directed

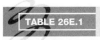 **TABLE 26E.1**	**Current Infectious Disease Risks from Blood Transfusions**

Pathogen	Risk per unit
Human immunodeficiency virus (HIV)	1 in 1,800,000
Hepatitis C virus (HCV)	1 in 1,600,000
Hepatitis A virus	1 in 1,000,000
Hepatitis B virus (HBV)	1 in 220,000
West Nile virus (WNV)	1 in 350,000
Human T-cell lymphotropic virus (HTLV)	1 in 3,000,000
Parvovirus B19	1 in 10,000

against antigens expressed on paternal erythrocytes or platelets, respectively. If a relative does donate blood components, the blood must be irradiated since it is at increased risk for causing TA-GVHD if the blood donors are first-degree blood relatives of the patient.

II. PACKED RED BLOOD CELLS (PRBCs)

A. General principles

1. **Mechanism.** Red blood cells (RBCs) provide oxygen-carrying capacity for patients whose blood lacks sufficient oxygen-carrying capacity owing to anemia, hemorrhage, or a hemoglobinopathy. Transfusion for hemoblobinopathies are unusual in the neonatal period when most patients will have significant amounts of fetal hemoglobin.

   Several types of PRBC units that vary in the preservatives added are available. Chemical additives delay storage damage to RBCs allowing for extended storage times. The types of units that are currently available in the United States are as follows:

   a. **Anticoagulant-preservative solution units.** These units contain approximately 250 mL of a concentrated solution of RBCs. The average hematocrit of these units is 70% to 80%. In addition, these units contain 62 mg of sodium, 222 mg of citrate, and 46 mg of phosphate. Three types of units are currently approved for use in the United States. These are as follows:

      i. **CPD.** This contains 773 mg of dextrose and has a 21-day shelf life.

      ii. **CP2D.** This contains 1,546 mg of dextrose and has a 21-day shelf life.

      iii. **CPDA-1.** This contains 965 mg of dextrose and 8.2 mg of adenine and has a 35-day shelf life. This is the most widely used of the anticoagulant-preservative solution units.

   b. **Additive solution units.** Most RBC units used in the United States are additive units. Three additive solutions are currently approved for use in the United States. Each of these units contains approximately 350 mL, has an average hematocrit of 50% to 60%, and has a 42-day shelf life. Contents of these units are shown in Table 26E.2 (9). For simple transfusions of 5 to 20 mL/kg, additive units can be used.

2. **The changes that occur in PRBCs during storage**

   a. The pH decreases from 7.4 to 7.55 to pH 6.5 to 6.6 at the time of expiration.

   b. Potassium is released from the RBCs. The initial plasma K+ concentration is approximately 4.2 mM and increases to 78.5 mM in CPDA-1 units at day 35 and 45 to 50 mM in additive solution units on day 42. CPDA-1 units contain approximately one third the plasma volume as additive units, so the total amount of extracellular potassium is similar in all units of the same age.

   c. 2,3-Diphosphoglycerol (2,3-DPG) levels drop rapidly during the first 2 weeks of storage. This increases the affinity of the hemoglobin for oxygen

| TABLE 26E.2 | Contents of Additive Solution RBC Units | | |

Contents (mg)	AS-1	AS-3	AS-5
Dextrose	2,973	2,645	1,673
Sodium	962	406	407
Citrate	222	711	222
Phosphate	46	233	46
Adenine	27	30	30
Mannitol	750	0	525

AS = additive solution.

and decreases its efficiency in delivering oxygen to tissue. The 2,3-DPG levels replenish over several hours after being transfused.

3. Toxicity. Although there are theoretic concerns that mannitol may cause a rapid diuresis and adenine may be a nephrotoxin in the premature infant, case reports and case series have found no risk associated with additive solution units. Hence, some hospitals transfuse additive solution units to neonates. In general, we prefer to use nonadditive solution units or washed additive solution units for larger transfusions such as exchange transfusions or transfusions for surgical procedures with substantial blood loss for young infants.

B. Indications/contraindications. The indications for transfusions and types of transfusions are described earlier in this chapter (see Chap. 26A).

C. Dosing and administration. The usual dose is 5 to 15 mL/kg transfused at a rate of approximately 5 mL/kg/hour. This may be adjusted depending on the severity of the anemia and/or the patient's ability to tolerate increases in intravascular volume.

D. Side effects

1. Acute transfusion reactions

a. Acute hemolytic transfusion reactions. These reactions are usually due to incompatibility of donor RBCs with antibodies in the patient's plasma. The antibodies usually responsible for acute hemolytic transfusion reactions are isohemagglutinins (anti-A, anti-B). These reactions are rare in neonates because they do not make isohemagglutinins until they are 4 to 6 months old. However, maternal isohemagglutinins can be present in the neonatal circulation.

i. Symptoms. Possible symptoms include hypotension, fever, tachycardia, infusion site pain, and hematuria.

ii. Treatment. Administer fluids and furosemide to protect kidneys. If necessary, treat hypotension with pressors and Disseminated intravascular coagulation (DIC). There might exist the need to transfuse compatible PRBCs.

b. Allergic transfusion reactions. These are unusual in neonates. Allergic reactions are due to antibodies in the patient's plasma that react with proteins in donor plasma.

i. Symptoms. Mild allergic reactions are characterized by hives and possibly wheezing. More severe reactions can present as anaphylaxis.

ii. Treatment. These reactions can be treated with antihistamines, bronchodilators, and corticosteroids as needed. These reactions are usually specific to individual donors. If they are serious or reoccur, RBCs and platelets can be washed.

c. Volume overload. Blood components have high oncotic pressure and rapid infusion can cause excessive intravascular volume. This can cause a sudden deterioration of vital signs.

d. **Hypocalcemia.** Rapid infusion of components, especially FFP, can cause transient hypocalcemia, usually manifested as hypotension.

e. **Hypothermia.** Cool blood can cause hypothermia. Transfusion through blood warmers can prevent this condition.

f. **Transfusion-associated acute lung injury (TRALI).** This is often due to antibodies in donor plasma that react with the patient's histocompatibility (HLA) antigens. These reactions present as respiratory compromise and are more likely to occur with blood components containing significant amounts of plasma such as platelets or FFP.

g. **Hyperkalemia.** Potassium leakage is not significant for simple transfusions of 5 to 20 mL/kg. However, hyperkalemia can be important in large transfusions such as exchange transfusions or transfusions for major surgery. This leakage is increased in whole blood. Ideally, fresher PRBC units can be provided for these transfusions. At Children's Hospital Boston, PRBCs <14 days old are transfused to children younger than 1 year undergoing surgery. If fresh PRBCs are unavailable, washing blood will temporarily remove the plasma potassium.

h. **Febrile nonhemolytic transfusion reactions** are usually due to cytokines released from leukocytes in the donor unit. These occur less frequently if the unit is leukoreduced.

i. **Bacterial contamination** can occur but is relatively rare with RBC transfusions.

j. **Transfusion-associated graft-versus-host disease (TA-GVHD).** Lymphocytes from donor blood components can mount an immune response against the patient. Patients are at risk if they are unable to mount immune responses against the transfused lymphocytes. Such patients include premature infants, infants with congenital immune deficiencies, and patients sharing HLA types with blood donors as often occurs when people donate blood for specific individuals. This can be prevented by irradiation. Leukoreduction filters do not remove enough lymphoctes to prevent TA-GVHD.

E. **Special considerations.** Donor exposures can be minimized by reserving a fresh unit of PRBCs for a neonate at his or her first transfusion and transfusion of aliquots of that unit for each subsequent transfusion (10). This is useful for premature infants who are expected to require multiple simple transfusions for anemia of prematurity.

III. FFP, THAWED PLASMA

A. **General principles.** The two frozen plasma products that are most frequently available are FFP and thawed plasma. Both components are used to administer all the clotting factors. The contents are as follows:

1. Each component has approximately 1 unit/mL of each coagulation factor except that thawed plasma may have approximately two thirds the levels of the unstable factors (V and VIII).

2. Sodium of 160 to 170 mEq/L and potassium of 3.5 to 5.5 mEq/L.

3. All plasma proteins including albumin and antibodies.

4. Sodium citrate of 1,440 g.

B. **Indications.** FFP and frozen plasma are indicated to correct coagulopathies due to factor deficiencies. Although plasma contains proteins and albumins, these components are not indicated for intravascular volume expansion or for antibody replacement since other components are safer and better for those indications.

C. **Dosing and administration.** A dose of 10 to 20 mL/kg is usually adequate, and this may need to be repeated every 8 to 1 hours depending on the clinical situation.

D. **Side effects.** The side effects of RBC can also occur with plasma transfusions, with some different risks when compared with RBC transfusions:

1. Hyperkalemia will not occur.

2. TRALI is more likely since more plasma containing antibodies is transfused.

3. Acute hemolytic reactions involving hemolysis of transfused RBCs are extremely unlikely. However, if the plasma contains incompatible antibodies (e.g., group O plasma transfused to a group A patient), an acute hemolytic reaction can

rarely occur. For this reason, transfused plasma should be compatible with the patient's blood group.

   4. Citrate induced hypocalcemia is a risk with plasma infusions. The amount of citrate is unlikely to cause transient hypocalcemia in most situations but this can happen with rapid infusions of large amounts of FFP.

IV. PLATELETS (see Chap. 26D)

   A. General principles. Platelets can be prepared from whole blood donations or collected by apheresis. If they are collected by apheresis, an aliquot is obtained for a neonatal transfusion. Often only a portion of a whole blood–derived platelet unit is transfused to neonates, but we do not find it worthwhile to aliquot whole blood–derived platelets.

   1. Contents. Each unit of whole blood–derived platelets contains at least 5×10^{10} platelets in 50 mL of anticoagulated plasma including proteins and electrolytes. Because platelets are stored at room temperature for up to 5 days, there may be low levels of the unstable coagulation factors, V and VIII.

   B. Indications. No good studies exist, but neonatal intensive care unit (NICU) patients at increased risk for intracranial hemorrhage should probably be maintained at a platelet count of 50,000 to 100,000 platelets/mm^3. For additional information, see Chapter 26D.

   C. Dosing and administration. (One tenth of a whole blood–derived platelet unit)/kg should **raise** the platelet count by 30,000/mm^3. This corresponds to approximately 5 mL/kg.

   D. Side effects. The side effects of FFP transfusions can also occur with platelet transfusions. Additionally, the following problems may occur:

   1. Platelets are more likely to be contaminated with bacteria, causing septic reactions since platelets are stored at room temperature. For this reason, many blood banks test platelet units for bacterial contamination.

   2. Inventory issues can limit the ability to match ABO types of platelets and patients. ABO-incompatible plasma in a platelet unit can rarely cause a hemolytic transfusion reaction. For this reason, Children's Hospital, Boston, routinely concentrates group O or B platelets transfused to group A patients.

   E. Special considerations. Platelets can be **concentrated** by centrifugation, resulting in a volume of 15 to 20 mL. This may damage the platelets.

V. GRANULOCYTES

   A. Indications. Granulocyte transfusions are a controversial therapy that may benefit patients with severe neutropenia or dysfunctional neutrophils and a bacterial or fungal infection not responding to antimicrobial therapy. Most granulocytes are given to patients who are neutropenic secondary to hematopoietic progenitor cell transplants. However, infants with septicemia having chronic granulomatous disease may also benefit from granulocyte transfusions. Granulocyte transfusions can only be used as a temporary therapy until the patient starts producing neutrophils or until another curative therapy can be instituted.

   B. Dosing and administration. The dose is 10 to 15 mL/kg. This may need to be repeated every 12 to 24 hours.

   C. Side effects. In addition to all the potential adverse effects associated with RBC transfusions, granulocyte transfusions can cause pulmonary symptoms and must be administered slowly to minimize the chances of severe reactions. Additionally, granulocytes can transmit CMV. Hence donors should be serologically negative for CMV if the patient is at risk for CMV disease.

   D. Special considerations. Granulocyte collections need to be specially scheduled and the granulocytes should be transfused as soon as possible after collection, and no later than 24 hours after the collection.

VI. WHOLE BLOOD

   A. General principles. Whole blood contains RBCs and plasma clotting factors. Few units are stored as whole blood. Whole blood can be reconstituted from a unit of RBCs and FFP.

   B. Indications. Exchange transfusions. Also, may be used as a substitute for blood components in priming circuits for extracorporeal membrane oxygenation (ECMO) or cardiopulmonary bypass, but this may cause increased fluid retention and longer postoperative recovery times (11). Whole blood may be useful for neonates immediately following disconnection from a cardiopulmonary bypass circuit for cardiac surgery (12).

C. Side effects. All of the adverse effects of individual blood components can occur with whole blood.

D. Special considerations. Whole blood should be transfused when it is relatively fresh since whole blood is stored at 1°C to 6°C and coagulation factors decay at this temperature. When used just after cardiopulmonary bypass, the blood should be no more than 2 to 3 days old. When used in other situations, the whole blood should be no more than 5 to 7 days old.

Platelets in whole blood will be cleared rapidly following transfusion and reconstituted whole blood lacks significant quantities of platelets.

VII. INTRAVENOUS IMMUNOGLOBULIN (IVIG)

A. General principles. IVIG is a concentrated purified solution of immunoglobulins with stabilizers such as sucrose. Most products contain >90% immunoglobulin G (IgG) with small amounts of immunoglobulin M (IgM) and immunoglobulin A (IgA). Several brands of IVIG are available.

B. Indications. IVIG can have an immunosuppressive effect that is useful for alloimmune disorders such as neonatal alloimmune thrombocytopenia and possibly alloimmune hemolytic anemia. Both of these disorders are due to maternal antibodies to antigens on the neonate's cells (13,14) (see Chaps. 18 and 26C).

IVIG can also be used to replace immunoglobulins for patients who are deficient in immunoglobulins as occurs with some congental immunodeficiency syndromes.

Some studies have attempted to determine whether IVIG is useful as a prophylaxis or treatment for neonatal sepsis. Results from these studies are mixed and not enough evidence exists for routine use of IVIG for general sepsis (15).

1. Hyperimmune immunoglobulins. High titer disease-specific immunoglobulins are available for several infectious agents including Varicella-zoster virus and respiratory syncytial virus (16,17). These immunoglobulins may be useful for infants at high risk for these infections.

C. Dosing and administration. IVIG (non–disease-specific) is usually given at a dose of 500 to 900 mg/kg. Doses for the disease-specific immunoglobulins should follow the manufacturer's recommendations.

D. Side effects. Rare complications include transient tachycardia or hypertension. Because of the purification processes, IVIG currently in use has a very low risk of transmitting infectious diseases.

References

1. Technical Manual Program Unit. *Technical manual*, 15th ed. Bethesda: AABB, 2005.
2. Busch MP, Kleinman SH, Nemo GJ. Current and emerging infectious risks of blood transfusions. *JAMA* 2003;289(8):959–962.
3. Dodd RY, Notari EP IV, Stramer SL. Current prevalence and incidence of infectious disease markers and estimated window-period risk in the American Red Cross blood donor population. *Transfusion* 2002;42(8):975–979.
4. Petersen LR, Epstein JS. Problem solved? West Nile virus and transfusion safety. *N Engl J Med* 2005;353(5):516–517.
5. Vamvakas EC. Is white blood cell reduction equivalent to antibody screening in preventing transmission of cytomegalovirus by transfusion? A review of the literature and meta-analysis. *Transfus Med Rev* 2005;19(3):181–199.
6. Llewelyn CA, Hewitt PE, Knight RS, et al. Possible transmission of variant Creutzfeldt-Jakob disease by blood transfusion. *Lancet* 2004;363(9407):417–421.
7. Peden AH, Head MW, Ritchie DL, et al. Preclinical vCJD after blood transfusion in a PRNP codon 129 heterozygous patient. *Lancet* 2004;364(9433):527–529.
8. Dzik WH. Leukoreduction of blood components. *Curr Opin Hematol* 2002;9(6):521–526.

9. Luban NL, Strauss RG, Hume HA. Commentary on the safety of red cells preserved in extended-storage media for neonatal transfusions. *Transfusion* 1991;31(3):229–235.

10. Strauss RG, Burmeister LF, Johnson K, et al. AS-1 red cells for neonatal transfusions: A randomized trial assessing donor exposure and safety. *Transfusion* 1996;36(10):873–878.

11. Mou SS, Giroir BP, Molitor-Krisch EA, et al. Fresh whole blood versus reconstituted blood for pump priming in heart surgery in infants. *N Engl J Med* 2004;351(16):1635–1644.

12. Manno CS, Hedberg KW, Kim HC, et al. Comparison of the hemostatic effects of fresh whole blood, stored whole blood, and components after open heart surgery in children. *Blood* 1991;77(5):930–936.

13. Kaplan C. Immune thrombocytopenia in the foetus and the newborn: diagnosis and therapy. *Transfus Clin Biol* 2001;8:3, 311–314.

14. Alcock GS, Liley H. Immunoglobulin infusion for isoimmune haemolytic jaundice in neonates. *Cochrane Libr* 2002;(3):CD003313.

15. Ohlsson A, Lacy JB. Intravenous immunoglobulin for suspected or subsequently proven infection in neonates. *Cochrane Libr* 2000;(2):CD001239.

16. Atkins JT, Karimi P, Morris BH, et al. Prophylaxis for respiratory syncytial virus with respiratory ssyncytial virus-immunoglobulin intravenous among preterm infants of thirty-two weeks gestation and less: reduction in incidence, severity of illness and cost. *Pediatr Infect Dis J* 2000;19:2, 138–143.

17. Huang YC, Tzou-Yien L, Yi-Jane L, et al. Prophylaxis of intravenous immunoglobulin and acyclovir in perinatal varicella. *Eur J Pediatr* 2001;160(2):91–94.

NEONATAL THROMBOSIS
Munish Gupta

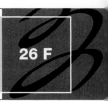

26 F

I. PHYSIOLOGY
A. Physiology of thrombosis
1. **Thrombin** is the primary procoagulant protein, converting fibrinogen into a fibrin clot. The intrinsic and extrinsic pathways of the coagulation cascade result in formation of active thrombin from prothrombin.
2. **Inhibitors of coagulation** include antithrombin, heparin cofactor I, protein C, protein S, and tissue factor pathway inhibitor (TFPI). Antithrombin activity is potentiated by heparin.
3. **Plasmin** is the primary fibrinolytic enzyme, degrading fibrin in a reaction that produces fibrin degradation products and D-dimers. Plasmin is formed from plasminogen by numerous enzymes, most important of which is tissue plasminogen activator (tPA).
4. In neonates, factors contributing to thrombus formation can affect blood flow, blood composition (leading to hypercoagulability), and vascular endothelial integrity.

B. Unique physiologic characteristics of hemostasis in neonates
1. *In utero,* coagulation proteins are synthesized by the fetus, and do not cross the placenta.
2. Both thrombogenic and fibrinolytic pathways are altered in the neonate compared with the older child and adult, resulting in increased vulnerability to both hemorrhage and pathologic thrombosis. However, under normal physiologic conditions, the hemostatic system in premature and term newborns is in balance,

and healthy neonates do not clinically demonstrate hypercoagulable or bleeding tendencies.

3. Concentrations of most procoagulant proteins are reduced in neonates compared with adult values, although fibrinogen levels are normal or even increased. Compared to adults, neonates have a decreased ability to generate thrombin, and values for the prothrombin time (PT) and the activated partial thromboplastin time (PTT) are prolonged.

4. Concentrations of most antithrombotic and fibrinolytic proteins are also reduced, including protein C, protein S, plasminogen, and antithrombin. Thrombin inhibition by plasmin is diminished compared with adult plasma.

5. Platelet number and lifespan appear to be similar to that of adults. The bleeding time, an overall assessment of platelet function, and interaction with vascular endothelium is shorter in neonates than in adults, suggesting more rapid platelet adhesion and aggregation.

II. EPIDEMIOLOGY AND RISK FACTORS

A. Epidemiology

1. Thrombosis occurs more frequently in the neonatal period than at any other age in childhood.

2. The presence of an **indwelling vascular catheter** is the single greatest risk factor for arterial or venous thrombosis. Indwelling catheters are responsible for >80% of venous and 90% of arterial thrombotic complications.

3. Autopsy studies show 20% to 65% of infants who expire with an umbilical venous catheter (UVC) in place are found to have a thrombus associated with the catheter. Venography suggests asymptomatic thrombi are present in 30% of newborns with a UVC.

4. **Umbilical arterial catheterization (UAC) appears to result in clinically severe symptomatic vessel obstruction requiring intervention in approximately 1% of patients.** Asymptomatic catheter-associated thrombi have been found in 3% to 59% of cases by autopsy and 10% to 90% of cases by angiography.

5. Other risk factors include infection, increased blood viscosity, polycythemia, dehydration, hypoxia, hypotension, maternal diabetes, and intrauterine growth restriction (IUGR).

6. Infants undergoing surgery involving the vascular system, including repair of congenital heart disease, are at increased risk for thrombotic complications. Diagnostic or interventional catheterizations also increase the risk for thombosis.

7. **Renal vein thrombosis (RVT)** is the most common type of noncatheter related pathologic thrombosis.

8. Registries from Canada, Germany, and the Netherlands have described series of cases of neonatal thrombosis.
   a. Incidence of clinically significant thrombosis were estimated as 2.4 per 1,000 admissions to the neonatal intensive care unit in Canada, 5.1 per 100,000 births in Germany, and 14.5 per 10,000 neonates aged 0 to 28 days in the Netherlands.
   b. Two series examined both venous and arterial thromboses. Among all thrombotic events, percentage of RVT, other venous thrombosis, and arterial thrombosis were 44%, 32%, and 24% respectively in one series, and 22%, 40%, and 34% in the other series.
   c. Excluding cases of RVT, 89% and 94% of venous thromboses were found to be associated with indwelling central lines in two of the studies.
   d. Other commonly identified risk factors included sepsis, perinatal asphyxia, congenital heart disease, and dehydration.
   e. Mortality was uncommon but present, and was generally restricted to very premature infants or infants with large arterial or intracardiac thromboses.

B. Inherited thrombophilias

1. **Inherited thrombophilias** are characterized by positive family history, early age of onset, recurrent disease, and unusual or multiple locations of thromboembolic

events. It is estimated that a genetic risk factor can be identified in approximately 70% of patients with thrombophilia.

2. Important inherited thrombophilias include the following:

   a. Deficiencies of protein C, protein S, and antithrombin, which appear to have the largest increase in relative risk for thromboembolic disease but are relatively rare.

   b. Activated protein C resistance, including the factor V Leiden mutation G1691A, and the prothrombin G20210A mutation, which have high incidence, particularly in certain populations, but appear to have low risk of thrombosis in neonates.

   c. Hyperhomocysteinemia, increased lipoprotein (a) levels, and homozygos C677T polymorphism in the methylene tetrahydrofolate reductase (MTHFR) gene, which are relatively common but the significance in neonatal thrombosis is still poorly understood.

   d. Increased levels of VIIIC and fibrinogen have been associated with neonatal thrombosis.

3. Multiple other defects in the anticoagulation, fibrinolytic, and antifibrinolytic pathways have been identified, including abnormalities in thrombomodulin, tissue factor pathway inhibitor (TFPI), fibrinogen, plasminogen, tPA, and plasminogen-activator inhibitors. The frequency and importance of these defects in neonatal thrombosis is poorly understood.

4. The incidence of thrombosis in patients heterozygous for most inherited thrombophilias is small; however, increasing evidence suggests that the presence of a second risk factor substantially increases the risk for thrombosis. This second risk factor can be an acquired clinical condition or illness, or another inherited defect. Patients with single defects for inherited prothrombotic disorders rarely present in neonatal period, unless another pathologic process or event occurs.

5. Patients who are homozygous for a single defect or double heterozygotes for different defects can present in the neonatal period, often with significant illness due to thrombosis. The classic presentation of homozygous prothrombotic disorders is **purpura fulminans** with homozygous protein C or S deficiency, which presents within hours or days of birth, often with evidence of *in utero* cerebral damage.

6. Overall, the importance of inherited thrombophilias as independent risk factors for neonatal thrombosis is still undetermined. It appears that the absolute risk of thrombosis in the neonatal period in all patients with inherited thrombophilia (nonhomozygous) is actually quite small; however, among neonates with thrombotic disease, the incidence of an inherited thrombophilia appears to be substantially increased compared with incidence in the general population.

C. Acquired thrombophilias

1. Newborns can acquire significant coagulation factor deficiencies because of placental transfer of maternal antiphospholipid antibodies, including the lupus anticoagulant and anticardiolipin antibody.

2. These neonates can present with significant thrombosis, including purpura fulminans.

III. SPECIFIC CLINICAL CONDITIONS

A. Venous thromboembolic disorders

1. General considerations

   a. Most venous thrombosis occurs secondary to **central venous catheters.** Spontaneous (i.e., noncatheter-related) venous thrombosis can occur in renal veins, adrenal veins, inferior vena cava, portal vein, hepatic veins, and the venous system of the brain.

   b. Spontaneous venous thrombi usually occur in the presence of another risk factor. Less than 1% of significant venous thromboembolic events in neonates are idiopathic.

   c. Thrombosis of the **sinovenous system of the brain** is an important cause of neonatal cerebral infarction.

    d. Short-term complications of venous catheter–associated thrombosis include loss of access, pulmonary embolism, superior vena cava syndrome, and specific organ impairment.

    e. It is likely that the frequency of pulmonary embolism in sick neonates is underestimated, as signs and symptoms would be similar to multiple other common pulmonary diseases.

    f. Long-term complications of venous thrombosis are poorly understood. Initial series suggest inferior vena cava thrombosis, if extensive, is associated with a high rate of persistent partial obstruction and symptoms such as leg edema, abdominal pain, lower extremity thrombophlebitis, varicose veins, and leg ulcers.

2. Major venous thrombosis — signs and symptoms

    a. Initial sign of catheter-related thrombosis is usually difficulty infusing through or withdrawing from the line.

    b. Signs of venous obstruction include swelling of the extremities, possibly including the head and neck, and distended superficial veins.

    c. The onset of **thrombocytopenia** in the presence of a central venous line (CVL) also raises the suspicion of thrombosis.

3. Major venous thrombosis — diagnosis

    a. Ultrasonography. Ultrasonography is diagnostic in most cases of significant venous thrombosis. In smaller infants or low flow states, however, the ultrasonography may not provide sufficient information about the size of the thrombus, and recent data suggest a significant false-negative rate for ultrasonographic diagnosis.

    b. Contrast studies. A radiographic line study can be helpful for diagnosis of catheter-associated thrombosis. Venography through peripheral vessels may be needed for diagnosis of thrombosis proximal to the catheter tip, for spontaneous thrombosis in the upper body, and for thrombosis not seen by other methods (see IV).

4. Prevention of catheter-associated venous thrombosis

    a. Heparin 0.5 units/mL is added to all infusions (compatability permitting) through CVLs.

    b. UVCs should be removed as soon as clinically feasible, and should not remain in place for longer than 10 to 14 days. Our usual practice is to place a peripherally inserted central catheter (PICC) line if anticipated need for central access is >7 days.

5. Management of major venous thrombosis

    a. Nonfunctioning CVL

        i. If fluid can no longer be easily infused through the catheter, remove the catheter unless the CVL is absolutely necessary.

        ii. If continued central access through the catheter is judged to be clinically necessary, clearance of the blockage with thrombolytic agents or HCl can be considered (see V.F).

    b. Local obstruction. If a small occlusive catheter-related thrombosis is documented, a low-dose infusion of thrombolytic agents through the catheter can be considered for localized site-directed thrombolytic therapy (see V.E). If infusion through the catheter is not possible, the CVL should be removed and heparin therapy considered.

    c. Extensive venous thrombosis. Consider leaving the catheter in place and attempting local site–directed thrombolytic therapy. Otherwise, remove the catheter and begin heparin therapy. Systemic thrombolytic therapy should be reserved for extensive noncatheter-related venous thrombosis and for venous thrombosis with significant clinical compromise.

B. Aortic or major arterial thrombosis

1. General Considerations

    a. Spontaneous arterial thrombi in the absence of a catheter is unusual but does occur in ill neonates.

    b. Acute complications of catheter-related and spontaneous arterial thrombi depend on location, and can include renal hypertension, intestinal necrosis, peripheral gangrene, and other organ failure.

    c. Thrombosis of cerebral arteries is an important cause of neonatal cerebral infarction.

    d. Long-term effects of symptomatic and asymptomatic arterial thrombi are not well studied, but may include increased risk for atherosclerosis at the affected area and chronic renal hypertension.

2. Aortic thrombosis — signs and symptoms

    a. Initial sign is often isolated dysfunction of umbilical artery catheter (UAC).

    b. Mild clinical signs include hematuria in absence of transfusions or hemolysis, hematuria with red blood cells (RBCs) on microscopic analysis, hypertension, and intermittent lower extremity decreased perfusion or color change.

    c. Strong clinical signs include persistent lower extremity color change or decreased perfusion, blood pressure differential between upper and lower extremities, decrease or loss of lower extremity pulses, signs of peripheral thrombosis, oliguria despite adequate intravascular volume, signs of necrotizing enterocolitis, and signs of congestive heart failure.

3. Aortic thrombosis — diagnosis

    a. Ultrasonography. Ultrasonography with Doppler flow imaging should generally be performed in all cases of suspected aortic thrombosis; if signs of thrombis are mild and resolve promptly after removal of the arterial catheter, an ultrasonograph may not be necessary. Ultrasonography is diagnostic in most cases, although recent data suggest a significant false-negative rate.

    b. Contrast study. If ultrasonograph is negative or inconclusive, and major arterial thrombosis is suspected, a radiographic contrast study can be performed, through the arterial catheter.

4. Prevention of catheter-associated arterial thrombosis

    a. Heparin 0.5 to 1 unit/mL is added to all infusions (compatability permitting) through arterial catheters; heparin infusion through arterial catheters has been shown to prolong patency and to likely reduce incidence of local thrombus, without risk of significant complications.

    b. Review of the literature suggests **"high" umbilical arterial lines** (tip in descending aorta below left subclavian artery and above diaphragm) are preferable to "low" lines (tip below renal arteries and above aortic bifurcation), with fewer clinically evident ischemic complications, an apparent trend to reduce incidence of thrombi, and no difference in serious complications such as necrotizing enterocolitis and renal dysfunction.

    c. Consider placing **peripheral arterial line** rather than umbilical in infants weighing >1,500 g.

    d. Monitor carefully for clinical evidence of thrombus formation when an umbilical arterial catheter is present.

        i. Monitor for evidence of UAC dysfunction, including waveform dampening and difficulty flushing or withdrawing blood.

        ii. Monitor lower extremity color and perfusion.

        iii. Check all urine for heme.

        iv. Check upper and lower extremity blood pressure three times daily.

        v. Monitor for hypertension and decreased urine output.

    e. Umbilical arterial catheters should be removed as soon as clinically feasible. Our general practice is to leave umbilical arterial catheters in place for no longer than 5 to 7 days, and to place a peripheral arterial line should continued arterial access be needed.

5. Management of aortic and major arterial thrombosis

    a. Minor aortic thrombi. Small aortic thrombi with limited mild symptoms can often be managed with prompt removal of the umbilical arterial catheter, with rapid resolution of symptoms.

b. **Large but nonocclusive thrombus.** For large thrombi that are nonocclusive to blood flow (as demonstrated by ultrasonography or contrast study) and that are not accompanied by signs of significant clinical compromise, the arterial catheter should be removed and anticoagulation with heparin considered. Close follow-up with serial imaging studies is indicated.

c. **Occlusive thrombus or significant clinical compromise.** Large occlusive aortic thrombi or thrombi accompanied by signs of significant clinical compromise including renal failure, congestive heart failure, necrotizing enterocolitis, and signs of peripheral ischemia, should be managed aggressively.

   i. If catheter is still present and patent, consider local thrombolytic therapy through the catheter (see V.E).

   ii. If catheter has already been removed or is obstructed, consider systemic thrombolytic therapy. The catheter should be removed if still in place and obstructed.

d. **Surgical thrombectomy is not indicated,** because the mortality and morbidity far exceed that of current medical management.

6. **Peripheral arterial thrombosis**

   a. Congenital occlusions of large peripheral arteries are seen, although rare, and can present with symptoms ranging from a poorly perfused pulseless extremity to a black, necrotic limb, depending on duration and timing of occlusion.

      i. Common symptoms include decreased perfusion, decreased pulses, pallor, and embolic phenomena that may manifest as skin lesions or petechiae.

      ii. Diagnosis can often be made by Doppler flow ultrasonography.

   b. Peripheral arterial catheters, including radial, posterior tibial, and dorsalis pedis catheters, are rarely associated with significant thrombosis.

      i. Poor perfusion to the distal extremity is frequently seen, and usually resolves with prompt removal of the arterial line.

      ii. We infuse heparin 0.5 to 1 unit/mL at 1 to 2 mL/hour through all peripheral arterial lines.

      iii. Treatment of significant thrombosis or persistently compromised extremity perfusion associated with a peripheral catheter should consist of heparin anticoagulation and consideration of systemic thrombolysis for extensive lesions. Close follow-up with serial imaging is indicated.

C. **RVT**

1. **RVT occurs primarily in newborns and young infants,** and most often presents in the first week of life. A significant proportion of cases appear to result from in utero thrombus formation.

2. **Affected neonates are usually term** and are often large for gestational age (LGA). There is an increased incidence among infants of diabetic mothers, and males are more often affected than females. Other associated conditions and risk factors include perinatal asphyxia, hypotension, polycythemia, increased blood viscosity, and cyanotic congenital heart disease.

3. **Presenting symptoms** in the neonatal period include flank mass, hematuria, proteinuria, thrombocytopenia, and renal dysfunction. Coagulation studies may be prolonged, and fibrin degradation products are usually increased.

4. Disease is often bilateral.

5. Some physicians suggest all patients with RVT should be screened for inherited prothrombotic disorders.

6. Diagnosis is usually by ultrasonography.

7. **Management is usually aggressive**

   a. Unilateral RVT without significant renal dysfunction and without extension into the inferior vena cava is often managed with supportive care alone.

   b. Unilateral RVT with renal dysfunction or extension into the inferior vena cava and bilateral RVT should be considered for anticoagulation with heparin.

   c. Bilateral RVT with significant renal dysfunction should be considered for thrombolysis.

IV. DIAGNOSTIC CONSIDERATIONS

A. Ultrasonography. Ultrasonography with Doppler flow analysis is the most commonly used diagnostic modality.

1. Advantages include relative ease of performance, noninvasiveness, and ability to perform sequential scans to assess progression of thrombosis or response to treatment.

2. Sensitivity of ultrasonography may be somewhat limited: several recent studies suggest that significant venous and arterial thrombi may be missed by ultrasonography. Ultrasonography remains our test of first choice, but if it is inconclusive or negative in the context of significant clinical suspicion of thrombosis, a contrast study should be considered.

B. Radiographic line study. Imaging after injection of contrast material through a central catheter often is diagnostic for catheter-associated thrombi, and has the advantage of relative ease of performance.

C. Venography. Venography with injection of contrast through peripheral vessels may be necessary when other diagnostic methods fail to demonstrate the extent and severity of thrombosis.

1. A contrast line study will not provide information on venous thrombosis proximal to catheter tip (i.e., along the length of the catheter).

2. Upper extremity and upper chest venous thromboses, either catheter-related or spontaneous, are particularly difficult to visualize with ultrasonography.

V. MANAGEMENT

A. Evaluation for thrombophilia

1. Consider evaluating for congenital or acquired thrombophilias those neonates with severe or unusual manifestations of thrombosis or with positive family histories of thrombosis. The benefit of evaluation in infants with known risk factors such as indwelling central catheters is uncertain.

2. Initial evaluation should include consideration of deficiencies of protein C, protein S, or antithrombin; presence of activated protein C resistance and the factor V Leiden mutation; presence of the prothrombin G20210A mutation; and passage of maternal antiphospholipid antibodies.

a. Protein C, protein S, and antithrombin deficiencies can be evaluated by measurement of antigen or activity levels. Results of testing of neonates should be compared with standard gestational age-based reference ranges, as normal physiologic values can be as low as 15% to 20% of adult values. In addition, levels will be physiologically depressed in the presence of active thrombosis, and may be difficult to interpret; we therefore generally wait until 2 to 3 months after the thrombotic episode before performing these measurements in the infant. Alternative to or in conjunction with testing of the neonate, parents can be tested for carrier status by measurement of protein C, protein S, and antithrombin levels.

b. Factor V Leiden and prothrombin G20210A mutations can be assayed by specific genetic tests in the neonate. Alternatively, parents can be tested for carrier status.

c. The mother can be tested for antinuclear antibodies, lupus anticoagulant, and anticardiolipin antibodies.

3. If all of the above are negative, subsequent specialized laboratory evaluation includes consideration of abnormalities or deficiencies of homocysteine, lipoprotein(a), MTHFR, plasminogen, and fibrinogen. Very rarely seen are abnormalities or deficiencies of heparin cofactor II, thrombomodulin, plasminogen-activator inhibitor-1, platelet aggregation, and tPA.

B. General considerations

1. Precautions

a. Avoid intramuscular (IM) injections and arterial punctures during anticoagulation or thrombolytic therapy.

b. Avoid indocin or other antiplatelet drugs during therapy.

c. Use minimal physical manipulation of patient (i.e., no physical therapy) during thrombolytic therapy.

    d. Thrombolytic therapy should not be initiated in the presence of active bleeding or significant risk for local bleeding, and should be carefully considered if there is a history of recent surgery of any type (particularly neurosurgery).

    e. Monitor clinical status carefully for signs of hemorrhage, including internal hemorrhage and intracranial hemorrhage.

    f. Consider giving fresh frozen plasma (FFP) 10 mL/kg to any patient who needs anticoagulation.

2. Guidelines for choice of therapy

    a. Small asymptomatic nonocclusive arterial or venous thrombi related to catheters can often be treated with catheter removal and supportive care alone.

    b. Large or occlusive venous thrombi can be treated with anticoagulation with heparin or low-molecular-weight (LMW) heparin; usually relatively short courses (7–14 days) of anticoagulation are sufficient, but occasionally long-term treatment may be necessary.

    c. Most arterial thrombi should be treated with anticoagulation with heparin or LMW heparin.

    d. In cases of massive venous thrombi or arterial thrombi with significant clinical compromise, treatment with local or systemic thrombolysis should be considered.

C. Heparin

1. General considerations

    a. Term newborns generally have increased clearance of heparin compared with adults, and therefore require relatively increased heparin dosage. This increased clearance is significantly diminished, however, in premature neonates.

    b. Heparin should be infused through a dedicated IV line that is not used for any other medications or fluids, if possible.

    c. Laboratory work. Before starting heparin therapy, obtain complete blood count (CBC), prothrombin time (PT), and PTT.

    d. Adjustment of heparin infusion rate is based on clinical response, serial evaluation of thrombus (usually by ultrasonography), and monitoring of laboratory parameters.

    e. Significant patient-to-patient variability in heparin dosage requirements is seen.

    f. Use of PTT to monitor heparin effect is problematic in neonates because of significant variability of coagulation factor concentrations and baseline prolongation of the PTT; **heparin activity level** is generally considered to be a more reliable marker.

    g. Therapeutic heparin activity for treatment of most thromboembolic events is considered to be an antifactor Xa level of 0.3 to 0.7 U/mL or a heparin level by protamine titration of 0.2 to 0.4 U/mL. Most laboratories report heparin activity levels as an antifactor Xa level.

    h. Follow CBC frequently while on heparin treatment to monitor for heparin-associated thrombocytopenia, which can be diagnosed by assay of heparin-associated antiplatelet antibodies.

    i. Heparin activity is dependent on presence of antithrombin. Consider administration of **FFP** (10 mL/kg) or antithrombin concentrate (one vial of 500 u) when effective anticoagulation with heparin is difficult to achieve.

      i. Antithrombin levels can be measured directly to aid in therapy, although administration of exogenous antithrombin can increase sensitivity to heparin even in patients with near normal antithrombin levels.

      ii. Note that measurement of heparin activity levels, unlike measurement of PTT, is independent of presence of antithrombin. Therefore, measured heparin activity levels may be therapeutic although effective anticoagulation is not seen due to antithrombin deficiency.

2. Dosing guidelines

    a. Heparin is given as an initial bolus of 75 units/kg, followed by a continuous infusion that is begun at 28 units/kg/hour. Slightly lower dosing can be used in premature infants under 36 weeks' gestation, with an initial bolus of 50 units/kg followed by a continuous infusion begun at 20 units/kg/hour.

b. Heparin activity levels and/or PTT should be measured 4 hours after initial bolus and 4 hours after each change in infusion dose, and every 24 hours once a therapeutic infusion dose has been achieved.

 Heparin Dosage Monitoring and Adjustment

PTT (s)	Heparin activity (U/mL)	Bolus (U/kg)	Hold	Rate	Recheck
<50	0–0.2	50	—	+10%	4 h
50–59	0.21–0.29	0	—	+10%	4 h
60–85	0.3–0.7	0	—	—	24 h
86–95	0.71–0.8	0	—	−10%	4 h
96–120	0.81–1.0	0	30 min	−10%	4 h
>120	>1	0	60 min	−15%	4 h

PTT = partial thromboplastin time.
PTT values may vary by laboratory depending on reagents used. Generally, PTT values of 1.5 to 2.5 × the baseline normal for a given laboratory correspond to heparin activity levels of 0.3 to 0.7 U/mL.
From Michelson, AD, Bovill, E, Andrew, M. Antithrombotic therapy in children. *Chest* 1995;108(suppl),506S–522S.

3. Duration of therapy. Anticoagulation with heparin may continue up to 10 to 14 days. Oral anticoagulants are generally not recommended in neonates; if long-term anticoagulation is needed, consult hematology.

4. Reversal of anticoagulation

a. Termination of heparin infusion will quickly reverse anticoagulation effects of heparin therapy, and is usually sufficient.

b. If rapid reversal is necessary, protamine sulfate may be given IV. Protamine can be given in a concentration of 10 mg/mL at a rate not to exceed 5 mg/minute. Hypersensitivity can occur in patients who have received protamine-containing insulin or previous protamine therapy.

c. Dosing. On the basis of total amount of heparin received in last 2 hours as follows.

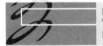 **Protamine Dosage to Reverse Heparin Therapy* Based on Total Amount Heparin Received in Prior 2 h**

Time since last heparin dose (min)	Protamine dose (mg/100 U heparin received)
<30	1.0
30–60	0.5–0.75
60–120	0.375–0.5
>120	0.25–0.375

*Maximum dosage is 50 mg. Maximum infusion rate is 5 mg/min of 10 mg/mL solution.
Adapted from Monagle P, et al. Antithrombotic therapy in children. *Chest* 2004;126:645S–687S.

D. LMW heparin
 1. General considerations
  a. Although data on LMW heparin usage in neonatal patients is limited, growing evidence of safety and efficacy in adult and pediatric patients has led to increased use in neonatal populations.
  b. Several **advantages of LMW heparins** over standard heparin exist: predictable pharmacokinetics; decreased need for laboratory monitoring; subcutaneous BID dosing; probable reduced risk of heparin-induced thrombocytopenia; and possible reduced risk of bleeding at recommended dosages.
  c. Therapeutic dosage of LMW heparins are titrated to antifactor Xa levels. **Target antifactor Xa levels** for treatment of most thromboembolic events are 0.50 to 1.0 U/mL, measured 4 to 6 hours after a subcutaneous injection. When used for prophylaxis, target levels are 0.2 to 0.4 U/mL. After therapeutic levels have been achieved for 24 to 48 hours, levels should be followed at least weekly.
  d. Infants younger than 2 months of age have a higher dose requirement than older children. In addition, some studies suggest premature infants may require higher doses than full term infants, up to 2 mg/kg/dose q12 hours.
  e. Several different LMW heparins are available, and the dosages are **not** interchangeable. **Enoxaparin (Lovenox)** has the most widespread pediatric usage and is generally preferred.
  f. Follow CBCs, as thrombocytopenia can occur.
 2. Dosing guidelines

Age	Initial treatment dose	Initial prophylactic dose
Initial Dosing of Enoxaprin, Age-dependent (in mg/kg/dose SQ)		
<2 mo	1.5 q12h	0.75 q12h
>2 mo	1.0 q12h	0.5 q12h

Preterm infants may require doses up to 2 mg/kg q12h to maintain target antifactor Xa levels.
Adapted from Young TE, Mangum B. *Neofax 2006* Acorn: Raleigh, 2006, and Monagle P, et al. Antithrombotic therapy in children. *Chest* 2004;126:645S–687S.

Monitoring and Dosage Adjustment of Enoxaparin Based on Antifactor XA Level Measured 4 h After Dose of Enoxaparin

Antifactor Xa level (U/mL)	Hold dose	Dose change	Repeat antiXa level
<0.35	—	+25%	4 h after next dose
0.35–0.49	—	+10%	4 h after next dose
0.5–1	—	—	24 h
1.1–1.5	—	−20%	Before next dose
1.6–2	3 h	−30%	Before next dose, then 4 h after next dose
>2	Until level is 0.5 U/mL	−40%	Before next dose; if level not <0.5 U/mL, repeat q12h

Adapted from Monagle P, et al. Antithrombotic therapy in children. *Chest* 2001;110:344–370S.

3. Reversal of anticoagulation
   a. Termination of subcutaneous injections is usually sufficient to reverse anticoagulation when clinically necessary.
   b. If rapid reversal is needed, protamine sulfate can be given within 3 to 4 hours of last injection, although protamine may not completely reverse anticoagulant effects. Administer 1 mg protamine sulfate per 1 mg LMW heparin given in last injection. See V.C.4 for administration guidelines.

E. Thrombolysis
 1. General considerations
   a. Thrombolytic agents act by converting endogenous plasminogen to plasmin. Plasminogen levels in neonates are reduced compared with adult values, and therefore effectiveness of thrombolytic agents may be diminished. Cotreatment with plasminogen can increase thrombolytic effect of these agents.
   b. Indications include recent arterial thrombosis, massive thrombosis with evidence of organ dysfunction or compromised limb viability, and life-threatening thrombosis. Thrombolytic agents can also be used to restore patency to thrombosed central catheters (see F), and local infusions of low-dose thrombolytic agents can be used for small to moderate occlusive thrombosis near a central catheter.
   c. Minimal data exist in newborn populations regarding all aspects of thrombolytic therapy, including appropriate indications, safety, efficacy, choice of agent, duration of therapy, use of heparin, and monitoring guidelines. Recommendations for use are generally based on small series and case reports, which overall suggest that thrombolytic therapy in neonates can be effective with limited significant complications.
   d. Consider evaluating all patients for intraventricular hemorrhage before initiating thrombolytic therapy.
   e. Contraindications to thrombolytic therapy include active bleeding, major surgery or hemorrhage within the last 7 to 10 days, neurosurgery within the last 3 weeks, severe thrombocytopenia, and generally, prematurity under 32 weeks.

 2. Treatment guidelines
   a. Preparation for thrombolytic therapy
      i. Place sign at head of bed indicating thrombolytic therapy.
      ii. Have topical thrombin available in unit refrigerator.
      iii. Notify blood bank to insure availability of cryoprecipitate.
      iv. Notify pharmacy to ensure availability of amino caproic acid (Amicar).
      v. Obtain good venous access; consider access to allow frequent blood draws to minimize need for phlebotomy.
      vi. Consider hematology consult.
   b. Thrombolysis can be achieved by local, site-directed administration of thrombolytic agents in low doses directly onto or near a thrombosis through a central catheter; or by **systemic** administration of thromobolytic agents in higher doses. Local therapy is generally limited to small or moderate-sized thromboses. Minimal data exist supporting one method over the other.
   c. Tissue plasminogen activator (tPA) versus streptokinase versus urokinase. Minimal data exist comparing safety, efficacy, and cost of different thrombolytic agents in children. **tPA has become the agent of choice,** although significantly more expensive, for several reasons:
      i. Streptokinase has the greatest potential for allergic reactions, whereas tPA has lowest.
      ii. tPA has the shortest half-life.
      iii. tPA theoretically has less stimulation of a systemic proteolytic state, because of its poor binding of circulating plasminogen and its maximal impact on fibrin-bound plasminogen.
      iv. The production of urokinase has faced difficulties in the past due to manufacturing concerns.

d. **Obtain CBC, platelets, PT, PTT, and fibrinogen** before initiating therapy.

e. **Monitor PT, PTT, and fibrinogen** every 4 hours initially, and then at least every 12 to 24 hours. Monitor hematocrit and platelets every 12 to 24 hours. Monitor thrombosis by imaging every 6 to 24 hours.

f. **Expect fibrinogen to decrease by 20% to 50%.** If no decrease in fibrinogen is seen, obtain d-dimers or fibrinogen split products to show evidence that a thrombolytic state has been initiated.

g. **Maintain fibrinogen level above 100 mg/dL** and **platelets above 50,000 to 100,000mm³** to minimize the risks of clinical bleeding. Administer cryoprecipitate 10 mL/kg (or 1 unit/5 kg) or platelets 10 mL/kg as needed. If fibrinogen level drops below 100, decrease the dose of thrombolytic agent by 25%.

h. If no improvement in clinical condition or thrombosis size is seen after initiating therapy, and if fibrinogen levels remain high, **consider giving FFP 10 mL/kg,** which may correct deficiencies of plasminogen and other thrombolytic factors.

i. **Duration of therapy.** Thrombolytic therapy is usually provided for a brief period, (i.e., 6–12 hours), but longer durations can be used for refractory thromboses with appropriate monitoring. Overall, therapy should balance resolution of the thrombus and improvement in clinical status against signs of clinical bleeding.

j. **Concomitant heparin therapy.** Heparin therapy, usually without the loading bolus dose, should be initiated during or immediately after completion of thrombolytic therapy.

3. **Dosing**

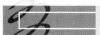

Systemic Thrombolytic Therapy

Agent	Load	Infusion	Notes
tPA	none	0.1–0.5 mg/kg/h for 6 h	Duration usually 6 h; can continue for 12 h or repeat after 24 h, although lysis of clot will continue for hours after infusion stops. Lower dose appears to be as effective as higher dose
Streptokinase	2,000 U/kg over 10 min	1,000–2,000 U/kg/h	Only one course should be given for 6 h. Consider premedication with tylenol and benadryl
Urokinase	4,400 U/kg over 10 min	4,400 U/kg/h for 6 h	Longer duration may be necessary based on clinical response

tPA, tissue plasminogen activator.
Consider concomitant heparin therapy at 5–20 U/kg/h without bolus dose for all three agents.
Optimal duration of therapy is uncertain, and can be individualized based on clinical response.

Local Site-directed Thrombolytic Therapy

Agent	Infusion	Notes*
tPA	0.03–0.05 mg/kg/h	Increase infusion rate up to 0.1 mg/kg/h if no clinical effect
Urokinase	150 U/kg/h	Increase infusion by 200 U/kg/h if no clinical effect

*Monitor laboratory studies as for systemic treatment.

4. Treatment of bleeding during thrombolytic therapy
   a. Localized bleeding: apply pressure, administer topical thrombin, and provide supportive care; thrombolytic therapy does not necessarily need to be stopped if bleeding is controlled.
   b. Severe bleeding: stop infusion and administer cryoprecipitate (1 unit/5 kg).
   c. Life-threatening bleeding: stop infusion, give cryoprecipitate, and infuse amino caproic acid (Amicar) (at usual dose of 100 mg/kg IV every 6 hours); consult hematology before giving Amicar.
5. Post-thrombolytic therapy. Consider initiating heparin therapy, but without the initial loading dose. Consider discontinuing heparin if no reaccumulation of the thrombus occurs after 24 to 48 hours.
F. Treatment of central catheter thrombosis
   1. Treatment guidelines
      a. Central catheters may become occluded because of thrombus or chemical precipitate, which is usually secondary to parenteral nutrition.
      b. Nonfunctioning central catheters should be removed whenever possible, unless continued access through that catheter is absolutely necessary.
      c. Thrombolytic agents may be used for thrombosis and hydrochloric acid (HCl) may be attempted for chemical blockage.
      d. General procedure
         i. Instill chosen agent at volume needed to fill catheter (up to 1–2 mL) with gentle pressure; agent should not be forced in if resistance is too high. If instillation is difficult, a three-way stopcock can be used to create a vacuum in the catheter: attach catheter, 10 mL empty syringe, and 1 mL syringe containing agent to the stopcock, and create vacuum by gently drawing back several mL in the 10-mL syringe while the stopcock is off to the 1-mL syringe. While holding pressure, turn stopcock off to the 10-mL syringe and allow vacuum in catheter to draw in infusate from the 1-mL syringe.
         ii. Use of HCl for catheter clearance in neonates is based on limited clinical data and experience, and should be performed with caution. Suggested volumes to use range from 0.1 mL to 1 mL of 0.1 molar solution. As severe tissue damage may result from peripheral administration or extravasation of HCl, consultation with a surgeon before HCl use should be considered.
         iii. Wait 1 to 2 hours for thrombolytic agents and 30 to 60 minutes for HCl and attempt to withdraw fluid through the catheter.
         iv. If unsuccessful, above steps can be repeated once. Urokinase can also be left in place for 8 to 12 hours if shorter intervals are unsuccessful.
         v. If clearance of catheter is not successful after two attempts or longer urokinase infusion, catheter should be removed or contrast study performed to delineate extent of blockage.
      e. Low-dose continuous infusion of thrombolytic agents can be considered for local thrombosis occluding catheter tip (see preceding text).

2. Dosing guidelines

Local Instillation of Agents for Catheter Blockage	
Agent	Dosing
tPA	0.5 mg/lumen diluted in NS to volume needed to fill line, to max 3 mL
Urokinase	5,000 U/mL, 1–2 mL/lumen; comes in unit doses prepared expressly for catheter clearance
HCl	0.1 M, 0.1–1 mL/lumen

tPA, tissue plasminogen activator; NS, normal saline; HCl, hydrochloric acid.

Suggested Readings

Andrew M, Monagle P, deVeber G, et al. Thromboembolic disease and antithrombotic therapy in newborns. *Hematology* 2001:358–374.

Barrington KJ. Umbilical artery catheters in the newborn: Effects of position of the catheter tip. *Cochrane Database Syst Rev* 1999;(1).

Chalmers EA. Epidemiology of venous thromboembolism in neonates and children. *Thromb Res* 2006;118:3–12.

Dix D, Andrew M, Marzinotto V, et al. The use of low molecular weight heparin in pediatric patients: A prospective cohort study. *J Pediatr* 2000;136:439–345.

Duffy LF, Kerzner B, Gebus V, et al. Treatment of central venous catheter occlusions with hydrochloric acid. *J Pediatr* 1989;114:1002–1004.

Gunther G, Junker R, Strater R, et al. Symptomatic ischemic stroke in full-term neonates: Role of acquired and genetic prothrombotic risk factors. *Stroke* 2000;31:2437–2441.

Hartmann J, Hussein A, Trowitzsch E, et al. Treatment of neonatal thrombus formation with recombinant tissue plasminogen activator: Six years experience and review of the literature. *Arch Dis Child Fetal Neonatal Ed* 2001;85:F18–F22.

Hausler M, Hubner D, Delhaas T, et al. Long-term complications of inferior vena cava thrombosis. *Arch Dis Child* 2001;85:228–233.

van Ommen H. Venous thromboembolism in childhood: A prospective two-year registry in the Netherlands. *J Pediatr* 2001;139:676–681.

Manco-Johnson MJ, Grabowski EF, Hellgreen M, et al. Laboratory testing for thrombophilia in pediatric patients. *Thromb Haemost* 2002;88:155–156.

Manco-Johnson MJ, Grabowski EF, Hellgreen M, et al. Recommendations for tPA thrombolysis in children. *Thromb Haemost* 2002;88:157–158.

Michaels LA, Gurian M, Hegyi T, et al. Low molecular weight heparin in the treatment of venous and arterial thromboses in the premature infant. *Pediatrics* 2004;114:703–707.

Monagle P, Andrew M. Developmental hemostasis: Relevance to newborns and infants. In: Nathan DG, Orkin SH, Ginsburg D, et al. eds. *Hematology of infancy and childhood.* Philadelphia: WB Saunders, 2003.

Monagle P, Chan A, Massicotte P, et al. Antithrombotic therapy in children. *Chest* 2004;126:645S–687S.

Nowak-Gottl U, von Kries R, Gobel U, et al. Neonatal symptomatic thromboembolism in Germany: Two year survey. *Arch Dis Child Fetal Neonatal Ed* 1997;76:F163–F167.

Luck RP, Maggiori L, Poujade O, et al. *Pediatr Rev* 2006;27:275–277. http://pedsinreview .aappublications.org

Schmidt B, Andrew M. Neonatal thrombosis: Report of a prospective Canadian and international registry. *Pediatrics* 1995;96:939–943.

Werlin SL, Lausten T, Jessen S, et al. Treatment of central venous catheter occlusions with ethanol and hydrochloric acid. *J Parent Ent Nutr* 1995;19:416–418.

Young TE, Mangum B. *Neofax 2006.* Raleigh: Acorn Publishing, 2006.

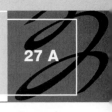

NEONATAL SEIZURES

Adré J. du Plessis

27 A

I. **INTRODUCTION.** Seizures are the most distinctive manifestation of neurologic dysfunction in the newborn infant. Moreover, neonatal seizures often herald potentially devastating forms of brain injury. Recent advances in diagnostic technology have provided important insights into neonatal seizures. Techniques such as bedside video-electroencephalogram (EEG) monitoring and magnetic resonance imaging (MRI) have challenged earlier beliefs and raised fundamental questions regarding the diagnosis, etiology, and management of seizures in the newborn infant. It is well known that most seizures in the newborn are symptomatic of a specific etiology; with these diagnostic advances, an etiology is increasingly identifiable. In addition, these advances have further highlighted the essential differences between seizures in newborn infants and older patients, including their response to conventional anticonvulsant agents. Such age-related differences in the manifestations and treatment response are due in large part to the immature developmental state of the newborn brain and the different etiologies involved. These are discussed in the following text.

In earlier reports, seizures occurred in up to 3 in 1,000 full-term infants and up to 60 in 1,000 premature infants. However, the reported incidence of neonatal seizures varies widely across studies, a variability that is primarily the result of inconsistent diagnostic criteria, as well as the often subtle clinical manifestations of neonatal seizures, and their potential confusion with nonepileptic neonatal behaviors (discussed in the subsequent text). Regardless of their precise incidence, it is clear that seizures are more common in the newborn period than at any other time in life, and that the tendency toward recurrent seizures and status epilepticus is far greater in the newborn.

The **decreased seizure threshold in the newborn** reflects the developmental events active in the immature brain. In essence, the newborn brain has a transient overdevelopment of excitatory systems compared to inhibitory systems. For example, the immature brain has a transient overexpression in the density of excitatory amino acid (primarily glutamate) receptors and a relative paucity of glutamate reuptake transporters. Together these features translate into more prolonged and intense contact of glutamate with postsynaptic receptors. Furthermore, these immature glutamate receptors are far more permissive of cationic influx, facilitating membrane depolarization and seizure activation. In contrast, inhibitory gamma-aminobutyric acid (GABA) ion channels are relatively underexpressed in the immature brain. In fact, in certain areas of the developing brain these immature GABA may be depolarizing (i.e., excitatory) rather than hyperpolarizing (i.e., inhibitory).

In addition to these cellular factors, differential development of neural systems may enhance the excitatory state of the immature brain and predispose to seizures. For example, the excitatory projections of the immature *substantia nigra* develop in advance of the inhibitory anticonvulsant pathways. By virtue of this relatively proconvulsant effect, the immature *substantia nigra* may actually function as an amplifier rather than inhibitor of epileptic discharges.

II. **DIAGNOSIS OF NEONATAL SEIZURES.** The clinical manifestations of neonatal seizures differ in many ways from those in older patients. The behavioral features of seizures in the newborn may be very subtle, in some cases confined to autonomic and subtle motor phenomena. In addition, the motor manifestations are often disorganized, and an orderly homunculus-based progression of convulsive activity (i.e., "Jacksonian march") is very uncommon. Furthermore, continuous video-EEG monitoring has shown an often inconsistent temporal association between clinical and electrographic seizures.

The peculiar clinical characteristics of seizures in the newborn infant likely reflect the immature state of brain development. In late gestation and early postnatal life, active but incomplete developmental processes include cortical organization, axonal and dendritic branching, and the development of synaptic connections. Myelination commences around term but at this stage is largely confined to the deep subcortical regions of the brain. The relatively underdeveloped organization of the cortex and undermyelination of axons likely underlies the disorganized convulsive activity and lack of orderly seizure propagation in the newborn. For the same reasons, primary generalized seizures are very rare in the newborn. In accordance with the caudal-to-rostral gradient of brain development, the cortical development of the deep limbic system, including its connections to the diencephalic and brainstem structures, is relatively advanced compared to the more rostral neocortex. This fact may underlie the prevalence of behaviors referable to the limbic system, diencephalon, and brainstem, such as the sucking and chewing oromotor automatisms, excessive drooling, oculomotor activity, and respiratory irregularities seen in subtle seizures.

A. Clinical diagnosis of neonatal seizures

1. **Clinical seizure subtypes.** Broadly speaking, clinical seizures may be defined as paroxysmal alterations of neurologic function, including behavioral, motor, and/or autonomic changes. Continuous video-EEG monitoring has demonstrated a number of important facts about seizures in the newborn. First, nonepileptic mimics of clinical seizures are common in the newborn. These seizure-like behavior patterns may occur in the normal newborn (e.g., non-nutritive sucking) and nonepileptic paroxysmal clinical changes are common in encephalopathic newborns.

   Given these diagnostic challenges, clinical seizure types may be categorized broadly into four groups: subtle seizures, clonic seizures, tonic seizures, and myoclonic seizures. In many cases, more than one type of seizure occurs in a newborn over time.

   a. **Subtle seizures** are the most common subtype, **comprising about half of all seizures in term and premature newborns.** Subtle seizures are rarely isolated and infants with subtle seizures will almost always have other seizure types as well. Subtle seizures include a broad spectrum of behavioral phenomena, occurring in isolation or in combination. Ocular phenomena are common and include tonic eye deviation, roving "nystagmoid" eye movements, and sudden sustained eye opening with apparent visual fixation. Tonic eye deviation is sometimes classified as a form of tonic seizure. Oro-bucco-lingual movements include chewing, sucking, or lip-smacking movements, and are often associated with a sudden increase in drooling. Various alternating limb movements ("progression movements") have been described, including pedaling, boxing, rowing, or swimming movements. Autonomic phenomena, including sudden changes in skin color and capillary size, may occur alone or in combination with various motor manifestations. Such autonomic paroxysms are usually associated with initial tachycardia, and if sustained, with later bradycardia and possibly apnea. Epileptic apnea is discussed in II.A.2.a. Uncommonly, and unlike clonic seizures, some cases of subtle seizures may be provoked or intensified by stimulation. Although the association between clinical and EEG events is variable, most subtle seizures are not associated with EEG seizures. Based on their inconsistent association with EEG seizures, as well as their poor response to conventional anticonvulsants, many consider these subtle seizures to be nonepileptic "brainstem release phenomena."

   b. **Clonic seizures** are stereotypic and repetitive biphasic movements with a fast contraction phase and a slower relaxation phase. The rhythm of clonic seizures tends to be slower in the newborn than in older patients. Clonic seizures may be unifocal, multifocal, or generalized. Clonic seizures that remain unifocal are usually not associated with loss of consciousness. **The most common cause for clonic seizures that remain unifocal is neonatal stroke** (see II.C.1.b). Other causes of unifocal seizures include focal traumatic contusions, subarachnoid hemorrhage, or metabolic disturbances. In the newborn, multifocal clonic seizures rarely follow a "Jacksonian march;" even when these multifocal seizures are sequential, they are rarely ordered in their progression. Each sequential seizure may appear independent with clinical and EEG features (e.g., rhythm and amplitude) that are different from the previous seizure. Primary generalized clonic seizures are extremely rare in the newborn, probably because of the inability of the immature brain to propagate highly synchronized discharges simultaneously to the entire brain. (One exception to this is benign familial neonatal seizures; see II.C.1.g.i.(a).)

   c. **Tonic seizures** have a sustained period (seconds) of muscle contraction without repetitive features. Tonic seizures may be generalized or focal. Generalized tonic seizures, which may closely mimic decerebrate or decorticate posturing, are **most common in premature infants with diffuse neurologic dysfunction or major intraventricular hemorrhage (IVH).** Generalized tonic seizures are often associated with other motor automatisms or with clonic seizures, as well. Typically, infants are lethargic or obtunded between these seizures. Certain features suggest that these seizures may be nonepileptic in origin. Specifically, they may be precipitated by tactile or other stimuli, suggesting reflex discharges, and may be abolished by repositioning or light restraint. Finally, the clinical events are typically not associated with electrographic seizure patterns. The background EEG pattern tends to have multifocal or generalized voltage depression and undifferentiated frequencies, and, in some cases, a markedly abnormal burst suppression pattern. Overall, **the prognosis of tonic seizures is very poor,** except in some cases of postasphyxial seizures where an outcome may be less grim.

   d. **Myoclonic seizures** are distinguished from clonic seizures by their lightning-fast contractions and nonrhythmic character. These seizures may occur in a multifocal or generalized pattern. Even when repetitive, myoclonic seizures tend to be irregular or erratic in nature. In some cases, myoclonic seizures may be elicited by tactile or auditory stimulation or suppressed by restraint. The electroclinical association of myoclonic seizures is variable, and when present, the myoclonic contraction is usually associated with a single high-voltage spike and followed by a slow-wave complex. Conversely, myoclonic movements in stimulus-sensitive myoclonic seizures or in those with chaotic fragmentary movement patterns are usually not associated with electrographic seizure activity. The EEG background activity tends to be low-voltage, slow-wave activity or a burst suppression pattern with focal sharp waves. These patterns may later evolve to a high-voltage, chaotic hypsarrhythmic pattern. Typically, **myoclonic seizures are associated with diffuse and usually serious brain dysfunction** resulting from etiologies such as perinatal asphyxia, inborn errors of metabolism, cerebral dysgenesis, or major brain trauma. **Myoclonic seizures are usually associated with a poor long-term outcome.**

2. **Seizure mimics.** In the newborn it may be difficult to distinguish between normal immature behaviors (e.g., non-nutritive sucking), abnormal but nonepileptic behaviors (e.g., "jitteriness"), and true epileptic manifestations. The following clinical guidelines may help distinguish true epileptic seizures from seizure mimics. These guidelines are most reliable with suspected clonic seizures but even then are not infallible.

   First, **true epileptic seizures are rarely stimulus-sensitive. Second, epileptic seizures cannot be abolished by passive restraint or repositioning of the infant. Third, epileptic seizures are often associated with autonomic changes or ocular phenomena.** "Jitteriness" (tremor) may be distinguished from clonic seizures by the equal amplitude and faster equiphasic rhythm, compared to the slower, fast-and-slow components of clonic seizures. Generally, normal nonepileptic behaviors are associated with a normal interictal examination. Conversely, abnormal but nonepileptic repetitive behaviors often occur in encephalopathic infants with an abnormal interictal exam.

A temporal association between repetitive clinical events and simultaneous repetitive EEG changes is the strongest supportive evidence for true epileptic seizures. However, using electrographic monitoring to confirm the epileptic nature of suspicious clinical events is more complicated and controversial in the newborn. This is particularly true when clinical seizure events are not accompanied by EEG changes, a situation most often seen with subtle seizures and generalized tonic seizures. There are two opposing views regarding electrically silent clinical "seizures," based on different interpretations of the same fundamental assumptions. In both views, cerebral hemispheric dysfunction results in "disconnection" between higher cortical regions and deeper brainstem areas, thereby causing the electroclinical dissociation in these "spells." On the one hand, these behavioral paroxysms are considered nonepileptic seizure mimics. In this model, the paroxysmal movements are considered to arise from "central pattern generators" in the brainstem. Normally, these brainstem centers are under tonic descending inhibitory input from higher cortical centers. However, injury to the more rostral hemispheric regions disconnects the inhibitory input to the brainstem, "releasing" the primitive reflex movement patterns. These released movements may include relatively complex progression movements, or simple tonic posturing that originates from the brainstem reticulospinal nuclei. Several features support the theory that these spells are disinhibited reflex movements. First, they can often be elicited by external stimuli (spontaneous events may be the result of endogenous stimuli). Second, there is often a temporal and spatial summation of these movements to stimulation, with repeated stimuli eliciting movements that radiate or spread to sites distant from the point of stimulation.

In contrast to this "reflex release" concept of electrically silent clinical seizures, others consider these events to have a true epileptic origin. According to this model, seizure discharges originating in the inferomedial cortex are transmitted to deep brainstem centers where they elicit paroxysmal behavioral phenomena. However, these deep discharges cannot be transmitted through the injured and dysfunctional hemispheric pathways to higher cortical regions, and therefore remain undetected by conventional EEG montages. Support for this model includes the fact that these clinical events with no EEG changes may at other times be coupled to EEG discharges in the same patient. To date, these difficult issues remain unresolved.

a. **Epileptic apnea in the newborn.** Apnea is not uncommon during neonatal seizures, but is rarely the only manifestation. Most infants with epileptic apnea will at some point in their course develop other seizure manifestations. Epileptic apnea may be difficult to distinguish from apnea due to other causes, such as neurologic depression, prematurity, sedative medications, and respiratory illness. However, there are several helpful distinguishing features. Neonatal epileptic apnea rarely lasts longer than 10 to 20 seconds. Bradycardia is often an early accompaniment of nonepileptic apnea, whereas in epileptic apnea, an initial tachycardia is more common, only followed in more prolonged seizures by later bradycardia. The EEG discharges that accompany epileptic apnea are often monorhythmic (most commonly α frequency); in addition, they are usually focal over the temporal regions, suggesting an epileptogenic focus in the limbic system. Conversely, nonepileptic apnea is not accompanied by EEG changes except for amplitude suppression that may develop during prolonged apnea.

b. **Benign neonatal sleep myoclonus** is a relatively common and sometimes dramatic nonepileptic form of myoclonus. This condition presents in the first week of life, and resolves spontaneously (i.e., without treatment) over weeks to months. The convulsive activity emerges during quiet non rapid eye movement (non-REM) sleep and is rapidly abolished by arousal. Myoclonic activity often builds up dramatically in both intensity and distribution over a period of minutes. Unlike other nonepileptic behaviors, this form of myoclonus may be precipitated in some cases by gentle rhythmic rocking or tactile stimuli, and gentle restraint may actually increase rather than abolish the myoclonus. These events never occur during wakefulness and the neurologic examination is normal. Immediately before and during the episodes, the EEG shows features of quiet sleep (sometimes open-eye sleep) with no ictal changes. The interictal EEG is unremarkable. The mechanism is unclear but may be related to a transient dysmaturity of the brainstem reticular-activating system. Anticonvulsants are not indicated, and, in fact, benzodiazepines may exacerbate the myoclonic jerks. The long-term outcome is normal and later epilepsy does not develop.

B. EEG diagnosis of neonatal seizures. By definition, an electrographic seizure is a repetitive series of electrical discharges that evolves in frequency, amplitude and topographic field. As with the clinical manifestations, the electrographic features of neonatal seizures differ in a number of ways from those in more mature patients. Unlike older patients, focal-onset seizures are the rule in the newborn, and primary generalized seizures are exceptionally rare. In addition, there are rhythmic EEG patterns that are normal at specific gestational ages. Abnormal but nonepileptic rhythmic changes may occur on abnormal EEG background in encephalopathic infants. Somewhat arbitrarily, the threshold criterion for the diagnosis of an electrographic seizure has been set at 10 seconds or more of repetitive electrographic discharges. Gestational age has an important influence on the electrographic expression of seizures in the newborn. Such EEG seizures are rare before 34 weeks of gestation; with increasing maturation, the frequency and duration of electrographic seizures increase.

Although the amplitude and frequency of an electrographic seizure tend to evolve as the focal seizure unfolds, the topographic field of seizure spread remains relatively circumscribed in the newborn. Even when several focal seizures develop in different brain regions at the same time, each seizure appears independent in frequency, amplitude, and morphology. Finally, unlike the interictal EEG in older patients with seizures, the neonatal EEG lacks interictal epileptiform patterns that reliably predict the risk for subsequent seizures; in fact, the development of electrographic seizures in the newborn has been described as an all-or-none phenomenon.

1. The role and timing of EEG studies in the newborn with suspected seizures. Ideally an EEG study should be recorded as soon as a seizure is first suspected, and preferably not later than 24 hours after. If such an EEG is normal, particularly if a suspected clinical event is captured during the EEG recording, then subsequent EEGs are only indicated if the clinical spells keep recurring. Whenever possible, several suspect events should be captured on EEG to confirm the true epileptic nature of the events. The absence of EEG changes during several clinical events, especially when the interictal EEG background is normal, is suggestive of a nonepileptic process.

If the initial EEG captures the features of seizure activity and antiepileptic drugs are started, a period of continuous video-EEG monitoring is recommended because anticonvulsant medications may abolish only the clinical manifestations, allowing ongoing and undetected EEG seizures to persist. Ideally, EEG monitoring should continue for 24 to 48 hours after the last recorded electrographic seizure. A repeat EEG after 1 week may have particular prognostic value. The need for subsequent EEG studies as a guide to discontinuation of anticonvulsant medications is controversial.

C. Etiologic diagnosis of neonatal seizures. At the first suspicion of neonatal seizures, the immediate focus should be the exclusion of rapidly correctable and potentially injurious processes, including hypoglycemia, hypocalcemia, and hypomagnesemia, among others. After seizures are confirmed and management has commenced, the etiology should be pursued through a rational and orderly approach, with a stepwise interpretation of the facts, and refocusing of the diagnostic plan. The evaluation should start with a careful history of pregnancy, labor and delivery, and family, followed by a detailed clinical examination for signs of dysmorphism, trauma, skin lesions, and unusual odors. The neurologic examination should include a careful and accurate clinical description of the seizure features,

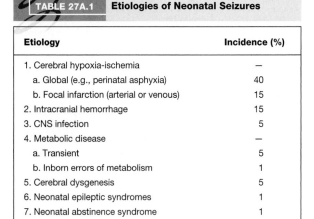

TABLE 27A.1 Etiologies of Neonatal Seizures

Etiology	Incidence (%)
1. Cerebral hypoxia-ischemia	—
a. Global (e.g., perinatal asphyxia)	40
b. Focal infarction (arterial or venous)	15
2. Intracranial hemorrhage	15
3. CNS infection	5
4. Metabolic disease	—
a. Transient	5
b. Inborn errors of metabolism	1
5. Cerebral dysgenesis	5
6. Neonatal epileptic syndromes	1
7. Neonatal abstinence syndrome	1
8. Unknown	10

the infant's mental status, and cranial nerve examination as well as interictal movements, muscle tone, and deep tendon and primitive reflexes. Certain clinical signs may suggest specific etiologies and may facilitate a more rapid etiologic diagnosis. Next, selected special diagnostic techniques may be necessary to pursue or confirm the etiology of seizures, including blood studies, cerebrospinal fluid (CSF) analysis, EEG recording, and neuroimaging studies. Using such an orderly and rational approach, most neonatal seizure etiologies should be identifiable. A list of these seizure etiologies is given in Table 27A.1.

1. Specific etiologies

  a. Hypoxic-ischemic encephalopathy (see Chap. 27C). The leading cause of neonatal seizures is cerebral hypoxia-ischemia, which may occur in the antenatal, intrapartum, or neonatal periods. Perinatal asphyxia is implicated in 25% to 40% of neonatal seizures. However, there is substantial variability in the reported incidence of this etiology, primarily because of the inconsistency of diagnostic criteria used in different reports. The advent of more sophisticated imaging techniques such as MRI and magnetic resonance (MR) spectroscopy have allowed the more precise *in vivo* diagnosis and timing of hypoxic-ischemic lesions. With such imaging, earlier (i.e., antepartum) hypoxic-ischemic lesions are diagnosed, even in cases without significant neonatal encephalopathy.

    Postasphyxial seizures occur in infants with moderate-to-severe grades of encephalopathy, that is, with obtundation, stupor, or coma. In addition, these infants tend to have muscle hypotonia, altered deep tendon reflexes and, in severe cases, brainstem abnormalities. **Intrapartum asphyxia should never be a diagnosis of exclusion,** and should satisfy certain criteria, including evidence of significant fetal distress, immediate postnatal "depression" at birth, and subsequent altered mental status. Significant fetal distress manifests with evidence of certain specific abnormal fetal heart rate patterns (e.g., loss of variability plus late decelerations; sustained bradycardia) and/or evidence of "significant" fetal metabolic acidosis. Although the absolute criteria for significant metabolic acidosis remain controversial, most agree that an umbilical artery pH <7.0 with a base deficit of >12 mEq reflects fetal asphyxia capable of causing neonatal encephalopathy and seizures. Commonly accepted criteria for immediate neonatal depression include an Apgar score of <5 at 5 minutes of life. In cases where there is a prolonged latency between a fetal asphyxial insult (e.g., an antepartum or early intrapartum insult) and delivery, the criteria in the preceding text may not be satisfied. In these cases, specialized MRI studies have demonstrated characteristic features of hypoxic-ischemic brain injury despite the absence of significant acidosis or immediate neonatal depression.

Most postasphyxial seizures in the newborn occur within the first 24 hours after the insult, 50% or more occurring within 12 hours of birth. The seizure onset in each case is likely influenced by the severity, duration, and onset of the intrauterine asphyxial insult. It is likely that more severe insults are followed by earlier onset seizures, but this is not firmly established.

b. Focal ischemic injury

i. Neonatal arterial stroke occurs in around 1 in 4,000 live births. In most cases, the etiology of neonatal strokes remains unknown; however, certain risk factors have been identified and are discussed elsewhere. **Seizures are the most common presentation of stroke in the newborn period, and stroke is the second most common cause of neonatal seizures,** accounting for 15% to 20% of cases. The onset of clinical seizures is variable and may be missed, because most strokes occur in otherwise well term infants, without previously known risk factors. These infants usually appear normal immediately before and after seizures. In fact, in the absence of identified seizures, the diagnosis of neonatal stroke may be delayed until the onset of infant hand use around 4 to 5 months when motor asymmetries become evident. These seizures are typically unifocal, with minimal spread. Because neonatal arterial stroke most commonly involves the left middle cerebral artery (MCA), right-sided clonic seizures are the most common clinical presentation. The clonic activity is generally slower than that in older patients. Poststroke seizures usually have a very good association between clinical and electrographic manifestations.

ii. Cerebral vein thrombosis usually occurs in the large dural sinuses, particularly the posterior aspects of the superior sagittal sinus. Although the presentation of cerebral vein thrombosis may be subtle, with lethargy often the only feature, approximately 60% of cases develop neonatal seizures. Unlike the relatively normal mental status of infants with arterial stroke and seizures, infants with cerebral vein thrombosis and seizures are more encephalopathic, with depressed mental status before and between seizures.

c. Intracranial hemorrhage (see Chap. 27B). Intracranial hemorrhage is implicated in approximately 10% of neonatal seizures. The location of hemorrhage and the clinical features of the seizures varies with gestational age. With term infants, posthemorrhagic seizures are most commonly associated with **primary subarachnoid hemorrhage** and less often with subdural hemorrhage (SDH). Primary subarachnoid hemorrhage occurs more frequently after difficult prolonged or traumatic labor, including forceps and vacuum deliveries. However, primary subarachnoid hemorrhage may occur after apparently uncomplicated labor (i.e., so-called parturitional hemorrhage). Such primary parturitional subarachnoid hemorrhage results in focal or multifocal seizures, usually starting on the second day of life, in infants who appear relatively well between seizures. These seizures often have good clinical and electrical association. **Infants with seizures associated with primary subarachnoid hemorrhage have a good long-term outcome in 90% of cases.**

About half of all subdural hemorrhages (SDH) diagnosed in the newborn are complicated by seizures, usually presenting in the first days of life. Neonatal SDH usually occurs in large babies, breech delivery, or difficult instrumented delivery, because of sheering forces and tears of the tentorium, falx, or cortical bridging veins. Infratentorial SDHs in the limited posterior fossa space demand urgent evaluation because potentially fatal brainstem dysfunction may evolve rapidly.

Posthemorrhagic seizures in the preterm infant have different features and a more ominous prognosis. These seizures are usually associated with **severe IVH,** or its parenchymal complication, periventricular hemorrhagic infarction (PVHI) (see Chap. 27B). Seizures following severe IVH usually present within the first 3 days of life in sick, very premature infants. The seizures are usually generalized tonic seizures with poor electroclinical association. They form part of a critical illness, which often evolves to coma and death in the acute phase. Seizures associated with PVHI tend to occur after the third day of life.

d. **Central nervous system infections** (see Chap. 23). Central nervous system infections from a variety of agents, including viral, bacterial, or other organisms such as toxoplasmosis, may have neonatal seizures as a prominent part of their presentation. These infections may originate in the fetus, for example, congenital encephalitis due to cytomegalovirus (CMV) and toxoplasmosis. When CMV encephalitis occurs in earlier gestation it may cause cerebral dysgenetic lesions, which may further increase the risk of seizures. Intrauterine infections with toxoplasmosis or CMV that are severe enough to cause neonatal seizures usually do so within the first 3 days of life. Other viral infections of importance are herpes simplex virus (HSV) infections that may become symptomatic in the first days of life after intrapartum infection [usually HSV type 2] or have a more delayed presentation (usually postnatal acquisition of HSV type 1). The development of bacterial meningitis, most commonly Group B streptococcal meningitis, may also have a biphasic appearance with early and late forms. The mechanism of seizures in central nervous system infections may be through direct cerebritis or vaso-occlusive injury with secondary seizures. The onset of infection-related seizures obviously depends on the various organisms and onset of infection. Of the bacterial infections, meningitis due to Group B *streptococcus* and *Escherichia coli* are the most common, and in these cases, seizures usually develop in the latter part of the first week or later.

e. **Metabolic disturbances** (see Chap. 29D). Two types of metabolic disturbances may result in neonatal seizures: (i) transient and rapidly correctable disturbances, and (ii) inherited and usually persistent causes.

i. **Transient metabolic disturbances** include disturbances of blood glucose and electrolyte disturbances such as hypoglycemia, hypocalcemia and hypomagnesemia. These conditions frequently occur in conjunction with other potentially epileptogenic conditions such as perinatal asphyxia.

a) **Hypoglycemia** (see Chap. 29A) is especially common in infants with intrauterine growth retardation, diabetic mothers, or perinatal asphyxia. Less commonly, hypoglycemia may be a prominent feature of certain inborn errors of metabolism (e.g., galactosemia, glycogen storage diseases) or hyperinsulinemic conditions (e.g., Beckwith–Wiedeman syndrome, nesidioblastosis). Glucose transporter deficiency is a more recently described condition in which blood glucose levels are normal but CSF glucose levels are low. The timing of seizures in neonatal hypoglycemia is usually on the second day of life, but the primary link between hypoglycemia and seizures may be difficult to establish. Because seizures usually develop after sustained hypoglycemia, these infants often have a poor outcome.

b) **Hypocalcemia** (see Chap. 29B) accounts for approximately 3% of neonatal seizures. Currently, hypocalcemic seizures are usually associated with perinatal asphyxia or endocrinopathies due to maternal neonatal hypoparathyroidism or deletion syndromes of chromosome 22, including the DeGeorge syndrome.

c) **Hyponatremic** seizures may develop in the setting of inappropriate antidiuretic hormone ([ADH]secretion), perinatal asphyxia, and inadvertent water intoxication (see Chap. 9).

ii. **Inborn errors of metabolism** (see Chap. 29D) are an uncommon cause of neonatal seizures; nevertheless, neonatal seizures have been described in a long list of such conditions (see partial list in Table 27A.2). Certain of these

TABLE 27A.2	Some of the Inborn Errors of Metabolism Presenting with Neonatal Seizures

Pyridoxine dependency
Nonketotic hyperglycinemia
Urea cycle defects
Sulfite oxidase deficiency
Glutaric aciduria type II
Maple syrup urine disease
Menkes disease
Molybdenum cofactor deficiency
Propionic aciduria
Methylmalonic aciduria
Mitochondrial diseases
Glucose transporter deficiency

conditions are more likely to be associated with seizures, including nonketotic hyperglycinemia, pyridoxine dependency, sulfate oxidase deficiency, glutaric aciduria type II, and urea cycle defects. The most common diagnostic abnormalities associated with these conditions include metabolic acidosis, hyperammonemia, hypoglycemia and ketosis. The clinical features and definitive diagnostic tests for these conditions are detailed in Chapter 29D. Most of these conditions are due to permanent enzyme defects, and are largely incurable. However, their recognition is important for two reasons. First, some metabolic disturbances have transient forms that resolve over time (e.g., nonketotic hyperglycinemia). Second, some of these conditions are treatable (e.g., pyridoxine dependency). In both these situations, early diagnosis and treatment may prevent or limit brain injury.

a) **Pyridoxine dependency results from impaired binding of the active form of pyridoxine to the enzyme glutamic acid decarboxylase (GAD).** This enzyme is responsible for the conversion of the excitatory amino acid neurotransmitter, glutamate, to the inhibitory neurotransmitter, GABA. Therefore, impaired GAD activity causes a marked increase in excitatory versus inhibitory neurotransmitter levels. Not only does this elevated excitatory state precipitate seizures, but high glutamate levels may be lethal to both neurons and oligodendroglia. Seizures in pyridoxine dependency often present early, that is, within the first hours of life or even in the fetus. The diagnosis is usually made by a therapeutic trial of intravenous pyridoxine with simultaneous EEG monitoring. Seizures cease after appropriate doses of pyridoxine (see III.B.d) and recur after it is withdrawn. Ongoing seizures after adequate dosing excludes the diagnosis. In addition, affected infants have low GABA levels and high glutamate levels in the CSF.

b) **Glycine encephalopathy (nonketotic hyperglycinemia)** is an autosomal recessive condition in which a deficiency in the glycine cleavage system results in very high levels of glycine in the brain and CSF. Glycine is a coagonist at the excitatory cerebral N-methyl-D-aspartate (NMDA) glutamate receptor, but is inhibitory in the brainstem and spinal cord. The marked elevation of glycine levels results in refractory myoclonic seizures (due to excitation of cortical NMDA receptors), stupor, respiratory disturbances, and hypotonia (due to brainstem inhibition). **The diagnosis is made by demonstrating markedly elevated glycine**

levels in the CSF, and may be missed if only serum or urine levels are measured because these may be normal or mildly elevated. The EEG background pattern typically shows burst suppression. Most infants with nonketotic hyperglycinemia die by 1 year of age, but a transient and potentially benign form may present with seizures in early neonatal life. Consequently, aggressive support is indicated until such a transient form is excluded. Antenatal diagnosis is possible by chorionic villus sampling.

c) **Folinic acid-responsive seizures** may present in the neonatal period, often within the first few hours as a severe neonatal epileptic encephalopathy with myoclonic, clonic, or apneic spells. Between seizures the infant may be irritable, jittery or comatose. The EEG may be discontinuous with multifocal discharges. Neuroimaging is normal at onset, but later shows white matter abnormalities and cerebral atrophy. The CSF shows an as yet unidentified compound; the true pathophysiology of this condition remains unknown. On occasion these seizures may respond initially to Phenobarbital (PB) or pyridoxine but eventually breakthrough seizures occur. Neonatal seizures of unknown etiology that persist after an adequate trial of anticonvulsant drugs and pyridoxine, warrant a 24- to 48-hour trial of enteral folinic acid (for dosing see III.B.e). Seizures usually cease within 24 hours of treatment.

f. **Cerebral dysgenesis.** A number of dysgenetic cerebral lesions may be associated with neonatal seizures. In many, but not all, cases these lesions can be demonstrated *in vivo* by computed tomography (CT) or MRI scan. Conditions most commonly associated with neonatal seizures are disorders of neuronal migration (e.g., heterotopias, lissencephalies) or disorders of neuronal organization (e.g., polymicrogyria). These ectopic or disorganized collections of neurons are abnormally prone to hyperexcitability and bursts of discharges leading to seizures. The genetic lesions causing these disorders are being uncovered. Occasionally cerebral dysgenesis may be associated with and possibly caused by inborn metabolic disturbances, such as 7-dehydrocholesterol deficiency in certain holoprosencephalies, and carbohydrate-deficient glycoprotein syndrome and nonketotic hyperglycinemia in some cases of agenesis of the corpus callosum. Infants with cerebral dysgenesis and fluctuating consciousness, vomiting, and apparent regression, should be evaluated for metabolic conditions that may cause ongoing neurodegeneration.

g. **Epileptic syndromes in the newborn infant**

i. There are two benign and three malignant epileptic syndromes presenting with seizures in the newborn infant.

a) **Benign familial neonatal seizures** is an autosomal dominant seizure disorder presenting in newborn infants without obvious risk factors for seizures. In this condition, seizures typically have their onset around the second to third day of life and may recur for days to weeks before gradually resolving. The interictal neurologic examination is normal, and **most cases have a normal long-term neurodevelopmental outcome.** Less than 10% of cases later develop epilepsy, usually in adulthood. Neither the number of neonatal seizures, nor their treatment, appears related to the long-term outcome. These features have suggested that aggressive anticonvulsant therapy may not be indicated in this condition.

Benign familial neonatal seizures are a rare form of primary generalized seizures in the newborn. The clinical phenomena are variable but include a brief initial phase of apnea, tachycardia, and tonic posturing (with abduction or adduction of the arms, flexion of the hips, and extension of the knees) followed by a phase of clonic activity. As such, this condition is one of the rare instances in which tonic–clonic seizures occur in the newborn. These seizures tend to occur mainly during active sleep and may be preceded by brief arousal. The ictal EEG features consist of a sudden brief period of generalized voltage attenuation (during the apneic and tonic phase) followed by a longer generalized discharge of repetitive spike and/or sharp waves (during the clonic phase). Rarely do benign familial neonatal seizures have a consistent EEG focus or a postictal phase. The interictal EEG is either normal or has occasional bursts of alternating θ-rhythmic activity (*theta pointu alternant*). All laboratory and imaging studies aimed at identifying an etiology are normal. Two separate genetic loci have been identified. Most families have a locus at chromosome 20q13.3, which encodes for a potassium channel, suggesting an impairment of potassium-dependent neuronal repolarization as the basis for the seizures. In other families, the locus is at chromosome 8q24.

b) **Benign idiopathic neonatal seizures** make up approximately 5% of seizures in term infants. Certain diagnostic criteria have been proposed, including: (i) birth after 39 weeks' gestational age; (ii) normal pregnancy and delivery; (iii) Apgar scores >8; (iv) normal neonatal course before the seizures; (v) seizure onset between days 4 and 6 of life; (vi) normal neurologic state before and between seizures; (vii) clonic and/or apneic (never tonic) seizures; (viii) normal diagnostic testing; (ix) an ictal EEG showing brief (1–3 minute) seizures (never α frequency) in the rolandic regions; and (x) a normal interictal EEG except for *theta pointu alternant* pattern (in 60% cases). The cause for these seizures remains unknown, but may be related to a transient zinc deficiency, because CSF zinc levels may be decreased. Several features distinguish these idiopathic seizures from benign familial seizures; these include: (i) absence of a family history; (ii) later seizure onset, around day 5 of life; (iii) convulsions that are clonic and/or apneic, but never tonic; (iv) multifocal clonic seizures that are never primary generalized; and (v) lack of the initial voltage attenuation on the ictal EEG. Instead, the ictal EEG shows lateralized or secondarily generalized rhythmic spikes and slow waves. The period of seizure activity is usually brief but intense, with frequent or serial seizures, and even status epilepticus. This phase is followed by gradual resolution, with seizures seldom persisting longer than 2 weeks. The long-term outcome is invariably favorable and later epilepsy does not occur.

ii. There are three early epileptic encephalopathies with associated with a poor prognosis.

a) **Neonatal myoclonic encephalopathy (NME)** presents with erratic and fragmentary partial seizures and massive **myoclonus.** These seizures typically start as focal motor seizures, and later evolve into typical infantile spasms. The most common etiologies associated with this condition are metabolic disorders (especially nonketotic hyperglycinemia). The ictal EEG shows high-amplitude EEG bursts coinciding with the massive myoclonic seizures. The interictal pattern shows a burst suppression pattern with complex bursts and sharp waves alternating with periods of low-amplitude quiescence. **The long-term outcome is universally poor,** with a high mortality in the first year and severe retardation in all survivors.

b) **Ohtahara syndrome** usually presents within the first 10 days of life but may present as late as 3 months. The seizures are typically numerous brief **tonic** spasms (and not clonic or fragmentary myoclonic). In contrast to the metabolic causes of NME, the causes of Ohtahara syndrome tend to be structural, with most being dysgenetic or, occasionally, destructive, such as hypoxic–ischemic injury. The interictal EEG is usually an invariant burst suppression pattern, with no sleep-wake cycling. Unlike the ictal EEG of NME, the tonic spasms tend to occur with a period of EEG suppression and not with the bursts. As in

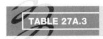

TABLE 27A.3	Acute Management of Neonatal Seizures

After each step, evaluate the infant for ongoing seizures. If seizures persist, advance to next step

Step 1. Stabilize vital functions

Step 2. Correct transient metabolic disturbances
- **a.** Hypoglycemia (target blood sugar 70–120 mg/dL)
  10% dextrose water IV bolus dose 2 mL/kg followed by a continuous infusion at 8 mg/kg/min
- **b.** Hypocalcemia 5% calcium gluconate IV at 4 mL/kg (need cardiac monitoring)
- **c.** Hypomagnesemia 50% magnesium sulfate IM at 0.2 mL/kg

Step 3. Phenobarbital 20 mg/kg IV load
   Cardiorespiratory monitoring
   5 mg/kg IV (may repeat to total dose of 40 mg/kg)
   Consider continuous EEG monitoring
   Consider intubation/ventilation

Step 4. Lorazepam   0.05 mg/kg IV (may repeat to total dose of 0.1 mg/kg)

Step 5. Phenytoin   20 mg/kg slow IV load
   (fosphenytoin)

                    5 mg/kg slow IV (may repeat to total dose of 30 mg/kg)

Step 6. Pyridoxine 50–100 mg/kg IV (with EEG monitoring)

Step 7. Other agents (see text)

EEG = electroencephalogram.

NME, **the prognosis of Ohtahara syndrome is universally grim,** with early death or, among survivors, severe handicap and frequently infantile spasms.

- c) **Migrating partial seizures of infancy (Coppola syndrome)** is an early onset epileptic encephalopathy starting between birth and 6 months of age, with no currently identifiable etiology and normal neuroimaging studies at the onset. The clinical seizures are partial clonic seizures often alternating between the two sides of the body. The seizures are typically multifocal on EEG and migrate independently and sequentially over both hemispheres. They are refractory to conventional antiepileptic medications and in most (but not all) cases develop marked hypotonia, severe neurodevelopmental retardation and cerebral atrophy over time. To date, extensive etiologic studies have not revealed a cause.

III. TREATMENT OF NEONATAL SEIZURES (see Table 27A.3). As a general rule, seizures in the newborn are less responsive to conventional anticonvulsants than are seizures in older patients. This is particularly true of seizures with electroclinical dissociation in which seizures may remain refractory to high doses and sometimes multiple anticonvulsants. The risk–benefit ratio of such high doses in the treatment of neonatal seizures has been questioned. Specifically, the potential for seizures to cause direct injury to the immature brain has to be weighed against the effect of high levels of anticonvulsants on the developing brain. These issues have triggered a vigorous but unresolved debate about the management of neonatal seizures.

A number of potentially deleterious effects on the systemic and cerebral systems support the treatment of neonatal seizures. First, seizures may cause significant hemodynamic and respiratory disturbances, which in the sick newborn, may complicate management and potentially extend brain injury. Seizures disrupt cerebral pressure autoregulation and cause wide fluctuations in blood pressure, a combination with potentially serious consequences for the immature brain. Second, massive amounts of cerebral energy are consumed during the repeated neuronal depolarization–repolarization associated with seizures. Neonatal seizures cause a rapid fall in cerebral glucose and rise in brain lactate, even with normal or elevated blood glucose levels. In the insulted brain, such energy depletion may seriously compromise recovery. Third, seizures release large amounts of glutamate, and, in conditions of cerebral energy failure, seizures inhibit the reuptake of glutamate. Together these mechanisms result in the accumulation of extracellular glutamate to toxic levels that are potentially lethal to postsynaptic neurons and immature oligodendrocytes.

In animal studies, the immature brain is remarkably resistant to even prolonged seizures induced by proconvulsant drugs. Conversely, in a model that mimics postasphyxial seizures in the human newborn, seizures preceded by an asphyxial insult cause extensive cellular loss in the immature brain. These studies suggest that seizures superimposed on insults that deplete or disrupt cerebral energetics are capable of causing or extending brain injury. Seizures may also disrupt protein and lipid metabolism of immature neurons, and activate genes that stimulate axonal growth and new synapse formation. These sublethal insults may result in aberrant neuronal pathways and a long-term reduction in seizure threshold. Together, these mechanisms likely contribute to the epilepsy, motor, and cognitive impairment seen in some survivors of neonatal seizures.

The lack of a single highly effective anticonvulsant regimen in the newborn has spawned many different approaches. However, the following protocol is used in many major centers, including our own (Table 27A.3). The initial steps in management consist of stabilization of the vital functions, exclusion or treatment of rapidly correctable conditions, and establishing the diagnosis of seizures by the clinical or EEG criteria detailed in the preceding text. Specific therapies against other treatable conditions (e.g., meningitis, narcotic withdrawal) should commence but should not delay the initiation of anticonvulsant therapy.

A. Reversing rapidly correctable causes

    1. Hypoglycemia (see Chap. 29A and Fig. 10.2). Even when other primary etiologies are identified for seizures, hypoglycemia should be excluded or corrected. In the newborn with seizures, the target goal for blood glucose should be 70 to 120 mg/dL. If the hypoglycemic infant is actively seizing, an IV loading dose of 10% dextrose at 2 mL/kg (0.2 g/kg) should be given, followed by a continuous infusion of up to 8 mg/kg/minute to achieve the target levels given in the preceding text. In rare cases where these measures do not achieve normoglycemia, glucagon or hydrocortisone may be necessary. Experimental studies show that (i) brain tissue levels of glucose may fall during seizures even when blood glucose is normal, and (ii) hyperglycemia may be neuroprotective. These data are interesting, but more data are required before supranormal blood glucose targets can be recommended.

    2. Hypocalcemia and hypomagnesemia (see Chap. 29B). Even if hypocalcemic seizures respond to antiepileptic medications, the low calcium levels should be corrected. An IV dose of 5% calcium gluconate at 2 mL/kg (18 mg of elemental calcium/kg) should be given under careful cardiac monitoring. Hypomagnesemia is best treated with an IM dose of 50% magnesium sulfate at 0.2 mL/kg. Infants treated for hypocalcemia should also receive magnesium because calcium administration increases renal magnesium excretion, and magnesium administration increases serum calcium levels. Of note, magnesium administration may result in transient weakness and hypotonia, even with normal serum levels.

B. Specific anticonvulsant agents (see Appendix A).

    1. Acute management. Once the diagnosis of seizures is strongly suspected or confirmed, anticonvulsant agents should be started. The administration of these agents should occur with careful cardiorespiratory monitoring.

        a. Phenobarbital should be started as an IV loading dose of 20 mg/kg given over 10 to 15 minutes. This usually achieves blood levels around 20 mg/dL, levels at which an anticonvulsant effect begins to be apparent in the newborn. If seizures persist, further bolus doses of 5 mg/kg should be given, up to a total dose of 40 mg/kg or control of seizures. At these levels, significant respiratory depression is usually not evident. However, in a recent randomized trial these levels achieved seizure control in less than half of infants. The use of higher levels has been advocated but remains controversial because additional therapeutic benefit may be outweighed by the risk of cardiorespiratory depression. In asphyxiated infants with hepatic dysfunction, the doses given in the preceding text may result in higher blood levels, with sedation that persists for days. For this reason, in the severely asphyxiated infant with hepatic dysfunction it may be advisable to add a second, less-sedating agent such as phenytoin if seizures persist after the first 20 mg/kg loading dose of phenobarbital.

b. Phenytoin the usual second-line agent, is given as an initial loading dose of 20 mg/kg, which usually produces therapeutic blood levels around 15 to 20 mg/dL. Phenytoin is given into normal saline (it precipitates in dextrose solutions) and not faster than 1 mg/kg/minute to avoid cardiac arrhythmias. If seizures persist, an additional dose of 5 mg/kg may be used. **Fosphenytoin** is a more recently developed prodrug form that is rapidly converted into phenytoin. This agent has several advantages over phenytoin including greater solubility in standard intravenous solutions (including dextrose-containing solutions), safe faster rates of infusion, safe IM dosing, and no tissue injury with IV infiltration. Initial studies have supported the use of this agent in the newborn.

c. Benzodiazepines. The combination of phenobarbital and phenytoin will control seizures in up to 85% of infants. For neonatal seizures that remain refractory to these measures, benzodiazepines may add further benefit. Lorazepam, diazepam, and midazolam have all demonstrated potent anticonvulsant effects in the newborn. Although all three agents gain rapid entry into the brain, important differences in their subsequent kinetics, efficacy, and adverse effect profile make lorazepam the preferred agent for neonatal seizures. Lorazepam has several advantages over diazepam. Specifically: (i) diazepam is rapidly redistributed after an IV dose and cleared from the brain within minutes; (ii) diazepam has greater respiratory and circulatory depressant effects (particularly when used with a barbiturate); (iii) the anticonvulsant effect of diazepam lasts minutes, whereas its sedative effect exceeds 24 hours; and (iv) sodium benzoate, the vehicle for IV diazepam, uncouples bilirubin from albumin, increasing the risk for kernicterus in jaundiced infants. **Lorazepam** at 0.05 mg/kg IV has an anticonvulsant onset within 2 to 3 minutes, which lasts between 6 and 24 hours (and much longer in infants with postasphyxial liver dysfunction). The dose may be repeated after several minutes to a total dose of 0.10 mg/kg. **Diazepam** is an effective anticonvulsant in the newborn and is given as an IV dose of 0.1 mg/kg increasing slowly up to 0.3 mg/kg given until the seizure stops. Because of their short anticonvulsant half-lives, both diazepam and **midazolam,** the newest benzodiazepine to be used as an anticonvulsant in the newborn, are most effective when given as a continuous infusion. Midazolam is given at an initial IV dose of 0.02 to 0.1 mg/kg, followed by a continuous infusion of 0.01 to 0.06 mg/kg/hour.

d. Pyridoxine. When neonatal seizures prove refractory to the preceding regimen, pyridoxine dependency should be excluded. This condition is diagnosed by the rapid (within minutes) cessation of EEG seizures to an IV dose of 50 to 100 mg pyridoxine. Because pyridoxine administration increases the cerebral synthesis of the inhibitory transmitter GABA, apnea and hypotonia may occasionally develop, necessitating close respiratory monitoring. If the diagnosis is made, maintenance oral doses of pyridoxine should be given at 10 to 100 mg/day, depending on the response.

e. Folinic acid. Infants that fail to respond to adequate doses of anticonvulsant drugs and pyridoxine warrant a trial of folinic acid for 24 to 48 hours. The starting dose is 2.5 mg of enteral folinic acid twice/day, but may have to be increased up to 8 mg/kg/day.

f. **Other agents.** Although not commonly used in the United States, **lidocaine** has been used in Europe as an effective adjunctive anticonvulsant for neonatal seizures, usually after failure of phenobarbital and diazepam. The anticonvulsant effects are seen within 10 minutes after starting an IV infusion of 4 to 6 mg/kg/hour, with or without a preceding loading dose. Once seizures are controlled, the lidocaine infusion is tapered over several days. In spite of its potential cardiac toxicity, the only adverse effect described in these reports is recurrence of seizures during the weaning period.

2. **Maintenance and withdrawal of anticonvulsant drugs.** Decisions regarding duration of therapy depend on the underlying etiology. Certain conditions, such as primary hypocalcemia, cause acute ("symptomatic") seizures with relatively low risk of later recurrent seizures, if the primary condition is appropriately managed. In these conditions discontinuation of anticonvulsant medications may be considered before intensive care unit (ICU) discharge. In conditions such as cerebral dysgenesis, the high risk for subsequent epilepsy warrants ongoing anticonvulsant treatment. Infants with postasphyxial seizures, have a 20% to 30% incidence of epilepsy, although subsequent seizures may present months to years later. If at the time of discharge from the neonatal intensive care unit (NICU) the infant's neurologic exam and EEG show good recovery towards normal, an early withdrawal of phenobarbital may be considered. Otherwise, the need for continued phenobarbital treatment should be reevaluated at 6- to 12-week intervals, maintaining interim blood levels around 20 mg/dL.

IV. **PROGNOSIS AFTER NEONATAL SEIZURES.** The overall prognosis for survival in neonatal seizures is around 85%, a significant improvement from earlier decades. Unfortunately, the prognosis for long-term neurodevelopmental outcome remains largely unchanged. Specifically, an adverse outcome occurs in approximately 50% of cases, with sequelae such as mental retardation, motor dysfunction, and seizures. The range of outcomes after neonatal seizures varies widely, with the three major predictors of long-term outcome being (i) the underlying etiology, (ii) the electrographic features, and (iii) gestational age. Other useful predictors include the neonatal neurologic examination and neuroimaging findings.

A. **Etiology as a prognostic factor** (see Table 27A.4). Neonatal seizures reflect significant brain dysfunction. The nature and severity of the insult causing these seizures might be expected to influence long-term brain function. Therefore, it is not surprising that in most studies the underlying etiology of neonatal seizures is the most powerful predictor of long-term outcome. Infants with hypoxic-ischemic encephalopathy, when accompanied by seizures, currently have an approximately

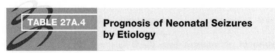

| TABLE 27A.4 | Prognosis of Neonatal Seizures by Etiology |

Etiology	Normal outcome (%)
Hypoxia-ischemia	50
Meningitis	50
Hypoglycemia	50
Subarachnoid hemorrhage	90
Early hypocalcemia	50
Late hypocalcemia	100
Intraventricular hemorrhage	10
Dysgenesis	0
Unknown	75

50% chance for normal development. Similarly, about half of infants with seizures due to bacterial meningitis have a favorable outcome. The overall outcome for infants with neonatal seizures after arterial or venous vaso-occlusive disease is relatively benign. However, there are certain features that predict a worse outcome. In arterial stroke, EEG and MRI studies may identify infants at risk for worse prognosis. Specifically, an abnormal interictal EEG background has a less favorable outcome. Likewise, an MRI study showing involvement of an entire vascular territory, for example, in the MCA with injury to the hemispheres, the basal ganglia, and the internal capsule, is associated with significant hemiparesis in the long term. Although uncommon, involvement of multiple arteries, especially if bilateral, predicts worse outcome. Approximately 75% of infants with cerebral vein thrombosis and seizures have a favorable outcome, and only 20% develop later epilepsy. Features that predict a worse outcome include the development of extensive hemorrhagic infarction, as well as venous occlusion that extends into the deep venous system. The outcome of intracranial hemorrhage depends on the degree of parenchymal injury and the gestational age. Most infants who develop seizures after primary subarachnoid (parturitional) hemorrhage have a good long-term outcome. Conversely, premature infants who develop seizures after IVH are usually critically ill and often have parenchymal hemorrhagic infarction; consequently, the outcome is significantly worse in these infants. Hypoglycemia severe and persistent enough to cause seizures is associated with a normal outcome in around 50% of cases. This prognosis is substantially worse when hypoglycemia complicates postasphyxial encephalopathy. The prognosis for infants with cerebral dysgenesis who develop seizures in the newborn period is universally dismal. If a thorough diagnostic evaluation fails to identify an etiology for neonatal seizures, the outcome is likely to be favorable.

B. Both the interictal and ictal EEG features have prognostic value. With severe interictal EEG background abnormalities, such as burst suppression, marked voltage suppression, and an isoelectric background, an adverse neurologic outcome occurs in 90% or more of cases. Conversely, a normal EEG background at presentation is associated with a favorable outcome. Although somewhat less reliable, the ictal EEG features may also be useful predictors of outcome. A better outcome may be expected when the clinical and EEG seizures are consistently correlated, whereas electrically silent clinical seizures or clinically silent EEG seizures are associated with a worse outcome. The EEG seizure morphology may also be helpful, with α-frequency seizures, seizures associated with electrodecremental changes, or myoclonic seizures coupled with spike bursts, having a worse prognosis. Others have associated an increased number and duration of EEG seizures (particularly seizures lasting >30 minutes) with a worse outcome.

C. Gestational age has prognostic significance with neonatal seizures in infants under 32 weeks' gestation having a high mortality up to 80% in some studies, and a significantly higher risk of adverse neurologic outcome in survivors, when compared to term infants.

Suggested Readings

Mizrahi E, Kellaway P. *The diagnosis and management of neonatal seizures.* Philadelphia: Lippincott-Raven, 1997.

Tekgul H, Gauvreau K, Soul JS, et al. The current etiologic profile and neurodevelopmental outcome of seizures in term newborn infants. *Pediatrics* 2006;117(4):1270–1280.

Volpe JJ, ed. Neonatal seizures. *Neurology of the newborn*, 4th ed. Philadelphia: WB Saunders, 2001:178–216.

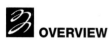

INTRACRANIAL HEMORRHAGE AND PERIVENTRICULAR LEUKOMALACIA

Janet S. Soul

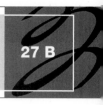

27 B

OVERVIEW

The incidence of intracranial hemorrhage (ICH) varies from 2% to >30% in newborns, depending on the gestational age (GA) at birth and the type of ICH. Bleeding within the skull can occur: (i) external to the brain into the epidural, subdural, or subarachnoid spaces; (ii) into the parenchyma of the cerebrum or cerebellum; or (iii) into the ventricles from the subependymal germinal matrix or choroid plexus (see Table 27B.1). The incidence, pathogenesis, clinical presentation, diagnosis, management, and prognosis of ICH varies according to the ICH location and size, and the infant's GA (1,2). There is often a combination of two or more types of ICH, as an ICH in one location often extends into an adjacent compartment; for example, extension of a parenchymal hemorrhage into the subarachnoid space or ventricles.

Diagnosis typically depends on clinical suspicion, when an infant presents with typical neurologic signs, such as seizures, irritability, or depressed level of consciousness, and/or with focal neurologic deficits referable either to the cerebrum or brainstem. Diagnosis is confirmed with an appropriate neuroimaging study. Management varies according to the size and location of the ICH and the presenting neurologic signs. In general, only very large hemorrhages with clinical signs require surgical intervention for removal of the ICH itself. With a large ICH, pressor support or volume replacement (with normal saline, albumin, or packed red blood cells) may be required because of significant blood loss. More commonly, management is focused on treating complications such as seizures or the development of posthemorrhagic hydrocephalus (PHH). In general, although a large ICH is more likely to result in greater morbidity or mortality than a small one, the presence and severity of parenchymal injury, whether due to hemorrhage, infarction, or other neuropathology, is usually the best predictor of outcome.

I. SUBDURAL HEMORRHAGE (SDH) AND EPIDURAL HEMORRHAGE (EH)

A. Etiology and pathogenesis. The pathogenesis of SDH relates to rupture of the draining veins and sinuses of the brain that occupy the subdural space. Vertical molding, fronto-occipital elongation, and torsional forces acting on the head during delivery may provoke laceration of dural leaflets of either the tentorium cerebelli or the falx cerebri. These lacerations can result in rupture of the vein of Galen, inferior sagittal sinus, straight sinus and/or transverse sinus, and usually a posterior fossa SDH. Breech presentation also predisposes to occipital osteodiastasis, a depressed fracture of the occipital bone or bones, which may lead to direct laceration of the cerebellum or rupture of the occipital sinus. Clinically significant SDH in the posterior fossa often results from trauma in the full-term infant, although small, inconsequential SDH may be fairly common in uncomplicated deliveries (the true incidence in apparently well newborns is unknown). SDH in the supratentorial space usually results from rupture of the bridging, superficial veins over the cerebral convexity. Other risk factors for SDH include factors that increase the likelihood of significant forces on the infant's head, such as large head size, rigid pelvis (e.g., in a primiparous or older multiparous mother), nonvertex presentation (breech, face, etc.), very rapid or prolonged labor or delivery, difficult instrumented delivery, or rarely, a bleeding diathesis.

B. Clinical presentation. When the accumulation of blood is rapid and large, as occurs with rupture of large veins or sinuses, the presentation follows shortly after birth and evolves rapidly. This is particularly true in infratentorial SDH, where compression

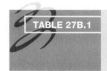

| TABLE 27B.1 | Illustrating Neonatal Intracranial Hemorrhage (ICH) by Location, and whether Each ICH Type Is Predominantly Primary (1°) or Secondary (2°) Source of Bleeding, and the Relative Incidence in Preterm (PT) or Term (T) Newborns |

Type (location) of hemorrhage	Principal source of ICH	Relative incidence in PT vs. T
1. Subdural and epidural hemorrhage	$1° > 2°$	T > PT
2. Subarachnoid hemorrhage (SAH)	$2° > 1°*$	?*
3. Intraparenchymal hemorrhage		
Cerebral	$2° > 1°$	PT > T
Cerebellar	$2° > 1°$	PT > T
4. Germinal matrix/intraventricular hemorrhage	$1° > 2°$	PT > T

*True incidence unknown, small primary SAH may be more common than is recognized.

of the brainstem may result in nuchal rigidity or opisthotonus; obtundation or coma; apnea; other abnormal respiratory patterns; and unreactive pupils and/or abnormal extraocular movements. With increased intracranial pressure (ICP), there may be a bulging fontanelle and/or widely split sutures. With large hemorrhages, there may be systemic signs of hypovolemia and anemia. When the sources of hemorrhage are small veins, there may be few clinical signs for up to 1 week, at which time either the hematoma attains a critical size, imposes on the brain parenchyma and produces neurologic signs, or hydrocephalus develops. Seizures may occur in up to half of neonates with SDH, particularly with SDH over the cerebral convexity. With cerebral convexity SDH, there may also be subtle focal cerebral signs and mild disturbances of consciousness, such as irritability. Subarachnoid hemorrhage (SAH) probably coexists in most cases of neonatal SDH, as demonstrated by a cerebrospinal fluid (CSF) examination (3). Finally, a chronic subdural effusion may gradually develop over months, presenting as abnormally rapid head growth, with the occipitofrontal circumference (OFC) crossing percentiles in the first weeks to months after birth.

C. **Diagnosis.** The diagnosis should be suspected on the basis of history and clinical signs and confirmed with a computed tomography (CT) scan. Although ultrasonography (US) may be valuable in evaluating the sick newborn at the bedside, **ultrasonic imaging of structures adjacent to bone (i.e., the subdural space) is often inadequate.** Magnetic resonance imaging (MRI) has proved to be quite sensitive to small hemorrhage and can help establish timing of ICH. MRI is also superior for detecting other lesions, such as contusion, thromboembolic infarction, or hypoxic-ischemic injury that may occur in some infants with severe hypovolemia/anemia or other risk factors for parenchymal abnormalities. However, a CT scan is much quicker to obtain and usually adequate in an unstable infant with elevated ICP who may require neurosurgical intervention. **When there is clinical suspicion of a large SDH, a lumbar puncture (LP) should not be performed until after the CT scan is obtained,** and the LP may be contraindicated if there is a large hemorrhage within the posterior fossa or supratentorial compartment. With a smaller SDH, an LP should be performed to rule out infection in the newborn with signs such as seizures, depressed mental status, or other systemic signs of illness.

D. **Management and prognosis.** Most infants with SDH do not require surgical intervention and can be managed with supportive care and treatment of any accompanying seizures. Infants with rapid evolution of a large infratentorial SDH require prompt stabilization with volume replacement (fluid and/or blood products), pressors, and respiratory support, as needed. An urgent CT scan of the head and neurosurgical consultation should be obtained in any infant with signs of progressive brainstem dysfunction (i.e., coma, apnea, cranial nerve dysfunction), opisthotonus, or tense, bulging fontanelle. Open surgical evacuation of the clot is the usual management for the minority of infants with large SDH in any location accompanied by such severe neurologic abnormalities or obstructive hydrocephalus. It has been suggested that when the clinical picture is stable and no deterioration in neurologic function or unmanageable increase in ICP exists, supportive care and serial CT examinations instead of surgical intervention should be used in the management of posterior fossa SDH (4). Laboratory testing to rule out sepsis or a bleeding diathesis should be considered with large SDH. The infant should be monitored for the development of hydrocephalus, which can occur in a delayed manner following SDH. Finally, chronic subdural effusions may occur rarely and can present weeks to months later with abnormally increased head growth. The outcome for infants with nonsurgical SDH is usually good, provided there is no other significant neurologic injury or disease. The prognosis for normal development is also good for cases in which prompt surgical evacuation of the hematoma is successful and there is no other parenchymal injury.

E. Epidural Hemorrhage. There are approximately 20 case reports of neonatal EH in the literature. EH appears to be correlated with trauma (e.g., difficult instrumented delivery), and a large cephalohematoma or skull fracture was found in approximately half the reported cases of EH. Removal or aspiration of the hemorrhage was performed in most cases, and the prognosis was quite good except when other ICH or parenchymal pathology was present.

II. SUBARACHNOID HEMORRHAGE (SAH)

A. Etiology and pathogenesis. SAH is a common form of ICH among newborns. Primary SAH (i.e., SAH not due to extension from ICH in an adjacent compartment) is probably frequent but clinically insignificant. In these cases, SAH may go unrecognized (the true incidence of small SAH remains unknown) because of a lack of clinical signs. For example, hemorrhagic or xanthochromic CSF may be the only indication of such a hemorrhage in infants who undergo a CSF exam to rule out sepsis. Small SAH probably results from the normal "trauma" associated with the birth process. The source of bleeding is usually ruptured bridging veins of the subarachnoid space or ruptured small leptomeningeal vessels (quite different from SAH in adults, where the source of bleeding is usually arterial and therefore produces a much more emergent clinical syndrome). SAH should be distinguished from subarachnoid extension of blood from a germinal matrix hemorrhage/intraventricular hemorrhage (GMH/IVH), which occurs most commonly in the preterm (PT) infant. SAH may also result from extension of SDH (e.g., particularly in the posterior fossa) or a cerebral contusion (parenchymal hemorrhage). Finally, subpial hemorrhage may occur, mostly in the otherwise healthy term newborn, and is usually a focal hemorrhage likely caused by local trauma resulting in venous compression or occlusion in the setting of a vaginal delivery (often instrumented) (5).

B. Clinical presentation. As with other forms of ICH, clinical suspicion of SAH may result because of blood loss or neurologic dysfunction. Only rarely is the volume loss large enough to provoke catastrophic results. More often, neurologic signs manifest as seizures, irritability, or other mild alteration of mental status, particularly with SAH or subpial hemorrhage occurring over the cerebral convexities.

C. Diagnosis. Seizures, irritability, lethargy, or focal neurologic signs should prompt investigation to determine whether there is an SAH (or other ICH). Often, babies with a small SAH may have seizures but appear otherwise quite well. The diagnosis is best established with a CT scan or MRI, or by LP to confirm or diagnose small SAH. CT scans are usually adequate to diagnose SAH, but an MRI may be useful to determine whether there is evidence of any other parenchymal pathology, because SAH may occur in the setting of hypoxia-ischemia or meningoencephalitis. Ultrasonography is not sensitive for the detection of small SAH, so should be used only if the patient is too unstable for transport to CT scan/MRI.

D. Management and prognosis. Management of SAH usually requires only symptomatic therapy, such as anticonvulsant therapy for seizures (see Chap. 27A) and nasogastric feeds or intravenous fluids if the infant is too lethargic to feed orally.

Most infants with small SAH do well without recognized sequelae. In rare cases, a very large SAH will result in a catastrophic syndrome with profound depression of mental status, seizures, and/or brainstem signs. In such cases, blood transfusions and cardiovascular support should be provided as needed, and neurosurgical intervention may be required. It is important to establish whether there is coexisting hypoxia-ischemia or other significant neuropathology (by MRI) that will be the crucial determinant of a poor outcome, to avoid performing a surgical procedure that will not improve outcome. Occasionally hydrocephalus will develop after a moderate–large SAH, and therefore follow-up CT or US scans should be performed in such infants, particularly if there are signs of increased ICP or abnormally rapid head growth.

III. INTRAPARENCHYMAL HEMORRHAGE (IPH)

A. Etiology and pathogenesis

1. Primary intracerebral IPH is uncommon in all newborns, whereas intracerebellar IPH is found in 5% to 10% of autopsy specimens in the premature infant. An intracerebral hemorrhage may occur rarely as a primary event related to rupture of an arteriovenous malformation or aneurysm, from a coagulation disturbance (e.g., hemophilia, thrombocytopenia), or from an unknown cause. More commonly, cerebral IPH occurs as a secondary event, such as hemorrhage into a region of hypoxic-ischemic brain injury. For example, IPH can occur in a region of arterial distribution infarction (term [T] >PT) or occasionally periventricular leukomalacia (PVL) (PT > T). IPH may also occur as a result of venous infarction (because venous infarctions are typically hemorrhagic) either in relation to a large GMH/IVH (PT >T, see IV), or as a result of sinus venous thrombosis (T >PT). IPH can also occur in infants undergoing extracorporeal membrane oxygenation (ECMO) therapy (as can GMH/IVH). Cerebral IPH may occur secondary to a large ICH in another compartment, such as large IVH, SAH, or SDH, as rarely occurs with significant trauma or coagulation disturbance.

2. **Intracerebellar hemorrhage** occurs more commonly in preterm than term newborns, and may be missed by routine cranial ultrasonography (CUS), because the reported incidence is significantly higher in neuropathologic than clinical studies. Intracerebellar IPH may be a primary hemorrhage or may result from venous hemorrhagic infarction or from extension of GMH/IVH (PT >T). It is often difficult to distinguish the primary source or etiology of such hemorrhages by CUS. Cerebellar IPH rarely occurs as an extension of large SAH/SDH in the posterior fossa related to a trauma (T >PT) (see I).

B. Clinical presentation.
The presentation of IPH is similar to that of SDH, where the clinical syndrome differs depending on whether the IPH is in the anterior or posterior fossa. In the preterm infant, IPH is often clinically silent in either intracranial fossa, unless the hemorrhage is quite large. In the term infant, intracerebral hemorrhage typically presents with focal neurologic signs such as seizures, hemiparesis, or gaze preference, along with irritability or depressed level of consciousness. A large cerebellar hemorrhage (±SDH/SAH) presents as described in **I**, and should be managed as for a large posterior fossa SDH.

C. Diagnosis.
CT scans or MRI are the best imaging studies for IPH, but CUS may be used in the preterm infant or when a rapid bedside imaging study is necessary. MRI is superior for demonstrating the extent and age of the hemorrhage and the presence of any other parenchymal abnormality. In addition, magnetic resonance (MR) angiography can be useful to demonstrate a vascular anomaly, lack of flow distal to an arterial embolus, or sinus venous thrombosis. Therefore, MRI is more likely than CT scan or CUS to establish the etiology of the IPH and to determine accurately the long-term prognosis for the term infant. For the preterm infant, CUS views through the mastoid and/or posterior fontanelle improve the detection of hemorrhage in the posterior fossa. Finally, an LP should be performed to rule out infection, unless there is significant mass effect or herniation.

D. Management and prognosis

1. The management of IPH is similar to that for SDH and SAH, where most small hemorrhages require symptomatic treatment and support, and only a large IPH

with severe neurologic compromise should prompt neurosurgical intervention. It is important to diagnose and treat any coexisting pathology, such as infection or sinus venous thrombosis, as these are more likely to have a significant impact on long-term outcome. A large IPH, especially in association with IVH or SAH/SDH, may cause hydrocephalus, and therefore head growth and neurologic status should be monitored for days to weeks following IPH. Follow-up imaging should usually be obtained in the case of large IPH, both to establish the severity and extent of injury and to rule out hydrocephalus or remaining vascular malformation.

2. The prognosis largely relates to location and size of the IPH and GA of the infant. A small IPH may have relatively few or no long-term neurologic consequences. A large cerebral IPH may result in a life-long seizure disorder, hemiparesis or other type of cerebral palsy, feeding difficulties, and cognitive impairments ranging from learning disabilities to mental retardation, depending on the location. Cerebellar hemorrhage in the term newborn often has a relatively good prognosis, although it may result in cerebellar signs of ataxia, hypotonia, tremor, nystagmus, and mild cognitive deficits. A large cerebellar IPH that destroys a significant portion of the cerebellum in a preterm newborn may result in severe cognitive and motor impairments, for those infants who survive the newborn period (such infants often die of systemic illness rather than IPH) (6).

IV. GERMINAL MATRIX HEMORRHAGE/INTRAVENTRICULAR HEMORRHAGE (GMH/IVH)

A. Etiology and pathogenesis

1. **GMH/IVH is found principally in the preterm infant,** where the incidence is currently 15% to 20% in infants born at <32 weeks' GA, but is uncommon in the term newborn. The etiology and pathogenesis are different for these two groups of infants. In the term newborn, primary IVH typically originates in the choroid plexus or in association with venous ($\pm$ sinus) thrombosis and thalamic infarction, although IVH may also occur in the small remnant of the subependymal germinal matrix. The pathogenesis of IVH in the term infant is more likely to be related to trauma (i.e., from a difficult delivery) or perinatal asphyxia. However, at least 25% of infants have no identifiable risk factors. One study utilizing CT imaging suggested that IVH might occur secondary to venous hemorrhagic infarction in the thalamus in 63% of term infants with clinically significant IVH (7).

2. **In the preterm infant, GMH/IVH originates from the fragile involuting vessels of the subependymal germinal matrix, located in the caudothalamic groove.** The pathogenesis of GMH/IVH in the preterm infant has been demonstrated to be related to numerous risk factors, which can be divided into intravascular, vascular, and extravascular factors (see Table 27B.2). The intravascular risk factors are probably the most important, and are also the factors most amenable to preventive efforts.

   The intravascular risk factors predisposing to GMH/IVH include ischemia/reperfusion, increases in cerebral blood flow (CBF), fluctuating CBF, and increases in cerebral venous pressure. Ischemia/reperfusion occurs commonly when hypotension due to disease or to iatrogenic intervention is corrected quickly. This scenario often occurs shortly after birth, when a premature infant may have hypovolemia or hypotension that is treated with infusion of colloid, normal saline, or hyperosmolar solutions such as sodium bicarbonate. Rapid infusions of such solutions are thought to be particularly likely to contribute to GMH/IVH. Indeed, studies of the beagle puppy model showed that ischemia/reperfusion (hypotension precipitated by blood removal followed by volume infusion) reliably produces GMH/IVH (8). Other causes of sustained increases in CBF that may contribute to GMH/IVH include pneumothorax, seizures, hypercarbia, anemia, and perhaps hypoglycemia, all of which result in a compensatory increase in CBF (9). Fluctuating CBF has also been demonstrated to be associated with GMH/IVH in preterm infants. In one study, infants with large fluctuations in CBF velocity by Doppler US were much more likely to develop GMH/IVH than infants with a stable pattern of CBF velocity (10). The

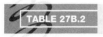

TABLE 27B.2	Factors in the Pathogenesis of GMH/IVH
Intravascular factors	Ischemia/reperfusion (e.g., volume infusion after hypotension)
	Fluctuating CBF (e.g., with mechanical ventilation)
	Increase in CBF (e.g., with hypertension, anemia, hypercarbia)
	Increase in cerebral venous pressure (e.g., with high intrathoracic pressure, usually from ventilator)
	Platelet dysfunction and coagulation disturbances
Vascular factors	Tenuous, involuting capillaries with large diameter lumen
Extravascular factors	Deficient vascular support
	Excessive fibrinolytic activity

GMH/IVH = germinal matrix hemorrhage/intraventricular hemorrhage; CBF = cerebral blood flow.

large fluctuations typically occurred in infants breathing out of synchrony with the ventilator, but such fluctuations have also been observed in infants with, for example, large patent ductus arteriosus or hypotension. Increases in cerebral venous pressure are also thought to contribute to GMH/IVH. Sources of such increases include ventilatory strategies where intrathoracic pressure is high (e.g., high continuous positive airway pressure), pneumothorax, tracheal suctioning, and both labor and delivery, where fetal head compression likely results in significantly increased venous pressure. Indeed, a higher incidence of GMH/IVH is found in preterm infants delivered vaginally compared with those delivered through caesarean section, and also in those with a longer duration of labor. In all of these intravascular factors related to changes in cerebral arterial and venous blood flow, the role of a **pressure-passive** cerebral circulation is likely to be important. Several studies have shown that preterm infants, particularly asphyxiated newborns, have an impaired ability to regulate CBF in response to blood pressure changes (hence "pressure-passive") (11,12). Such impaired autoregulation puts the infant at increased risk of rupture of the fragile germinal matrix vessels in the face of significant increases in cerebral arterial or venous pressure, and particularly when ischemia precedes such increased pressure. Finally, impaired coagulation and platelet dysfunction are also intravascular factors that can contribute to the pathogenesis of GMH/IVH.

Vascular factors that contribute to GMH/IVH include the fragile nature of the involuting vessels of the germinal matrix. There is no muscularis mucosa and little adventitia in this area of relatively large diameter, thin-walled vessels; all of these factors make the vessels particularly susceptible to rupture. Extravascular risk factors for GMH/IVH include deficient extravascular support and likely excessive fibrinolytic activity.

B. Pathogenesis of complications of GMH/IVH. There are two major complications of GMH/IVH, namely **periventricular hemorrhagic infarction (PVHI)** and **PHH**; the pathogeneses of these two complications are discussed here.

    1. PVHI has previously been considered an extension of a large IVH, hence referred to as a grade 4 IVH (this designation is still used in much of the literature). However, careful neuropathologic studies have shown that the finding of a large, often unilateral or asymmetric hemorrhagic lesion dorsolateral to the lateral ventricle **is not an extension of the original IVH.** Rather, neuropathologic studies demonstrate the fan-shaped appearance of a typical hemorrhagic venous infarction in the distribution of the medullary veins that drain into the terminal vein, resulting from obstruction of flow in the terminal vein by the large ipsilateral IVH. Evidence supporting this view includes the observation that PVHI occurs on the side of the larger IVH, and Doppler US studies show markedly decreased or absent flow in the terminal vein on the side of the large IVH (13). Further neuropathologic evidence that **PVHI is a separate lesion from the original IVH** is that the ependymal lining of the lateral ventricle between the IVH and the PVHI has been observed to remain intact in some cases, demonstrating that the IVH did not extend into the adjacent cerebral parenchyma. Risk factors for the development of PVHI include low birth GA, low Apgar scores, early life acidosis, patent ductus arteriosus, pneumothorax, pulmonary hemorrhage, and need for significant respiratory or blood pressure support (14).

2. **Posthemorrhagic ventricular dilation (PVD), or PHH,** may occur days to weeks following the onset of GMH/IVH. Not all ventricular dilation progresses to established hydrocephalus that requires treatment, hence the terms are used with slightly different meanings (see IV.C.3 for clinical course of PVD). The pathogenesis of PHH likely relates at least in part to impaired CSF resorption and/or obstruction of the aqueduct or the foramina of Luschka or Magendie by particulate clot (15). Recent work suggests that other mechanisms may play a role in the pathogenesis of PVD. High levels of TGF-β1 are found in the CSF following IVH, particularly in infants with PHH; TGF-β1 upregulates genes for extracellular matrix proteins that elaborate a "scar" which may obstruct CSF flow and/or CSF reabsorption (16). In addition, restricted arterial pulsations (e.g., due to decreased intracranial compliance) have been proposed to underlie chronic hydrocephalus in hydrodynamic models of hydrocephalus (17). The **pathogenesis of the brain injury resulting from PHH** is probably related in large part to regional hypoxia-ischemia and mechanical distension of the periventricular white matter, based on animal and human studies (18–21). In addition, the presence of nonprotein-bound iron in the CSF of infants with PHH may lead to the generation of reactive oxygen species that in turn contribute to the injury of immature oligodendrocytes in the white matter (22). The brain injury associated with PHH is principally a bilateral cerebral white matter injury similar to periventricular leukomalacia (PVL) with regard to both its neuropathology and long-term outcome (21,23–25).

C. **Clinical presentation**
1. **GMH/IVH in the preterm newborn is usually a clinically silent syndrome** and is therefore recognized only when a routine CUS is performed. However, some infants present with decreased levels of consciousness and spontaneous movements, hypotonia, abnormal eye movements, or skew deviation. Rarely, an infant will present with a rapid and severe neurologic deterioration with obtundation or coma, severe hypotonia and lack of spontaneous movements, and generalized tonic posturing that is often thought to be seizure (but does not have an electrographic correlate by electroencephalogram).
2. **The term newborn with IVH typically presents with signs such as seizures, apnea, irritability or lethargy, vomiting with dehydration, or a full fontanelle.** Ventriculomegaly is often present at the time of IVH diagnosis in a term newborn. It is rare to find a catastrophic presentation unless there is another ICH, such as a large SDH or parenchymal hemorrhage.
3. **PVD may develop over days to weeks following IVH,** particularly in premature infants, and may present with increasing head growth (crossing percentiles on the growth chart), bulging fontanelle, splitting of sutures, decreased level of consciousness, impaired upgaze or sunsetting sign, apnea, worsening respiratory status, or feeding difficulties. However, PVD may be relatively asymptomatic in preterm newborns, as ICP is often normal in this population, particularly with slowly progressive dilation. Therefore, serial CUS scans are critical for diagnosis of PVD in preterm infants with known IVH. A study of infants with birth weight <1,500 g who developed IVH and survived at least 14 days showed that 50% of such infants will not show ventricular dilation, 25% will develop nonprogressive ventricular dilation (or stable ventriculomegaly), and the remaining 25% will develop PVD (26). The incidence of PVD increases with increasing severity of GMH/IVH; it is uncommon with grades 1 to 2 IVH (up to 5 to 12%), but occurs in up to 75% of infants with grade 3 IVH ± PVHI. The incidence of PHH is also higher with

younger GA at birth. Ventricular dilation may proceed rapidly (over a few days) or slowly (over weeks). Approximately 40% of infants with PVD will have spontaneous resolution of PVD without any treatment. The remaining 60% generally require medical and/or surgical therapy (~15% of this latter group do not survive).

D. Diagnosis

1. **The diagnosis of GMH/IVH is almost invariably made by real-time portable CUS in the premature infant.** Routine CUS studies should be performed in all infants born at <32 weeks' GA. In addition, CUS may be considered in older infants born at >32 weeks' GA who have risk factors such as perinatal asphyxia or pneumothorax, or who present with abnormal neurologic signs as described in the preceding text. We perform routine CUS studies on or around days 3, 7, 30, and 60 (or just before discharge) for infants born at <32 weeks' GA (or birth weight <1,500 g). Recently, in stable infants in whom the CUS will not change management, we have eliminated the day 3 CUS. However, in a very sick, very low birth weight infant, consideration should be given to performing a first CUS within 24 hours of birth, as a large IVH with/without other intracranial pathology (e.g., PVHI) may be an important factor in considering redirection of care. Also, a large IVH in this population may require earlier follow-up CUS studies to determine whether there is rapidly progressive ventricular dilation. Infants found to have GMH/IVH require more frequent CUS to monitor for complications of GMH/IVH such as PHH and PVHI, and for other lesions such as PVL (see IV.E.4.). In addition, any infant who develops abnormal neurologic signs or a significant risk factor for IVH at any point (such as pneumothorax, sepsis, sudden hypotension or volume loss of any etiology) should undergo CUS.

2. **Grading of GMH/IVH is important for determining management and prognosis.** Two systems are widely used for grading GMH/IVH, as outlined in Table 27B.3. Grading of GMH/IVH should be assigned based on the earliest CUS obtained when the IVH itself is of maximal size. Specifically, ventricular dilation that occurs days to weeks following GMH/IVH is not a grade 3 IVH; it represents either PHH or ventriculomegaly secondary to parenchymal volume loss. Given the variability in grading systems and in CUS interpretation, a detailed

TABLE 27B.3   Grading of Germinal Matrix Hemorrhage/Intraventricular Hemorrhage (GMH/IVH)

Grading system	Severity of GMH/IVH	Description of findings
Papile (27) (by CT scan)	I	Isolated GMH (no IVH)
	II	IVH without ventricular dilatation
	III	IVH with ventricular dilatation
	IV	IVH with parenchymal hemorrhage
Volpe (1) (by CUS)	I	GMH with no or minimal IVH (<10% ventricular volume)
	II	IVH occupying 10%–50% of ventricular area on parasagittal view
	III	IVH occupying >50% of ventricular area on parasagittal view, usually distends lateral ventricle **(at time of IVH diagnosis)**
	Separate notation	Periventricular echodensity (location and extent)

CT = computed tomography; CUS = cranial ultrasonography.

description of the CUS findings should be reported. Specifically, the description should include the following:

a. Presence or absence of blood in the germinal matrix.

b. Laterality (or bilaterality) of the hemorrhage.

c. Presence or absence of blood in each ventricle, including volume of blood in relation to ventricle size.

d. Presence or absence of blood in cerebral parenchyma, with specification of location.

e. Presence or absence of ventricular dilation, with measurements of ventricles when dilated.

f. Presence or absence of other any other hemorrhage (e.g., SAH) or parenchymal abnormalities.

3. **In the term newborn, IVH is usually diagnosed when a head CT or CUS is performed because of seizures, apnea, or abnormal mental status.** A brain MRI is superior for the demonstration of other lesions that may be associated with IVH in full-term newborns, such as thalamic hemorrhagic infarction, hypoxic-ischemic brain injury, or sinus venous thrombosis.

E. Management and prognosis

1. **Prevention of GMH/IVH should be the primary goal;** the decreased incidence of GMH/IVH since the 1980s is likely related to numerous improvements in maternal and neonatal care. Although antenatal administration of **glucocorticoids** has clearly been shown to decrease the incidence of GMH/IVH, antenatal phenobarbital, vitamin K, and magnesium sulfate have not been conclusively demonstrated to prevent GMH/IVH. Postnatal prevention of GMH/IVH should be directed toward minimizing risk factors outlined in IV.A. In particular, infusions of colloid or hyperosmolar solutions should be given slowly, and all efforts should be directed to avoiding hypotension and large fluctuations or sustained increases in arterial blood pressure or cerebral venous pressure. Elimination of CBF fluctuation related to mechanical ventilation may be achieved by administration of sedative or paralytic medication. This recommendation is based on the randomized trial that showed a marked reduction in the incidence of GMH/IVH in premature infants with fluctuating CBF who were paralyzed for the first 72 hours after birth, compared with infants who were not paralyzed (28).

2. **Management of GMH/IVH in the premature newborn largely consists of supportive care** of the infant, and monitoring for and treatment of complications of GMH/IVH. An increase in the size of GMH/IVH may occur; therefore appropriate early care may prevent enlargement of the IVH. Supportive care should be directed toward maintaining stable cerebral perfusion by maintaining normal blood pressure, circulating volume, electrolytes and blood gases. Transfusions of packed red blood cells may be required in cases of large IVH to restore normal blood volume and hematocrit. Thrombocytopenia or coagulation disturbances should be corrected.

3. **Management of IVH in the term newborn is directed at supportive care of the infant and treatment of seizures during the acute phase.** However, as symptomatic IVH in this group of newborns is frequently large, PHH develops in many infants, and **may require serial LPs and/or eventual ventriculoperitoneal (VP) shunt placement in up to 50% of such infants.** Outcome in this group of infants likely relates to factors other than IVH alone, as uncomplicated IVH has a good prognosis. Infants with a history of trauma or perinatal asphyxia, or with neuroimaging evidence of thalamic hemorrhagic infarction or hypoxic-ischemic brain injury, are at risk for significant cognitive and/or motor deficits.

4. **Management of PHH consists of careful monitoring of ventricle size by serial CUS and appropriate intervention when needed to reduce CSF accumulation, such as serial LPs to remove CSF, surgical interventions to divert CSF flow, and rarely, medications to reduce CSF production (see Fig. 27B.1).** The goals of therapy are to reduce ventriculomegaly and remove blood products, both of which may contribute to the pathogenesis

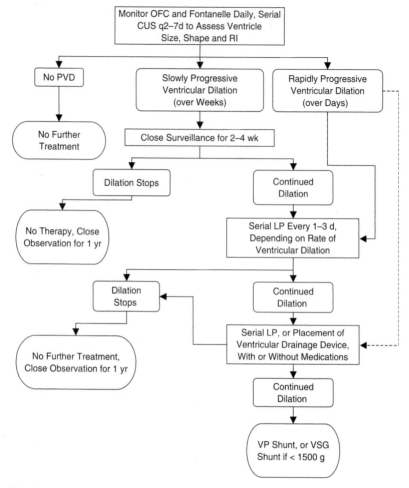

Figure 27B.1. Suggested algorithm for management of posthemorrhagic ventricular dilation (PVD) following intraventricular hemorrhage (IVH). OFC = occipital-frontal circumference; CUS = cranial ultrasonography; RI = resistive index; LP = lumbar puncture; VP = ventriculoperitoneal; VSG = ventriculosubgaleal.

of brain injury (see IV.B.2), and potentially to prevent need for a permanent shunt. CSF removal has been shown to improve cerebral perfusion, metabolism, and neurophysiologic function in infants with PVD (18,29–31). Evidence from numerous animal studies and some human data suggest that earlier treatment of PHH can improve neurologic outcome (24,32–34).

a. In cases of **slowly progressive PHH** (over weeks), close monitoring of clinical status (particularly OFC, fontanelle and sutures) and ventricle size (by CUS) may be sufficient. Many such cases will have spontaneous resolution of PHH without intervention or will prove to have stable ventriculomegaly. **It is critical to determine by serial CUS which infants have progressive dilation requiring therapy, versus which infants have stable ventriculomegaly due to other causes (such as atrophy due to PVL).**

b. **When serial CUS show persistent PVD, intervention is usually required, particularly if the infant shows clinical signs related to the PVD (e.g., worsening clinical status, bulging fontanelle, widening sutures, rapid increase in OFC). We typically begin therapy when progressive dilation persists for approximately 2 weeks in infants with clinical signs,** although the rate of ventricular dilation and size of ventricles will need to be assessed in each case to decide whether therapy should be initiated sooner or later. One retrospective study suggested that treatment initiated before ventricle size reached the 97th percentile +4 resulted in improved long-term neurologic outcome (34). We usually rely on a combination of measures of ventricle size, rate of PVD, resistive index (RI) (see subsequent text) and the infant's clinical course to decide when to initiate treatment, rather than using a single measure of ventricle size as an upper limit (e.g., 97th percentile +4 mm) (35). Therapy should begin with spinal (or ventricular) taps performed every 1 to 3 days, depending on the rate of ventricular dilation and the effect of CSF removal on ventricle size. The opening pressure should be measured whenever possible. A CUS performed before and after removal of 10 to 15 mL of CSF per kg body weight is often helpful in establishing the diagnosis of PHH and determining the effect of CSF removal in decreasing ventricle size. If PVD is rapidly progressive, daily taps or early surgical intervention may be needed (see IV.E.4.f)

c. **Measurement of the RI can be helpful in guiding management of PHH.** The RI is a measure of resistance to blood flow (see formula in the subsequent text), and therefore a high RI may indicate low intracranial compliance and risk of decreased cerebral perfusion. Because decreases in cerebral perfusion may result in ischemic brain injury, we have used the measurement of RI to help guide treatment of PHH. **RI is obtained by measuring systolic and diastolic blood flow velocities** by Doppler US (usually in the anterior cerebral artery), and calculating the RI as given by the formula:

$$RI = \frac{(systolic - diastolic)}{systolic}$$

where "systolic" refers to systolic blood flow velocity and "diastolic" refers to diastolic blood flow velocity.

A significant rise in RI from baseline RI values when gentle fontanelle compression is applied may indicate hemodynamic compromise and the need to remove CSF. We typically consider a >30% increase in RI with compression compared to baseline RI, or a baseline RI >0.9, as an indication for the need for CSF removal (36).

d. A combination of the infant's clinical status, ventricular size and shape by serial CUS, measurement of ICP by manometry, RI by Doppler US, and response to CSF removal should be used to determine **the need for and frequency of CSF removal procedures** or other interventions to reduce intraventricular CSF volume (Fig. 27B.1).

e. **If the foregoing medical therapy does not successfully reduce ventricle size, and/or PHH is rapidly progressive, surgical intervention is indicated. A ventriculosubgaleal shunt (VSG), ventricular access device (reservoir), or external ventricular drain** should be placed. We prefer to insert a VSG because (like a ventricular drain) it offers continuous CSF drainage and hence the potential to maintain normal ventricle size and cerebral perfusion, as opposed to intermittent CSF removal by spinal or ventricular taps. A VSG may be sufficient for adequate CSF drainage into the subgaleal space, although often only for a matter of days to weeks (37). If the VSG is insufficient to drain CSF adequately, CSF may be removed intermittently by a needle placed in the reservoir of the VSG (or ventricular access device) every 1 to 3 days, as for serial LPs. External ventricular drains are less favored by many neurosurgeons because of the high incidence of infection, especially if the catheter is not tunneled subcutaneously.

f. **Acetazolamide and furosemide are carbonic anhydrase inhibitors that can be used to decrease CSF production. However, their combined use often produces electrolyte disturbances and nephrocalcinosis, and may be associated with a worse long term neurologic outcome** (38,39). **For these reasons, the use of acetazolamide and furosemide together has fallen out of favour.** The use of acetazolamide alone may be considered, because it was shown to be effective as monotherapy in three of five infants in one small study (40). Acetazolamide could be used in cases where intermittent CSF removal is inadequate, or to reduce the frequency of intermittent CSF removal procedures, for example in very small or critically ill infants in whom a tap or surgical procedure has an unacceptably high risk. It should be noted that the safety and efficacy of acetazolamide monotherapy for PHH has not been demonstrated in large studies. Pharmacotherapy alone is usually ineffective in most severe cases of PHH.

   i. **Logistics.** Accepted diuretic therapy includes acetazolamide (25–150 mg/kg/day, given every 6 hours, administered intravenously or orally, starting dose of 25 mg/kg/day increased by 25 mg/kg/day to a maximum of 150 mg/kg/day); furosemide (1–3 mg/kg/day, given every 6–12 hours, administered intravenously or orally, starting dose of 1 mg/kg/day); or glycerol (4–8 mg/kg/day, given every 6 hours). The lowest effective dose of acetazolamide and furosemide should be used because of concerns about potentially toxic effects of high doses of acetazolamide. As glycerol can result in dramatic osmotic changes, it is currently used only in crises. We rarely use any of these agents in our current therapy of PHH.

   ii. **Side effects and risks.** There are a number of common and significant side effects and risks associated with use of these agents. Side effects include metabolic acidosis, electrolyte abnormalities, dehydration, gastrointestinal upset, and hypercalciuria with a risk of nephrocalcinosis. As a result, careful monitoring and specific treatment of these side effects is necessary. Infants who receive prolonged acetazolamide therapy usually require replacement of sodium, potassium, and bicarbonate, most conveniently provided in the form of tricitrates oral solution (PolyCitra, ALZA) (Na citrate, K citrate, and citric acid 2 mEq/mL based on the citrate). The starting dose is 1 to 3 mEq/kg/day divided into 3 or 4 doses. If K is not needed, then Bicitra (ALZA) (Na citrate and citric acid 1 mEq Na and the equivalent of 1 mEq of bicarbonate $(HCO_3)/$ mL) is used. The starting dose is 2 to 4 mEq/kg/day divided into 3 to 4 doses. The goal is to keep the serum HCO_3 >10 mEq/mL.

   Infants receiving prolonged furosemide therapy should be monitored for nephrocalcinosis with serial renal US scans. The urine Ca^{2+}: Cr ratios should be intermittently measured, with a ratio of >0.21 suggesting a degree of hypercalciuria that might promote nephrocalcinosis. The diagnosis of hypercalciuria and nephrocalcinosis, made by either renal ultrasonographic scan or Ca^{2+}: Cr ratio requires discontinuation of diuretic therapy. Nephrocalcinosis is a reversible condition; therefore, diuretic therapy may be reinstituted at a decreased dose if there are no other options for treating the PHH. Finally, because the physiologic nadir of the hematocrit tends to coincide with progression of PHH and the total blood volume in these tiny infants is small, monitoring of electrolytes in these infants can result in anemia and increased need for transfusion with blood products.

g. Fibrinolytic therapy alone has not been demonstrated to prevent PHH in five separate studies of different fibrinolytic agents (41). A single nonrandomized trial of continuous drainage, irrigation, and fibrinolytic therapy in 24 infants with PHH showed an apparent reduction in mortality, need for permanent shunt, and disability compared with historical controls (42). However, this radical high-risk therapy requires experienced clinicians and very intensive monitoring, and hence needs testing in larger trials before it is widely applied as routine therapy for infants with PHH.

h. **If PHH has persisted for >4 weeks despite medical therapy as described in the preceding text, a permanent shunt will usually be needed.** However, a permanent VP shunt can usually only be placed once infants weigh >1,500 to 2,000 g and are stable enough to undergo this surgery. If the infant weighs <1,500 g, a VSG, external drain or ventricular access device will be needed (if not already placed) until the infant has gained sufficient weight to undergo VP shunt placement.

i. **Rarely, PHH will recur weeks to months later despite apparent resolution in the neonatal period.** (43) Monitoring of head growth and fontanelle should continue after discharge home.

5. The long-term prognosis for infants with GMH/IVH varies considerably depending on the severity of IVH, complications of IVH or other brain lesions, the birth weight/GA, and other significant illnesses that affect neurologic outcome. Several recent studies suggest that preterm infants with grade 1–2 IVH have an increased risk of cerebral palsy and/or cognitive impairment compared to those without IVH (44–46). However, as many as 50% of children born at <32 weeks' GA have school difficulties whether or not they had IVH, although the risk is clearly higher among children and adolescents with a history of IVH and lower birth GA/weight (47,48). These cognitive impairments likely relate in part to coexisting cerebral white matter injury (i.e., PVL), which has many of the same risk factors as GMH/IVH. Infants with ventriculomegaly by CUS with or without GMH/IVH have been shown to be at increased risk of long-term neurologic impairments, likely because mild ventriculomegaly is a consequence of white matter injury (49,50). Studies thus far have been unable to determine definitively the separate contributions of small GMH/IVH and cerebral white matter injury, especially as these lesions frequently coexist and the latter is often missed by CUS. Infants with grade 3 IVH are at increased risk of cognitive and motor impairments; however, these infants frequently have complications of IVH or other neuropathologic lesions such as PVL that likely contribute significantly to their neurologic outcome. Notably, infants with grade 3 IVH and those with PVHI ("grade 4 IVH") are often grouped together in outcome studies. Recent work shows that MRI is superior to CUS in improving detection, classification and hence prognosis of GMH/IVH and its associated complications and other neuropathologic lesions such as periventricular white matter injury (51–53).

Infants with the two major complications of IVH, namely PVHI and PHH, are at much higher risk of neurologic impairments than those with IVH alone. Infants with PHH requiring significant intervention often manifest spastic diparesis and cognitive impairments due to bilateral periventricular white matter injury. Infants with a localized, unilateral PVHI may develop a spastic hemiparesis affecting the arm and leg with minimal or mild cognitive impairments (51). Quadriparesis and significant cognitive deficits (including mental retardation) are more likely if the PVHI is extensive or bilateral, or if there is also coexisting PVL (54). In addition to cognitive and motor impairments, infants with severe PHH and/or PVHI are at risk for developing cerebral visual impairment and epilepsy (54).

V. PERIVENTRICULAR LEUKOMALACIA (PVL)

A. **Etiology and pathogenesis.** Periventricular leukomalacia is a lesion found predominantly in the preterm infant, and is probably the neuropathologic lesion underlying much of the cognitive, motor, and sensory impairments and disabilities in children born prematurely. However, white matter injury with a similar imaging pattern to PVL in the preterm infant has also been reported in infants born at term (55) and in term newborns who underwent surgical repair of congenital heart disease (56).

The **characteristic neuropathology** of PVL was first described in detail by Banker and Larroche in their 1962 report detailing the histologic findings in 51 autopsy specimens (57). They described the classic features of PVL to include bilateral areas of focal necrosis, gliosis, and disruption of axons, with the so-called "retraction clubs and balls." The topographical distribution of the lesions was noted to be in the periventricular white matter dorsolateral to the lateral ventricles, primarily anterior to the frontal horn (at the level of the foramen of Monro) and lateral to the occipital horns. They noted that a severe "anoxic" episode occurred in 50 of 51 infants, that the lesions were consistently observed in the location of the border zone of the vascular supply, and that 75% of the group had been born prematurely. They therefore suggested two key features of the pathogenesis of PVL, namely (i) hypoxia-ischemia affecting the watershed regions of the white matter, and (ii) a particular vulnerability of the periventricular white matter of the premature brain. Further neuropathologic studies have extended these initial observations, demonstrating that in many cases PVL consists of areas of both focal necrosis (which become cystic) and a diffuse white matter lesion. The diffuse white matter lesion consists of hypertrophic astrocytes and loss of oligodendrocytes, and is followed by an overall decrease in the volume of cerebral white matter myelin. Interestingly, volumetric MRI analysis has demonstrated a significant reduction in cortical and subcortical gray matter volumes in newborns and children born prematurely (58–60). Despite the significant gray matter volume reductions measured by MRI, there are few neuropathologic data demonstrating overt neuronal injury in premature infants with PVL (61). One reason is that autopsy studies have a disproportionate representation of infants with severe PVL, IVH, PHH and/or PVHI, rather than mild or moderate PVL. In addition, the neuronal abnormality may be an impairment of cortical and subcortical neuronal development resulting from injury to axons or subplate neurons in the white matter (62), which may have a subtle histologic appearance requiring sophisticated microstructural and immunocytochemical studies to demonstrate the abnormality.

This distinctive lesion of PVL found in the immature white matter of premature newborns likely results from the interaction of multiple pathogenetic factors. **Several major factors have been identified to date: (i) vascular anatomic factors, (ii) pressure-passive cerebral circulation, (iii) intrinsic vulnerability of cerebral white matter of the premature newborn, and (iv) infection/inflammation** (63). These major factors will be discussed briefly, as follows. Banker and Larroche originally suggested that PVL occurred in the regions of vascular border zones in the cerebral white matter, and that ischemia would therefore be expected to preferentially affect these zones (57). Subsequent authors have further defined these zones using postmortem injection of the blood vessels to demonstrate the presence of vascular border and end zones in the periventricular white matter, where PVL is found (64,65). Second, there is evidence to suggest the presence of a pressure-passive circulation in a subset of premature infants (11,66). Furthermore, one study of 32 infants showed a higher incidence of PVL (as well as IVH) in infants who demonstrated evidence of a pressure-passive circulation (67). Third, a maturational vulnerability of the periventricular white matter is suggested by the finding that PVL occurs much more commonly in the premature than term newborn. Specifically, the observation that the diffuse lesion of PVL affects the oligodendrocyte (with resulting myelin loss) with relative preservation of other cellular elements suggests that the immature oligodendrocyte is the cell most vulnerable to injury. Immature oligodendrocytes are susceptible to injury and apoptotic cell death by free radical attack (68,69) and by glutamate receptor-mediated excitotoxic mechanisms (70). Notably, apoptosis is postulated to be the mechanism of cell death by a moderate ischemic insult; necrosis results from severe ischemic insults. Therefore, there is cellular and biochemical evidence to support the original postulate that the preterm infant's white matter displays a maturational vulnerability to hypoxic-ischemic injury which results in PVL. Finally, epidemiological and experimental studies suggest a role for infection and inflammation in the pathogenesis of PVL. Epidemiologic studies have shown an association between maternal infection, prolonged rupture of membranes, cord blood interleukin-6 levels, and an increased incidence of PVL (71), leading to the hypothesis that maternal infection may be an etiologic factor in the development of PVL (72). Experimental work has shown that certain cytokines, such as interferon-γ, have a cytotoxic effect on immature oligodendrocytes (73). However, cytokines may also be secreted in the setting of hypoxia-ischemia (in the absence of infection).

Moreover, infection and/or cytokines may lead to ischemia-reperfusion, which may cause further injury to oligodendrocytes. Therefore, there are multiple pathways by which infection/inflammation may contribute to the pathogenesis of PVL. In most cases, the pathogenesis of PVL probably involves the interaction of more than one of the pathogenetic mechanisms described earlier.

B. **Clinical presentation and diagnosis.** PVL is typically a clinically silent lesion, evolving over days to weeks with few or no outward neurologic signs until weeks to months later when spasticity is first detected, or at an even later age when children present with cognitive difficulties in school. With severe PVL, spasticity in the lower extremities may be detected by the careful observer by term age or earlier. However, **PVL is usually diagnosed in the neonatal period by CUS, or less commonly by MRI** (74). The evolution of echogenicity in the periventricular white matter over the first few weeks after birth, with or without cysts (which are echolucent), is the classical description of PVL by ultrasonographic imaging. Ventriculomegaly due to atrophy of the periventricular white matter (i.e., volume loss) is often present within weeks. Notably, isolated ventriculomegaly is associated with an increased risk of CP (49), suggesting that ventriculomegaly without radiologically evident white matter abnormalities may also indicate the presence of PVL. Studies correlating ultrasonography and autopsy data have demonstrated that the incidence of PVL is underestimated by cranial ultrasonography, the technique most widely used to diagnose brain abnormalities in the preterm infant (75,76). Several studies have shown that MRI is more sensitive than CUS for the detection of PVL, especially for the noncystic form of PVL (74,77,78). However, the true incidence of PVL is difficult to determine, as one recent study reported abnormal signal intensity within the white matter by MRI exam at term age in 80% of infants born at 23 to 30 weeks' GA (79). It has not been shown that this diffuse excessive high signal intensity on T2-weighted MRI correlates with neuropathologically proved PVL, although there was some correlation between this MRI finding and mild developmental delay at 18 months of age (79). The routine use of MRI scans for all premature infants has not been recommended (80), although it may be useful in some high-risk premature infants. It is probably most useful to perform an MRI scan close to term age, if an MRI scan is to be obtained during the newborn period. A brain MRI may be useful to confirm clinically suspected PVL in an older infant or child born prematurely who presents with cognitive, motor and/or sensory impairments.

C. **Management.** There are currently no medications or treatments available for the specific treatment of PVL during the newborn period. Current efforts are directed at prevention, based on knowledge of the various risk factors and pathogenetic mechanisms described earlier. Maintenance of normal cerebral perfusion should be attempted by careful management of systemic hemodynamics (e.g., blood pressure), intravascular volume, oxygenation and ventilation, and avoidance of sudden changes in systemic hemodynamics. It should be noted that there is controversy about the management of blood pressure in the premature infant, and that a normal blood pressure does not necessarily imply normal cerebral perfusion, given the known impairments of cerebral pressure autoregulation in some premature infants (66). Avoidance and prompt treatment of infection may also minimize PVL, although no studies have shown conclusively any effect of such interventions. Management of PVL after discharge from the NICU is directed at identification of any cognitive, sensory or motor impairments, and appropriate therapies for any such impairments, as described in the subsequent text. Promising studies of neuroprotective strategies to prevent or minimize PVL are being conducted in animal models (68,70), but human trials of such agents are probably still years away.

D. **Prognosis. PVL is the principal cause of the cognitive, behavioral, motor and sensory impairments found in children born at <32 weeks' GA** (81). There is an approximately 10% incidence of CP and up to 50% incidence of school difficulties in children born prematurely that is largely due to PVL, with PVHI being the other cerebral lesion that contributes significantly to neurologic disabilities. The incidence of neurologic impairments increases with lower GA at birth. For example, one study of extremely low birthweight infants (<1000 g) showed that only 30% of such children were performing at grade level without extra support at 8 years of age (47). Similarly, the incidence of CP is much higher in children born extremely prematurely, occurring in approximately 20% of children born at ≤26 weeks' GA but in only 4% of children born at 32 weeks' GA (45,82). Spastic diparesis is the most common form of CP in children born prematurely (45), because PVL typically affects the periventricular white matter closest to the ventricles. The axons subserving the lower extremities are located closest to the ventricle, the axons of the upper extremities are situated lateral to them, and the axons of the facial musculature are located farthest from the ventricle. Therefore, PVL produces abnormal tone (usually spasticity) and weakness predominantly in the lower extremities, with the upper extremities and face demonstrating milder abnormalities. Vision may also be affected by PVL, since the optic radiations subserving the lower visual field pass through the white matter dorsolateral to the occipital horns that is frequently affected by PVL (83). Some premature infants have retinopathy of prematurity affecting their vision, but PVL and other cerebral lesions alone can result in strabismus, nystagmus, visual field deficits, and perceptual difficulties, which may not be recognized until school age or later (84). Finally, children with severe PVL may develop epilepsy, although epilepsy is more commonly related to PVHI.

References

1. Volpe JJ. Intracranial hemorrhage: Germinal matrix-intraventricular hemorrhage of the premature infant. *Neurology of the newborn*. Philadelphia: WB Saunders, 2001: 428–496.
2. Volpe JJ. Intracranial hemorrhage: Subdural, primary subarachnoid, intracerebellar, intraventricular (term infant), and miscellaneous. *Neurology of the newborn*. Philadelphia: WB Saunders, 2001:397–427.
3. Chamnanvanakij S, Rollins N, Perlman JM. Subdural hematoma in term infants. *Pediatr Neurol* 2002;26:301–304.
4. Perrin RG, Rutka JT, Drake JM, et al. Management and outcomes of posterior fossa subdural hematomas in neonates. *Neurosurgery* 1997;40:1190–1199; discussion 1199–1200.
5. Huang AH, Robertson RL. Spontaneous superficial parenchymal and leptomeningeal hemorrhage in term neonates. *AJNR Am J Neuroradiol* 2004;25:469–475.
6. Bodensteiner JB, Johnsen SD. Cerebellar injury in the extremely premature infant: Newly recognized but relatively common outcome. *J Child Neurol* 2005;20:139–142.
7. Roland EH, Flodmark O, Hill A. Thalamic hemorrhage with intraventricular hemorrhage in the full-term newborn. *Pediatrics* 1990;85:737–742.
8. Goddard-Finegold J, Armstrong D, Zeller RS. Intraventricular hemorrhage, following volume expansion after hypovolemic hypotension in the newborn beagle. *J Pediatr* 1982;100:796–799.
9. Hill A, Perlman JM, Volpe JJ. Relationship of pneumothorax to occurrence of intraventricular hemorrhage in the premature newborn. *Pediatrics* 1982;69:144–149.
10. Perlman JM, McMenamin JB, Volpe JJ. Fluctuating cerebral blood-flow velocity in respiratory-distress syndrome. Relation to the development of intraventricular hemorrhage. *N Engl J Med* 1983;309:204–209.
11. Lou H, Lassen N, Friis-Hansen B. Impaired autoregulation of cerebral blood flow in the distressed newborn infant. *J Pediatr* 1979;94:118–121.
12. Pryds O, Greisen G, Lou H, et al. Heterogeneity of cerebral vasoreactivity in preterm infants supported by mechanical ventilation. *J Pediatr* 1989;115:638–645.
13. Taylor GA. Effect of germinal matrix hemorrhage on terminal vein position and patency. *Pediatr Radiol* 1995;25(Suppl 1):S37–S40.
14. Bassan H, Feldman HA, Limperopoulos C, et al. Periventricular hemorrhagic infarction: Risk factors and neonatal outcome. *Pediatr Neurol* 2006;35:85–92.
15. Larroche JC. Post-haemorrhagic hydrocephalus in infancy anatomical study. *Biol Neonate* 1972;20:287–299.
16. Whitelaw A, Thoresen M, Pople I. Posthaemorrhagic ventricular dilatation. *Arch Dis Child Fetal Neonatal Ed* 2002;86:F72–F74.

17. Greitz D. Radiological assessment of hydrocephalus: New theories and implications for therapy. *Neurosurg Rev* 2004;27:145–165.

18. Bejar R, Saugstad OD, James H, et al. Increased hypoxanthine concentrations in cerebrospinal fluid of infants with hydrocephalus. *J Pediatr* 1983;103:44–48.

19. da Silva M, Drake J, Lemaire C, et al. High-energy phosphate metabolism in a neonatal model of hydrocephalus before and after shunting. *J Neurosurg* 1994;81:544–553.

20. da Silva MC, Michowicz S, Drake JM, et al. Reduced local cerebral blood flow in periventricular white matter in experimental neonatal hydrocephalus-restoration with CSF shunting. *J Cereb Blood Flow Metab* 1995;15:1057–1065.

21. Del Bigio MR, Zhang YW. Cell death, axonal damage, and cell birth in the immature rat brain following induction of hydrocephalus. *Exp Neurol* 1998;154:157–169.

22. Savman K, Nilsson UA, Blennow M, et al. Non-protein-bound iron is elevated in cerebrospinal fluid from preterm infants with posthemorrhagic ventricular dilatation. *Pediatr Res* 2001;49:208–212.

23. Fukumizu M, Takashima S, Becker L. Neonatal posthemorrhagic hydrocephalus: Neuropathologic and immunohistochemical studies. *Pediatr Neurol* 1995;13:230–234.

24. du Plessis AJ. Posthemorrhagic hydrocephalus and brain injury in the preterm infant: Dilemmas in diagnosis and management. *Semin Pediatr Neurol* 1998;5:161–179.

25. Whitelaw A, Rosengren L, Blennow M. Brain specific proteins in posthaemorrhagic ventricular dilatation. *Arch Dis Child Fetal Neonatal Ed* 2001;84:F90–F91.

26. Murphy BP, Inder TE, Rooks V, et al. Posthaemorrhagic ventricular dilatation in the premature infant: Natural history and predictors of outcome. *Arch Dis Child Fetal Neonatal Ed* 2002;87:F37–F41.

27. Papile LA, Burstein J, Burstein R, et al. Incidence and evolution of subependymal and intraventricular hemorrhage: A study of infants with birth weights less than 1,500 gm. *J Pediatr* 1978;92:529–534.

28. Perlman JM, Goodman S, Kreusser KL, et al. Reduction in intraventricular hemorrhage by elimination of fluctuating cerebral blood-flow velocity in preterm infants with respiratory distress syndrome. *N Engl J Med* 1985;312:1353–1357.

29. Ehle A, Sklar F. Visual evoked potentials in infants with hydrocephalus. *Neurology* 1979;29:1541–1544.

30. De Vries LS, Pierrat V, Minami T, et al. The role of short latency somatosensory evoked responses in infants with rapidly progressive ventricular dilatation. *Neuropediatrics* 1990;21:136–139.

31. Soul JS, Eichenwald E, Walter G, et al. CSF removal in infantile posthemorrhagic hydrocephalus results in significant improvement in cerebral hemodynamics. *Pediatr Res* 2004;55:872–876.

32. Del Bigio MR, Kanfer JN, Zhang YW. Myelination delay in the cerebral white matter of immature rats with kaolin-induced hydrocephalus is reversible. *J Neuropathol Exp Neurol* 1997;56:1053–1066.

33. del Bigio MR, Crook CR, Buist R. Magnetic resonance imaging and behavioral analysis of immature rats with kaolin-induced hydrocephalus: Pre- and postshunting observations. *Exp Neurol* 1997;148:256–264.

34. de Vries LS, Liem KD, van Dijk K, et al. Early versus late treatment of posthaemorrhagic ventricular dilatation: Results of a retrospective study from five neonatal intensive care units in The Netherlands. *Acta Paediatr* 2002;91:212–217.

35. Levene MI. Measurement of the growth of the lateral ventricles in preterm infants with real-time ultrasound. *Arch Dis Child* 1981;56:900–904.

36. Taylor GA, Madsen JR. Neonatal hydrocephalus: Hemodynamic response to fontanelle compression—correlation with intracranial pressure and need for shunt placement. *Radiology* 1996;201:685–689.

37. Rahman S, Teo C, Morris W, et al. Ventriculosubgaleal shunt: A treatment option for progressive posthemorrhagic hydrocephalus [see comments]. *Childs Nerv Syst* 1995; 11:650–654.

38. International PHVD Drug Trial Group. International randomised controlled trial of acetazolamide and furosemide in posthaemorrhagic ventricular dilatation in infancy. *Lancet* 1998;352:433–440.

39. Kennedy CR, Ayers S, Campbell MJ, et al. Randomized, controlled trial of acetazolamide and furosemide in posthemorrhagic ventricular dilation in infancy: Follow-up at 1 year. *Pediatrics* 2001;108:597–607.

40. Mercuri E, Faundez JC, Cowan F, et al. Acetazolamide without frusemide in the treatment of post-haemorrhagic hydrocephalus. *Acta Paediatr* 1994;83:1319–1321.

41. Haines SJ, Lapointe M. Fibrinolytic agents in the management of posthemorrhagic hydrocephalus in preterm infants: The evidence. *Childs Nerv Syst* 1999;15:226–234.

42. Whitelaw A, Pople I, Cherian S, et al. Phase 1 trial of prevention of hydrocephalus after intraventricular hemorrhage in newborn infants by drainage, irrigation, and fibrinolytic therapy. *Pediatrics* 2003;111:759–765.

43. Perlman JM, Lynch B, Volpe JJ. Late hydrocephalus after arrest and resolution of neonatal post- hemorrhagic hydrocephalus. *Dev Med Child Neurol* 1990;32:725–729.

44. Sherlock RL, Anderson PJ, Doyle LW. Neurodevelopmental sequelae of intraventricular haemorrhage at 8 years of age in a regional cohort of ELBW/very preterm infants. *Early Hum Dev* 2005;81:909–916.

45. Ancel PY, Livinec F, Larroque B, et al. Cerebral palsy among very preterm children in relation to gestational age and neonatal ultrasound abnormalities: The EPIPAGE cohort study. *Pediatrics* 2006;117:828–835.

46. Patra K, Wilson-Costello D, Taylor HG, et al. Grades I-II intraventricular hemorrhage in extremely low birth weight infants: Effects on neurodevelopment. *J Pediatr* 2006;149:169–173.

47. Bowen JR, Gibson FL, Hand PJ. Educational outcome at 8 years for children who were born extremely prematurely: A controlled study. *J Paediatr Child Health* 2002;38:438–444.

48. van de Bor M, den Ouden L. School performance in adolescents with and without periventricular-intraventricular hemorrhage in the neonatal period. *Semin Perinatol* 2004;28:295–303.

49. Allan WC, Vohr B, Makuch RW, et al. Antecedents of cerebral palsy in a multicenter trial of indomethacin for intraventricular hemorrhage [see comments]. *Arch Pediatr Adolesc Med* 1997;151:580–585.

50. Vollmer B, Roth S, Riley K, et al. Neurodevelopmental outcome of preterm infants with ventricular dilatation with and without associated haemorrhage. *Dev Med Child Neurol* 2006;48:348–352.

51. De Vries LS, Groenendaal F, van Haastert IC, et al. Asymmetrical myelination of the posterior limb of the internal capsule in infants with periventricular haemorrhagic infarction: An early predictor of hemiplegia. *Neuropediatrics* 1999;30:314–319.

52. Valkama AM, Paakko EL, Vainionpaa LK, et al. Magnetic resonance imaging at term and neuromotor outcome in preterm infants. *Acta Paediatr* 2000;89:348–355.

53. Woodward LJ, Anderson PJ, Austin NC, et al. Neonatal MRI to predict neurodevelopmental outcomes in preterm infants. *N Engl J Med* 2006;355:685–694.

54. Bassan H, Benson CB, Limperopoulos C, et al. Ultrasonographic features and severity scoring of periventricular hemorrhagic infarction in relation to risk factors and outcome. *Pediatrics* 2006;117:2111–2118.

55. Kwong KL, Wong YC, Fong CM, et al. Magnetic resonance imaging in 122 children with spastic cerebral palsy. *Pediatr Neurol* 2004;31:172–176.

56. Galli KK, Zimmerman RA, Jarvik GP, et al. Periventricular leukomalacia is common after neonatal cardiac surgery. *J Thorac Cardiovasc Surg* 2004;127:692–704.

57. Banker B, Larroche J. Periventricular leukomalacia of infancy. *Arch Neurol* 1962;7:386–410.

58. Peterson BS, Vohr B, Staib LH, et al. Regional brain volume abnormalities and long-term cognitive outcome in preterm infants. *JAMA* 2000;284:1939–1947.

59. Abernethy LJ, Cooke RW, Foulder-Hughes L. Caudate and hippocampal volumes, intelligence, and motor impairment in 7-year-old children who were born preterm. *Pediatr Res* 2004;55:884–893.

60. Inder TE, Warfield SK, Wang H, et al. Abnormal cerebral structure is present at term in premature infants. *Pediatrics* 2005;115:286–294.

61. Marin-Padilla M. Developmental neuropathology and impact of perinatal brain damage. II: white matter lesions of the neocortex. *J Neuropathol Exp Neurol* 1997;56:219–235.

62. Volpe JJ. Encephalopathy of prematurity includes neuronal abnormalities. *Pediatrics* 2005;116:221–225.

63. Volpe JJ. Neurobiology of periventricular leukomalacia in the premature infant. *Pediatr Res* 2001;50:553–562.

64. Takashima S, Tanaka K. Development of cerebrovascular architecture and its relationship to periventricular leukomalacia. *Arch Neurol* 1978;35:11–16.

65. De Reuck JL. Cerebral angioarchitecture and perinatal brain lesions in premature and full-term infants. *Acta Neurol Scand* 1984;70:391–395.

66. Soul JS, Hammer PE, Tsuji M, et al. Fluctuating pressure-passivity is common in the cerebral circulation of sick premature infants. *Pediatr Res* 2007;61:467–473.

67. Tsuji M, Saul JP, du Plessis A, et al. Cerebral intravascular oxygenation correlates with mean arterial pressure in critically ill premature infants. *Pediatrics* 2000;106:625–632.

68. Oka A, Belliveau MJ, Rosenberg PA, et al. Vulnerability of oligodendroglia to glutamate: pharmacology, mechanisms, and prevention. *J Neurosci* 1993;13:1441–1453.

69. Back SA, Gan X, Li Y, et al. Maturation-dependent vulnerability of oligodendrocytes to oxidative stress-induced death caused by glutathione depletion. *J Neurosci* 1998;18:6241–6253.

70. Follett PL, Deng W, Dai W, et al. Glutamate receptor-mediated oligodendrocyte toxicity in periventricular leukomalacia: a protective role for topiramate. *J Neurosci* 2004;24:4412–4420.

71. Yoon BH, Romero R, Yang SH, et al. Interleukin-6 concentrations in umbilical cord plasma are elevated in neonates with white matter lesions associated with periventricular leukomalacia. *Am J Obstet Gynecol* 1996;174:1433–1440.

72. Dammann O, Leviton A. Maternal intrauterine infection, cytokines, and brain damage in the preterm newborn. *Pediatr Res* 1997;42:1–8.

73. Baerwald KD, Popko B. Developing and mature oligodendrocytes respond differently to the immune cytokine interferon-gamma. *J Neurosci Res* 1998;52:230–239.

74. Maalouf EF, Duggan PJ, Counsell SJ, et al. Comparison of findings on cranial ultrasound and magnetic resonance imaging in preterm infants. *Pediatrics* 2001;107:719–727.

75. Hope PL, Gould SJ, Howard S, et al. Precision of ultrasound diagnosis of pathologically verified lesions in the brains of very preterm infants. *Dev Med Child Neurol* 1988;30:457–471.

76. Carson SC, Hertzberg BS, Bowie JD, et al. Value of sonography in the diagnosis of intracranial hemorrhage and periventricular leukomalacia: a postmortem study of 35 cases. *AJNR Am J Neuroradiol* 1990;11:677–683.

77. Roelants-van Rijn AM, Groenendaal F, Beek FJ, et al. Parenchymal brain injury in the preterm infant: comparison of cranial ultrasound, MRI and neurodevelopmental outcome. *Neuropediatrics* 2001;32:80–89.

78. Inder TE, Anderson NJ, Spencer C, et al. White matter injury in the premature infant: a comparison between serial cranial sonographic and MR findings at term. *AJNR Am J Neuroradiol* 2003;24:805–809.

79. Dyet LE, Kennea N, Counsell SJ, et al. Natural history of brain lesions in extremely preterm infants studied with serial magnetic resonance imaging from birth and neurodevelopmental assessment. *Pediatrics* 2006;118:536–548.

80. Ment LR, Bada HS, Barnes P, et al. Practice parameter: neuroimaging of the neonate: report of the Quality Standards Subcommittee of the American Academy of Neurology and the Practice Committee of the Child Neurology Society. *Neurology* 2002;58:1726–1738.

81. Volpe JJ. Cerebral white matter injury of the premature infant-more common than you think. *Pediatrics* 2003;112:176–180.

82. Wood NS, Marlow N, Costeloe K, et al. Neurologic and developmental disability after extremely preterm birth. EPICure Study Group. *N Engl J Med* 2000;343:378–384.

83. Jacobson L, Lundin S, Flodmark O, et al. Periventricular leukomalacia causes visual impairment in preterm children. A study on the aetiologies of visual impairment in a

population-based group of preterm children born 1989-95 in the county of Varmland, Sweden. *Acta Ophthalmol Scand* 1998;76:593–598.

84. Jacobson L, Ygge J, Flodmark O, et al. Visual and perceptual characteristics, ocular motility and strabismus in children with periventricular leukomalacia. *Strabismus* 2002;10:179–183.

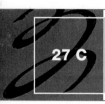

27 C PERINATAL ASPHYXIA
Lisa M. Adcock and Lu-Ann Papile

I. PERINATAL ASPHYXIA refers to a condition of impaired gas exchange that leads, if persistent, to fetal hypoxemia and hypercarbia. It occurs during the first and second stage of labor and is identified by fetal acidosis, as measured in umbilical arterial blood. The umbilical artery pH that defines asphyxia of a sufficient degree to cause brain injury is unknown. Although the most widely accepted definition is a pH <7.0, even with this degree of acidosis the likelihood of brain injury is low. The following terms may be used in evaluating a term infant at risk for brain injury in the perinatal period:

- **A. Neonatal depression** is a general term used to describe an infant who has a prolonged transition from an intrauterine to an extrauterine environment. These infants usually have low 1- and 5-minute Apgar scores.
- **B. Neonatal encephalopathy** is a clinical term used to describe an abnormal neurobehavioral state that consists of a decreased level of consciousness with abnormalities in neuromotor tone. It characteristically begins within the first postnatal day and may be associated with seizure-like activity, hypoventilation or apnea, depressed primitive reflexes and the appearance of brain stem reflexes. It does **not** imply a specific etiology, nor does it imply irreversible neurologic injury.
- **C. Hypoxic-ischemic encephalopathy (HIE)** is an abnormal neurobehavioral state in which the predominant pathogenic mechanism is impaired cerebral blood flow.
- **D. Hypoxic-ischemic brain injury** refers to neuropathology attributable to hypoxia and/or ischemia as evidenced by biochemical (such as serum creatine kinase brain bound [CK-BB]), electrophysiologic (EEG), neuroimaging (head ultrasonography [HUS], magnetic resonance imaging [MRI], computed tomography [CT]), or postmortem abnormalities.

II. INCIDENCE. The frequency of perinatal asphyxia is approximately 1% to 1.5% of live births in the Western Hemisphere and is inversely related to gestational age and birth weight. It occurs in 0.5% of live born infants >36 weeks' gestation and accounts for 20% of perinatal deaths (50% if stillborns are included). A higher incidence is noted in term infants of diabetic or toxemic mothers, infants with intrauterine growth restriction, breech presentation, and postdates infants.

III. ETIOLOGY. In term infants, 90% of asphyxial events occur in the antepartum or intrapartum period as a result of impaired gas exchange across the placenta that leads to the inadequate provision of oxygen (O_2) and removal carbon dioxide (CO_2) and H^+ from the fetus. The remainder of these events occurs in the postpartum period and is usually secondary to pulmonary, cardiovascular, or neurologic abnormalities.

- **A.** Factors that increase the risk of perinatal asphyxia include the following:
  - **1.** Impairment of maternal oxygenation.
  - **2.** Decreased blood flow from mother to placenta.

3. Decreased blood flow from placenta to fetus.
4. Impaired gas exchange across the placenta or at the fetal tissue level.
5. Increased fetal O_2 requirement.

B. Etiologies of perinatal hypoxia-ischemia include the following:

1. Maternal factors: hypertension (acute or chronic), infection, diabetes, hypotension, vascular disease, drug use, and hypoxia due to pulmonary, cardiac, or neurologic disease.
2. Placental factors: infarction, fibrosis, abruption, or hydrops.
3. Uterine rupture.
4. Umbilical cord accidents: prolapse, entanglement, true knot, compression.
5. Abnormalities of umbilical vessels.
6. Fetal factors: anemia, infection, cardiomyopathy, hydrops, severe cardiac/circulatory insufficiency.
7. Neonatal factors: severe neonatal hypoxia due to cyanotic congenital heart disease, persistent pulmonary hypertension of the newborn (PPHN), cardiomyopathy, other forms of neonatal cardiogenic and/or septic shock.

IV. PATHOPHYSIOLOGY

A. Events that occur during the normal course of labor cause most babies to be born with little O_2 reserve. These include the following:

1. Decreased blood flow to placenta due to uterine contractions, some degree of cord compression, maternal dehydration, maternal alkalosis due to hyperventilation.
2. Decreased O_2 delivery to the fetus as a result of the reduction of placental blood flow.
3. Increased O_2 consumption in both mother and fetus.

B. During labor complicated by a hypoxic-ischemic challenge, the following changes may occur:

1. With **brief asphyxia,** there is a transient increase, followed by a decrease in heart rate (HR), mild elevation in blood pressure (BP), an increase in central venous pressure (CVP), and essentially no change in cardiac output (CO). This is accompanied by a redistribution of CO with an increased proportion going to the brain, heart and adrenal glands (diving reflex).
2. With **prolonged asphyxia** cerebral blood flow becomes dependent on systemic BP (loss of cerebral vascular autoregulation). A decrease in CO leads to hypotension and impaired cerebral blood flow resulting in anaerobic metabolism and eventual intracellular energy failure due to an increase in the utilization of glucose in the brain and a fall in the concentration of glycogen, phosphocreatine, and adenosine triphosphate (ATP).
3. Hypoxia-induced vascular dilatation increases glucose availability, at least transiently; and anaerobic metabolism produces lactic acid.

C. Cellular changes occur due to diminished oxidative phosphorylation and ATP production. This energy failure impairs ion pump function, causing accumulation of intracellular Na^+, Cl^-, H_2O, and Ca^{2+}; extracellular K^+; and excitatory amino acid (EAA) neurotransmitters (e.g., glutamate). Impairment of oxidative phosphorylation can occur during the primary asphyxial episode as well as during a secondary energy failure that usually occurs approximately 6 to 24 hours after the initiating insult. Cell death can be either immediate or delayed, and either apoptotic or necrotic.

1. **Immediate neuronal death** can occur due to intracellular osmotic overload of Na^+ and Ca^{2+}, as seen with excessive EAA acting on inotropic glutamate receptors (such as the N-methyl-D-aspartate [NMDA] receptor])
2. **Delayed neuronal death** occurs secondary to uncontrolled activation of enzymes and second messenger systems within the cell (e.g., Ca^{2+}-dependent lipases, proteases, and caspases); perturbation of mitochondrial respiratory electron chain transport; generation of free radicals and leukotrienes; generation of nitric oxide (NO) through NO synthase; or depletion of energy stores.
3. EAA also can activate α-3-hydroxy-5-methyl-isoxazole (AMPA) receptor channels, leading to **oligodendrocyte progenitor cell death.**

4. **Reperfusion** of previously ischemic tissue may cause injury as it can promote the formation of excess reactive oxygen species (e.g., superoxide, hydrogen peroxide, hydroxyl, singlet oxygen), which can overwhelm the endogenous scavenger mechanisms, thereby causing damage to cellular lipids, proteins, and nucleic acids, as well as to the blood–brain barrier. This may result in an influx of neutrophils that, along with activated microglia, release injurious cytokines (e.g., interleukin 1-ß [IL-1 ß] and tumor necrosis factor α [TNF-α]).

V. DIAGNOSIS

A. **Perinatal assessment of risk** includes awareness of preexisting maternal or fetal problems that may predispose to perinatal asphyxia (see preceding list) and of changing placental and fetal conditions (see Chap. 1) ascertained by ultrasonographic examination, biophysical profile, nonstress tests, measurement of urinary estriol.

B. **Clinical presentation** can be variable. Common clinical scenarios include a postdates infant with asphyxia, meconium aspiration, pulmonary hypertension, pneumothorax, or birth trauma.

C. **Low Apgar scores** and need for resuscitation in the delivery room are common but nonspecific findings. Many features of the Apgar score relate to cardiovascular integrity and **not** neurologic function.

1. In addition to perinatal asphyxia, the differential diagnosis for a term infant with an Apgar score ≤3 for >5 minutes includes depression from maternal anesthesia or analgesia; trauma; metabolic or infectious insults; neuromuscular disorders; and central nervous system (CNS), cardiac, or pulmonary malformations

2. If the Apgar score is >6 by 5 minutes, perinatal asphyxia is not likely.

D. Umbilical cord or first **blood gas** determination.

The specific blood gas criteria that define asphyxia causing brain damage are uncertain.

1. In a population-based cohort of 17,000 term infants, the average umbilical cord arterial pH was 7.24 ± 0.07 and BE was -5.6 ± 0.3 mmol/L. Umbilical arterial pH <7.0 was present in only 0.4%. Of these, 5-minute Apgar score was <7 in 31% and <3 in 8.5%. The risk of adverse outcome was more likely if the acidosis is purely metabolic or mixed.

2. In another study, base deficit was measured in term infants who had persistent hemodynamic, respiratory, or neurologic abnormalities at 30 minutes of age. Metabolic acidosis with base deficit of 14 mmol/L or more had a sensitivity of 73.2% and a specificity of 82% in predicting moderate or severe neonatal encephalopathy. In two large randomized clinical trials of hypothermia for neonatal hypoxic/ischemic encephalopathy, severe acidosis was defined as pH of 7.0 or less or base deficit of ≥16 mmol/L.

VI. HIE.
The diagnosis of perinatal HIE requires an abnormal neurologic examination on the first day following birth. It is important to note that no significant neurologic abnormality diagnosed later in childhood (e.g., cerebral palsy [CP]) can be ascribed to perinatal asphyxia in the absence of evidence in the immediate neonatal period of neurologic abnormality and severe multiorgan dysfunction.

A. The clinical spectrum of HIE is described as mild, moderate and severe (see Table 27C.1 Sarnat Stages of HIE). Infants can progress from mild to moderate and/or severe encephalopathy over the 72 hours following the hypoxic-ischemic insult.

B. The diagnosis of neonatal encephalopathy includes a number of etiologies in addition to perinatal hypoxia-ischemia. Asphyxia may be suspected and HIE reasonably included in the differential diagnosis of term neonatal depression, coma, or neurologic dysfunction if the following have been documented:

1. Apgar score ≤3 at >5 minutes.

2. Fetal HR <60 beats/minute.

3. Prolonged (>1 hour) antenatal acidosis.

4. Seizures within first 24 to 48 hours after birth (50% of seizures are **not** asphyxial in etiology).

5. Burst-suppression pattern electroencephalography (EEG).

TABLE 27C.1	Sarnat and Sarnat Stages of Hypoxic-Ischemic Encephalopathy[*]		
Stage	**Stage 1 (Mild)**	**Stage 2 (Moderate)**	**Stage 3 (Severe)**
Level of consciousness	Hyperalert; irritable	Lethargic or obtunded	Stuporous, comatose
Neuromuscular control:	Uninhibited, overreactive	Diminished spontaneous movement	Diminished or absent spontaneous movement
Muscle tone	Normal	Mild hypotonia	Flaccid
Posture	Mild distal flexion	Strong distal flexion	Intermittent decerebration
Stretch reflexes	Overactive	Overactive, disinhibited	Decreased or absent
Segmental myoclonus	Present or absent	Present	Absent
Complex reflexes:	Normal	Suppressed	Absent
Suck	Weak	Weak or absent	Absent
Moro	Strong, low threshold	Weak, incomplete high threshold	Absent
Oculovestibular	Normal	Overactive	Weak or absent
Tonic neck	Slight	Strong	Absent
Autonomic function:	Generalized sympathetic	Generalized parasympathetic	Both systems depressed
Pupils	Mydriasis	Miosis	Midposition, often unequal; poor light reflex
Respirations	Spontaneous	Spontaneous; occasional apnea	Periodic; apnea
Heart rate	Tachycardia	Bradycardia	Variable
Bronchial and salivary secretions	Sparse	Profuse	Variable
Gastrointestinal motility	Normal or decreased	Increased diarrhea	Variable
Seizures	None	Common focal or multifocal (6 to 24 hours of age)	Uncommon (excluding decerebration)
Electroencephalographic findings	Normal (awake)	Early: generalized low-voltage, slowing (continuous delta and theta)	Early: periodic pattern with isopotential phases
		Later: periodic pattern (awake); seizures focal or multifocal; 1.0 to 1.5 Hz spike and wave	Later: totally isopotential
Duration of symptoms	<24 hours	2 to 14 days	Hours to weeks
Outcome	About 100% normal	80% normal; abnormal if symptoms more than 5 to 7 days	About 50% die; remainder with severe sequelae

[*]The stages in this table are a continuum reflecting the spectrum of clinical states of infants over 36 weeks' gestational age.
Source: From Sarnat H. B., Sarnat M. S. Neonatal encephalopathy following fetal distress: A clinical and electroencephalographics study. *Arch Neurol* 1976;33:696.

6. Need for positive pressure ventilation for >1 minute or first cry delayed >5 minutes.

VII. OTHER NEUROLOGIC CONSIDERATIONS

A. Increased intracranial pressure (ICP), defined as >10 mm Hg, or cerebral edema should be regarded as an **effect** rather than a **cause** of brain damage. Cerebral edema peaks at 36 to 72 hrs after the insult. It often reflects extensive prior cerebral necrosis rather than swelling of intact cells, making this finding consistent with a uniformly poor prognosis. Efforts to reduce ICP and cerebral edema (high-dose phenobarbital, steroids, mannitol, and other hypertonic solutions) do not affect outcome.

B. Seizures are described in 20% to 50% of infants with HIE, and usually start between 6 and 24 hours after the insult. They are most often seen in Sarnat stage 2 HIE, rarely in Sarnat stage 3, and almost never in Sarnat stage 1 HIE.

1. Seizures in HIE are usually subtle, tonic, or multifocal clonic. Generalized seizures are uncommon due to comparatively immature myelinization and synaptogenesis of the neonatal brain. Distinguishing between multifocal seizures and jitteriness (rhythmic segmental myoclonus) in stages 1 and 2 HIE may be difficult. They can be differentiated by holding the affected extremity and changing the tension on the muscle stretch receptor by slightly flexing or extending the joint. This should arrest clonus, whereas in true seizures, convulsive movements continue to be felt in the examiner's hand.

2. Seizures may be associated with increased cerebral metabolic rate, which could lead to further cerebral injury.

3. Seizures can compromise ventilation and oxygenation, especially in infants who are not on mechanical ventilation. In infants on musculoskeletal blockade for mechanical ventilation, seizures may be manifested by abrupt changes in BP, HR and oxygenation.

4. Seizures associated with HIE are often very difficult to control. Whether seizures alone, in the absence of metabolic or cardiopulmonary abnormalities, lead to brain injury is controversial.

VIII. MULTIORGAN DYSFUNCTION. Other organ systems in addition to the brain usually exhibit evidence of asphyxial damage.

A. In some cases, the brain may be the only organ exhibiting dysfunction following asphyxia. In one series of 57 infants, HIE occurred without other system involvement in 14 (24.5%).

B. The gamut of organ involvement in perinatal asphyxia varies among series, depending in part upon the definitions used for asphyxia and organ dysfunction.

1. In a retrospective study of 130 term infants with asphyxia, the proportion of those with organ dysfunction was: renal 70%, cardiovascular 62%, pulmonary 86%, hepatic 85%. Infants were diagnosed with asphyxia if they needed mechanical ventilation at birth, exhibited encephalopathy, and had one or more of the following: (i) 5-minute Apgar score <5, (ii) Base deficit 16 or more mmol/L documented within first hour of life, and (iii) delayed respiratory effort for 5 or more minutes of life.

2. In another series of 152 asphyxiated term infants followed prospectively, neurologic and systemic complications occurred in 43% and 57%, respectively. Organ dysfunction included respiratory abnormalities 39%, infection 17%, gastrointestinal intolerance 15%. Infants were considered to have asphyxia if they had fetal distress, were depressed at birth, and exhibited a metabolic acidosis.

C. Multiorgan dysfunction is theorized to be secondary to the "diving reflex" (see IV B 1).

1. The **kidney** is the most common organ to be affected in perinatal asphyxia. The proximal tubule of the kidney is especially affected by decreased perfusion, leading to acute tubular necrosis (ATN) (see Chap. 31).

2. **Cardiac** dysfunction is caused by transient myocardial ischemia. The ECG may show ST depression in the midprecordium and T-wave inversion in the left precordium. Echocardiographic findings include decreased left ventricular

contractility, especially of posterior wall; elevated ventricular end-diastolic pressures; tricuspid insufficiency and pulmonary hypertension due to poor ventricular function. In severely asphyxiated infants, dysfunction more commonly affects the right ventricle. A fixed HR may raise suspicion of clinical brain death.

3. **Gastrointestinal effects** include an increased risk of bowel ischemia and necrotizing enterocolitis (see Chap. 32).

4. **Hematologic effects** include disseminated intravascular coagulation due to damage to blood vessels, poor production of clotting factors due to liver dysfunction, and poor production of platelets by the bone marrow.

5. **Liver involvement** may be manifested by isolated elevation of hepatocellular enzymes. More extensive damage may occur, leading to DIC, inadequate glycogen stores with resultant hypoglycemia, or altered detoxification or elimination of drugs.

6. **Pulmonary effects** include increased pulmonary vascular resistance leading to PPHN, pulmonary hemorrhage, pulmonary edema due to cardiac dysfunction, secondary RDS due to failure of surfactant production, and meconium aspiration.

IX. LABORATORY EVALUATION OF EFFECTS OF ASPHYXIA

A. Cardiac evaluation

1. **Cardiac troponin I (cTNI) and cardiac troponin T (cTnT),** cardiac regulatory proteins that control the calcium-mediated interaction of actin and myosin, are markers of myocardial damage. Normal values in the neonate are troponin $I = 0 - 0.28 \pm 0.42$ μg/L and troponin $T = 0 - 0.097$ μg/L. Elevated levels of these proteins have been described in infants with clinical and laboratory evidence of asphyxia.

2. An elevation of **serum creatine kinase myocardial bound** (CK-MB) fraction of >5% to 10% may indicate myocardial injury.

B. Brain injury.

1. **Serum CK-BB.** This may be increased in asphyxiated infants within 12 hours of the insult, but has not been correlated with long-term neurodevelopmental outcome. CK-BB is also expressed in placenta, lungs, gastrointestinal tract, and kidneys.

2. In one report, measurement of protein S-100 (>8.5 μg/L) plus elevated CK-BB, or elevated CK-BB and low cord blood arterial pH had sensitivity of 71% each and specificity of 95% and 91% respectively in predicting moderate to severe encephalopathy.

C. Renal evaluation

1. Blood urea nitrogen (BUN) and serum creatinine (Cr) may be elevated in perinatal asphyxia. Typically elevation is noted 2 to 4 days after the insult.

2. Fractional excretion (FE) of Na^+ or renal failure index may help confirm renal insult (see Chap. 31).

3. Urine levels of β-2-microglobulin have been used as an indicator of proximal tubular dysfunction, although not routinely. This low molecular weight protein is freely filtered through the glomerulus and reabsorbed almost completely in the proximal tubule.

4. Renal sonographic abnormalities correlate with the occurrence of oliguria.

X. CRANIAL IMAGING

A. Cranial sonographic examination is less useful than other imaging modalities in assessing edema, subtle midline shift, superficial cortical or posterior fossa hemorrhage, and ventricular compression.

B. Computed tomography (CT) may be useful for determining the extent of cerebral edema, especially when performed 2 to 4 days after the insult.

C. Magnetic resonance imaging (MRI). T1- and T2-weighted MRI has been considered the best modality for imaging the neonatal brain; however, standard MRI may not detect hyoxic-ischemic changes during the first few days after the insult. High signal on T2-weighted images represents vasogenic edema.

1. **Diffusion-weighted images (DWI)** can show abnormalities within hours of the insult that may yield prognostic information. By detecting differences in rates

of diffusion of water protons, DWI reveals restricted water diffusion, reflecting cytotoxic edema that is not apparent on conventional MRI. However, DWI does not distinguish cytotoxic edema from cell death, especially in global diffuse injuries, during the first hours following a hypoxic-ischemic insult.

2. Localized **magnetic resonance spectroscopy (MRS),** also called *proton-MRS or ¹H-MRS,* measures the relative concentrations of various metabolites in tissue. Elevated lactate and abnormal ratios of choline to total creatine and N-acetylaspartate (NAA) to total creatine have been described following neonatal hypoxic-ischemic brain injury and may yield prognostic information.

XI. **EEG** is used both to evaluate for seizure activity and also to define abnormal background activity such as burst-suppression, continuous low voltage, or isoelectric patterns. When expertise in interpretation of neonatal EEGs is not readily available, amplitude integrated EEG (aEEG) has been used to evaluate for seizures and to define abnormal background patterns. This method consists of a single-channel EEG from biparietal electrodes. There is selective filtering of specific channels (<2 Hz and >15 Hz), then integration of the signal amplitude and semilogarithmic recording of the processed signal.

XII. **PATHOLOGIC FINDINGS OF BRAIN INJURY**
   A. Specific neuropathology may be seen after moderate or severe asphyxia.
   1. Focal or multifocal cortical necrosis affecting all cellular elements can result in cystic encephalomalacia and/or ulegyria (attenuation of depths of sulci) due to loss of perfusion in one or several vascular beds.
   2. Watershed infarcts occur in boundary zones between cerebral arteries, particularly following severe hypotension. They reflect poor perfusion of the vulnerable periventricular border zones in the centrum semiovale and produce predominantly white matter injury. In the term infant, this typically results in bilateral parasagittal cortical and subcortical white matter injury or injury to the parieto-occipital cortex.
   3. Selective neuronal necrosis is the most common type of injury seen following perinatal asphyxia. It is due to differential vulnerability of specific cell types; for example, neurons are more easily injured than glia. Specific regions at increased risk are CA1 region of hippocampus, Purkinje cells of cerebellum in term infants, and brainstem nuclei. Necrosis of thalamic nuclei and basal ganglia (status marmoratus) can be considered a subtype of selective neuronal necrosis.
   B. Neuropathology may reflect the type of asphyxial episode, although the precise pattern is not predictable.
   1. Prolonged partial episodes of asphyxia tend to cause diffuse cerebral (especially cortical) necrosis. Expected clinical findings usually include seizures and paresis.
   2. Acute total asphyxia tends to spare the cortex although affecting primarily the brainstem, thalamus, and basal ganglia. Expected clinical findings usually include disturbances in consciousness, respiration, HR, BP, and temperature control; disorders of tone and reflexes; cranial nerve palsies.
   3. Partial prolonged asphyxia followed by a terminal acute asphyxial event (combination) is probably present in most cases.

XIII. **TREATMENT**
   A. **Perinatal management of high-risk pregnancies**
   1. Fetal HR and rhythm abnormalities may provide supporting evidence of asphyxia, especially if accompanied by presence of thick meconium. However, they provide no information concerning duration or severity of an asphyxial event.
   2. Measurement of fetal scalp pH is a better determinant of fetal oxygenation than Po_2. With intermittent hypoxia-ischemia, Po_2 may improve transiently whereas the pH progressively falls. Fetal scalp blood lactate has been suggested as easier and more reliable than pH, but has not gained wide acceptance.
   3. Close monitoring of progress of labor with awareness of other signs of *in utero* stress.

4. The presence of a constellation of abnormal findings may indicate the need to mobilize the perinatal team for a newborn that could require immediate intervention. Alteration of delivery plans may be indicated and guidelines for intervention in cases of suspected fetal distress should be designed and in place in each medical center (see Chap. 1).

B. Delivery room management (see Chaps. 4, 17, and 24).

The initial management of the hypoxic-ischemic infant in the delivery room is described in Chapter 4.

C. Postnatal management of neurologic effects of asphyxia

1. **Ventilation.** CO_2 should be maintained in the normal range. Hypercapnia can cause cerebral acidosis and cerebral vasodilation. This may result in more flow to uninjured areas and relative ischemia to damaged areas ("steal phenomenon"). Excessive hypocapnia (CO_2 <25 mm Hg) may decrease CBF.

2. **Oxygenation.** Oxygen levels should be maintained in the normal range, although poor peripheral perfusion may limit the accuracy of continuous noninvasive monitoring. Hypoxemia should be treated with supplemental O_2 and/or ventilation. Hyperoxia may cause decreased CBF or exacerbate free radical damage.

3. **Temperature** should be maintained in the normal range and hyperthermia should be avoided.

4. **Perfusion.** Cardiovascular stability and adequate mean systemic arterial BP are important in order to maintain adequate cerebral perfusion pressure.

5. **Maintain physiologic metabolic state**
   a. Hypocalcemia is a common metabolic alteration after neonatal asphyxia. It is important to maintain calcium in the normal range, because hypocalcemia can compromise cardiac contractility and may cause seizures (see Chap. 29B, Hypocalcemia, Hypercalcemia, and Hypermagnesemia Glucose); (see Chaps. 27A).
   b. Hypoglycemia is often seen in asphyxiated infants.
      Blood glucose level should be maintained in the normal range for term infants. Hyperglycemia may lead to an increase in brain lactate, damage to cellular integrity, increased edema, or further disturbance in vascular autoregulation. Hypoglycemia may potentiate excitotoxic amino acids.

6. **Judicious fluid management** is needed and fluid overload should be avoided. Two processes predispose to fluid overload in asphyxiated infants:
   a. Syndrome of inappropriate secretion of antidiuretic hormone (SIADH) (see Chap. 9) is often seen 3 to 4 days after the hypoxic-ischemic event. It is manifested by hyponatremia and hypo-osmolarity in combination with inappropriately concentrated urine (elevated urine specific gravity, osmolarity, and Na^+).
   b. ATN (see Chap. 31) can result from the "diving reflex" (see preceding text).
   c. Fluid restriction may aid in minimizing cerebral edema although the effect of fluid restriction on long-term outcome in infants who are not in renal failure is not known.

7. **Control of seizures.** Seizures secondary to asphyxia are generally self-limited to the first few postnatal days. Because they are extremely difficult to control, it may not be possible to eliminate them completely. Once levels of conventional anticonvulsants are maximized, there is little utility in eliminating every "twitch" or electrographic seizure unless there is cardiopulmonary compromise from the seizures. In infants on musculoskeletal blockade, seizures may be manifested by abrupt changes in BP, HR, and oxygenation. Whether seizures, *per se*, cause brain injury is unknown. There is inadequate evidence to support the continued use of anticonvulsants in the absence of clinical or electrical (EEG) seizures. Metabolic perturbations such as hypoglycemia, hypocalcemia, hyponatremia, should be excluded before initiating anticonvulsant therapy.

a. Acute use of anticonvulsants

i. Phenobarbital is the initial drug of choice. It is given as a loading dose of 20 mg/kg IV. If seizures continue, an additional loading dose of 10 to 20 mg/kg IV may be given. A maintenance dose of 3 to 5 mg/kg/day PO or IV divided BID should be started 12 to 24 hours after the loading dose. Intramuscular (IM) is avoided because absorption is too slow. During initiation, the infant needs to be monitored closely for respiratory depression. Therapeutic serum levels are 20 to 40 mg/dL. Because a prolonged serum half-life due to renal compromise may result in drug accumulation, serum levels need to be monitored closely and the maintenance dose adjusted accordingly.

ii. Phenytoin is usually added when seizures are not controlled by phenobarbital. The loading dose is 15 to 20 mg/kg IV followed by a maintenance dose of 4 to 8 mg/kg/day. In many centers, **phosphenytoin** is used in place of parent drug (phenytoin) because the risk of hypotension is less and extravasation has no adverse effects. Dosage is calculated and written in terms of phenytoin equivalents to avoid medication errors. Therapeutic serum level is typically 20 mg/dL.

iii. Benzodiazapenes are considered third-line drugs and include lorazepam 0.05 to 0.1 mg/kg/dose IV.

b. Long-term anticonvulsant management. Anticonvulsant therapy can be weaned when the clinical exam and EEG indicate that the infant is no longer having seizures. If the infant is receiving more than one anticonvulsant, weaning should be in the reverse order of initiation, with phenobarbital being weaned last. Phenobarbital is then tapered over several weeks. If there is EEG evidence of seizure activity, phenobarbital should be continued for 3 to 6 months. Approximately 25% of infants will need ongoing anticonvulsant therapy. Infants who have a high risk of recurring seizures in infancy or childhood are those with persistent neurologic deficit (50%) and those with an abnormal EEG between seizures (40%)

8. Management of other target organ injury

a. Cardiac dysfunction should be managed with correction of hypoxemia, acidosis, and hypoglycemia and avoidance of volume overload. Diuretics may or not be helpful if concomitant renal impairment is present. Infants will require continuous monitoring of systemic mean arterial BP, CVP (if available), and urine output. Infants with cardiovascular compromise may require inotropic drugs such as dopamine (see Chap. 17) and may need afterload reduction with a peripheral β-antagonist (e.g., isoproterenol) or phosphodiesterase inhibitor (e.g., milrinone) to maintain BP and perfusion.

i. Arterial BP should be maintained in the normal range to support adequate cerebral perfusion.

ii. Monitoring of CVP may be helpful to assess adequacy of preload (i.e., that the infant is not hypovolemic due to vasodilatation or third spacing); a reasonable goal is 5 to 8 mm Hg in term infants.

b. Renal dysfunction should be monitored by measuring urine output, and with urinalysis, urine specific gravity, paired urine/serum osmolarity and serum electrolytes.

i. In the presence of oliguria or anuria avoid fluid overload by limiting free water administration to replacement of insensible losses and urine output ($\sim$60 mL/kg/day) and consider using low-dose dopamine infusion ($\leq$5 μg/kg/min) (see Chaps. 9 and 31).

ii. Volume status should be evaluated before instituting strict fluid restriction. If there is no or low urine output, a 10 to 20 mL/kg fluid challenge followed by a loop diuretic such as furosemide may be helpful.

iii. To avoid fluid overload, as well as hypoglycemia, concentrated glucose infusions delivered through a central line may be needed. Glucose levels should be monitored closely and rapid glucose boluses avoided. Infusions should be weaned slowly to avoid rebound hypoglycemia.

- **c. Gastrointestinal effects.** Feeding should be withheld until good bowel sounds are heard and stools are negative for blood and/or reducing substances (see Chap. 32).

- **d.** Hematologic abnormalities (see Chap. 26). Coagulation profile is monitored with partial thromboplastin time (PTT) and prothrombin time (PT), fibrinogen, and platelets. Abnormalities may need to be corrected with fresh frozen plasma, cryoprecipitate, and/or platelet infusions.

- **e.** Liver function should be monitored with measurement of transaminases (ALT, AST), clotting (PT, PTT, fibrinogen), albumin, bilirubin, and ammonia. Levels of drugs that are metabolized or eliminated through the liver must be monitored.

- **f. Lung** (see Chap. 24). Management of the pulmonary effects of asphyxia depends on the specific condition.

XIV. NEUROPROTECTIVE STRATEGIES. A number of neuroprotective strategies have been proposed.

- **A.** Agents tested in animals with little data in human newborns include antagonists of excitotoxic neurotransmitter receptors such as NMDA receptor blockade with ketamine or MK-801; free radical scavengers such as allopurinol, superoxide dismutase, and vitamin E; Ca^{2+}-channel blockers such as magnesium sulfate, nimodipine, nicardipine; cyclooxygenase inhibitors such as indomethacin; benzodiazepine receptor stimulation such as midazolam; and enhancers of protein synthesis such as dexamethasone.

- **B.** Mild induced hypothermia used under strict experimental protocols may be a potentially useful treatment for acute perinatal asphyxia based on short-term outcomes (18 months) in two randomized clinical trials. However, the results of ongoing trials and long-term efficacy and safety need to be established before this therapeutic modality can be considered standard of care.

XV. OUTCOME IN PERINATAL ASPHYXIA

- **A.** The overall mortality rate is 10% to 30%. The frequency of neurodevelopmental sequelae in surviving infants is approximately 15% to 45%.

- **B.** The risk of CP in survivors of perinatal asphyxia is 5% to 10% compared to 0.2% in the general population. **Most CP is not related to perinatal asphyxia, and most perinatal asphyxia does not cause CP.** Only 3% to 13% of infants with CP have evidence of intrapartum asphyxia.

- **C.** Specific outcomes depend on the severity of the encephalopathy, the presence or absence of seizures, EEG results, and neuroimaging findings

  - **1.** Severity of encephalopathy can be ascertained using the **Sarnat clinical stages of HIE** (Table 27C.1).

    - **a.** Stage 1 HIE: 98% to 100% of infants will have a normal neurologic outcome and <1% mortality.

    - **b.** Stage 2 HIE: 20% to 37% die or have abnormal neurodevelopmental outcomes. Infants who exhibit Stage 2 signs for >7 days have poorer outcomes. In one study, half of the 42 surviving infants who had Sarnat stage 2 encephalopathy had normal neurodevelopment at 1 year of age; approximately 10% had a normal neurologic exam and mild developmental delay and one-third were diagnosed with CP.

    - **c.** Stage 3 HIE: 50% to 89% die and all survivors have major neurodevelopmental impairment.

    - **d.** Prognosis is considered to be good if an infant does not progress to and/or remains in stage 3 and if total duration of stage 2 is <5 days.

    - **e.** Some neurologically normal survivors of perinatal asphyxia have problems in school. In one study, all stage 1 HIE and 65% to 82% of stage 2 HIE children performed at expected grade level at 8 years. In another study, children 8 to 13 years' old who had neonatal encephalopathy plus Apgar score <4 had increased risk of problems with mathematics (3.3 times higher), problems with reading (4.6 times higher), epilepsy (7 times higher), minor motor problems (13 times greater), attention deficit-hyperactivity disorder (14 times greater) compared to unaffected children.

2. The presence of seizures increases an infant's risk of CP 50 to 70 fold. Mortality risk is highest for seizures that begin within 12 hours of birth (53%). In one study, infants whose seizure duration was 1 day had a 7% rate of CP and 11% had epilepsy on follow-up. If seizures lasted for >3 days, the rates of CP and epilepsy were 46% and 40% respectively.

3. The detection of low voltage activity, electrocerebral inactivity or burst-suppression patterns on **EEG** is a better prognostic indicator of poor outcome than is the finding of epileptiform activity. In particular, 93% of neonates with extreme burst suppression activity have poor outcomes. Persistent burst suppression is associated with an 86% to 100% risk of death or severe neurodevelopmental sequelae.

4. Normal findings on DWI MRI between 2 and 18 days of age are associated with normal neuromotor outcome at 12 to 18 months. Abnormalities of deep gray matter that are detected early have the worse motor and cognitive outcomes. In one study, abnormal DWI of the basal ganglia noted within 10 days of a hypoxic-ischemic insult was associated with a 93% risk of abnormal neurodevelopmental outcome at 9 months to 5 years.

Suggested Readings

ACOG Task Force on Neonatal Encephalopathy and Cerebral Palsy. *Neonatal encephalopathy and cerebral palsy: Defining the pathogenesis and pathophysiology.* Washington, DC: American College of Obstetricians and Gynecologists, 2003.

Blackmon LR, Stark AR. Hypothermia: A neuroprotective therapy for neonatal hypoxic-ischemic encephalopathy. *Pediatrics* 2006;117:942–948.

Edwards AD, Azzopardi DV. Therapeutic hypothermia following perinatal asphyxia. *Arch Dis Child Fetal Neonatal Ed* 2006;91:F127–F131.

Higgins RD, Raju TNK, Perlman J, et al. Hypothermia and perinatal asphyxia: Executive summary of the National Institute of Child Health and Human Development Workshop. *J Pediatr* 2006;148:170–175.

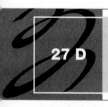

NEURAL TUBE DEFECTS

27 D

John A. F. Zupancic

I. DEFINITIONS AND PATHOLOGY. Neural tube defects constitute one of the most common congenital malformations in newborns. The term refers to a group of disorders that is heterogeneous with respect to embryologic timing, involvement of specific elements of the neural tube and its derivatives, clinical presentation, and prognosis.

A. Types of neural tube defects

1. Primary neural tube defects. These constitute approximately 95% of all neural tube defects. They are due to primary failure of closure of the neural tube or disruption of an already closed neural tube between 18 and 25 days' gestation. The resulting abnormality usually consists of two anatomic lesions: an exposed (open or *operta*) neural placode along the midline of the back caudally, and rostrally, the Arnold-Chiari II malformation (malformation of pons and medulla, with downward displacement of cerebellum, medulla, and fourth ventricle into the upper cervical region), with associated aqueductal stenosis, and hydrocephalus.

- a. **Myelomeningocele.** This is the most common primary neural tube defect. It involves a saccular outpouching of neural elements (neural placode), typically through a defect in the bone and the soft tissues of the posterior thoracic, sacral, or lumbar regions, the latter comprising 80% of lesions. Dura and arachnoid are typically included in the sac (meningo-), which contains visible neural structures (myelo-), and the skin is usually discontinuous over the sac. Hydrocephalus occurs in 84% of these children; Arnold-Chiari II malformation occurs in approximately 90%. Various associated anomalies of the central nervous system are noted, most important, cerebral cortical dysplasia in up to 92% of cases.
- b. **Encephalocele.** This defect of anterior neural tube closure is an outpouching of dura with or without brain, noted in the occipital region in 80% of cases, and less commonly in the frontal or temporal regions. It may vary in size from a few millimeters to many centimeters.
- c. **Anencephaly.** In the most severe form of this defect, the cranial vault and posterior occipital bone are defective, and derivatives of the neural tube are exposed, including both brain and bony tissue. The defect usually extends through the foramen magnum and involves the brainstem. It is not compatible with long-term survival.

2. **Secondary neural tube defects.** Five percent of all neural tube defects result from abnormal development of the lower sacral or coccygeal segments during secondary neurulation. This leads to defects primarily in the lumbosacral spinal region. These heterogeneous lesions are rarely associated with hydrocephalus or the Arnold-Chiari II malformation, and the skin is typically intact over the defect.

- a. **Meningocele.** This is an outpouching of skin and dura without involvement of the neural elements. Meningoceles may be associated with bone and contiguous soft tissue abnormalities.
- b. **Lipomeningocele.** A lipomeningocele is a lipomatous mass usually in the lumbar or sacral region, occasionally off the midline, typically covered with full-thickness skin. Adipose tissue frequently extends through the defect into the spine and dura and adheres extensively to a distorted spinal cord or nerve roots.
- c. **Sacral agenesis/dysgenesis, diastematomyelia, myelocystocele.** These and others all may have varying degrees of bony involvement. Although rarely as extensive as with primary neural tube defects, neurologic manifestations may be present representing distortion or abnormal development of peripheral nerve structures. These lesions may be inapparent on physical examination of the child, resulting in the use of the term *occulta* to describe them (see Chap. 2A).

B. **Etiologies.** The exact cause of failed neural tube closure remains unknown, and proposed etiologies for both primary and secondary neural tube defects are heterogeneous. Factors implicated include folic acid deficiency, maternal ingestion of the anticonvulsants carbamazepine and valproic acid and folic acid antagonists such as aminopterin; maternal diabetes; and disruptive influences such as prenatal x-irradiation; maternal hyperthermia and amniotic band disruption. There is concordance for neural tube defect in monozygotic twins and an increased incidence with consanguinity and with a positive family history. Neural tube defects can occur with trisomies 13 and 18, triploidy, and Meckel syndrome (autosomal recessive syndrome of encephalocele, polydactyly, polycystic kidneys, cleft lip, and palate), as well as other chromosome disorders. Although specific genes (particularly those in the folate-homocysteine pathway) have been implicated as risk factors, the genetics are likely complex and multifactorial.

C. **Epidemiology and recurrence risk.** The incidence of neural tube defects varies significantly with geography and ethnicity. In the United States, the overall frequency of neural tube defects is approximately 1 in 2,000 live births. A well-established increased incidence is known among individuals living in parts of Ireland and Wales, and carries over to descendants of these individuals who live elsewhere in the world. This may be true also for other ethnic groups, including Sikh Indians and certain groups in Egypt. The literature may underestimate the true prevalence, because of the effects of prenatal diagnosis and termination of affected fetuses. More than 95% of all neural tube defects occur to couples with no known family history. Primary neural tube defects carry an increased empiric recurrence risk of approximately 2% to 3% for couples with one affected pregnancy, with the risk increasing further if more than one sibling was affected. Similarly, affected individuals have a 3% risk of having one offspring with a primary neural tube defect. Recurrence risk is strongly affected by the level of the lesion in the index case, with risks as high as 7.8% for lesions above T11. In 5% of cases, neural tube defects may be associated with uncommon disorders; some, such as Meckel syndrome, are inherited in an autosomal recessive manner, resulting in a 25% recurrence risk. Secondary neural tube defects are generally sporadic and carry no increased recurrence risk. In counseling families for recurrence, however, it is critical to obtain a careful history of drug exposure and/or family history.

D. Prevention. Controlled, randomized clinical studies of prenatal multivitamin administration both for secondary prevention in mothers with prior affected offspring and for primary prevention in those without a prior history suggest a much lower recurrence risk than in control groups. The Centers for Disease Control of the U.S. Public Health Service recommends that women of childbearing age who are capable of becoming pregnant should consume 0.4 mg of folic acid per day to reduce their risks of having a fetus affected with spina bifida or other neural tube defects. Higher doses are recommended for women with prior affected offspring. In addition, folate supplementation of enriched cereal-grain products has been mandated by the U.S. Food and Drug Administration (FDA); however, the level of folate intake from this source is not high enough to forgo additional supplementation in the large majority of women.

II. DIAGNOSIS

A. Prenatal diagnosis. The combination of maternal serum α-fetoprotein (AFP) determinations and prenatal ultrasonography, along with AFP and acetylcholinesterase determinations on amniotic fluid where indicated, greatly improves the ability to make a prenatal diagnosis and to distinguish from abdominal wall defects. Maternal serum AFP measurements of 2.5 multiples of the median (MoM) in the second trimester (16 to 18 weeks) have a sensitivity of 80% to 90% for myelomeningocele. The exact timing of this measurement is critical as AFP levels change throughout pregnancy. Karyotype may also be performed at the time of amniocentesis to detect associated chromosomal abnormalities. Ultrasonographic diagnosis through direct visualization of the spinal defect or through indirect signs related to Arnold Chiari malformation has a sensitivity of >90%. Determining the prognosis based on prenatal ultrasonography remains difficult, except in obvious cases of encephalocele or anencephaly (see Chap. 1), although fetal magnetic resonance imaging (MRI) holds promise to improve the prognostic accuracy through delineation of level of lesion, presence of other anomalies, and characterization of the Chiari malformation.

B. Postnatal diagnosis. Except for some secondary neural tube defects, most neural tube defects, especially meningomyelocele, are immediately obvious at birth. Occasionally some saccular masses, including sacrococcygeal teratomas, are confused with these. These are usually in the low sacrum.

III. EVALUATION

A. History. Obtain a detailed family history. Ask about the occurrence of neural tube defects, and other congenital anomalies or malformation syndromes. Note should be made of any of the risk factors described in the preceding text, including maternal medication use in the first trimester or maternal diabetes.

B. Physical examination. It is important to do a thorough physical examination, including a neurologic examination. The following are portions of the examination likely to reveal abnormal conditions.

1. **General newborn assessment.** Without exception, evaluate all newborns with neural tube defects for the presence of congenital heart disease, renal malformation, and structural defects of the airway, gastrointestinal tract, ribs, and hips. Although uncommon in primary neural tube defects, these can be encountered and should be considered before beginning surgical treatment or before discharge from the hospital. Other findings of associated chromosomal anomalies may be noted. In addition, plan an ophthalmologic examination and hearing evaluation during the hospitalization or following discharge.

2. **Back.** Inspect the defect and note if it is leaking cerebrospinal fluid (CSF). Use a sterile nonlatex rubber glove when touching a leaking sac (in most circumstances, only the neurosurgeon needs to touch the back). Note the location, shape, and size of the defect, and observe the size of the cutaneous defect or thin "parchment-like" skin, although it has little relation to the size of the sac. Often the sac is deflated and has a wrinkled appearance. It is important to note the curvature of the spine and the presence of a bony gibbus underlying the defect. Occasionally, there is more than one meningomyelocele.

3. **Head.** Record the head circumference and plot daily throughout the first hospitalization. At birth, some infants will have macrocephaly because of hydrocephalus, and still more will develop hydrocephalus after closure of the defect on the back.

4. **Intracranial pressure (ICP).** Assess the ICP by palpating the anterior fontanel and tilting the head and torso forward until the midportion of the anterior fontanel is flat. The fontanels may be quite large and the calvarial bones widely separated. (see Chap. 27B).

5. **Eyes.** Abnormalities in conjugate movement of the eyes are common and include esotropias, esophorias, and abducens paresis.

6. **Lower extremities.** Look for deformities and evidence of muscle weakness. Abnormalities in the lower extremities, some representing deformations, are common. Look at thigh positions and skinfolds, and perform the Ortolani and Barlow maneuvers, for evidence of congenital dislocation of the hips. Dislocation of the hips can be diagnosed clinically and by ultrasonography (see Chap. 28).

7. **Neurologic examination.** Observe the child's spontaneous activity and response to sensory stimuli in all extremities. Predicting ambulation and muscle strength based on the "level" of the neurologic deficit can be misleading, and very often the anal reflex, or "wink," will be present at birth and absent postoperatively, owing to spinal shock and edema. Repeating neurologic examinations at periodic intervals is more helpful in predicting functional outcome than a single newborn examination. Similarly, sensory examination of the newborn can be misleading because of the potential absence of a motor response to pinprick. Carefully examine deep tendon reflexes (see Table 27D.1).

8. **Bladder and kidneys.** Observe bladder function, particularly for the possibility of inadequate emptying. Palpate the abdomen for evidence of kidney enlargement. Observe the pattern of urination, and check the child's response to the Credé maneuver by monitoring residual urine in the bladder.

IV. **CONSULTATION.** The care of infants with neural tube defects requires the coordinated efforts of a number of medical and surgical specialists as well as specialists in nursing, physical therapy, and social service. If follow-up is by a myelodysplasia team, follow their protocols. If not, the following specialties represent the areas needing careful assessment:

A. **Specialty consultations**

1. **Neurosurgery.** The initial care of the child with a neural tube defect is predominantly neurosurgical. The neurosurgeon is responsible for assessment and surgical closure of the defect, and for control and treatment of elevated ICP.

2. **Pediatrics.** A thorough evaluation before surgical procedures is important, particularly for detecting other abnormalities, such as congenital cardiac anomalies, that might influence surgical risk.

3. **Clinical genetics.** Begin a complete dysmorphology evaluation and genetic counseling during the first hospitalization and follow-up during outpatient visits.

4. **Urology.** Consult a urologist on the day of birth because of the risk of obstructive uropathy.

5. **Orthopaedics.** The pediatric orthopaedic surgeon is responsible for the initial assessment of musculoskeletal abnormalities and long-term management of ambulation, seating, and spine stability. Clubfeet, frequently encountered in these newborns, should be assessed and may be managed during this hospitalization.

6. **Physical therapy.** Perform a thorough muscle examination as early as possible and involve physical therapists in planning for outpatient physical therapy programs.

7. **Social service.** Arrange for a social worker familiar with the special needs of children with neural tube defects to meet the parents as early as possible. Children with meningomyelocele may require a considerable amount of parents' time and resources, thereby placing considerable strain on parents and siblings.

B. **Diagnostic tests.** During the first hospitalization, the following tests should be done on most children with meningomyelocele. Scheduling these tests will vary depending on each situation.

1. **Radiographs**
   a. **Chest.** Rib deformities are common; cardiac malformations may also be identified.
   b. **Spine.** Abnormalities in vertebral bodies, absent or defective posterior arches, and evidence of kyphosis are common.
   c. **Hips.** Evidence of dysplasia of hips is common, and some children with neural tube defects are born with dislocated hips. As noted, ultrasonographic examination of the hips can be very helpful to the orthopaedic surgeon (see Chap. 28).

2. **Serum creatinine** level should be measured if voiding patterns appear initially abnormal. Occasionally, potassium levels may be elevated in the nonvoiding newborn.

3. **Ultrasonography of the urinary tract** is useful to assess possible hydronephrosis and/or structural abnormalities of the upper urinary tract.

4. **Urodynamic study** should be done early in the hospitalization or shortly after discharge to document the status of the bladder and urinary sphincter function and innervation and to serve as a basis for comparison later in life.

5. Consider a **voiding cystourethrogram** if there is an abnormality seen on ultrasonographic or urodynamic study or in the setting of a rising serum creatinine level.

6. **Computed tomography (CT) scan or MRI of the head** is usually not necessary before repair of the defect on the back, but should generally be done soon thereafter, even if there is no clinical evidence of hydrocephalus. If ultrasonography is available and can accurately evaluate the presence of hydrocephalus, this may be a useful alternative to an initial CT. MRI is particularly valuable in assessment of the posterior fossa and syringomyelia.

V. MANAGEMENT

A. **Fetal surgery.** *In utero* repair has been used in humans as early as 1994. Observational studies have suggested that *in utero* repair is associated with lower rates of ventriculoperitoneal (VP) shunting and consistent reversal of hindbrain herniation. Long-term effects remain uncertain. A multicenter randomized controlled trial of *in utero* surgical correction with standard management is currently in progress (www.spinabifidamoms.com). Until those results are available, all *in utero* repairs should be completed under a study protocol.

B. **Perinatal.** Consideration should be given to cesarean section as evident from observational studies of possibly improved survival and neuromotor outcomes with operative delivery. At birth, the very thin sac is often leaking. Keep the newborn in the prone position, with a sterile saline-moistened gauze sponge placed over the defect. This reduces bacterial contamination and damage related to dehydration. Administer intravenous antibiotics (ampicillin and gentamicin) to diminish the risk of meningitis, particularly that due to group B streptococci. Children with an open

Lesion	Segmental innervation	Cutaneous sensation	Motor function	Working muscles	Sphincter function	Reflex	Potential for ambulation
Cervical/Thoracic	Variable	Variable	None	None	—	—	Poor, even in full braces
Thoracolumbar	T12	Lower abdomen	None	None	—	—	Full braces, long-term ambulation unlikely
	L1	Groin	Weak hip flexion	Iliopsoas	—	—	
	L2	Anterior upper thigh	Strong hip flexion	Iliopsoas and sartorius	—	—	
Lumbar	L3	Anterior distal thigh and knee	Knee extension	Quadriceps	—	Knee jerk	
	L4	Medial leg	Knee flexion and hip abduction	Medial hamstrings	—	Knee jerk	May ambulate with braces and crutches
Lumbosacral	L5	Lateral leg and medial knee	Foot dorsiflexion and eversion	Anterior tibial and peroneals	—	Ankle jerk	Ambulate with or without short leg braces
	S1	Sole of foot flexion	Foot plantar	Gastrocnemius, soleus, and posterior tibial	—	Ankle jerk	
Sacral	S2	Posterior leg and thigh	Toe flexion	Flexor hallucis	Bladder and rectum	Anal wink	Ambulate without braces
	S3	Middle of buttock	—	—	Bladder and rectum	Anal wink	
	S4	Medial buttock	—	—	Bladder and rectum	Anal wink	

Source: From Noetzel MJ. Myelomeningocele: Current concepts of management. *Clin Perinatol* 1984;6:318.

spinal defect can receive a massive inoculation of bacteria directly into the nervous system at the time of vaginal delivery or even *in utero* if the placental membranes rupture early. Meningitis is a particularly devastating complication. Because of the potential for allergy to latex rubber and possible anaphylaxis, no latex equipment should be used.

C. Surgical treatment. The initial neurosurgical treatment of an open meningomye-locele consists of (i) closing the defect to prevent infection and (ii) reducing the elevated ICP. The back should be closed on the first day of life or as soon thereafter as safely possible to minimize bacterial contamination and the risk of infection. Techniques are available to close rapidly even very large cutaneous defects without skin grafting. Intracranial hypertension can be initially controlled by continuous ventricular drainage. Typically, once the back is sealed, a VP shunt catheter can be placed. Some neurosurgeons may elect to insert the catheter at the time of back closure. If a shunt is to be placed as a second procedure after back closure, careful monitoring of head circumference should be done because ICP often increases following closure of the back in unshunted patients.

Children whose defect is covered with skin and whose nervous system is therefore not at risk of bacterial contamination can undergo elective repair. This may be done at the age of 1 month or later.

D. Parents. Keep parents accurately informed of their child's condition. The involvement of multiple specialists heightens the importance of the identification of a primary care provider to coordinate the flow of information.

VI. PROGNOSIS

A. Survival. Nearly all children with neural tube defects, even those severely affected, can survive for many years. In a recent large observational study, the 1-year survival rate for children with myelomeningocele was approximately 91%, whereas for encephalocele it was 79%. Survival rates appear to have increased since folic acid fortification of the US grain supply was started, possibly because of a general decrease in severity or location of lesions. It should also be noted that survival rates are significantly influenced by selection bias of prenatal diagnosis and termination of severely affected fetuses, and by decisions to intervene or to withhold aggressive medical and surgical care in the early neonatal period. Most deaths occur in the most severely affected children and are likely related to brainstem dysfunction.

B. Motor and intellectual outcome

1. Motor outcome. This depends more on the level of paralysis and surgical intervention than it does on congenital hydrocephalus. In a long-term study of children with spina bifida, 46% of young adults were ambulatory, 13% were partially ambulatory and the remainder required wheelchair assistance. Among individuals with sacral level lesions, 93% were exclusively ambulatory without assistance. There is a likelihood that there will be a delay in motor progress in most children with neural tube defects, but appropriate bracing, physical therapy interventions, and monitoring and treatment of kyphosis and scoliosis can mitigate this. Factors such as obesity, frequent hospitalizations, tethering of the spinal cord, and decubitus ulcers may also contribute to motor delays.

2. Intellectual outcome. Three identifiable subgroups are at risk for mental retardation: those with severe hydrocephalus at birth, those who develop infection in the central nervous system early in life, and those whose intracranial hypertension is not properly controlled. True mental retardation is encountered most commonly in children who have high thoracic level lesions, a history of central nervous system infection, and hydrocephalus with <1 cm of cortical mantle. Formal developmental testing is critical, because visual/perceptual deficits and fine motor difficulties may interfere with intellectual functioning. In the study cited in the preceding text, 85% of individuals with myelomeningocele were attending or had graduated from secondary school or college. Some 37% required additional assistance with school work or attended special education classes. Complex partial seizures were noted in 23%. Seizures may contribute to impaired intellectual function and should be considered in children, especially school-age children who have lost cognitive milestones.

C. Morbidity. The number of hospitalizations, of days in the hospital, and of operations required are much lower for children with sacral level lesions and much higher for those with thoracic lesions. In the long-term study in the preceding text, 86% of children had undergone VP shunting, and the large majority of these had required additional shunt revision. Release of tethered cord was required in 32%, and scoliosis was noted in 49%, of whom approximately half required a spinal fusion procedure. Approximately 85% of the cohort requires clean intermittent catheterization for bladder dysfunction, and 80% achieve social bladder continence, and half have some degree of bowel incontinence. Latex hypersensitization may be seen in one-third of children, and may be associated with life-threatening anaphylaxis.

Approximately 5% of newborns with open neural tube defects develop symptoms related to the Arnold-Chiari II malformation. These pontomedullary symptoms include stridor, ophthalmoplegia, apnea, abnormal gag, and vomiting (often confused with gastroesophageal reflex). These symptoms may indicate shunt malfunction but frequently disappear without treatment. If they persist, especially in association with cyanosis, the prognosis is poor, with the risk of respiratory failure and death. Posterior fossa decompression and cervical laminectomy are surgical options but are often not successful.

Suggested Readings

American Academy of Pediatrics, Committee on Genetics. Folic acid for the prevention of neural tube defects. *Pediatrics* 1999;104:325–327.

Bol KA, Collins JS, Kirby RS. The National Birth Defects Prevention Network. Survival of infants with neural tube defects in the presence of folic acid fortification. *Pediatrics* 2006;117:803.

Bowman RM, McLone DG, Grant JA, et al. Spina bifida outcome: A 25-year prospective. *Pediatr Neurosurg* 2001;34(3):114–120.

Cowchock S, Ainbender E, Prescott G. The recurrence risk for neural tube defects in the United States: A collaborative study. *Am J Obstet Gynecol* 1984;149:744.

Czeizel AE, Duds I. Prevention of the first occurrence of neural tube defects by periconceptual vitamin supplementation. *N Engl J Med* 1992;327:1832.

Feuchtbaum LB, Currier RJ, Riggle S, et al. Neural tube defect prevalence in California (1990–1994): Eliciting patterns by type of defect and maternal race/ethnicity. *Genet Test* 1999;3:265.

Goh YI, Bollano E, Einerson TR, et al. Prenatal multivitamin supplementation and rates of congenital anomalies: A meta-analysis. *J Obstet Gynaecol Can* 2006;28:680.

Jobe AH. Fetal surgery for myelomeningocele. *N Engl J Med* 2002;347:4–6.

Johnson MP, Gerdes M, Rintoul N, et al. Maternal-fetal surgery for myelomeningocele: Neurodevelopmental outcomes at 2 years of age. *Am J Obstet Gynecol* 2006;194:1145.

Mitchell LE, Adzick NS, Melchionne J. Spina bifida. *Lancet* 2004;364:1885.

MRC Vitamin Study Research Group. Prevention of neural tube defects: Results of the medical research council vitamin study. *Lancet* 1991;338:131.

Volpe JJ. Human brain development. In: Volpe JJ, ed. *Neurology of the Newborn*, 4th ed. Philadelphia: WB Saunders, 2001:3.

Walsh DS, Adzick NS. Foetal surgery for spina bifida. *Semin Neonatol* 2003;8(3):197–205.

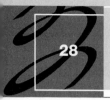

28 ORTHOPAEDIC PROBLEMS
James R. Kasser

$\mathscr{T}$his chapter considers common musculoskeletal abnormalities that may be detected in the neonatal period. Consultation with an orthopaedic surgeon is often required to provide definitive treatment after the initial evaluation.

I. CONGENITAL MUSCULAR TORTICOLLIS (CMT)

A. CMT is a disorder characterized by limited motion of the neck, asymmetry of the face and skull, and a tilted position of the head. It is usually caused by shortening of the **sternocleidomastoid (SCM) muscle** but may be secondary to muscle adaptation from an abnormal *in utero* position of the head and neck.

1. The etiology of the shortened SCM muscle is unclear; in many infants it is due to an abnormal *in utero* position, and in some it may be due to stretching of the muscle at delivery. The result of the latter is a contracture of the muscle associated with fibrosis. One hypothesis is that the SCM abnormality is secondary to a compartment syndrome occurring at the time of delivery.

2. Clinical course. The limitation of motion is minimum at birth, but increases over the first few weeks. At 10 to 20 days, a mass is frequently found in the SCM muscle. This mass gradually disappears, and the muscle fibers are partially replaced by fibrous tissue, which contracts and limits head motion. Because of the limited rotation of the head, the infant rests on the ipsilateral side of the face in the prone position and on the contralateral side when supine. The pressure from resting on one side of the face and the opposite occipital bone contributes to the facial and skull asymmetry. The ipsilateral zygoma is depressed and the contralateral occiput flattened.

3. Treatment. Most infants will respond favorably to positioning the head in the direction opposite to that produced by the tight muscle. Padded bricks or sandbags can be used to help maintain the position of the head until the child is able to move actively to free the head. Passive stretching by rotating the head to the ipsilateral side and tilting it toward the contralateral side also may help. The torticollis in most infants resolves by the age of 1. Patients who have asymmetry of the face and head and limited motion after 1 year should be considered for surgical release of the SCM muscle.

B. Differential diagnosis. Torticollis with limited motion of the neck may be due to a congenital abnormality of the cervical region of the spine. Some infants with this disorder also have a tight SCM muscle. These infants are likely to have significant limitation of motion at birth, generally not seen in CMT. Radiologic evaluation of the cervical region is necessary to make this diagnosis. Infection in the retropharangeal area may present with torticollis. The neck mass seen in torticollis in the SCM muscle may be differentiated from other cervical lesions by ultrasound.

II. POLYDACTYLY

A. Duplication of a digit may range from a small cutaneous bulb to an almost perfectly formed digit. Treatment of this problem is variable. Syndromes associated with polydactyly include Laurence-Moon-Biedl syndrome, chondroectodermal dysplasia, Ellis-van Creveld syndrome, and trisomy 13. Polydactyly is generally inherited in an autosomal dominant manner with variable penetrance.

B. Treatment
1. The small functionless skin bulb without bone or cartilage at the ulnar border of the hand or lateral border of the foot can be ligated and allowed to develop necrosis for 24 hours. The part distal to the suture should be removed. The residual stump should have an antiseptic applied twice a day to prevent infection. Do not tie off digits on the radial side of the hand (thumb) or the medial border of the foot.
2. When duplicated digits contain bone or muscle attached by more than a small bridge of skin, treatment is delayed until the patient is evaluated by an orthopedist or hand surgeon. In general, polydactyly is managed surgically in the first year of life after 6 months of age. X-rays can be delayed until necessary for definitive management.

III. FRACTURED CLAVICLE (see Chap. 20)
A. The clavicle is the site of the most common fracture associated with delivery.
B. Diagnosis is usually made soon after birth, when the infant does not move the arm on the affected side or cries when that arm is moved. There may be tenderness, swelling, or crepitance at the site. Occasionally, the bone is angulated. Diagnosis can be confirmed by radiographic examination. A "painless" fracture discovered by radiography of the chest is more likely a congenital pseudarthrosis (nonunion). All pseudarthroses occur on the right side unless associated with dextrocardia.
C. The clinical course is such that clavicle fractures heal without difficulty. **Treatment** consists of providing comfort for the infant. If the arm and shoulder are left unprotected, motion occurs at the fracture site when the baby is handled. We usually pin the infant's sleeve to the shirt and put a sign on the baby to remind personnel to decrease motion of the clavicle. No reduction is necessary. If the fracture appears painful, a wrap to decrease motion of the arm is useful.

IV. CONGENITAL AND INFANTILE SCOLIOSIS
A. Congenital scoliosis is a lateral curvature of the spine secondary to a failure either of formation of a vertebra or of segmentation. Scoliosis in the newborn may be difficult to detect; by bending the trunk laterally in the prone position, however, a difference in motion can usually be observed. Congenital scoliosis is differentiated from **infantile scoliosis,** in which no vertebral anomaly is present. Infantile scoliosis often improves spontaneously, although the condition may be progressive in infants who have a spinal curvature of >20 degrees. If the scoliosis is progressive, treatment is indicated and magnetic resonance imaging (MRI) of the spine looking for spinal cord pathology should be done. Rarely, severe congenital scoliosis may be termed *thoracic insufficiency syndrome* and be associated with pulmonary compromise.
B. Clinical course. Congenital scoliosis will increase in many patients. Bracing of congenital curves is usually not helpful. Surgical correction with chest expansion or limited fusion may be indicated before the curve becomes severe. Many patients with congenital curves have renal or other visceral abnormalities. Abdominal ultrasonography is used to screen all such patients.

V. DEVELOPMENTAL DISLOCATION OF THE HIP (DDH). Most (but not all) hips that are dislocated at birth can be diagnosed by a careful physical examination (see Chap. 3A). The U.S. Preventive Services Task Force has recommended against generalized ultrasound screening of infants for DDH. Such screening is common in Europe but not in the United States. Ultrasonographic examination of the hip is useful for diagnosis in high-risk cases. In general, ultrasonography is delayed as a screening technique until 1 month of age to avoid a high incidence of false-positive examinations. X-ray examination will not lead to a diagnosis in the newborn because the femoral head is not calcified but will reveal an abnormal acetabular fossa seen with hip dysplasia. There are three types of congenital dislocations.
A. The classic DDH is diagnosed by the presence of Ortolani sign. The hip is unstable and dislocates on adduction and also on extension of the femur but readily relocates when the femur is abducted in flexion. No asymmetry of the pelvis is seen. This type of dislocation is more common in females and is usually unilateral, but it may be bilateral. Hips that are unstable at birth often become stable after a few days.

The infant with hips that are unstable after 5 days of life should be treated with a splint that keeps the hips flexed and abducted. The **Pavlik harness** has been used effectively to treat this group of patients, with approximately 80% success rate. Ultrasonography is used to monitor the hip during treatment as well as to confirm the initial diagnosis.

  B. The **teratologic type of dislocation** occurs very early in pregnancy. The **femoral head does not relocate on flexion and abduction;** that is, Ortolani sign is not present. If the dislocation is unilateral, there may be asymmetry of the gluteal folds and asymmetric motion with limited abduction. In bilateral dislocation, the perineum is wide and the thighs give the appearance of being shorter than normal. This may be easily overlooked, however, and requires an extremely careful physical examination. Treatment of the teratologic hip dislocation is by open reduction. Exercise to decrease contracture is indicated but use of the Pavlik harness is not beneficial.

  C. The **third type of dislocation** occurs late, is unilateral, and is associated with a **congenital abduction contracture** of the contralateral hip. The abduction contracture causes a pelvic obliquity. The pelvis is lower on the side of the contracture, which is unfavorable for the contralateral hip, and the acetabulum may not develop well. After the age of 6 weeks, infants with this type of dislocation develop an apparent short leg and have asymmetric gluteal folds. Some infants will develop a dysplastic acetabulum, which may eventually allow the hip to subluxate. Treatment of the dysplasia is with the Pavlik harness, but after the age of 8 months, other methods of treatment may be necessary.

VI. GENU RECURVATUM, or hyperextension of the knee, is not a serious abnormality and is easily recognized and treated. It must be differentiated, however, from subluxation or dislocation of the knee, which also may present with hyperextension of the knee. The latter two abnormalities are more serious and require more extensive treatment.

  A. Congenital genu recurvatum is secondary to *in utero* position with hyperextension of the knee. This can be treated successfully by repeated cast changes, with progressive flexion of the knee until it reaches 90 degrees of flexion. Minor degrees of recurvatum can be treated with passive stretching exercises.

  B. All infants with **hyperextension of the knee** should have a radiographic examination to differentiate genu recurvatum **from true dislocation of the knee.** In congenital genu recurvatum, the tibial and femoral epiphyses are in proper alignment except for the hyperextension. In the subluxed knee with dislocation, the tibia is completely anterior or anterolateral to the femur. The tibia is shifted forward in relation to the femur and is frequently lateral as well.

      Congenital fibrosis of the quadriceps is frequently associated with the fixed dislocated knee and open reduction is essential, as attempted treatment of the dislocated knee by stretching or by repeated cast changes is hazardous and may result in epiphyseal plate damage.

  C. Treatment. Hyperextended or subluxed knees are treated with manipulation and splinting after delivery with progressive knee flexion and reduction.

VII. DEFORMITIES OF THE FEET

  A. Metatarsus adductus (MTA) is a condition in which the metatarsals rest in an adducted position, but the appearance does not always reveal the severity of the condition. Whether treatment is necessary is determined by the difference in the degree of structural change in the metatarsals and tarsometatarsal joint.

    1. Most infants with MTA have **positional deformities** that are probably caused by *in utero* position. The positional type of MTA is flexible and the metatarsals can be passively corrected into abduction with little difficulty. **This condition does not need treatment.**

    2. The **structural MTA** has a relatively fixed adduction deformity of the forefoot and the metatarsals cannot be abducted passively. The etiology has not been definitely identified but is probably related to *in utero* position. This is seen more commonly in the firstborn infant and in pregnancies with oligohydramnios. Most infants with the structural types of MTA have a valgus deformity of the hindfoot. **The structural deformity needs to be treated with manipulation**

and immobilization in a shoe or cast until correction occurs. Although there is no urgency to treat this condition, it is more easily corrected earlier than later and should be done before the child is of walking age.

B. **Calcaneovalgus deformities** result from an *in utero* position of the foot that holds the ankle dorsiflexed and abducted. At birth, the top of the foot lies up against the anterior surface of the leg. Structural changes in the bones do not seem to be present. The sequela to this deformity appears to be a valgus or pronated foot that is more severe than the typical pronated foot seen in toddlers. Whether this disorder is treated or not is variable, and no study supports either course. **Treatment consists of either exercise or application of a short leg cast** that will keep the foot plantar flexed and inverted. If the foot cannot be plantar flexed to a neutral position, casts are indicated. Casts are changed appropriately for growth and maintained until plantar flexion and inversion are equal to those of the opposite foot. Generally, the foot is held in plaster for approximately 6 to 8 weeks. Feet that remain in the calcaneovalgus position for several months may be more likely to have significant residual *pes valgus*; a fixed or rigid calcaneovalgus deformity probably represents a congenital vertical talus.

C. **Congenital clubfoot** is a deformity with a multifactorial etiology. A first-degree relative of a patient with this deformity has 20 times the risk of having a clubfoot than does the normal population. The risk in subsequent siblings is 3% to 5%. The more frequent occurrence in the firstborn and the association with oligohydramnios suggest an influence of *in utero* pressure as well. Sometimes clubfoot is part of a syndrome. Infants with neurologic dysfunction of the feet (spina bifida) often have clubfoot.

1. **There are three and sometimes four components to the deformity.** The foot is in equinus, cavus, and varus position, with a forefoot adduction; therefore the clubfoot is a talipes equinocavovarus with metatarsal adduction. Each of these deformities is sufficiently rigid to prevent passive correction to a neutral position by the examiner. The degree of rigidity is variable in each patient.

2. **Treatment** should be started early, within a few days of birth. An effective method of treatment **consists of manipulation and application of either tapes, or plaster or fiberglass casts that are changed every few days.** If conservative treatment does not successfully correct the deformities, the Ponseti method of management with serial casting followed by heel cord tenotomy is commonly used. Treatment should begin when the child is medically stable in the first weeks of life. Physical therapy and splinting are used in a newborn with complex medical problems as initial management.

Suggested Readings

Cooperman DR, Thompson GH. Neonatal orthopaedics. In: Fanatoff AA, Martin RJ, eds. *Neonatal perinatal medicine*, 6th ed. St. Louis: Mosby, 1997:1709.

Jones KL. *Smith's recognizable patterns of human malformation*, 5th ed. Philadelphia: WB Saunders, 2002.

Lovell WW, Winter RB, eds. *Pediatric orthopaedics*. Philadelphia: Lippincott Williams & Wilkins, 2006.

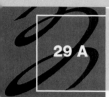

HYPOGLYCEMIA AND HYPERGLYCEMIA
Richard E. Wilker

*H*ypoglycemia is one of the most common metabolic problems seen in both the newborn nursery and neonatal intensive care unit (NICU). However, its definition, clinical significance, and management remain controversial. Blood-glucose levels are frequently lower in newborn babies than in older children or adults, but confirming a diagnosis of clinically significant hypoglycemia requires that one interpret the blood-glucose level within the clinical context. Most cases of neonatal hypoglycemia are transient, respond readily to treatment, and are associated with an excellent prognosis. Whereas persistent hypoglycemia is more likely to be associated with abnormal endocrine conditions and possible neurologic sequelae, a recent systematic review by Boluyt did not identify any study that validly quantifies the effects of neonatal hypoglycemia on subsequent neurodevelopment.

Hyperglycemia is very rarely seen in the newborn nursery, but frequently occurs in very low birth weight (VLBW) babies in the NICU.

I. HYPOGLYCEMIA. Glucose provides the fetus with approximately 60% to 70% of its energy needs. Almost all fetal glucose derives from the maternal circulation by the process of transplacental-facilitated diffusion that maintains fetal glucose levels at approximately two-thirds of maternal levels. The severing of the umbilical cord at birth abruptly interrupts the source of glucose, and to maintain adequate glucose levels, the newborn must rapidly respond by glycogenolysis of hepatic stores, inducing gluconeogenesis, and utilizing exogenous nutrients from feeding. During this transition, newborn glucose levels fall to a low point in the first 1 to 2 hours of life, and then increase and stabilize at mean levels of 65 to 70 mg/dL by the age of 3 to 4 hours.

A. Incidence. The reported incidence of hypoglycemia varies with its definition, but it has been estimated to occur in approximately 16% of large-for-gestational-age (LGA) infants and 15% of small-for-gestational-age (SGA) babies.

B. Definition. Discussion of the incidence, effects, and treatment of hypoglycemia has been hampered by lack of agreement on its definition.

1. Historical definitions

a. Epidemiologic definition

i. Early definitions of normal neonatal glucose levels were derived by measuring glucose levels in populations of infants, some of whom were not being fed or given other sources of glucose. The statistical definition of normal, values that are within two standard deviations of the mean, resulted in the acceptance of glucose levels in the range of 20 to 30 mg/dL.

This definition was affected by clinical practice at the time, and did not define "optimal" glucose level in newborns. This definition is no longer generally accepted.

b. Clinical definition (**Whipple triad**) requires the following:

i. Reliable measurement of a low glucose level.

ii. Signs and symptoms consistent with hypoglycemia. **Development of clinical signs or symptoms may be a late sign of hypoglycemia**.

iii. Resolution of signs and symptoms after blood-glucose level is restored to normal range.

2. Operational threshold. Cornblath recommended use of an **operational threshold** for blood-sugar management in newborn infants. The operational threshold is an indication for action and is not diagnostic of disease.

    a. Defines glucose level at which intervention should be considered on the basis of current knowledge.

    b. Differs from therapeutic goal.

    c. Depends on clinical state and age.

    d. Does not define normal or abnormal.

    e. Provides margin of safety.

    f. Operational thresholds as suggested by Cornblath et al.

        i. Healthy full-term infant.

           a) Less than 24 hours of age—30 to 35 mg/dL may be acceptable once, but raised to 45 mg/dL if the level persists after feeding or recurs in first 24 hours.

           b) After 24 hours, threshold should be increased to 45 to 50 mg/dL.

        ii. Infant with abnormal signs or symptoms—45 mg/dL.

        iii. Asymptomatic infants with risk factors for low blood sugar—36 mg/dL. Close surveillance is required and intervention is needed if plasma glucose remains below this level, it does not increase after feeding, or if abnormal clinical signs are seen.

        iv. For any baby, if glucose levels are <20 to 25 mg/dL, IV glucose is needed to raise the plasma glucose to >45 mg/dL.

3. The significance of a given glucose level depends on the method of measurement, the infant's gestational age, chronological age, and other risk factors.

4. The absence of overt symptoms at low glucose levels does not rule out central nervous system (CNS) injury. There is no evidence indicating that the premature or young infant is protected from the effects of inadequate glucose delivery to the CNS.

5. There is no single value below which brain injury definitely occurs.

6. A glucose level <40 mg/dL at any time in any newborn requires follow-up glucose measurements to document normal values.

7. Within the first hours of life, normal asymptomatic babies may have transient glucose levels in the 30s (mg/dL) that will increase either spontaneously or in response to feeding. These babies have an excellent prognosis.

8. On the basis of recent developmental, neuroanatomic, metabolic, and clinical studies, our goal is to maintain the glucose value >45 mg/dL in the first day, and >50 mg/dL thereafter.

C. Etiology

1. Increased utilization of glucose: hyperinsulinism

    a. Diabetic mothers (see Chap. 2A).

    b. LGA infants. Current prenatal obstetric care includes testing women for glucose intolerance, and the number of undiagnosed infants of gestational diabetic mothers has decreased. There is a 16% incidence of hypoglycemia in LGA infants of nondiabetic mothers and routine glucose screening of these babies is recommended.

    c. Erythroblastosis (hyperplastic islets of Langerhans) (see Chaps. 18 and 26A).

    d. Islet-cell hyperplasia, hyperfunction, focal hyperinsulinism, or diffuse hyperinsulinism (mutations of *SUR1* [high-affinity sulfonylurea receptor] or K_{IR} 6.2 [potassium-channel gene]).

    e. Beckwith-Weidemann syndrome (macrosomia, mild microcephaly, omphalocele, macroglossia, hypoglycemia, and visceromegaly).

    f. Insulin-producing tumors (nesidioblastosis, islet-cell adenoma, or islet-cell dysmaturity).

    g. Maternal tocolytic therapy with β-sympathomimetic agents (terbutaline).

    h. Maternal chlorpropamide therapy (Diabinese); possibly maternal thiazide diuretics (chlorothiazide).

    i. Malpositioned umbilical artery catheter used to infuse glucose in high concentration into the celiac and superior mesenteric arteries T11 to 12, stimulating insulin release from the pancreas.

    j. Abrupt cessation of high-glucose infusion.

    k. After exchange transfusion with blood containing high-glucose concentration.

      i. Exaggerated response to neonatal transition.

2. Decreased production/stores

    a. Prematurity.

    b. Intrauterine growth restriction (IUGR).

    c. Inadequate caloric intake.

    d. Delayed onset of feeding.

3. Increased utilization and/or decreased production. Any baby with one of the following conditions should be evaluated for hypoglycemia; parenteral glucose may be necessary for the management of these infants.

    a. Perinatal stress

      i. Sepsis.

      ii. Shock.

      iii. Asphyxia.

      iv. Hypothermia (increased utilization).

      v. Respiratory distress.

      vi. Post resuscitation.

    b. Exchange transfusion with heparinized blood that has a low glucose level in the absence of a glucose infusion; reactive hypoglycemia after exchange with relatively hyperglycemic citrate-phosphate-dextrose (CPD) blood.

    c. Defects in carbohydrate metabolism (see Chap. 29D)

      i. Glycogen storage disease.

      ii. Fructose intolerance.

      iii. Galactosemia.

    d. Endocrine deficiency

      i. Adrenal insufficiency.

      ii. Hypothalamic deficiency.

      iii. Congenital hypopituitarism.

      iv. Glucagon deficiency.

      v. Epinephrine deficiency.

    e. Defects in amino acid metabolism (see Chap. 29D)

      i. Maple syrup urine disease.

      ii. Propionic acidemia.

      iii. Methylmalonic acidemia.

      iv. Tyrosinemia.

      v. Glutaric acidemia type II.

      vi. Ethylmalonic adipic aciduria.

    f. Polycythemia. Hypoglycemia may be due to higher glucose utilization by the increased mass of red blood cells. The decreased amount of serum per drop of blood may cause a reading consistent with hypoglycemia on whole-blood measurements, but may yield a normal glucose level on laboratory analysis of serum.

    g. Maternal therapy with β-blockers (e.g., labetalol or propranolol). Possible mechanisms include the following:

      i. Prevention of sympathetic stimulation of glycogenolysis.

      ii. Prevention of recovery from insulin-induced decreases in free fatty acids and glycerol.

      iii. Inhibition of epinephrine-induced increases in free fatty acids and lactate after exercise.

D. Diagnosis

  1. Symptoms that have been attributed to hypoglycemia are nonspecific.

    a. Tremors, jitteriness, or irritability.

    b. Seizures, coma.

    c. Lethargy, apathy, and limpness.

    d. Poor feeding, vomiting.

    e. Apnea.

    f. Weak or high-pitched cry.

g. Cyanosis.

h. Some infants may have no symptoms.

2. **Screening.** Serial blood-glucose levels should be routinely measured in infants who have risk factors for hypoglycemia and in infants who have symptoms that could be due to hypoglycemia (see I.C and I.D.1).

a. Babies with risk factors should have their glucose levels measured within the first 1 to 2 hours after birth. The period for which screening should be continued depends on the glucose levels measured and the etiology of hypoglycemia (see I).

i. Infants of diabetic mothers usually develop hypoglycemia in the first hours of life and should have frequent early measurements of blood-glucose level (see Chap. 2A, Maternal Conditions That Affect the Fetus).

ii. Preterm and SGA infants should have blood-glucose measurements soon after birth and also during the first 3 to 4 postnatal days.

iii. Infants with erythroblastosis fetalis should have blood-glucose levels measured after exchange transfusions with CPD blood.

iv. Infants with symptoms should be evaluated for hypoglycemia when the symptoms are present.

3. **Reagent strips with reflectance meter.** Although in widespread use as a screening tool, reagent strips are of unproven reliability in documenting hypoglycemia in neonates.

a. Reagent strips measure whole-blood glucose, which is 15% lower than plasma levels.

b. Reagent strips are subject to false-positive and false-negative results, even when used with a reflectance meter.

c. A valid confirmatory laboratory glucose determination is required before one can diagnose hypoglycemia.

d. If a reagent strip reveals a concentration <45 mg/dL, treatment should not be delayed while one is awaiting confirmation of hypoglycemia using laboratory analysis. If an infant has either symptoms that could be due to hypoglycemia and/or a low glucose level as measured by reagent strip, treatment should be initiated immediately after the confirmatory blood sample is obtained.

4. New point of care devices are being developed to allow for the accurate and rapid determination of glucose levels on small volume samples.

5. **Laboratory diagnosis**

a. The laboratory sample must be obtained and analyzed promptly to avoid the measurement being falsely lowered by glycolysis. The glucose level can fall 18 mg/dL/hour in a blood sample that awaits analysis.

6. **Clinical confirmation** of the diagnosis of symptomatic hypoglycemia requires both of the following:

a. A laboratory-determined serum glucose level of <40 mg/dL at the time symptoms are present.

b. Prompt resolution of the symptoms with the administration of IV glucose and correction of the hypoglycemia.

7. **Additional testing.** When the hypoglycemia is refractory and severe or if the need for large glucose infusions lasts over 1 week, evaluation of some of the rare causes of hypoglycemia should be considered (see I.C.1). At that time an endocrine consultation may be helpful and measurements of the following should be considered:

a. Insulin.

b. Growth hormone.

c. Cortisol.

d. Adrenocorticotropic hormone (ACTH).

e. Thyroxine (T_4).

f. Thyroid-stimulating hormone (TSH).

g. Glucagon.

h. Plasma amino acids.

i. Urine ketones.

      j. Urine-reducing substance.

      k. Urine amino acids.

      l. Urine organic acids.

  8. Differential diagnosis. The symptoms mentioned in I.D can be due to many other causes with or without associated hypoglycemia. If symptoms persist after the glucose concentration is in the normal range, other etiologies should be considered. Some of these are as follows:

      a. Sepsis.

      b. CNS disease.

      c. Toxic exposure.

      d. Metabolic abnormalities

         i. Hypocalcemia.

         ii. Hyponatremia or hypernatremia.

         iii. Hypomagnesemia.

         iv. Pyridoxine deficiency.

      e. Adrenal insufficiency.

      f. Heart failure.

      g. Renal failure.

      h. Liver failure.

E. Management. Anticipation and prevention, when possible, are key to the management of infants at risk of hypoglycemia.

  1. Well infants who are at risk for hypoglycemia (see I.C) should have serial blood-glucose levels measured. **Infants of diabetic mothers** should have glucose measured, and be treated, according to the protocol in Chap. 2A.

  2. Other **asymptomatic** infants who are at risk for hypoglycemia should have blood glucose measured in the first 1 to 2 hours of life. Immediately after birth and as soon as their condition allows they should be nursed or given formula per the mother's preference. This feeding should be repeated every 2 to 3 hours.

  3. The interval between measurement of glucose levels requires clinical judgment. If the glucose concentration is as low as 20 to 25 mg/dL, the baby should be treated with IV glucose with a goal of maintaining the glucose at a level of >45 mg/dL in the first 24 hours, and >50 mg/dL thereafter.

  4. Feeding. Some asymptomatic infants with early glucose levels in the 30s (mg/dL) will respond to feeding (breast or bottle). A follow-up blood-glucose measurement should be done within 1 hour of the feeding. If the glucose level does not rise, a more aggressive therapy may be needed. While early feeding of glucose water will transiently raise the serum glucose level, there is often an associated rebound hypoglycemia, within 1 to 2 hours of feeding glucose water. The early introduction of milk feeding is preferable and will often result in raising glucose levels to normal, maintaining normal stable levels, and avoiding problems with rebound hypoglycemia. Sometimes it is useful to add Polycose (4 kcal/oz) to feedings in infants who feed well but have marginal glucose levels.

  5. Breast-feeding. Babies who are breast-fed have lower glucose levels but higher ketone body levels compared with those who are formula-fed. The use of alternate fuels may be an adaptive mechanism during the first days of life as breast-feeding is developing. Early breast-feeding enhances gluconeogenesis and increases the production of gluconeogenic precursors. Some infants will have difficulty in adapting to breast-feeding, and development of symptomatic hypoglycemia has been reported in breast-fed babies after hospital discharge. It is important to document that breast-fed babies are latching on and appear to be sucking milk, but there is no need to routinely monitor glucose levels in healthy full-term breast-fed babies who do not have additional risk factors.

  6. IV therapy

      a. Indications

         i. Inability to tolerate oral feeding.

         ii. Symptoms.

         iii. Oral feedings do not maintain normal glucose levels.

         iv. Glucose levels <25 mg/dL.

b. Urgent treatment

   i. Administration of 200 mg/kg of glucose over 1 minute, to be followed by continuing therapy as in the following text. This is equivalent to 2 mL/kg of dextrose 10% in water (10% D/W) infused intravenously over 1 minute.

c. Continuing therapy

   i. Infusion of glucose at a rate of 6 to 8 mg of glucose/kg/minute.

   ii. Administration of 10% D/W at a rate of 86.4 mL/kg/day or 3.6 mL/kg/hour gives 6 mg/kg/minute of glucose. Glucose infusion rate (GIR) may be calculated using the following formula:

$$\text{GIR in mg/kg/min} = \frac{\text{dextrose\%concentration} \times \text{mL/kg/day}}{144}$$

For example, in an infant receiving 10% D/W at 80 mL/kg/day, the GIR would be $\frac{10 \times 80}{144} = 5.6$ mg/kg/min.

   Many hospitals now have computerized provider order entry systems that automatically calculate the GIR.

   iii. Recheck glucose level after 20 to 30 minutes and hourly until stable, to determine if additional therapy is needed.

   iv. Additional bolus infusions of 2 mL/kg of 10% D/W may be needed.

   v. If glucose is stable and in acceptable range, feedings may be continued and the glucose infusion tapered as permitted by glucose measurements before feeding.

d. For most infants, intravenous 10% D/W at daily maintenance rates will provide adequate glucose. The required concentration of dextrose in the IV fluids will depend on the daily water requirement. It is suggested that calculation of both glucose intake (i.e., milligrams of glucose per kilogram per minute) and water requirements be done each day, or more frequently if glucose levels are unstable. For example, on the first day, the fluid requirement is generally approximately 80 mL/kg/day, or 0.055 mL/kg/minute; therefore, 10% D/W provides 5.6 mg of glucose/kg/minute, and 15% D/W, at 80 mL/kg/day provides 8.33 mg of glucose/kg/minute.

e. Some infants with hyperinsulinism and infants with IUGR will require 12 to 15 mg of dextrose/kg/minute (often as 15% or 20% D/W).

f. The concentration of glucose and the rate of infusion are increased as necessary to maintain a normal blood-glucose level. A central venous catheter may be necessary to give adequate glucose (15%–20% D/W) in an acceptable fluid volume. Taper GIR and concentration, monitoring glucose levels; and wean IV slowly while feedings are advanced.

7. Consider adding **hydrocortisone,** 10 mg/kg/day intravenously in two divided doses, if the infant remains hypoglycemic despite receiving >12 mg of glucose/kg/minute. Hydrocortisone reduces peripheral glucose utilization, increases gluconeogenesis, and increases the effects of glucagon. The hydrocortisone will usually result in stable and adequate glucose levels, and it can then be rapidly tapered over the course of a few days. **Before administering hydrocortisone,** obtain a blood sample for measurements of glucose, insulin, and cortisol levels at a time when the serum sugar is low. Cortisol levels can be used to screen for the integrity of the hypothalamic–pituitary–adrenal axis.

8. Unless there is a suspicion of a metabolic defect, feedings of mothers milk or formula can be started and advanced as the clinical situation allows. As the feedings are advanced and the IV glucose infusion is tapered, it is important to continue to monitor glucose levels before feeding.

9. Glucagon 0.025–0.3 mg/kg intramuscularly (maximum 1 mg) may be given to hypoglycemic infants with good glycogen stores but it is only a temporizing measure to mobilize glucose for 2 to 3 hours in an emergency until IV glucose can be given. The glucose level will often fall after the effects of glucagon have worn off, and it remains important to obtain IV access to adequately treat these babies. For infants of diabetic mothers, the dose is 0.3 mg/kg (maximum dose is 1 mg) (see Chap. 2A).

10. **Diazoxide** (2–5 mg/kg per dose orally given q8h) may be given for infants who are persistently hyperinsulinemic. It inhibits insulin release by acting as a specific adenosine triphosphate (ATP)-sensitive potassium-channel agonist in normal pancreatic β cells, decreasing insulin release. A positive response is usually seen in 48 to 72 hours if it is going to occur.

11. **Other.** Epinephrine and growth hormone are used rarely and only in the treatment of persistent hypoglycemia. Surgical subtotal pancreatectomy may be necessary for insulin-secreting tumors.

12. **Additional evaluation.** Most hypoglycemia will resolve in 2 to 3 days. A requirement of >8 mg of glucose/kg/minute suggests increased utilization due to hyperinsulinism. This is usually transient as in infants of diabetic mothers. If it lasts >7 days, endocrine evaluation may be necessary to rule out excess insulin secretion from an insulin-secreting tumor or other cause as listed in I.C.

   a. A sample drawn to determine insulin level at the time of low blood glucose will document an inappropriate secretion of insulin.

   b. If the insulin level is normal for the blood-glucose level, other causes of persistent hypoglycemia such as defects in carbohydrate metabolism (see I.C.3.c), endocrine deficiency (see I.C.3.d), and defects in amino acid metabolism (see I.C.3.e) should be considered.

   c. **In severe endocrine or metabolic deficiency, the glucose level will often remain low despite glucose infusions at >10 mg/kg/minute. Diagnosing hyperinsulinemia requires measuring an insulin level that is inappropriately high for a simultaneous serum glucose.** Evaluation requires drawing blood for insulin, cortisol, and amino acids at a time when the glucose level is <40 mg/dL. Many evaluations are not productive because they are done too early in the course of a transient hypoglycemic state or the samples to determine hormone levels are drawn when the glucose level is normal.

   d. Genetic testing is available for various mutations such as *SUR1* and K_{iR} 6.2.

II. **HYPERGLYCEMIA** is usually defined as a whole-blood glucose level >125 mg/dL or plasma glucose values >145 mg/dL. This problem is commonly encountered in low birth weight premature infants receiving parenteral glucose but it is also seen in other infants who are sick. There are usually no specific symptoms associated with neonatal hyperglycemia, but the major clinical problems associated with hyperglycemia are hyperosmolarity and osmotic diuresis. Osmolarity of >300 mOsm/L usually leads to osmotic diuresis (each 18 mg/dL rise in blood-glucose concentration increases serum osmolarity by 1 mOsm/L). Subsequent dehydration may occur rapidly in small premature infants with large insensible fluid losses.

The hyperosmolar state, an increase of 25 to 40 mOsm or a glucose level of >450 to 720 mg/dL, can cause water to move from the intracellular compartment to the extracellular compartment. The resultant contraction of the intracellular volume of the brain may be a cause of intracranial hemorrhage.

Although rarely seen in the first months of life, diabetes mellitus, can present with severe clinical symptoms including polyuria, dehydration, and ketoacidosis that require prompt treatment. The genetic basis of neonatal diabetes is beginning to be understood and has implications for its treatment.

A. **Etiology**

1. **Exogenous parenteral glucose.** Administration of >4 to 5 mg/kg/minute of glucose in preterm infants weighing <1,000 g may be associated with hyperglycemia.

2. **Drugs.** The most common association is with steroids. Other drugs associated with hyperglycemia are caffeine, theophylline, phenytoin, and diazoxide.

3. **VLBW infants** (<1,000 g), possibly due to variable insulin response, persistent endogenous hepatic glucose production despite significant elevations in plasma insulin, or insulin resistance that may in part be due to immature glycogenolysis enzyme systems. VLBW infants will often be treated with fluids in excess of 200 mL/kg/day. A minimum glucose concentration of dextrose 5% must be used to avoid infusing a hypotonic solution and when this fluid is administered the infant may present with an excessive glucose load.

4. **Lipid infusion.** Free fatty acids are associated with increased glucose levels.
5. **Sepsis,** possibly due to depressed insulin release, cytokines, or endotoxin, resulting in decreased glucose utilization. Stress hormones such as cortisol and catecholamines are elevated in sepsis. In an infant who has normal glucose levels and then becomes hyperglycemic without an excess glucose load, sepsis should be the prime consideration.
6. **"Stressed" premature infants** requiring mechanical ventilation or other painful procedures, from persistent endogenous glucose production due to catecholamines and other "stress hormones." Insulin levels are usually appropriate for the glucose level.
7. **Hypoxia,** possibly due to increased glucose production in the absence of a change in peripheral utilization.
8. **Surgical procedures.** Hyperglycemia in this setting is possibly due to the secretion of epinephrine, glucocorticoids, and glucagon as well as excess administration of glucose-containing IV fluids.
9. **Neonatal diabetes mellitus.** In this rare disorder, infants present with significant hyperglycemia that requires insulin treatment in the first months of life. They are characteristically SGA term infants, they have no gender predilection, and a third have a family history of diabetes mellitus. They present with marked glycosuria, hyperglycemia (240–2,300 mg/dL), polyuria, severe dehydration, acidosis, mild or absent ketonuria, reduced subcutaneous fat, and failure to thrive. Insulin values are either absolutely or relatively low for the corresponding blood-glucose elevation. Approximately half of the infants have a transient need for treatment but are at risk of recurrence of diabetes in the second or third decade. Many of the patients with permanent diabetes have mutations involving regulation of the ATP-sensitive potassium channels of the pancreatic beta cells. Activating mutations of either the *KCNJ11* gene that encodes the Kir6.2 subunit or the *ABCC8* gene that encodes the SUR1 have been implicated in the cause of neonatal diabetes. **Treatment** consists of rehydration, and most of the patients require insulin (regular 0.5–3 units/kg/day subcutaneously divided q6h or 0.01–0.1 units/kg/hour by constant infusion). Start with the IV dose, and then switch to the subcutaneous dose. Monitor serum electrolytes, glucose, and acid–base balance. Repeated plasma insulin values are necessary to distinguish transient from permanent diabetes mellitus. Molecular genetic diagnosis can help distinguish the infants with transient diabetes from those with permanent diabetes, and it may also be important for determining which babies are likely to respond to treatment with sulfonylureas.
10. **Diabetes due to pancreatic lesions** such as pancreatic aplasia, or hypoplastic or absent pancreatic β cells is usually seen in SGA infants who may have other congenital defects. They usually present soon after birth and rarely survive.
11. **Transient hyperglycemia associated with ingestion of hyperosmolar formula.** Clinical presentation may mimic transient neonatal diabetes with glycosuria, hyperglycemia, and dehydration. A history of inappropriate formula dilution is the key. Treatment consists of rehydration, discontinuation of the hyperosmolar formula, and appropriate instructions for mixing concentrated or powder formula. Insulin has been used briefly but cautiously.
12. **Hepatic glucose production** can persist despite normal or elevated glucose levels.
13. **Immature development of glucose transport proteins,** such as GLUT-4.

B. **Treatment.** The primary goal is prevention and early detection of hyperglycemia by carefully adjusting GIRs, and frequently monitoring blood-glucose levels and urine for glycosuria. If present, evaluation and possible intervention are indicated.
1. Measure glucose levels in premature infants or infants with abnormal symptoms.
2. Extremely low birth weight premature infants (<1,000 g) should start with an IV glucose concentration no >5%. If hyperglycemia is documented, parenteral glucose intake is reduced to 4 to 6 mg of glucose/kg/minute by adjusting the concentration or the rate (or both) of glucose infusion and monitoring the

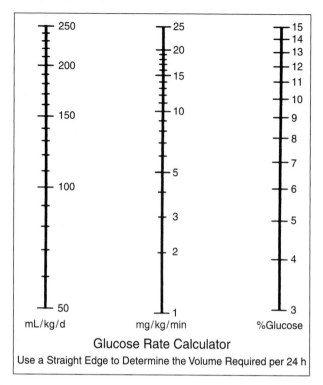

Figure 29A.1. Interconversion of glucose infusion units. (From Klaus MH, Faranoff AA, eds. *Care of the high-risk neonate*, 2nd ed. Philadelphia: WB Saunders, 1979:430.)

falling blood-glucose level. Hypotonic fluids (solutions <dextrose 5%) should be avoided.

3. If appropriate, decrease the glucose infusion by 2 mg/kg/minute every 4 to 6 hours (see Fig. 29A.1).

4. Begin parenteral nutrition as soon as possible in low birth weight infants. Some amino acids promote insulin secretion.

5. Feed if condition allows; feeding can promote the secretion of hormones that promote insulin secretion.

6. Many small infants will initially be unable to tolerate a certain glucose load (e.g., 6 mg/kg/minute) but will eventually develop tolerance if they are presented with just enough glucose to keep their glucose level high yet not enough to cause glycosuria.

7. Exogenous insulin therapy has been used when glucose values exceed 250 mg/dL despite efforts to lower the amount of glucose delivered or when prolonged restriction of parenterally administered glucose would substantially decrease the required total caloric intake. **Neonates may be extremely sensitive to the effects of insulin. It is desirable to decrease the glucose level gradually to avoid rapid fluid shifts.** Very small doses of insulin are used and the actual amount delivered may be difficult to determine because some of the insulin is adsorbed on the plastic surfaces of the IV tubing.

a. Insulin infusion

   i. The standard dilution is 15 units regular human insulin added to 150 mL D10W, D5W, or normal saline for a concentration of 0.1 units/mL.

ii. Flush the IV tubing with a minimum of 25 mL of this insulin solution to saturate binding sites.

iii. Bolus insulin infusion.

    a) Dose 0.05 to 0.1 units/kg q4–6h PRN.

    b) Infuse over 15 minutes through syringe pump.

iv. Continuous insulin infusion.

    a) Rate of infusion is 0.01 to 0.2 units/kg/hour. (Usual starting dose is 0.05 units/kg/hour.)

$$\text{Flow rate (mL/hour)} = \frac{\text{dose (units/kg/hour)} \times \text{weight (kg)}}{\text{concentration (units/mL)}}$$

For example:

Ordered dose: 0.05units/kg/hour and infant weighs 600 g (0.6 kg)

0.05units/kg/hour × 0.6 kg = 0.03units/hour

Concentration is 0.1 units/mL

Infusion rate is: $\dfrac{0.03\text{units/hour}}{0.1\text{mL}} = 0.3 \text{ mL/hour}$

    b) Check glucose levels every 30 minutes until stable to adjust the infusion rate.

    c) If glucose level remains at >180 mg/dL, titrate in increments of 0.01 unit/kg/hour.

    d) If hypoglycemia occurs, discontinue insulin infusion and administer IV bolus of 10% D/W at 2 mL/kg × 1dose.

8. Monitor for rebound hyperglycemia.

  a. Subcutaneous insulin

    i. This is **rarely used except in neonatal diabetes.** Dose is 0.1 to 0.2 unit/kg every 6 hours Monitor glucose level at 1, 2, and 4 hours.

    ii. Monitor potassium level every 6 hours initially.

Suggested Readings

Babenko AP, Polak M, Cave H, et al. Activating mutation in the *ABCC8* gene in neonatal diabetes mellitus. *N Engl J Med* 2006;355:456–466.

Bolouyt N, van Kempen A, Offringa M. Neurodevelopment after neonatal hypoglycemia: A systematic review and design of an optimal future study. *Pediatrics* 2006;117:2231–2243.

Cornblath M, Hawdon JM, Williams AF, et al. Controversies regarding definition of neonatal hypoglycemia: Suggested operational thresholds. *Pediatrics* 2000;105:1141–1145.

Cornblath M, Ichord R. Hypoglycemia in the neonate. *Semin Perinatol* 2000;24:136–149.

Cowett RM, Farrag HM. Selected principles of perinatal-neonatal glucose metabolism. *Semin Neonatol* 2004;9:37–47.

Duvanel CB, Fawer CL, Cotting J, et al. Long-term effects of neonatal hypoglycemia on brain growth and psychomotor development in small-for-gestational-age preterm infants. *J Pediatr* 1999;134:492–498.

Eidelman A. Hypoglycemia and the breastfed neonate. *Pediatr Clin North Am* 2001;48:377–387.

Moore AM, Perlman M. Symptomatic hypoglycemia in otherwise healthy, breastfed newborns. *Pediatrics* 1999;103:837–839.

Pearson ER, Flechtner I, Njolstad PR, et al. Switching from insulin to oral sulfonylureas in patients with diabetes due to Kir6.2 mutations. *N Engl J Med* 2006;355:467–477.

Sperling MA, Menon RK. Differential diagnosis and management of neonatal hypoglycemia. *Pediatr Clin North Am* 2004;51:703–723.

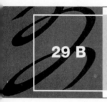

ABNORMALITIES OF SERUM CALCIUM AND MAGNESIUM

29 B

Steven A. Abrams

I. HYPOCALCEMIA
A. General principles
1. **Definition.** Neonatal hypocalcemia is defined as a total serum calcium concentration of <7 mg/dL or an ionized calcium concentration of <4 mg/dL (1 mmol/L). In very low birth weight (VLBW) infants, ionized calcium values of 0.8 to 1 mmol/L are common and not usually associated with clinical symptoms. In larger infants, and in infants of >32 weeks gestation, symptoms may more readily occur with an ionized calcium concentration of <1 mmol/L.
2. **Pathophysiology**
   a. Calcium ions (Ca^{2+}) in cellular and extracellular fluid (ECF) are essential for many biochemical processes. Significant aberrations of serum calcium concentrations are frequently observed in the neonatal period.
      i. **Hormonal regulation of calcium homeostasis.** Regulation of serum and ECF-ionized calcium concentration within a narrow range is critical for blood coagulation, neuromuscular excitability, cell membrane integrity and function, and cellular enzymatic and secretory activity. The principal calcitropic or calcium-regulating hormones are parathyroid hormone (PTH) and 1,25-dihydroxyvitamin D, ($1,25(OH)_2D$, also referred to as *calcitriol*).
      ii. When ECF-ionized calcium level declines, parathyroid cells secrete PTH. PTH mobilizes calcium from bone, increases calcium resorption in the renal tubule, and stimulates renal production of $1,25(OH)_2D$. PTH secretion causes the serum calcium level to rise and the serum phosphorus level to be maintained or to fall.
      iii. Vitamin D is synthesized from provitamin D in the skin after exposure to sunlight and is also ingested in the diet. Vitamin D is transported to the liver, where it is converted to $25(OH)D$ (the major storage form of the hormone). This is transported to the kidney, where it is converted to the biologically active hormone, $1,25(OH)_2D$ (calcitriol). Calcitriol increases intestinal calcium and phosphate absorption and mobilizes calcium and phosphate from bone. There is evidence that calcitriol production and utilization is relatively inefficient in preterm babies and possibly in the first weeks of life in full-term infants.
3. **Etiology**
   a. **Prematurity.** Preterm infants are capable of mounting a PTH response to hypocalcemia, but target-organ responsiveness to PTH may be diminished.
   b. Infants of diabetic mothers (IDMs) have a 25% to 50% incidence of hypocalcemia if maternal control is poor. Hypercalcitoninemia, hypoparathyroidism, abnormal vitamin D metabolism, and hyperphosphatemia have been implicated, but the etiology remains uncertain.
   c. Severe neonatal birth depression is frequently associated with hypocalcemia and hyperphosphatemia. Decreased calcium intake and increased endogenous phosphate load are likely causes.
   d. Congenital. Parathyroids may be absent in DiGeorge sequence (hypoplasia or absence of the third and fourth branchial pouch structures) as an isolated defect in the development of the parathyroid glands, or as part of the Kenny-Caffey syndrome.
   e. **Pseudohypoparathyroidism.** Maternal hyperparathyroidism.

    f. Magnesium deficiency (including inborn error of intestinal magnesium transport) impairs PTH secretion.

    g. Vitamin D deficiency (rarely a cause in the first weeks of life).

    h. Alkalosis and bicarbonate therapy.

    i. Rapid infusion of citrate-buffered blood (exchange transfusion) chelates ionized calcium.

    j. Shock or sepsis.

    k. Phototherapy may be associated with hypocalcemia by decreasing melatonin secretion and increasing uptake of calcium into the bone.

    l. For late-onset hypocalcemia, high phosphate intakes lead to excess phosphorus and decreased serum calcium.

B. Diagnosis

1. Clinical presentation

    a. Hypocalcemia increases cellular permeability to sodium ions and increases cell membrane excitability. The signs are usually nonspecific: apnea, seizures, jitteriness, increased extensor tone, clonus, hyperreflexia, and stridor (laryngospasm).

    b. Early-onset hypocalcemia in preterm newborns is often asymptomatic but may show apnea, seizures, or abnormalities of cardiac function.

    c. Late-onset syndromes, in contrast, may present as hypocalcemic seizures. Often it must be differentiated from other causes of newborn seizures, including "fifth-day" fits.

2. History

    a. For late-onset presentation, mothers may report partial breast-feeding. Abnormal movements and lethargy may precede obvious seizure activity. Rarely, use of goat's milk or whole milk of cow may be reported. Symptoms are usually described beginning from the third to fifth days of life.

3. Physical examination

    a. General physical findings associated with seizure disorder in the newborn may be present in some cases. Usually there are no apparent physical findings.

4. Laboratory studies

    a. There are three definable fractions of calcium in serum: (i) ionized calcium ($\sim$50% of serum total calcium); (ii) calcium bound to serum proteins, principally albumin ($\sim$40%); and (iii) calcium complexed to serum anions, mostly phosphates, citrate, and sulfates ($\sim$10%). Ionized calcium is the only biologically available form of calcium.

    b. Assessment of calcium status using ionized calcium is preferred, especially in the first week of life. Use of correction nomagrams to convert total calcium into ionized calcium are not reliable.

    c. Calcium concentration reported as milligrams per deciliter can be converted to molar units by dividing by 4 (e.g., 10 mg/dL converts to 2.5 mmol/L).

    d. Postnatal changes in serum calcium concentrations. At birth, the umbilical serum calcium level is elevated (10–11 mg/dL). In healthy term babies, calcium concentrations decline for the first 24 to 48 hours; the nadir is usually 7.5 to 8.5 mg/dL. Thereafter, calcium concentrations progressively rise to the mean values observed in older children and adults.

5. Monitoring

    a. Suggested schedule for monitoring calcium levels in infants such as VLBW, IDM, and birth depression who are at risk for developing hypocalcemia:

        i. Ionized calcium: at 12, 24, and 48 hours of life.

        ii. Total serum phosphorus and total serum magnesium for infants with hypocalcemia.

        iii. Other lab tests, including PTH, 25(OH)D, and 1,25(OH)$_2$D are not usually needed unless neonatal hypocalcemia does not readily resolve with calcium therapy

        iv. A prolonged electrocardiographic QTc interval is a traditional indicator that is typically not clinically useful in the newborn period.

6. Imaging

a. Absence of a thymic shadow on a chest radiograph and the presence of conotruncal cardiac abnormalities may suggest a diagnosis of 22q11 syndrome, also known as *CATCH22* or *DiGeorge sequence*.

C. Treatment

1. Medications

a. Therapy with calcium is usually adequate for most cases. In some cases (see the following text), concurrent therapy with magnesium is indicated.

b. Rapid intravenous infusion of calcium can cause a sudden elevation of serum calcium level, leading to bradycardia or other dysrhythmias. Intravenous calcium should only be "pushed" for treatment of hypocalcemic crisis (e.g., seizures) and done with careful cardiovascular monitoring.

c. Infusion by means of the umbilical vein may result in hepatic necrosis if the catheter is lodged in a branch of the portal vein.

d. Rapid infusion by means of the umbilical artery can cause arterial spasms and, at least experimentally, intestinal necrosis and is generally not indicated.

e. Intravenous calcium solutions are incompatible with sodium bicarbonate, since calcium carbonate will precipitate.

f. Extravasation of calcium solutions into subcutaneous tissues can cause severe necrosis and subcutaneous calcifications.

g. Calcium preparations. Calcium gluconate 10% solution is preferred for intravenous use. Calcium glubionate syrup (Neo-Calglucon) is a convenient oral preparation. However, the high sugar content and osmolality may cause gastrointestinal irritation or diarrhea and is generally not used with early hypocalcemia or in VLBW infants during the first weeks of life.

i. If the ionized calcium level drops to 1 mmol/L or less (>1,500 g) or 0.8 mmol/L or less (<1,500 g), a continuous intravenous calcium infusion may be commenced. For infants with early hypocalcemia, this may be done using Total parenteral nutrition (TPN). For use without other TPN components, a dose of 40 to 50 mg/kg/day of elemental calcium is typical.

ii. It may be desirable to prevent the onset of hypocalcemia for newborns who exhibit cardiovascular compromise (e.g., severe respiratory distress syndrome, asphyxia, septic shock, and persistent pulmonary hypertension of the newborn). Use a continuous calcium infusion, preferably by means of a central catheter, to maintain an ionized calcium 1 to 1.4 mmol/L (<1,500 g) or 1.2 to 1.5 mmol/L (>1,500 g).

iii. Emergency calcium therapy (active seizures or profound cardiac failure thought to be associated with severe hypocalcemia) consists of 100 to 200 mg/kg of 10% calcium gluconate (9–18 mg of elemental calcium/kg) by intravenous infusion over 10 to 15 minutes.

h. Monitor heart rate and rhythm and the infusion site throughout the infusion.

i. Repeat the dose in 10 minutes if there is no clinical response.

j. Following the initial dose(s), maintenance calcium should be given through continuous intravenous infusion.

k. Hypocalcemia associated with hyperphosphatemia presenting after day of life (DOL)#3.

i. The goal of initial therapy is to reduce renal phosphate load while increasing calcium intake. Reduce phosphate intake by feeding the infant human milk or a low-phosphorus formula (Similac PM 60/40 is most widely used).

ii. Avoid the use of preterm formulas, lactose-free or other special formulas or transitional formulas as these have high levels of phosphorus or may be more limited in calcium bioavailability.

iii. Increase the oral calcium intake using supplements (e.g., 20–40 mg/kg/day of elemental calcium added to Similac PM 60/40). Phosphate binders are generally not necessary and may not be safe for use, especially in premature infants.

iv. Gradually wean calcium supplements over 2 to 4 weeks. Monitor serum calcium and phosphorus levels 1 to 2 times weekly.

    I. Rare defects in vitamin D metabolism are treated with vitamin D analogs, for example, dihydrotachysterol (Hytakerol) and calcitriol (Rocaltrol). The rapid onset of action and short half-life of these drugs lessen the risk of rebound hypercalcemia.

II. HYPERCALCEMIA

A. General principles

1. Definition

    a. Neonatal hypercalcemia (serum total calcium level >11 mg/dL, serum ionized calcium level >1.5 mmol/L) may be asymptomatic and discovered incidentally during routine screening. Alternatively, the presentation of severe hypercalcemia (>14 mg/dL) can be dramatic and life-threatening, requiring immediate medical intervention.

2. Etiology

    a. Imbalance in intake or use of calcium.

    b. Clinical adjustment of TPN by removing the phosphorus (due to, e.g., concern about excess sodium or potassium intake) can rapidly lead to hypercalcemia, especially in VLBW infants.

    c. Hyperparathyroidism

        i. Congenital hyperparathyroidism associated with maternal hypoparathyroidism usually resolves over several weeks.

        ii. Neonatal severe primary hyperparathyroidism (NSPHP). The parathyroids are refractory to regulation by calcium, producing marked hypercalcemia (frequently 15–30 mg/dL).

        iii. Self-limited secondary hyperparathyroidism associated with neonatal renal tubular acidosis.

    d. Hyperthyroidism. Thyroid hormone stimulates bone resorption and bone turnover.

    e. Hypophosphatasia, an autosomal recessive bone dysplasia, produces severe bone demineralization and fractures.

    f. Increased intestinal absorption of calcium.

    g. Hypervitaminosis D may result from excessive vitamin D ingestion by the mother (during pregnancy) or the neonate. Since vitamin D is extensively stored in fat, intoxication may persist for weeks to months (see Chap. 10).

    h. Decreased renal calcium clearance.

    i. Familial hypocalciuric hypercalcemia, a clinically benign autosomal dominant disorder, can present in the neonatal period. The gene mutation is on chromosome 3q21-24.

    j. Idiopathic neonatal/infantile hypercalcemia occurs in the constellation of Williams syndrome (hypercalcemia, supravalvular aortic stenosis or other cardiac anomalies, "elfin" facies, psychomotor retardation) and in a familial pattern lacking the Williams phenotype. Increased calcium absorption has been demonstrated; increased vitamin D sensitivity and impaired calcitonin secretion are proposed as possible mechanisms.

    k. Subcutaneous fat necrosis is a sequela of trauma or asphyxia. Only the more generalized necrosis seen in asphyxia is associated with significant hypercalcemia. Granulomatous (macrophage) inflammation of the necrotic lesions may be a source of unregulated $1,25(OH)_2D_3$ synthesis.

    l. Acute renal failure, usually during the diuretic or recovery phase.

B. Diagnosis

1. Clinical presentation

    a. Hyperparathyroidism—includes hypotonia, encephalopathy, poor feeding, vomiting, constipation, polyuria, hepatosplenomegaly, anemia, and extraskeletal calcifications, including nephrocalcinosis.

    b. Milder hypercalcemia may present as feeding difficulties or poor linear growth.

2. History

    a. Maternal/family history of hypercalcemia or hypocalcemia, parathyroid disorders, nephrocalcinosis.

    b. Family history of hypercalcemia or familial hypocalciuric hypercalcemia.

    c. Manipulations of TPN.

3. Physical examination

    a. Small for dates (hyperparathyroidism, Williams syndrome).

    b. Craniotabes, fractures (hyperparathyroidism), or characteristic bone dysplasia (hypophosphatasia).

    c. "Elfin" facies (Williams syndrome).

    d. Cardiac murmur (supravalvular aortic stenosis and peripheral pulmonic stenosis associated with Williams syndrome).

    e. Indurated, bluish-red lesions (subcutaneous fat necrosis).

    f. Evidence of hyperthyroidism.

4. Laboratory evaluation

    a. The clinical history, serum and urine mineral levels of phosphorus, and the urinary calcium:creatinine ratio ([U_{Ca}/U_{Cr}]) should suggest a likely diagnosis.

       i. Very elevated serum calcium level (>15 mg/dL) usually indicates primary hyperparathyroidism or, in VLBW infants, phosphate depletion.

       ii. Low serum phosphorus level indicates phosphate depletion, hyperparathyroidism, or familial hypocalciuric hypercalcemia.

       iii. Very low U_{Ca}/U_{Cr} suggests familial hypocalciuric hypercalcemia.

    b. Specific serum hormone levels (PTH, 25(OH)D, 1,25(OH)$_2$D) will confirm the diagnostic impression in cases where obvious manipulations of diet/TPN are not apparent.

    c. A level very low serum alkaline phosphatase activity suggests hypophosphatasia (confirmed by increased urinary phosphoethanolamine level).

    d. Radiography of hand/wrist may suggest hyperparathyroidism (demineralization, subperiosteal resorption) or hypervitaminosis D (submetaphyseal rarefaction).

C. Treatment

  1. Emergency medical treatment (symptomatic or calcium >14 mg/dL).

    a. Volume expansion with isotonic saline solution. Hydration and sodium promote urinary calcium excretion. If cardiac function is normal, infuse normal saline solution (10–20 mL/kg) over 15 to 30 minutes.

    b. Furosemide (1 mg/kg q6–8h intravenously) induces calciuria.

  2. Inorganic phosphate may lower serum calcium levels in hypophosphatemic patients by inhibiting bone resorption and promoting bone mineral accretion.

    a. Glucocorticoids are effective in hypervitaminosis A and D and subcutaneous fat necrosis by inhibiting both bone resorption and intestinal calcium absorption; they are ineffective in hyperparathyroidism.

       i. Other therapies.

    b. Low-calcium, low-vitamin D diets are an effective adjunctive therapy for hypervitaminosis A or D, subcutaneous fat necrosis, and Williams syndrome.

    c. Calcitonin is a potent inhibitor of bone resorption. The antihypercalcemic effect is transient but may be prolonged if glucocorticoids are used concomitantly. There is little reported experience in neonates.

    d. Parathyroidectomy with autologous reimplantation may be indicated for severe persistent neonatal hyperparathyroidism.

III. DISORDERS OF MAGNESIUM: HYPO AND HYPERMAGNESEMIA

A. Etiology

  1. Hypermagnesemia is usually due to an exogenous magnesium load exceeding renal excretion capacity.

    a. Magnesium sulfate therapy for maternal preeclampsia or preterm labor.

    b. Administration of magnesium-containing antacids to the newborn.

    c. Excessive magnesium in parenteral nutrition.

    d. Hypomagnesemia is uncommon but is often seen with late onset hypocalcemia.

B. Diagnosis

  1. Elevated serum magnesium level (>3 mg/dL) suggests hypermagnesemia. Low serum magnesium level of <1.6 mg/dL suggests hypomagnesemia.

    2. Severe hypermagnesemic symptoms are unusual in neonates with serum magnesium level <6 mg/dL. The common curariform effects include apnea, respiratory depression, lethargy, hypotonia, hyporeflexia, poor suck, decreased intestinal motility, and delayed passage of meconium.

    3. Hypomagnesemic symptoms can also include apnea and poor motor tone. Hypomagnesemia is usually seen along with hypocalcemia in the newborn.

C. Treatment

    1. Hypocalcemic seizures with concurrent hypomagnesemia should include treatment for the hypomagnesemia.

        a. The preferred preparation for treatment is magnesium sulfate. The 50% solution contains 500 mg, or 4 mEq/mL.

        b. Correct severe hypomagnesemia (<1.6 mg/dL) with 50 to 100 mg/kg of magnesium sulfate intravenously given over 1 to 2 hours. When administering intravenously, infuse slowly and monitor heart rate. The dose may be repeated after 12 hours. Obtain serum magnesium levels before each dose.

    2. Often the only intervention necessary for hypermagnesemia is removal of the source of exogenous magnesium.

    3. Exchange transfusion, peritoneal dialysis, and hemodialysis are not used in the newborn period.

    4. For hypermagnesemic babies, begin feedings only after suck and intestinal motility are established. Rarely, respiratory support may be needed.

Suggested Readings

De Marini S, Mimouni FB, Tsang RC, et al. Disorders of calcium, phosphorus, and magnesium metabolism. In: Fanaroff AA, Mouton RJ, eds. *Neonatal–perinatal medicine*, 6th ed. St. Louis: Mosby, 1997.

Tsang RC Calcium, phosphorus, and magnesium metabolism. In: Polin RA, Fox WW, eds. *Fetal and neonatal physiology*. Philadelphia: WB Saunders, 1992.

OSTEOPENIA (METABOLIC BONE DISEASE) OF PREMATURITY

29 C

Steven A. Abrams

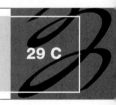

I. GENERAL PRINCIPLES

A. Definition

    1. Osteopenia is defined as postnatal bone mineralization that is inadequate to fully mineralize bones. Osteopenia occurs commonly in very low birth weight (VLBW) infants. Prior to the use of high-mineral containing diets for premature infants–which is the current practice–significant radiographic changes were seen in about half of infants with birth weight <1,000 g.

    2. The current incidence is unknown and likely closely associated with the severity of overall illness and degree of prematurity.

B. Etiology

    1. Deficiency of calcium and phosphorus is the principal cause. Demands for rapid growth in the third trimester are met by intrauterine mineral accretion rates of approximately 120 mg of calcium and 60 mg of phosphorus/kg/day. Poor mineral intake and absorption after birth result in undermineralized new and remodeled bone.

    a. Diets low in mineral content predispose preterm newborns to metabolic bone disease.

    b. Unsupplemented human milk.

    c. Long-term use of parenteral nutrition.

    d. Formulas not designed for use in preterm infants (e.g., full-term, elemental, soy-based).

    e. Furosemide therapy causes renal calcium wasting. It is not likely the principal contributor to osteopenia however for most preterm infants.

    f. Long-term steroid use.

    g. Renal phosphorus wasting.

2. Vitamin D deficiency. Human milk has a total antirachitic sterol content of only 25 to 50 IU/L, insufficient for maintaining normal 25-hydroxyvitamin D ($25(OH)D_3$) levels in preterm infants. However, when vitamin D intake is adequate, even VLBW newborns can synthesize 1,25-dihydroxyvitamin D ($1,25(OH)_2D_3$), although synthesis may be minimal in the first few weeks of life.

    a. Maternal vitamin D deficiency can cause congenital rickets.

    b. Inadequate vitamin D intake or absorption produces nutritional rickets but this is not the primary cause of osteopenia in preterm infants.

    c. Hepatobiliary rickets results largely from vitamin D malabsorption.

    d. Chronic renal failure (renal osteodystrophy).

    e. Chronic use of phenytoin or phenobarbital increases 25(OH)D metabolism.

    f. Hereditary pseudo–vitamin D deficiency: type I (abnormality or absence of 1-α-hydroxylase activity) or type II (tissue resistance to $1,25(OH)_2D_3$).

II. DIAGNOSIS

A. Clinical presentation

    1. Osteopenia ("washed out" or undermineralized bones) develops during the first postnatal weeks. Signs of rickets (epiphyseal dysplasia and skeletal deformities) usually become evident after 6 weeks postnatal age or by term-corrected gestational age. The risk of bone disease is greatest for the sickest, most premature infants.

B. History

    1. A history of VLBW, especially <26 weeks or 1,000 g birth weight, and use of fluid restriction, prolonged parenteral nutrition, or long-term steroids is very common.

    2. Rapid increase in alkaline phosphatase value is common.

    3. A history of a fracture noticed by caregivers or incidentally on x-rays taken for other purposes may be seen.

C. Physical examination

    1. Clinical signs include respiratory insufficiency or failure to wean from a ventilator, hypotonia, pain on handling due to pathologic fractures, decreased linear growth with sustained head growth, frontal bossing, enlarged anterior fontanel and widened cranial sutures, craniotabes (posterior flattening of the skull), "rachitic rosary" (swelling of costochondral junctions), Harrison grooves (indentation of the ribs at the diaphragmatic insertions), and enlargement of wrists, knees, and ankles.

D. Laboratory studies

    1. Laboratory evaluation. The earliest indications of osteopenia are often a decreased serum phosphorus concentration, typically <3.5 to 4 mg/dL (1.1–1.3 mmol/L), and an increased alkaline phosphatase activity. Alkaline phosphatase values >800 IU/L are worrisome, especially if combined with serum phosphorus values <4 mg/dL (1.3 mmol/L). However, it is often difficult to distinguish the normal rise in alkaline phosphatase activity associated with rapid bone mineralization from the pathologic increase related to early osteopenia. In this circumstance, decreased bone mineralization observed on a radiograph confirms the diagnosis.

    a. Serum calcium level (low, normal, or slightly elevated) is generally not a good indicator of the presence or severity of metabolic bone disease.

    b. Serum alkaline phosphatase level (an indicator of osteoclast activity) is often but not invariantly correlated with disease severity (>1,000–1,200

IU/L in severe rickets). Note the following about alkaline phosphatase activity.

   c. Normal neonatal range may be up to 4 times the adult upper limit. Values of 400 to 600 are common in VLBW infants with no evidence of osteopenia.

   d. Hepatobiliary disease also elevates alkaline phosphatase level. Determining bone isoenzymes may be helpful but is not usually clinically necessary.

   e. Solitary elevated alkaline phosphatase level rarely occurs in the absence of bone or liver disease (transient hyperphosphatasemia of infancy).

   f. Serum $25(OH)D_3$ levels are usually normal if liver function is normal and do not need to be routinely assessed.

   g. Reserve measurement of serum $1,25(OH)_2D_3$ or parathyroid hormone (PTH) for complicated or refractory cases.

E. Imaging

  1. Radiographic signs include widening of epiphyseal growth plates; cupping, fraying, and rarefaction of the metaphyses; subperiosteal new-bone formation; osteopenia, particularly of the skull, spine, scapula, and ribs; and occasionally osteoporosis or pathologic fractures.

   a. A loss of up to 40% of bone mineralization can occur without radiographic changes. Chest films may show osteopenia and sometimes rachitic changes.

   b. Wrist or knee films can be useful. Generally if marked abnormalities are present, films should be obtained again 3 to 4 weeks later.

   c. Measurement of bone mineral content by densitometry or ultrasonography remains investigational.

III. TREATMENT

A. Management

  1. In VLBW infants, early enteral feeding significantly enhances the establishment of full-volume enteral intake, leading to increased calcium accumulation and decreased osteopenia.

  2. Mineral-fortified human milk or "premature" formulas are the appropriate diets for preterm infants weighing <1,800 to 2,000 g; their use at 120 kcal/kg/day can prevent and treat metabolic bone disease of prematurity.

  3. Bone formation is dependent on adequate calcium and phosphorus availability; hence calcium supplementation alone may not prevent rickets.

  4. Small for gestational infants weighing <1,800 to 2,000 g will usually also benefit from human milk fortification or use of premature infant formula regardless of gestational age.

  5. Elemental mineral supplementation of human milk is less desirable than the use of prepackaged fortifiers containing calcium and phosphorus because of concern over medication error and potential hyperosmolarity. The addition of both calcium and phosphorus supplements directly to milk or formula should be avoided, as it may lead to the formation of a precipitate.

  6. The long-term use of specialized formulas in VLBW infants, including soy and elemental formulas should be discouraged as it may increase the risk for osteopenia.

  7. In special circumstances, including babies with radiologic evidence or rickets not responding to fortified human milk or premature formula, smaller amounts of calcium (usually up to 40 mg of elemental calcium/kg/day) and/or sodium or potassium phosphate (usually up to 20 mg of elemental phosphorus) can be provided. This is usually needed in babies whose birth weights were <800 g or who had a prolonged hospital course including long-term Total parenternal nutrition (TPN), fluid restrictions, or bronchopulmonary dysplasia.

  8. Ensure adequate vitamin D stores by an intake of 150 to 400 IU/day.

  9. High doses of vitamin D have not been shown to have short or long-term benefits. Some prefer to give 800 IU/day. This is unlikely to be harmful, but there is no evidence of benefit.

  10. Rare defects in vitamin D metabolism may respond better to dihydrotachysterol (DHT) or calcitriol.

11. Furosemide-induced renal calcium wasting can be lessened by adding a thiazide diuretic or by alternate-day administration. Benefits of these approaches are not well established in neonates.

12. Avoid nonessential handling and vigorous chest physiotherapy in preterm infants with severely undermineralized bones. Recent data suggests that daily passive physical activity (range of motion, 5–10 minutes) may enhance both growth and bone mineralization.

13. Infants receiving human milk with added fortifier or premature formula should have serum calcium, phosphorus, and alkaline phosphate levels monitored periodically. Measurement of vitamin D metabolite levels and PTH levels are rarely useful in this setting.

14. Human milk fortification or the use of premature infant formula can usually be discontinued after the infant weighs approximately 2,000 to 2,200 g and tolerating enteral feeds well. It may be continued longer for infants who are fluid restricted or have a markedly elevated alkaline phosphatase activity or radiologic evidence of osteopenia.

15. At hospital discharge, infants with birth weight <1,500 g who are formula-fed may benefit from the use of a transitional formula that has calcium and phosphorus contents midrange between that of preterm formulas and formulas designed for full-term infants.

16. Former LBW infants discharged from hospital and who are on unsupplemented mother's milk are at risk for persistent osteopenia. They should be provided vitamin D supplementation based an American Academy of Pediatrics (AAP) guidelines for full-term infants (200 IU/day) or higher (many would recommend 400 IU/day for this population). This patient population may be candidates for a follow-up measurement of serum phosphorus and alkaline phosphatase activity at 4 to 8 weeks postdischarge.

Suggested Readings

Atkinson SA, Tsang RC. Calcium, magnesium, phosphorus, and Vitamin D. In: Tsang RC, Uauy R, Koletzko B, et al. eds. *Nutrition of the preterm infant: Scientific basis and practical guidelines*, 2nd ed. Cincinnati: Digital Educational Publishing, Inc, 2005:135.

Hawthorne KM, Abrams SA. Safety and efficacy of human milk fortification for very-low-birth-weight infants. *Nutr Rev* 2004;62:482–485.

Hsu HC, Levine MA. Perinatal calcium metabolism: Physiology and pathophysiology. *Semin Neonatol* 2004;9:23–36.

Ziegler EE, O'Donnell AM, Nelson SE, et al. Body composition of the reference fetus. *Growth* 1976;40:329.

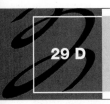

INBORN ERRORS OF METABOLISM

29 D

Sule U. Cataltepe and Harvey L. Levy

Infants with inborn errors of metabolism (IEM) are usually normal at birth. In those disorders that present symptomatically in the neonatal period, the signs often develop in hours to days after birth. Since the newborn infant has a limited repertoire of responses to acute illness, the manifestations of IEM are common to several other neonatal conditions, such as infections and cardiopulmonary dysfunction. Therefore, in the face of such nonspecific features, it is important to maintain a high index of suspicion of IEM in sick neonates since most of these disorders can be lethal unless diagnosed and treated immediately. Even if the disorder is not treatable, establishing the diagnosis in the index case is crucial for prenatal diagnosis in subsequent pregnancies.

I. **INCIDENCE.** Although IEM are individually rare, their overall incidence is as high as 1 in 2,000. About 100 different IEM may present clinically in the neonatal period.

II. **INHERITANCE.** Most IEM are transmitted as autosomal recessive genetic traits. A history of parental consanguinity, unexplained neonatal deaths, or severe illness in the immediate family should alert the clinician to the possibility of an IEM. Some IEM, such as the urea cycle disorder ornithine transcarbamylase (OTC) deficiency, are X-linked. As in any X-linked disorder, the severely affected family member could have been a maternal uncle, or a brother, or perhaps a mildly affected mother, sister, or maternal aunt.

III. **CLINICAL PRESENTATION**

A. **Pregnancy.** Women carrying fetuses with long-chain 3-hydroxyacyl-coenzyme A (CoA) dehydrogenase deficiency (LCHADD) as well as other disorders of fatty acid oxidation are predisposed to developing acute fatty liver of pregnancy and the syndrome of hemolysis, elevated liver enzymes, and low platelet counts (the HELLP syndrome). In most IEM, however, the pregnancy is normal.

B. **Time and pattern of onset.** IEM can be divided into two groups on the basis of the timing and pattern of presentation in the newborn infant. In the **intoxication type**, the typical course is that of a newborn infant who is born healthy and deteriorates clinically after an initial symptom-free period. The first signs are usually poor feeding and vomiting followed by neurological deterioration with lethargy, apnea, seizures, and coma. The organic acidemias and urea cycle defects (UCDs) classically present in this manner. In **energy deficiencies**, the most common presentation is an overwhelming neurologic illness with apnea, seizures, and coma without an apparent symptom-free period. The diseases in this group include mitochondrial and peroxisomal disorders, nonketotic hyperglycinemia (NKH), molybdenum cofactor deficiency, and primary lactic acidosis.

C. **Patterns of presentation.** Newborns with IEM present with one or more of the following manifestations:

1. **Neurological abnormalities. Encephalopathy, seizures, and tone abnormalities.** Encephalopathy and seizures are commonly seen in organic acidemias, UCDs, maple syrup urine disease (MSUD), fatty acid oxidation defects, and congenital lactic acidosis. Seizures may be the presenting symptom in pyridoxine-dependent seizures, folinic acid–responsive seizures, NKH, sulfite oxidase deficiency, and peroxisomal disorders. A few IEM present as predominant hypotonia in the neonatal period. These disorders include NKH, sulfite oxidase deficiency, peroxisomal disorders, and respiratory chain disorders.

2. **Disorders of acid–base status.** Metabolic acidosis with a raised anion gap is an important laboratory feature of many IEM. A flowchart for the investigation of metabolic acidosis with anion gap in patients with suspected IEM is presented in Fig. 29D.1. The organic acidemias, fatty acid oxidation defects, and primary lactic acidemias (defects of gluconeogenesis, glycogenolysis, pyruvate metabolism, Krebs cycle, and respiratory chain) cause metabolic acidosis with an increased anion gap. Measurement of lactate/pyruvate ratio can be helpful to differentiate various causes of primary lactic acidosis (Fig. 29D.1). Respiratory alkalosis can be associated with hyperammonemia syndromes.

3. **Hypoglycemia.** Hypoglycemia, a frequent finding in neonates, should raise a suspicion of IEM if it is severe and persistent without any other etiology. Hypoglycemia associated with metabolic acidosis suggests an organic acidemia or a defect of gluconeogenesis, such as glycogen storage disease type I or fructose 1,6-diphosphatase deficiency. Nonketotic hypoglycemia is the hallmark of defects of fatty acid oxidation.

A flowchart for the evaluation of persistent hypoglycemia is presented in Fig. 29D.2.

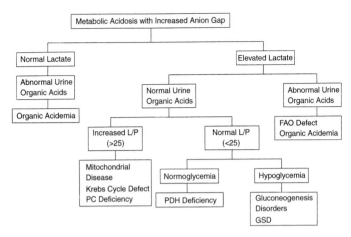

Figure 29D.1. Approach to the investigation of neonatal metabolic acidosis. L/P = lactate/pyruvate ratio; FAO = fatty acid oxidation; PC = pyruvate carboxylase; PDH = pyruvate dehydrogenase; GSD = glycogen storage disease.

4. **Liver dysfunction.** Galactosemia is the most common metabolic cause of liver disease in the neonate. Hepatomegaly with hypoglycemia and seizures suggest glycogenosis type I or III, gluconeogenesis defects, or hyperinsulinism. Hereditary fructose intolerance (when there is ingestion of fructose or sucrose, in the neonate usually a soy formula), tyrosinemia type I, neonatal hemochromatosis, and mitochondrial diseases can also present predominantly with liver dysfunction in the neonate. Cholestatic jaundice with failure to thrive is observed primarily in alpha-1-antitrypsin deficiency, Byler disease, and Niemann-Pick disease type C.
5. **Dysmorphic features.** Several IEM can present with facial dysmorphism (see Table 29D.1). Congenital disorders of glycosylation and some lysosomal storage diseases can present with hydrops fetalis (see Table 29D.2).

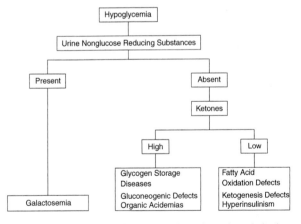

Figure 29D.2. Approach to the investigation of persistent hypoglycemia in the newborn with suspected inborn errors of metabolism (IEM).

TABLE 29D.1 Inborn Errors of Metabolism Associated with Dysmorphic Features

Disorder	Dysmorphic features
Peroxisomal disorders Zellweger syndrome	Large fontanelle, prominent forehead, flat nasal bridge, epicanthal folds, hypoplastic supraorbital ridges
Pyruvate dehydrogenase deficiency	Epicanthal folds, flat nasal bridge, small nose with anteverted flared alae nasi, long philtrum
Glutaric aciduria type II	Macrocephaly, high forehead, flat nasal bridge, short anteverted nose, ear anomalies, hypospadias, rocker-bottom feet
Cholesterol biosynthetic defects Smith-Lemli-Opitz syndrome	Epicanthal folds, flat nasal bridge, toe 2/3 syndactyly, genital abnormalities, cataracts
Congenital disorders of glycosylation	Inverted nipples, lipodystrophy
Lysosomal storage disorders I-cell disease	Hurler-like phenotype

6. **Cardiac disease.** Long-chain fatty acid oxidation defects and mitochondrial respiratory chain defects can present with cardiomyopathy, arrhythmias, and hypotonia in neonates (see Table 29D.3). The neonatal form of Pompe disease, a lysosomal disorder with glycogen storage, presents with generalized hypotonia, failure to thrive, and cardiomyopathy.

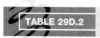

TABLE 29D.2 Inborn Errors of Metabolism Associated with Hydrops Fetalis

Lysosomal disorders
Mucopolysaccharidosis types I, IVA, and VII
GM1 gangliosidosis
Gaucher disease
Niemann-Pick disease type C
Sialidosis
Galactosialidosis
Farber disease

Hematologic disorders
Glucose-6-phosphate dehydrogenase deficiency
Pyruvate kinase deficiency
Glucosphosphate isomerase deficiency

Others
Congenital disorders of glycosylation
Neonatal hemochromatosis
Respiratory chain disorders
Glycogen storage disease type IV

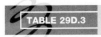

TABLE 29D.3	Inborn Errors of Metabolism Associated with Neonatal Cardiomyopathy

Disorders of fatty acid oxidation
 Carnitine uptake deficiency
 Carnitine–acylcarnitine translocase (CAT) deficiency
 Carnitine palmitoyltransferase II (CPT II) deficiency
 Long-chain 3-hydroxyacyl-CoA dehydrogenase deficiency (LCHADD)
 Trifunctional protein deficiency
 Very long chain acyl-CoA dehydrogenase deficiency (VLCADD)

Mitochondrial respiratory chain disorders

Tricarboxylic acid cycle defects
 α-Ketoglutarate dehydrogenase deficiency

GSDs
 Pompe disease (GSD type II)
 Phosphorylase b kinase deficiency

Lysosomal storage disorders
 I-cell disease

GSD = glycogen storage disorder.

---

   7. Abnormal urine odor. Abnormal urine odors can best be detected in a drying filter paper or by opening a container that has been closed at room temperature for a few minutes. Table 29D.4 lists IEM associated with characteristic odors.

IV. INITIAL EVALUATION OF A NEONATE WITH SUSPECTED IEM. Initial screening of a sick newborn infant with a suspected underlying metabolic disease should include the investigations listed in Table 29D.5. The first line laboratory studies can be performed by any clinical laboratory and should be obtained immediately once IEM is suspected. The results of these simple tests can provide important information about the underlying disease and help to narrow down the specialized tests required for definitive diagnosis.

   A. Initial evaluation

   1. The complete blood cell count should include examination of cell morphology as well as differential cell count. Neutropenia and thrombocytopenia may be associated with a number of organic acidemias (isovaleric acidemia [IVA], methylmalonic acidemia [MMA], and propionic acidemia [PPA]). Neutropenia

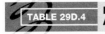

TABLE 29D.4	Inborn Errors of Metabolism Associated with Abnormal Urine Odor in Newborns

Inborn error of metabolism	**odor**
Glutaric acidemia (type II)	Sweaty feet
Isovaleric acidemia	Sweaty feet
Maple syrup urine disease	Maple syrup
Hypermethioninemia	Boiled cabbage
Multiple carboxylase deficiency	Tomcat urine

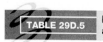

TABLE 29D.5	Laboratory Studies for a Newborn Suspected of Having an Inborn Error of Metabolism

First line laboratory studies
Complete blood count with differential
Serum electrolytes, calcium, magnesium
Blood glucose
Blood gases
Plasma ammonia
Plasma lactate, pyruvate
Liver function tests
Urine-reducing substances
Urine ketones if acidosis or hypoglycemia present

Second line laboratory studies
Plasma amino acids, quantitative
Urine organic acids
Plasma carnitine and acylcarnitine profile
Plasma uric acid
Cerebrospinal fluid (CSF) amino acids
Peroxisomal function tests
Plasma and urine for storage at 20°C

may also be found with glycogen storage disease type 1b and respiratory chain defects, such as Barth syndrome and Pearson syndrome.

2. **Electrolytes and blood gases** are required to determine whether an acidosis or alkalosis is present and, if so, whether the abnormality is associated with an increased anion gap. The organic acidemias and the primary lactic acidosis cause metabolic acidosis with a raised anion gap in early stages. Most metabolic conditions result in acidosis in late stages as encephalopathy and circulatory disturbances progress. A persistent metabolic acidosis with normal tissue perfusion may suggest an organic acidemia or a congenital lactic acidosis. A mild respiratory alkalosis in nonventilated babies suggests hyperammonemia. However, in late stages of hyperammonemia, vasomotor instability and collapse can cause metabolic acidosis.

3. **Glucose.** Hypoglycemia is a critical finding in some IEM. Ketones are useful in developing a differential diagnosis for newborns with hypoglycemia (Fig. 29D.2). Nonketotic hypoglycemia is the hallmark of defects of fatty acid oxidation. Hypoglycemia associated with metabolic acidosis and ketones suggests an organic acidemia or defect of gluconeogenesis (glycogen storage disease type I or fructose 1,6-biphosphatase deficiency).

4. **Plasma ammonia level** should be determined in all sick neonates, especially those with unexplained lethargy and neurologic intoxication. Early recognition of severe neonatal hyperammonemia is crucial since irreversible damage can occur within hours.

5. **Plasma lactate level.** A high plasma lactate can be secondary to hypoxia, cardiac disease, infection, or seizures, whereas primary lactic acidosis may be caused by disorders of pyruvate metabolism and respiratory chain defects. Some IEM (fatty acid oxidation disorders, organic acidemias, and UCDs) may also be associated with a secondary lactic acidosis. Persistent increase of plasma lactate above 3 mmol/L in a neonate who did not suffer from asphyxia and who has no evidence of other organ failure should lead to further investigation for an

IEM (Fig. 29D.1). Specimens for lactate measurement should be obtained from a central line or through an arterial stick since use of tourniquet during venous sampling may result in a spurious increase in lactate.

6. **Liver function tests (LFTs).** Galactosemia is the most common metabolic cause of liver dysfunction in the newborn period. Other causes of abnormal LFTs in the newborn include tyrosinemia, alpha-1-antitrypsin deficiency, neonatal hemochromatosis, mitochondrial respiratory chain disorders, and Niemann-Pick disease type C.

7. **Urine ketones.** The presence of ketonuria is abnormal in neonates. Excessive urinary excretion of ketones (acetone and acetoacetate) can be investigated with the Acetest or Ketostix reactions. The dinitrophenylhydrazine (DNPH) test screens for the presence of α-ketoacids, such as those seen in MSUD.

8. **Urine-reducing substances.** Urine specimens should be tested for reducing substances. The Clinitest reaction detects excess excretion of galactose and glucose, but not fructose. A positive reaction with the Clinitest should be investigated further with the Clinistix reaction (glucose oxidase) that is specific for glucose.

B. **Second line evaluations**

1. **Plasma amino acid analysis.** Plasma amino acid analysis is indicated for any infant suspected of having IEM. A biochemical geneticist who is informed of the patient's clinical presentation and nutritional status should evaluate the results.

2. **Urine organic acid analysis** is indicated for patients with unexplained metabolic acidosis, seizures, hyperammonemia, hypoglycemia, and/or ketonuria.

3. **Plasma carnitine and acylcarnitine profile.** Carnitine transports long-chain fatty acids across the inner mitochondrial membrane. An elevation of carnitine esters may be seen in fatty acid oxidation defects, organic acidemias, and ketosis. In addition to patients with inherited disorders of carnitine biosynthesis, low carnitine levels are common in preterm infants and neonates receiving total parenteral nutrition (PN) without adequate carnitine supplementation. Several metabolic diseases may cause secondary carnitine deficiency.

4. **Plasma uric acid** test is a convenient screen for the few IEM that are associated with either hyperuricemia (type I glycogen storage disease) or hypouricemia (xanthine dehydrogenase deficiency).

5. **Cerebrospinal fluid (CSF) amino acids.** NKH is diagnosed by the presence of an elevated CSF to plasma glycine ratio.

6. **Peroxisomal function tests** include plasma very long chain fatty acids (VLCFAs), phytanic acid, and erythrocyte plasmalogen levels.

V. **IEM THAT ARE POTENTIALLY LETHAL IN THE NEWBORN.** Information on diagnosis and acute management of many of these disorders is available at web site www.metabolicprotocols.org.

A. **Galactosemia**

1. **Inheritance and enzyme deficiency.** Galactosemia is inherited as an autosomal recessive trait and develops because of the deficiency of galactose-1-phosphate uridyl transferase (GALT).

2. **Clinical manifestations.** Typical symptoms of galactosemia in the newborn develop after ingestion of lactose (a disaccharide of glucose and galactose) through a standard formula or breast milk. Clinical manifestations include jaundice, hepatosplenomegaly, feeding difficulties and vomiting, hypoglycemia, lethargy, irritability, seizures, cataracts, and increased risk of *Escherichia coli* neonatal sepsis. Delayed diagnosis results in cirrhosis and mental retardation.

3. **Laboratory findings.** The preliminary diagnosis is made by demonstrating non–glucose-reducing substance in urine while the patient is receiving lactose-containing formula or breast milk. The reducing substance is found in urine by Clinitest and can be specifically identified by chromatography or by specific enzymatic test for galactose. The Clinistix urine test results are negative because these tests are based on the action of glucose oxidase and are therefore specific for glucose and are nonreactive with galactose. Semiquantitative assay of blood for galactose-1-phosphate uridyltransferase (GALT), known as the

Beutler test, can be performed on a newborn screening blood specimen by the newborn screening program. Almost all newborn screening programs screen for galactosemia. Newborns with galactosemia who have received a lactose-free formula from birth, however, may be missed on screening programs that test only for galactose but do not measure the GALT enzyme. Conversely, screening programs that depend on the GALT assay (Beutler test) will report the result as normal if the infant has received a blood transfusion.

4. **Management** consists of substituting a lactose-free formula for breast-feeding or for a standard formula, and, later, a galactose-free diet.

B. **Hereditary fructose intolerance**
1. **Inheritance and enzyme deficiency.** Autosomal recessive inheritance, deficiency of fructose 1,6-biphosphate aldolase (aldolase B).
2. **Clinical manifestations** develop when the neonate is exposed to fructose (from the sucrose, which is a glucose–fructose disaccharide, in soy-based formulas or later from fruits) in the diet. Early manifestations include hypoglycemia, jaundice, hepatomegaly, vomiting, lethargy, irritability, seizures, and abnormal LFTs.
3. **Laboratory findings.** The presence of galactosemia is suspected on the basis of hypoglycemia and clinical manifestations that may suggest galactosemia. However, the diagnosis of galactosemia is eliminated when reducing substance is absent in urine and blood GALT activity is normal. Definitive diagnosis is made by assay of fructaldolase activity in the liver or by deoxyribonucleic acid (DNA) analysis of point mutations in the *aldolase B* gene.
4. **Management** is done by elimination of sucrose, fructose, and sorbitol from the diet.

C. **MSUD**
1. **Inheritance and enzyme deficiency.** Autosomal recessive, deficiency of branched-chain α-ketoacid dehydrogenase.
2. **Manifestations.** Poor feeding and vomiting during the first week of life; lethargy, seizures and coma, hypertonicity and muscular rigidity with severe opisthotonus, maple syrup odor in body fluids.
3. **Laboratory findings.** High plasma and urine levels of leucine, isoleucine, alloisoleucine, valine, and their respective ketoacids. These ketoacids may be qualitatively detected in urine by adding a few drops of 2,4-DNPH reagent (0.1% in 0.1N HCl) to the urine; a yellow precipitate of 2,4-dinitrophenyl-hydrazone is formed in a positive test. Many newborn screening programs include MSUD.
4. **Management** is aimed at quick removal of the branched-chain amino acids and their metabolites from the tissues and body fluids. Hemodialysis is the most effective means of therapy in the sick neonate with ketoacidosis and markedly increased leucine and should be promptly initiated. Treatment after recovery from the acute state requires a special low branched-chain amino acid diet. Patients with MSUD should remain on the diet for the rest of their lives.

D. **Organic acidemias.** Branched-chain organic acidemias are a group of disorders that result from a deficiency of any of the degradative enzymes involving the catabolism of branched-chain amino acids valine, leucine, and isoleucine. Collectively, IVA, PPA, and MMA are the most commonly encountered organic acidemias in the neonatal period. These disorders have similar clinical and biochemical findings.
1. **IVA**
   a. **Inheritance and enzyme deficiency.** Autosomal recessive, deficiency of isovaleryl-CoA dehydrogenase.
   b. **Manifestations.** Vomiting (sometimes severe enough to suggest pyloric stenosis) and severe acidosis in the first few days of life, followed by lethargy, convulsions, coma, and death if proper therapy is not initiated. The characteristic unpleasant odor of "sweaty feet" may be present.
   c. **Laboratory findings.** Laboratory findings are severe ketoacidosis, neutropenia, thrombocytopenia, and occasionally pancytopenia, hyperammonemia,

and hypocalcemia. **Diagnosis** is established by demonstrating elevations of isovalerylcarnitine in blood and isovalerylglycine in urine. Measuring the enzyme in cultured skin fibroblasts or DNA analysis for mutations in the gene confirms the diagnosis. Newborn screening programs that have expanded metabolic screening include IVA. Antenatal diagnosis has been accomplished by measuring isovalerylglycine in amniotic fluid or by enzyme assay in cultured amniocytes.

d. **Management** of the acute attack is aimed at hydration, sodium bicarbonate infusion, and removal of the excess isovaleric acid. Glycine (250 mg/kg per 24 hours) and carnitine (100 mg/kg per 24 hours) administration is recommended to enhance excretion of isovaleric acid in urine. Hemodialysis may be needed if above measures fail. Chronic treatment includes a special low leucine diet.

2. PPA

a. **Inheritance and enzyme defect.** Autosomal recessive deficiency of propionyl-CoA carboxylase.

b. **Manifestations.** Poor feeding, vomiting, hypotonia, lethargy, dehydration, and clinical signs of acidosis progress rapidly to coma and death.

c. **Laboratory findings.** Laboratory findings are severe metabolic acidosis with a large anion gap, ketosis, neutropenia, thrombocytopenia, hypoglycemia, hyperglycinemia (ketotic hyperglycinemia due to inhibition of glycine cleavage enzyme by the high levels of accumulated organic acid) and hyperammonemia, elevated plasma propionylcarnitine, and plasma and urine concentrations of propionic acid and methylcitric acid. Newborn screening programs that have expanded metabolic screening include PPA.

d. **Management** of acute attacks include rehydration, correction of acidosis, and prevention of catabolic state by provision of adequate calories through parenteral hyperalimentation. To control the possible production of propionic acid by intestinal bacteria, sterilization of the intestinal tract flora by antibiotics (e.g., oral neomycin, metronidazole) should be promptly initiated. In patients with concomitant hyperammonemia, measures to reduce blood ammonia should be employed. Chronic treatment includes a special diet with only very small amounts of the offending amino acids and related metabolites.

3. MMA

a. **Inheritance and enzyme deficiency.** Autosomal recessive deficiency of methylmalonyl-CoA mutase or its B_{12} coenzyme adenosylcobalamin.

b. **Manifestations.** Identical to PPA in the sick neonate. The fulminant neonatal form is more common in patients with MMA than with PPA.

c. **Laboratory findings.** Large quantities of methylmalonic acid are detected in body fluids. Propionic acid and its metabolites 3-hydroxypropionate and methylcitrate are also found in urine. Newborn screening programs that have expanded metabolic screening include MMA.

d. **Management** is similar to PPA, except that large doses of vitamin B_{12} are used.

E. **Hyperammonemia syndromes.** Figure 29D.3 summarizes the approach to neonatal hyperammonemia.

1. Transient hyperammonemia is manifested in premature babies by respiratory distress during the first 24 hours of life and may progress to seizures and coma within 48 hours. Ammonia levels may exceed 1,000 μmol/L and require vigorous treatment. Asymptomatic transient hyperammonemia (range 40–72 μmol/L), on the other hand, is not associated with any short-term or long-term neurologic deficits.

2. UCDs

a. **Inheritance.** Besides the X-linked OTC deficiency, UCD are inherited as autosomal recessive traits. There are six disorders in the urea cycle, each due to a specific enzyme deficiency.

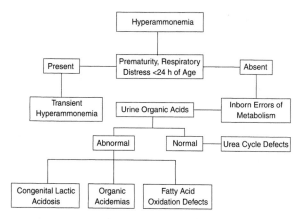

Figure 29D.3. Approach to neonatal hyperammonemia.

b. **Manifestations.** Infants with complete urea cycle enzyme deficiencies present with poor feeding, vomiting, lethargy, hypotonia, and hyperventilation between 1 and 5 days of age. These patients may develop seizures, apnea, coma, and increased intracranial pressure unless hyperammonemia is diagnosed and treated promptly. Since almost all neonates with UCD are initially thought to be septic, the plasma ammonia level should be measured in all septic-appearing patients without microbiologic evidence of infection.

c. **Laboratory findings.** In neonatal-onset UCD, ammonia levels are usually higher than 300 μmol/L and are often in the range of 500 to 1,500 μmol/L. Respiratory alkalosis secondary to hyperventilation is an important initial clue for the diagnosis of a UCD. Other laboratory abnormalities may include mild serum liver enzyme elevations and coagulopathy. Before initiation of therapy, samples should be sent for plasma amino acid analysis and for urinary amino acid, organic acid, and orotic acid determination. Plasma and urine should be frozen for future testing. These tests will help identify the cause of hyperammonemia (see Figs. 29D.3 and 29D.4). Newborn screening programs that have expanded metabolic screening include some of the UCD.

d. **Management.** All neonates with symptomatic hyperammonemia should be transferred to a level III neonatal unit with hemodialysis facilities. Dialysis is the only means for rapid removal of ammonia from blood in acute neonatal hyperammonemia, and hemodialysis is preferred over peritoneal dialysis because it is much more effective. All feedings containing protein should be discontinued and administration of intravenous (IV) 10% glucose and fluids should be started before transport. Calories should be provided as IV glucose and lipids. IV therapy with ammonia-scavenging drugs should be started when ammonia elevation causes any central nervous system symptoms. For acute neonatal hyperammonemic coma from carbamyl phosphate synthetase I (CPS) and OTC deficiency, give a loading dose of 200 mg/kg L-arginineHCL and 2.5 mL/kg Ammonul (contains sodium benzoate 100 mg and sodium phenylacetate 100 mg/mL) in 25 mL/kg of 10% dextrose solution over a 90-minute period and then the same doses daily for sustained infusion. For citrullinemia and argininosuccinic acidemia, give the same except increase the L-arginineHCl dose to 600 mg/kg for loading and sustained infusions. For arginase deficiency, use the same regimen of Ammonul for loading and sustained infusions, but omit L-arginineHCl. For argininosuccinic acidemia, if the neonate is not critically ill and the hyperammonemia is only mild,

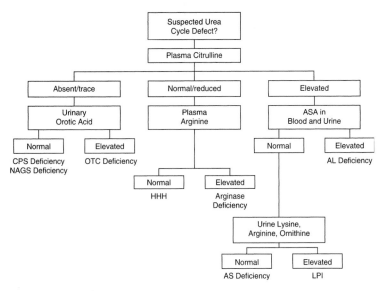

Figure 29D.4. Approach to differential diagnosis of suspected urea cycle defect. ASA = argininosuccinic acid; CPS = carbamyl phosphate synthetase I; NAGS = N-acetyl glutamate synthase; OTC = ornithine transcarbamylase; AL = argininosuccinic acid lyase; AS = argininosuccinic acid synthetase; LPI = lysinuric protein intolerance; HHH = hyperornithinemia, hyperammonemia, homocitrullinuria. (Adapted from protocol of Korson M. Boston: New England Medical Center, Tufts University.)

arginine therapy alone may suffice. IV therapy with ammonia-scavenging drugs for all of the urea cycle disorders should be continued while dialysis is being performed. A repeat loading dose of ammonia-scavenging drugs should be given only in neonates with very severe illness who are receiving dialysis. Toxicity is associated with high drug doses (750 mg/kg/day and higher).

F. Nonketotic hyperglycinemia (NKH)
    1. Inheritance and enzyme deficiency. Autosomal recessive deficiency of the glycine cleavage complex characterized by defective glycine degradation and glycine accumulation in tissues.
    2. Clinical manifestations. Patients with neonatal form of NKH present with lethargy, hypotonia, and poor feeding within a few days of birth. Seizures, hiccups, and apneic episodes are common. Electroencephalogram (EEG) shows the characteristic burst-suppression pattern. Most of these infants die within a few weeks of life; survivors develop severe psychomotor retardation. In transient NKH, which is secondary to the immaturity of glycine cleavage enzymes, laboratory and clinical abnormalities return to normal by 2 to 8 weeks of age.
    3. Laboratory findings. Diagnosis is established by the findings of elevated glycine levels in body fluids and an elevated CSF/plasma glycine ratio. Measurement of glycine cleavage system activity in hepatocytes confirms the diagnosis.
    4. Management. There is no known effective treatment for NKH. However, large amounts of sodium benzoate may reduce the seizure frequency.

G. Holocarboxylase synthetase (HCS) deficiency (multiple carboxylase deficiency — infantile or early form)
    1. Inheritance and enzyme deficiency. HCS is inherited as an autosomal recessive trait. HCS catalyzes the binding of biotin with the inactive apocarboxylases, leading to carboxylase activation. Deficiency of this enzyme causes malfunction of all carboxylases and is fatal unless diagnosed and treated rapidly.

2. **Clinical manifestations.** Affected infants become symptomatic in the first few weeks of life with respiratory distress, hypotonia, seizures, vomiting, and failure to thrive. The urine may have a peculiar odor (tomcat urine). Skin manifestations include generalized erythematous rash with exfoliation and alopecia totalis. These infants may also have an immunodeficiency manifested by a decrease in the number of T cells.

3. **Laboratory findings** include metabolic acidosis, ketosis, organic aciduria, and hyperammonemia. Diagnosis is confirmed by measuring the enzyme activity in lymphocytes or cultured fibroblasts. Prenatal diagnosis is available.

4. **Management.** Almost all patients respond to treatment with very large amounts of biotin (10–80 mg/day), although in some affected neonates the response may be only partial.

H. **Mitochondrial disorders.** The principal function of mitochondria is to produce adenosine triphosphate (ATP) from the oxidation of fatty acids and sugars through the electron transport chain. Therefore, tissues that are more dependent on aerobic metabolism, such as brain, muscle, and heart, are more likely to be affected in these disorders. Relatively common mitochondrial disorders with potentially lethal presentations in the neonate fall into three main subgroups:

1. **Defects in the carnitine cycle.** Carnitine is required for the transfer of long-chain fatty acids into the mitochondrial matrix for their oxidation. Defects include primary carnitine deficiency and deficiencies in carnitine palmitoyltransferase I (CPTI), carnitine–acylcarnitine translocase, and carnitine palmitoyltransferase II (CPTII). Each of these defects can cause neonatal onset of seizures, cardiac arrhythmias, and apnea. Laboratory studies show nonketotic hypoglycemia, and in some cases hyperammonemia. The plasma free carnitine level is high in CPTI deficiency and low in the other defects.

2. **Defects of fatty acid oxidation**
   a. Very long chain acyl-CoA dehydrogenase deficiency (VLCADD) and LCHADD can present in the neonatal period with hypotonia, cardiomyopathy, and hypoketotic hypoglycemia.
   b. Medium chain acyl-CoA dehydrogenase deficiency (MCADD) can present acutely in the neonate with hypoketotic hypoglycemia, metabolic acidosis, hyperammonemia, and hepatomegaly with abnormal LFTs.

3. **Defects of pyruvate metabolism**
   a. Pyruvate dehydrogenase complex (PDHC) deficiency can present with severe lactic acidosis, hypotonia, feeding and breathing abnormalities, seizures, dysmorphic facial features (Table 29D.2), agenesis of corpus callosum, and white matter abnormalities. Diagnosis is confirmed by measuring PDH activity in cultured fibroblasts. It is usually an X-linked disorder with the most severe illness in male babies.
   b. Pyruvate carboxylase deficiency can present with lactic acidosis, profound hypotonia, and seizures in the neonatal period.

I. **Peroxisomal disorders.** Zellweger syndrome, neonatal adrenoleukodystrophy (ALD), and infantile Refsum disease represent a continuum, with the Zellweger syndrome being the most severe one. In all three disorders, the basic defect is the failure of peroxisomal biogenesis, that is, to assemble peroxisomes. Newborn infants with Zellweger syndrome have dysmorphic facies (Table 29D.2), severe weakness and hypotonia, neonatal seizures, and eye abnormalities. Patients with neonatal ALD show fewer dysmorphic features. Neonatal seizures are common. The diagnosis is established by measurement of VLCFAs and other metabolites that are elevated secondary to the defect in peroxisome structure.

VI. **MANAGEMENT OF INFANT AT RISK FOR A METABOLIC DISORDER**

A. When a sibling has had symptoms consistent with a metabolic disorder, or has died of a metabolic disorder, the following steps should be taken:

1. **Preliminary considerations before or during subsequent pregnancy**
   a. Old hospital charts and postmortem material should be reviewed.
   b. There should be a prenatal discussion of possible diagnoses, and the parents and relatives should be screened for possible clues to diagnosis.

    c. When a diagnosis is known, intrauterine diagnosis by measurement of abnormal metabolites in the amniotic fluid or by enzyme assay or DNA analysis of amniocytes obtained by amniocentesis should be considered.

    d. The new baby should be delivered in a facility equipped to handle potential metabolic or other complications, preferably closely associated with a laboratory capable of performing or arranging the necessary diagnostic tests.

2. Initial evaluation includes a careful physical examination, seeking any of the signs described in III. All nonmetabolic causes of symptoms such as infection or asphyxia should be excluded. Careful examination of the eyes, skin, and liver should also be performed. The newborn screening program should be contacted for the results of the screening and for a list of the disorders screened. Tests should be targeted toward the hereditary anomaly, if it is known. Blood and urine tests should be obtained as summarized in Table 29D.5. It is important to obtain these specimens at the time of presentation before starting treatment for metabolic disease. The specimens can be frozen (plasma, urine) and analysis performed later. Enzyme assay of red blood cells, or enzyme and DNA analysis of white blood cells, fibroblasts, or liver tissue may be done for confirmation of diagnosis. DNA analysis can sometimes be performed on a dried blood specimen (Guthrie blood spot).

3. Initial feedings for the asymptomatic infant at risk for metabolic disease will vary with the diagnosis; for example, in disorders of protein metabolism, the infant may be given IV glucose or fed 10% glucose or dextrose polymer (Polycose, Ross Laboratories, Columbus, OH) as tolerated. This may be followed by fat in the form of medium chain triglycerides (e.g., Product 80056, Mead Johnson Laboratories, Evansville, IN). However, before feeding medium chain triglycerides, it is very important to be certain that the infant does not have a short chain or medium chain fatty acid oxidation disorder (SCADD or MCADD); otherwise these triglycerides could provoke a very severe metabolic reaction. If the results of tests performed at 48 hours are all negative, protein may be introduced in the form of breast milk or any low-protein milk.

    The tests are repeated after 48 hours of protein intake. If no abnormalities are found, the child may be cautiously fed. If metabolic abnormalities are found, the specific problem should be identified and the appropriate diet or treatment started.

    The initial feeding will vary with the type of suspected disorder. Many special products are available for various metabolic diseases. More information about these products is available through the following companies' web sites:

        http://www.meadjohnson.com/app/iwp/HCP/Content2.do?dm=mj&id=/HCP_Home/Product_Information/Product_Descriptions

        http://www.ross.com/productHandbook/metabolic.asp (Ross Products)

        http://www.shsna.com/pages/products.htm

        http://www.medicalfood.com (Applied Nutrition Corp.)

B. When an infant has signs or symptoms of an acute metabolic disease, the condition should be managed as follows:

    1. Other causes of the symptoms should be ruled out, for example, asphyxia, infection, or intracranial hemorrhage. Even when one of these is the likely cause, if an inborn error cannot be ruled out, obtain acute specimens and keep frozen.

    2. Tests as described in IV should be performed. The newborn screening program should be immediately contacted for the newborn screening results and for a list of disorders screened. Note that organic acids and ammonia are toxic to the brain, and accumulation of these substances may result in cerebral edema. Caution should be exercised when the need for lumbar puncture is considered in a situation where sepsis should be ruled out.

    3. The therapy for acute metabolic decompensation in these disorders includes the following:

        a. Hydration.

b. Correction of the biochemical abnormalities (metabolic acidosis, hyperammonemia, hypoglycemia).

c. Reversal of catabolism/promotion of anabolism.

d. Elimination of toxic metabolites, for example, by hemodialysis.

e. Treatment of the precipitating factor when possible (e.g., infection, excess protein ingestion).

f. Cofactor supplementation.

4. The infant should be adequately hydrated, and provided with glucose (and in some cases lipids) to prevent catabolism and with alkali to treat acidosis.

   a. The patient should be kept nothing by mouth (NPO) for 1 to 2 days and with IV glucose in high doses. Added insulin should be considered if metabolic stability cannot be achieved (see Chap. 29A). If a diagnosis is not available, a protein source at 0.5 g/kg/day by PN or enteral formula is given with other non-nitrogenous caloric supplements (carbohydrates and fats).

   In galactosemia, the infant can be fed a lactose-free formula immediately. Ringer lactate should not be used for fluid or electrolyte therapy in a child with a known or suspected metabolic disorder.

   b. In undiagnosed cases of acidosis, when the lactate and pyruvate are markedly elevated, the possibility of a **disorder of pyruvate metabolism** must be considered. In pyruvate dehydrogenase deficiency specifically, excess glucose will make the acidosis worse. Glucose and lactate levels should be monitored. In this disorder, lipids are given to prevent catabolism. Small amounts of glucose are given only to keep the blood glucose normal.

5. If the infant is acidotic (pH <7.22) or the bicarbonate level is <14 mEq/L, give $NaHCO_3$ (1 mEq/kg) as a bolus followed by a continuous infusion of bicarbonate. If hypernatremia is a problem, use potassium acetate as part of the solution.

6. **Correct hypoglycemia** (see Chap. 29A).

7. **Lipids.** Intralipid may be given to supply extra calories. Intralipid is composed of even-chain fatty acids, so it is not contraindicated in PPA and MMA.

8. **Calories.** Caloric consumption during a period of decompensation, in order to support anabolism, should be at least 20% greater than that needed for ordinary maintenance. One must remember that withholding natural protein from the diet also eliminates this source of calories, which should be replaced using other dietary or nutritional (non-nitrogenous) sources.

9. **Insulin.** Insulin is a potent anabolic hormone, promoting protein and lipid synthesis. It will allow extra glucose to be metabolized and prevent hyperglycemia (see Chap. 29A).

10. **Protein.** All natural protein (containing amino acids) should be withheld for 48 to 72 hours while the patient is acutely ill. Afterward, amino acid therapy may be very beneficial in facilitating clinical improvement, but it should be implemented only under the supervision of a physician/nutritionist with expertise in metabolic management. Special parenteral amino acid solutions and specialized formulas are available for many disorders.

11. **Elimination of toxic metabolites.** Correction of acute metabolic perturbations (acidosis, hypoglycemia, dehydration) may help clear some of the factors contributing to the encephalopathy associated with acute metabolic crisis. However, large quantities of toxic intermediate metabolites, believed to be toxic to the brain as well, are not cleared with glucose or bicarbonate. Hydration promotes renal excretion of toxins. Consideration should be given for providing the means to facilitate the excretion of these compounds.

    a. L-Carnitine. Free carnitine levels are low in the organic acidemias because of increased esterification with organic acid metabolites. Whereas the benefit of carnitine supplementation is controversial, there is evidence that carnitine facilitates excretion of these metabolites. If administered, it should be mixed in 10% glucose and given as an infusion to provide 25 to 100 mg/kg per 24-hour period. When oral fluids are tolerated, carnitine may be administered PO at a dose of 100 to 400 mg/kg/day. Diarrhea is the primary adverse effect of oral carnitine.

    b. Antibiotics. For certain organic acidemias (e.g., PPA, MMA), gut bacteria are a significant source of organic acid synthesis (e.g., propionic acid). Eradicating the gut flora with a short course of a broad-spectrum antibiotic (e.g., neomycin, metronidazole) orally or intravenously may speed the recovery of a patient in acute crisis. In a newborn with galactosemia, there is a significant risk of sepsis, particularly gram-negative sepsis due to *E. coli.* Acute PPA and MMA are often associated with neutropenia as well as thrombocytopenia.

    c. In hyperammonemia due to a urea cycle disorder, a mixture of sodium benzoate and sodium phenylacetate may be used in addition to glucose, lipids, and electrolytes to facilitate the removal of ammonia (see V.E.2d). Arginine is given in all the UCDs except arginase deficiency to prevent arginine deficiency and to stimulate further excretion of waste nitrogen by stimulating the activity of ornithine transcarboxylase. When ammonia levels exceed 500 to 600 mg/dL, hemodialysis is far more effective in reducing them.

    d. Hemodialysis is indicated in cases of intractable metabolic acidosis, unresponsive hyperammonemia ($>500–600$ mg/dL), coma, or severe (usually iatrogenic) electrolyte disturbances.

  12. Treatment of precipitating factors. Infection should be treated vigorously when possible. Neutropenia (and thrombocytopenia) frequently accompanies metabolic decomposition. Bone marrow recovery can be expected once the levels of toxic metabolites have diminished significantly.

  13. Cofactor supplementation. Pharmacologic doses of appropriate cofactors may be useful in cases of vitamin-responsive enzyme deficiencies.

  14. Monitoring the patient. The patient should be monitored closely for any mental status changes, overall fluid balance, evidence of bleeding (if thrombocytopenic), and symptoms of infection (if neutropenic). Biochemical parameters including electrolytes, measured CO_2, glucose, ammonia, blood gases, Complete blood cell count (CBC) with differential, platelets, urine for ketones, and urine specific gravity at every voiding should be followed.

  15. Recovery. The patient should be kept NPO until his or her mental status is more stable. Anorexia, nausea, and vomiting during the acute crisis period make significant oral intake unlikely. If the patient is not significantly neurologically compromised, consideration should be given to providing the patient (PO or by nasogastric [NG] tube) with a modified formula preparation containing all but the offending amino acids. When the infant is able to take oral feedings, a specific diet must be used. The diet will be individualized for each child and his or her metabolic defect.

VII. POSTMORTEM DIAGNOSIS. If an infant is dying or has died of what may be a metabolic disease, it is very important to make a specific diagnosis in order to help the parents with genetic counseling for future reproductive planning. Sometimes families that will not permit a full autopsy will allow the collection of some premortem or immediately postmortem specimens that may help in diagnosis. Specimens that should be collected include the following:

  A. Blood, both clotted and heparinized. The specimen should be centrifuged and the plasma frozen. Lymphocytes may be saved for culture.

  B. Urine, refrigerated.

  C. Spinal fluid, refrigerated.

  D. Skin biopsy for fibroblast culture to be used for chromosomal analysis or enzyme assay. Two samples should be taken from a well-perfused area in the torso. The skin should be well cleaned, but any residual cleaning solution should be washed off with sterile water. The skin can be placed briefly in sterile saline until special media are available.

E. Liver biopsy samples, both premortem samples and generous-size postmortem samples, should be flash-frozen to preserve enzyme integrity as well as tissue histology.

F. Others. Depending on the nature of the disease, other tissues such as skeletal muscle, cardiac muscle, brain, and kidney should be preserved.

Photographs should be taken and a full skeletal radiologic screening done of any infant with dysmorphic features. A full autopsy should be done if permitted. Information on the proper handling of the tissue should be obtained from one of the regional information centers (see VIII).

VIII. REGIONAL INFORMATION CENTERS. Metabolic problems in the newborn are complicated and require sophisticated diagnosis and treatment. There are regional centers for assistance with these problems. More information about regional centers can be found at the following web addresses:

http://www.meadjohnson.com/app/iwp/HCP/Content2.do?dm=mj&id=
/HCP_Home/Product_Information/Product_Descriptions
http://www.geneclinics.org.

IX. ROUTINE NEWBORN SCREENING. Each state in the United States mandates its own newborn screening program. Recent advances have enabled tandem mass spectrometry (MS/MS) to be applied to the newborn screening specimen. This technique is currently being used in several states to offer screening for many treatable IEM. Routine newborn screening always includes phenylketonuria and congenital hypothyroidism, almost always includes MSUD, galactosemia, and sickle cell disease, and very often includes congenital adrenal hyperplasia and biotinidase deficiency. Information about abnormal newborn screening findings, possible disorders represented by each abnormality, and basic information about each disorder can be found in the article by James and Levy cited in the reference list. Very useful information for follow-up of newborn screening ("ACT Sheets") and for confirmation of a disorder identified by newborn screening ("Algorithms") is available on the web site of the American College of Medical Genetics: www.acmg.net/resources/policies/ACT/condition-analyte-links.htm

Suggested Readings

Behrman ER, Kliegman R, Jensen H, et al. eds. Metabolic diseases. *Nelson textbook of pediatrics*, 16th ed. Philadelphia: WB Saunders, 2000.

Browning MF, Levy HL, Wilkins-Haug LE, et al. Fetal fatty acid oxidation defects and maternal liver disease in pregnancy. *Obstet Gynecol* 2006;107:115.

Burton BK. Inborn errors of metabolism in infancy: A guide to diagnosis. *Pediatrics* 1998;102:e69.

Chakrapani A, Cleary MA, Wraight JE. Detection of inborn errors of metabolism in the newborn. *Arch Dis Child Neonatal Ed* 2001;84:205.

Enns GM, Packman S. Diagnosing inborn errors of metabolism in the newborn: Clinical features. *NeoReviews* 2001;2:183.

Enns GM, Packman S. Diagnosing inborn errors of metabolism in the newborn: Laboratory investigations. *NeoReviews* 2001;2:192.

James PM, Levy HL. The clinical aspects of newborn screening: Importance of newborn screening follow-up. *MRDD Res Rev* 2006;12:246–254.

Leonard JV, Morris AAM. Inborn errors of metabolism around time of birth. *Lancet* 2000;356:583.

Scaglia F, Longo N. Primary and secondary alterations in neonatal carnitine metabolism. *Semin Perinatol* 1999;23:152.

Scriver CR, Beaudet AL, Sly WS, et al. eds. *The metabolic and molecular bases of inherited disease*, Vols. I–IV. New York: McGraw-Hill, 2001.

Sue CM, Hirano M, DiMauro S, et al. Neonatal presentations of mitochondrial metabolic disorders. *Semin Perinatol* 1999;23:113.

Summar M, Tuchman M. Proceedings of a consensus conference for the management of patients with urea cycle disorders. *J Pediatr* 2001;138:S6.

The Urea Cycle Disorders Conference Group. Consensus statement from a conference for the management of patients with urea cycle disorders. *J Pediatr* 2001;138:S1.

Zinn AB. Inborn errors of metabolism. In: Fanaroff AA, Martin RJ, eds. *Neonatal-perinatal medicine*, 6th ed. St. Louis: Mosby, 1997.

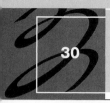

DISORDERS OF SEX DEVELOPMENT

Elizabeth T. Rosolowsky and Norman P. Spack

I. DEFINITION AND NOMENCLATURE. The term *disorders of sex development* (DSD) is preferred over older terms such as *ambiguous genitalia, pseudohermaphroditism,* and *intersex* to connote atypical development of genetic, gonadal, and phenotypic sex (see Table 30.1). The normal full-term male infant has a phallus length of at least 2.5 cm measured stretched from the pubic ramus to the tip of the glans (see Fig. 30.1). Testes usually migrate into the scrotum during the last 6 weeks of gestation. The normal full-term female infant has a clitoris <1 cm in length.

   A. Examples of DSD presenting in the newborn period include the infant with the following:

   1. A phallus and bilaterally nonpalpable testes.

   2. Unilateral cryptorchidism and hypospadias.

   3. Penoscrotal or perineoscrotal hypospadias, with or without microphallus, even if the testes are descended.

   4. Discordance of external genitalia compared with prenatal karyotype.

   5. Apparently female appearance with enlarged clitoris or inguinal hernia.

   6. Overt genital ambiguity such as cloacal exstrophy.

   7. Asymmetry of labioscrotal folds, with or without cryptorchidism.

   The internal genital anatomy, karyotype, and sex for rearing cannot be determined from the baby's external appearance; a thorough evaluation is required. The evaluation must be expedited because of conditions such as salt-losing congenital adrenal hyperplasia (CAH) that could be life-threatening in the first 2 to 4 weeks of life.

II. ASSIGNMENT OF A SEX FOR REARING. Rapidity in the determination of sex assignment is essential for the parents' peace of mind but must be balanced against prematurely drawing conclusions about gender. Most causes can be clarified in 2 to 4 days, although some cases may take 1 to 2 weeks or longer. Sex assignment depends on anatomy, functional prenatal and postnatal endocrinology, and the potential for sexual functioning and fertility, which may be independent of chromosomal sex. Until a gender assignment is made, gender-specific names or references should be withheld. Inappropriate statements may have profound psychosocial consequences for families. After the infant's genitalia are examined in their presence, the parents should be told about the process of genital differentiation; that their child's genitalia are incompletely or variably formed; and that further tests will clarify the problem and provide the necessary information to be able to assign the gender. If future hormonal therapy is necessary, parents should be told that it will help their child to live as normally as possible. Options for surgery on the internal and/or external genitalia should be discussed in the context of a team approach consisting of a pediatrician/neonatologist, pediatric endocrinologist, pediatric surgeon, and/or pediatric urologist, geneticist, and a counselor experienced in dealing with DSD. No guarantees should be made about fertility.

III. NORMAL SEXUAL DEVELOPMENT. The process of gonadal and genital differentiation is described in Fig. 30.2. Sex determination progresses in stages. At fertilization, **genetic sex** is determined. Under the influence of specific genes such as SRY (which encodes for testis-determining factor) located on the short arm of the Y chromosome, **gonadal sex** is determined by the seventh week of gestation. Specific ovarian-determining genes have also been identified. The 46,XX males and 46,XY females result from aberrant X-Y interchange during paternal meiosis.

TABLE 30.1	Proposed Revised Nomenclature
Previous	**Proposed**
Intersex	DSD
Male pseudohermaphrodite	46, XY DSD
Undervirilization of an XY male	"
Undermasculinization of an XY male	"
Female pseudohermaphrodite	46, XX DSD
Overvirilization of an XX female	"
Masculinization of an XX female	"
True hermaphrodite	Ovotesticular DSD
XX male or XX sex reversal	46, XX testicular DSD
XY sex reversal	46, XY complete gonadal dysgenesis

DSD = disorders of sex development.
From Hughes IA, Houk C, Ahmed SF, et al. LWPES Consensus Group, ESPE Consensus Group. Consensus statement on management of intersex disorders. *Arch Dis Child* 2006;91(7):554–563.

The testis secretes two hormones critical for genital formation: anti-müllerian hormone (AMH) from the Sertoli cells, which causes regression of the müllerian ducts (which would otherwise become uterus, fallopian tubes, and upper vagina), and testosterone from the Leydig cells, which promotes development of the Wolffian ducts (into the vas deferens, seminal vesicles, and epididymis). Müllerian duct regression and Wolffian duct development require high **local** concentrations of AMH and testosterone, respectively. Failure of a testis to develop on one side may result in

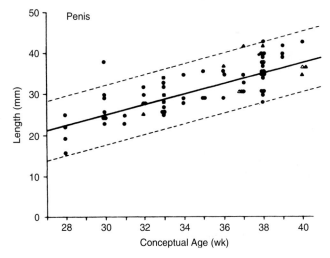

Figure 30.1. Stretched phallic length of normal premature and full-term babies (closed circles), showing lines of mean 2 standard deviations. Correlation coefficient is 0.80. Superimposed are data for two small-for-gestational-age infants (open triangles), seven large-for-gestational infants (closed triangles), and four twins (closed boxes), all of whom are in the normal range. (From Feldman KW, Smith DW. Fetal phallic growth and penile standards for newborn male infants. *J Pediatr* 1975;86:395.)

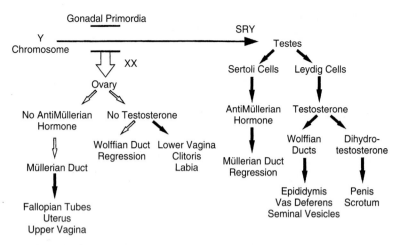

Figure 30.2. The process of gonadal, internal, and genital differentiation. (From Holm IA. Ambiguous genitalia in the newborn. In: Emans SJ, Laufer M, and Goldstein D, eds. *Pediatric and adolescent gynecology*. Philadelphia: Lippincott Williams & Wilkins, 1998:53.)

ipsilateral retention of müllerian structures and regression of Wolffian structures. The enzyme 5α-reductase, in high concentration in genital skin, converts testosterone to dihydrotestosterone (DHT), which is responsible for masculinizing of the genital tubercle and labioscrotal folds to form the penis and scrotum, respectively. Formation of normal male internal and external genitalia requires that the target tissues contain functional androgen receptors.

The time course of fetal sexual differentiation is depicted in Fig. 30.3 and Table 30.2. **Phenotypic sex** is established at the end of the first trimester. If a female infant is exposed to excessive androgens during the first trimester, her clitoris and labioscrotal folds will virilize and may appear indistinguishable from a normal male phallus and scrotum, although the latter will be empty. Exposure to testosterone during the second and third trimesters lead to clitoral enlargement and darkening and rugation of labioscrotal folds, but not labial fusion. Testosterone synthesis during the first trimester in the male fetus is stimulated primarily by placental human chorionic gonadotropin (hCG) due to its LH-like action. In the second and third trimesters, male phallic growth and scrotal maturation are dependent on testicular androgens stimulated by gonadotropins from the fetal pituitary. Endogenous growth hormone also contributes to penile growth. High intrauterine concentrations of testosterone may influence the brain in terms of later behavior and **gender identity** formation.

IV. NURSERY EVALUATION OF A NEWBORN WITH SUSPECTED DSD
A. History
1. **Family history** of hypospadias, CAH, cryptorchidism, infertility, consanguinity, or genetic syndromes.
2. **Maternal drug exposure** in pregnancy such as to synthetic androgens (e.g., Danazol), antiseizure medication (e.g., phenytoin, trimethadione), antiandrogens (e.g., finasteride, spironolactone), estrogens, or progestins.
3. **Maternal virilization** in pregnancy (maternal adrenal hyperplasia; virilizing adrenal or ovarian tumor; fetal aromatase deficiency).
4. **Neonatal deaths.** Death from vomiting/dehydration of a male sibling in early infancy, possibly from undiagnosed CAH. Genital manifestations of CAH from 21-hydroxylase deficiency in a male are subtle.
5. **Placental insufficiency** hCG initiates first-trimester synthesis of testosterone in the fetal testis.

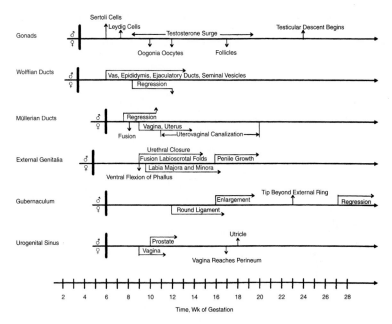

Figure 30.3. Timelines for five aspects of sexual differentiation. (From White PC, Speiser PW. Congenital adrenal hyperplasia due to 21-hydroxylase deficiency. *Endocr Rev.* 2000;21(3):245–291. Adapted from Barthold JS, Gonzalez R. Intersex states. In: Gonzalez ET, Bauer SB, eds. *Pediatric urology practice.* Philadelphia: Lippincott Williams & Wilkins, 1999;547–578.)

B. Physical examination
1. The examiner should note the stretched phallic length, width of the corpora, engorgement, presence of chordee, position of the urethral orifice, presence of a vaginal opening, and pigmentation and symmetry of the scrotum or labioscrotal folds. Posterior fusion of the labioscrotal folds is defined as an increased "anogenital ratio," which is determined by measuring the distance between the anus and posterior fourchette divided by the distance between the

TABLE 30.2	Timetable of Sexual Development

Days after conception	Events of sexual development
19	Primordial germ cells migrate to the genital ridge
40	Genital ridge forms an undifferentiated gonad
44	Müllerian ducts appear; testes develop
62	Müllerian inhibitor (from testes) becomes active
71	Testosterone synthesis begins (induced by placental chorionic gonadotropin)
72	Fusion of the labioscrotal swellings
73	Closure of the median raphe
74	Closure of the urethral groove
77	Müllerian regression is complete

anus and base of the clitoris. An anogenital ratio >0.5 is indicative of early intrauterine androgen exposure.

2. Gonadal size, position, and descent should be carefully noted. A gonad below the inguinal ligament is usually a testis, but an ovotestis and a uterus may present as a hernia. Genital ambiguity with clitoromegaly or an apparently well-formed phallus and an empty scrotum should raise immediate concern that the infant is a female virilized by CAH.

3. Bimanual rectal examination may reveal müllerian structures, e.g., a palpable cervix or uterus in the midline.

4. Associated anomalies: dysmorphic features suggest a more generalized disorder. Denys-Drash syndrome (Wilms tumor and nephropathy) or WAGR (**W**ilms tumor, **A**niridia, **G**enitourinary anomalies, and mental **R**etardation) syndrome can affect both 46,XY and 46,XX infants and are due to mutations of the WT1 gene on 11p13. Other syndromes associated with genital ambiguity include Smith-Lemli-Opitz, Robinow and Goldenhar syndromes, and trisomy 13.

5. Circumcision is contraindicated until a determination is made concerning the need for surgical reconstruction.

C. Diagnostic tests

1. **Laboratory tests** are tailored to the differential diagnosis, although baseline serum electrolytes, blood urea nitrogen (BUN), creatinine, 17-hydroxyprogesterone, creatinine, 17-hydroxyprogesterone, plasma renin activity, testosterone, gonadotropins, and AMH are included or considered. **Chromosome analysis** on peripheral blood can be performed using standard techniques within 72 hours and more rapidly through fluorescent *in situ* hybridization (FISH). A standard karyotype may reveal 46,XX, but portions of the Y chromosome containing the SRY gene may be translocated to an X chromosome. FISH techniques may be required to locate or confirm Y material.

2. **Pelvic ultrasonography,** especially when the bladder is full, can determine whether a uterus is present. Testes can often be visualized, ovaries less well. Magnetic resonance imaging (MRI) may be needed to locate intra-abdominal testes.

3. **Vesicourethrogram (VCUG) or genitogram.** These studies may reveal a vagina with cervix at its apex or a utricle (a müllerian duct remnant).

V. 46,XX DSD (VIRILIZED 46,XX FEMALES). The infant has normally developed müllerian structures and no Wolffian structures but has evidence of external genital virilization.

A. The most common form of genital ambiguity is a female infant with CAH from 21-hydroxylase (21-OH in Fig. 30.4) deficiency due to mutations in the gene CYP21. Virilization may occur in other adrenogenital syndromes: 11β-hydroxylase (11-OH or CYP11B1) deficiency or 3β-hydroxysteroid dehydrogenase (3β-HSD or HSD3B2) deficiency. CYP11B1 deficiency also presents with hypertension, whereas CYP21 and HSD3B2 deficiency may progress to hypovolemic shock if diagnosis is delayed.

1. State newborn screening programs may include screening for CYP21 deficiency. Blood spot measurements on filter-paper of 17-hydroxyprogesterone (17-OHP) are ideally performed between 48 and 72 hours postnatal age. An abnormal test is flagged when 17-OHP levels exceed **50 ng/mL (5,000 ng/dL)** 24 hours after birth in affected full-term infants. Normal values must be determined for each individual program because they depend on the filter-paper thickness and the radioimmunoassay used. In 90% of infants with adrenogenital syndrome, the 17-OHP will be elevated. Worldwide newborn screening programs for 17-OHP show an incidence of 1:15,000 births; the incidence varies markedly by country. Salt-losers outnumber simple virilizers by 3:1. The male:female sex ratio is 1:1. The diagnosis of CYP21 deficiency in boys is difficult to make by phenotype alone, although hyperpigmentation of the scrotum can be a clue. False-positive results occur in sick, premature, and low birth weight infants. Rapid turnaround of results is critical to avert salt-wasting crises. Abnormal results should be confirmed by serum measurements of 17-OHP on the second or third day

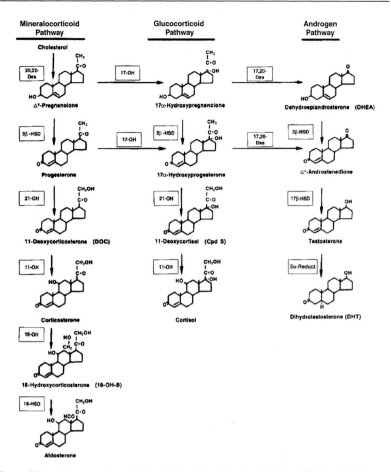

Figure 30.4. Pathways of steroid biosynthesis. (From Esoterix, 4301 Lost Hills Road, Calabasas Hills, CA 91301.)

of age. Measurements of plasma renin activity and aldosterone may also help differentiate between the salt-wasting and simple-virilizing forms. Serum electrolytes should be monitored at least every other day until salt-wasting status is determined. Levels of 11-deoxycorticosterone would be elevated and hypertension present in an infant with CYP11B1 deficiency. A female infant virilized from HSD3B2 deficiency would not be expected to have elevated 17-OHP on newborn screen.

2. Virilized females suspected of 21-hydroxylase deficiency should be started on hydrocortisone 20 mg/m²/day, divided into q8h dosing, after the laboratory tests mentioned in the preceding text have been obtained. Salt-wasting crises usually do not develop until the fifth to 14th day of life (and as late as 1 month) and may occur in affected infants whose virilization is not severe. Weight, fluid balance, and electrolytes must be monitored closely with blood samples at least every 2 days to detect hyponatremia or hyperkalemia during the first few weeks of life. If salt-wasting occurs, salt loss should be replaced with intravenous normal saline with glucose added. Once the infant is stabilized, NaCl 2 to 3 g/day, divided into q6h dosing, should be added to the formula.

Fludrocortisone acetate (Florinef) 0.05 to 0.2 mg/day should be given for mineralocorticoid replacement.

3. In a virilized 46,XX female suspected of having a form of CAH, who has equivocal 17-OHP levels, an ACTH (Cortrosyn) stimulation test may be necessary to demonstrate the adrenal enzyme defect (Fig. 30.4).

B. Placental aromatase deficiency. The hallmark of this disorder is that both mother and baby are virilized due to an inability to convert androgens to estrogens.

C. Maternal hyperandrogenic conditions. CAH or virilizing tumors of the adrenal or ovary.

VI. **46,XY DSD (UNDERVIRILIZED 46,XY MALES).** Even if the chromosomes contain Y material, the parents should not be hastily told that the child should be raised as a male. In addition, only 50% of 46, XY children with DSD will receive a definitive diagnosis.

A. Environmental disorders. maternal drug ingestion (finasteride, phenytoin, spironolactone).

B. Hereditary disorders. Usually at least one gonad is palpable and there are no müllerian structures because of AMH secreted from the testes.

1. Partial or complete end-organ resistance to testosterone leading to partial androgen insensitivty syndrome (PAIS) or complete androgen insensitivity syndrome (CAIS) (X-linked recessive mutations of the androgen receptor gene).

2. Enzyme defects in testosterone synthesis: deficiencies of 17β-hydroxysteroid dehydrogenase type 3 also known as 17-ketosteroid reductase (17β-HSD in Fig. 30.4 or HSD17B3), 3β-hydroxysteroid dehydrogenase (3β-HSD or HSD3B2), 17α-hydroxylase/17,20-lyase (17-OH or CYP17), and isolated 17,20-lyase (17,20 Des in Fig. 30.4).

3. Defects in testosterone metabolism (5α-reductase type 2 or SRD5A2 deficiency). Though generally uncommon, the Dominican Republic and Middle East have a higher prevalence.

C. Laboratory evaluation. Sampling of serum electrolytes may reveal hyperkalemia and hyponatremia in HSD3B2 deficiency or hypokalemia in CYP17 deficiency. Additional laboratory evaluation is focused on determining whether the cause of undervirilization is due to a defect in testosterone synthesis, metabolism, or action.

1. Obtain blood samples for measurement of electrolytes, follicle-stimulating hormone (FSH), luteinizing hormone (LH), testosterone, DHT, AMH, 17-hydroxyprogesterone, androstenedione, and dehydroepiandrosterone (DHEA). Measurement of 17-OH pregnenolone, 11-deoxycorticosterone, and plasma renin activity may help define the type of enzyme deficiency. If the results in the preceding text do not lead to a diagnosis, hCG, 500 IU, is given intramuscularly every alternate day for a total of three doses. This stimulation test should preferably take place within the first 2 to 3 months of life when the hypothalamic-pituitary-gonadal axis is active. Measurements of DHEA, androstenedione, testosterone, and DHT concentrations are repeated 24 hours after the final dose. Inability to increase the testosterone level in response to hCG is characteristic of a biosynthetic defect in testosterone synthesis, LH receptor insensitivity, or gestational loss of testicular tissue ("vanishing testes"). An elevated testosterone: DHT ratio (>20:1) after hCG stimulation suggests 5α-reductase deficiency.

2. An ACTH stimulation test may be necessary to define earlier enzyme defects in testosterone synthesis such as salt-losing (HSD3B2) or salt-retaining (CYP17) deficiencies, which also produce cortisol insufficiency and CAH (Fig. 30.4)

3. If the initial laboratory tests show high levels of testosterone that do not increase when hCG is given and the ratios of testosterone: androstenedione and testosterone: DHT are normal, the infant probably has PAIS. This can be further evaluated by the monthly administration of 25 to 50 mg of intramuscular depot testosterone for 3 months. Failure of the stretched phallus length to increase by 2.0 ± 0.6 cm supports the suspicion of PAIS. In the past, infants with PAIS were given a female gender assignment and underwent gonadectomy and feminizing genitoplasty. This practice has become controversial. When a testis is retained,

these patients will virilize to a variable degree during puberty but will develop gynecomastia and will not achieve normal adult phallic size on their own. It is not possible, however, to predict the extent to which an infant with PAIS will respond to exogenous testosterone.

Newborns with the **complete** form of androgen resistance have normal-appearing female genitalia and absent müllerian and Wolffian structures. They may be identified by an antepartum 46,XY karyotype (amniocentesis) or the presence of an apparent inguinal hernia that proves to be a testis. Infants with CAIS should be raised female. Their gender identities are invariably female.

D. Other causes of microphallus (<2.5 cm in a full-term infant) with or without cryptorchidism include: hypothalamic-pituitary disorders of fetal gonadotrophin production such as septo-optic dysplasia or Kallmann Syndrome. Infants with panhypopituitarism often have neonatal hypoglycemia and direct hyperbilirubinemia. Among the many syndromes associated with microphallus are: CHARGE association, Prader-Willi, Robinow, Klinefelter, Carpenter, Meckel-Gruber, Noonan, de Lange, trisomy 21, Fanconi, and fetal hydantoin. Treatment with testosterone enanthate 25 mg given intramuscularly monthly for 3 months may produce substantial increase in penile length in these patients.

E. Bilateral cryptorchidism. Bilateral cryptorchidism at birth occurs in 3:1,000 infants, most of whom are premature. By 1 month of life, the testes are still undescended in 1:1,000.

Either ultrasonography or MRI may reveal inguinal or abdominal testes, although MRI is more sensitive for locating the latter. If testicular tissue cannot be found, serum FSH, LH, and testosterone levels should be measured. These hormones rise shortly after birth, are elevated until approximately 6 months of age in boys, and therefore should be measurable. If gonadotropins and testosterone levels are low, then three doses of hCG 500 IU can be given intramuscularly every alternate day and serum testosterone remeasured 24 hours after the final dose to determine the presence and responsiveness of testicular tissue. Elevated serum gonadotropins and a low basal testosterone concentration that fails to rise suggest absent or nonfunctioning testes. Undetectable AMH is indicative of bilateral anorchia rather than undescended testes (see subsequent text). A urologist should be consulted and, if surgery is indicated, orchidopexy should be performed by 1 year of life. If abdominal testes cannot be brought into the scrotum, they should be removed because of the 3- to 10-fold increased risk of germ cell cancer in cryptorchid testes.

The presence of any of the following physical findings also merits evaluation for a disorder of sex development.

1. Unilateral cryptorchidism and hypospadias, especially proximal (e.g., perineal and penile) hypospadias.

2. Unilateral cryptorchisim with microphallus.

Cryptorchidism occurs in congenital ichthyosis, anencephaly, neural tube defects, Prader-Willi, Bardet-Biedl, Aarskog, Cockayne, Fanconi, Noonan, trisomy 21, and Klinefelter syndromes.

VII. GONADAL DIFFERENTIATION DISORDERS

A. Ovotesticular DSD (true hermaphroditism). Less than 10% are 46,XY; 50% are 46,XX; and the remainder show mosaicism (45,X/46,XY or 46,XY/47,XXY) or are chimeric for 46,XX/46,XY. Laparotomy, gonadal biopsy, or both, may be required to diagnose the rare ovotesticular DSD. Diagnosis is based on the histology of the gonads, which, by definition, contain both testicular and follicle-containing ovarian tissue. Whether the internal structures contain Wolffian or müllerian elements depends on the local presence of testosterone and AMH on that side of the abdomen. The external genitalia may appear normal or may show incomplete labioscrotal fusion, asymmetric labioscrotal folds, and hypospadias. Sex assignment should be based on the external and internal genitalia and the degree of intrauterine androgen exposure. An hCG stimulation test that produces a rise in serum testosterone concentration confirms the presence of Leydig cells, whereas a measurable AMH level indicates the presence of Sertoli cells. Dysgenetic

Y chromosome–containing gonads should be removed. If a male sex assignment is made, müllerian structures should be removed.

B. Mixed gonadal dysgenesis (MGD). The hallmark of MGD is the presence of testis on one side of the body and either a streak or dysgenetic testis on the other side. This disorder has a 45,X/46,XY chromosomal complement. Often the Y chromosome is abnormal, or Y-material may have been translocated to an autosome. The combination of asymmetric external genitals with one palpable testis in the labioscrotal fold is almost certainly MGD, although the appearance can range from completely male to completely female. The gonad governs the differentiation of the ipsilateral internal duct. A fallopian tube and uterus are frequently present, and these structures can herniate into a labioscrotal fold. Gender assignment is discretionary because of the marked phenotypic and hormonal variability. Approximately two-thirds are raised as girls. If AMH is measurable or an hCG stimulation test causes a significant rise in serum testosterone concentration indicative of testicular tissue, the testis should be sought and either removed if female sex assignment is made, or brought into the scrotum for close observation if a male sex assignment is made. Gonadal neoplasia (gonadoblastoma) may arise in the first 20 years of life in up to 20% of these children. Therefore, streak and dysgenetic gonads should be removed in infancy. MGD is one type of gonadal dysgenesis disorder, with Turner syndrome (45,XO or 45,X/46,XX) being the classic example of absent or lack of full gonadal differentiation. Children with MGD may have features of Turner syndrome: webbed neck, lymphedema, short stature, and occasional cardiac defects, specifically coarctation of the aorta. They should be considered early candidates for growth hormone treatment.

C. 46,XX or 46,XY "complete" gonadal dysgenesis (CGD). The 46,XY CGD has also been referred to as *complete sex reversal*. Most do not have genital ambiguity at birth; in fact, these children appear female. Infants with 46,XY gonadal dysgenesis fail to masculinize, owing to incomplete testicular differentiation as a result of abnormal functioning of the SRY gene or of transcription factors that regulate the gene's activity. Bilateral streak gonads are present. The external genitalia usually appear female, but clitoromegaly may occur if "gonadal" hilus cells secrete testosterone. Up to 30% of patients with 46,XY gonadal dysgenesis may develop gonadoblastoma or germinoma. These gonads should be removed in infancy. Internal structures are female due to inadequate production of AMH and testosterone from the undifferentiated gonads. These patients are usually raised female and may not be diagnosed until they fail to initiate puberty and exhibit high gonadotropins consistent with gonadal failure. With gonads retained, these patients may virilize at puberty. Individuals with 46,XX sex reversal appear phenotypically male. At puberty, they resemble patients with Klinefelter syndrome (small testes, azoospermia, eunochoid body habitus, gynecomastia) due to testosterone deficiency. A loss of Y chromosome during early embryogenesis, a cryptic mosaicism with Y-bearing cell line, or translocation of Y chromosomal material to the X chromosome may be responsible.

VIII. Table 30.3 summarizes causes and Figs. 30.5 and 30.6 describe an approach to patients with ambiguous genitalia.

USE OF AMH. The hCG stimulation test can be cumbersome and expensive and occasionally requires protracted dosing to stimulate a refractory testis. AMH is produced in a sexually dimorphic manner. Starting at birth, AMH from Sertoli cells rises to a peak of 115 ng/mL at 6 months and declines during adolescence to an adult level of 4 ng/mL; in contrast, granulosa cells of the ovary do not make any significant amounts of AMH until puberty when levels also reach approximately 4 ng/mL.

    Measuring AMH by enzyme-linked immunosorbent assay (ELISA) can distinguish between absent and present testicular tissue. AMH in the normal or detectable range has a 100% positive predictive value that testicular tissue is present; the negative predictive value for anorchia is 94% if AMH is undetectable.

IX. ISSUES OF GENDER ASSIGNMENT. In the past, a primary criterion for male gender assignment was phallic size adequate for sexual function. This issue is currently being debated. Infants with 46,XY born with little or no penile tissue have usually been

TABLE 30.3   **Causes of Ambiguous Genital Development (Intersex)**

| Disorder | Phenotype | | Karyotype |
	External Genitalia	Gonads	
Disorders of gonadal differentiation			
True hermaphroditism	Ambiguous	Ovarian and testicular tissue	46, XX; 46, XY; 46, XX/46, XY chmerism or mosaic
"Pure" gonadal dysgenesis	Female	Streak gonads or hypoplastic ovaries	46, XX
	Female or ambiguous	Dysgenetic testes or dysgenetic testes and streak gonads	46, XY
Mixed gonadal dysgenesis	Ambiguous	Streak gonad and dysgenetic testis	45, X/46, XY; 46, XYp-
Female pseudohermaphroditism (masculinization of the genetic female)			
Congenital adrenal hyperplasia			
21α-hydroxylase deficiency	Ambiguous	Ovaries	46, XX
11β-hydroxylase deficiency	Ambiguous	Ovaries	46, XX
3β-OH steroid dehydrogenase deficiency	Ambiguous	Ovaries	46, XX
Transplacental synthetic progestogens	Ambiguous	Ovaries	46, XX
Maternal androgen excess	Ambiguous	Ovaries	46, XX
Male pseudohermaphroditism (incomplete masculinization of the genetic male)			
Testicular unresponsiveness to HCG and LH (Leydig cell hypoplasia or agenesis)	Ambiguous	Testes	46, XY
Disorders of testosterone synthesis	Ambiguous	Testes	46, XY
Side chain cleavage enzyme deficiency			
17α-hydroxylase deficiency			
3β-OH steroid dehydrogenase deficiency			
17-lyase deficiency			
17-ketosteroid reductase deficiency			

(continued)

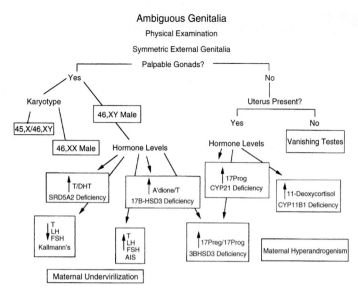

Figure 30.5. Algorithm for the evaluation of symmetrical genital ambiguity. A'dione = androstenedione; AIS = androgen insensitivity syndrome; DHT = dihydrotestosterone; FSH = follicle-stimulating hormone; LH = luteinizing hormone; 17 Preg = 17-hydroxypregnenolone; 17 Prog = 17-hydroxyprogesterone; T = testosterone. (From Witchel SS, Lee PA. Ambiguous genitalia. In: Sperling MA, ed. *Pediatric endocrinology.* Philadelphia: WB Saunders, 1996:31–49.)

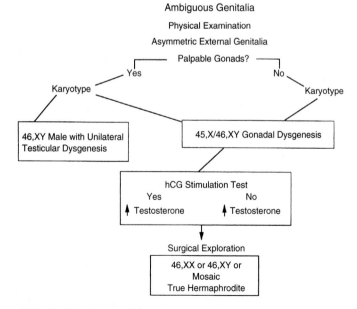

Figure 30.6. Algorithm for the evaluation of asymmetrical genital ambiguity. (From Witchel SS, Lee PA. Ambiguous genitalia. In: Sperling MA, ed. *Pediatric endocrinology.* Philadelphia: WB Saunders, 1996:31–49.)

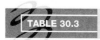 **TABLE 30.3** *(Continued)*

| Disorder | Phenotype | | Karyotype |
	External Genitalia	Gonads	
End-organ resistance to testosterone			
Complete testicular feminization	Female	Testes	46, XY
Incomplete testicular feminization	Ambiguous	Testes	46, XY
Disorder of testosterone metabolism			
5α-reductase deficiency	Ambiguous	Testes	46, XY
Vanishing testes syndrome	Variable	Absent gonads	46, XY
Lack of Müllerian inhibiting substance	Male	Testes, uterus, fallopian tubes	46, XY

Source: From Wolfsdorf J.I., Muglia L., Endocrine Disorders. In: Graef J.W. (Ed.), *Manual of Pediatric Therapeutics*. Philadelphia: Lippincott-Raven, 1997:381–413.
HCG = human chorionic gonadotropin; LH = luteinizing hormone.

given female sex assignment and surgically and hormonally feminized by means of genitoplasty early in life and estrogen treatment at the age of puberty. The decision to assign gender is, however, complicated by evidence that the prenatal hormonal environment may influence gender identity formation and gender role behavior. During the second trimester, the normal fetal testis produces levels of testosterone comparable to an adult male. The 46,XY neonate born with minimal penile tissue, who is not androgen resistant and who has been exposed to normal intrauterine testosterone concentrations, may retain a male gender identity regardless of gender assignment. Fueling the debate are the new techniques such as intracytoplasmic sperm injection (ICSI) which makes fertilization possible without penetration or ejaculation.

Likewise, the issue of gender assignment in the case of the most severely virilized 46,XX newborns with CAH who have completely fused labioscrotal folds and a phallic urethra is also under debate. A minority opinion recommends male assignment and gonadectomy, thereby eliminating the need for feminizing genitoplasty. Nevertheless, most geneticists and endocrinologists continue to recommend female assignment to preserve fertility.

Whether and when to perform genital surgery, particularly clitoral reduction in virilized females, is also the subject of controversy. Whereas some adults with DSD view their genital surgery as mutilation, most parents prefer surgery so that their child's genitalia appear more consistent with the gender of rearing. One-stage surgical procedures that preserve the neurovascular bundle can be done in infancy and are much improved compared to the clitorectomies routinely performed several decades ago.

Parents require a thorough explanation of their child's condition as the laboratory and imaging data become available. They should participate with the interdisciplinary team in the decision-making as the options for medical and surgical therapy and future prospects for genital appearance, gender identity, sexual functioning, and fertility are evaluated. Long-term, unbiased studies of gender identity and sexual functioning in individuals born with various forms of DSD are needed to provide insight for the difficult task of assigning an appropriate gender.

Suggested Readings

American Academy of Pediatrics. Committee on Genetics. Evaluation of the newborn with developmental anomalies of the external genitalia. *Pediatrics* 2000;106:138.

Anhalt H; Neely E.K and Hintz R.L. Ambiguous genitalia. *Pediatr Rev* 1996;17:213.

Berenbaum SA. Effects of early androgens on sex-typed activities and interests in adolescents with congenital adrenal hyperplasia. *Horm Behav* 1999;35:102.

Creighton SM, Minto CL, Steele SJ. Objective cosmetic and anatomical outcomes at adolescence of feminising surgery for ambiguous genitalia done in childhood. *Lancet* 2001;358:124.

Diamond M, Sigmundson HK. Management of intersexuality: Guidelines for dealing with persons with ambiguous genitalia. *Arch Pediatr Adolesc Med* 1997;151:1046.

Drummon-Borg M, Pagon RA, Bradley CM, et al. Nonfluorescent dicentric Y in males with hypospadias. *J Pediatr* 1988;113:469.

Federman DD, Donahoe PK. Ambiguous genitalia—etiology, diagnosis and therapy. *Adv Endocrinol Metab* 1995;6:91.

Grumbach MM, Hughes IA, Conte FA. Disorders of sex differentiation. In: Larsen, K, Melmed P, eds. *Williams textbook of endocrinology*, 10th ed. Chapter 22 by Copyright USA: Elsevier Science: 2003.

Hawkins JR. The SRY gene. *Trend Endocrinol Metab* 1993;4:328.

Hawkins JR, Taylor A, Goodfellow PN, et al. Evidence for increased prevalence of SRY mutations in XY females with complete rather than partial gonadal dysgenesis. *Am J Hum Genet* 1992;51:1979.

Hughes IA, Houk C, Ahmed SF, et al. LWPES Consensus Group, ESPE Consensus Group. Consensus statement on management of intersex disorders. *Arch Dis Child* 2006; 91:554–563.

Lee PA. Fertility in cryptorchidism: Does treatment make a difference? *Endocrinol Metab Clin North Am* 1993;22:479.

Lee MM. MIS/AMH in the assessment of cryptorchidism and intersex conditions. *Mol Cell Endocrinol* 2003;211:91–98.

New MI. Inborn errors of adrenal steroidogenesis. *Mol Cell Endocrinol* 2003;211:75–83.

Neri G. Syndromal (and nonsyndromal) forms of male pseudohermaphrodism. *Am J Med Genet* 1999;89:201–9.

Page DC, Brown LG, de la Chapelle A. Exchange of terminal portions of X- and Y- chromosomal short arms in human XX males. *Nature* 1987;328:437.

Pang S, Clark A. Congenital adrenal hyperplasia due to 21 hydroxylase deficiency: Newborn screening and its relationship to the diagnosis and treatment of the disorder. *Screening* 1993;2:105.

Papadimitriou DT. Puberty in subjects with complete androgen insensitivity syndrome. *Horm Res* 2006;65(3):126–131.

Pritchard-Jones K, Fleming S, Davidson D, et al. The candidate Wilms' tumour gene is involved in genitourinary development. *Nature* 1990;346:194.

Reiner WG. Assignment of sex in neonates with ambiguous genitalia. *Curr Opin Pediatr* 1999;11:363.

Saenger P. Male pseudohermaphroditism. *Pediatr Ann* 1981;10:15.

Savage MO, Lowe DG. Gonadal neoplasia and abnormal sexual differentiation. *Clin Endocrinol* 1990;32:519.

Schnitzer JJ, Donahoe PK. Surgical treatment of congenital adrenal hyperplasia. *Endocrinol Metab Clin North Am* 2001;30:137.

Styne DM. The testes: Disorders of sexual differentiation and puberty. In: Sperling MA, ed. *Pediatric endocrinology*. Philadelphia: Saunders, 1996:424.

Therell BL. Newborn screening for congenital adrenal hyperplasia. *Endocrinol Metab Clin North Am* 2001;30:15.

Vainio S, Heikkila M, Kispert A, et al. Female development in mammals is regulated by Wnt-4 signalling. *Nature* 1999;397:405.

Warne GL, Zajac JD. Disorders of sexual differentiation. *Endocrinol Metab Clin North Am* 1998;27:945.

Witchel SS, Lee PA. Ambiguous genitalia. In: Sperling MA, ed. *Pediatric endocrinology*. Philadelphia: WB Saunders, 1996:32.

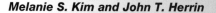

RENAL CONDITIONS
Melanie S. Kim and John T. Herrin

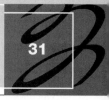

*R*enal problems in the neonate may be the result of specific inherited, developmental abnormalities or the result of acquired events either in the prenatal or postnatal period. For this reason evaluation includes a detailed review of the history (family history, gestational history, and the neonatal events) as well as a review of the presenting clinical features and relevant laboratory findings. An understanding of the developmental process and the differences in renal physiology in the neonatal period compared to that at later ages is necessary for evaluation.

I. RENAL EMBRYOGENESIS AND FUNCTIONAL DEVELOPMENT

A. Embryology

1. Three paired renal systems develop from the nephrogenic ridge of the mesoderm.

2. The first two systems, the **pronephros** and the **mesonephros,** have limited function in the human being and are transient. The mesonephric tubules and duct form the efferent ductules of the epididymis, the vas deferens, the ejaculatory ducts, and the seminal vesicles in men. In women they result in the vestigial epoophoron and the paroophoron.

3. The **metanephros** is the third and final excretory system and appears in the fifth week of gestation. The metanephros is made up of two different cell types. These differentiate into the **pelvicalyceal** system, which is well delineated by the 13th or 14th week, and the **nephrons,** which continue to form up to the 25th week of gestation to a final complement of 1 million nephrons per kidney. Urine is produced by the 12th week.

4. Parallel development of the lower urinary tract occurs with opening of the mesonephric duct to the allantois and cloaca at 5 weeks' gestation. Shortly thereafter at 6 weeks, the urorectal fold forms as a septum dividing the gastrointestinal (GI) tract (posterior compartment) from the anterior genitourinary (GU) compartment—the urogenital sinus. At 7 weeks, separate vesicoureteral openings form and the allantois degenerates to a cord that becomes the urachus and the upper bladder, although the trigone develops from the Wolffian duct remnant. Müllerian system development produces a ureterovaginal cord, which in women becomes the vaginal vestibule, vagina, and uterine cervix. In men, müllerian system regression leads to the prostatic urethra.

5. Disruption of normal renal development may lead to renal malformations such as renal agenesis, renal hypoplasia, renal ectopy, renal dysplasia, and cystic disease.

B. Functional development.
At birth, the kidney replaces the placenta as the major homeostatic organ, maintaining fluid and electrolyte balance and removing harmful waste products. This transition occurs with changes in renal blood flow (RBF), glomerular filtration rate (GFR), and tubular functions. The level of renal function relates more closely to the postnatal age than to the gestational age at birth.

1. **RBF** remains low in the fetus, accounting for only 2% to 3% of cardiac output. At birth, RBF rapidly increases to 15% to 18% of cardiac output because of (i) a decrease in renal vascular resistance, which is proportionally greater in the kidney compared to other organs, (ii) an increase in systemic blood pressure, and (iii) increase in inner to outer cortical blood flow.

2. **Glomerular filtration** begins soon after the first nephrons are formed and GFR increases in parallel with body and kidney growth (approximately

587

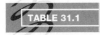

| TABLE 31.1 | Commonly Used Equations and Formulas |

CrCl (mL/min/1.73 m^2) = K × Length (cm)/P_{Cr}

K = 0.34 in premature infants <34 wk and 0.44 in infants from 35 wk to term

CrCl (mL/min/1.73 m^2) = U_{Cr} × U_{vol} × 1.73/P_{Cr} × BSA

FeNa = 100 × (U_{Na+} × P_{Cr})/(P_{Na+} × U_{Cr})

TRP = 100 × (1 − ((U_P × P_{Cr})/(P_P × U_{Cr})))

Calculated $P_{osm} \geq 2$ × plasma [Na$^+$] + [glucose]/18 + BUN/2.8

Plasma anion gap = [Na$^+$] − [Cl$^-$] − [HCO$_3^-$]

BSA = body surface area; CrCl = creatinine clearance; FeNa = fractional excretion of sodium; P_{Cr} = plasma creatinine; P_{osm} = plasma osmolarity; P_{Na} = plasma sodium; TRP = tubular reabsorption of phosphorus; U_{Cr} = urinary creatinine; U_{vol} = urinary volume per minute.

1 mL/minute/kg of body weight). Once all the glomeruli are formed by 34 weeks' gestation, the GFR continues to increase until birth because of decreases in renal vascular resistance. After birth, the GFR rises quickly, doubling by 2 weeks of age and reaching adult levels by 1 year of age. The rate of GFR maturation is not altered by premature birth and increases in response to solute load. GFR is less well autoregulated in the neonate. It is controlled by maintenance of glomerular capillary pressure by the greater vasoconstrictive effect of angiotension II at the efferent then afferent arteriole where the effect is attenuated by concurrent prostglandin induced vasodilatation.

3. **Tubular function**
   a. **Sodium (Na$^+$) handling.** The capacity to reabsorb Na$^+$ is developed by 24 weeks' gestation. However, tubular resorption of Na$^+$ is low until 34 weeks' gestation, with fractional excretion of sodium (FeNa; see Table 31.1) ranging from 5% to 10%. In severely ill infants, urinary Na$^+$ losses can be very high, with FeNa reaching 15%. Very premature infants cannot conserve Na$^+$ even when Na$^+$ balance is negative. Hence premature infants below 34 weeks' gestation receiving formula or breast milk without Na$^+$ supplementation can develop hyponatremia. After 34 weeks' gestation, Na$^+$ reabsorption becomes more efficient, so that 99% of filtered Na$^+$ can be reabsorbed, resulting in an FeNa of <1%. Full-term neonates can retain Na$^+$ when in negative Na$^+$ balance but, like premature infants, are also limited in their ability to excrete a Na$^+$ load because of their low GFR.
   b. **Water handling.** The newborn infant has a limited ability to concentrate urine due to limited urea concentration within the interstitium because of low protein intake and anabolic growth. The resulting decreased osmolality of the interstitium leads to a decreased capacity to reabsorb water and concentrating ability of the neonatal kidney. The maximal urine osmolality is 500 mOsm/L in premature infants and 800 mOsm/L in term infants. Although this is of little consequence in infants receiving appropriate amounts of water with hypotonic feeding, it can become clinically relevant in infants receiving high osmotic loads. In contrast, both premature and full-term infants can dilute their urine with a minimal urine osmolality of 25 to 35 mOsm/L. Their low GFR, however, limits their ability to handle water loads.
   c. **Potassium (K$^+$) handling.** The limited ability of premature infants to excrete large K$^+$ loads is related to decreased distal tubular K$^+$ secretion, a result of decreased aldosterone sensitivity, low Na$^+$–K$^+$ adenosine triphosphatase (ATPase) activity, and low GFR.
   d. **Acid and bicarbonate handling** are limited by a low serum bicarbonate threshold in the proximal tubule (14 to 16 mEq/L in premature infants, 18 to

21 mEq/L in full-term infants) which improves as maturation of $Na^+ - K^+$ ATPase and $Na^+ - H$ transporter occurs. In addition, the production of ammonia in the distal tubule and proximal tubular glutamine synthesis are decreased. The lower rate of phosphate excretion limits the generation of titratable acid, further limiting their ability to eliminate an acid load. Very low birth weight infants can develop mild metabolic acidosis during the second to fourth week after birth that may require administration of additional sodium bicarbonate if the infant is not thriving.

e. **Calcium and phosphorous** handling in the neonate is characterized by a pattern of increased phosphate retention associated with growth. The intake and filtered load of phosphate, parathyroid hormone (PTH), and growth factors modulate phosphate transport. The higher phosphate level and higher rate of phosphate reabsorption are not explained by a low GFR or tubular unresponsiveness to extrarenal factors (PTH, vitamin D). More likely, there is a developmental mechanism that favors renal conservation of phosphate in part due to growth hormone effects, as well as a growth-related Na^+-dependent phosphate transporter, so that a positive phosphate balance for growth is maintained. Tubular reabsorption of phosphate (TRP) is also altered by gestational age, increasing from 85% at 28 weeks to 93% at 34 weeks and 98% by 40 weeks.

Calcium levels in the fetus and cord blood are higher than those in the neonate. Calcium levels fall in the first 24 hours, but low levels of PTH persist. This relative hypoparathyroidism in the first few days after birth may be the result of this physiologic response to hypercalcemia in the normal fetus. Although plasma Ca^+ values <8 mg/dL in premature infants are common, they are usually asymptomatic, because the ionized calcium level is usually normal. Factors that favor this normal ionized Ca^+ fraction include lower serum albumin and the relative metabolic acidosis in the neonate.

Urinary calcium excretion is lower in premature infants and correlates with gestational age. At term, calcium excretion rises and persists until approximately 12 months of age. The urine calcium excretion in premature infants varies directly with Na^+ intake, urinary Na^+ excretion, and inversely with plasma Ca^{2+}. Neonatal stress and therapies such as aggressive fluid use or furosemide administration increase Ca^{2+} excretion, aggravating the tendency to hypocalcemia.

f. Fetal urine contribution to amniotic fluid volume is minimal (10 mL/hour) in the first half of gestation but increases significantly to an average of 50 mL/hour and is a necessary contribution to pulmonary development. Oligohydramnios or polyhydramnios may reflect dysfunction of the developing kidney.

II. CLINICAL ASSESSMENT OF RENAL FUNCTION. Assessment of renal function is based on the patient's history, physical examination, and appropriate laboratory and radiologic tests.

A. **History**

1. **Prenatal history** includes any maternal illness, drug use, or exposure to known and potential teratogens.

   a. Maternal use of captopril or indomethacin decreases glomerular capillary pressure and GFR and has been associated with neonatal renal failure.

   b. Oligohydramnios may indicate a decrease in fetal urine production. It is often associated with renal agenesis, renal dysplasia, polycystic kidney disease, or severe obstruction of the urinary-tract system. Polyhydramnios may be a result of renal tubular dysfunction with inability to fully concentrate urine.

   c. Elevated serum and amniotic fluid α-fetoprotein have been associated with congenital nephrotic syndrome.

2. **Family history.** The risk of renal disease is increased if there is a family history of urinary-tract anomalies, polycystic kidney disease, consanguinity, or inherited renal tubular disorders. Familial diseases may be recognized *in utero* (congenital nephrotic syndrome, autosomal recessive polycystic disease of kidney

[ARPKD]), at birth (renal anomalies, congenital nephrotic syndrome) or remain asymptomatic until later life (autosomal dominant polycystic disease of the kidney [ADPKD]).

3. **Delivery history.** Fetal distress, perinatal asphyxia, or shock due to volume loss may lead to ischemic or anoxic injury, resulting in acute tubular necrosis.

4. **Micturition.** Seventeen percent of newborns void in the delivery room, approximately 90% void by 24 hours, and 99% void by 48 hours. The rate of urine formation ranges from 0.5 to 5.0 mL/kg/hour at all gestational ages. The most common cause of delayed or decreased urine production is inadequate perfusion of the kidneys; however, delay in micturition may be due to intrinsic renal abnormalities or obstruction of the urinary tract.

B. **Physical examination.** Careful examination will detect abdominal masses in 0.8% of neonates. Most of these masses are either renal in origin or related to the GU system. It is important to consider in the differential diagnosis whether the mass is unilateral or bilateral (see Table 31.2). Edema may be present in infants with congenital nephrotic syndrome, renal failure, or fluid overload. Concentrating defects or tubular defects with salt wasting may cause dehydration.

Other congenital anomalies detected by physical examination which are associated with renal abnormalities include low-set ears, ambiguous genitalia, anal atresia, abdominal wall defect, vertebral anomalies, aniridia, meningomyelocele or tethered cord, pneumothorax, hemihypertrophy, persistent urachus, hypospadias, and cryptorchidism (see Table 31.3). Spontaneous pneumothorax may be associated with an increased risk of renal abnormalities.

C. **Laboratory evaluation.** Renal function tests must be interpreted in relation to gestational and postnatal age (see Tables 31.4 and 31.5).

1. Urinalysis reflects the developmental stages of renal physiology.
   a. **Specific gravity.** Full-term infants have a limited concentrating ability with a maximum specific gravity of 1.021 to 1.025.
   b. **Protein excretion** varies with gestational age. Urinary protein excretion is higher in premature infants and decreases progressively with postnatal age. In normal full-term infants, protein excretion is minimal after the second week of life.

TABLE 31.2	Abdominal Masses in the Neonate

Type of mass	Total percentage
Renal	55
Hydronephrosis	
Multicystic dysplastic kidney	
Polycystic kidney disease	
Mesoblastic nephroma	
Renal ectopia	
Renal vein thrombosis	
Nephrobastomatosis	
Wilms tumor	
Genital	15
Hydrometrocolpos	
Ovarian cyst	
Gastrointestinal	20

From Pinto E, Guignard JP. Renal masses in the neonate. *Biol Neonate* 1995;68:175–184.

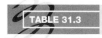
TABLE 31.3   **Congenital Syndromes with Renal Components**

Dysmorphic disorders, sequences, and associations	General features	Renal abnormalities
Oligohydramnios sequence (Potter syndrome)	Altered facies, pulmonary hypoplasia, abnormal limb and head position	Renal agenesis, severe bilateral obstruction, severe bilateral dysplasia, autosomal recessive polycystic kidney disease
Vater and Vacterl syndrome	Vertebral anomalies, anal atresia, tracheo esophageal fistula, radial dysplasia, cardiac and limb defects	Renal agenesis, renal dysplasia, renal ectopia
MURCS association and Rokitansky sequence	Failure of paramesonephric ducts, vaginal and uterus hypoplasia/atresia, cervicothoracic somite dysplasia	Renal hypoplasia/ agenesis, renal ectopia, double ureters
Prune belly	Hypoplasia of abdominal muscle, cryptorchidism	Megaureters, hydro nephrosis, dysplastic kidneys, atonic bladder
Spina bifida	Meningomyelocele	Neurogenic bladder, vesicoureteral reflux, hydronephrosis, double ureter, horseshoe kidney
Caudal dysplasia sequence (caudal regression syndrome)	Sacral (and lumbar) hypoplasia, disruption of the distal spinal cord	Neurogenic bladder, vesicoureteral reflux, hydrone phrosis, renal agenesis
Anal atresia (high imperforate anus)	Rectovaginal, rectovesical, or rectourethral fistula tethered to the spinal cord	Renal agenesis, renal dysplasia
Hemihypertrophy	Hemihypertrophy	Wilms tumor, hypospadias
Aniridia ✓	Aniridia, cryptorchidism	Wilms tumor
Drash syndrome	Ambiguous genitalia	Mesangial sclerosis, Wilms tumor
Small deformed or low-set ears		Renal agenesis/ dysplasia

(continued)

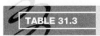

TABLE 31.3 *(Continued)*

Hereditary disorders	General features	Renal abnormalities
Autosomal recessive		
Cerebrohepatorenal syndrome (Zellweger syndrome)	Hepatomegaly, glaucoma, brain anomalies, chondrodystrophy	Cortical renal cysts
Jeune syndrome (thoracic asphyxiating dystrophy)	Small thoracic cage, short ribs, abnormal costochondral junctions, pulmonary hypoplasia	Cystic tubular dysplasia, glomerulosclerosis, hydronephrosis, horseshoe kidneys
Meckel-Gruber syndrome (dysencephalia splanchnocystica)	Encephalocele, microcephaly, polydactyly, cryptorchidism, cardiac anomalies, liver disease	Polycystic/dysplastic kidneys
Johanson-Blizzard syndrome	Hypoplastic alae nasi, hypothyroidism, deafness, imperforate anus, cryptorchidism	Hydronephrosis, caliectasis
Schinzel-Giedon syndrome	Short limbs, abnormal facies, bone abnormalities, hypospadias	Hydronephrosis, megaureter
Short rib–polydactyly syndrome	Short horizontal ribs, pulmonary hypoplasia, polysyndactyly, bone and cardiac defects, ambiguous genitalia	Glomerular and tubular cysts
Bardet-Biedl syndrome	Obesity, retinal pigmentation, polydactyly	Interstitial nephritis
Autosomal dominant		
Tuberous sclerosis	Fibrous-angiomatous lesions, hypopigmented macules, intracranial calcifications, seizures, bone lesions	Polycystic kidneys, renal angiomyolipoma
Melnick-Fraser syndrome (branchio-otorenal [BOR] syndrome)	Preauricular pits, branchial clefts, deafness	Renal dysplasia, duplicated ureters
Nail-patella syndrome (hereditary osteo-onychodysplasia)	Hypoplastic nails, hypoplastic or absent patella, other bone anomalies	Proteinuria, nephrotic syndrome
Townes syndrome	Thumb, auricular and anal anomalies	Various renal abnormalities
X-Linked		
Oculocerebrorenal syndrome (Lowe's syndrome)	Cataracts, rickets, mental retardation	Fanconi syndrome
Oral–facial–digital (OFD) syndrome, type I	Oral clefts, hypoplastic alae nasi, digital asymmetry (X-linked, lethal in men)	Renal microcysts

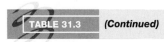 **TABLE 31.3** *(Continued)*

Chromosomal abnormalities	General features	Renal abnormalities
Trisomy 21 (Down syndrome)	Abnormal facies, brachy cephaly, congenital heart disease	Cystic dysplastic kidney and other renal abnormalities
X0 syndrome (Turner syndrome)	Small stature, congenital heart disease, amenorrhea	Horseshoe kidney, duplications and malrotations of the urinary collecting system
Trisomy 13 (Patau syndrome)	Abnormal facies, cleft lip and palate, congenital heart disease	Cystic dysplastic kidneys and other renal anomalies
Trisomy 18 (Edwards syndrome)	Abnormal facies, abnormal ears, overlapping digits, congenital heart disease	Cystic dysplastic kidneys, horse-shoe kidney, or duplication
XXY, XXX syndrome (Triploidy syndrome)	Abnormal facies, cardiac defects, hypospadias and cryptorchidism in men, syndactyly	Various renal abnormalities
Partial trisomy 10q	Abnormal facies, microcephaly, limb and cardiac abnormalities	Various renal abnormalities

   c. **Glycosuria** is commonly present in premature infants of <34 weeks' gestation. The tubular resorption of glucose is <93% in infants born before 34 weeks' gestation compared with 99% in infants born after 34 weeks' gestation. Glucose excretion rates are highest in infants born before 28 weeks' gestation.

   d. **Hematuria** is abnormal and may indicate intrinsic renal damage or result from a bleeding or clotting abnormality (see III.G).

   e. **The sediment examination** will usually demonstrate multiple epithelial cells (thought to be urethral mucosal cells) for the first 24 to 48 hours. In infants with asphyxia, there is an increase in epithelial cells and transient microscopic hematuria with leukocytes is common. Further investigation is necessary if these sediment findings persist. Hyaline and fine granular casts are common in dehydration or hypotension. Uric acid crystals are common in deyhdration states and concentrated urine samples. They may be seen as pink or reddish brown diaper staining (particularly with the newer absorptive diapers).

2. **Method of collection**

   a. **Suprapubic aspiration** is the most reliable method of detecting urinary-tract infection (UTI).

   b. **Bladder catheterization** is used if an infant has failed to pass urine by 36 to 48 hours and is not apparently hypovolemic (see III.B), or if urine volume, flow, or sedimentary examination is important.

   c. **Bag collections** are adequate for most studies such as determinations of specific gravity, pH, electrolytes, protein, glucose, and sediment but not urine culture. It is the preferred method for detecting red blood cells in the urine.

   d. **Diaper urine specimens** are reliable for estimation of pH and qualitative determination of the presence of glucose, protein, and blood.

TABLE 31.4	Normal Urinary and Renal Values in Term and Preterm Infants				
	Preterm infants <34 wk	Term infants at birth	Term infants 2 wk	Term infants 8 wk
GFR (mL/min/1.73 m^2)	13–58	15–60	63–80	
FeNa (%) (oliguric patient)	>1%	<1%	<1%	<1%
Bicarbonate threshold (mEq/L)	14–18	21	21.5	
TRP (%)	>85%	>95%		
Protein excretion (mg/m^2/24 h) (mean ± 1 SD)	60 ± 96	31 ± 44		
Maximal concentration ability (mOsmol/L)	500	800	900	1,200
Maximal diluting ability (mOsmol/L)	25–30	25–30	25–30	25–30
Specific gravity	1.002–1.015	1.002–1.020	1.002–1.025	
Dipstick				
pH	5.0–8.0	4.5–8.0	4.5–8.0	4.5–8.0
Proteins	Neg to ++	Neg to +	Neg	Neg
Glucose	Neg to ++	Neg	Neg	Neg
Blood	Neg	Neg	Neg	Neg
Leukocytes	Neg	Neg	Neg	Neg

Neg = negative.

TABLE 31.5	Normal Serum Creatinine Values in Term and Preterm Infants (Mean ± SD)			
Age (d)	**<28 wk**	**28–32 wk**	**32–37 wk**	**>37 wk**
3	1.05 ± 0.27	0.88 ± 0.25	0.78 ± 0.22	0.75 ± 0.2
7	0.95 ± 0.36	0.94 ± 0.37	0.77 ± 0.48	0.56 ± 0.4
14	0.81 ± 0.26	0.78 ± 0.36	0.62 ± 0.4	0.43 ± 0.25
28	0.66 ± 0.28	0.59 ± 0.38	0.40 ± 0.28	0.34 ± 0.2

From Rudd PT, Hughes EA, Placzek MM, et al. Reference ranges for plasma creatinine during the first month of life. *Arch Dis Child* 1983;58:212–215; Van den Anker JN, de Groot, R, Broerse HM, et al. Assessment of glomerular filtration rate in preterm infants by serum creatinine: Comparison with insulin clearance. *Pediatrics* 1995;96: 1156–1158.

3. **Evaluation of renal function**
   a. **Serum creatinine** at birth reflects maternal renal function. In infants, serum creatinine levels after a transient rise over the first 24 to 36 hours (particularly in premature infants), and fall quickly from 0.8 mg/dL at birth to 0.5 mg/dL at 5 to 7 days and reach a stable level of 0.3 to 0.4 mg/dL by 9 days. The rate of decrease in serum creatinine in the first few weeks is slower in younger gestational age infants with lower GFR (Table 31.5).
   b. **Blood urea nitrogen (BUN)** is a useful indicator of renal function. However, BUN can be elevated as a result of increased production of urea nitrogen in hypercatabolic states, sequestered blood, tissue breakdown, hemoconcentration, or increased protein intake. Renal insufficiency is suspected if BUN is >20 mg/dL or rises at a rate of 5 mg/dL/day or higher.
   c. **GFR** can be measured by clearance studies of either exogenous substances (insulin, Cr-EDTA [chromium ethylene diamine tetra-acetic acid], sodium iothalamate) or endogenous substances such as creatinine. Practical considerations such as frequent blood sampling, urine collection, or infusion of an exogenous substance limit their use. GFR can be estimated from serum creatinine and body length (Table 31.1).
   d. **Measurement of serum and urine electrolytes** is used to guide fluid and electrolyte management and in assessing renal tubular function.
D. **Radiological studies**
   1. **Ultrasonography** is the initial imaging study to delineate renal parenchymal architecture. Color Doppler flow techniques can estimate RBF. The length of the kidneys in millimeters is approximately the gestational age in weeks. The renal cortex has echogenicity similar to that of the liver or spleen in the neonate, in contrast to the hypoechoic renal cortex seen in adults and older children. In addition, the medullary pyramids in the neonate are much more hypoechoic than the cortex and hence are more prominent in appearance.
   2. **Intravenous pyelography (IVP)** is rarely used in the newborn period, because the neonate has a limited concentrating ability and difficulty in excreting a highly osmolar load.
   3. **Voiding cystourethography (VCUG),** with fluoroscopy, is indicated in infants with UTIs or with renal anomalies on ultrasound to rule out vesicoureteral reflux (VUR), and in neonates with obstructive uropathy to define associated reflux and define lower-tract anatomy more specifically. Radionuclide cystography is often used to evaluate VUR because of its lower radiation dose. However, VCUG produces better static imaging for anatomical defects and is preferred for the initial evaluation of obstructive uropathy.
   4. **Radionuclide scintography** is useful in demonstrating the position and relative function of the kidneys. Isotopes such as technetium-99m-diethylene triamine

pentacetic acid (DTPA) or mercaptoacetyltriglycine (MAG 3) are handled by glomerular filtration and can be used to assess RBF and renal function. In conjunction with intravenously administered furosemide, it can help differentiate obstructive from nonobstructive hydronephrosis. Isotopes that bind to the renal tubules, such as technetium-99m-dimercaptosuccinic acid (DMSA), produce static images of the renal cortex. This may be helpful for assessing acute pyelonephritis and renal scarring from renal artery emboli, or renal vascular disorders and to quantify the amount of renal cortex in patients with renal dysplasia and hypoplasia.

III. COMMON CLINICAL RENAL PROBLEMS

A. Prenatal ultrasonography. Routine maternal ultrasonographic screening detects an incidence of fetal GU abnormalities of 0.3 to 0.5%.

  1. The most common finding is **hydronephrosis,** reported in >80% of the cases. Approximately 75% of these are confirmed postnatally.

   a. Initial management of a newborn with prenatally identified hydronephrosis depends on the clinical condition of the patient and the suspected nature of the lesion.

   b. Unilateral hydronephrosis is more common and is not associated with systemic or pulmonary complications if the contralateral kidney is normal. Postnatal ultrasonographic confirmation may be carried out electively at approximately 1 month, depending on severity. It is important to not perform the ultrasonographic examination in the first few days after birth, when hydronephrosis may not be detected because of physiologic dehydration.

   c. Bilateral hydronephrosis is more worrisome, especially if oligohydramnios or pulmonary disease is present. In the male infant, postnatal evaluation (VCUG and ultrasonography) should be performed within the first day to rule out the possibility of posterior urethral valves (PUV). With postbladder obstruction such as PUV, ultrasonography will often demonstrate a trabeculated and thickened bladder wall.

   d. Prophylactic antibiotics (amoxicillin 20 mg/kg orally everyday) is recommended before VCUG is performed, as hydronephrosis may be due to VUR.

  2. Routine prenatal ultrasonography has increased the diagnosis of multicystic dysplastic kidney (MCDK) especially with unilateral involvement. Infants with unilateral MCDK are usually asymptomatic, and the affected kidney has no renal function as demonstrated by DMSA renal scan. There is general agreement that surgical removal is indicated in cases with associated hypertension or infection, or with respiratory compromise secondary to abdominal compression by the abnormal kidney. Although surgical removal had been suggested to decrease the potential of renal cell carcinoma, there is no evidence that surgical removal of asymptomatic MCDK improves long-term outcomes. In asymptomatic patients, medical observation is the current practice and surgical removal is reserved only if symptoms develop.

  3. Renal abnormalities may be associated with other congenital anomalies including neural tube defects, congenital heart lesions, intestinal obstructive lesions, abdominal wall defects, central nervous system (CNS) or spinal abnormailites, and urological abnormalities of the lower urinary tract.

B. Acute renal failure may be secondary to prenal, intrinsic, or postrenal disorders (see Table 31.6). **Prerenal failure** is due to hypoperfusion to the kidneys. This is the most common cause of renal failure in the neonate, and if not corrected it may lead to intrinsic renal damage. **Intrinsic renal failure** implies direct damage to the kidneys from an insult or congenital anomaly. **Postrenal failure** results from obstruction to urinary flow in both kidneys. In boys, the most common lesion is PUV. Renal function may be abnormal even after correction of the obstruction.

  1. Diagnosis and management should proceed simultaneously to correct the defect as quickly as possible, so that compromise of the kidney will be limited.

   a. Suspect renal failure if oliguria is present (urine flow <0.5 mL/kg/hour) and/or if serum creatinine is elevated 2 standard deviations above the mean value for gestational age (Table 31.5) or rising (0.3 mg/dL/day).

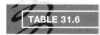

TABLE 31.6	Causes of Renal Failure in the Neonatal Period

Prerenal
  Reduced effective circulatory volume
    Hemorrhage
    Dehydration
    Sepsis
    Necrotizing enterocolitis
    Congenital heart disease
    Hypoalbuminemia
  Increased renal vascular resistance
    Polycythemia
    Indomethacin
    Adrenergic drugs (e.g., tolazoline)
  Hypoxia/asphyxia
Intrinsic or renal parenchymal
  Sustained hypoperfusion leading to acute tubular necrosis
  Congenital anomalies
    Agenesis
    Hypoplasia/dysplasia
    Polycystic kidney disease
  Thromboembolic disease
    Bilateral renal vein thrombosis
    Bilateral renal arterial thrombosis
  Nephrotoxins
    Aminoglycosides
    Radiographic contrast media
    Maternal use of captopril or indomethacin
Obstructive
  Urethral obstruction
    Posterior urethral valves
    Stricture
  Ureterocele
  Ureteropelvic/ureterovesical obstruction
  Extrinsic tumors
  Neurogenic bladder
  Megacystis or megaureter syndrome

    b. Evaluate history for oligohydramnios, perinatal asphyxia, bleeding disorders, polycythemia, thrombocytosis, thrombocytopenia, or maternal drug use.
    c. Identify abdominal mass or congenital anomaly.
    d. Perform ultrasonographic examination of GU system.
    e. Catheterize the bladder to rule out lower urinary-tract obstruction, measure residual urine volume, collect urine for analysis, and monitor subsequent urinary flow rate.
    f. To rule out prerenal failure, give a fluid challenge of normal saline 10 to 20 mL/kg over 1 hour if there is no evidence of heart failure or volume

TABLE 31.7	Renal Failure Indices in the Oliguric Neonate	
Indices	**Prerenal failure**	**Intrinsic renal failure**
Urine sodium (mEq/L)	10–50	30–90
Urine/plasma creatinine	29.2 ± 1.6	9.7 ± 3.6
FeNa*	0.9 ± 0.6	4.3 ± 2.2

*Fractional excretion of sodium defined in Chap. 9.
Modified from Mathew OP, Jones AS, James E, et al. Neonatal renal failure: Usefulness of diagnostic indices. *Pediatrics* 1980;65:57.

overload, and administer a diuretic (furosemide, 1 mg/kg). No response suggests intrinsic or postrenal failure. An infusion of low-dose dopamine ($\sim$2.5 μg/kg/min) may improve RBF and increase urine output.

- **g.** Table 31.7 lists laboratory tests that are helpful in differentiating prerenal from intrinsic renal failure in the oliguric patient. Test samples should be obtained before fluid challenge or diuretic administration if possible.

2. Management of renal failure. (see Chap. 9)

- **a.** Discontinue or minimize potassium (K^+) intake. Low-K^+ formula such as Similac PM 60/40 or K^+-free IV solution is used. Treatment of hyperkalemia (K^+ >6 mEq/L) is as follows:
  - **i. Sodium polystyrene sulfonate (Kayexalate)** is administered rectally in a dose of 1.0 to 1.5 g/kg (dissolved in normal saline at 0.5 g/mL saline) or orally in a dose of 1.0 g/kg (dissolved in dextrose 10% in water) every 4 to 6 hours. The enema tube, a thin Silastic feeding tube, is inserted 1 to 3 cm. If possible, we avoid using Kayexalate in low birth weight infants. Kayexalate 1 g/kg of removes 1 mEq/L of potassium.
  - **ii. Calcium** is given as 1 to 2 mL/kg of calcium gluconate 10% over 2 to 4 minutes while the electrocardiogram (ECG) is monitored.
  - **iii. Sodium bicarbonate.** 1 mEq/kg given intravenously over 5 to 10 minutes, will decrease serum potassium by 1 mEq/L.
  - **iv. Glucose and insulin.** Begin with a bolus of regular human insulin (0.05 units/kg) and dextrose 10% in water (2 mL/kg) followed by a continuous infusion of dextrose 10% in water at 2 to 4 mL/kg/hour and human regular insulin (10 units/100 mL) at 1 mL/kg/hour. Monitor blood glucose level frequently. Maintain a ratio of 1 or 2 units of insulin to 4 g glucose.
  - **v. Furosemide.** Furosemide 1 mg/kg is given when renal function is adequate or as a trial to establish urine flow as kaliuresis as well as natriuresis occurs with this diuretic.
  - **vi. Dialysis** is considered when hyperkalemia cannot be controlled or if anuria is present. All modes of dialysis—hemodialysis (HD), peritoneal dialysis (PD), continuous venovenous hemoperfusion (CVVH)—can be used, however, special expertise is needed in this age-group (see j).
- **b.** Fluid management is based on the patient's fluid status and should be limited to replacement of insensible losses and urine output (see Chap. 9).
- **c.** Sodium (Na^+) is restricted and Na^+ concentration is monitored, accounting for fluid balance. Hyponatremia is usually secondary to excess free water. Close monitoring of electrolytes especially sodium is needed during diuretic therapy or with dialysis.
- **d.** Phosphorus is restricted by using a low-phosphorus formula (e.g., Similac PM 60/40). Oral calcium carbonate can be used as a phosphate-binding agent.
- **e.** Calcium supplementation is given if ionized calcium is decreased or the patient is symptomatic. In infants with chronic renal failure, 1,25-dihydroxyvitamin

D or its analog is given to maximize Ca^{2+} absorption and prevent renal osteodystrophy (see Chap. 29).

f. Metabolic acidosis is usually mild unless there is (i) significant tubular dysfunction with decreased ability to reabsorb bicarbonate, or (ii) increased lactate production due to decreased perfusion due to heart failure or volume loss from hemorrhage (see III.B). Use sodium bicarbonate or sodium citrate to correct severe metabolic acidosis.

g. Nutrition is limited by severe fluid restriction. Infants who can take oral feeding are given a low-phosphate formula with a low renal solute load (e.g., Similac PM 60/40). Caloric density is increased to a maximum of 50 kcal/oz with glucose polymers (Polycose) and corn oil. Parenteral nutrition is given when oral feeding is not tolerated. Protein is limited to 0.5 g/kg/day and is increased as tolerated.

h. Hypertension (see III. D).

i. Drugs that are renally excreted must have their dosing schedule adjusted in accordance with the patient's renal function. Potential nephrotoxic drugs such as indomethacin and aminoglycosides should be avoided.

j. Dialysis is indicated when conservative management has been unsuccessful in correcting severe fluid overload, hyperkalemia, acidosis, and uremia. Inadequate nutrition because of severe fluid restriction in the anuric infant is a relative indication. Because the technical aspects and the supportive care is specialized and demanding, this procedure must be performed in centers where the staff have experience with dialysis in infants and neonates.

C. Congenital anomalies may be defined by prenatal or postnatal ultrasonography. Common lesions are hydronephrosis and MCDK. Differential diagnosis includes other renal masses (Table 31.2). The clinician should evaluate the infant for other potential renal problems such as poor urinary stream or dribbling, UTI, hematuria, and fever.

D. Blood pressure in the newborn is related to weight and gestational age. Blood pressure rises with postnatal age, 1 to 2 mm Hg/day during the first week and 1 mm Hg/week during the next 6 weeks in both the preterm and full-term infant.

1. Normative values of blood pressure are shown for full-term infants and premature infants in Tables 31.8–31.10.

2. Hypertension is defined as persistent blood pressure >2 standard deviations above the mean. Premature infants with bronchopulmonary dysplasia or who have undergone umbilical artery catheterization are at increased risk for hypertension. The clinical signs and symptoms, which may be absent or nonspecific, include cardiorespiratory abnormalities such as tachypnea, cardiomegaly, or

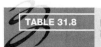

TABLE 31.8 **Normal Longitudinal Blood Pressure in Full-term Infants (mm Hg)**

Age	Boys		Girls	
	Systolic	Diastolic	Systolic	Diastolic
1st d	67 ± 7	37 ± 7	68 ± 8	38 ± 7
4th d	76 ± 8	44 ± 9	75 ± 8	45 ± 8
1 mo	84 ± 10	46 ± 9	82 ± 9	46 ± 10
3 mo	92 ± 11	55 ± 10	89 ± 11	54 ± 10
6 mo	96 ± 9	58 ± 10	92 ± 10	56 ± 10

From Gemeilli M, Managanaro R, Mami C, et al. Longitudinal study of blood pressure during the 1st year of life. *Eur J Pediatr* 1990;149:318.

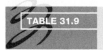

| TABLE 31.9 | Systolic and Diastolic Blood Pressure Ranges in Infants of 500–2,000 Grams Birth Weight at 3–6 h of Life |

Birth weight (g)	Systolic (mm Hg)	Diastolic (mm Hg)
501–750	50–62	26–36
751–1,000	48–59	23–36
1,001–1,250	49–61	26–35
1,251–1,500	46–56	23–33
1,501–1,750	46–58	23–33
1,751–2,000	48–61	24–35

From Hegyi T, Carbone MT, Anwar M, et al. Blood pressure ranges in premature infants. 1. The first hours of life. *J Pediatr* 1994;124:627–633.

heart failure; neurologic findings such as irritability, lethargy, or seizure; failure to thrive; or GI difficulties.

3. Neonatal hypertension has many causes (see Table 31.11), which may be determined by history and physical examination and a review of fluid status, medications, use and location of umbilical arterial catheter, maternal history, and other clinical findings such as intracranial hemorrhage and chronic lung disease. If a particular cause is suspected, proceed with appropriate evaluation. Otherwise, the initial evaluation is focused on renovascular and renal causes, which are most commonly responsible for neonatal hypertension. Urinalysis, renal function studies, serum electrolyte levels, and renal ultrasonographic examination should also be obtained. Color Doppler flow studies may detect aortic or renal vascular thrombosis. A DMSA renal scan may detect segmental renal arterial infarctions. Plasma renin levels are difficult to interpret in newborns because of the lack of normative values for gestational age and postnatal age.

4. Management is directed at correcting the underlying cause whenever possible. Antihypertensive therapy (see Table 31.12) is administered for sustained hypertension not related to volume overload or medications.

E. **Renal vascular thrombosis** (see Chap. 26F)

1. **Renal artery thrombosis (RAT)** is often related to the use of indwelling umbilical artery catheters. Management is controversial. The options include surgical

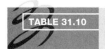

| TABLE 31.10 | Mean Arterial Blood Pressure (MAP) in Infants of 500–1,500 Grams Birth Weight |

	MAP ± SD (mm Hg)		
Birth weight (g)	Day 3	Day 17	Day 31
501–750	38 ± 8	44 ± 8	46 ± 11
751–1,000	43 ± 9	45 ± 7	47 ± 9
1,001–1,250	43 ± 8	46 ± 9	48 ± 8
1,251–1,500	45 ± 8	47 ± 8	47 ± 9

From Klaus MH, Fanaroff AA, eds. *Care of the High-risk Neonate.* Philadelphia: WB Saunders, 1993;497.

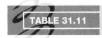

TABLE 31.11 **Causes of Hypertension in the Neonate**

Vascular
  Renal artery thrombosis
  Renal vein thrombosis
  Coarctation of the aorta
  Renal artery stenosis
  Idiopathic arterial calcification
Renal
  Obstructive uropathy
  Polycystic kidney disease
  Renal insufficiency
  Renal tumor
  Wilms tumor
  Glomerulonephritis
  Pyelonephritis
Endocrine
  Congenital adrenal hypoplasia
  Primary hyperaldosteronism
  Hyperthyroidism
Neurologic
  Increased intracranial pressure
  Cushing's disease
  Neural crest tumor
  Cerebral angioma
  Drug withdrawal
Pulmonary
  Bronchopulmonary dysplasia
Drugs
  Corticosteroids
  Theophylline
  Adrenergic agents
  Phenylephrine
Other
  Fluid/electrolyte overload
  Abdominal surgery
  Associated with extracorporeal membrane oxygenation (ECMO)

thrombectomy, thrombolytic agents, and conservative medical care including antihypertensive therapy. The surgical renal salvage rate is no better than medical management, and carries a considerable mortality rate of 33%. Patients with unilateral RAT who received conservative medical treatment are usually normotensive by 2 years of age, no longer receiving antihypertensive medications, and have normal creatinine clearance, although some have unilateral renal atrophy with compensatory contralateral hypertrophy. There have been reports of long-term complications with hypertension and/or proteinuria and progression to renal failure in adolescence.

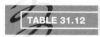

TABLE 31.12	**Antihypertensive Agents for the Newborn (See Appendix A for Specific Dosing Recommendations)**

	Dose	Comment
Diuretics		
Furosemide	0.5–1.0 mg/kg/dose IV, IM, PO	May cause hyponatremia, hypokalemia, hypercalciuria
Chlorothiazide	20–40 mg/kg/day PO; divided q12h	May cause hyponatremia, hypokalemia, hypochloremia
	2–8 mg/kg/day IV divided q12h	
Vasodilators		
Hydralazine	1–8 mg/kg/day; divided q 6–8 h	May cause tachycardia
Nitroprusside	0.2–6 μg/kg/min continuous IV infusion	Monitor isothiocyanate levels
Calcium channel blockers		
Nifedipine	0.2 mg/kg/dose SL, PO	Limited in neonates; may cause tachycardia
Basal receptor antagonist		
Propranolol	0.5–5.0 mg/kg/day PO; divided q 6–8 h	May cause bronchospasm
α/β-receptor antagonist		
Labetalol	0.5–1.0 mg/kg/dose IV, q 4–6 h	Limited use in neonates
ACE inhibitor		
Captopril	0.15–2.0 mg/kg/day PO, divided q 8–12 h	May cause oliguria, hyperkalemia, renal failure
Enalapril	5–10 μg/kg/dose IV, 8–24 h	May cause oliguria, hyperkalemia, renal failure

ACE = angiotensin-converting enzyme.

2. **Renal vein thrombosis (RVT)** has the predisposing conditions of hyperosmolarity, polycythemia, hypovolemia, and hypercoagulable states and is therefore commonly associated with infant of diabetic mothers, or use of umbilical venous catheters. Cases of interuterine renal venous thrombosis have been described and present with calcification of the clot in the inferior vena cava (IVC). The clinical findings include gross hematuria often with clots, enlarged kidneys, hypertension, and thrombocytopenia. Other symptoms include vomiting, shock, lower extremity edema, and abdominal distention. The diagnosis of RVT is confirmed by ultrasonography, which typically shows an enlarged kidney with diffuse homogenous hyperechogenicity; Doppler-flow studies may detect thrombi in the IVC or renal vein. Differential diagnosis include renal masses or hemolytic uremic syndrome.

   The management of RVT is also controversial. Initial therapy should focus on the maintenance of circulation, fluid, and electrolyte balance while examining for underlying predisposing clinical conditions. Assessment of the coagulation status includes platelet count, prothrombin time (PT), partial thromboplastin time (PTT), fibrinogen, and fibrin split products and, if suggested by maternal history, lupus antiphospholipid antibodies.

   No consensus exists on the use of heparin. Our approach depends on the patient's clinical status. If there is unilateral involvement without evidence of disseminated intravascular coagulation (DIC), we use conservative management. If there is bilateral involvement and evidence of DIC, we initiate heparin therapy with an initial bolus of 50 to 100 units/kg followed by continuous infusion at 25 to 50 units/kg to maintain PTT of 1.5 times normal. Antithrombin III (AT III) activity should be reassessed before heparin therapy is instituted as AT III is required for the anticoagulant action of heparin. Heparin-induced hyperkalemia is a risk, hence monitoring K^+ is necessary. Recently, low-molecular-weight heparin has been used both as initial treatment for thrombosis and as prophylactic therapy after recannulization of the occluded vessel. In the treatment of patients with thrombosis, dosages of 200 to 300 anti-Fxa U/kg are reported to reach a therapeutic level of 0.5–1.0 anti-Fxa U/mL. Reported dosages range from 45 to 100 anti-Fxa units/kg to reach prophylactic levels of 0.2 to 0.4 anti-Fxa U/mL.

Thrombolytic therapy with streptokinase and urokinase have been used in both RAT and RVT, with variable success (see Chap. 26) but are no longer commercially available. There is limited experience with the use of thromboplastin activator (TPA). This is used in low dose (0.02–0.03 mg/kg) if there is evidence of bleeding, and titrated to PTT value of 1.5 times normal. Plasma infusion may be necessary to provide thromboplastin activation. Protamine and e-caproic acid should be present at the bedside because significant bleeding can occur. Surgical intervention should be considered if there has been an indwelling umbilical vein catheter, the thrombosis is bilateral, and involves the main renal renal veins leading to renal failure. This type of thrombosis is likely to have started in the IVC rather than intrarenal and hence is more likely amenable to surgical attention.

F. Proteinuria in newborns is frequently normal. After the first week, persistent proteinuria >250 mg/m^2/day should be investigated (Table 31.4).

1. In general, **mild proteinuria** reflects a vascular or tubular injury to the kidney. Administration of large amounts of colloid can exceed the reabsorptive capacity of the neonatal renal tubules and may result in mild proteinuria.

2. **Massive proteinuria** (>1.5 g/m^2/day), hypoalbuminemia with serum albumin levels <2.5 g/dL, and edema are all components of congenital nephrotic syndrome. A renal biopsy is often required for final diagnosis. Prenatal diagnosis of Finnish-type nephrotic syndrome is possible before the 20th week of gestation by detection of elevated maternal and amniotic α-fetoprotein levels.

3. No specific treatment is required for mild proteinuria. Treat the underlying disease and monitor the proteinuria until resolved.

4. Glomerular disease is rare and usually associated with congenital nephrotic syndrome if presentation is in the nursery.

G. Hematuria is defined as >5 red blood cells per high-power field. It is uncommon in newborns and should always be investigated.

1. Hematuria has many causes (see Table 31.13) including hemorrhagic disease of the newborn if vitamin K supplementation has not been given. The differential diagnosis for hematuria includes urate staining of the diaper, myoglobinuria, or hemoglobinuria. A negative dipstick with benign sediment suggests urates, whereas a positive dipstick with negative sediment for red blood cells (RBCs) indicates the presence of globin pigments. Vaginal bleeding ("pseudomenses") in girls or a severe diaper rash is also a possible cause of blood in the diaper or positive dipstick for heme.

2. Evaluation of neonatal hematuria depends on the clinical situation. In most cases, the initial investigation includes the following tests: urinalysis with examination of the sediment, urine culture, ultrasonography of the upper and lower urinary tract, evaluation of renal function (serum creatinine and BUN), and coagulation studies.

H. UTI. (see Chap. 5)

1. Infections of the urinary tract in newborns can result in asymptomatic bacteriuria or can lead to pyelonephritis and/or sepsis. A urine culture should be obtained from every infant with fever, poor weight gain, poor feeding, unexplained prolonged jaundice, or any clinical signs of sepsis.

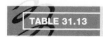

TABLE 31.13	Etiology of Hematuria in the Newborn

Acute tubular necrosis
Cortical necrosis
Vascular diseases
   Renal vein thrombosis
   Renal artery thrombosis
Bleeding and clotting disorders (including hemorrhagic disease of newborn)
   Disseminated intravascular coagulation
   Severe thrombocytopenia
   Clotting factors deficiency
Urological anomalies
Urinary-tract infection
Glomerular diseases (see F)
Tumors
   Wilms tumor
   Neuroblastoma
   Angiomas
Nephrocalcinosis
Trauma
   Suprapubic bladder aspiration
   Urethral catheterization

2. The diagnosis is confirmed by positive urine culture obtained by suprapubic bladder aspiration or catheterized specimen with a colony count exceeding 1,000 colonies per millimeter. A blood culture should also be obtained, even from asymptomatic infants. Although most newborns with UTIs have leukocytes in the urine, an infection can be present in the absence of leukocyturia.

3. *Escherichia coli* accounts for approximately 75% of the infections. The remainder are caused by other gram-negative bacilli (Klebsiella, Enterobacter, Proteus) and by gram-positive cocci (enterococci, *Staphylococcus epidermidis*, *Staphylococcus aureus*).

4. Evaluation of the urinary tract by ultrasonography is required emergently to rule out obstructive uropathy or neurogenic bladder with inability to empty the bladder. Adequate drainage or relief of obstruction is necessary for antibiotic control of the infection. VCUG is needed to detect reflux and define lower-tract abnormalities. VUR occurs in 40% of neonates with UTIs and predominates slightly in boys. If a renal abnormality is detected, a renal scan is done to assess renal cortex and function. Inadequate therapy, particularly in the presence of urological abnormalities, could lead to renal scarring with potential development of hypertension and loss of renal function.

5. The initial treatment is antibiotics, usually a combination of ampicillin and gentamicin, given parenterally. The final choice of antibiotic is based on the sensitivity of the cultured organism. Treatment is continued for 10 to 14 days, and amoxicillin prophylaxis (20 mg/kg/day) is administered until a VCUG is performed. If VUR is present, prophylactic treatment should continue until the reflux has resolved. For later onset infections (>7 days) in hospitalized infants, some experts would suggest using vancomycin rather than ampicillin to cover the possibility of hospital acquired organisms until definitive culture results are available.

I. Tubular disorders

1. **Fanconi syndrome** is a group of disorders with generalized dysfunction of the proximal tubule resulting in excessive urinary losses of amino acids, glucose, phosphate, and bicarbonate. The glomerular function is usually normal.

   a. **Clinical and laboratory findings** include the following:

      i. Hypophosphatemia due to the excessive urinary loss of phosphate. In these patients the TRP is abnormally low. Rickets and osteoporosis are secondary to hypophosphatemia and can appear in the neonatal period.

      ii. Metabolic acidosis is secondary to bicarbonate wasting (proximal renal tubular acidosis [RTA]).

      iii. Aminoaciduria and glycosuria do not result in significant clinical signs or symptoms.

      iv. These infants are often polyuric and therefore at risk for dehydration.

      v. Hypokalemia, due to increased excretion by the distal tubule to compensate for the increased sodium reabsorption, is also frequent and sometimes profound.

   b. **Etiology.** The primary form of Fanconi syndrome is rare in the neonatal period and is a diagnosis of exclusion. Although familial cases (mainly autosomal dominant) have been reported, it is generally sporadic. Most secondary forms of the syndrome in the neonatal period are related to inborn errors of metabolism, including cystinosis, hereditary tyrosinemia, hereditary fructose intolerance, galactosemia, glycogenosis, Lowe syndrome (oculocerebrorenal syndrome), and mitochondrial disorders. Cases associated with heavy metal toxicity have also been described.

2. **RTA** is defined as metabolic acidosis resulting from the inability of the kidney to excrete hydrogen ions or to reabsorb bicarbonate. Poor growth may result from RTA.

   a. **Distal RTA (type I)** is caused by a defect in the secretion of hydrogen ions by the distal tubule. The urine cannot be acidified below 6 pH. It is frequently associated with hypokalemia and hypercalciuria. Nephrocalcinosis (NC) is common later in life. In the neonatal period, distal RTA may be primary, due to a genetic defect, or secondary to several disorders including NC, obstructive uropathies, drugs such as amphotericin B, heavy metals, and hereditary elliptocytosis.

   b. **Proximal RTA (type II)** is a defect in the proximal tubule with reduced bicarbonate reabsorption leading to bicarbonate wasting. Serum bicarbonate concentration falls until the abnormally low threshold for bicarbonate reabsorption is reached in the proximal tubule (generally <16 mEq/L). Once this threshold has been reached, no significant amount of bicarbonate reaches the distal tubule, and the urine can be acidified at that level. Proximal RTA can occur as an isolated defect or in association with Fanconi syndrome (see III.I).

   c. **Hyperkalemic RTA (type IV)** is a result of a combined impaired ability of the distal tubule to excrete hydrogen ions and potassium. In the neonatal period, this disorder is seen in infants with aldosterone deficiency, adrenogenital syndrome, reduced tubular responsiveness to aldosterone, or associated obstructive uropathies. It can also be induced by treatment with angiotensin-converting enzyme (ACE) inhibitors or spironolactone.

   d. **The treatment of RTA** is based on correction of the acidosis with alkaline therapy. Bicitra or sodium bicarbonate, 2 to 3 mEq/kg/day in divided doses, is usually sufficient to treat type I and type IV RTA. The treatment of proximal RTA requires larger doses sometimes as high as 10 mEq/kg/day bicarbonate. In secondary forms of RTA, the treatment of the primary cause often results in the resolution of the RTA.

J. Nephrocalcinosis (NC) is detected by renal ultrasound examinations (see Chap. 29).

1. NC is generally associated with a hypercalciuric state. Drugs that are associated with NC and increased urinary calcium excretion include loop diuretics such as furosemide, methylxanthines, glucocorticoids, and vitamin D in

pharmacologic doses. In addition, hyperoxaluria, often associated with parenteral nutrition, and hyperphosphaturia facilitate the deposition of calcium crystals in the kidney.

2. Renal stones and NC secondary to primary hyperoxaluria/oxalosis, RTA, or UTIs are rare in newborns.

3. Few follow-up studies of NC in premature infants are available. In general, renal function is not significantly impaired, and 75% cases resolve spontaneously often within the first year of life as demonstrated by ultrasonography but resolution may take up to 5 to 7 years. However, significant tubular dysfunction at 1 to 2 years of age has been reported.

4. It is unclear whether NC requires a specific treatment. If possible, drugs that cause hypercalciuria should be discontinued. Change to or addition of thiazide diuretics and supplemental magnesium in patients with bronchopulmonary dysplasia with a need for long-term diuretic therapy may be helpful. Monitoring of urinary calcium excretion (urine calcium:creatinine ratio) help in determining response to therapy.

K. **Cystic disease of the kidney** may result from abnormalities in development, such as multicystic dysplasia, or from genetically induced diseases. The principal differential diagnosis of bilateral cystic kidney disease in the newborn includes autosomal recessive polycystic kidney disease (**ARPKD**), the infantile form of autosomal dominant polycystic kidney disease (ADPKD), and glomerulocystic kidney disease (which in some affected families represents a variant of ADPKD).

1. In ARPKD, the genetic defect has been mapped to chromosome 6p21, which encodes a novel protein product named fibrocystin or polyductin. In infants with ARPKD, the kidneys appear markedly enlarged and hyperechogenic by ultrasonography, with a typical "snowstorm" appearance with concurrent liver fibrosis and/or dilated bile ducts. In contrast, macroscopic cysts are usually detected in cases of ADPKD and glomerulocystic disease and the liver is spared. The clinical findings of ARPKD are variable and include bilateral smooth enlarged kidneys, varying degrees of renal insufficiency, which usually progresses to renal failure over time and severe renin-mediated hypertension. Infants with more severe involvement may have oligohydramnios with pulmonary hypoplasia and Potter syndrome but those patients who survive the neonatal period can be carried to renal transplantation in later childhood or adolescence. ARPKD is always associated with liver involvement, which may progress to liver failure requiring transplantation in adolescence. The diagnosis is confirmed by renal and liver biopsy, unless the family history is certain.

2. In ADPKD, an abnormal gene PKD1 has been identified and located on the short arm of chromosome 16, and a second gene PKD2 located on the long arm of chromosome 4. These two genes account for most of the ADPKD patients. Clinical manifestations include bilateral renal masses that are usually less symmetrical than in ARPKD. Hypertension is also less common than ARPKD.

3. Other hereditary syndromes that can manifest as renal cystic disease include tuberous sclerosis, von Hippel-Lindau disease, Jeune asphyxiating thoracic dysplasia, oral-facial-digital syndrome type 1, brachymesomelia-renal syndrome, and trisomy 9, 13, and 18.

L. The decision for circumcision is based primarily on cultural or ethnic background. Data on risk of UTIs, penile cancer, and protection from sexually transmitted diseases in circumcised and uncircumcised men are insufficient to recommend routine circumcisions. Medical indications for circumcision include urinary retention due to adhesions of the foreskin or to tight phimosis. Circumcision should be avoided in cases of hypospadias, ambiguous genitalia, and bleeding disorders (see Chap. 23B).

M. Renal tumors are rare in the neonatal period. These include mesoblastic nephroma and nephroblastomatosis. The differential diagnosis includes other causes of renal masses (Table 31.2).

Suggested Readings

Bailie MD, ed. Renal function and disease. *Clin Perinatol* 1992;19(1):91–92.

Guignard JP, Drukker A. Clinical neonatal nephrology. In: Barratt TM, Avner ED, Harmon WE, eds. *Pediatric nephrology*. Philadelphia: Lippincott Williams & Wilkins, 1999.

Moghal NE, Embleton ND. Management of acute renal failure in the newborn. *Semin Fetal Neonatal Med* 2006;11;207–213.

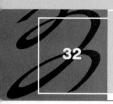

32

NECROTIZING ENTEROCOLITIS
Eric C. Eichenwald

I. **BACKGROUND. NECROTIZING ENTEROCOLITIS (NEC)** is an acute intestinal necrosis syndrome of unknown etiology. Its pathogenesis is complex and multifactorial. Our understanding of the pathophysiology is increasing as we learn more about the crucial role of inflammatory mediators. Current clinical practice is directed toward prompt, early diagnosis and rapid institution of proper intensive care management.

A. **Epidemiology.** NEC is the most common serious surgical disorder among infants in a neonatal intensive care unit (NICU) and is a significant cause of neonatal morbidity and mortality.

1. The **incidence** of NEC varies from center to center and from year to year within centers. There are endemic and epidemic occurrences. An estimated 0.3 to 2.4 cases occur in every 1,000 live births. In most centers, NEC occurs in 2% to 5% of all NICU admissions and 5% to 10% of very low birth weight (VLBW) infants. If VLBW infants who die early are excluded and only infants who have been fed included, the incidence is approximately 15%.

2. Sex, race, geography, climate, and season do not appear to play any determining role in the incidence or course of NEC.

3. **Prematurity** is the single greatest risk factor. Decreasing gestational age is associated with an increased risk for NEC. The mean gestational age of infants with NEC is 30 to 32 weeks, and the infants generally are weight appropriate for gestational age. Approximately 10% of infants with NEC are full-term. The postnatal age at onset is inversely related to birth weight and gestational age, with a mean age at onset of 12 days. More than 90% of infants have been fed before the onset of this disease.

4. Infants exposed to cocaine have a 2.5 times increased risk of developing NEC. The vasoconstrictive and hemodynamic properties of cocaine may promote intestinal ischemia (see Chap. 19).

5. The overall **mortality** is 9% to 28% regardless of surgical or medical intervention. The mortality for infants weighing <1,500 g can be as high as 45%; for those weighing <750 g, it may be much higher. The introduction of standardized therapeutic protocols with criteria for medical management and surgical intervention, a high index of suspicion for the disease, and general improvements in neonatal intensive care, have decreased the mortality rate. Infants exposed to cocaine who develop NEC have a significantly higher incidence of massive gangrene, perforation, and mortality than do infants not exposed.

6. Case-controlled epidemiologic studies have revealed that almost all previously described risk factors for NEC, including maternal disorders (e.g., toxemia), the infant's course (e.g., asphyxia, patent ductus arteriosus [PDA]), and the type of management (e.g., umbilical artery catheterization [UAC]), simply describe a population of high-risk neonates. Excluding cocaine exposure, no maternal or neonatal factors other than prematurity are known to increase the risk of NEC. This suggests that immaturity of the gastrointestinal (GI) tract is the greatest risk factor.

B. **Pathogenesis**
1. The **causes** of NEC are not well defined. NEC is likely a heterogeneous disease resulting from complex interactions between mucosal injury secondary to a variety of factors (including ischemia, luminal substrate, and infection) and poor host protective mechanism(s) in response to injury.

2. The concept of a **hypoxic or hemodynamic insult,** resulting in splanchnic vasoconstriction and reduced mesenteric flow, inducing bowel mucosal hypoxia and rendering the intestine susceptible to injury, has long been considered a contributing factor in the pathogenesis of NEC. The pathologic findings of NEC resemble those seen in older individuals with gut vascular compromise. However, in a significant number of cases no hypoxic or ischemic problems can be identified, and the temporal sequence of events does not support an ischemic event alone.

3. **Enteral feedings** have been implicated in the pathogenesis of NEC, as almost all babies who develop NEC have been fed. Factors that have been considered include osmolality of formula, the lack of immunoprotective factors in formula, and the timing, volume, and rate of feeding. Breast milk has been shown to have protective factors; however, breast milk alone does not prevent development of NEC. Some studies have shown that very slow introduction of feedings and avoidance of large day-to-day volume increases may lower the incidence of NEC. However, the exact rate of feeding increment that predisposes infants to NEC has not been identified, and the mechanism by which excessive volumes predispose to the development of NEC is not known.

4. The **microbiologic flora** involved in NEC are not unique but represent the predominant bowel organisms present in the infant at the time of onset. Various bacterial and viral agents have been included in the microbial picture that is sometimes associated with NEC, especially with epidemic NEC, but none has yet been proved to be causal. Release of endotoxin and cytokines by proliferation of colonizing bacteria, and bacterial fermentation with gaseous distension, may play a role.

5. Evidence supports a critical role for **platelet activating factor (PAF)** and other inflammatory mediators in the pathophysiology of NEC. Animal studies show that exogenous administration or endogenous increased production of PAF causes ischemic bowel necrosis pathologically similar to NEC. Several factors may promote (e.g., leukotrienes, oxygen radicals, tumor necrosis factor) or inhibit (e.g., acetylhydrolase, steroids, nitric oxide, prostacyclin) PAF-induced intestinal injury. PAF antagonists, including dexamethasone and PAF acetylhydrolase, prevent this histologic necrosis. All the NEC risk factors—prematurity, hypoxia, feeding, and bacteria—tend to increase the concentration of circulating or local PAF. The high biosynthetic activity of intestinal tissue for inflammatory mediators (especially PAF), make it particularly susceptible to necrosis.

6. **Histopathologic examination** of tissue after surgery or autopsy shows that the terminal ileum and ascending colon are the most frequently involved areas, but in the most severe cases the entire bowel may be involved. This localization has implications for long-term sequelae (see IV). The pathologic lesions consist of coagulation necrosis, bacterial overgrowth, inflammation, and reparative changes. These suggest that the disease is initiated by subtotal ischemia and gradual tissue compromise that results in bacterial invasion and inflammation.

7. Use of **H2 blockers** have been implicated in a higher risk of NEC in extremely low birth weight (ELBW) infants, suggesting that an acidic GI environment may be protective.

II. DIAGNOSIS. Early diagnosis of NEC is the most important factor in determining outcome. This is accomplished by careful clinical observation for nonspecific signs in infants at risk.

A. Clinical characteristics. There is a broad spectrum of disease manifestations. The clinical features of NEC can be divided into systemic and abdominal signs. Most infants have a combination of both.

1. **Systemic signs.** Respiratory distress, apnea and/or bradycardia, lethargy, temperature instability, irritability, poor feeding, hypotension (shock), decreased peripheral perfusion, acidosis, oliguria, bleeding diathesis.

2. **Abdominal (enteric) signs.** Bloody stools, abdominal distension or tenderness, gastric aspirates (feeding residuals), vomiting (of bile, blood, or both), ileus

(decreased or absent bowel sounds), abdominal wall erythema or induration, persistent localized abdominal mass, or ascites.

3. The **course of the disease** varies among infants. Most frequently, it will appear (i) as a fulminant, rapidly progressive presentation of signs consistent with intestinal necrosis and sepsis or (ii) as a slow, paroxysmal presentation of abdominal distension, ileus, and possible infection. The latter course will vary with the rapidity of therapeutic intervention and require consistent monitoring and anticipatory evaluation (see III).

B. Laboratory features. The diagnosis is suspected from clinical presentation but must be confirmed by diagnostic radiographs, surgery, or autopsy. No laboratory tests are specific for NEC; nevertheless, some tests are valuable in confirming diagnostic impressions.

1. Radiology studies. The abdominal radiograph will often reveal an abnormal gas pattern consistent with ileus. Both anteroposterior (AP) and cross-table lateral or left lateral decubitus views should be included. These films may reveal bowel wall edema, a fixed-position loop on serial studies, the appearance of a mass, pneumatosis intestinalis (the radiologic hallmark used to confirm the diagnosis), portal or hepatic venous air, pneumobilia, or pneumoperitoneum. Isolated intestinal perforation (IP) may present with pneumoperitoneum without other clinical signs.

2. Blood studies. Thrombocytopenia, persistent metabolic acidosis, and severe refractory hyponatremia constitute the most common triad of signs and help to confirm the diagnosis. Serial measurements of C-reactive protein (CRP) may also be helpful in the diagnosis and assessment of response to therapy of severe NEC.

3. Analysis of stool for blood and carbohydrate has been used to detect infants with NEC based on changes in intestinal integrity. Although grossly bloody stools may be an indication of NEC, occult hematochezia does not correlate well with NEC. Carbohydrate malabsorption, as reflected in a positive stool Clinitest result, can be a frequent and early indicator of NEC within the setting of signs noted in A.

C. Bell staging criteria with the Walsh and Kleigman modification allow for uniformity of diagnosis and treatment based on severity of illness.

1. Stage I (suspect) clinical signs and symptoms, nondiagnostic radiographs.

2. Stage II (definite) clinical signs and symptoms, pneumatosis intestinalis on radiograph.
   a. Mildly ill.
   b. Moderately ill with systemic toxicity.

3. Stage III (advanced) clinical signs and symptoms, pneumatosis intestinalis on radiograph, and critically ill.
   a. Impending IP.
   b. Proven IP.

D. Differential diagnosis

1. Pneumonia and sepsis are common and frequently associated with an intestinal ileus. The abdominal distension and tenderness characteristic of NEC will be absent, however, in infants with ileus not due to NEC.

2. Surgical abdominal catastrophes include malrotation with obstruction (complete or intermittent), malrotation with midgut volvulus, intussusception, ulcer, gastric perforation, and mesenteric vessel thrombosis (see Chap.26F). The clinical presentation of these disorders may overlap with that of NEC. Occasionally, the diagnosis is made only at the time of exploratory laparotomy.

3. Isolated IP is a distinct clinical entity which occurs in approximately 2% of ELBW infants. It often presents as asymptomatic pneumoperitoneum, although other clinical and laboratory abnormalities may be present. IP tends to occur at an earlier postnatal age then NEC, and is not associated with feeding. The risk of IP is increased with early glucocorticoid exposure and indomethacin treatment for PDA. Concurrent treatment with glucocorticoids and indomethacin substantially increases the risk of IP.

4. **Infectious enterocolitis** is rare in this population but must be considered if diarrhea is present. Campylobacter species have been associated with bloody diarrhea in the newborn. These infants lack any other systemic or enteric signs of NEC.

5. Severe forms of **inherited metabolic disease** (e.g., galactosemia with *Escherichia coli* sepsis) may lead to profound acidosis, shock, and vomiting and may initially overlap with some signs of NEC.

6. Severe **allergic colitis** can present with abdominal distension and bloody stools. Usually these infants are well appearing, and have normal abdominal radiographs and laboratory studies.

7. **Feeding intolerance** is a common but ill-defined problem in premature infants. Despite adequate GI function *in utero*, some premature infants will have periods of gastric residuals and abdominal distension associated with advancing feedings. The differentiation of this problem from NEC can be difficult. Cautious evaluation by withholding enteral feedings and administering intravenous fluids and antibiotics for 48 to 72 hours may be indicated until this benign disorder can be distinguished from NEC.

E. **Additional diagnostic considerations**

1. Since the early features are often nonspecific, **a high index of suspicion** is the most reliable approach to early diagnosis. The entire picture of history, physical examination, and laboratory features must be considered in the context of the particular infant's course. Isolated signs or laboratory values often indicate the need for a careful differential diagnosis, despite the obvious concern over NEC.

2. **Diarrhea** is an uncommon presentation of NEC in the absence of bloody stools. This sign should point away from NEC.

3. **Radiographic findings** can often be subtle and confusing. For example, perforation of an abdominal viscus will not always cause pneumoperitoneum, and conversely, pneumoperitoneum does not necessarily indicate abdominal perforation from NEC. Serial review of the radiographs with a pediatric radiologist is indicated to assist in interpretation and to plan for further appropriate studies.

III. MANAGEMENT

A. **Immediate medical management** (Table 32.1). Treatment should begin promptly when signs suggestive of NEC are present. Therapy is based on intensive-care measures and the anticipation of potential problems.

1. **Respiratory function.** Rapid assessment of ventilatory status (physical examination, arterial blood gases) should be made, and supplemental oxygen and mechanical ventilatory support should be provided as needed.

2. **Cardiovascular function.** Rapid assessment of circulatory status (physical examination, blood pressure) should be made, and circulatory support should be provided as needed. Volume in the form of normal saline or fresh frozen plasma (dose 10 mL/kg) may be used. Pharmacologic support may be necessary; in this case, we use low doses of dopamine (3 to 5 μg/kg per minute) to optimize the effect on splanchnic and renal blood flow. Impending circulatory collapse will often be reflected by poor perfusion and oxygenation, although arterial blood pressure may be maintained. Intra-arterial blood pressure monitoring is often necessary, but the proximity of the umbilical arteries to the mesenteric circulation precludes the use of these vessels. In fact, any umbilical artery catheter should be promptly removed and peripheral artery catheters used. Further monitoring of central venous pressure (CVP) may become necessary if additional pharmacologic support of the circulation or failing myocardium is needed (see Chap. 17).

3. **Metabolic function.** Severe metabolic acidosis will generally respond to volume expansion but may require treatment with sodium bicarbonate (2 mEq/kg). The blood pH and lactate level should be carefully monitored; in addition, serum electrolyte levels and liver function should be measured. Blood glucose levels should be monitored as well.

4. **Nutrition.** All GI feedings are discontinued, and the bowel is decompressed by suctioning through a nasogastric tube. Parenteral nutrition (PN) is given

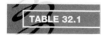

Bell staging criteria	Diagnosis	Management (usual attention to respiratory, cardiovascular and hematologic resuscitation presumed)
Stage I (suspect)	Clinical signs and symptoms Nondiagnostic radiograph	NPO with IV fluids Nasogastric drainage CBC, lytes, KUB q6–8 h × 48 h Blood culture Stool heme test and Clinitest Ampicillin and gentamicin × 48 hours
Stage II (definite)	Clinical signs and symptoms Pneumatosis intestinalis on radiograph	NPO with parenteral nutrition (by CVL once sepsis ruled out) Nasogastric drainage CBC, lytes, KUB (AP and lateral) q6–8 h × 48–72 h, then prn Blood culture Stool heme test and Clinitest Ampicillin, gentamicin and clindamycin × 14 days Surgical consultation
Stage III (Advanced)	Clinical signs and symptoms Critically ill Pneumatosis intestinalis or pneumoperitoneum on radiograph	NPO with parenteral nutrition (by CVL once sepsis ruled out) Nasogastric drainage CBC, lytes, KUB (AP and lateral) q6–8 h × 48–72 h, then prn Stool heme test and Clinitest Ampicillin, gentamicin, and clindamycin × 14 days Surgical consultation with intervention, if indicated: Resection with enterostomy or primary anastomosis In selected cases (usually <1,000 g and unstable), bedside drainage under local anesthesia

TABLE 32.1 Management of Necrotizing Enterocolitis

AP = anteroposterior; CBC = complete blood count, CVL = central venous line; KUB = kidney, urethra, bladder x-ray; NPO = nothing by mouth.

through a peripheral vein as soon as possible, with the aim of providing 90 to 110 cal/kg per day once amino acid solutions and intralipid are both tolerated. A central venous catheter is almost always necessary to provide adequate calories in the VLBW infant. We wait to place a central catheter for this purpose until the blood cultures are negative for 2 to 5 days, during which time adaptation to peripheral PN can take place.

5. **Infectious disease.** Blood, urine, stool, and cerebrospinal fluid (CSF) specimens are obtained, examined carefully for indications of infection, and sent for culture and sensitivity. We routinely begin broad-spectrum antibiotics as soon as possible, utilizing ampicillin, gentamicin, and clindamycin to cover most enteric flora. Piperacillin-tazobactam (Zosyn) has recently been used due to its broad spectrum and the ability to use as a single agent. With changing antibiotic sensitivities, one must be aware of the predominant NICU flora,

the organisms associated with NEC, and their resistance patterns and adjust antibiotic coverage accordingly. Stool should be tested for aminoglycoside-resistant organisms. Antibiotic therapy is adjusted on the basis of culture results, but only 10% to 40% of blood cultures will be positive, necessitating continued broad coverage in most cases. In infants requiring surgery, peritoneal fluid cultures may also help target appropriate antibiotic treatment. Treatment is generally maintained for 14 days. There is no evidence to support the use of enteral antibiotics.

6. **Hematologic aspects.** Analysis of the complete blood count and differential, with examination of the blood smear, is always indicated. We use platelet transfusions to correct severe thrombocytopenia and packed red blood cells (PRBCs) to maintain the hematocrit above 35%. The prothrombin time, partial thromboplastin time, fibrinogen, and platelet count should be evaluated for evidence of disseminated intravascular coagulation. Fresh-frozen plasma is used to treat coagulation problems.

7. **Renal function.** Oliguria often accompanies the initial hypotension and hypoperfusion of NEC; measurement of urine output is essential. In addition, serum blood urea nitrogen (BUN), creatinine, and serum electrolyte levels should be monitored. Impending renal failure from acute tubular necrosis, coagulative necrosis, or vascular accident must be anticipated, and fluid therapy must be adjusted accordingly (see Chap. 31).

8. **Neurologic function.** Evaluation of the infant's condition is difficult given the degree of illness, but one must be alert to the problems of associated meningitis and intraventricular hemorrhage. Seizures may occur secondary to either of these problems or from the metabolic perturbations associated with NEC. These complications must be anticipated and promptly recognized and treated.

9. **GI function.** Physical examination and serial (every 6 to 8 hours during the first 2 to 3 days) radiographs are used to assess ongoing GI damage. Unless perforation occurs or full-thickness necrosis precipitates severe peritonitis, management remains medical. The evaluation for surgical intervention, however, is an important and complex management issue (see III.B).

10. **Family support.** Any family of an infant in the NICU may be overwhelmed by the crisis. Infants with NEC present a particular challenge because the disease often causes sudden deterioration for "no apparent reason." Furthermore, the impending possibility of surgical intervention and the high mortality and uncertain prognosis make this situation most difficult for parents. Careful anticipatory sharing of information must be utilized by the staff to establish a trusting alliance with the family.

B. **Surgical intervention**
1. **Prompt consultation** should be obtained with a pediatric surgeon. This will allow the surgeon to become familiar with the case and will provide an additional evaluation by another skilled individual. If a pediatric surgeon is not available, the infant should be transferred to a site where one is.

2. **GI perforation** is generally agreed on as an indication for intervention. Unfortunately, there is no reliable or absolute indicator of imminent perforation; therefore, careful monitoring is necessary. Perforation occurs in 20% to 30% of patients, usually 12 to 48 hours after the onset of NEC, although it can occur later. In some cases, the absence of pneumoperitoneum on the abdominal radiograph can delay the diagnosis, and paracentesis may aid in establishing the diagnosis. In general, an infant with increasing abdominal distension, an abdominal mass, a worsening clinical picture despite medical management, or a persistent fixed loop on serial radiographs may have a perforation and may require operative intervention.

3. **Full-thickness necrosis of the GI tract** may require surgical intervention, although this diagnosis is difficult to establish in the absence of perforation. In most cases, the infant with bowel necrosis will have signs of peritonitis, such as ascites, abdominal mass, abdominal wall erythema, induration, persistent thrombocytopenia, progressive shock from third-space losses, or refractory

metabolic acidosis. Paracentesis may help to identify these patients before perforation occurs.

4. The mainstay of **surgical treatment** is resection with enterostomy although resection with primary anastomosis is useful in selected cases. At surgery, the goal is to excise necrotic bowel although preserving as much bowel length as possible. Peritoneal fluid is examined for signs of infection and sent for culture, necrotic bowel is resected and sent for pathologic confirmation, and viable bowel ends are exteriorized as stomas. All sites of diseased bowel are noted, whether or not removal is indicated. If there is extensive involvement, a "second look" operation may be done within 24 to 48 hours to determine whether any areas that appeared necrotic are actually viable. The length and areas of removed bowel are recorded. If large areas are resected, the length and position of the remaining bowel are noted, as this will affect the long-term outcome. In approximately 14% of infants with this condition, NEC totalis (bowel necrosis from duodenum to rectum) is found. In these cases mortality is almost certain.

5. More recently, **peritoneal drainage** has been considered in a select group of infants. In ELBW infants (<1,000 g) and extremely unstable infants, peritoneal drainage under local anesthesia may be a management option. In many cases, this temporizes laparotomy until the infant is more stable and in some cases no further operative procedure is required. A recent randomized trial of laparotomy versus peritoneal drainage in NEC with perforation showed no significant differences in survival, duration of PN or length of hospital stay between the two procedures. However, other studies have suggested worse long term outcome in infants with NEC treated with peritoneal drains alone, so optimal surgical therapy remains controversial.

C. **Long-term management.** Once the infant has been stabilized and effectively treated, feedings can be reintroduced. We generally begin this process after 2 weeks of treatment by stopping nasogastric decompression. If infants can tolerate their own secretions, feedings are begun very slowly while parenteral alimentation is gradually tapered. No conclusive data are available on the best method or type of feeding, but breast milk may be better tolerated and is preferred. The occurrence of strictures may complicate feeding plans. The incidence of recurrent NEC is 4% and appears to be independent of type of management. Recurrent disease should be treated as before and will generally respond similarly. If surgical intervention was required and an ileostomy or colostomy was created, intestinal reanastomosis can be electively undertaken after an adequate period of healing. Before reanastomosis, a contrast study of the distal bowel is obtained to establish the presence of a stricture that can be resected at the time of ostomy closure.

IV. **PROGNOSIS.** Few detailed and accurate studies are available on prognosis. In uncomplicated cases of NEC, the long-term prognosis may be comparable with that of other low birth weight infants; however, those with stage IIB and stage III NEC have a higher incidence of growth delay (delay in growth of head circumference is of most concern). NEC requiring surgical intervention may have more serious sequelae, including increased morbidity and mortality secondary to infection, respiratory failure, PN—associated hepatic disease, rickets, and significant developmental delay.

A. **Sequelae** of NEC can be directly related to the disease process or to the long-term NICU management often necessary to treat it. GI sequelae include strictures, enteric fistulas, short bowel syndrome, malabsorption and chronic diarrhea, dumping syndromes related to loss of terminal ileum and ileocecal valve, fluid and electrolyte losses with rapid dehydration, and hepatitis or cholestasis related to long-term PN. Strictures occur in 25% to 35% of patients with or without surgery and are most common in the large bowel. Not all strictures are clinically significant. Short bowel syndrome occurs in approximately 10% to 20% following surgical treatment. Metabolic sequelae include failure to thrive, metabolic bone disease, and problems related to central nervous system (CNS) function in the VLBW infant.

B. **Prevention of NEC is the ultimate goal.** Unfortunately, this can best be accomplished only by preventing premature birth. If prematurity cannot be avoided, several preventive strategies may be of benefit.

1. **Induction of GI maturation.** The incidence of NEC is significantly reduced after prenatal steroid therapy.
2. **Alteration of the immunologic status of the intestine.** Oral immunoglobulins may have potential benefit, and in one study immunoglobulin A (IgA) and immunoglobulin G (IgG) supplementation of feedings reduced the incidence of NEC. Breast milk contains many immunoprotective factors; however, no study has convincingly demonstrated that breast milk alone can prevent NEC, although its incidence is lower in premature infants fed only breast milk.
3. **Optimization of enteral feedings** (see Chap. 10). Very slow introduction of feedings may be useful, but more data are required. Feeds with polyunsaturated fatty acids have been shown to be protective in animal models.
4. **Reduction or antagonism of inflammatory mediators.** Because many of the factors associated with NEC promote increased PAF concentrations and the subsequent inflammatory cascade resulting in bowel injury, trials of oral PAF antagonists may reduce the incidence and severity of NEC.
5. **Enterally fed probiotics** are a promising new approach to the prevention of NEC. Probiotics fed to preterm infants may help to normalize intestinal microflora colonization. Small randomized trials have shown decreased incidence and severity of NEC in infants fed probiotics (e.g., *Lactobacillus acidophilus, Bifidobacterium infantis, Streptococcus thermophilus, Bifidobacterium bifidus*) compared with controls. Studies are ongoing to determine which organisms are most effective, and the short and long-term safety of this approach.

Suggested Readings

Hammerman C, Kaplan M. Germ warfare: Probiotics in defense of the premature gut. *Clin Perinatol* 2004;31:489–500.

Moss, R, Dimmitt RA, Barnhart DC, et al. Laparotomy versus peritoneal drainage for necrotizing enterocolitis and perforation. *N Engl J Med* 2006;354:2225–2234.

Muguruma K., Gray PW, Tjoelker LW, et al. The central role of PAF in necrotizing enterocolitis development. *Adv Exp Med Biol* 1997;407:379.

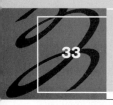

SURGICAL EMERGENCIES IN THE NEWBORN

33

Steven A. Ringer and Anne R. Hansen

I. FETAL SURGICAL DISORDERS

A. Polyhydramnios (amniotic fluid volume >2L) occurs in 1 in 1,000 births.

1. Gastrointestinal (GI) obstruction (including esophageal atresia (EA)) is the most frequent surgical cause of polyhydramnios.

2. Other causes of polyhydramnios include abdominal wall defects (omphalocele and gastroschisis), anencephaly, diaphragmatic hernia, maternal diabetes with consequent fetal hyperglycemia and glucosuria and other conditions impairing the fetus' ability to concentrate urine, tight nuchal cord and other causes of impaired fetal swallowing, and fetal death.

3. All women with suspected polyhydramnios should have an ultrasonographic examination. In experienced hands, this is the study of choice for the diagnosis of intestinal obstruction, abdominal wall defects, diaphragmatic hernia, as well as abnormalities leading to an inability of the fetus to swallow.

4. If intestinal obstruction is diagnosed antenatally and there is no concern for dystocia, vaginal delivery is acceptable. Pediatric surgical consultation should be obtained before delivery.

B. Oligohydramnios is associated with amniotic fluid leak, intrauterine growth restriction, postmaturity, fetal distress, renal dysgenesis or agenesis (Potter syndrome; see Chap. 31). If the duration of oligohydramnios is prolonged, it is important to anticipate respiratory compromise in these infants, as adequate amniotic fluid volume is generally necessary for normal pulmonary development, particularly during the second trimester of gestation. Severity of pulmonary hypoplasia correlates with degree and duration of oligohydramnios.

C. Meconium peritonitis can be diagnosed prenatally by ultrasonography, typically seen as areas of calcification scattered throughout the abdomen. Postnatally, calcifications are confirmed by plain film of the abdomen. It is usually due to antenatal perforation of the intestinal tract. Therefore it is most commonly seen in association with a congenital lesion causing intestinal obstruction, either anatomic or functional. (see V.A).

D. Fetal ascites (see VII) is usually associated with urinary tract anomalies (e.g., lower urinary tract obstruction due to posterior urethral valves). Other causes include hemolytic disease of the newborn, any severe anemia (e.g., α-thalassemia), peritonitis, thoracic duct obstruction, cardiac disease, hepatic or portal vein obstruction, hepatitis, and congenital infection (e.g., TORCH infections; see Chap. 23) as well as other causes of hydrops fetalis (see Chap. 18). After birth, ascites may be seen in congenital nephrotic syndrome. Accurate prenatal ultrasonography is important in light of the potential for fetal surgery to minimize renal parenchymal injury by decompressing either the bladder or a hydronephrotic kidney (see Chap. 1 and 31).

E. Dystocia may result from fetal hydrocephalus, intestinal obstruction, abdominal wall defect, genitourinary anomalies, or fetal ascites (see I.D).

F. Fetal surgery. The potential for surgical intervention during fetal life continues to develop. It depends heavily on the availability of precise prenatal diagnostic techniques and experience in accurately characterizing disorders including the use of ultrasonography and fast magnetic resonance imaging (MRI).

Advances in obstetric and anesthesia management have also contributed to the feasibility of performing *in utero* procedures. The mother must be carefully managed through what is often a long and unpredictable anesthesia course.

Medications that reduce uterine irritability have been developed that maximally ensure that the uterus can be maintained without contractions during and after the procedure. The criteria for consideration of a procedure include the following:

1. Ethical considerations are important, including balancing the risk to the fetus versus potential pain or harm to the mother, and the impact on the family as a whole.

2. Technical feasibility

3. Severity of fetal condition. Initially most cases dealt with conditions that were life threatening either because they caused death *in utero*, or the inability to survive postnatal life if born unrepaired. Currently cases are considered when a condition is not life threatening, but is severe and either the condition itself is progressive (such as the growth of a large tumor partially obstructing the fetal airway), or the consequences of the condition worsen progressively (such as worsening hydrops due to a large teratoma).

4. Necessary resources. The care of the mother, fetus and potential baby during surgery, in the immediate postoperative period, and after birth must all be available in seamless proximity to the institution where the surgery is performed.

Fetal surgery has been successfully used for removal or an enlarging chest mass, such as an adenomatoid malformation of the lung or a bronchopulmonary sequestration. Other mass lesions such as sacrococcygeal teratoma, when diagnosed *in utero*, have been treated with excision or by fetoscopically guided laser ablation of the feeder vessels, resulting in involution. Progressive fetal urethral obstruction has been ameliorated by the use of shunts or fulguration of posterior urethral valves. Similar fetoscopic laser ablation of connecting vessels has been used successfully in the treatment of twin–twin transfusion syndrome or twin reversed arterial perfusion (TRAP). Fetal surgical correction of meningomyelocele is a rapidly evolving area of endeavor.

Successful fetal procedures that we are currently performing include **ex utero intrapartum treatment** (EXIT) procedures for complex airway obstructions and complex congenital diaphragmatic hernia, aortic valve dilation for critical aortic stenosis, atrial septostomy, or stent placement for intact atrial septum with hypoplastic left heart syndrome, vascular photocoagulation for twin–twin transfusion syndrome or TRAP syndrome, and percutaneous bladder shunt for bladder outlet obstruction. Indications for fetal intervention continue to evolve and change.

II. POSTNATAL SURGICAL DISORDERS

A. Respiratory distress (see IV.B and C; Chaps. 4 and 24). Although most etiologies of respiratory distress are treated medically, some respiratory disorders do require surgical therapies.

1. Diaphragmatic hernia (see IV.B).

2. Choanal atresia. (see IV.C.6).

3. Laryngotracheal clefts (see IV.C.3).

4. Tracheal agenesis.

5. EA with or without tracheoesophageal fistula (TEF) (see IV.A).

6. Congenital lobar emphysema.

7. Cystic adenomatoid malformation of the lung.

8. Biliary tracheobronchial communication (extremely rare).

B. Scaphoid abdomen

1. Diaphragmatic hernia (see IV.B).

2. EA without TEF (see IV.A).

C. Excessive mucus and salivation: EA with or without TEF (see IV.A).

D. Abdominal distention: can be due to pneumoperitoneum or intestinal obstruction (mechanical or functional).

1. Pneumoperitoneum: any perforation of the bowel may cause pneumoperitoneum (Chapter 32).

    a. Any portion of the GI tract can potentially perforate for a variety of reasons including poor bowel wall integrity (e.g. necrotizing enterocolitis or localized ischemia of the stomach associated with some medications such as indomethacin), excessive pressure (e.g., obstruction, TEF or instrumentation [i.e., with a nasogastric tube]). Perforated stomach is associated with large amounts of free intra-abdominal air. Active airleak requires urgent surgical closure. It may be necessary to aspirate air from the abdominal cavity to relieve respiratory distress before definitive surgical repair.

    b. Air from a pulmonary air leak may dissect into the peritoneal cavity of infants receiving mechanical ventilation. Treatment of pneumoperitoneum transmitted from pulmonary airleak should focus on managing the pulmonary air leak.

  2. Intestinal obstruction

    a. EA with TEF (see IV.A) can present as abdominal distension. Obstruction of proximal bowel (e.g. complete duodenal atresia) causes rapid distension of the left upper quadrant. Obstruction of distal bowel causes more generalized distension, varying with location of obstruction.

    b. The normal progression of the air column seen on an x-ray film of the abdomen is as follows: 1 hour after birth the air is past the stomach into the upper jejunum; 3 hours after birth it is at the cecum; by 8 to 12 hours after birth it is at the rectosigmoid. This progression is slower in the premature infant.

E. Vomiting. The causes of vomiting can be differentiated by the presence or absence of bile.

  1. Bilious emesis. The presence of bile-stained vomit in the newborn should be treated as a life-threatening emergency, with at least 20% of such infants requiring surgical intervention immediately after evaluation. Surgical consultation should be obtained immediately. Unless the infant is clinically unstable, a contrast study of the upper gastrointestinal tract should be obtained as quickly as possible.

    Intestinal obstruction may result from malrotation with or without volvulus; duodenal, jejunal, ileal, or colonic atresias; annular pancreas; Hirschsprung disease; aberrant superior mesenteric artery; preduodenal portal vein; peritoneal bands, persistent omphalomesenteric duct; or duodenal duplication.

    Bile-stained emesis is occasionally seen in infants without intestinal obstruction who have decreased motility (see 2c). In these cases the bile-stained vomiting will only occur one or two times and will present without abdominal distention. However, a nonsurgical condition is a diagnosis of exclusion: bilious emesis is malrotation until proved otherwise.

  2. Nonbilious emesis

    a. Feeding excessive volume.

    b. Milk (human or formula) intolerance.

    c. Decreased motility.

      i. Prematurity

      ii. Antenatal exposure to $MgSO_4$ or narcotics.

      iii. Sepsis with ileus.

      iv. Central nervous system (CNS) lesion.

    d. Lesion above ampulla of Vater.

      i. Pyloric stenosis.

      ii. Upper duodenal stenosis.

      iii. Annular pancreas (rare).

F. Failure to pass meconium. Can occur in sick and/or premature babies with decreased bowel motility. It also may be the result of the following disorders.

  1. Imperforate anus.

G. Failure to develop transitional stools after the passage of meconium

  1. Volvulus.

  2. Malrotation.

H. Hematemesis or hematochezia

  1. Nonsurgical conditions: many patients with hematemesis, and most patients with **hematochezia** (bloody stools), have a nonsurgical condition. Differential diagnosis includes the following:

   a. Milk intolerance/allergy (usually cow's milk protein allergy).
   b. Instrumentation (e.g., nasogastric tube, endotracheal tube).
   c. Swallowed maternal blood.
      i. Maternal blood is sometimes swallowed by the newborn during labor and delivery. This can be diagnosed by an Apt test performed on blood aspirated from the infant's stomach (see XI.C and Chap. 26A).
      ii. In breast-fed infants, if blood obtained from the infant's stomach is adult blood, inspection of the mother's breasts or her expressed milk may reveal the source of blood. Aspirating the contents of the baby's stomach after a feeding is most likely to yield milk for testing. In breast-fed infants, either micro- or macroscopic blood noted several days after birth in either emesis or stool may be due to swallowed blood during breast feeding in setting of cracked maternal nipples. Inspecting the mother's breasts or expressed milk is usually diagnostic. If not, aspirate the contents of the baby's stomach after a feeding and send the recently swallowed milk for an Apt test.
   2. Surgical conditions resulting in hematemesis and bloody stool
      a. Necrotizing enterocolitis (most frequent cause of hematemesis and bloody stool in premature infants; see Chap. 32).
      b. Gastric or duodenal ulcers (due to stress, steroid therapy).
      c. Coagulation disorders including disseminated intravascular coagulation (DIC), lack of postnatal vitamin K injection (see Chap. 26B).
      d. GI obstruction: late sign, concerning for threatened or necrotic bowel.
      e. Volvulus.
      f. Intussusception.
      g. Polyps, hemangiomas.
      h. Meckel diverticulum.
      i. Duplications of the small intestine
      j. Cirsoid aneurysm.
 I. Abdominal masses (see IX).
   1. Genitourinary anomalies including distended bladder (see VII and Chap. 31).
   2. Hepatosplenomegaly: may be confused with other masses; requires medical evaluation.
   3. Tumors (see VIII).
 J. Birth trauma (see Chap. 20).
   1. Fractured clavicle/humerus (see Chap. 28).
   2. Intracranial hemorrhage (see Chap. 27B).
   3. Lacerated solid organs—liver, spleen.
   4. Spinal cord transection with quadriplegia.
III. LESIONS CAUSING RESPIRATORY DISTRESS
   A. EA and TEF. At least 85% of infants with EA also have TEF. Pure Esophagel Atresia GEAL and Tracheo-esophagel fistula GEAL with proximal TEF may be suspected on prenatal ultrasonography by the absence of a stomach bubble.
   1. Postnatal presentation depends on the presence or absence as well as location of a TEF.
      a. Infants often present with excessive salivation and vomiting soon after feedings. They may develop respiratory distress due to the following:
         i. Airway obstruction by excess secretions.
         ii. Compromised pulmonary capacity due to diaphragmatic elevation secondary to abdominal distension.
         iii. Reflux of gastric contents up the distal esophagus into the lungs through the fistula.
      b. If there is no fistula, or if it connects the trachea to the esophagus proximal to the atresia, no GI gas will be seen on x-ray examination, and the abdomen will be scaphoid. Respiratory difficulties are less acute.
      c. TEF without EA (H-type fistula) is extremely rare and usually presents after the neonatal period. The diagnosis is suggested by a history of frequent pneumonias or respiratory distress temporally related to meals.

2. **Diagnosis**
   a. **EA** itself is diagnosed by the inability to pass a catheter into the stomach. The catheter is passed into the esophagus until resistance is met. Air is then injected into the catheter while listening (for lack of air) over the stomach. The diagnosis is confirmed by x-ray studies showing the catheter coiled in the upper esophageal pouch. Plain x-ray films may demonstrate a distended blind upper esophageal pouch filled with air that is unable to progress into the stomach. (The plain films may also show associated vertebral anomalies of the cervical or upper thoracic region of the spine.) Pushing 50 mL of air into the catheter under fluoroscopic examination may show dilatation and relaxation of the upper pouch, thereby avoiding the need for contrast studies.
   b. **H-type fistula.** This disorder can often be demonstrated with administration of nonionic water-soluble contrast medium (Omnipaque) during cinefluoroscopy. The definitive examination is combined fiberoptic bronchoscopy and esophagoscopy with passage of a fine balloon catheter from the trachea into the esophagus. The H-type fistula is usually high in the trachea (cervical area).
3. **Associated issues and anomalies.** Babies with TEF and EA are often of low birth weight. Approximately 20% of these babies are premature (five times the normal incidence), and another 20% are small for gestational age (eight times the normal incidence). Other anomalies may be present, including chromosomal abnormalities and the VACTERL association: Vertebral defects, imperforate **A**nus, **C**ardiac defects, **TE**F with EA, **R**enal dysplasia or defects and **L**imb anomalies.
4. **Management.** Preoperative management focuses on minimizing the risk of aspiration and avoiding gaseous distension of the GI tract with positive pressure crossing from the trachea into the esophagus.
   a. A multiple end-hole suction catheter (Replogle) should be placed in the proximal pouch and put to intermittent suction immediately after the diagnosis is made.
   b. The head of the bed should be elevated 45 degrees to diminish reflux of gastric contents into the fistula and aspiration of oral secretions that may accumulate in the proximal esophageal pouch.
   c. If possible, mechanical ventilation of these babies should be avoided until the fistula is controlled because the positive pressure may cause severe abdominal distension compromising ventilation. If intubation is required, the case should be considered an emergency. Guidelines for intubation are the same as for other types of respiratory distress (see Chap. 36). The endotracheal tube should be advanced to just above the carina in the hopes of obstructing airflow through the fistula. Most commonly, the fistula connects to the trachea near the carina. Care must be taken to avoid accidental intubation of the fistula. Optimally, if mechanical ventilation is required, it should be done using a relatively high rate and low pressure to minimize GI distention. Heavy sedation should be avoided because the patient's spontaneous respiratory effort generates negative intrathoracic pressure, minimizing passage of air through the fistula into the esophagus.
   d. Surgical therapy usually involves immediate placement of a gastrostomy tube. As soon as the infant can tolerate further surgery, the fistula is divided, and if possible, primary repair of the esophagus is performed.
   e. Many infants with EA are premature or have other defects that make it advisable to delay primary repair. Mechanical ventilation and nutritional management may be difficult in these infants because of the TEF. These babies need careful nursing care to prevent aspiration, and gastrostomy with G tube feedings to allow growth until repair is possible. In some cases, the fistula can be divided, with deferral of definitive repair.
   f. If the infant has cardiac disease that requires surgery, it is usually best to repair the fistula first. If not, the postoperative ventilatory management can be very difficult.

B. Diaphragmatic Hernia (DH)

1. **Anatomy.** The most common site is the left hemithorax, with the defect in the diaphragm being posterior (foramen of Bochdalek) in 70% of infants. It can also occur on the right, with either an anterior or a posterior defect.

2. **Incidence.** Occurs in approximately 1 in 4,000 live births. Fifty percent of these hernias are associated with other malformations, especially cardiac, neural tube, intestinal, skeletal, and renal defects Diaphragmatic hernia has been associated with trisomies 13 and 18, and 45 XO, and has been reported as part of Goldenhar, Beckwith-Wiedemann, Pierre Robin, Goltz-Gorlin, and the Rubella syndromes. In some cases diaphragmatic hernia is familial.

3. **Symptoms.** Infants with large diaphragmatic hernias usually present at birth with cyanosis, respiratory distress, a scaphoid abdomen, decreased or absent breath sounds on the side of the hernia, and heart sounds displaced to the side opposite the hernia. Small hernias, right-sided hernias, sac type hernias and substernal hernias of Morgagni may have a more subtle presentation, manifested as feeding problems and mild respiratory distress.

4. **Diagnosis**

   a. **Prenatal Dx.** DH's often occur after the routine 16-week prenatal ultra-sonography; therefore many of these cases are not diagnosed until postnatally. The development of polyhydramnios can prompt a later fetal ultrasonography that will detect DH. Diagnosis earlier in gestation may correlate with a poorer prognosis due to severity of condition. However, the prognostic advantage of prenatal diagnosis is that it generally leads to delivery in a center equipped to optimize chances for survival. If delivery before term is likely, fetal lung maturity should be assessed to evaluate the need for maternal betamethasone therapy (see Chap. 24). Presence of liver in the thorax correlates with increased severity and poorer prognosis. Lung-to-head ratio (LHR) can be measured prenatally, and in skilled hands, can help predict severity of involvement, and help guide initial therapy. In our institution, there are no reported survivors with an LHR <1. An LHR >1.4 has a100% survival rate and a LHR between 1 and 1.4, has a 38% survival rate with a high need for ECMO. Early work suggests that relative lung volumes, as measure by MRI, may have an important role in predicting the risk of morbidity and mortality. The lower the percent predicted lung volume (PPLV), the higher the risk.

   b. **Postnatal Dx.** The diagnosis is made or confirmed by radiograph. Because of the possibility of marked cardiothymic shift, a radiopaque marker should be placed on one side of the chest to aid interpretation of the x-ray film.

5. **Treatment**

   a. Severe cases that have been diagnosed before birth may be best managed with delivery by the EXIT procedure, with immediate institution of extra-corporeal membrane oxygenation (ECMO) (see Chap. 24). This requires a multidisciplinary team consisting of surgeons, obstetricians, neonatologists, specialized anesthesiologists, nurses, respiratory therapists and ECMO technicians to be assembled at a specialized center. Deep general anesthesia is established in the mother, ensuring fetal anesthesia. Maternal laparotomy is performed, with exposure of the uterus, which should be extremely hypotonic because of the anesthesia. Bleeding is minimized by using a special device to open the uterus that simultaneously cuts a full-thickness uterine incision and places hemostatic clips along the incision.

   The fetus is then partially delivered through the uterine opening. A pulse oximeter probe is placed on the fetal hand to permit direct monitoring of heart rate and oxygen saturation, with the oxygen saturation maintained at fetal levels of approximately 60%. If the saturation gets too high, the umbilical vessels will constrict and umbilical blood supply will diminish. Monitoring may be augmented by palpation of the umbilical pulse.

   The fetus is then intubated and assessed. A decision is then made whether delivery should be completed at that point, and further care continued as detailed in (5.b.). If the fetal condition does not improve upon intubation or if the diaphragmatic hernia is known to be severe, the EXIT procedure may be used as a bridge to immediate initiation of ECMO. Once the fetus is partially delivered, the surgeons can expose the major vessels of the neck and insert the ECMO catheters. Portable ECMO equipment brought to the operating room is then used during transport to the intensive care unit or during subsequent surgery on the delivered newborn.

- b. **Intubation.** All infants should be intubated immediately after delivery if the diagnosis has been made antenatally, or at the time of postnatal diagnosis. Bag and mask ventilation is contraindicated. Immediately after intubation, a large sump nasogastric tube should be inserted and attached to **continuous** suction. Care must be taken with assisted ventilation to keep inspiratory pressures low to avoid damage or rupture of the contralateral lung. Peripheral venous and arterial lines are preferable, as umbilical lines may need to be removed during surgery. However, if umbilical lines are the only practical access, these should be placed initially. Heavy sedation should be avoided as spontaneous respiratory effort enables the use of the assist control mode of ventilation which we have found to induce the least barotrauma.
- c. **Preoperative management** is focused on avoiding barotrauma and minimizing pulmonary hypertension. Permissive hypercapnia is the preferred respiratory approach, although the mode of ventilation remains controversial, including the role for high-frequency ventilation. Avoidance of hypoxia and acidosis will aid in minimizing pulmonary hypertension. Inhaled nitric oxide has not been shown to reduce the need for ECMO, but its role in reducing right heart strain may be beneficial.

6. **Surgical repair** is through either the abdomen or the chest, with reduction of intestine into the abdominal cavity.

7. **Mortality and prognosis**
- a. **Mortality** from diaphragmatic hernias is largely related to associated defects, especially pulmonary hypoplasia and congenital heart disease. Our local survival is now >90% for infants without associated congenital heart disease (CHD). Repair of the defect itself is relatively straightforward; the underlying pulmonary hypoplasia and pulmonary hypertension are largely responsible for overall mortality (see Chap. 24F).
- b. **Prognosis.** Early oxygen tension (Po_2) and carbon dioxide tension (Pco_2) are predictive of prognosis. In addition, the later the onset of postnatal symptoms, the higher the survival rate. Extracorporeal membrane oxygenation and nitric oxide inhalation therapy offer the hope of improved survival (see Chap. 24D).

C. **Other mechanical causes for respiratory distress**
1. **Choanal atresia.** Bilateral atresia presents in the delivery room as respiratory distress that resolves with crying. Infants are obligate nasal breathers until approximately 4 months of age. An oral airway is effective initial treatment. Definitive therapy includes opening a hole through the bony plate, which can be accomplished with a laser in some settigs.
2. **Robin anomaly** (Pierre Robin syndrome) consists of a hypoplastic mandible associated with a secondary U-shaped midline cleft palate. Often the tongue occludes the airway causing obstruction. Prone positioning or forcibly pulling the tongue forward will relieve the obstruction. These infants often improve after placement of a nasopharyngeal or endotracheal tube. If the infant can be supported for a few days, he or she will sometimes adapt, and aggressive procedures can be avoided. In some cases, a procedure to adhere the tongue to the lip can avoid the need for tracheostomy. A specialized feeder (Breck) facilitates PO feeding the infant, but sometimes a gastrostomy is necessary. Severely affected babies will require tracheostomy and gastrostomy.
3. **Laryngotracheal clefts.** The length of the cleft determines the symptoms. The diagnosis is made by instillation of contrast material into the esophagus and

is confirmed by bronchoscopy. Very ill newborns should undergo immediate bronchoscopy without contrast studies.

4. **Laryngeal web occluding the larynx.** Perforation of the web by a stiff endotracheal tube or bronchoscopy instrument may be lifesaving.

5. **Tracheal agenesis.** This rare lesion is suspected when a tube cannot be passed down the trachea. The infant ventilates by way of bronchi coming off the esophagus. Diagnosis is by use of contrast material in the esophagus and by endoscopy. Prognosis is poor as tracheal reconstruction is difficult.

6. **Congenital lobar emphysema** may be due to a malformation, a cyst in the bronchus, or a mucous or meconium plug in the bronchus. These lesions cause air trapping, compression of surrounding structures, and respiratory distress. There may be a primary malformation of the lobe (polyalveolar lobe). Overdistension from mechanical ventilation may cause lobar emphysema. Extrinsic pressure on a bronchus can also cause obstruction. Lower lobes are generally relatively spared. Diagnosis is by chest x-ray studies.

   a. **High-frequency ventilation** may enable the lobar emphysema to recover (see Chap. 24).

   b. **Selective intubation.** After consultation with a surgeon, selective intubation of the opposite bronchus may be attempted in an effort to decompress the emphysematous lobe if overinflation is thought to be the cause. It should generally be viewed as a temporizing therapy and should not be employed for more than few hours. Many infants will not tolerate this procedure, due to both overdistension of the ventilated lung, and profound $\dot{V}/\dot{Q}$ mismatch; therefore it must be carefully considered and monitored. Rarely, selective intubation is successful and the lobar emphysema does not recur. Much more commonly, even if the selective intubation is initially helpful, the baby goes on to develop progressive atelectasis and further respiratory compromise. Occasionally, selective suctioning of the bronchus on the side of the emphysema may remove obstructing mucus or meconium.

   c. **Bronchoscopy, resection.** If the baby is symptomatic and conservative measures fail, bronchoscopy should be performed to remove any obstructing material or rupture a bronchogenic cyst. If this procedure fails, surgical resection of the involved lobe should be considered.

7. **Cystic adenomatoid malformation and pulmonary sequestration** may be confused with a diaphragmatic hernia. Respiratory distress is related to the effect of the mass on the uninvolved lung. This malformation can cause shifting of the mediastinal structures.

8. **Vascular rings.** The symptomatology of vascular rings is related to the anatomy of the ring. Both respiratory (stridor) and GI (vomiting, difficulty swallowing) symptoms may occur. Barium swallow radiography is diagnostic.

IV. **LESIONS CAUSING INTESTINAL OBSTRUCTION.** The most critical lesion to rule out is malrotation with midgut volvulus. All patients with suspected intestinal obstruction should have a nasogastric sump catheter placed to continuous suction without delay. Any baby with a GI obstruction is at increased risk of hyperbilirubinemia due to increased enterohepatic circulation.

A. **Congenital mechanical obstruction**

1. Intrinsic types include atresia, stenosis, hypertrophic pyloric stenosis, meconium ileus (most commonly associated with cystic fibrosis), small left colon syndrome, cysts within the lumen of the bowel and imperforate anus.

2. Extrinsic forms of congenital mechanical obstruction include congenital peritoneal bands with or without malrotation, annular pancreas, duplications of the intestine, aberrant vessels (usually the mesenteric artery or preduodenal portal vein), hydrometrocolpos, and obstructing bands (persistent omphalomesenteric duct).

B. **Acquired mechanical obstruction**

1. Malrotation with volvulus.

2. Intussusception.

3. Peritoneal adhesions.

      a. After meconium peritonitis.

      b. After abdominal surgery.

      c. Idiopathic.

  4. Mesenteric thrombosis.

  5. Strictures secondary to necrotizing enterocolitis.

  6. Incarcerated hernia (common in premature infants).

  7. Formation of abnormal intestinal concretions not associated with cystic fibrosis.

C. Functional intestinal obstruction constitutes the major cause of intestinal obstruction seen in the neonatal unit.

  1. Immaturite bowel motility.

  2. Defective innervation (Hirschsprung disease) or other intrinsic defects in the bowel wall.

  3. Paralytic ileus.

      a. Induced by medications.

        i. Narcotics (pre- or postnatal exposure).

        ii. Hypermagnaesemia due to prenatal exposure to magnesium sulfate.

      b. Septic ileus.

  4. Meconium and mucous plugs.

  5. Endocrine disorders (e.g. hypothyroidism).

D. The more **common etiologies** of GI obstruction warrant more detailed discussion.

  1. Pyloric stenosis: typically presents with nonbilious vomiting after the age of 2 to 3 weeks, but it has been seen in the first week of life. Radiographic examination will show a large stomach with little or no gas below the duodenum. Often the pyloric mass, or "olive," cannot be felt in the newborn. The infant may have associated jaundice and hematemesis. Diagnosis can be confirmed by ultrasonography. Some centers confirm diagnosis by upper GI series, but the consequent radiation exposure makes this a less attractive option.

  2. Duodenal atresia: 70% of cases have other associated malformations, including Down syndrome, cardiovascular (CVR) anomalies, and such GI anomalies as annular pancreas, EA, malrotation of the small intestine, small-bowel atresias, and imperforate anus.

      a. There may be a history of polyhydramnios.

      b. Commonly diagnosed prenatally by ultrasonography.

      c. Vomiting of bile-stained material usually begins a few hours after birth.

      d. Abdominal distention is limited to the upper abdomen.

      e. The infant may pass meconium in the first 24 hours of life; then bowel movements cease.

      f. The diagnosis is suggested if aspiration of the stomach yields >30 mL of gastric contents before feeding.

      g. A plain radiograph of the abdomen will show air in the stomach and upper part of the abdomen ("double bubble") with no air in the small or large bowel. Contrast radiographs of the upper intestine are not mandatory.

      h. Preoperative management includes decompression with nasogastric suction.

  3. Jejunal and ileal atresias: It is not widely appreciated that 15% to 30% are associated with CF; these patents should be screened (see 4. c).

  4. Meconium ileus is a frequent cause of meconium peritonitis. Unlike most other etiologies of obstruction in which flat and upright x-ray films will demonstrate fluid levels, in cases of nonperforated meconium ileus the distended bowel may be granular in appearance or may show tiny bubbles mixed with meconium.

      a. No meconium will pass through the rectum, even after digital stimulation.

      b. Ninety percent of babies with meconium have cystic fibrosis. Blood sample or cheek brushing for DNA analysis can be used to screen for cystic fibrosis. If the results are negative or equivocal, or if the baby weighs >2 kg and is older than 2 weeks ideally (but certainly older than 3 days) a sweat test should be performed. Sweat tests on babies who are younger or smaller risk both false positive results due to the high NaCl content of the sweat of new born babies and false negative or uninterprettable results when an inadequate volume of sweat can be obtained. Some couples will have received prenatal CF genetic testing. Increasingly, states include CF in the newborn screen. A family history can provide rapid information regarding expected risk.

    c. Rare cases (both familial and nonfamilial) of meconium ileus are not associated with cystic fibrosis.

    d. Decompression with continuous nasogastric suction will minimize further distention. Contrast enemas can be both diagnostic and therapeutic. Meglumine diatrizoate (Gastrografin) or diatrizoate sodium (Hypaque) can be used in an adequately hydrated infant. Meglumine diatrizoate is often diluted 1:4 before use. Both of these contrast agents are hypertonic. Therefore, the baby should start the procedure well hydrated, and careful attention should be paid to fluid balance after the procedure. If the diagnosis is certain and the neonate stable, repeat therapeutic enemas may be administered in an effort to relieve the impaction.

    e. Surgical therapy is required if the contrast enema fails to relieve the obstruction.

    f. Microcolon distal to the atresia will generally dilate spontaneously with use.

5. Imperforate anus. Fifty percent have anomalies including those in the VACTERL association. Infants with imperforate anus may pass meconium if a rectovaginal or rectourinary fistula exists; in these infants, the diagnosis may be delayed. The presence or absence of a visible fistula at the perineum is the critical distinctions in the diagnosis and management of imperforate anus.

    a. Perineal fistula. Meconium may be visualized on the perineum. It may be found in the rugal folds or scrotum in boys, and in the vagina in girls. This fistula may be dilated to allow passage of meconium to temporarily relieve intestinal obstruction. When the infant is beyond the newborn period, the imperforate anus can generally be primarily repaired.

    b. No perineal fistula present. There may be a fistula that enters the urinary tract or, for girls, the vagina. The presence of meconium particles in the urine is diagnostic of a rectovesicular fistula. Vaginal examination with a nasal speculum or cystoscope may reveal a fistula. A cystogram may show a fistula and document the level of the distal rectum. Ultrasonography is often helpful in defining the distal level of the rectum. A temporary colostomy may be necessary in neonates with an imperforate anus without a perineal fistula. Primary repair of these infants without a colostomy is now being performed at some institutions.

6. Volvulus with or without malrotation of the bowel.

    a. Malrotation may be associated with other GI abnormalities such as diaphragmatic hernia, annular pancreas, and bowel atresias, and is always seen with omphalocele.

    b. If this condition develops during fetal life, it may cause the appearance of a large midabdominal calcific shadow on x-ray examination; this results from calcification of meconium in the segment of necrotic bowel.

    c. After birth, there is a sudden onset of bilious vomiting in an infant who has passed some normal stools. Malrotation as the cause of intestinal obstruction is a surgical emergency because intestinal viability is at stake. **Bileous emesis is malrotation until proved otherwise.**

    d. If the level of obstruction is high, there may not be much abdominal distension.

    e. Signs of shock and sepsis are often present.

    f. Plain x-rays will often show a dilated small bowel. A normal x-ray does not rule out malrotation, which can be intermittent.

    g. If a malrotation is present, barium enema may show failure of barium to pass beyond the transverse colon or may show the cecum in an abnormal position.

    h. An upper GI series should be obtained, specifically looking for an absent or abnormal position of the ligament of Treitz that confirms the diagnosis of malrotation.

7. Annular pancreas may be nonobstructing but associated with duodenal atresia or stenosis. It presents as a high intestinal obstruction.

8. Hydrometrocolpos. In this rare condition, a membrane across the vagina prevents fluid drainage and the consequent accumulation causes distension of the uterus and vagina.

    a. The hymen bulges.

    b. Accumulated secretions in the uterus may cause intestinal obstruction by bowel compression.

    c. This intestinal obstruction may, in turn, cause meconium peritonitis or hydronephrosis.

    d. Edema and cyanosis of the legs may be observed.

    e. If hydrometrocolpos is not diagnosed at birth, the secretions will decrease, the bulging will disappear, and the diagnosis will be delayed until puberty.

9. Meconium and mucous plug syndrome Seen in babies who are premature or sick (see IV.D.3), and those with functional immaturity of the bowel with a small left colon as seen in infants of diabetic mothers or those with Hirschsprung disease (see V.D.9), which should always be considered when a newborn has difficulty passing stools. Cystic fibrosis should also be ruled out. Treatment consists of glycerin suppository, warm half normal saline enemas (5 to 10 mL/kg), and rectal stimulation with soft rubber catheter. If these maneuvers fail, a contrast enema with a hyperosmolar contrast material may be both diagnostic and therapeutic. A normal stooling pattern should follow evacuation of a plug.

10. Hirschsprung disease Should be suspected in any newborn who fails to pass meconium spontaneously by 24 to 48 hours after birth and who develops distension relieved by rectal stimulation. This is especially so if the infant is neither premature nor born to a diabetic mother. The diagnosis should be considered until future development shows sustained normal bowel function.

    a. When the diagnosis is suspected, every effort should be made to rule the condition in or out. If the diagnosis is considered but seems very unlikely, parents taking the newborn home must specifically understand the importance of immediately reporting any obstipation, diarrhea, poor feeding, distention, lethargy, or fever. Development of a toxic megacolon may be fatal.

    b. Barium enema frequently does not show the characteristic transition zone in the newborn.

    c. Rectal biopsy is obtained to confirm the diagnosis. If suspicion is relatively low, a suction biopsy is useful, as presence of ganglion cells in the submucosal zone rules out the diagnosis. If the index of suspicion is high, or the suction biopsy is positive, formal full-thickness rectal biopsy is the definitive method for diagnosis. Absence of ganglion cells and hypertrophic nonmyelinated axons is diagnostic. Histochemical tests of biopsy specimens show an increase in acetylcholine.

    d. Obstipation can be relieved by gentle rectal irrigations with warm saline solution. If the patient has a barium enema, gentle rectal saline washes are helpful in removing trapped air and barium.

    e. Babies require surgical intervention when the diagnosis is made. A primary pull through procedure is possible in some cases. Otherwise, a colostomy is made and definitive repair is postponed until the infant is of adequate size and stability.

    f. Late complications include constipation, encopresis and enterocolitis.

V. OTHER SURGICAL PROBLEMS

    A. Appendicitis: extremely rare in newborns. Its presentation may be that of pneumoperitoneum. The appendix usually perforates before the diagnosis; therefore, the baby may present with intestinal obstruction, sepsis, or even DIC related to the intra-abdominal infection. Rule out Hirschsprung disease.

B. Omphalocele. The sac may be intact or ruptured. The diagnosis is often made by prenatal ultrasonography. Cesarean section may prevent rupture of the sac, but is not specifically indicated unless the defect is large (>5 cm) or contains liver.

1. Intact sac. Emergency treatment includes the following.

a. Use latex-free products, including gloves.

b. Provide continuous nasogastric sump suction

c. It is preferable to encase intestinal contents in a bowel bag (e.g., Vi Drape Isolation Bag) as it is the least abrasive. Otherwise, cover the sac with warm saline soaked gauze, then wrap the sac on abdomen with Kling gauze and cover with plastic wrap so as to support the intestinal viscera on the abdominal wall, taking great caution to ensure no kinking of the mesenteric blood supply.

d. Do not attempt to reduce the sac because this can rupture it, interfere with venous return from the sac or cause respiratory compromise.

e. Bowel viability may be compromised with a small abdominal wall defect and an obstructed segment of eviscerated intestine. In these circumstances, before transfer, the defect must be enlarged by incising the abdomen cephalad or caudad to relieve the strangulated viscera.

f. Keep the baby warm, including thoroughly wrapping in warm blankets to prevent heat loss.

g. Place a reliable intravenous line in an upper extremity.

h. Monitor temperature and pH.

i. Start broad-spectrum antibiotics (ampicillin and gentamicin).

j. Obtain a surgical consultation; definitive surgical therapy should be delayed until the baby is stabilized. In the presence of other more serious abnormalities (respiratory or cardiac), definitive care can be postponed as long as the sac remains intact.

2. Ruptured sac. As in the preceding text for intact sac except surgery is more emergent.

3. As up to 80% will have associated anomalies, physical examination should include a careful search for phenotypic features of chromosomal defects as well as congenital heart disease, genitourinary defects such as cloacal extrophy, craniofacial, musculoskeletal, vertebral, or limb anomalies. The Beckwith-Wiedemann syndrome includes omphalocele, macroglossia, hemihypertrophy, and hypoglycemia.

C. Gastroschisis [15], by definition, contains no sac and the intestine is eviscerated.

1. Preoperative management as per omphalocele with ruptured sac (V,B).

2. Obtain immediate surgical evaluation.

3. Ten percent of infants with gastroschisis have intestial atresia.

4. Unlike omphalocele, gastroschesis is not commonly associated with anomalies unrelated to the GI tract.

VI. RENAL DISORDERS (see Chap. 31)

A. Genitourinary abnormalities should be suspected in babies with abdominal distention, ascites, flank masses, persistently distended bladder, bactiuria, pyuria or poor growth. Male infants exhibiting the symptoms listed in the preceding text should be observed for the normal forceful voiding pattern. First void should be noted in all infants. Approximately 90% of babies void in the first 24 hours of life, and 99% within the first 48 hours of life.

1. Posterior urethral valves may cause obstruction.

2. Renal vein thrombosis should be considered in the setting of hematuria with a flank mass.

a. Renal ultrasonography will initially show a large kidney on the side of the thrombosis. Kidney will return to normal size over ensuing weeks to months.

b. Doppler ultrasonography will show diminished or absent blood flow to involved kidney.

c. Current treatment in most centers starts with medical support in the hope of avoiding surgery. Heparin is generally not indicated, but its use has been advocated by some (see Chaps. 31 and 26F).

3. Extrophy of the bladder. Ranges from an epispadias to complete extrusion of the bladder onto the abdominal wall. Most centers attempt bladder turn-in within the first 48 hours of life.

a. Preoperative management

  i. Use moist, fine-mesh gauze or petroleum jelly–impregnated gauze to cover the exposed bladder.

  ii. Transport the infant to a facility for definitive care as soon as possible.

  iii. Obtain renal ultrasonography.

b. Intraoperative management. Surgical management of an extrophied bladder includes turn-in of the bladder to preserve bladder function. The symphysis pubis is approximated. The penis is lengthened. Iliac osteotomies are not necessary if repair is accomplished within 48 hours. No attempt is made to make the bladder continent at this initial procedure.

4. Cloacal extrophy is a complex GI and genitourinary anomaly that includes vesicointestinal fissure, omphalocele, extrophied bladder, hypoplastic colon, imperforate anus, absence of vagina in women, and microphallus in men.

a. Preoperative management

  i. Gender assignment. It is surgically easier to create a phenotypic woman, regardless of genotype. Understanding of the long-term psychological effects of this practice has made this decision extremely controversial. Endocrine consultation is critical when deciding phenotypic gender assignment (see chap. 30).

  ii. Nasogastric suction relieves partial intestinal obstruction. The baby excretes stool through a vesicointestinal fissure that is often partially obstructed.

  iii. A series of complex operations is required in stages to achieve the most satisfactory results.

b. Surgical management

  i. The initial procedure includes division of the vesicointestinal fissure and establishment of fecal and urinary stomas.

  ii. The bladder can be closed during the initial procedure if the baby is stable.

  iii. Subsequent procedures are designed to reduce the number of stomas and create genitalia.

VII. TUMORS

A. Teratomas are the most common tumor in the neonatal period. Although they are most commonly found in the sacrococcygeal area, they can arise anywhere, including the retroperitoneal area or the ovaries. Approximately 10% contain malignant elements. Prenatal diagnosis is often made by ultrasonography. Dystocia and airway compromise should be considered prenatally. Masses compromising the airway have been successfully managed by the EXIT procedure (see IV.B.5a) with establishment of an airway before complete delivery of the baby.

After delivery, evaluation may include rectal examination, ultrasonography, computed tomography (CT), MRI, as well as serum α-fetoprotein and β-human chorionic gonadotropin measurements are used in evaluation. Calcifications are often seen on x-ray films. Excessive heat loss and platelet trapping are possible complications.

B. Neuroblastoma is the most common malignant neonatal tumor, accounting for approximately 50%. It is irregular, stony hard, and ranges in size from minute to massive. There are many sites of origin; the adrenal-retroperitoneal area is the most common. On rare occasions this tumor can cause hypertension or diarrhea by the release of tumor by-products, especially catecholamines or vasointestinal peptides. Serum levels of catecholamines and their metabolites should be measured. Calcifications can often be seen on plain radiographs. Ultrasonography is the most useful diagnostic test. Prenatal diagnosis by ultrasonography is associated with improved prognosis. Of note, many neuroblastomas diagnosed prenatally resolve spontaneously before birth.

C. **Wilms tumor** is the second most common malignant tumor in the newborn. It presents as a smooth flat mass and may be bilateral. One should palpate gently to avoid rupture. Ultrasonography is the most useful diagnostic test.

D. **Sarcoma botryoides.** This grape-like tumor arises from the edge of the vulva or vagina. It may be small and therefore be confused with a normal posterior vaginal tag. IVP is an important test preoperatively, especially to avoid confusing the lesion with an obstructing ureterocele.

E. **Other** tumors include hemangiomas, lymphangiomas, hepatoblastomas, hepatomas, hamartomas, and nephromas

VIII. ABDOMINAL MASSES

A. **Renal** masses (see VII and Chap. 31) are the most common etiology: polycystic kidneys, multicystic dysplastic kidney, hydronephrosis, renal vein thrombosis

B. **Other** causes of abdominal masses include tumors (see VIII), adrenal hemorrhage, ovarian tumor or cysts, pancreatic cyst, choledochal cyst, hydrometrocolpos, mesenteric or omental cyst, and intestinal duplications, hepatosplenomegally.

IX. INGUINAL HERNIA is found in 5% of premature infants weighing <1,500 gm, and as many as 30% of infants weighing <1,000 gm at birth. It is more common in small-for-gestational-age infants and male infants. In women the ovary is often in the sac.

A. **Surgical repair.** Inguinal hernia repair is the most common operation performed on premature infants. In general, hernias in this patient population can be repaired shortly before discharge home if they are easily reducible and cause no other problems.

1. **Repair before discharge.** In a term infant, repair should be scheduled when the diagnosis is made. An incarcerated hernia can usually be reduced with sedation, steady firm pressure, and elevation of the feet. If a hernia has been incarcerated, it should be repaired as soon as the edema has resolved. The operation may be difficult and should be performed by an experienced pediatric surgeon. The use of spinal anesthesia has simplified the postoperative care of the infants with respiratory problems. As these infants often develop postoperative apnea, they should be monitored for at least 24 hours, and not be sent home on the day of surgery.

2. **Repair after discharge.** Infants with significant pulmonary disease, such as bronchopulmonary dysplasia, are often best repaired at a later time when their respiratory status has improved. We have occasionally had well-instructed parents bring their babies home, and then have them readmitted later for repair. The risks and benefits of this option must be weighed carefully as there is a real risk of the hernia incarcerating at home.

X. ACUTE SCROTAL SWELLING

A. Differential diagnosis includes the following:

1. **Testicular torsion.** Approximately 70% of the cases of testicular torsion that are diagnosed in the newborn period occur prenatally. In the newborn, testicular torsion is generally extravaginal (the twist occurs outside the tunica vaginalis) and is caused by an incomplete attachment of the gubernaculum to the testis, allowing torsion and infarction.

   a. **Diagnosis is made be physical examination.** The testicle is generally nontender, firm, indurated, and swollen with a slightly bluish or dusky cast of the affected side of the scrotum. If the torsion is acute, rather than longstanding, it will be extremely tender to palpation. The testicle can have a transverse lie or be high riding. The overlying skin, limited to the scrotum itself, may be erythematous or edematous. Transillumination is negative and the cremasteric reflex is absent. Ultrasonography employing Doppler flow studies can be helpful if available, but testing should not delay referral for surgery if there is a possibility that the torsion is recent.

   b. **Treatment.** In the vast majority of cases, the torsed testicle is already necrotic at birth, therefore surgical intervention will not salvage the testicle.

However, if there is *any possibility* that the torsion occurred recently, and the infant is otherwise healthy, emergency surgical exploration and de-torsion should be performed within 4–6 hours. This may result in salvage of the torsed testicle. Because there have been reports of bilateral testicular torsion, surgical exploration should include contralateral orchiopexy. Even if emergency exploration is not indicated because of definitive evidence of chronicity of torsion, exploration should be performed on a nonemergent basis to rule out a tumor with clinical and imaging findings identical to testicular torsion.

  c. Prognosis. Testicular protheses are available. Oligospermia has been reported after unilateral testicular torsion.

2. Trauma/scrotal hematoma. Most commonly secondary to breech delivery. This is generally bilateral, and may present with hematocele, scrotal swelling, and ecchymoses. Rarely transilluminates. Resolution is usually spontaneous but severe cases may require surgical exploration, evacuation of the hematocele and repair of the testes.

3. Torsion of the testicular appendage. Swelling is usually less marked, and may present on palpation or as a blue dot on the scrotum. The cremasteric reflexes are preserved, and Doppler flow ultrasonography may be helpful in ruling out testicular torsion. No treatment is needed.

4. Incarcerated hernia

5. Spontaneous idiopathic scrotal hemorrhage. Most common in large-for-gestational-age (LGA) infants. Distinguishable from torsion by the appearance of a small but distinct ecchymosis over the superficial inguinal ring.

6. Tumor. These are usually nontender, solid, and firm. Transillumination is negative.

7. Meconium peritonitis.

XI. COMMON TESTS used in the diagnosis of surgical conditions include the following

A. Abdominal x-ray examinations. A flat plate radiograph of the abdomen kidney-ureter-bladder (KUB) is sufficient for assessing intraluminal gas patterns and mucosal thickness. A left lateral decubitus or cross table lateral radiograph is obtained to ascertain the presence of free air in the abdomen.

  1. Contrast enema may be diagnostic in suspected cases of Hirschsprung disease. It may reveal microcolon in the infant with complete obstruction of the small intestine and may show a narrow segment in the sigmoid in the infant with meconium plug syndrome due to functional immaturity.

  2. Upper GI series with meglumine diatrizoate may be used to demonstrate obstructions of the upper gastrointestinal tract.

  3. In patients with suspected malrotation, a combination of contrast studies may be necessary, starting with a contrast swallow/upper GI. In combination with air or contrast media, an upper GI series will determine the presence or absence of the normally placed ligament of Treitz. A barium enema may show malposition of the cecum but will not always rule out malrotation. Neonates with intestinal obstruction presumed secondary to malrotation require urgent surgery to relieve possible volvulus of the midgut.

B. Ultrasonography is the preferred method of evaluating abdominal masses in the newborn. It is useful for defining the presence of masses, together with their size, shape, and consistency.

C. CT is an excellent modality to evaluate abdominal masses as well as their relation to other organs. Contrast enhancement can outline the intestine, blood vessels, kidneys, ureter, and bladder.

D. MRI is useful to better define the anatomy and location of masses.

E. IVP use should be restricted to evaluating genitourinary anatomy if other modalities (ultrasonography and contrast CT) are not available. The IVP dye is poorly concentrated in the newborn.

F. Radionuclide scan of the kidneys can aid in determining function. This is especially useful in assessing complex genitourinary anomalies and in evaluating the contribution of each kidney to renal function.

G. **The Apt test** differentiates maternal from fetal blood. A small amount of bloody material is mixed with 5 mL of water and centrifuged. One part 0.25N sodium hydroxide is added to five parts of pink supernatant. The fluid remains pink in the presence of fetal blood but rapidly becomes brown if maternal blood is present. The test is useful only if the sample is not contaminated by pigmented material (e.g., meconium/stool) (see chap. 26A).

H. **Blood or cheek brush sampling** for DNA analysis is the initial test for cystic fibrosis, and will detect most cases. When the test result is negative but clinical suspicion remains high, a sweat test should be done. Ideally, the baby should be older than 2 weeks (certainly older than 3 days) and weigh >2 kg to avoid both false positive results due to the relatively high chloride content of newborn infants' sweat, as well as false negative or be uninterpretable results if <100 mg of sweat can be collected. It may be necessary to repeat the test when the infant is 3 to 4 weeks old if an adequate volume of sweat cannot be collected.

XII. PREOPERATIVE MANAGEMENT BY PRESENTING SYMPTOM

A. **Vomiting without distention**

1. The mechanics of feeding the baby should be observed. Rapid feeding, intake of excessive volume and lack of burping are all causes of nonbilious vomiting without distention.

2. Functional and mechanical causes must be ruled out. Often a history, physical examination, and observation of feedings is sufficient. An abdominal x-ray may be useful.

3. If the baby's general condition is good, feedings of dextrose water should be attempted. If this is tolerated, milk should be tried again. If vomiting recurs and there is a family history of milk allergy, blood in the stool, or elevated percentage of eosinophils on the complete blood count (CBC), consider a trial of non–cow's milk-based formula (e.g. soy based or elemental).

B. **Nonbilious vomiting with distention.** An overall assessment of the well versus sick appearance of the baby as well as the degree of the abdominal distention is critical in determining the evaluation and management of nonbileous vomiting and distention. In general, there should be a low threshold to assess for mechanical and functional obstruction, starting with history, physical examination, abdominal radiographs, and ± contrast studies depending on the clinical presentation. If no source of obstruction is identified, many babies with nonbilious vomiting and mild distention respond to glycerin suppositories, half-strength saline enemas (5 mL/kg body weight), rectal stimulation with a soft rubber catheter, or a combination of these measures. Limited feedings, stimulation to the rectum, and care for the general condition of the baby will solve most of these problems.

C. **Bilious vomiting and abdominal distension**

1. While instituting treatment recommendations in the subsequent text, concurrently proceed aggressively with diagnostic evaluation to rule out malrotation with midgut volvulous.

2. **Enteral feedings should be discontinued.** Continuous gastric decompression with a sump catheter is mandatory if intestinal obstruction is suspected. All babies with presumed intestinal obstruction should be transported with a nasogastric suction catheter in place, attached to a catheter-tip syringe for continuous aspiration of gastric contents. Failure to decompress the stomach could lead to gastric rupture, aspiration, or respiratory compromise secondary to excessive diaphragmatic convexity into the thorax. This is especially important in infants who are to be transported by air, because loss of cabin pressure would create a high-risk setting for the rupture of an inadequately drained viscus.

3. Shock, dehydration, and electrolyte imbalance should be prevented, or treated if present (see Chap. 9 and 17).

4. Broad-spectrum antibiotics (ampicillin and gentamicin) should be initiated if there is suspicion of volvulus or any question about bowel integrity. Clindamycin should be added if perforation is high risk or documented.

5. Studies that should be performed include the following:

   a. Monitoring of oxygen saturation, blood pressure, and urine output
   b. Blood tests, as follows:
      i. CBC with differential and blood culture.
      ii. Electrolytes.
      iii. Blood gas and pH.
      iv. Clotting studies (e.g., prothrombin time, partial thromboplastin time).
   c. Contrast study (start with upper GI) to rule out malrotation.
D. Masses. The following steps may be taken to determine the etiology of abdominal masses.
   1. Complete blood cell count with differential.
   2. Determination of the level of catecholamines and their metabolites.
   3. Urinalysis.
   4. X-ray examination of the chest and abdomen with the infant supine and upright.
   5. Abdominal ultrasonography.
   6. Contrast-enhanced CT.
   7. MRI.
   8. Angiography; venous and arterial.
   9. Surgical consultation.
XIII. GENERAL INTRAOPERATIVE MANAGEMENT
   A. Monitoring devices
      1. Temperature probe.
      2. Electrocardiogram (ECG) and/or CVR monitor.
      3. Pulse oximetry responds rapidly to changes in patient condition, but is subject to artifacts.
      4. Transcutaneous Po_2 (see Chap. 24C) is helpful if pulse oximetry is unavailable, but can be inaccurate in the setting of anesthetic agents that dilate skin vessels.
      5. Arterial cannula to monitor blood gases and pressure.
   B. Well-functioning intravenous line. Babies with omphalocele or gastroschesis should have the intravenous line in the upper extremities, neck or scalp.
   C. Maintenance of body temperature
      1. Warmed operating room.
      2. Humidified, warmed anesthetic agents.
      3. Warmed blood and other fluids used intraoperatively.
      4. Cover exposed parts of the baby, especially the head (with a hat).
   D. Fluid replacement
      1. Replace loss of >15% of total blood volume with warmed packed red blood cells.
      2. Replace ascites loss with normal saline mL/mL to maintain normal blood pressure.
      3. The neonate loses approximately 5 mL of fluid per kilogram for each hour that the intestine is exposed. This should generally be replaced by Ringers lactate.
   E. Anesthetic management of the neonate is reviewed in Chapter 37.
   F. Postoperative pain management is discussed Chapter 37.
   G. Postoperatively, the newborn fluid requirement must be monitored closely, including replacement of estimated losses due to bowel edema as well as losses through drains.

Suggested Readings

Achildi O, Grewal H. Congenital anomalies of the esophagus. *Otolaryngol Clin North Am* 2007;40:219–244.

Adzick NS, Nance ML. Medical progress: Pediatric surgery: Second of two parts. *N Engl J Med* 2000;342:1726.

American Academy of Pediatrics, Committee on Bioethics. Fetal therapy: Ethical considerations. *Pediatrics* 1999;103:1061.

Chandler JC, Gauderer MWL. The neonate with an abdominal mass. *Pediatr Clin North Am* 2004;51:979–997.

Glick RD, Hicks MJ, Nuchtern JG, et al. Renal tumors in infants <6 months of age. *J Pediatr Surg* 2004;39:522–525.

Hansen A, Puder M. *Manual of surgical neonatal intensive care.* Hamilton: BC Decker, 2003.

Irish MS, Pearl RH, Caty MG, et al. The approach to common abdominal diagnosis in infants and children. *Pediatr Clin North Am* 1998;45(4):729–772.

Johnson MP, Burkowski TP, Reitleman C, et al. In utero surgical treatment of fetal obstructive uropathy: A new comprehensive approach to identify appropriate candidates for vesicoamniotic shunt therapy. *Am J Obstet Gynecol* 1994;170:1770.

Jona JZ. Advances in neonatal surgery. *Pediatr Clin North Am* 1998;45:605–617.

Keckler SJ, St Peter SD, Valusek PA, et al. VACTERL anomalies in patients with esophageal atresia: An updated delineation of the spectrum and review of the literature. *Pediatr Surg Int* 2007;4:309–313.

Kunisaki SM, Barnewolt CE, Barnewolt CE, et al. Ex utero intrapartum treatment with extracorporeal membrane oxygenation for severe congenital diaphragmatic hernia. *J Pediatr Surg* 2007;42:98–104.

Liechty KW, Crombleholme TM, Flake AW, et al. Intrapartum airway management for giant fetal neck masses: The exit (ex utero intrapartum treatment) procedure. *Am J Obstet Gynecol* 1997;177:870.

Nakayama D, Bose C, Chescheir N, et al. *Critical care of the surgical newborn.* Armonk: Futura Publishing, 1997.

Nuchtern JG. Perinatal neuroblastoma. *Semin Pediatr Surg* 2006;15:10–16.

Parad RB. Buccal cell DNA mutation analysis for diagnosis of cystic fibrosis in newborns and infants inaccessible to sweat chloride measurement. *Pediatrics* 1998;101:851–855.

Reiner WG, Gearhart JP. Discordant sexual identity in some genetic males with cloacal extrophy assigned to female sex at birth. *N Engl J Med* 2004;350:333–341.

Ringer SA, Stark AS. Management of neonatal emergencies in the delivery room. *Clin Perinatol* 1989;16:23.

Sheldon CA. The pediatric genitourinary examination: Inguinal, urethral, and genital diseases. *Pediatr Clin North Am* 2001;48:1339–1380.

Stone KT, Kass EJ, Cacciarelli AA, et al. Management of suspected antenatal torsion: What is the best strategy? *J Urol* 1995;153:782–784.

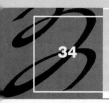

SKIN CARE
34
Caryn E. Douma

I. INTRODUCTION. The skin performs a vital role in the newborn period. It provides a protective barrier that assists in the prevention of infection, facilitates thermoregulation, and helps control insensible water loss and electrolyte balance. Other functions include tactile sensation and protection against toxins. The neonatal intensive care unit (NICU) environment presents numerous challenges to maintaining skin integrity. Routine care practices including bathing, application of monitoring devices, intravenous (IV) insertion and removal, tape application, and exposure to potentially toxic substances disrupt normal barrier function and predispose both premature and term newborns to skin injury. This chapter will address basic physiologic differences that affect newborn skin integrity, describe skin care practices in the immediate newborn period and common disorders.

II. ANATOMY. The three main layers of the skin are the epidermis, dermis, and the subcutaneous layer. The epidermis is the outermost layer providing the first line of protection against injury. It performs a critical barrier function, retaining heat and fluid, and providing protection from infection and environmental toxins. Its structural development has generally occurred by 24 weeks' gestation, but epidermal barrier function is not complete until after birth. Maturation typically takes 2 to 4 weeks following exposure to the extrauterine environment. The epidermis is composed primarily of keratinocytes, which mature to form the stratum corneum. The dermis is composed of collagen and elastin fibers that provide elasticity and connect the dermis to the epidermis. Blood vessels, nerves, sweat glands, and hair follicles are another integral part of the dermis. The subcutaneous layer, composed of fatty connective tissue, provides insulation, protection and calorie storage.

The premature infant has significantly fewer layers of stratum corneum than term infants and adults, which can be seen by the transparent, ruddy appearance of their skin. Infants born at <30 weeks may have <2 to 3 layers of stratum corneum compared with 10 to 20 in adults and term newborns. The maturation of the stratum corneum is accelerated following premature birth and improved barrier function and skin integrity is generally present within 10 to 14 days. Other differences in skin integrity in premature infants include decreased cohesion between the epidermis and dermis, less collagen, and a marked increase in transepidermal water loss.

III. SKIN CARE PRACTICES. Routine assessment, identification, and avoidance of harmful practices combined with early treatment can eliminate or minimize neonatal skin injury. The identification of potential risk factors for injury and the development of skin care policies and guidelines are an essential part of providing care to both premature and term newborns.

An evidence-based neonatal skin care guideline was created through the collaboration of the National Association of Neonatal Nurses (NANN) and the Association of Women's Health, Obstetric and Neonatal Nurses (AWHONN) (2001) in an effort to provide clinical practice recommendations for practitioners caring for newborns from birth to 28 days of age. This guideline provides a comprehensive reference for developing unit based skin care policies.

A. Prevention of injury
   1. Daily inspection and assessment of all skin surfaces.
   2. Avoidance of practices known to cause injury.
   3. Identification of risk factors.
       a. Prematurity.
       b. Use of monitoring equipment.

    c. Adhesives used to secure central and peripheral access lines, endotracheal tubes.

    d. Immobility secondary to extracorporeal membrane oxygenation (ECMO), Pavulon, high frequency ventilation, which can cause pressure necrosis.

    e. Use of high risk medications (vasopressors, calcium, sodium bicarbonate etc.).

    f. Avoidance of thermal injury. Temperature of any product in contact with the skin should not be higher than $41°C/105°F$.

B. Bathing

1. Initial bath should be performed 2 to 4 hours after admission when temperature has been stabilized to prevent risk of hypothermia. Provide a controlled environment utilizing warming lights and warm blankets. Bathing is often deferred for the first 24 hours in infants <36 weeks.
2. Use mild nonalkaline soap.
3. Daily bathing is not indicated. Warm sterile water is sufficient for premature infants during the first few weeks of life. No more than 2 or 3 times per week is preferred.

C. Adhesives

1. Minimize use of adhesives and tape.
2. Use nonadhesive products in conjunction with transparent dressings and double backed tape to secure IV catheters.
3. Avoid use of adhesive bonding agents that can be absorbed easily through the skin.
4. Use warm sterile water to remove adhesives from the skin to prevent epidermal stripping. Adhesive removers contain hydrocarbon derivatives or petroleum distillates that can result in toxicity in the preterm population.
5. Pectin barriers should be applied to skin before application of adhesives when securing umbilical lines, endotracheal tubes, feeding tubes, nasal cannulae and urine bags. Remove carefully using soft gauze or cotton balls soaked in warm water.

D. Cord care

1. Clean umbilical cord area with mild soap and water during first bath. Keep clean and dry. Wipe gently with water if area becomes soiled with stool or urine.
2. Routine application of alcohol is no longer recommended and may delay cord separation.
3. The routine use of antibiotic ointments and creams are not recommended.
4. Assess for signs of swelling or redness at base of cord.

E. Humidity

1. Consider the use of humidified incubator care in infants <32 weeks' gestation and/or <1,200 g to decrease transepidermal water loss, maintain skin integrity, decrease fluid requirements, and minimize electrolyte imbalance. Strict equipment cleaning protocols must be in place during humidification.
2. Recommended relative humidity (RH) is 75% to 80% for the first 7 days, decreasing to 50% to 60% RH during the second week until 30 to 32 weeks post-menstrual age (PMA).
3. Most infants will require humidity only for the first 2 weeks of life.

F. Circumcision care

1. Maintain dressing with petroleum gauze for the first 24 hours.
2. Keep site clean and dry using water for the first few days.

G. Disinfectants

1. Minimize use of isopropyl alcohol and alcohol-based disinfectants in preterm infants.
2. Use povidone iodine or chlorhexidine, removing with sterile saline following procedure. Evidence is currently inconclusive for chlorhexidine use in low birth weight infants. Prolonged or frequent exposure to iodine containing solutions in premature infants may affect thyroid function.

H. Emollients

1. Emollients are used to prevent and treat skin breakdown and dryness.
2. Emollients should not be used routinely in extremely premature infants because their use may increase the risk of systemic infection.
3. Single use or patient specific containers should be used to minimize risk of contamination.
4. Product should not contain perfumes, dyes, or preservatives.

IV. WOUND CARE. Wounds acquired in the immediate newborn period are most commonly related to surgical procedures, trauma, contact dermatitis, or excoriation. Skin care protocols and careful attention to positioning can prevent many of the common wounds requiring treatment. Epidermal stripping is common and can be avoided by minimizing adhesive use and utilizing protective barriers. Routine assessment and prompt treatment maximizes healing.

A. Common causes of neonatal wounds

1. Surgical procedures.
2. Trauma.
3. Pressure necrosis.
4. IV extravasation.
5. Prolonged contact with moisture or chemicals.

B. Three phases of wound healing

1. **Inflammatory**
   a. Occurs when the wound is created and is characterized by erythema, swelling and warmth.
2. **Proliferative**
   a. Characterized by granulation and tissue regeneration.
3. **Maturation**
   a. Shape of the wound is contracted and scar tissue is visible.

C. Treatment. Accurate assessment followed by immediate, effective treatment promotes wound healing and prevents further damage. Individualized, multidisciplinary care plans should be developed and implemented considering the etiology, type of wound, and the gestational age of the infant. Most neonatal wounds are caused by trauma or surgical procedures. Optimal wound treatment is achieved through proper assessment, cleansing, and dressing choice. Multiple wound care products are currently available to optimize healing and prevent further injury.

1. **Wound assessment**
   a. Assess wound for color, thickness, and exudates using unit developed tools to provide consistent, objective documentation
2. **Wound cleansing**
   a. Avoid the use of antiseptics in open wounds. Sterile normal saline (NS) is the preferred cleanser to remove debris and necrosed tissue, using gentle friction or irrigation.
   b. Clinical signs of infection may require culture and treatment with local or systemic antibiotics.
3. **Common wound dressings and products**
   a. Occlusive, nonadherent dressings provide a moist environment to promote healing and protect the site from further injury.
   b. Gauze.
   c. Hydrocolloids.
   d. Hydrogels.
   e. Barrier creams.

V. INTRAVENOUS EXTRAVASATIONS AND INFILTRATION. Intravenous extravasations and infiltration injuries can be prevented with frequent site assessment and prompt intervention.

A. Prevention

1. Hourly site assessment and documentation of integrity of IV site.
2. Peripheral IV infusions should not exceed 12.5% dextrose concentrations.
3. Use central access whenever possible for vasopressors and other high-risk medications.

B. Treatment

1. When an infiltration or extravasation occurs, stop the infusion immediately and elevate the extremity. Do not apply heat or cold as further tissue damage may occur. Pharmacologic intervention should be administered as soon as possible but no later than 12 to 24 hours from time of injury.

2. Hyaluronidase is used to treat infiltration or extravasation of hyperosmolar or extremely alkaline solutions. Administer as a 150 unit/mL solution in NS. Inject 0.2 mL subcutaneously in five separate sites around the leading edge of the infiltrate using a 25- or 27-gauge needle. Change the needle after each skin entry.

3. Phentolomine is used to treat injury caused by extravasation of vasoconstrictive agents such as dopamine, epinephrine, or dobutamine. Use a 1 mg/mL solution of phentolamine diluted in NS. Inject 0.2 mL subcutaneously in five separate sites around the leading edge of the infiltrate using 25- or 27-gauge needle. Change the needle after each skin entry.

4. Consider consultation with plastic surgery for severe injury.

VI. COMMON SKIN LESIONS.

Transient cutaneous lesions are common in the neonatal period. Among the most common are the following:

A. Erythema toxicum.

1. Scattering of macules, papules, and even some vesicles, or small white or yellow pustules which usually occur on the trunk, but also frequently appear on the extremities and face. It occurs in up to 70% of term newborns; occurs rarely in premature infants.

2. Unknown etiology.

3. Vesicle contents when smeared and stained with Wright stain will show a predominance of eosinophils.

4. No treatment necessary.

B. Diaper dermatitis

1. Most often caused by sensitivity to chemicals contained in detergent, clothing or diapers.

2. Prevention is the best treatment, keeping diaper area clean with warm water and barrier products if needed.

3. Use of powder is not recommended.

C. Milia

1. Multiple pearly white or pale yellow papules or cysts mainly found on the nose, chin, and forehead in term infants.

2. Consists of epidermal cysts up to 1 mm in diameter that develop in connection with the pilosebaceous follicle.

   a. Disappear within the first few weeks requiring no treatment.

D. Sebaceous gland hyperplasia

1. Similar to milia with smaller more numerous lesions primarily confined to the nose, upper lip and chin.

2. Rarely occurs in preterm infants.

3. Related to maternal androgen stimulation.

4. Disappears within the first few weeks.

VII. VASCULAR ABNORMALITIES.

Vascular abnormalities occur in up to 40% of newborns. Hemangiomas appear on 1% to 3% of newborns at birth and develop in another 10% within the first few weeks of life. Premature infants have a higher incidence of developing hemangiomas, especially those born at <1,000 g. Most completely resolve by age 12 and do not require intervention unless they interfere with vital functions.

A. Cavernous hemangioma

1. Deep strawberry hemangioma often present at birth. The lesion grows during the first year but regression is often not complete. They can be associated with significant complications including hemorrhage due to platelet trapping (Kasabach-Merritt syndrome), hypertrophy of involved structures (Klippel-Trenaunay syndrome), heart failure (due to arteriovenous anastomoses) and infection. Treatment may involve surgery, occlusion, laser therapy, steroids or alpha interferon.

B. **Nevus simplex (salmon patch or macular hemangioma)**
   1. Flat, pink macular lesion found on the forehead, upper eyelid, nasolabial area, glabella, or nape of the neck. It is the most common vascular lesion found in the newborn, occurring in 30% to 40% of infants. Often referred to as a stork bite, it consists of distended dermal capillaries. Most resolve by 1 year of age, excluding those found on the neck.

C. **Nevus flammeus (port-wine stain)**
   1. Flat or mildly elevated reddish purple lesion most commonly found on the face. The lesion is a vascular malformation of dilated capillary—like vessels that do not involute. They are often unilateral and may be associated with hemangiomas of the underlying structures. The association of nevus flammeus in the region of the first branch of the trigeminal nerve with cortical lesions of the brain is known as the Sturge Weber syndrome.

D. **Strawberry hemangioma**
   1. May be present at birth or present as a pale macule with irregular margins. More common in the head, neck and trunk, they can occur anywhere. Most grow rapidly during the first 6 months and continue to grow for the first year. The majority involute completely by age 4 to 5.

E. **Disorders of lymphatic vessels**
   1. Lymphangiomas.
   2. Cystic hygroma.
   3. Lymphedema.

VIII. **PIGMENTATION ABNORMALITIES.** Pigmentary lesions may be present at birth and are most often benign. Some of the most common are briefly described in the subsequent text. A diffuse pattern of hyperpigmentation presenting in the newborn period is unusual and may indicate a variety of hereditary, nutritional, or metabolic disorders. Hypopigmentation presenting in a diffuse pattern may be linked to endocrine, metabolic, or genetic disease.

A. **Mongolian spots**
   1. Benign pigmented lesions found in 70% to 90% of black, Hispanic, and Asian infants. The lesions may be small or large, grayish blue or bluish black in color.
   2. Caused by the increased presence of melanocytes, most commonly found in the lumbosacral region.

B. **Café au lait spots**
   1. Flat, brown, round, or oval lesions with smooth edges occurring in 10% of normal infants.
   2. Usually of little or no significance but may indicate neurofibromatosis if larger than 4 to 6 cm or >6 are present

C. **Albinism**
   1. Most commonly an autosomal recessive condition involving abnormal melanin synthesis leading to a deficiency in pigment production. The only effective treatment is protection from light.

D. **Piebaldism (partial albinism)**
   1. Autosomal dominant disorder present at birth characterized by off-white macules on the scalp and forehead extending to the extremities. The hair may be involved as well. A white "forelock," as in Waardenberg's syndrome, is a feature of this disorder.

E. **Junctional nevi**
   1. Brown or black, flat or slightly raised lesions present at birth occurring at the junction of the dermis and epidermis. They are benign lesions requiring no treatment.

F. **Compound nevi**
   1. Larger than junctional nevi, involving the dermis and epidermis. Removal is recommended to decrease possibility of later progression to malignant melanoma.

G. **Giant hairy nevi**
   1. Present at birth, they may involve 20% to 30% of the body surface, with other pigmentary abnormalities frequently present. Brown to black and leathery in appearance, also known as bathing trunk nevi, they have a large amount of

hair and may include central nervous system involvement. Surgical removal is indicated for cosmetic reasons, and because they can progress to malignant melanoma.

IX. DEVELOPMENTAL ABNORMALITIES OF THE SKIN

A. Skin dimples and sinuses can occur on any part of the body, but they are most common over bony prominences such as the scapula, knee joint, and hip. They may be simple depressions in the skin of no pathologic significance or actual sinus tracts connecting to deeper structures.

1. A pilonidal dimple or sinus may occur in the sacral area. A sinus that is deep but does not communicate with the underlying structures is usually insignificant.

2. Some deep sinuses connect to the central nervous system. Occasionally a dimple, sometimes accompanied by a nevus or hemangioma may signify an underlying spinal disorder. These usually require ultrasonography, computed tomography (CT) or magnetic resonance imaging (MRI) scans for diagnosis.

3. Dermal sinuses or cysts along the cheek or jawline or extending into the neck, may represent remnants of the branchial cleft structures of the early embryo.

4. A preauricular sinus is the most common, and may be unilateral or bilateral. It appears in the most anterior upper portion of the tragus of the external ear. They rarely cause problems in the newborn period, but may require later excision due to infection.

B. Small skin tags can occur on the chest wall near the breast, and are of no significance.

C. Aplasia cutis (congenital absence of the skin) occurs most frequently in the midline of the posterior part of the scalp. Treatment involves protection from trauma and infection. It can occur in trisomy 13 and 18.

X. OTHER SKIN DISORDERS.
Complete identification and description of all dermatologic disorders is beyond the scope of this chapter. Refer to the suggested reading list for resources. Several of the more common developmental and hereditary disorders are mentioned in the subsequent text.

A. Scaling disorders

1. Most common causes of scaling in neonatal period are related to desquamation found in post mature and dysmature infants. The condition is time limited and transient without long-term consequences.

2. Less common scaling disorders that occur within the first month of life include Harlequin ichthyosis, Collodion baby, X-linked ichthyosis, Bullous ichthyosis and others.

B. Vesicobullous eruptions

1. Epidermolysis bullosa is characterized by lesions that appear at birth or within the first few weeks. Severity of symptoms ranges from simple nonscarring bullae to more severe forms with large numerous lesions that result in scarring, contractions, and loss of large areas of epidermis. Prevention of infection and protection of fragile skin surfaces is the goal of treatment. Various forms include Epidermolysis bullosa simplex, Epidermolysis bullosa lethalis, Epidermolysis bullosa dystrophica (both autosomal dominant and recessive)

C. Infection

1. Infections caused by bacterial (especially staphylococcal, *pseudomonas, Listeria*, viral (herpes simplex) or fungal (e.g., candidal) may also cause vesicular, bullous or other skin manifestations.

Suggested Readings

Lund C, Kuller J, Lane A, et al. Neonatal skin care: The scientific basis for practice JOGNN. *J Obstet Gynecol Neonatal Nurs* 1999;28(3):241–254.

Lund CH, Kuller J, Lane AT, et al. Neonatal skin care: Evaluation of the AWHONN/NANN research-based practice project on knowledge and skin care practices. Association of Women's Health, Obstetric and Neonatal Nurses/National Association of Neonatal Nurses JOGNN. *J Obstet Gynecol Neonatal Nurs* 2001;30(1):30–40. Neonatal Skin Care. *Evidence-based clinical practice guideline.* The Association of Women's Health, Obstetric and Neonatal Nurses, National Association of Neonatal Nurses, 2001.

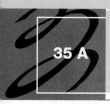

RETINOPATHY OF PREMATURITY
Deborah K. VanderVeen and John A.F. Zupancic

 GENERAL PRINCIPLES

I. DEFINITION. RETINOPATHY OF PREMATURITY (ROP) is a multifactorial vasoproliferative retinal disorder that increases in incidence with decreasing gestational age. Approximately 65% of infants with a birth weight <1,250 g and 80% of those with a birth weight <1,000 g will develop some degree of ROP.

II. PATHOGENESIS

A. Normal development. After the sclera and choroid have developed, retinal elements, including nerve fibers, ganglion cells, and photoreceptors, migrate from the optic disc at the posterior pole of the eye and move toward the periphery. The photoreceptors have progressed 80% of the distance to their resting place at the ora serrata by 28 weeks gestation. Before the retinal vessels develop, the avascular retina receives its oxygen supply by diffusion across the retina from the choroid vessels. The retinal vessels, which arise from the spindle cells of the adventitia of the hyaloid vessels at the optic disc, begin to migrate outward at 16 weeks gestation. Migration is complete by 36 weeks on the nasal side and by 40 weeks on the temporal side.

B. Possible mechanisms of injury. Clinical observations suggest that the onset of ROP consists of two stages.

1. The **first stage** involves an initial insult or insults, such as hyperoxia, hypoxia, or hypotension, at a critical point in retinal vascularization that results in vasoconstriction and decreased blood flow to the developing retina with a subsequent arrest in vascular development. The relative hyperoxia after birth is hypothesized to downregulate the production of growth factors such as vascular endothelial growth factor that are essential for the normal development of the retinal vessels.

2. During the **second stage,** neovascularization occurs. This aberrant retinal vessel growth is thought to be driven by excess angiogenic factors (such as vascular endothelial growth factor) released by the ischemic relatively hypoxic avascular retina. New vessels grow through the retina into the vitreous. These vessels are permeable and hemorrhage and edema can occur. Extensive and severe extraretinal fibrovascular proliferation can lead to retinal detachment and abnormal retinal function. In most affected infants, however, the disease process is mild and regresses spontaneously.

C. Risk factors. ROP has been consistently associated with low gestational age, low birth weight, and prolonged oxygen exposure. In addition, potential or confirmed risk factors include lability in oxygen requirement as well as markers of neonatal illness severity, such as mechanical ventilation, systemic infection, blood transfusion, and intraventricular hemorrhage.

III. DIAGNOSIS

A. Screening. Because no early clinical signs or symptoms indicate developing ROP, early and regular retinal examination is necessary. The timing of the occurrence of ROP is related to the maturity of retinal vessels and therefore postnatal age. In the Cryotherapy for Retinopathy of Prematurity (CRYO-ROP) Study, for infants <1,250 g the median postnatal ages at the onset of stage 1 ROP, prethreshold disease, and threshold disease were 34, 36, and 37 weeks, respectively. At the time of the first examination, 17% of infants had ROP, and prethreshold ROP has been reported as early as 29 weeks gestational age. Because ROP that meets treatment criteria may be reached at any postnatal age, all preterm infants who meet screening criteria and are discharged before they show resolution of the ROP or have mature retinal vasculature must continue to have ophthalmologic examinations on an out-patient basis.

B. Diagnosis. ROP is diagnosed by retinal examination with indirect ophthalmoscopy; this should be performed by an ophthalmologist with expertise in ROP screening. The current recommendation is to screen all infants with a birth weight <1,500 g or gestational age <30 weeks. Infants who are born after 30 weeks gestational age may be considered for screening if they have been ill (e.g., those who have had severe respiratory distress syndrome, hypotension requiring pressor support, or surgery in the first several weeks of life). Because the timing of ROP is related to postnatal age, infants who are born at <26 weeks gestation are examined at the postnatal age of 6 weeks, those born at 27 to 28 weeks at the postnatal age of 5 weeks, those born at 29 to 30 weeks are examined at the postnatal age of 4 weeks, and those >30 weeks at the postnatal age of 3 weeks. Patients are examined every 2 weeks until their vessels have grown out to the ora serrata and the retina is considered mature. If ROP is diagnosed, the frequency of examination depends on the severity and rapidity of progression of the disease.

IV. CLASSIFICATION AND DEFINITIONS

A. Classification. The International Classification of Retinopathy of Prematurity (ICROP) is used to classify ROP. This classification system consists of four components (see Fig. 35A.1).

1. **Location** refers to how far the developing retinal blood vessels have progressed. The retina is divided into three concentric circles or zones.

   a. **Zone 1** consists of an imaginary circle with the optic nerve at the center and a radius of twice the distance from the optic nerve to the macula.

   b. **Zone 2** extends from the edge of zone 1 to the equator on the nasal side of the eye and approximately half the distance to the ora serrata on the temporal side.

   c. **Zone 3** consists of the outer crescent-shaped area extending from zone 2 out to the ora serrata temporally.

2. Severity refers to the **stage** of disease.

   a. **Stage 1.** A demarcation line appears as a thin white line that separates the normal retina from the undeveloped avascular retina.

   b. **Stage 2.** A ridge of fibrovascular tissue with height and width replaces the line of stage 1. It extends inward from the plane of the retina.

   c. **Stage 3.** The ridge has extraretinal fibrovascular proliferation. Abnormal blood vessels and fibrous tissue develop on the edge of the ridge and extend into the vitreous.

   d. **Stage 4.** Partial retinal detachment may result when scar tissue pulls on the retina. Stage 4A is partial detachment outside the macula, so that there is still a chance for good vision. Stage 4B is partial detachment that involves the macula, thereby limiting the likelihood of good vision in that eye.

   e. **Stage 5.** Complete retinal detachment occurs. The retina assumes a funnel-shaped appearance and is described as open or narrow in the anterior and posterior regions.

3. **Plus disease** is an additional designation that refers to the presence of vascular dilatation and tortuosity of the posterior retinal vessels in at least two quadrants. This indicates a more severe degree of ROP, and may also be associated with iris vascular engorgement, pupillary rigidity, and vitreous haze. **Preplus disease** describes vascular abnormalities of the posterior pole (mild venous dilatation or arterial tortuosity) that are present but are insufficient for the diagnosis of plus disease.

4. **Extent** refers to the circumferential location of disease and is reported as clock hours in the appropriate zone.

Figure 35A.1. Sample of form for ophthalmologic consultation.

B. Definitions

1. **Aggressive posterior ROP** (previously referred to as *Rush disease*) is an uncommon, rapidly progressing, severe form of ROP characterized by its posterior location (usually zone 1), and prominence of plus disease out of proportion to the peripheral retinopathy. Stage 3 ROP may appear as a flat, intraretinal network of neovascularization. When untreated, this type of ROP usually progresses to stage 5.

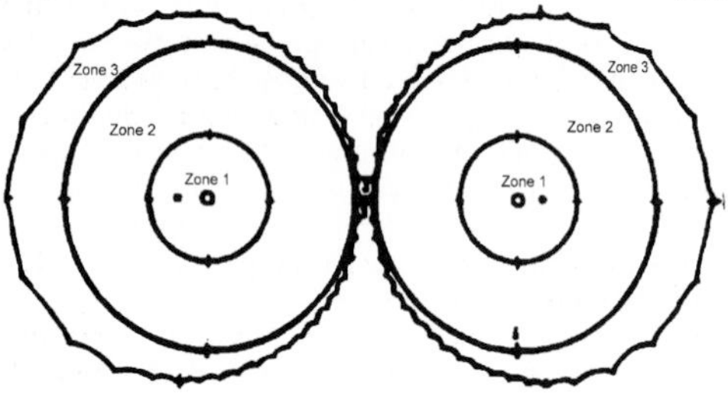

2. **Threshold ROP** is present if 5 or more contiguous or 8 cumulative clock hours (30-degree sectors) of stage 3 with plus disease in either zone 1 or 2 are present. This is the level of ROP at which the risk of blindness is predicted to be at least 50%, and at which the CRYO-ROP study showed that the risk of blindness could be reduced to approximately 25%

3. **Prethreshold ROP** is any of the following: zone 1 ROP of any stage less than threshold; zone 2 ROP with stage 2 and plus disease; zone 2 ROP with stage 3 without plus disease; or zone 2 ROP with stage 3 with plus disease with fewer than the threshold number of sectors of stage 3. The early treatment for ROP study showed that for eyes with high risk prethreshold ROP, early treatment may reduce the risk of blindness to approximately 15% (see section V).

V. TIMING OF TREATMENT

A. Current recommendations are to consider treatment for "type 1" prethreshold ROP, which includes in zone 1, eyes with any ROP and plus disease or stage 3 with or without plus disease, and in zone 2, stage 2 or 3 with plus disease. Observation is recommended for "type 2" prethreshold ROP, which includes zone 1, stage 1 or 2 ROP without plus disease, or zone 2, stage 3 ROP without plus disease.

B. Treatment should be considered for an eye with type 2 ROP when progression to type 1 status or threshold ROP occurs.

VI. PROGNOSIS

A. **Short-term prognosis.** Risk factors for ROP requiring treatment include posterior location (zone 1 or posterior zone 2), presence of ROP on the first examination, increasing severity of stage, circumferential involvement, the presence of plus disease, and rapid progression of disease. Most infants with stage 1 or 2 ROP will experience spontaneous regression. In the CRYO-ROP study of infants weighing <1,250 g at birth, the overall incidence of ROP was 66%; stage 1 was the highest stage reached in 25% and stage 2 was the highest stage in 22%. Prethreshold ROP was reached in 18% and threshold in 6%. Any zone 3 disease has an excellent prognosis for complete recovery.

B. **Long-term prognosis.** Infants with significant ROP have an increased risk of high myopia, anisometropia and other refractive errors, strabismus, amblyopia, astigmatism, late retinal detachment, and glaucoma. **Cicatricial disease** refers to residual scarring in the retina and may be associated with retinal detachment years later. The prognosis for stage 4 ROP depends on the involvement of the macula; the chance for good vision is greater when the macula is not involved. Once the retina has detached, the prognosis for good vision is poor even with surgical reattachment, although some useful vision may be preserved. All premature infants who meet screening criteria regardless of the diagnosis of ROP are at risk for long-term vision problems, from either ocular or neurologic abnormalities. We recommend a follow-up evaluation by an ophthalmologist with expertise in neonatal sequelae at approximately 1 year of age, or sooner if ocular or visual abnormalities have been noted.

VII. PREVENTION.

Currently no proven methods are available to prevent ROP. Multiple large clinical trials to prevent ROP have been performed evaluating the use of prophylactic vitamin E therapy, reduction in exposure to bright light, and administration of penicillamine, but none of these have shown clear benefit. Nonrandomized studies have suggested that lower or more tightly regulated oxygen saturation limits early on in the neonatal course may reduce the severity of ROP without adverse effects on mortality, bronchopulmonary dysplasia, or neurologic sequelae. Several multicenter randomized trials to formally test this hypothesis are now underway, but results are not expected for several years.

VIII. TREATMENT

A. **Laser therapy.** Laser photocoagulation therapy for ROP is the preferred initial treatment in most centers. Laser treatment is delivered through an indirect ophthalmoscope and is applied to the avascular retina anterior to the ridge of extraretinal fibrovascular proliferation for 360 degrees. An average of 1,000 spots are placed in each eye, but the number may range from a few hundred to approximately 2,000. Both argon and diode laser photocoagulation have been successfully used in infants with severe ROP. The procedure can be performed in the newborn intensive care unit, and usually can be performed with local anesthesia and sedation, avoiding some of the adverse effects of general anesthesia. Clinical observations and comparative studies suggest that laser therapy is as at least as effective as cryotherapy in achieving favorable visual outcomes. The development of cataracts, glaucoma, or anterior segment ischemia following laser surgery or cryotherapy has been reported.

B. Cryotherapy. A cryoprobe is applied to the external surface of the sclera and areas peripheral to the ridge of the ROP are frozen until the entire anterior avascular retina has been treated. Approximately 35–75 applications are made in each eye. The procedure is usually done under general anesthesia. Cryotherapy causes more inflammation and requires more analgesia than laser therapy, but may be necessary in special cases, such as when there is poor pupillary dilation or vitreous hemorrhage, both of which prevent adequate delivery of laser therapy.

C. Retinal reattachment. Once the macula detaches in stage 4B or 5 ROP, retinal surgery is usually performed in an attempt to reattach the retina. This may include vitrectomy with or with out lensectomy, and membrane peeling if necessary, to remove tractional forces causing the retinal detachment. A scleral buckling procedure may be useful for more peripheral detachments, with drainage of subretinal fluid, for effusional detachments. Reoperations for redetachment of the retina are common. Even if the retina can be successfully attached, with rare exception the visual outcome is in the range of legal blindness. Despite the low vision measure, however, children find any amount of vision useful, and untreated stage 5 ROP eventually leads to no light perception vision. The achievement of even minimal vision can result in a large difference in a child's overall quality of life.

D. Supplemental oxygen. A large clinical trial was performed to determine whether supplemental oxygen given to infants with prethreshold ROP would limit the progression from prethreshold to threshold ROP. This showed no significant reduction in the number of infants that progressed to threshold ROP. In a subgroup analysis, however, it appeared that supplemental oxygen therapy may be beneficial for infants with prethreshold ROP without plus disease.

Suggested Reading

American Academy of Pediatrics, Section on Ophthalmology. Screening examination of premature infants for retinopathy of prematurity. *Pediatrics* 2006;117:572–576; Errata: *Pediatrics* 2006;117:572–576.

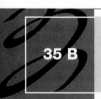

35 B

HEARING LOSS IN NEONATAL INTENSIVE CARE UNIT GRADUATES

Jane E. Stewart and Jeffrey W. Stolz

I. DEFINITION. Neonatal intensive care unit (NICU) graduates are at high risk of developing hearing loss. When undetected, hearing loss can result in delays in language, communication, and cognitive development. Hearing loss falls into four major categories:

A. Sensorineural loss is the result of abnormal development or damage to the cochlear hair cells (sensory end organ) or auditory nerve.

B. Conductive loss is the result of interference in the transmission of sound from the external auditory canal to the inner ear. The most common cause for conductive hearing loss is fluid in the middle ear or middle ear effusion. Less common are anatomic causes such as microtia, canal stenosis, or stapes fixation that often occur in infants with craniofacial malformations.

C. **Auditory dyssynchrony or auditory neuropathy.** In this less common type of hearing loss, the inner ear or cochlea appears to receive sounds normally; however, the transfer of the signal from the cochlea to the auditory nerve is abnormal. The etiology of this disorder is not well understood; however, babies who have severe hyperbilirubinemia, prematurity, hypoxia and immune disorders are at increased risk. There is also a reported genetic predisposition to auditory dyssynchrony.

D. **Central hearing loss.** In this type of hearing loss there is an intact auditory canal and inner ear and normal neurosensory pathways but abnormal auditory processing at higher levels of the central nervous system.

II. **INCIDENCE.** The overall incidence of severe congenital hearing loss is 1 to 3 in 1,000 live births. However, 2 to 4 per 100 infants surviving neonatal intensive care have some degree of sensorineural hearing loss.

III. **ETIOLOGY**

A. **Genetic.** Approximately 50% of congenital hearing loss is thought to be of genetic origin, 70% recessive, 15% autosomal dominant and 15% with other types of genetic transmission. The most common genetic cause of hearing loss is a mutation in the **connexin 26(Cx26) gene**, located on chromosome 13q11–12. The carrier rate for this mutation is 3% and it causes approximately 20% to 30% of congenital hearing loss. Deletion of the **mitochondrial gene** 12SrRNA, A1555G, is associated with a predisposition for hearing loss after exposure to aminoglycoside antibiotics. **Other mutations,** such as those of the SLC26A4 gene and Connexin 30 (Cx30) gene, are associated with newborn hearing loss. Approximately 30% of infants with hearing loss have other associated medical problems that are part of a **syndrome**. More than 400 syndromes are known to include hearing loss (e.g., Alport, Pierre Robin, Usher, Waardenburg Syndrome, Trisomy 21).

B. **Nongenetic.** In approximately 25% of childhood hearing loss, a nongenetic cause is identified. Hearing loss is thought to be secondary to injury to the developing auditory system in the intrapartum or perinatal period. This injury may be due to infection, hypoxia, ischemia, metabolic disease, ototoxic medication, or hyperbilirubinemia. Preterm infants and term infants who require newborn intensive care are often exposed to these factors.

1. **Cytomegalovirus (CMV)** congenital infection is the most common cause of nonhereditary sensorineural hearing loss. Approximately 1% of all infants are born with CMV infection. Of these (~40,000 infants/year), 10% have clinical signs of infection at birth (small for gestational age, heopatosplenomegaly, jaundice, thrombocytopenia, neutropenia, intracranial calcifications, skin rash), and 50% to 60% of these infants develop hearing loss. Although most (90%) of infants born with CMV infection have no clinical signs of infection, hearing loss still develops in 10% to 15% of these infants. Because there is no established treatment for CMV in the newborn, prevention of hearing loss is not possible. Treatment with the antiviral agent ganciclovir is being studied and preliminary data indicate that it may prevent the development and/or progression of hearing loss.

C. **Risk factors.** The Joint Committee on Infant Hearing listed the following risk indicators for progressive or delayed-onset sensorineural and/or conductive hearing loss.

1. Parental or caregiver concern regarding hearing, speech, language, or developmental delay.

2. Family history of permanent childhood hearing loss.

3. Stigmata or other findings associated with a syndrome known to include a sensorineural or conductive hearing loss or eustacian tube dysfunction.

4. Postnatal infections associated with sensorineural hearing loss, including bacterial meningitis.

5. *In utero* infections such as CMV, herpes, rubella, syphilis, human immunodeficiency virus (HIV), and toxoplasmosis.

6. Neonatal indicators: specifically, hyperbilirubinemia at a serum level requiring exchange transfusion (some centers use a level of $\geq$20 mg/dL as a general guideline for risk), persistent pulmonary hypertension of the newborn associated with mechanical ventilation, conditions requiring the use of extracorporeal membrane oxygenation (ECMO), and prolonged treatment with mechanical ventilation.
7. Syndromes associated with progressive hearing loss such as neurofibromatosis, osteopetrosis, and Usher syndrome.
8. Neurodegenerative disorders, such as Hunter syndrome, or sensory motor neuropathies, such as Friedreich's ataxia and Charcot-Marie-Tooth syndrome.
9. Head trauma.
10. Recurrent or persistent otitis media with effusion for at least 3 months.

However, a substantial proportion of infants with congenital hearing loss have no identified risk factors. New recommendations for identifying infants at risk for late-onset hearing loss and progressive hearing loss are expected from the Joint Committee on Newborn Hearing Screening in the near future.

D. Detection. Universal newborn hearing screening is recommended to detect hearing loss as early as possible. The Joint Committee on Infant Hearing and the American Academy of Pediatrics endorse a goal that 100% of infants be tested during their hospital birth admission. The implementation of this recommendation is under way; many states have passed legislation to ensure this goal is achieved promptly.

IV. SCREENING TESTS. The currently acceptable methods for physiologic hearing screening in newborns are auditory brainstem response and evoked otoacoustic emissions (EOAEs). A threshold of $\geq$35 dB has been established as a cutoff for an abnormal screen, which prompts further testing.

A. Auditory brainstem responses (ABR). ABR measures the electroencephalographic waves generated by the auditory system in response to clicks through three electrodes placed on the infant's scalp. The characteristic waveform recorded from the electrodes becomes more well defined with increasing postnatal age. ABR is reliable after 34 weeks postnatal age. The automated version of ABR allows this test to be performed quickly and easily by trained hospital staff. At present, because of the increased risk of injury to the auditory pathway beyond the cochlea (auditory nerve) including auditory dyssynchrony, ABR is the preferred screening method to evaluate hearing loss in the NICU graduate.

B. EOAEs. This records acoustic "feedback" from the cochlea through the ossicles to the tympanic membrane and ear canal following a click stimulus. EOAE is even quicker to perform than ABR. However, EOAE is more likely to be affected by debris or fluid in the external and middle ear, resulting in higher referral rates. Furthermore, EOAE is unable to detect some forms of sensorineural hearing loss including auditory dyssynchrony. EOAE is often combined with automated ABR in a two-step screening system.

V. FOLLOW-UP TESTING. Infants with abnormal screening ABRs should have follow-up testing. Infants who are abnormal in both ears should have a diagnostic auditory brainstem response performed within 2 weeks of their initial test. Infants with unilateral abnormal results should have follow-up testing within 3 months. Testing should include a full diagnostic frequency-specific ABR to measure hearing threshold. Evaluation of middle ear function, observation of the infant's behavioral response to sound, and parental report of emerging communication and auditory behaviors should also be included.

A. Definitions of the degree and severity of hearing loss are listed in this table.

Mild	15–30 dB HL
Moderate	30–50 dB HL
Severe	50–70 dB HL
Profound	70+ dB HL

B. Infants who have risk factors for progressive or delayed-onset sensorineural and/or conductive hearing loss require continued surveillance, even if the initial newborn screening results are normal. Current recommendations are that audiologic testing be performed at least every 6 months for the first 3 years of age. As noted in the preceding text, these specific recommendations will be modified with the Joint Committee's newest statement.

C. Infants with **mild or unilateral hearing loss** should also be monitored closely as they are at increased risk for both progressive hearing loss and delayed and abnormal development of language and communication skills.

D. All infants should be monitored by their primary care providers for normal hearing and language development.

VI. MEDICAL EVALUATION. An infant diagnosed with true hearing loss should have the following additional evaluations.

A. Complete evaluation should be performed by an otolaryngologist or otologist who has experience with infants. Referral for radiologic imaging with computed tomography (CT) or magnetic resonance imaging (MRI) should occur when needed.

B. Genetic evaluation and counseling should be provided for all infants with true hearing loss.

C. Examination should be performed by a pediatric ophthalmologist to detect eye abnormalities that may be associated with hearing loss.

D. Developmental pediatrics, neurology, cardiology, and nephrology referral should be made as indicated.

VII. HABILITATION/TREATMENT. Infants with true hearing loss should be referred for early intervention services to enhance the child's acquisition of developmentally appropriate language skills. Infants who are appropriate candidates and whose parents have chosen to utilize personal amplification systems should be fitted with hearing aids as soon as possible. Children with severe to profound bilateral hearing loss may be candidates for cochlear implants by the end of the first year of age. Early intervention resources and information for parents to make decisions regarding communication choices should also be provided as promptly as possible.

VIII. PROGNOSIS. The prognosis depends largely on the extent of hearing loss, as well as on the time of diagnosis and treatment. For optimal auditory brain development, normal maturation of the central auditory pathways depends on the early maximizing of auditory input. The earlier habilitation starts, the better the child's chance of achieving age-appropriate language and communication skills. Fitting of hearing aids by the age of 6 months has been associated with improved speech outcome. Initiation of early intervention services before 3 months of age has been associated with improved cognitive developmental outcome at 3 years. Language and communication outcomes for children receiving early cochlear implants and the accompanying intensive multidisciplinary team therapy are also extremely promising.

ONLINE RESOURCES

Boystown National Research Center: http://www.babyhearing.org

Center for Disease Control: http://www.cdc.gov/ncbddd/ehdi/default.htm

Marion Downs National Center for Infant Hearing: http://www.colorado.edu/slhs/mdnc/

National Center for Hearing Assessment and Management: http://www.infanthearing.org/

American Academy of Audiology: http://www.audiology.org

American Speech-Language-Hearing Association: http://www.asha.org

National Association of the Deaf: http://www.nad.org

Hands & Voices: http://www.handsandvoices.org/

Harvard Medical School Center for Hereditary Deafness: http://hearing.harvard.edu

National Deaf Education Network and Clearinghouse: http://clerccenter.gallaudet.edu/Clearinghouse/

Better Hearing Institute: http://www.betterhearing.org/

Suggested Readings

AAP Task Force on Newborn Hearing and Infant Screening. Newborn and infant hearing loss: Detection and intervention. *Pediatrics* 1999;103: 527–530, www.aap.org/policy /re9846.html.

Kaye CI. The AAP Committee on Genetics. Newborn screening fact sheets. *Pediatrics* 2006;118:e934–e963.

NIH Joint Committee on Infant Hearing. Year 2000 position statement: Principles and guidelines for early hearing detection and intervention programs. *Pediatrics* 2000;106:798–817.

Weichbold V, Nekahm-Heis D, Welzl-Mueller K. Universal newborn hearing screening and postnatal hearing loss. *Pediatrics* 2006;117(4):e631–e636.

COMMON NEONATAL PROCEDURES

Steven A. Ringer and James E. Gray

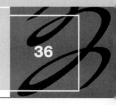

36

$\int$nvasive procedures are a necessary but potentially risk-laden part of newborn intensive care. To provide maximum benefit, these techniques must be performed in a manner that both accomplishes the task at hand and maintains the patient's general well-being.

I. GENERAL PRINCIPLES

   A. Consideration of alternatives. For each procedure, all alternatives should be considered and risk–benefit ratios evaluated. Many procedures involve the placement of indwelling devices made of plastic. Polyvinylchloride-based devices leach a plasticizer, Di (2-ethylhexyl)-phthalate (DEHP) which may be toxic over long-term exposure. Alternatives exist and devices that are DEHP-free should be used for procedures on neonates whenever possible.

   B. Monitoring and homeostasis. Care providers should always maintain their primary focus on the patient, rather than on the procedure being performed. They must assess cardiorespiratory and thermoregulatory stability throughout the procedure, and apply interventions when needed. Continuous monitoring can be accomplished through a combination of invasive (e.g., arterial blood pressure monitoring) or noninvasive (e.g., oximeter) techniques. Whenever possible, the operator should delegate the responsibility for monitoring and managing the patient to another care provider during the procedure.

   C. Pain control. Treatment of procedure-associated discomfort can be accomplished with pharmacologic or nonpharmacologic approaches (see Chap. 37). The potential negative impact of any medication on the patient's cardiorespiratory status should be considered. Oral sucrose (0.2–0.4 mL/kg) is very effective in reducing pain of minor procedures and blood drawing. It can also be used as adjunctive therapy for more painful procedures when the patient can tolerate oral medication. Morphine or fentanyl are commonly administered before beginning potentially painful procedures. The use of neonatal pain scales to assess the need for medication is recommended.

   D. Informing the family. Other than during true emergencies, we notify parents of the need for invasive procedures in their child's care before we perform them. We discuss the indications for and possible complications of each procedure. In addition, alternative procedures, where available, are also discussed.

   E. Precautions. The operator should use universal precautions, including use of gloves, impermeable gowns, barriers, and eye protection to prevent exposure to blood and bodily fluids that may be contaminated with infectious agents.

   F. The safety pause. Before beginning any procedure, the entire team should take a "safety pause" and ascertain that it is the correct patient, the correct procedure and if appropriate, that the procedure is being done on the correct side (e.g., thoracostomy tube, central venous catheter placement).

   G. Education and supervision. Individuals should be trained in the conduct of procedures before performing the procedure on patients. This training should include a discussion of indications, possible complications and their treatment, alternatives, and the techniques to be used. Experienced operators should be available at all times to provide further guidance and needed assistance.

   H. Documentation. Careful documentation of procedures enhances patient care. For example, noting difficulties encountered at intubation or the size and positioning of an endotracheal tube used provides important information if the procedure must be repeated. We routinely write notes after all procedures, including unsuccessful attempts. We document the date and time, indications, techniques used, difficulties encountered, complications (if any), and results of any laboratory tests performed. The safety pause is documented.

II. BLOOD DRAWING. The preparations for withdrawing blood depend somewhat on the blood studies that are required.

    A. Capillary blood is drawn when there is no need for many serial studies in close succession.

        1. Applicable blood studies include hematocrit, blood glucose (using glucometers or other point-of-care testing methods), bilirubin levels, and electrolyte determinations, and occasionally blood gas studies.

        2. Techniques

            a. The extremity to be used should be warmed to increase peripheral blood flow.

            b. Spring-loaded lancets minimize pain while ensuring a puncture adequate for obtaining blood. The blood should flow freely, with minimal or no squeezing. This will ensure the most accurate determination of laboratory values.

            c. Capillary punctures of the foot should be performed on the lateral side of the sole of the heel, avoiding previous sites if possible.

            d. The skin should be cleaned carefully with povidone-iodine and alcohol before puncture to avoid infection of soft tissue or underlying bone.

    B. Catheter blood samples

        1. Umbilical artery or radial artery catheters are often used for repetitive blood samples, especially for blood gas studies.

        2. Techniques

            a. A needleless system for blood sampling from arterial catheters **should be used.** Specific techniques for use vary with the product and the manufacturer's guidelines should be followed.

            b. For **blood gas studies,** a 1-mL preheparinized syringe, or a standard 1-mL syringe rinsed with 0.5 mL of heparin is used to withdraw the sample. The rate of sample withdrawal should be limited to 1.5 mL/minute to avoid altering downstream arterial perfusion.

            c. The catheter must be adequately cleared of infusate before withdrawing samples, **to avoid false readings.** After the sample is drawn, blood should be cleared with a small volume of heparinized saline-flushing solution.

    C. Venous blood for blood chemistry studies, blood cultures, and other laboratory studies **is usually obtained from either the antecubital vein, the external jugular vein, or the saphenous vein.** For blood cultures, the area should be cleaned with an iodine-containing solution; if the position of the needle is directed by using a sterile gloved finger, the finger should be cleaned in the same way. A new sterile needle should be used to insert the blood into the culture bottles.

III. BLADDER TAP

    A. Because bladder taps are most often used to obtain urine for culture, **a sterile technique is crucial.** Careful cleaning with iodine and alcohol solution over the prepubic region is essential.

    B. Technique. Bladder taps are done with a 5- to 10-mL syringe attached to a 22- or 23-gauge needle or to a 23-gauge butterfly needle. Before the tap, one should try to determine that the baby has not recently urinated. Ultrasonographic guidance is useful. One technique is as follows:

        1. The pubic bone is located by touch.

        2. The needle is placed in the midline, just superior to the pubic bone.

        3. The needle is slid in, aimed at the infant's coccyx.

        4. If the needle goes in >3 cm and no urine is obtained, one should assume that the bladder is empty and wait before attempting again.

IV. INTRAVENOUS THERAPY. The insertion and management of intravenous catheters require great care. As in older infants, hand veins are used most often, but veins in the scalp, foot, and ankle can be used. Transillumination of an extremity can help identify a vein, and newer devices that enhance the detection of veins may be even more useful.

V. ARTERIAL PUNCTURES are usually carried out by using the radial artery or posterior tibial artery. Rarely, the brachial artery is used. Radial artery punctures are most easily done using a 25- to 23-gauge butterfly needle, and transillumination often aids in locating the vessel. The radial artery is visualized and entered with the bevel of the needle facing up and at a 15-degree angle against the direction of flow. The artery is transfixed, and then the needle is slowly withdrawn and the syringe filled.

VI. LUMBAR PUNCTURE
   A. Technique
   1. The infant should be placed in the lateral decubitus position or in the sitting position with legs straightened. The assistant should hold the infant firmly at the shoulders and buttocks so that the lower part of the spine is curved. Neck flexion should be avoided so as not to compromise the airway.
   2. A sterile field is prepared and draped with towels.
   3. A 22- to 24-gauge spinal needle with a stylet should be used. Use of a No. 25 butterfly needle may introduce skin into the subarachnoid space and is to be avoided.
   4. The needle is inserted in the midline into the space between the fourth and fifth lumbar spinous processes. The needle is advanced gradually in the direction of the umbilicus, and the stylet is withdrawn frequently to detect the presence of spinal fluid. Usually a slight "pop" is felt as the needle enters the subarachnoid space.
   5. The cerebrospinal fluid **(CSF)** is collected into three or four tubes, each with a volume of 0.5 to 1.0 mL.
   B. Examination of the spinal fluid. CSF should be inspected immediately for turbidity and color. In many newborns normal CSF may be mildly xanthochromic, but it should always be clear.
   1. **Tube 1.** Cell count and differential should be determined from the unspun fluid in a counting chamber. The unspun fluid should be stained with methylene blue; it should be treated with concentrated acetic acid if there are numerous red blood cells (RBCs). The centrifuged sediment should be stained with Gram stain and Wright stain.
   2. **Tube 2.** Culture and sensitivity studies should be obtained.
   3. **Tube 3.** Glucose and protein determinations should be obtained.
   4. **Tube 4.** The cells in this tube also should be counted if the fluid is bloody. The fluid can be sent for other tests such as polymerase chain reaction amplification for herpes simplex virus (HSV), etc.).
   C. Information obtainable
   1. When the CSF is collected in three or four separate containers, an **RBC count** can be done on the first and last tubes to see if there is a difference in the number of RBCs/mm^3 between these specimens. In fluid obtained from a traumatic tap, the final tube will have fewer RBCs than the first; more equal numbers suggest the possibility of an intracranial hemorrhage. CSF in the newborn may normally contain up to 600 to 800 RBCs/mm^3.
   2. **White blood cell (WBC) count.** The normal number of WBCs/mm^3 in newborns is a matter of controversy. We accept up to 5 to 8 lymphocytes or monocytes as normal if there are no polymorphonuclear WBCs. Others accept as normal up to 25 WBCs/mm^3, including several polymorphonuclear cells. Data obtained from high-risk newborns without meningitis (see Table 36.1) show 0 to 32 WBCs/mm^3 in term infants and 0 to 29 WBCs/mm^3 in preterm infants with approximately 60% polymorphonuclear cells to be within the normal range. Higher WBC counts are generally seen with gram-negative meningitis than with group B streptococcal disease; as high as 50% of the latter group will have 100 WBCs/mm^3 or less. Because of the overlap between

TABLE 36.1	Cerebrospinal Fluid Examination in High-risk Neonates without Meningitis	
Determination	**Term**	**Preterm**
White blood cell count (cells/mL)		
No. of infants	87	30
Mean	8.2	9.0
Median	5	6
Standard deviation	7.1	8.2
Range	0–32	0–29
±2 Standard deviations	0–22.4	0–25.4
Percentage of polymorphonuclear cells	61.3%	57.2%
Protein (mg/dL)		
No. of infants	35	17
Mean	90	115
Range	20–170	65–150
Glucose (mg/dL)		
No. of infants	51	23
Mean	52	50
Range	34–119	24–63
Glucose in cerebrospinal fluid divided by blood glucose (%)		
No. of infants	51	23
Mean	81	74
Range	44–248	55–105

From Sarff LD, Platt LH, McCracken GH. Cerebrospinal fluid evaluation in neonates: comparison of high-risk neonates with and without meningitis. *J Pediatrics* 1976;88:473.

normal infants and those with meningitis, the presence of polymorphonuclear leukocytes in CSF deserves careful attention. Ultimately, the diagnosis depends on culture results and clinical course.

3. Data on **glucose and protein levels** in CSF from high-risk newborns are shown in Table 36.1. Normally the CSF glucose level is approximately 80% of the blood glucose level for term infants and 75% for preterm infants. If the blood glucose level is high or low, there is a 4- to 6-hour equilibration period with the CSF glucose.

The normal level of CSF protein in newborns may vary over a wide range. In full-term infants, levels below 100 mg/dL are acceptable. In premature infants, the acceptable level can be as high as 180 mg/dL. Values for high-risk infants are shown in Table 36.1. The level of CSF protein in the premature infant appears to be related to the degree of prematurity.

No single parameter can be used to rule out or rule in meningitis. Meningitis may occur in the absence of positive blood cultures (see Chap 23).

VII. INTUBATION

A. **Endotracheal intubation.** In most cases an infant can be adequately ventilated by bag and mask so that endotracheal intubation can be done as a controlled procedure.

1. **Tube size and length.** The correct tube size (see Chap. 4) and length (see Fig. 36.1) can be estimated from the infant's weight.

2. **Route.** Contradictory data exist over the preferred route for endotracheal intubation (i.e., oral versus nasal). In most circumstances local practice should

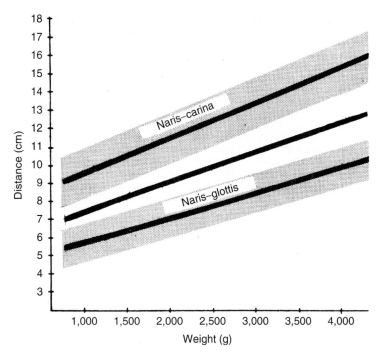

Figure 36.1. The relation of naris–carina and naris–glottis distance with body weight. The middle line represents the distance from naris to midtrachea. (Modified from Coldiron J. American Academy of Pediatrics. Estimation of nasotracheal tube length in neonate. *Pediatrics* 1968;41:823.)

guide this selection with two exceptions. First, oral intubation should be performed in all emergent situations, as it is generally easier and quicker than nasal intubation. Second, a functioning endotracheal tube should never be electively changed simply to provide an alternate route.

3. **Technique**
   a. **The patient should be preoxygenated** to ensure that the patient has normal oxygen saturations before laryngoscopy. Laryngoscopy and intubation of an active, unmedicated patient is more difficult for the operator, more uncomfortable for the patient, and the risk of complications may be increased. Whenever possible, the patient should be premedicated with a narcotic or short-acting benzodiazepine, unless the patient's condition is a contraindication (see Chap. 37).
   b. Throughout the intubation procedure, **observation of the patient and monitoring of the heart rate are mandatory.** Pulse oximetry should also be used when available. Electronic monitoring with an audible pulse rate frees personnel to attend to other tasks. If bradycardia is observed, especially if accompanied by hypoxia, the procedure should be stopped and the baby ventilated with bag and mask. An anesthesia bag attached to the tube adapter can deliver oxygen to the pharynx during the procedure or free-flow oxygen at 5 L/min can be given from a tube placed one half inch from the infant's mouth.
   c. **The baby's head should be slightly lifted anteriorly** (the "sniffing" position) with the baby's body aligned straight. The operator should stand looking down the midline of the body.

    d. The **laryngoscope** is held between the thumb and first finger of the left hand, with the second and third fingers holding the baby's chin and stabilizing the head.

    e. The **laryngoscope blade** is passed into the right side of the mouth and then to the midline, sweeping the tongue up and out of the way. The blade tip should be advanced into the vallecula, and the handle of the laryngoscope raised to an angle of approximately 60 degrees. The blade should then be lifted with care being taken not to rock or lever the laryngoscope blade. Visualization of the vocal cords may be improved by pushing down slightly on the larynx with the fourth or fifth finger of the left hand (or having an assistant do it) to displace the trachea posteriorly.

    f. The **endotracheal tube** is held with the right hand and inserted between the vocal cords to approximately 2 cm below the glottis (less in extremely small infants). During nasotracheal intubation, the tube can be guided by moving the baby's head slightly, or with small Macgill-type forceps. If a finger is pressing on the trachea, the tube can be felt passing through.

    g. The anatomic structures of the larynx and pharynx have different appearances. The esophagus is a horizontal posterior muscular slit; it should never be accidentally or mistakenly intubated if this is kept clearly in mind. The glottis, in contrast, consists of an anterior triangular opening formed by the vocal cords meeting anteriorly at the apex. This orifice lies directly beneath the epiglottis, which is lifted away by gentle upward traction with the laryngoscope.

    h. The **tube position** is checked by auscultation of the chest to ensure equal aeration of both lungs and observation of chest movement with positive-pressure inflation. If air entry is poor over the left side of the chest, the tube should be pulled back until it becomes equal to the right side. The insertion length of an oral tube is generally between 6 and 7 cm when measured at the lip for the smallest babies, and 8 and 9 cm for term or near-term babies (Fig. 36.1). The tube will "steam up" if it is correctly placed in the trachea. The baby should show improved oxygenation.

  4. Once correct position is ascertained, the tube should be held against the palate with one finger, until it can be taped securely in place; the position of the tube should be confirmed by radiograph when possible.

  5. Commonly observed errors

    a. Focus is placed on the procedure and not the patient.

    b. The baby's neck is hyperextended. This displaces the cords anteriorly and obscures visualization or makes the passing of the endotracheal tube difficult.

    c. Excessive pressure is placed on the infant's upper gum by the laryngoscope blade. This results from the tip of the laryngoscope blade being tilted or rocked upward instead of traction being exerted parallel to the baby.

    d. The tube is inserted too far and the position not assessed, resulting in continued intubation of the right mainstem bronchus.

B. Nasal continuous positive airway pressure (CPAP). Continuous distending pressure can be applied using nasal prongs as part of the ventilator circuit. These are simple to insert and are held on by a Velcro-fastened headset. In unusual circumstances, CPAP can be delivered through an appropriately sized endotracheal tube passed nasally and advanced to a pharyngeal position just inferior to the uvula. This tube is then connected to the ventilator circuit as in the preceding text.

VIII. THORACENTESIS AND CHEST TUBE PLACEMENT (see Chap. 24E)

IX. VASCULAR CATHETERIZATION (see Figs. 36.2 and 36.3 for diagrams of the newborn venous and arterial systems).

  A. Types of catheters

    1. Umbilical artery catheters (UALs) are used (i) for frequent monitoring of arterial blood gases, (ii) as a stable route for infusion of parenteral fluids, and (iii) for continuous monitoring of arterial blood pressure.

    2. Peripheral artery catheters are used when frequent blood gas monitoring is still required and an umbilical artery catheter is contraindicated, cannot be

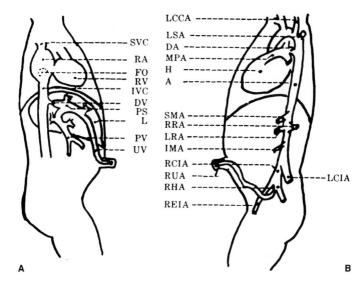

Figure 36.2. A: Diagram of the newborn umbilical venous system (SVC = superior vena cava; RA = right atrium; FO = foramen ovale; RV = right ventricle; IVC = inferior vena cava; DV = ductus venosus; PS = portal sinus; L = liver; PV = portal vein; UV = umbilical vein). **B:** Diagram of the newborn arterial system, including the umbilical artery (LCCA = left common carotid artery; LSA = left subclavian artery; DA = ductus arteriosus; MPA = main pulmonary artery; H = heart; A = aorta; SMA = superior mesenteric artery; RRA = right renal artery; LRA = left renal artery; IMA = inferior mesenteric artery; LCIA = left common iliac artery; RCIA = right common iliac artery; RUA = right umbilical artery; RHA = right hypogastric artery; REIA = right external iliac artery). (From Kitterman JA, Phibbs RH, Tooley WH. Catheterization of umbilical vessels in newborn infants. *Pediatr Clin North Am* 1970;17:898.)

placed, or is removed because of complications. Peripheral artery catheters must not be used to infuse alimentation solution or medications. They require that motion of the infant's arm be kept restricted.

3. **Umbilical vein catheters (UVC)** are used for exchange transfusions, monitoring of central venous pressure, infusion of fluids (when passed through the ductus venous and near the right atrium), and emergency vascular access for infusion of fluid, blood, or medications.

4. **Central venous catheters,** used largely for prolonged parenteral nutrition and occasionally to monitor central venous pressure, also can be placed percutaneously through the external jugular, subclavian, basilic, or saphenous vein.

B. Umbilical artery catheterization

1. **Guidelines.** In general, only seriously ill infants should have an umbilical artery catheter placed. If only a few blood gas measurements are anticipated, peripheral arterial punctures should be performed together with noninvasive oxygen monitoring, and a peripheral intravenous route should be used for fluids and medications.

2. **Technique**

a. **Sterile technique is used.** Before preparing cord and skin, make external measurements to determine how far the catheter will be inserted (see Figs. 36.3–36.5). For a high UAC, the distance is usually (umbilicus-to-shoulder) +2 cm, plus the length of the stump. In a high setting, the catheter tip is placed between the eighth and tenth thoracic vertebrae; in a low setting, the tip is between the third and fourth lumbar vertebrae.

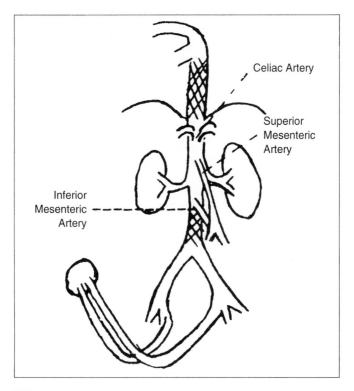

Figure 36.3. Localization of umbilical artery catheters. The cross-hatched areas represent sites in which complications are least likely. Either site may be used for placement of the catheter tip.

   b. **The cord stump is suspended with forceps.** It and the surrounding area
      are washed carefully with an antiseptic solution. In infants the preferred
      choice of agent is not clear. It is important to avoid chemical burns caused
      by iodine solution by carefully cleaning the skin (including the back and
      trunk) with sterile water after the solution has dried. Following this, the
      abdomen is draped with sterile towels.
   c. **Umbilical (twill) tape** should be placed as a simple tie around the base of
      the cord itself. In unusual circumstances it is necessary to place the tape on
      the skin itself. If this is done, care must be taken to loosen the tie after the
      procedure. The tape is used to gently constrict the cord to prevent bleeding.
      The cord is then cut cleanly with a scalpel to a length of 1.0 to 1.5 cm.
   d. **The cord is stabilized** with a forceps or hemostat, and the two arteries are
      identified.
   e. The open tip of an iris forceps is inserted into the artery lumen and gently
      used to **dilate the vessel;** and then the closed tip is inserted into the lumen
      of an artery to a depth of 0.5 cm. Tension on the forceps tip is released, and
      the forceps is left in place to dilate the vessel for approximately 1 minute.
      This pause may be the most useful step in insertion of the catheter.
   f. **The forceps is withdrawn,** and a sterile saline-filled 3.5F or 5F umbil-
      ical vessel catheter with an end hole is threaded into the artery. The
      smaller catheter is generally used for infants weighing <1,500 g. A slightly
      increased resistance will be felt as the catheter passes through the base of

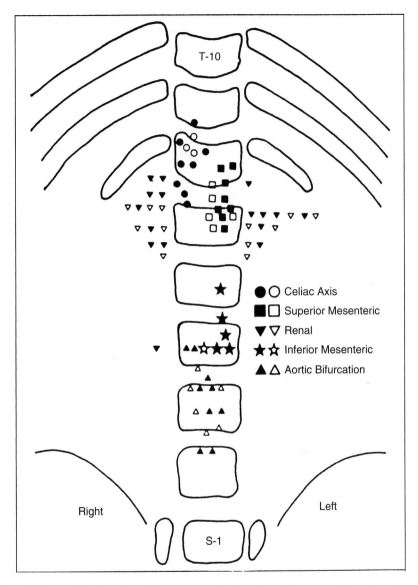

Figure 36.4. Distribution of the major aortic branches found in 15 infants by aortography as correlated with the vertebral bodies. Filled symbols represent infants with cardiac or renal anomalies (or both); open symbols represent those without either disorder. Major landmarks appear at the following vertebral levels: diaphragm, T12 interspace; celiac artery, T12; superior mesenteric artery, L1 interspace; renal artery, L1; inferior mesenteric artery, L3; aortic bifurcation, L4. (From Phelps DL, Lachman RS, Leake RD et al. The radiologic localization of the major aorta tributaries in the newborn. *J Pediatr* 1972;81:336.)

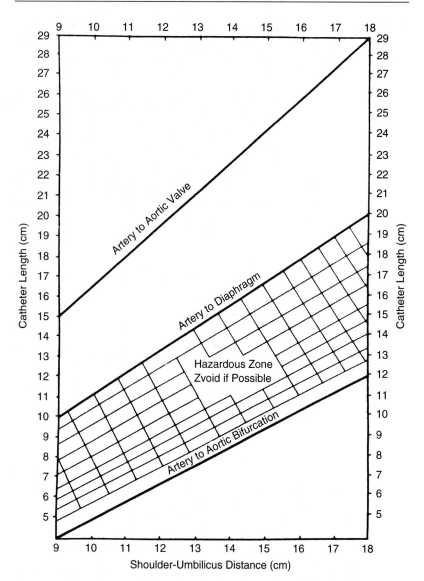

Figure 36.5. Distance from shoulder to umbilicus measured from above the lateral end of the clavicle to the umbilicus, as compared with the length of umbilical artery catheter needed to reach the designated level. (From Dunn PM. Localization of the umbilical catheter by postmortem measurement. *Arch Dis Child* 1969;41:69.)

the cord and as it navigates the umbilical artery–femoral artery junction. In approximately 5% to 10% of attempted umbilical artery catheterizations, one of the following problems may occur.

   i. The catheter will not pass into the abdominal aorta. Sometimes a double-catheter technique will allow successful cannulation in this situation.

   ii. The catheter may pass into the aorta but then loop caudad back down the contralateral iliac artery or out one of the arteries to the buttocks. There may be difficulty advancing the catheter and cyanosis or blanching of the leg or buttocks may occur. This happens more frequently when a small catheter (3.5 Fr) is placed in a large baby. Sometimes using a larger, stiffer catheter (5 Fr) will allow the catheter to advance up the aorta. Alternatively, retracting the catheter into the umbilical artery, rotating it, and readvancing it into the aorta will result in aortic placement. If this fails, the catheter should be removed and placement attempted through the other umbilical artery. Sometimes the catheter goes up the aorta and then loops back on itself. This also happens more frequently in a large baby when a small catheter is used. The catheter may also enter any of the vessels coming off the aorta. If the catheter cannot be advanced to the desired position, the tip should be pulled to a low position or the catheter removed.

   iii. There is persistent cyanosis, blanching, or poor distal extremity perfusion. This may be improved by warming the contralateral leg, but if there is no improvement the catheter should be removed. Hematuria is an indication for catheter removal.

   g. When the catheter is advanced the appropriate distance, placement should be confirmed by x-ray examination.

   h. The catheter should be fixed in place with a purse-string suture using silk thread, and a tape bridge added for further stability (see Chap. 34).

3. Catheter removal

   a. The umbilical artery catheter should be removed when either of the following criteria are met.

   i. The infant improves so that continuous monitoring and frequent blood drawings are no longer necessary.

   ii. A maximum dwell time of 7 days is recommended to reduce infectious and thrombotic complications.

   iii. Complications are noted.

   b. Method of catheter removal. The catheter is removed slowly over a period of 30 to 60 seconds, allowing the umbilical artery to constrict at its proximal end while the catheter is still occluding the distal end. This usually prevents profuse bleeding. Old sutures should be removed.

4. Complications associated with umbilical artery catheterization. Significant morbidity can be associated with complications of umbilical artery catheterization. These complications are mainly due to vascular accidents, including thromboembolic phenomena to the kidney, bowel, legs, or rarely the spinal cord. These may manifest as hematuria, hypertension, signs of necrotizing enterocolitis or bowel infarction, and cyanosis or blanching of the skin of the back, buttocks, or legs. Other complications seen are infection, disseminated intravascular coagulation, and vessel perforation. All these complications are indications for catheter removal. Close observation of the skin, monitoring of the urine for hematuria, measuring blood pressure, and following the platelet count may give clues to complications.

   a. We perform doppler ultrasonographic examination of the aorta and renal vessels in infants in whom we are concerned about complications. If thrombi are observed, the catheter is removed.

   b. If there are small thrombi without symptoms or with increased blood pressure alone, we usually remove the catheter, follow resolution of the thrombi by ultrasonographic examination, and treat hypertension if necessary (see

Chap. 31). If there are signs of emboli or loss of pulses, or coagulopathy, and no intracranial hemorrhage is present, we consider heparinization, maintaining the partial thromboplastin time (PTT) at double the control value. Published data to guide practice are limited. If there is a large clot with impairment of perfusion, we consider the use of fibrinolytic agents (see Chap. 26F). Surgical treatment of thrombosis is not generally effective.

    c. Blanching of a leg following catheter placement is the most common complication noted clinically. Although this often occurs transiently, it deserves careful attention. One technique that may reverse this finding is to warm the opposite leg. If the vasospasm resolves, the catheter may be left in place. If there is no improvement, the catheter should be removed.

5. Other considerations
    a. Use of heparin for anticoagulation to prevent clotting. Whether the use of heparin in the infusate decreases the incidence of thrombotic complications is not known. We use dilute heparin 0.5 unit/mL of infusate.

    b. Positioning of the catheter tip. Little helpful information convincingly supports the choice between high and low placement of UALs. A higher complication rate has been reported in infants with the catheter tip at L3 to L4, compared with T7 to T8, owing to more episodes of blanching and cyanosis of one or both legs. No difference between the high- and low-position groups was seen in the rate of complications requiring catheter removal. Renal complications and emboli to the bowel may be more common with catheter tips placed at T7 to T8 while catheters placed low (L3–L4) are associated with complications such as cyanosis and blanching of the leg, which are easier to observe.

    c. Indwelling time. The incidence of complications associated with umbilical artery catheterization appears to be directly related to the length of time the catheter is left in place.

6. Infection and use of antibiotics. We do not use prophylactic antibiotics for placement of UALs. In infants with UALs, we use antibiotics whenever infection is suspected and after appropriate cultures have been obtained.

C. Umbilical vein catheterization (see Figs. 36.2 and 36.6).

1. Indications. We use umbilical vein catheterization for emergency vascular access and exchange transfusions; in these cases, the venous catheter is replaced by a peripheral intravenous catheter or other access as soon as possible. In critically ill and extremely premature infants, we also use an umbilical vein catheter to infuse vasopressors and as the primary route of venous access in the first several days after birth.

2. Technique
    a. The site is prepared as for umbilical artery catheterization after determining the appropriate length of catheter to be inserted (Fig. 36.6).

    b. Any clots seen are removed with a forceps, and the umbilical vein is gently dilated as with the umbilical artery in IX. C.

    c. The catheter (3.5 Fr or 5 Fr), is prepared by filling the lumen with heparinized saline solution, 1 unit/mL of saline solution through an attached syringe. The catheter should never be left open to the atmosphere because negative intrathoracic pressure could cause an air embolism.

    d. The catheter is inserted while gentle traction is exerted on the cord. Once the catheter is in the vein, one should try to slide the catheter cephalad just under the skin, where the vein runs very superficially. If the catheter is being placed for an exchange transfusion, it should be advanced only as far as is necessary to establish good blood flow (usually 2–5 cm). If the catheter is being used for continuous infusion or to monitor central venous pressure, it should be advanced through the ductus venosus into the inferior vena cava and its position verified by x-ray.

    e. Only isotonic solutions should be infused until the position of the catheter is verified by x-ray studies. If the catheter tip is in the inferior vena cava, hypertonic solutions may be infused.

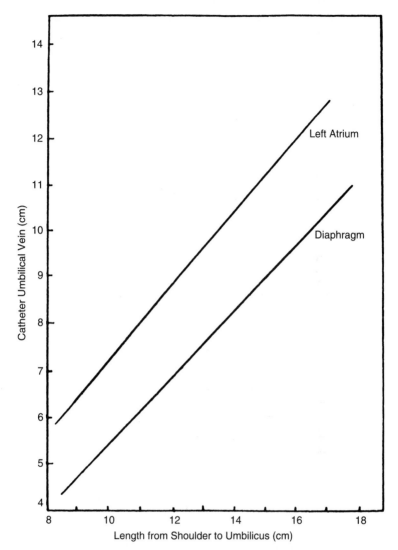

Figure 36.6. Catheter length for umbilical vein catheterization. The catheter tip should be placed between the diaphragm and the left atrium. (From Dunn PM. Localization of the umbilical catheter by postmortem measurements. *Arch Dis Child* 1966;41:69.)

  f. If no other access is available catheters may be left in place for up to 14 days, after which the increased risk of infectious or other complications increases. In very low birth weight infants, our practice is to change access to a peripherally placed central venous catheter by 7 to 8 days if possible.

D. Multiple-lumen catheters for umbilical venous catheterization

 1. Indications. Placement of a double- or triple-lumen catheter into the umbilical vein provides additional venous access for administration of incompatible solutions (e.g., those containing vasopressor agents, sodium bicarbonate, or calcium). The use of a multiple-lumen catheter significantly reduces the need for multiple peripheral intravenous catheters and skin punctures, and is preferred in very low birth weight infants.

2. Technique

   a. Direct placement. Multiple-lumen catheters can be placed directly following the outline provided for single-lumen catheters. The increased pliability of many of the multiple-lumen catheters makes passage into the hepatic veins more likely.

   b. Modified Seldinger technique. In patients with an indwelling single-lumen catheter, a wire exchange technique may be used to change to a multiple-lumen catheter. Although this method decreases the probability of catheter loss during exchange, it entails the risks of wire passage including cardiac dysrhythmias and perforation, and should be attempted only by those familiar with the Seldinger technique.

3. Usage. Where possible, infusions that should not be interrupted (e.g., vasopressors) are placed in the proximal lumen to allow measurement of central venous pressure from the distal port.

E. Percutaneous radial artery catheterization. Placement of an indwelling radial artery catheter is a useful alternative to umbilical artery catheterization for monitoring blood gas levels and blood pressure.

1. Advantages

   a. Accessibility (when the umbilical artery is inaccessible or has been used for a long period).

   b. Reflection of preductal flow (if the right radial artery is used).

   c. Avoidance of thrombosis of major vessels, which is sometimes associated with umbilical vessel catheterization.

2. Risks are usually small if the procedure is performed carefully, but infection, air embolus, inadvertent injection of incorrect solution, and arterial occlusion may occur.

3. Equipment required includes a 22- or 24-gauge intravenous cannula with stylet, a T-connector, heparinized saline flushing solution (0.5–1.0 unit of heparin per milliliter of solution), and an infusion pump.

4. Method of catheterization

   a. The adequacy of the ulnar collateral flow to the hand must be assessed. The radial and ulnar arteries should be simultaneously compressed, and the ulnar artery should then be released. The degree of flushing of the blanched hand should be noted. If the entire hand becomes flushed while the radial artery is occluded, the ulnar circulation is adequate.

   b. The hand may be secured on an arm board with the wrist extended, leaving all fingertips exposed, to observe color changes.

   c. The wrist is prepared with an iodine-containing solution, and the site of maximum arterial pulsation is palpated.

   d. The intravenous cannula is inserted through the skin at an angle <30 degrees to horizontal and is slowly advanced into the artery. Transillumination may help delineate the vessel and its course. If the artery is entered as the catheter is advanced, the stylet is removed and the catheter is advanced in the artery. If there is no blood return, the artery may be transfixed. The stylet is then removed, and the catheter is slowly withdrawn until blood flow occurs; then it is advanced into the vessel.

5. Caution. Only heparinized saline solution (0.45%–0.9%) is infused into the catheter. The minimum infusion rate is 0.8 mL/h; the maximum is 2 mL/h.

F. Percutaneous central venous catheterization is useful for long-term venous access for intravenous fluids, particularly parenteral nutrition.

1. Peripheral or **external jugular vein catheterization** is useful in infants weighing <1,500 g. This is the primary method of central venous access.

   a. The equipment required includes a 1.1 Fr or 1.9 Fr silicone or double-lumen polyurethane catheter cut to the appropriate length, a splittable introducer needle, and iris forceps.

b. **Technique.** The infant is sedated and placed supine. An appropriate vein of entry is selected. This may be a basilic, greater saphenous, or external jugular vein. The cephalic vein should be avoided, as central placement is more difficult. The site is prepared with an antiseptic solution, and the introducer needle is inserted into the vein until blood flows freely. The silicone catheter is inserted through the needle with forceps and is slowly advanced the predetermined distance for central venous positioning. The introducer needle is removed, the extra catheter length is coiled on the skin near the insertion site, and the site is covered with transparent surgical covering. The catheter tip is positioned at the junction of the vena cava and right atrium, as confirmed by radiography. Some physicians inject a small amount of isotonic contrast material to make visualization easier.

c. **Complications** include hemorrhage during insertion, infection, and thrombosis of the catheter, but these are unusual. Some babies will develop a thrombophlebitis, usually within 24 hours of catheter placement. Care must be taken when flushing or infusing to minimize the pressure on the catheter, which could cause rupture. By using a larger syringe (10 mL) infusion pressure is reduced over that obtained with a smaller (3 mL) syringe.

2. **Subclavian vein catheterization** may be useful in infants weighing >1,200 g.

a. The equipment required includes a 3 Fr catheter with introducer needle and guidewire. Double-lumen 4 Fr catheters may be used in larger infants (>2.5 kg).

b. **Technique.** The infant is sedated and placed supine with a roll between the scapulae. Generally, the patient should be ventilated and muscle relaxed to afford maximum chance of success. The head is turned away from the side of insertion. The shoulders should drop posteriorly. The skin is prepared with an iodine-containing solution and infiltrated with local anesthetic. The introducer needle is inserted through the skin and immediately beneath the clavicle, a third of the way from the shoulder to the midline. The needle should be almost parallel to the chest wall and aimed at the sternal notch. When blood flow is established, the guidewire is passed and the catheter is placed over the wire. Catheter position is determined radiographically. The catheter tip should lie at the junction of the superior vena cava and right atrium.

c. **Complications** include pneumothorax, hemothorax, and inadvertent subclavian artery puncture. The potential severity of these complications dictates that only those thoroughly familiar with this technique should attempt this form of venous cannulation.

X. ABDOMINAL PARACENTESIS FOR REMOVAL OF ASCITIC FLUID

A. Indications

1. Therapeutic indications include respiratory distress resulting from abdominal distension (e.g., hydropic infants, infants with urinary ascites) for which removal of ascitic fluid will ameliorate respiratory symptoms. In addition, interference with urine production or lower extremity perfusion resulting from increased intra-abdominal pressure may be improved by paracentesis.

2. Diagnostic indications include the evaluation of suspected peritonitis.

B. Technique

1. The equipment needed includes an 18- to 22-gauge intravenous catheter, three-way stopcock, and a 10- to 50-mL syringe.

2. The lower abdomen is prepared with povidone-iodine solution and the area is draped. If the bladder is distended, it is drained with manual pressure or a urinary catheter. A local anesthetic such as 1% lidocaine (Xylocaine) is infiltrated into the subcutaneous tissues when possible. The catheter is inserted just lateral to the rectus sheath one-third of the distance between the umbilicus and the symphysis pubis. Alternatively the catheter can be inserted in the midline, during aspiration with the syringe. The catheter is advanced approximately 1 cm until the resistance of passing through the abdominal wall diminishes or fluid is obtained. Five to 10 mL of fluid is removed for diagnostic

paracentesis while 10 to 20 mL/kg should be removed for therapeutic effects. The catheter is removed and the site bandaged.

C. Potential complications

   1. Cardiovascular effects, including tachycardia, hypotension, and decreased cardiac output, may result from rapid redistribution of intravascular fluid to the peritoneal space following removal of large amounts of ascites.

   2. Bladder or intestinal aspiration may occur more frequently in the presence of a dilated bladder or bowel. These puncture sites usually heal spontaneously and without significant clinical findings.

Suggested Readings

Fletcher MA, McDonald MG, Avery GB, eds. *Atlas of procedures in neonatology*. Philadelphia: JB Lippincott Co, 1994.

Garges HP, Moody MA, Cotton CM, et al. Neonatal meningitis: What is the correlation among cerebrospinal fluid cultures, blood cultures, and cerebrospinal fluid parameters? *Pediatrics* 2006;117:1094–1100.

Garland JS, Henrickson K, Maki DG. The 2002 hospital infection control practices advisory committee centers for disease control and prevention guideline for prevention of intravascular device-related infection. *Pediatrics* 2002;110:1009–1013.

Green R, Hauser R, Calafat AM, et al. Use of di(2-ethylhexyl) phthalate-containing medical products and urinary levels of mono(2-ethylhexyl) phthalate in neonatal intensive care unit infants. *Environ Health Perspect* 2005;113(9):1222–1225.

Latini G. Potential hazards of exposure to Di-(2-Ethylhexyl)-phthalate in babies. *Biol Neonate* 2000;78:269–276.

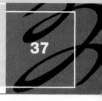

PREVENTING AND TREATING PAIN AND STRESS AMONG INFANTS IN THE NEWBORN INTENSIVE CARE UNIT

37

Linda J. Van Marter and Corinne Cyr Pryor

I. **BACKGROUND.** Recognition that both premature and full term infants experience pain has led to increasing appreciation of the prevalent problem of under-treatment of stress and pain of infants hospitalized in the newborn intensive care unit. Both humanitarian considerations and scientific principles favor improved management strategies to prevent pain and stress whenever possible and, when discomfort is unavoidable, to provide prompt and appropriate treatment.

A. **Fetal and neonatal physiologic responses to pain.** Because sensory nerve terminals exist on all body surfaces by 22–29 weeks of gestation, the fetus is capable of sensing painful stimuli. Early in development, overlapping nerve terminals create local hyperexcitable networks, enabling even low-threshold stimuli to produce an exaggerated pain response. Fetal wounds heal more quickly and with less scarring than those of infants, children or adults. The process, in part, involves sprouting of sensory nerve endings in and near the wound. Although it seems to enhance wound healing, hyperinnervation results in hypersensitivity to painful stimuli that persists after wound healing has occurred. Repeated noxious stimuli further alter sensitivity to painful stimuli appear to lower the pain threshold, slow recovery, and adversely affect long-term outcomes.

Physiologic responses to painful or stressful stimuli include increases in circulating catecholamines, increased heart rate and blood pressure, and elevated intracranial pressure. The fetus is capable of mounting a stress response beginning at approximately 23 weeks of gestation. The autonomic and other markers of the stress response of the immature fetus or preterm infant, however, are less competent than that of the more mature infant or child. Therefore, among immature infants, neither the common vital sign changes associated with pain or stress (e.g, tachycardia, hypertension) nor behaviorial cues (e.g., agitation) are reliable indicators of painful stimuli. Even when the infant's stress response is intact, persistence of painful stimuli for hours or days fatigues or deactivates the sympathetic nervous system response, obscuring signs of pain or discomfort.

B. **Medical and developmental outcomes**

1. **Neonatal medical and surgical outcomes.** Neonatal responses to pain contribute to compromised physiologic states such as hypoxia, hypercarbia, acidosis, hyperglycemia, respiratory dyssynchrony and pneumothorax. Early studies of surgical responses showed more stable intraoperative course and improved postoperative recovery among infants who received perioperative analgesia and anesthesia. Changes in intrathoracic pressure due to diaphragmatic splinting and vagal responses produced in response to pain following invasive procedures precipitate hypoxemic events and alterations in oxygen delivery and cerebral blood flow.

2. **Neurodevelopmental outcomes.** Behavioral and neurologic studies suggest that preterm infants who experience repeated painful procedures and noxious stimuli are less responsive to painful stimuli at 18 months corrected age. However, at 8 to 10 years of age, unlike their normal birth weight peers, infants born at or below 1,000 grams birth weight rate medical pain intensity greater than measures of psychosocial pain. These data provide evidence that neonatal pain and stress influence neurodevelopment and affect later perceptions of painful stimuli and behavioral responses and that prevention and control of pain are likely to benefit infants. There are few large randomized clinical trials of pain management. One such trial (i.e., NEOPAIN Trial) evaluated preemptive

665

analgesia with morphine infusion up to 14 days among ventilated preterm infants and showed no difference overall in the primary composite outcome (i.e., neonatal death, severe intraventricular hemorrhage [IVH], or periventricular leukomalacia [PVL]) between placebo and preemptive morphine treated groups. Post hoc analyses however revealed an increased risk of severe IVH among morphine infusion treated babies in the subgroup born at 27–29 weeks of gestation. Further, the addition of open-label morphine was found to be associated with increased risk of severe IVH among the morphine infusion treated infants as well as with increased risk of all three morbidities (i.e., severe IVH, PVL and neonatal death) among the placebo group. Subsequent analyses suggested the adverse outcomes were limited to infants who were hypotensive before morphine therapy was initiated. These data suggest that treatment with morphine infusion might best be limited to infants who are normotensive.

II. PRINCIPLES OF PREVENTION AND MANAGEMENT OF NEONATAL PAIN AND STRESS

A. Principles of pain management. The initial management guideline of the Committee on the Fetus and Newborn of the American Academy of Pediatrics (AAP) offered a number of principles relevant to newborn pain and stress. These include the following:

- Neuroanatomic components and neuroendocrine systems of the neonate are sufficiently developed to allow transmission of painful stimuli.
- Exposure to prolonged or severe pain may increase neonatal morbidity.
- Infants who have experienced pain during the neonatal period respond differently to subsequent painful events.
- Severity of pain and effects of analgesia can be assessed in the neonate using validated instruments.
- Newborn infants usually are not easily comforted when analgesia is needed.
- A lack of behavioral responses (including crying and movement) does not necessarily indicate the absence of pain.

B. Current AAP recommendations. In 2006, the Committee on the Fetus and Newborn of the AAP provided the following expanded guidelines for assessment and management of pain and stress in the newborn.

1. Assessment of pain and stress in the newborn

a. Caregivers should be trained to assess neonates for pain using multidimensional tools.

b. Neonates should be assessed for pain routinely and before and after procedures.

c. The chosen pain scales should help guide caregivers in the provision of effective pain relief.

2. Reducing pain from bedside care procedures

a. Care protocols for neonates should incorporate a principle of minimizing the number of painful disruptions in care as much as possible.

b. Use of a combination of oral sucrose/glucose and other nonpharmacologic pain-reduction methods (nonnutritive sucking, kangaroo care, facilitated tuck, swaddling, developmental care) should be used for minor routine procedures.

c. Topical anesthetics can be used to reduce pain associated with venipuncture, lumbar puncture, and intravenous catheter insertion when time permits but are ineffective for heel-stick blood draws and repeated use of topical anesthetics should be limited.

d. The routine use of continuous infusion of morphine, fentanyl, or midazolam in chronically ventilated preterm neonates is not recommended because of concern about short-term adverse effects and lack of long-term outcome data.

3. Reducing pain from surgery

a. Any health care facility providing surgery for neonates should have an established protocol for pain management. Such a protocol requires a coordinated, multidimensional strategy and should be a priority in perioperative management.

   b. Sufficient anesthesia should be provided to prevent intraoperative pain and stress responses to decrease postoperative analgesic requirements.

   c. Pain should be routinely assessed using a scale designed for postoperative or prolonged pain in neonates.

   d. Opioids should be the basis for postoperative analgesia after major surgery in the absence of regional anesthesia.

   e. Postoperative analgesia should be used as long as pain-assessment scales document that it is required.

   f. Acetaminophen can be used after surgery as an adjunct to regional anesthetics or opioids, but there are inadequate data on pharmacokinetics at gestational ages <28 weeks to permit calculation of appropriate dosages.

4. Reducing pain from other major procedures

   a. Analgesia for chest-drain insertion comprises all of the following:

   i. general nonpharmacologic measures;

   ii. slow infiltration of the skin site with a local anesthetic before incision unless there is a life-threatening instability; and

   iii. systemic analgesia with a rapidly acting opiate such as fentanyl

   b. Analgesia for chest drain removal comprises the following

   i. general nonpharmacologic measures and

   ii. short-acting, rapid onset systemic analgesia

   c. Although there are insufficient data to make a specific recommendation, retinal examinations are painful and pain-relief measures should be used. A reasonable approach would be to administer local anesthetic eye drops and oral sucrose

   d. Retinal surgery should be considered major surgery, and effective opiate-based pain relief should be provided.

III. EVALUATING NEONATAL PAIN AND STRESS. There are a number of validated and reliable scales of pain assessment. Behavioral indicators (e.g., facial expression, crying, body/extremity movement) as well as physiologic indicators (e.g., tachycardia or bradycardia, hypertension, tachypnea or apnea, oxygen desaturation, palmar sweating, vagal signs, plasma cortisol or catecholamine levels) often are useful in assessing the infant's level of comfort or discomfort.

   Physiologic responses to painful stimuli include release of circulating catecholamines, heart rate acceleration, blood pressure increase, and a rise in intracranial pressure. Because the stress response of the immature fetus or preterm infant is less competent than that of the more mature infant or child, gestational age must be considered in evaluating the pain response. Among preterm infants experiencing pain, the vital signs associated with the stress response (e.g., tachycardia, hypertension) and agitation are not consistently evident. Even among infants with an intact response to pain, a painful stimulus that persists for hours or days exhausts sympathetic nervous system output and obscures the clinician's ability to objectively assess the infant's level of discomfort.

A. Recommended assessment tools.

   Selecting the most appropriate tool for evaluation of neonatal pain assessment must take into consideration the infant's gestational age and other clinical factors, such as severity of illness. A number of useful tools exist; we recommend three.

   1. Intensive care infants. Pain assessment must consider the influence of gestational age on the pain response. The **premature infant pain profile (PIPP)**, a method that includes assessment of facial expression as well as physiologic measures in the context of gestational age and neonatal state, is the only method that has been validated for assessment of pain among preterm infants.

   2. Intermediate care or well nursery infants. For full-term or growing former preterm infants, there are a number of pain assessment scales. We recommend the **behavioral pain score (BPS)**, a method that assesses motor activity, cry, consolability and sleep. An alternative is the **neonatal infant pain scale (NIPS)**, a research tool that has been used to assess pre- and post-intervention pain.

IV. MANAGEMENT: PAIN PREVENTION AND TREATMENT

A. Environmental and behavioral approaches. Painful or stressful procedures should be minimized and coordinated with other necessary aspects of the newborn's care.

1. During the procedure, the following environmental and developmentally-supportive measures might prove useful to reduce infant pain and stress:

- Clustering painful interventions before a comforting event (e.g., feeding)
- Swaddling during the procedure
- Nonnutritive sucking; pacifier
- Use of mechanical lancets for heel-stick blood draws

2. Following the procedure, other measures are helpful:

- Reducing noise and light
- Touch or massage
- Parent-infant skin-to-skin contact or Kangaroo care
- Holding the baby following the procedure
- Positional "nesting" or containment using blanket rolls

B. Physiologic interventions. There are two primary approaches to physiologic pain management. These are sucrose analgesia and competitive stimulation.

1. Sucrose analgesia (0.12–0.36 grams) (0.5–1.5 mL of 24% sucrose solution) given orally approximately 2 minutes before the painful procedure

2. Competitive stimulation (e.g., gently rubbing, tapping, or vibrating one extremity **before** and/or **during** painful stimulus to another extremity)

C. Pharmacologic management. A number of considerations are relevant to the pharmacologic management of neonatal pain.

1. Complementary therapies: Environmental and behavioral interventions should be applied to all infants experiencing painful stimuli. These measures and sucrose analgesia often are useful in conjunction with pharmacologic treatments.

2. Prophylaxis versus pain treatment: Narcotic analgesia given prophylactically on a scheduled basis results in a lower total dose and improved pain control compared with "as needed" dosing.

3. Gestational maturity: A prophylactic approach is appropriate in the immature acutely ill infant who must be assumed to be incapable of mounting a stress response to signal his/her discomfort. The inability of the infant to mount an appropriate response is especially relevant when the infant is extremely immature or the painful stimulus is severe and/or prolonged.

4. No long-term adverse effects of the use of opioid analgesia among ventilated infants have been reported. These include long-term studies assessing intelligence, motor function, and behavior.

V. PHARMACOLOGIC TREATMENT OF PROCEDURE-RELATED PAIN (see Tables 37.1–37.4)

A. Analgesia for minimally-invasive procedures. When the infant is full-term, sucrose analgesia is recommended for once or twice-daily blood draws, at a dose of: sucrose 0.12–0.36 grams total dose (24% sucrose solution 0.5–1.5 mL) approximately 2 minutes before the procedure. Studies of sucrose analgesia are largely limited to full-term infant populations. Evidence is limited regarding the use of sucrose analgesia among premature infants and one investigator raised caution concerning the use of sucrose analgesia among infants below 31 weeks of gestation. However, some centers use smaller doses of sucrose solution to treat moderately preterm infants (30–36 weeks gestational age) who were undergoing minimally invasive procedures. Among preterm infants, we recommend lower doses: sucrose 24% solution, 0.1 to 0.5 mL (0.024–0.12 grams), with the option to repeat this dose 2 minutes before and after the procedure. Guidelines are listed in Table 37.1.

B. Analgesia for invasive procedures. Narcotics (e.g., morphine or fentanyl) and sedatives (e.g., midazolam or phenobarbital) are useful in treating critically ill newborns undergoing invasive or very painful procedures. Alleviating pain is the most important goal. Therefore, treatment with analgesics is recommended in preference to sedation without analgesia. The addition of a short-acting muscle relaxant might decrease the time and number of attempts needed for intubation and reduce the rate of severe oxygen desaturation. Guidelines are listed in Table 37.2.

TABLE 37.3 Perioperative Analgesia

Procedures	Intubated and ventilated infants	Nonintubated infants
Preoperative (i.e., intubated infants under-going general anesthesia)	Consider Fentanyl* 1–3 µg/kg IV 1 h before transfer to the operating room for the procedure	N/A
Laser surgery	2 h before the procedure: tylenol 15 mg/kg **and** During the procedure: Morphine 0.05–0.1 mg/kg Q 1–2 h **or** fentanyl* 1–3 µg/kg Q 1–2 h PRN **and,** if ≥34 wks PMA: Midazolam 0.1 mg/kg Q 1–2 h PRN	N/A
Circumcision	N/A	24% sucrose 0.5–1.5 mL/kg PO **and** tylenol 10–15 mg/kg 2 h PO/PG before and Q 6 h after the procedure (× 24 h) **and** Ring block (Lidocaine 0.5%) (max.: 0.5 mL/kg) **or** dorsal penile block (Lidocaine 0.5%) **or** if ≥34 wks PMA and >1.8 kg: topical EMLA
Herniorraphy	Acetaminophen 10–15 mg/kg PO/PG/PR Q 4–6 h fentanyl* 2–3 µg/kg Q 2–4 h PRN **or** morphine 0.05–0.1 mg/kg Q 2–4 h PRN	Acetaminophen 10–15 mg/kg PO/PG/PR Q 6 h **or** fentanyl* 0.25–0.5 µg/kg Q 4 h PRN **or** morphine 0.025–0.05 mg/kg IV or SQ Q 4 h PRN

Laparotomy	First 24 h: Fentanyl* 1–3 μg/kg Q 4–6 h **or** morphine 0.1 mg/kg Q 4–6 h Then: Morphine 0.05–0.1 Q 2–4 h PRN **or** fentanyl* 1–3 μg/kg Q 2–4 h PRN	Fentanyl* 0.25–0.5 μg/kg Q 4 h PRN **or** morphine 0.025–0.05 mg/kg IV or SQ Q 4 h PRN
Thoracotomy	First 24 h: Fentanyl* 1–3 μg/kg Q 4 h **or** morphine 0.05–0.1 mg/kg Q 4 h Then: Morphine 0.05–0.1 mg/kg Q 2–4 h PRN **or** fentanyl* 1–3 μg/kg Q 2–4 h PRN	Acetaminophen 10–15 mg/kg Q 6 h Q 6 h PRN **or** fentanyl* 0.25–0.5 μg/kg Q 4 h PRN **or** morphine 0.025–0.05 mg/kg IV or SQ Q 4 h PRN
Laser surgery	Acetaminophen 15 mg/kg PG/PR 2 h before and acetaminophen 10 mg/kg Q 6 h after procedure (× 24 h); then Q 6 h PRN	Acetaminophen 10 mg/kg Q 6 h after the procedure (× 24 h); then Q 6 h PRN
Neurosurgery (cranial)	Fentanyl* 1–3 μg/kg Q 2–4 h PRN **or** morphine 0.05–0.1 mg/kg Q 2–4 h PRN	Acetaminophen 10–15 mg/kg Q 6 h PRN **or** fentanyl* 0.25–0.5 μg/kg Q 4 h PRN **or** morphine 0.025–0.05 mg/kg IV or SQ Q 4 h PRN
Neurosurgery (lumbar)	Fentanyl* 1–3 μg/kg Q 2–4 h PRN **or** morphine 0.05–0.1 mg/kg Q 2–4 h PRN	Acetaminophen 10–15 mg/kg Q 6 h Q 4 h PRN **or** fentanyl* 0.25–0.5 μg/kg (over 2 min) **or** morphine 0.025–0.05 mg/kg IV or SQ Q 4 h PRN

*Fentanyl should be infused at ≤1 μg/kg/min (e.g., 3 μg/kg infused over ≥3 min).

TABLE 37.4 Commonly used Analgesic, Sedative and Local Anesthetic Agents

Local anesthetics	Use	Maximum dose
Buffered Lidocaine 0.5%*		5 mg/kg SQ (1.0 mL/kg of 0.5% solution, 0.5 mL/kg of 1% solution)
Topical EMLA 5% Cream†	33–37 wk postmenstrual age (PMA) and >1.8 kg	0.5 g for 1–2 h (then remove excess)
	>37 wk PMA and >2.5 kg	1.0 g for 1–2 h (then remove excess)

Analgesics	Single dose‡	Infusion§
Morphine‖	Intubated: 0.05–0.15 mg/kg IV or SQ	0.01–0.03 mg/kg/h
	Nonintubated: 0.025–0.05 mg/kg IV or SQ	Not recommended
Fentanyl¶	Intubated: 1–3 μg/kg (over 5 min) IV	0.2–0.5 μg/kg/h
	Nonintubated: 0.25–1.0 μg/kg (over 5 min) IV	Not recommended
Acetaminophen	10–15 mg/kg PO/PG/PR every 6 h PRN; maximum dose 40 mg/kg/24 h	

Sedatives	Dose
Short-term	
Midazolam**	0.05–0.1 mg/kg IV or intranasal
Chloral hydrate††	20–30 mg/kg PO or PG
Long-term	
Phenobarbital	loading dose: 5–15 mg/kg PO, PG or IV
	Maintenance dose: 3–4 mg/kg PO, PG or IV

EMLA, eutectic mixture of local anesthetic; IV, intravenous; PG, per gastric tube; PMA, postmenstrual age; PO, by mouth; PR, per rectum; PRN, as needed; SQ, subcutaneous.
*Lidocaine toxicity may cause cardiac arrhythmia or seizure.
Lidocaine 0.5% solution can be made by 1:1 dilution of 1% Lidocaine with normal saline.
† topical EMLA should be limited to a **single dose** per day and it must be removed within 2 h. It takes 40–60 min following application to achieve the maximum effect of topical EMLA. Prilocaine (in topical EMLA) may cause methemoglobinemia. Local edema associated with the use of topical EMLA might distort anatomical structures.
‡ May repeat dosing at 10–15 min intervals until initial therapeutic effect is achieved.
§ May titrate above this dosing range to achieve a therapeutic effect.
‖ Morphine may cause hypotension.
¶ Rapid infusion of fentanyl may cause chest-wall rigidity. Fentanyl in repeated doses of by infusion might be associated with tachyphylaxis.
** Midazolam is recommended for use only in full-term infants. Abnormal movements have been described in preterm infants treated with midazolam.
†† Chloral hydrate is metabolized to trichloroethanol, which competes for glucuronidation and may exacerbate hyperbilirubinemia.

adverse effects without exacerbating pain. If the baby's clinical status permits, an alternative approach is to titrate administration of naloxone, giving it in increments of 0.05 mg/kg until the side effects are reversed.

Suggested Readings

American Academy of Pediatrics Committee on Fetus and Newborn and Section on Surgery and Canadian Paediatric Society Fetus and Newborn Committee. Prevention and management of pain in the neonate: An update. *Pediatrics* 2006;118:2231–2241.

Anand KJ, Aranda JV, Berde CB, et al. Summary proceedings from the neonatal pain-control group. *Pediatrics* 2006;117:S9–S22.

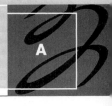
 ACETAMINOPHEN

Classification: Analgesic; antipyretic. Indication: analgesia.
Dosage/administration: 32 weeks postmenstrual age (PMA): 10 to 15 mg/kg/dose q12h PO/PR, PRN >32 weeks PMA: 10 to 15 mg/kg/dose q8h PO/PR PRN. Term: 10 to 15 mg/kg/dose q6h PO/PR PRN.
Precautions: Rectal suppositories associated with erratic release.
Contraindications: G6PD deficiency.
Monitoring: Complete blood count (CBC), liver function tests (LFTs).
Adverse reactions: Blood dyscrasias (thrombocytopenia, leukopenia, pancytopenia, and neutropenia). Adverse reactions are associated with excessive dosages.
Acute effects: Hepatic necrosis, transient azotemia, and renal tubular necrosis.
Chronic effects: Anemia, renal damage, and gastrointestinal (GI) disturbances.

 ACETAZOLAMIDE

Classification: Diuretic, carbonic anhydrase inhibitor.
Indication: To slow the progression of hydrocephalus.
Dosage/administration: 5 mg/kg/dose orally or intravenously every 6 hours. If desired may increase by 25 mg/kg/day up to a maximum of 100 mg/kg/day if tolerated. Usual concentration for infusion is 25 mg/mL up to a maximum of 100 mg/mL. Maximum infusion rate is 500 mg/minute.
Precautions: Adjust dose for renal impairment. Intramuscular administration painful because of alkaline pH. Tolerance to diuretic effect occurs with long-term administration.
Monitoring: Acid–base status, daily intake/output, weight, and weekly head circumference.
Adverse reactions: Hyperchloremic metabolic acidosis, hypokalemia, and bone marrow suppression.

 ACYCLOVIR

Classification: Antiviral agent.
Indications: Treatment of herpes simplex infections, varicella zoster infections with central nervous system (CNS) and pulmonary involvement, and herpes simplex encephalitis.
Dosage/administration: (see Table A.1)
Do not refrigerate because it can cause precipitation of the drug. Infuse by syringe pump over >1 hour.
Precautions: Reduce dosage for impaired renal function.
Monitoring: Renal and hepatic function.
Adverse reactions: Nephrotoxicity, bone marrow suppression, fever, thrombocytosis, and transitory increase of serum creatinine and liver enzymes. Rare encephalopathy associated with rapid intravenous administration (lethargy, obtundation, agitation, tremor, seizure, and coma).

TABLE A.1

Indication	Dosage
Localized HSV infection	20 mg/kg/dose IV q8h for 14 d
	Infusion concentration must be <7 mg/mL, usual infusion concentration = 5 mg/mL
Disseminated or CNS infections	20 mg/kg/dose IV q8h for 21 d
Varicella	20 mg/kg/dose PO q6h for 5 d
	Initiate therapy within the first 24 h of disease onset.

HSV = herpes simplex virus; IV = intravenous; CNS = central nervous system; q8h = every 8 hours; q6h = every 6 hours; PO = orally.

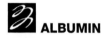

ALBUMIN

Classification: Plasma volume expander.
Indications: Hypovolemia, hypoproteinemia.
Dosage/administration: (see Table A.2)

TABLE A.2

Indication	IV Dosage	Administration
Hypovolemia	0.5–1 g/kg/dose	Infuse **5% albumin** over >60 min, may be infused more rapidly (10–20 min) in hypovolemic shock, repeat PRN
Hypoproteinemia	0.5–1 g/kg/dose	Infuse **5% albumin** over >2 h, repeat q1–2 d. Dilutions may be made with NS or D5W in cases of sodium restriction

IV = intravenous; PRN = as needed; NS = normal saline.

Precautions: There is no clinical advantage to using albumin as a volume expander compared to using NS. Maximum dose: 6 g/kg/day. Infuse using a 5-micron filter or larger. Use within 4 hours after opening vial. If >6 g/24 hours is required, consider blood products for treatment of hypovolemia. Albumin is contraindicated in patients with severe anemia or congestive heart failure (CHF). **Albumin 25% is contraindicated in preterm neonates due to increased risk of intraventricular hemorrhage (IVH).**
Monitoring: Observe for signs of hypervolemia, pulmonary edema, and cardiac failure.
Adverse reactions: Chills, fever, and urticaria. Rapid infusion (>1 g/minute) may precipitate CHF and pulmonary edema due to fluid overload.

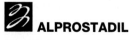

ALPROSTADIL

Classification: Prostaglandin.
Indications: Temporary maintenance of patent ductus arteriosis (PDA), in neonates with ductal-dependent congenital heart disease.

Dosage/administration:
Initial: 0.01 µg/kg/minute.
Maintenance: 0.01 to 0.4 µg/kg/minute; titrate to effective dosage with therapeutic response. Alprostadil is usually given at an infusion rate of 0.05 µg/kg/minute as a continuous intravenous infusion on a syringe pump (central venous access preferred). Dilute with dextrose or normal saline (NS). Recommended concentration is 10 µg/mL.
Precautions: Use cautiously in neonates with bleeding tendencies. If hypotension or pyrexia occurs, reduce infusion until symptoms subside. Severe hypotension, apnea, or bradycardia require drug discontinuation with cautious reinstitution at a lower dose. Apnea occurs in approximately 10% of neonates with congenital heart defects (especially in those weighing <2 kg at birth) and usually appears during the first hour of drug infusion. **Be prepared to intubate and resuscitate.**
Contraindications: Respiratory distress syndrome (RDS), persistent pulmonary hypertension, coagulation abnormalities.
Adverse reactions: Apnea, respiratory depression, flushing, bradycardia, fever, seizure-like activity, systemic hypotension, hypocalcemia, hypoglycemia, and cortical proliferation of long bones has been seen with long-term infusions; diarrhea, gastric-outlet obstruction secondary to antral hyperplasia (occurrence related to duration of therapy and cumulative dose), inhibition of platelet aggregation.

 AMINOPHYLLINE

Classification: Respiratory stimulant, bronchodilator.
Dosage/administration:
Loading dose: 5 to 6 mg/kg IV or PO. IV loading dose should be given >20 minutes on a syringe pump.
Maintenance dose: 2 mg/kg/dose q6 to 8h IV or PO. **Increase dose by 20% when changing from IV to PO route.** Maintenance IV doses are given >5 minutes on a syringe pump.
Precautions: Intramuscular administration causes intense local pain and sloughing.
Monitoring: Heart rate, blood glucose periodically during loading-dose therapy, agitation, feeding intolerance. Withhold dose for heart rate >180 beats/minute. Monitor serum trough levels before the fifth dose. Consider checking earlier if toxicity is suspected or spells increase in number or severity. If level is low, give a partial bolus of 1 mg/kg for each desired 2 µg/mL in serum theophylline concentration.
Therapeutic ranges: Apnea of prematurity: 7 to 10 µg/mL; bronchospasm: 10 to 20 µg/mL.
Adverse reactions: Gastrointestinal upset, arrhythmias, seizures, tachycardia (heart rate >180 beats/minute) warrants determination of serum levels to detect excessive aminophylline levels.

 AMPHOTERICIN-B LIPOSOME (AMBISOME)

Classification: Systemic antifungal agent.
Indication: Treatment of suspected or proven systemic fungal infections.
Dosage/administration: 5 mg/kg IV q24h infused over >2 hours. Maximum concentration for infusion is 2 mg/mL. Average duration of therapy is 2 to 4 weeks.
Precautions: Concurrent use with other nephrotoxic medications may lead to additive nephrotoxicity. Corticosteroids may increase the potassium depletion caused by amphotericin. May intensify toxicity to neuromuscular blocking agents (e.g., pancuronium) secondary to hypokalemia. Use with caution in patients with electrolyte instabilities. **Do not confuse with conventional amphotericin-B or other lipid–based forms of amphotericin.**
Contraindications: Do not dilute with NS or mix with any other medication that is diluted in NS. Do not mix with any other medication or electrolytes to avoid precipitation.
Adverse reactions: Hypokalemia, nephrotoxicity, LFT abnormalities, thrombocytopenia, and tachycardia.

Monitoring: Blood urea nitrogen (BUN), serum creatinine, LFTs, serum electrolytes, CBC, vitals, inputs and outputs, monitor electrocardiogram (EKG) changes for signs of hypokalemia.

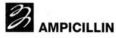 AMPICILLIN

Classification: Semisynthetic penicillinase-sensitive penicillin.
Indications: Combined with either an aminoglycoside or cephalosporin for the prevention and treatment of infections with group B *streptococci* and *Listeria monocytogenes*.
Dosage/administration: (see Table A.3)

TABLE A.3

Age	Weight	Dosing
<7 d		150 mg/kg/dose q12h
>7 d	<1,200 g	100 mg/kg/dose q12h
>7 d	1,200–2,000 g	50 mg/kg/dose q8h
>7 d	>2,000 g	50 mg/kg/dose q6h

q12h = every 12 hours; q8h = every 8 hours; q6h = every 6 hours;

Infused over >15 minutes on syringe pump. Maximum final concentration for administration is 100 mg/mL in NS. Intramuscular administration associated with sterile abscess formation.
Precautions: Dosage adjustment for renal impairment.
Drug interactions: Blunting of peak aminoglycoside concentration if administered simultaneously with ampicillin. Administer after aminoglycoside level is drawn.
Adverse reactions: Diarrhea, hypersensitivity reaction (rubella-like rash and fever), nephritis (typically preceded by eosinophilia), elevated transaminases, and penicillin encephalopathy (CNS excitation and seizure activity associated with large or rapidly administered doses).

 ATROPINE SULFATE

Classification: Anticholinergic agent.
Indications: Prolonged cardiopulmonary resuscitation unresponsive to epinephrine.
Dosage/administration: Intravenous: 0.01 to 0.03 mg/kg/dose, every 10 to 15 minutes, for two to three doses as needed. Endotracheal tube: 0.01 to 0.03 mg/kg/dose. Administer undiluted form for intravenous and endotracheal tube administration.
Clinical considerations: Effective oxygenation and ventilation must precede atropine treatment of bradycardia. Low doses (<0.1 mg) may cause paradoxical bradycardia secondary to central action. Monitor heart rate.
Contraindications: Tachycardia, narrow-angle glaucoma, thyrotoxicosis, GI or genitourinary obstruction.
Precautions: Spastic paralysis or CNS damage.
Adverse reactions: Tachycardia, mydriasis, cycloplegia, abdominal distention/ileus, urinary retention, arrhythmias, esophageal reflux.
Antidote: Physostigmine.

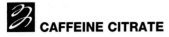 **CAFFEINE CITRATE**

Classification: Respiratory stimulant.
Indications: Apnea of prematurity. Caffeine given to infants <1,250 g in the first 10 days of life may decrease the risk of developing bronchopulmonary dysplasia (BPD).
Dosage/administration:
Loading dose: 20 mg/kg intravenously. Infuse over >30 minutes on syringe pump.
Maintenance dose: 5 to 12 mg/kg intravenously or orally daily, starting 24 hours after loading dose. May increase maintenance dose by 1 mg/kg/day every 72 hours up to a maximum of 12 mg/kg/day. Minibolus = 5 mg/kg/dose. Infuse intravenous maintenance dose over >10 minutes on a syringe pump. A small loading dose of caffeine citrate (10 mg/kg) is required when switching from aminophylline/theophylline to caffeine citrate due to approximately 1 week for caffeine citrate to reach steady-state levels because of its long half-life. **Do not push intravenous doses of caffeine citrate.**
Precautions: Do not use caffeine-base formulations because of different dosage requirements. Do not use caffeine preparations that contain sodium benzoate.
Adverse reactions: Cardiac arrhythmias, tachycardia (withhold dose for heart rate >180), insomnia, restlessness, irritability, nausea, vomiting, diarrhea. Consider a decrease in dose to treat the CNS or/and GI side effects.
Monitoring parameters: Monitor heart rate, number and severity of apnea spells.

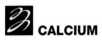 **CALCIUM**

Classification: Electrolyte supplement; calcium salt.
Indication: Treatment and prevention of hypocalcemia.
Dosage/administration: Calcium glubionate(PO)—1,200 mg/kg/day, PO divided q3–4 h. Maximum 9 g/day. Elemental calcium (using 10% calcium gluconate IV): 10 to 20 mg/kg/dose (1–2 mL/kg/dose) 100 to 200 mg/kg/dose (1–2 mL/kg/dose) of 10% calcium gluconate IV. Infuse over a **minimum** of 30 minutes on a syringe pump. May need to decrease infusion rate (10 minutes) for persistent bradycardia. Not for IM or subcutaneous (SC) administration, for IV administration only.
Precautions: Rapid administration is associated with bradycardia. Extravasation may cause tissue necrosis. Use hyaluronidase to treat extravasation. Bolus infusion by umbilical arterial catheter (UAC) has been associated with intestinal bleeding and lower-extremity tissue necrosis.
Contraindications: Hypercalcemia, renal calculi, ventricular fibrillation. Adverse reactions: Arrhythmias and deterioration of cardiovascular function. Extravasation may cause skin sloughing. May potentiate digoxin-related arrhythmias.
Monitoring parameters: Monitor serum calcium levels. Avoid hypercalcemia during treatment. Correct hypomagnesemia if present. Observe IV infusion site closely for extravasation. Observe IV tubing for precipitates.

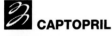 **CAPTOPRIL**

Classification: Angiotensin-converting enzyme inhibitor.
Indication: Antihypertensive agent, treatment of CHF.
Dosage/administration:
Initial dose: Premature newborns: 0.01 to 0.05 mg/kg/dose PO q8–12 h. Term newborns: 0.05 to 0.1 mg/kg/dose PO q8–24 h.
Maximum recommended dose: 0.5 mg/kg/dose PO q6–24 h. Titrate dose and frequency to effect. Administer on an empty stomach 1 hour before or 2 hours after feedings if possible. Food decreases absorption by approximately 50%. Administration times need to be consistent.

Precautions: Use with caution and modify dosage in patients with renal impairment.
Contraindications: Angioedema, bilateral renal artery stenosis, hyperkalemia, renal failure.
Adverse reactions: Hypotension, rash, fever, eosinophilia, neutropenia, GI disturbances, cough, dyspnea, acute renal failure, hyperkalemia. Development of jaundice or elevated hepatic enzymes is reason for immediate drug withdrawal.
Monitoring parameters: Monitor blood pressure (BP) for hypotension within 1 hour after first dose or after a new higher dose, BUN, serum creatinine, renal function, urine dipstick for protein, CBC with differential, serum potassium.

 CEFOTAXIME SODIUM

Classification: Third-generation cephalosporin.
Indications: Reserved for suspected or documented gram-negative meningitis or sepsis. Combine with ampicillin or aqueous penicillin G for empiric therapy.
Dosage/administration: (see Table A.4)

 TABLE A.4

Age	Weight	Dosage (IV/IM)
All neonates	<1,200 g	50 mg/kg/dose IV/IM q12h
Postnatal age <7 d	1,200–2,000 g	50 mg/kg/dose IV/IM q12h
Postnatal age <7 d	>2,000 g	50 mg/kg/dose IV/IM q8h
Postnatal age >7 d	1,200–2,000 g	50 mg/kg/dose IV/IM q8h
Postnatal age >7 d	>2,000 g	50 mg/kg/dose IV/IM q6h

IM = intramuscularly; IV = intravenously; q6h = every 6 hours; q8h = every 8 hours; q12h = every 12 hours.

Maximum concentration for infusion is 100 mg/mL in dextrose 5% water (D5W), dextrose 10% water (D10W), or NS. Infuse over >30 minutes on syringe pump. Maximum concentration for intramuscular dose is 300 mg/mL.
Precautions: Dosage modification for impaired renal function.
Monitoring: CBC, BUN, creatinine, LFTs.
Drug interactions: Blunting of peak aminoglycoside concentration if administered over <2 hours before/after cefotaxime.
Adverse reactions: Leukopenia, granulocytopenia, pseudomembranous colitis, positive direct Coombs' test, serum–sickness-like reaction, and transient elevation of BUN, creatinine, eosinophils, and liver enzymes.
Clinical considerations: Routine or frequent use of cephalosporins in the neonatal intensive care unit will quickly result in the emergence of resistant enteric organisms.

 CEFTAZIDIME

Classification: Third-generation cephalosporin.
Indications: Broad-spectrum cephalosporin and the only antipseudomonal cephalosporin. Treatment of gram-negative meningitis.
Dosage/administration: (see Table A.5)
Final concentration for infusion is 100 mg/mL in dextrose 5% water (D5W) or NS. Infuse over >30 minutes on syringe pump.

TABLE A.5

Age	Weight	Dosage (IV/IM)
All neonates	<1,200 g	50 mg/kg/dose IV/IM q12h
Postnatal age <7 d	1,200–2,000 g	50 mg/kg/dose IV/IM q12h
Postnatal age <7 d	>2,000 g	50 mg/kg/dose IV/IM q8h
Postnatal age >7 d	>1,200 g	50 mg/kg/dose IV/IM q8h

IM = intramuscularly; IV = intravenously; q8h = every 8 hours; q12h = every 12 hours.

Clinical considerations: Treat serious pseudomonal infections with ceftazidime in combination with an aminoglycoside.
Precautions: Modify dosage for renal impairment.
Drug interaction: Blunting of peak aminoglycoside concentration if administered simultaneously with ceftazidime.
Monitoring: CBC, renal, and LFTs.
Adverse reactions: Transient leukopenia and bone marrow suppression, positive direct Coombs' test, candidiasis, hemolytic anemia, pseudomembranous colitis, and transient elevation of eosinophils, platelets, renal, and LFTs.

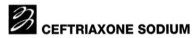

CEFTRIAXONE SODIUM

Classification: Third-generation cephalosporin.
Indications: Good activity against both gram-negative and gram-positive organisms except for *Pseudomonas spp.*, *enterococci*, methicillin-resistant *staphylococci*, and *L. monocytogenes*. Indicated for treatment of gonococcal meningitis and conjunctivitis. Not recommended for use in neonates with hyperbilirubinemia. Use cefotaxime instead.
Dosage/administration: (see Table A.6)

TABLE A.6

Age	Weight	Dosage (IV/IM)
Postnatal age <7 d	All weights	50 mg/kg/dose IV/IM q24h
Postnatal age >7 d	<2,000 g	50 mg/kg/dose IV/IM q24h
Postnatal age >7 d	>2,000 g	75 mg/kg/day IV/IM q24h

IM = intramuscularly; IV = intravenously; q24h = every 24 hours.

Gonococcal prophylaxis: 25 to 50 mg/kg IV/IM as a single dose (dose not to exceed 125 mg).
Gonococcal infection: 25 to 50 mg/kg/day (maximum dose: 125 mg) IV/IM q24h for 7 days, up to 10 to 14 days if meningitis is documented. Uncomplicated gonococcal ophthalmia = 50 mg/kg IV/IM (maximum = 125 mg) single dose.
Maximum concentration for intravenous administration is 100 mg/mL in dextrose or saline. Infused over >30 minutes on syringe pump. Reconstitute intramuscular doses with 1%

lidocaine without epinephrine to reduce pain at injection site. Maximum concentration for intramuscular administration is 350 mg/mL.

Precautions: Do not use in gallbladder, biliary tract, liver, or pancreatic disease. Consider cefotaxime or ceftazidime instead.

Clinical considerations: Do not use as sole therapy for staphylococcal or pseudomonal infections. Combine with ampicillin for initial empiric therapy of meningitis. Ceftriaxone displaces bilirubin from albumin binding sites, leading to increased free-serum bilirubin levels. In newborns with hyperbilirubinemia, use cefotaxime instead of ceftriaxone. Clinicians are advised to use aminoglycosides combined with ampicillin or penicillin for initial empiric therapy of suspected or proven neonatal sepsis.

Monitoring: CBC, electrolytes, and renal/ LFTs.

Adverse reactions: Leukopenia, anemia, GI intolerance, and rash. Transient increase in eosinophils, platelets, bleeding time, free serum bilirubin concentration, and renal/LFTs. Transient formation of gallbladder precipitates characterized by vomiting and cholelithiasis. GI tract bacterial or fungal overgrowth.

 CHLORAL HYDRATE

Classification: Sedative, hypnotic.

Indications: Sedative/hypnotic.

Dosage/administration: 25 to 50 mg/kg/dose orally (PO) or rectally (PR), every 6 to 8 hours as needed.

Maximum dose: 50 mg/kg/dose. To reduce gastric irritation, dilute in feedings or administer after feedings.

Precautions: Rectal suppositories are not recommended because of unreliable release characteristics. Use caution with concurrent administration of furosemide and anticoagulants.

Clinical considerations: No analgesic properties. Excitation may occur instead of sedation in infants with pain. Assess level of sedation. Accumulation of the toxic metabolite (trichloroethanol) and direct hyperbilirubinemia occur with repeated doses.

Contraindications: Hepatic or renal impairment.

Adverse reactions: Paradoxical excitation, GI intolerance, allergic manifestations, leukopenia, eosinophilia, vasodilation, cardiopulmonary depression (especially when coadministered with barbiturates and opiates), cardiac arrhythmias.

 CHLOROTHIAZIDE

Classification: Thiazide diuretic, loop diuretic.

Indications: Fluid overload, pulmonary edema, BPD, CHF, and hypertension.

Dosage/administration: 20 to 40 mg/kg/day orally, divided every 12 hours. Intravenously 2 to 8 mg/kg/day, divided every 12 hours. When converting from oral to intravenous dose, use one-half of the oral dose. Intramuscular and SC administration not recommended because of local pain and irritation.

Contraindications: Anuria or hepatic dysfunction.

Drug interactions: Reduced antihypertensive effect with concurrent nonsteroidal anti-inflammatory drug use.

Monitoring: Serum electrolytes, calcium, blood glucose, urine output, BP, and daily weight.

Adverse reactions: Hypochloremic alkalosis, prerenal azotemia, volume depletion, blood dyscrasias, decreased serum potassium and magnesium levels, and increased levels of glucose, uric acid, lipids, bilirubin, and calcium.

 CITRATE MIXTURES, ORAL

Classification: Electrolyte supplement.

Indications: Metabolic acidosis.

Dosage/administration: 0.5 to 1 mEq/kg/dose, orally 3 or 4 times/day. Give with feedings. Adjust dose to maintain desired urine pH. One mEq citrate equivalent to 1 mEq HCO_3 (see Table A.7).

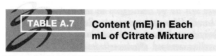

Citrate mixtures	Na^+	K^+	Citrate
Polycitra	1	1	2
Polycitra-K	0	2	2
Bicitra	1	0	1
Oracit	1	0	1

TABLE A.7 Content (mE) in Each mL of Citrate Mixture

Precautions: Use with caution in infants receiving potassium supplements.
Adverse reactions: Laxative effect.

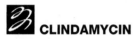

CLINDAMYCIN

Classification: Anaerobic antibiotic.
Indications: Treatment of *B. fragilis* septicemia, peritonitis, necrotizing enterocolitis (NEC). Not indicated for meningitis.
Dosage/administration: (see Table A.8)

TABLE A.8

Age	Dosage
Postmenstrual age <29 wk	7.5 mg/kg/dose IV q12h
Postmenstrual age >29 wk	7.5 mg/kg/dose IV q8h
IV = intravenously; q8h = every 8 hours; q12h = every 12 hours.	

Final concentration of 10 mg/mL in dextrose 5% water or NS. Infuse over >30 minutes on syringe pump. Maximum concentration for infusion is 18 mg/mL. Intramuscular administration associated with sterile abscess formation.
Contraindications: Hepatic impairment.
Warnings: Can cause severe and possibly fatal pseudomembranous colitis characterized by severe persistent diarrhea and possibly the passage of blood and mucus.
Drug interactions: Potentiates neuromuscular blockade of tubocurarine, pancuronium.
Adverse reactions: *Pseudomembranous colitis*, Stevens-Johnson syndrome, glossitis, pruritus, granulocytopenia, thrombocytopenia, hypotension, and increased LFTs.

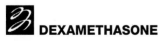

DEXAMETHASONE

Classification: Adrenal corticosteroid, anti-inflammatory agent.
Indications: Anti-inflammatory glucocorticoid used to facilitate extubation and improve lung mechanics.

Dosage/administration: Acetate injection is not for IV use. Administer IV through syringe pump over >5 minutes. Maximum concentration 1 mg/mL. Maximum dose: 1 mg/kg/day IV/PO.

Extubation/airway edema dosing: 0.25 to 0.5 mg/kg × 1. May repeat q8–12 h for total of four doses.

Begin dosing 6 to 8 hours before extubation and continue 4 to 6 hours post extubation (see Table A.9).

	Dosing	**Frequency**	**Duration**
Day 1	0.1 mg/kg	q12h	× Two total doses
Day 2	0.075 mg/kg	q12h	× Two total doses
Day 3	0.05 mg/kg	q12h	× Two total doses

TABLE A.9   **Chronic Lung Disease Dosing**

q12h = every 12 hours.

Precautions: Hyperglycemia and glycosuria occur frequently after the first few doses. Increase in BP is common. Edema, hypertension, pituitary–adrenal axis suppression, growth suppression, glucose intolerance, hypokalemia, alkalosis, Cushing syndrome, peptic ulcer, immunosuppression.

Monitoring: Hemoglobin, occult blood loss, BP, serum potassium and glucose; IOP with systemic use >6 weeks; weight and height.

Adverse reactions: Facial flushing, ↑ BP, tachycardia, agitation, hyponatremia, hyperglycemia, poor growth, bone demineralization, protein catabolism, secondary adrenal suppression, nausea, dyspepsia, vomiting, pain at injection site, itchy or light sensitive eyes, rhinitis, upper respiratory infections, nose bleed, nasal congestion. **Dexamethasone given for treatment or prevention of BPD has been associated with a higher risk of cerebral palsy and neurodevelopmental abnormalities. Its use should be avoided except under exceptional clinical circumstances (maximal ventilatory support or high risk of mortality).**

 DIAZOXIDE

Classification: Antihypoglycemic agent.
Indications: Hyperinsulinemic hypoglycemia.
Dosage/administration: 8 to 15 mg/kg/day, orally, divided every 8 to 12 hours.
Clinical considerations: Used only for glucose-refractory hypoglycemia.
Contraindications: Compensatory hypertension associated with aortic coarctation or arteriovenous (AV) shunts.
Precautions: Diabetes mellitus, renal, or liver disease. May displace bilirubin from albumin.
Monitoring: BP, CBC, serum uric acid levels.
Drug interactions: Phenytoin.
Adverse reactions: Hyperglycemia (insulin reverses diazoxide-induced hyperglycemia), ketoacidosis, sodium and water retention, hypotension, hyponatremia, extrapyramidal symptoms, seizures, arrhythmias, leukopenia, thrombocytopenia, and hyperosmolar coma.

 DIGOXIN

Classification: Antiarrhythmic agent, inotrope.
Indications: Heart failure, paroxysmal atrioventricular nodal tachycardia, atrial fibrillation/flutter.

Dosage/administration: (see Table A.10)

TABLE A.10

Age	Total digitalizing dose		Maintenance dose	
	PO	IV	PO	IV
<37 wk	20–30 mg/kg/d	15–25 mg/kg/d	5–7.5 mg/kg/d	4–6 mg/kg/d
≥37 wk	25–35 mg/kg/d	20–30 mg/kg/d	6–10 mg/kg/d	5–8 mg/kg/d
IV = intravenously; PO = orally.				

Reserve total digitalizing dose (TDD) for treatment of arrhythmias and acute CHF. Administer TDD over 24 hours in three divided doses: first dose is one-half TDD, second dose is one-fourth TDD administered 8 hours after first dose, and third dose is one-fourth TDD administered 8 hours after second dose. Administer intravenous doses over >10 minutes on syringe pump. Utilize maintenance dose schedule for nonacute arrhythmia and CHF conditions. Do not administer intramuscularly. The pediatric intravenous formulation (100 μg/mL) may be given undiluted. The pediatric oral elixir is 50 μg/mL.

Precautions: Reduce dose for renal and hepatic impairment. Cardioversion or calcium infusion may precipitate ventricular fibrillation in the digoxin-treated neonate (may be prevented by lidocaine pretreatment).

Monitoring: Heart rate/rhythm for desired effects and signs of toxicity, serum calcium, magnesium (especially in neonates receiving diuretics and amphotericin-B, both of which predispose to digoxin toxicity).

Therapeutic levels: 0.8 to 2 ng/mL. Neonates may have falsely elevated digoxin levels as a result of maternal digoxin-like substances.

Contraindications: Atrioventricular block, idiopathic hypertrophic subaortic stenosis, ventricular dysrhythmias, atrial fibrillation/flutter with slow ventricular rates, or constrictive pericarditis.

Drug interactions: Amiodarone, erythromycin, cholestyramine, indomethacin, spironolactone, quinidine, verapamil, and metoclopramide.

Adverse reactions: Persistent vomiting, feeding intolerance, diarrhea, and lethargy, shortening of QT_c interval, sagging ST segment, diminished T-wave amplitude, bradycardia, prolongation of PR interval, sinus bradycardia or S-A block, atrial or nodal ectopic beats, ventricular arrhythmias. Toxicity enhanced by hypokalemia. Treat life-threatening digoxin toxicity with Digoxin Immune Fab.

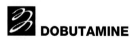

DOBUTAMINE

Classification: Sympathomimetic, adrenergic agonist agent.

Indications: Treatment of hypoperfusion, hypotension, short-term management of cardiac decompensation.

Dosage/administration: 5 to 25 μg/kg/minute continuous intravenous infusion on intravenous pump. Begin at a low dose and titrate to obtain desired mean arterial pressure. Central *venous* access is preferred. **Do not administer through UAC.** Maximum concentration is 90 mg/100 mL = 900 μg/mL in NS or dextrose.

Precautions: Hypovolemia should be corrected before use. Infiltration causes local inflammatory changes. Extravasation may cause dermal necrosis. Use phentolamine to treat extravasation.

Contraindications: Idiopathic hypertrophic subaortic stenosis.

Adverse reactions: Hypotension if hypovolemic, arrhythmias, tachycardia (with high doses), cutaneous vasodilation, increased BP and dyspnea.
Monitoring: Continuous heart rate and arterial BP.

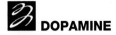
DOPAMINE

Classification: Sympathomimetic, adrenergic agonist agent.
Indications: Treatment of hypotension.
Dosage/administration: 2.5 to 25 μg/kg/minute through continuous intravenous infusion on intravenous pump. Once 20 to 25 μg/kg/minute is reached, consideration should be given to adding a second pressor. Clinical benefits have been noted at doses of up to 40 μg/kg/minute. Begin at a low dose and titrate to obtain desired mean arterial pressure. Central *venous* access preferred. **Do not administer through UAC.** Maximum concentration is 90 mg/100 mL = 900 μg/mL mixed in NS or dextrose.
Precautions: Hypovolemia should be corrected before use. Extravasation may cause tissue necrosis. Treat dopamine extravasation with phentolamine.
Contraindications: Pheochromocytoma, tachyarrhythmias, or hypovolemia may increase pulmonary artery pressure. Use with caution in neonates with pulmonary hypertension.
Adverse reactions: Arrhythmias, tachycardia, vasoconstriction, hypotension, widened QRS complex, bradycardia, hypertension, excessive diuresis and azotemia, reversible suppression of prolactin and thyrotropin secretion.
Monitoring parameters: Continuous heart rate and arterial BP, urine output, peripheral perfusion.

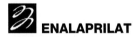
ENALAPRILAT

Classification: Angiotensin-converting enzyme inhibitor, antihypertensive.
Indications: Hypertension, CHF.
Dosage/administration:
Neonatal hypertension: Enalaprilat: 5 to 10 μg/kg/dose (0.005–0.01 mg/kg/dose), intravenously every 8 to 24 hours.
CHF: Enalapril maleate: Initial dose: 0.1 mg/kg/day orally every 24 hours; may be given without regard to feeding times; increased according to response, every 3 to 4 days, to a maximum of 0.43 mg/kg/day. Oral suspension prepared by dissolving a crushed 2.5-mg tablet in 12.5 mL of sterile water, yielding final concentration of 0.2 mg/mL (200 μg/mL). Use immediately, discard remaining portion.
Precautions: Impaired renal function.
Monitoring: BP, renal function, serum electrolytes. Hold for mean arterial pressure <30 and heart rate <100.
Adverse reactions: Transient or prolonged episodes of hypotension, oliguria, mild nonoliguric renal failure, hypotension in volume-depleted neonates, and hyperkalemia in neonates receiving potassium supplements and/or potassium-sparing diuretics.

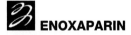
ENOXAPARIN

Classification: Low-molecular-weight heparin, anticoagulant.
Indication: Prophylaxis and treatment of thromboembolic disorders.
Dosage/administration: Prophylaxis: 0.75 mg/kg/dose subcutaneously every 12 hours. Treatment: 1.5 mg/kg/dose subcutaneously every 12 hours.
Clinical considerations: Adjust dose to maintain antifactor Xa level between 0.5 and 1 U/mL. Peak antifactor Xa activity is obtained 4 hours after dose (see Table A.11).
For SC administration only. To minimize bruising, do not administer intramuscularly or intravenously; do not rub injection site.
Precautions: Reduce dose by 30% in severe renal impairment.

| TABLE A.11 | Monitoring Parameters |

Antifactor Xa	Dose titration	Time to repeat antifactor Xa level
<0.35 units/mL	↑ Dose by 25%	4 h after next dose
0.350.49 units/mL	↑ Dose by 10%	4 h after next dose
0.51 units/mL	Keep same dose	Next day, then 1 wk later (4 h after dose) Adjust dose for weight gain
1.1 – 1.5 units/mL	↓ Dose by 20%	Before next dose
1.6 – 2 units/mL	Hold dose for 3 h, then ↓ dose by 30%	Before next dose, then 4 h after dose
>2 units/mL	Hold all doses until antifactor Xa is 0.5 units/mL; then ↓ dose by 40%	Before next dose and q12h until antifactor Xa <0.5 units/mL

↑ = increasing; ↓ = decreasing; q12h = every 12 hours.

Contraindications: Avoid in infants who require spinal puncture to minimize risk of epidural/spinal hematoma.
Adverse effects: Fever, edema, hemorrhage, thrombocytopenia, pain/erythema at injection site.

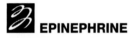

EPINEPHRINE

Classification: Adrenergic agent.
Indications: Cardiac arrest, refractory hypotension, bronchospasm.
Dosage/administration: (see Table A.12)

| TABLE A.12 | | |

Indication	Dose	Comments
Severe bradycardia and hypotension	**IV push:** 0.1 to 0.3 mL/kg of **1:10,000** concentration (equal to 0.01–0.03 mg/kg or 10–30 μg/kg) **Endotracheal tube:** 0.3 to 1 mL/kg of **1:10,000** concentration (equal to 0.03–0.1 mg/kg or 30–100 μg/kg)	May repeat 2–3 q3–5min if heart rate remains below 60 beats/min
Continuous IV	Start at 0.1 μg/kg/min. Adjust dose to desired response, to a maximum of 1 μg/mg/min	Use the **1:1,000** formulation for mixing continuous IV preparations. Maximum IV concentration = 1 mg/50 mL

IV = intravenous; q = every.

Monitoring: Continuous heart rate and BP monitoring.
Drug interactions: Incompatible with alkaline solutions (sodium bicarbonate).
Precautions: Note the differences in concentration for emergency administration and continuous intravenous epinephrine doses. High doses of preservative-containing epinephrine will necessitate caution in selection of epinephrine preparations. Always use a 1:10,000 concentration (0.1 mg/mL) for individual doses, endotracheal tube doses, and for emergency administration (IV and endotracheal). Use the 1:1000 concentration for preparation of continuous infusions. Correction of acidosis before administration of catecholamines enhances their effectiveness.
Contraindications: Hyperthyroidism, hypertension, and diabetes.
Adverse reactions: Ventricular arrhythmias, tachycardia, pallor and tremor, severe hypertension with possible intraventricular hemorrhage, myocardial ischemia, hypokalemia, and decreased renal and splanchnic blood flow. Intravenous infiltration may cause tissue ischemia and necrosis (consider treatment with phentolamine).

 EPINEPHRINE RACEMIC

Classification: Adrenergic agonist.
Indications: Treatment of postextubation stridor.
Dosage/administration: 0.25 to 0.5 mL of 2.25% **racemic epinephrine** solution diluted in 3 mL NS. Given by nebulizer every 2 hours as needed.
Clinical considerations: Observe closely for rebound airway edema. Closely monitor heart rate (hold for heart rate >180 beats/minute) and BP during administration.
Adverse reactions: Tachyarrhythmias, hypokalemia.

 ERYTHROMYCIN

Classification: Macrolide antibiotic.
Indications: Treatment of infections caused by chlamydia, mycoplasma, and ureaplasma; treatment and prophylaxis of *Bordetella pertussis* and ophthalmia neonatorum; also used as a prokinetic agent.
Dosage/administration: (see Table A.13)
Precautions: Do not administer intramuscularly (causes pain and necrosis). Cholestatic jaundice occurs with erythromycin estolate. Hepatotoxicity can occur with pre-existing liver impairment.
Contraindications: Pre-existing hepatic dysfunction.
Drug interactions: Increased blood levels of carbamazepine, digoxin, cyclosporine, warfarin, methylprednisolone, and theophylline.
Test interactions: False-positive urine catecholamines.
Monitoring: LFTs, CBC (eosinophilia).
Adverse reactions: Anaphylaxis, rash, stomatitis, candidiasis, hepatotoxicity, ototoxicity (high-dose erythromycin), intrahepatic cholestasis, and vomiting.

 FAMOTIDINE

Classification: H-2 blocker.
Indications: Short-term therapy and treatment of duodenal ulcer, gastric ulcer, gastroesophageal reflux disease (GERD), control of gastric pH in critically ill patients (like ranitidine, famotidine does not significantly interfere with cytochomes P-450, thereby reducing its potential for drug interactions). Famotidine has little antiandrogenic effect.
Dosage/administration:
IV: 0.5 mg/kg/dose, q24h. Administer IV dose over >10 minutes on syringe pump.
PO: 0.5 mg/kg/dose, q24h. Precautions: Use with caution and modify dose in patients with renal impairment. Avoid injection formulations that contain benzyl alcohol.
Monitoring: Gastric pH, BUN, creatinine, urine output, bilirubin, LFTs and CBC.

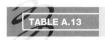

TABLE A.13

Indication	Dosage	Comment
Systemic infections	Erythromycin estolate (Ilosone): 10 mg/kg/dose PO q8h. Erythromycin ethylsuccinate (ESS, EryPed): 10 mg/kg/dose PO q6h	Administer with feeding to enhance absorption of Erythromycin ethylsuccinate and to reduce possible GI upset
Severe systemic infections or PO route unavailable	5–10 mg/kg/dose, IV q6h. (Dilute to 1–5 mg/mL and infuse >1 h)	Use only preservative-free IV erythromycin formulations
Opthalmia neonatorum	Prophylaxis: 0.5–1 cm ribbon of 0.5% ointment into each conjucntival sac × 1	Administered at birth
Chlamydia conjunctivitis	0.5–1 cm ribbon of 0.5% ointment into each conjunctival sac q6h × 7 d	PO therapy is preferable to topical therapy for eradication of nasopharyngeal carrier state Treat mother and her sexual partner
Prokinetic agent	**Initial:** 3 mg/kg/ IV >60 min, followed by 20 mg/kg/d PO in 3–4 divided doses 30 min before meals	
Ureaplasma urealyticum	5–10 mg/kg/dose PO or IV q6h and treat for 10–14 d	

GI = gastrointestinal; IV = intravenously; PO = orally; q6h = every 6 hours; q8h = every 8 hours.

Adverse reactions: Dry mouth, constipation, thrombocytopenia, agranulocytosis, neutropenia, and elevated liver enzymes. Use of H-2 blockade in very low birth-weight (VLBW) infants has been associated with a higher risk of nectrotizing enterocolitis.

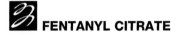

FENTANYL CITRATE

Classification: Narcotic analgesic.
Indication: Analgesia, sedation, anesthesia.
Dosage/administration:
Sedation/analgesia: Intravenous: 1 to 5 μg/kg/dose every 2 to 4 hours over >10 minutes on syringe pump. Maximum concentration for continuous intravenous infusion is 10 μg/mL in NS or dextrose.
Bolus: 1 to 2 μg/kg; then 1 to 5 μg/kg/hours titrate as needed.
Intravenous bolus: Mix 1 mL of 100 μg/2 mL fentanyl in 9 mL NS, mixture = 10 μg/mL of fentanyl.
Anesthesia: 5 to 50 μg/kg/dose.
Precautions: Give intravenous bolus dose over >10 minutes on syringe pump to avoid apnea and fentanyl-induced decreased total lung and chest wall compliance.
Contraindications: Increased intracranial pressure, severe respiratory depression, severe liver or renal insufficiency.
Adverse reactions: CNS and respiratory depression, skeletal/thoracic muscle rigidity, vomiting, constipation, peripheral vasodilation, miosis, biliary or urinary tract spasms and

antidiuretic hormone release; tolerance develops in association with continuous intravenous infusions for >5 days.

Monitoring: Respiration rate (RR), heart rate, BP, abdominal status, muscle rigidity. Adherence to extracorporeal membrane oxygenation (ECMO) membranes may necessitate increased dose.

 FERROUS SULFATE

Classification: Oral mineral supplement.

Indication: Prophylaxis for prevention of iron-deficiency anemia in preterm newborns.

Dosage/administration: 2 to 4 mg of elemental iron/kg/day orally every day. Ferrous sulfate drops contain 25 mg elemental iron/mL. Iron supplements are available in different concentrations. When ordering, specify exact amount in mg to avoid over- or underdosing. Iron supplementation may increase hemolysis if adequate vitamin E therapy is not supplied. Start iron therapy no later than 2 months of age.

Clinical considerations: Absorption is variable.

Contraindications: Peptic ulcer disease, ulcerative colitis, enteritis, hemochromatosis, and hemolytic anemia.

Drug interactions: Decreased absorption of both iron and tetracycline when given together. Antacids and chloramphenicol decrease iron absorption.

Monitoring: Hemoglobin and reticulocyte counts during therapy. Observe stools (may color the stool black and cause false-positive guaiac test for blood), and monitor for constipation.

Adverse reactions: Constipation, diarrhea, and GI irritation.

Overdose: Serum iron level >300 µg/dL usually requires treatment because of severe toxicity; acute GI irritation, erosion of GI mucosa, hematemesis, lethargy, acidosis, hepatic and renal dysfunction, circulatory collapse, coma, and death. Antidote is deferoxamine chelation therapy. Gastric lavage with 1% to 5% sodium bicarbonate or sodium phosphate solution prevents additional absorption of iron.

 FLUCONAZOLE

Classification: Systemic antifungal agent.

Indications: Treatment of systemic fungal infections, meningitis, and severe superficial mycoses. Alternative to amphotericin-B in patients with pre-existing renal impairment or when concomitant therapy with other potentially nephrotoxic drugs is required. Recently used as prophylaxis against invasive fungal infections in VLBW infants.

Dosage/administration: Daily dose of fluconazole is the same for oral and IV administration. See Table A.14 for interval.

TABLE A.14

Postmenstrual age	Postnatal age	Dosing interval
≤29 wk	0–14 d	72 h
	>14 d	48 h
30–36 wk	0–14 d	48 h
	>14 d	24 h
>37–44 wk	0–7 d	48 h
	>7 d	24 h
>45	All ages	24 h

Systemic infections, including meningitis: 12 mg/kg loading dose, then 6 mg/kg/dose IV infusion by syringe pump over >60 minutes, or PO.

Thrush: 6 mg/kg on day 1, then 3 mg/kg/dose q24 hours PO.

Prophylaxis: 3 mg/kg/dose once daily 3 times weekly for first 2 weeks, then every other day for total of 4 to 6 weeks (longer duration for infants with birth-weight <1,000 g). Administer intravenous dose on syringe pump for 60 minutes.

Clinical considerations: Well-absorbed orally. Good cerebrospinal fluid penetration by both intravenous and oral routes.

Precautions: Adjust dosage for impaired renal function.

Drug interactions: Warfarin, phenytoin, rifampin. Possible interference with metabolism of caffeine and theophylline.

Food interactions: Food decreases the rate but not its extent of absorption.

Monitoring: Renal and LFTs.

Adverse reactions: Vomiting, diarrhea, exfoliative skin disorders, and reversible increased aspartate aminotransferase, alanine aminotransferase (ALT), alkaline phosphatase.

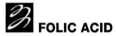 FOLIC ACID

Classification: Vitamin, mineral, nutritional supplement.

Indication: Treatment of megaloblastic and macrocytic anemias as a result of folate deficiency.

Dosage/administration: 15 μg/kg/dose or up to maximum of 50 μg/day. May be given orally/intramuscularly/intravenously/subcutaneously. The parenteral form may be diluted to a concentration of 0.1 mg/mL (100 μg/mL) and administered orally. Administer deeply if intramuscular route is used. The oral form may be given without regard to feeds.

Clinical considerations: May mask hematologic defects of vitamin B_{12} deficiency, but will not prevent progression of irreversible neurologic abnormalities, despite the absence of anemia.

Precautions: The injection contains benzyl alcohol (1.5%) as a preservative; avoid using in preterm infants.

Contraindications: Pernicious, aplastic, and normocytic anemias.

Drug interactions: May decrease phenytoin serum concentrations.

Monitoring parameters: Hematocrit, hemoglobin, reticulocyte.

Adverse effects: GI upset, slight flushing but generally well tolerated.

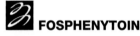 FOSPHENYTOIN

Classification: Anticonvulsant.

Indications: Management of generalized convulsive status epilepticus refractory to phenobarbital. For short term (<5 days) parenteral (intravenous or intramuscular) administration when other means of phenytoin administration are unavailable, inappropriate, or less advantageous.

Dosage/administration: PE: phenytoin equivalent. Fosphenytoin 1 mg PE = Phenytoin 1 mg = Fosphenytoin 1.5 mg.

Loading dose: 15 to 20 mg PE/kg intramuscularly or intravenously. Infuse loading dose over >10 minutes on syringe pump.

Maintenance dose: 4 to 8 mg PE/kg intramuscularly or intravenously, slow push every 24 hours. Begin maintenance dose 24 hours after the loading dose. Modify dose in infants with hepatic or renal impairment. Maximum concentration for intravenous or intramuscular administration is 25 mg PE/mL. Flush intravenous line with NS before/after administration.

Precautions: To avoid medication errors, always prescribe and dispense fosphenytoin in mg of PE. Consider the amount of phosphate delivered by fosphenytoin in infants who require phosphate restriction. Each 1 mg PE fosphenytoin delivers 0.0037 mmol of phosphate. Use with caution in infants with hyperbilirubinemia. Fosphenytoin and bilirubin compete with phenytoin and displace phenytoin from plasma protein-binding sites. This results in an increased serum concentration of free phenytoin. Use with caution in hypotension and myocardial insufficiency.

Contraindications: Heart block, sinus bradycardia.

Adverse reactions: Hypotension, vasodilation, tachycardia, bradycardia, fever, hyperglycemia, neutropenia, thrombocytopenia, megaloblastic anemia, osteomalacia.

Monitoring considerations: Monitor BP, EKG during intravenous loading doses.

Monitoring parameters: Therapeutic levels: 10 to 20 mg/L total phenytoin **or** 1 to 2 mg/L unbound phenytoin only.

Guidelines for obtaining levels: Obtain phenytoin levels 2 hours after end of intravenous infusion or 4 hours after intramuscular dose. Obtain the first level 48 hours after the loading dose.

 FUROSEMIDE

Classification: Loop diuretic.

Indications: Management of pulmonary edema. To provide diuresis and improve lung function when a greater diuretic effect than produced by Chlorothiazide (Diuril) is needed.

Dosage/administration:

Intravenous: 1 mg/kg/dose.

Oral: 2 mg/kg/dose. For long-term use, consider alternate day therapy or longer (every 48–72 hours) in order to prevent toxicities. Give with feeds to reduce GI irritation. Give the alcohol and sugar-free product to neonates. Intravenous form may be used orally.

Monitoring: Follow daily weight changes, urine output, serum phosphate, and serum electrolytes. Closely monitor potassium levels in neonates receiving digoxin.

Precautions: Use with caution in hepatic and renal disease.

Adverse reactions: Fluid and electrolyte imbalance, hypokalemia, hypocalcemia/hypercalciuria, hypochloremic alkalosis, nephrocalcinosis (associated with long-term therapy), potential ototoxicity (especially if receiving aminoglycosides), prerenal azotemia, hyperuricemia, agranulocytosis, anemia, thrombocytopenia, interstitial nephritis, pancreatitis, and cholelithiasis (in BPD or CHF and long-term total parenteral nutrition and furosemide therapy).

 γ-GLOBULIN

Classification: Immune globulin.

Indications: Alloimmune thrombocytopenia and immune hemolysis causing hyperbilirubunemia.

Dosage/administration: 0.5 to 1 g/kg intravenously for 1 to 2 doses given over >2 to 3 hours. Usual concentration for intravenous administration is 5% to 10% (50–100 mg/mL). Maximum concentration for infusion is 12% (12% concentration should be given through central line).

Precautions: Delay immunizations with live virus vaccines until 3 to 11 months after intravenous immunoglobulin administration.

Monitoring: Continuous heart rate and BP monitoring during administration.

Adverse reactions: Transient hypoglycemia, tachycardia, and hypotension (resolved with cessation of infusion). Tenderness, erythema, and induration at injection site and allergic manifestations. Rare hypersensitivity reactions reported with rapid intravenous administration.

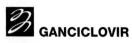 **GANCICLOVIR**

Classification: Antiviral agent.

Indications: Treatment or prophylaxis of cytomegalovirus (CMV) infections.

Dosages/administration: For congenital CMV infection, 10 to 15 mg/kg/day divided every 12 hours for 3 to 6 weeks; infuse over >1 hour on syringe pump. Maximum concentration for infusion must not exceed 10 mg/mL in dextrose or NS. **Administer through central line to minimize risk of phlebitis.** If central line is not available, it may be administered peripherally at a concentration no greater than 2 mg/mL. Do not administer intramuscularly or subcutaneously to avoid severe tissue irritation that is due to its high pH.

Precautions: Treat ganciclovir as **cytotoxic** drug. **Avoid all contact** with skin and mucous membranes. Wear impervious protective gown, nonlatex procedure gloves, and mask. Priming of intravenous set should not allow any drug to be released into the environment.

Contraindications: For infants with neutropenia with an absolute neutrophil count <500 or thrombocytopenia with a platelet count <25,000. Consider treatment with G-CSF (Neupogen) in patients with neutropenia. Adjust dose in renal impairment. Avoid dehydration during therapy.

Adverse reactions: Neutropenia, thrombocytopenia, anemia. Thrombocytopenia is usually reversible and responds to a decreased dose. Inflammation at intravenous site. Increased LFTs, increased BUN/serum creatinine, decrease dosage if renal function worsens.

Monitoring considerations: Obtain daily CBC with differential and platelet count. Obtain weekly BUN, serum creatinine. At the first sign of significant renal dysfunction, the dose of ganciclovir should be adjusted by either reducing the number of mg/dose or by prolonging the dosing interval.

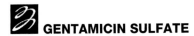

GENTAMICIN SULFATE

Classification: Aminoglycoside, antibiotic.

Indications: Active against gram-negative aerobic bacteria, some activity against coagulase-positive *staphylococci*, ineffective against anaerobes, *streptococci*.

Dosage/administration: (see Table A.15)

TABLE A.15

Age	IV Dosage
<35 wk postmenstrual age	3 mg/kg/dose q24h
≥35 wk postmenstrual age	4 mg/kg/dose q24h
IV = intravenous; q24h = every 24 hours.	

Administer intravenous infusion on syringe pump over >30 minutes. Intravenous route preferred because intramuscular absorption is variable.

Precautions: Modify dosage in patients with renal impairment.

Drug interactions: Indomethacin decreases gentamicin clearance and prolongs its half-life. Increased neuromuscular blockade is observed when aminoglycosides are used with neuromuscular blocking agents (e.g., pancuronium). The risk of aminoglycoside-induced ototoxicity and/or nephrotoxicity is increased when used concurrently with loop diuretics (e.g., furosemide, bumetanide) or vancomycin. Penicillins, cephalosporins, amphotericin-B, blunt gentamicin serum peak concentration if administered <1 hour before/after these agents. Neuromuscular weakness or respiratory failure may occur in infants with hypermagnesemia.

Adverse reactions: Vestibular and auditory ototoxicity (associated with high trough levels) and renal toxicity (occurs in the proximal tubule, associated with high trough levels, usually reversible). Treat extravasation with hyaluronidase around periphery of affected area.

Monitoring considerations: Assess renal function.

Guidelines for obtaining levels: Draw trough levels within 30 minutes before the next dose. Draw peak levels at 30 minutes after the end of a 30-minute infusion or 1 hour after an intramuscular injection.

Monitoring parameters: For all infants, **obtain blood levels pre- and post-third dose. Trough:** Less than 1.5 µg/mL.

Peak: 6 to 15 µg/mL.

Dose adjustment: For trough levels between 1.5 and 2 µg/mL, obtain another trough with next dose. For trough >2 µg/mL, increase interval by 12 hours. For peak <6 µg/mL, increase dose by 20% to 25% to achieve peak of 6 to 15. For peak >15 µg/mL, decrease dose by 20% to 25% to achieve peak of 6 to 15.

GLUCAGON

Classification: Antihypoglycemic agent.

Indications: Treatment of hypoglycemia in cases of documented glucagon deficiency.

Dosage/administration: 25 to 300 µg/kg/dose (0.025–0.3 mg/kg/dose) intravenous push/ intramuscular/SC every 20 minutes as needed.

Maximum dose: 1 mg.

Continuous intravenous: Administer in dextrose 10% water solution, starting at 0.5 mg/ kg/day. Add hydrocortisone if no response within 4 hours. Further dosage increases >2 mg/day unlikely to be effective. After effect seen, slowly taper over at least 24 hours. Compatible with dextrose solutions.

Contraindications: Should not be used in small-for-gestational-age infants.

Precautions: Do not delay starting glucose infusion while awaiting effect of glucagon. Use caution in infants with history of insulinoma or pheochromocytoma. Incompatible with electrolyte-containing solutions.

Monitoring: Serum glucose.

Adverse reactions: Vomiting, tachycardia, hypertension, and GI upset.

HEPARIN SODIUM

Classification: Anticoagulant.

Indications: Line flushing for heparin locks and to maintain patency of single- and double-lumen central catheters.

Dosage/administration: (see Table A.16)

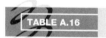
TABLE A.16

Indication	Dosage	Comment
Heparin lock for peripheral IV, central lines	1–2 mL of 10 U/mL solution q4–6h and PRN	To keep line open
Continuous infusion for central venous and/or arterial line U/mL	Add heparin to make a final concentration of 0.5–1	To keep line open

IV = intravenous; PRN = as needed; q4–6h = every 4 to 6 hours.

Contraindications: Platelet count <50,000/mm^3, suspected intracranial hemorrhage, GI bleeding, shock, severe hypotension, and uncontrolled bleeding.

Precautions: Risk factors for hemorrhage include intramuscular injections, venous and arterial blood sampling, and peptic ulcer disease. Use preservative-free heparin in neonates. To avoid systemic heparinization in small neonates, use more dilute (0.5 U/mL) heparin flush concentrations.

Monitoring: Follow platelet counts every 2 to 3 days. Assess for signs of bleeding and thrombosis.
Drug interactions: Thrombolytic agents and intravenous nitroglycerin.
Adverse reactions: Heparin-induced thrombocytopenia reported in some heparin-exposed newborns. Other adverse reactions include hemorrhage, fever, urticaria, vomiting, increased LFTs, osteoporosis, and alopecia.
Antidote: Protamine sulfate (1 mg/100 U of heparin given in the previous 4 hours).

 HYALURONIDASE

Classification: Antidote, extravasation.
Indications: Prevention of tissue injury caused by intravenous extravasation of hyperosmolar or extremely alkaline solutions.
Dosage/administration: SC or intradermal: Dilute to 150 U/mL in NS. Inject five separate 0.2-mL injections into the leading edge of the infiltrate. Use a 25- or 27-gauge needle, and change after each injection. Elevate the extremity. Do not apply heat and do not administer intravenously. Best results are obtained when used within 1 hour of extravasation. May repeat if necessary.
Clinical considerations: Some agents for which hyaluronidase is effective include aminophylline, amphotericin, calcium, diazepam, erythromycin, gentamicin, methicillin, nafcillin, oxacillin, phenytoin, potassium chloride, sodium bicarbonate, tromethamine, vancomycin, total parenteral nutrition, and concentrated intravenous solutions.
Warnings: Hyaluronidase is neither effective nor indicated for treatment of extravasations of vasoconstrictive agents (phentolamine is the preferred agent for treatment of extravasation with vasoconstrictive agents).

 HYDRALAZINE

Classification: Antihypertensive, vasodilator.
Indication: BP reduction in neonatal hypertension. After load reduction in CHF.
Dosage/administration:
Initial dose: 0.1 to 0.5 mg/kg/dose intravenously every 6 to 8 hours. Increase gradually to a maximum of 2 mg/kg/dose intravenously every 6 hours as required for BP control. Usual concentration for intravenous administration is 1 mg/mL. Maximum concentration for intravenous administration is 20 mg/mL.
Oral dose: 0.25 to 1 mg/kg/dose orally every 6 to 8 hours. Administer with food to enhance absorption.
Maximum dose: 7 mg/kg/day. Double the dose when changing from intravenous to oral because hydralazine is only approximately 50% absorbed.
Precautions: Use with caution in severe renal and cardiac disease.
Clinical considerations: May cause reflex tachycardia. Concurrent β-blocker therapy recommended to reduce the magnitude of reflex tachycardia and to enhance antihypertensive effect. Maximum effect occurs in 3 to 4 days. Tachyphylaxis reported with chronic therapy.
Drug interactions: Concurrent use with other antihypertensives allows reduced dosage requirements of hydralazine to <0.15 mg/kg/dose.
Monitoring: Daily monitoring of heart rate, BP, urine output, and weight. Guaiac all stools, and obtain CBC at least twice weekly.
Adverse reactions: Tachycardia, vomiting, diarrhea, orthostatic hypotension, edema, GI irritation and bleeding, anemia, and agranulocytosis.

HYDROCORTISONE

Classification: Adrenal corticosteroid.
Indication: Vasopressor resistant hypovolemic shock; treatment of cortisol insufficiency.

Dosage/administration: Initial dose may be given as a slow push over >3 to 5 minutes. Administer subsequent doses over >30 minutes on syringe pump (see Table A.17).

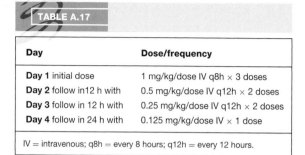

TABLE A.17

Day	Dose/frequency
Day 1 initial dose	1 mg/kg/dose IV q8h × 3 doses
Day 2 follow in12 h with	0.5 mg/kg/dose IV q12h × 2 doses
Day 3 follow in 12 h with	0.25 mg/kg/dose IV q12h × 2 doses
Day 4 follow in 24 h with	0.125 mg/kg/dose IV × 1 dose

IV = intravenous; q8h = every 8 hours; q12h = every 12 hours.

If BP improves and other pressors have been weaned off, may stop after 24 hours. Final concentration for infusion is 1 mg/mL in dextrose or saline. Maximum infusion concentration is 10 mg/mL. Use preservative-free hydrocortisone sodium succinate formulation for intravenous dosing.
Precautions: Acute adrenal insufficiency may occur with abrupt withdrawal following long-term therapy or during periods of stress.
Adverse reactions: Hypertension, edema, cataracts, peptic ulcer, immunosuppression, hypokalemia, hyperglycemia, dermatitis, Cushing syndrome, and skin atrophy.

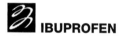 **IBUPROFEN**

Classification: Nonselective cyclo-oxygenase enzyme inhibitor. Inhibitor of prostaglandin synthesis. Nonsteroidal anti-inflammatory agent.
Indications: Pharmacologic closure of ductus arteriosus.
Dosage/administration:
Initial dose: 10 mg/kg IV × 1, then 5 mg/kg IV at 24 and 48 hours after initial dose.
Precautions: Avoid use with steroids to decrease incidence of GI bleed. Use with caution in patients with decreased renal or hepatic function, dehydration, CHF, hypertension, history of GI bleed, or those receiving anticoagulants.
Monitoring: BUN and serum creatinine, CBC, occult blood loss, liver enzymes; echocardiogram, heart murmur.
Adverse reactions: Edema, peptic ulcer, GI bleed, GI perforation, neutropenia, anemia, agranulocytosis, inhibition of platelet aggregation, acute renal failure.

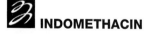 **INDOMETHACIN**

Classification: Cardiovascular agent.
Indications: Pharmacologic alternative to surgical closure of PDA.
Dosage/administration: (see Table A.18)
Intravenous dosing only—oral dosing not recommended. Give by intravenous syringe pump over >30 minutes, three doses/course with a usual maximum of two courses, given at 12 to 24 hour intervals. Some infants require a longer treatment course (0.2 mg/kg every 24 hours for 5–7 days).
Clinical considerations: Hold enteral feeds until 12 hours after last indomethacin dose.
Contraindications: Impaired renal function (BUN >30 mg/dL, urine output <0.6 mL/kg/hour for preceding 8 hours, and creatinine >0.8 mg/dL), active bleeding, ulcer disease, NEC or stool hema test >3+, platelet count <60,000/ mm³, and coagulation defects.

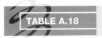
TABLE A.18

Age at first dose	First dose (mg/kg/dose IV)	Second dose (mg/kg/dose IV)	Third dose (mg/kg/dose IV)
<48 h	0.2	0.1	0.1
2–7 d	0.2	0.2	0.2
>7 d	0.2	0.25	0.25
IV = intravenous.			

Precautions: Use with caution in neonates with cardiac dysfunction and hypertension. Because indomethacin causes a decrease in renal and GI blood flow, withhold enteral feedings during therapy. Reduction in cerebral flow reported with intravenous infusions of <5 minutes' duration.

Monitoring: Urine output (keep >0.6 mL/kg/hour), serum electrolytes, serum BUN and creatinine, platelet count. Closely assess pulse pressure, cardiopulmonary status, and PDA murmur for evidence of success/failure of therapy. Guaiac all stools and test gastric aspirates to detect GI bleeding. Observe for prolonged bleeding from puncture sites.

Drug interactions: Concurrent administration with digoxin and/or with aminoglycosides results in increased plasma concentrations of these respective agents.

Adverse reactions: Decreased platelet aggregation, ulcer, GI intolerance, hemolytic anemia, bone marrow suppression, agranulocytosis, thrombocytopenia, ileal perforation, transient oliguria, electrolyte imbalance, hypertension, hypoglycemia, indirect hyperbilirubinemia, and hepatitis.

 INSULIN, REGULAR

Classification: Pancreatic hormone, hypoglycemic agent.

Indication: Hyperglycemia, hyperkalemia.

Dosage/administration: (see Table A.19)
For intravenous bolus and intravenous infusion, use regular human insulin. Mix 15 units regular insulin in 150 mL intravenous bag NS or dextrose 5% water (D5W) = 10 U/100 mL or 0.1 U/mL. Maximum recommended concentration is 1 U/mL.

Monitoring: Follow blood glucose concentration every 30 minutes to 1 hour after starting infusion and after changes in infusion rate. Follow these parameters every 2 to 4 hours after achieving a stable euglycemic state.

Clinical considerations: Reduce loss of insulin that is due to adsorption to the plastic tubing by flushing tubing with minimum of 25 mL of insulin solution before beginning the infusion.

Precaution: Only regular insulin may be administered intravenously.

Adverse reactions: Hyperglycemic rebound, urticaria, anaphylaxis; may rapidly induce hypoglycemia. Insulin resistance may develop with prolonged use and necessitate an increased dose.

 LEVOTHYROXINE SODIUM

Classification: Thyroid hormone.

Indications: Replacement or supplementary therapy for hypothyroidism.

Dosage/administration: To avoid differences in bioavailability, use the same brand of thyroid hormone (100 mg levothyroxine = 65 mg thyroid USP).

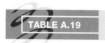

TABLE A.19

Indication	Dosage	Administration	Comment
Bolus	0.05–0.1 U/kg q4–6h PRN	Give as IV bolus	Monitor glucose every 30 min
Continuous IV infusion	0.05–0.2 U/kg/h	If BG remains >180 mg/dL, titrate in increments of 0.01 U/kg/h If hypoglycemia occurs, D/C insulin infusion and give D10W at 2 mL/kg (0.2 g/kg)	Before start of infusion, purge IV tubing with minimum of 25 mL of the infusion solution to saturate plastic binding sites. Titrate to maintain euglycemia
Hyperkalemia	First administer calcium gluconate 50 mg/kg/dose IV then sodium bicarbonate 1 mEq/kg/dose IV Calcium gluconate *is not compatitbile* with NaHCO₃ Flush IV lines between infusions	Follow with dextrose 300–600 mg/kg/dose + regular insulin 0.2 U/kg/dose IV	May repeat dose in 30 to 60 minutes or begin dextrose infusion at 0.25 g/kg/h with regular insulin 0.1 U/kg/h. g/kg/h with regula insulin 0.1 U/kg/h

IV = intravenously; PRN = as needed; BG = blood glucose; D/C = discontinue; q4–6h = every 4 to 6 hours.

Initial oral dose: 10 to 15 µg/kg/day every 24 hours; adjust in 12.5-µg increments every 2 weeks until T_4 is 10 to 15 µg/dL and thyroid-stimulating hormone (TSH) is <15 mU/L.

Maintenance dose: Term infant 37.5 to 50 µg/day. Administer oral dose on an empty stomach.

Initial intravenous dose: 5 to 10 µg/kg/day, every 24 hours, increase every 2 weeks by 5 to 10 µg. When switching from oral to intravenous, intravenous dose should be 80% of the oral dose/day. Use only NS to reconstitute intravenous preparations. Use immediately after mixing. Do not add to any other solution. Usual concentration for infusion is 20 to 40 µg/mL. Maximum concentration for infusion is 100 µg/mL. Administer as a slow push. May also be given intramuscularly.

Clinical considerations: Oral route preferred: use intravenous when oral route unavailable or with myxedema stupor/coma.

Contraindications: Thyrotoxicosis and uncorrected adrenal insufficiency.

Precautions: Use with caution in infants receiving anticoagulants. In infants with cardiac disease, begin with one-fourth of usual maintenance dose and increase weekly. Do not use the intravenous form orally because it crystallizes when exposed to acid. **Do not administer iron or zinc within 4 hours of levothyroxine dose.**

Monitoring: Adjust dosage based on clinical status and serum T_4 and TSH. Serum T_4 and TSH levels should be measured every 1 to 2 months or 2 to 3 weeks after any change in dose. Obtain serum T_4, free T_4 index, and TSH levels. Adequate therapy should suppress TSH values to 15 mU/L within 3 to 4 months of starting therapy. Assess for signs of hypothyroidism: lethargy, poor feeding, constipation, intermittent cyanosis, and prolonged neonatal jaundice. Also closely assess for signs of thyrotoxicosis: hyperreactivity, tachycardia, tachypnea, fever, exophthalmos, and goiter. Periodically assess growth and bone-age development.

Adverse reactions: Hyperthyroidism, rash, weight loss, diarrhea, tachycardia, cardiac arrhythmias, tremors, fever, and hair loss. Prolonged over treatment can produce premature craniosynostosis and acceleration of bone age.

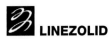 **LINEZOLID**

Classification: Antibiotic, oxazolidinone.
Indications: Treatment of bacteremia caused by susceptible vancomycin-resistant *Enterococcus faecium* (VREF).
Dosage/administration: 10 mg/kg/dose IV/PO q8h. Preterm newborns <7 days old: 10 mg/kg/dose IV/PO q12h. Infuse IV dose over >60 minutes.
Precautions: There have been reports of vancomycin-resistant *E. faecium* and *Staphilococcus aureus* (methicillin-resistant) developing resistance to linezolid during its clinical use.
Monitoring: CBC; platelet counts and hemoglobin, particularly in patients at increased risk for bleeding, patients with pre-existing thrombocytopenia or myelosuppression, or concomitant medications that decrease platelet count or function or produce bone marrow suppression, and inpatients requiring >2 weeks of therapy; number and type of stools/day for diarrhea.
Adverse reactions: Elevated ALT; diarrhea; thrombocytopenia, anemia.

 LORAZEPAM

Classification: Benzodiazepine, anticonvulsant, sedative hypnotic.
Indication: Status epilepticus refractory to conventional therapy.
Dosage/administration:
Initial dose: 0.05 to 0.1 mg/kg/dose, intravenously over >5 minutes; repeat in 10 to 15 minutes if necessary.
Maximum dose: 4 mg/dose.
Maintenance dose: 0.05 mg/kg/dose intravenously/intramuscularly/orally/rectally, every 6 to 24 hours, depending on response. Reduce dosage in hepatic or renal impairment. The intravenous formulation may be given orally. May administer with feeds to decrease GI distress.
Contraindications: Pre-existing CNS depression or severe hypotension.
Warning: Stereotypic movements have been observed in preterm infants.
Precautions: Some preparations contain 2% benzyl alcohol and may be hazardous to neonates in high doses. Dilute before intravenous use with equal volume of NS or sterile water (to minimize benzyl alcohol content). Use with caution in infants with renal or hepatic impairment or myasthenia gravis.
Monitoring: Respiratory status during and after administration.
Adverse reactions: CNS depression, bradycardia, circulatory collapse, respiratory depression, BP instability, and GI symptoms. Discontinue therapy if syncope and paradoxic CNS stimulation occur.

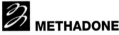 **METHADONE**

Classification: Narcotic, analgesic.
Indications: Treatment of neonatal opiate withdrawal.
Dosage/administration:
Initial dose: 0.05 to 0.2 mg/kg/dose, oral or slow intravenous push, every 12 to 24 hours. Titrate dose based on neonatal abstinence score (NAS). Wean dose by 10% to 20%/week over a 4 to 6 week period.
Clinical considerations: Tapering is difficult because of its long elimination half-life. Consider alternative agents. Reserve for use in infants born to methadone-treated mothers only.
Monitoring: Respiratory and cardiac status.
Drug interactions: Methadone metabolism accelerated by rifampin and phenytoin; this may precipitate withdrawal symptoms.
Adverse reactions: Respiratory depression, ileus, delayed gastric emptying.

METOCLOPRAMIDE

Classification: Antiemetic, prokinetic agent.
Indications: Improve gastric emptying and GI motility.
Dosage/administration: GI dysmotility: 0.4 to 0.8 mg/kg/day divided every 6 hours intravenously/orally; orally administer 30 minutes before feeds. Orally available as 0.1 mg/mL and 1 mg/mL. Administer intravenous over >30 minutes on syringe pump. Maximum concentration for intravenous infusion is 5 mg/mL (usual concentration: 1 mg/mL) in NS or dextrose. Intravenous form may be given orally.
Contraindications: GI obstruction, pheochromocytoma, history of seizure disorder.
Monitoring: Measure gastric residuals.
Adverse reactions: Drowsiness, restlessness, agitation, diarrhea, methemoglobinemia, and extrapyramidal symptoms (usually occur following intravenous administration of large doses and within 24 to 48 hours of starting therapy; responds rapidly to Benadryl and subsides within 24 hours after stopping metoclopramide).
Overdose: Associated with doses greater than 1 mg/kg/day, characterized by drowsiness, ataxia, extrapyramidal reactions, seizures, and methemoglobinemia (treat with methylene blue).

 MIDAZOLAM

Classification: Benzodiazepine, sedative hypnotic, anticonvulsant.
Indications: Sedation.
Dosage/administration: 0.05 to 0.15 mg/kg/dose every 2 to 4 hours as needed. Infuse over >15 minutes on syringe pump. Final infusion concentration is 0.5 mg/mL in NS or dextrose.
Contraindications: Pre-existing CNS depression or shock.
Precautions: CHF and renal impairment. Some formulations may contain 1% benzyl alcohol (minimize neonate exposure by diluting the 5 mg/mL concentration to 0.5 mg/mL).
Monitoring: RR, heart rate, BP.
Drug interactions: CNS depressants, anesthetic agents, cimetidine, and theophylline. Decrease midazolam dose by 25% during prolonged concurrent narcotic administration.
Adverse reactions: Sedation, respiratory depression, apnea, cardiac arrest, hypotension, bradycardia, and seizures (following rapid bolus administration and in neonates with underlying CNS disorders). Encephalopathy reported in several infants sedated for 4 to 11 days with midazolam and fentanyl.

 MILRINONE

Classification: Phosphodiesterase inhibitor.
Indications: Effective inotropic agent indicated for the short-term intravenous treatment of CHF. In infants with decreased myocardial function, milrinone increases cardiac output, decreases pulmonary capillary wedge pressure, and decreases vascular resistance. It increases myocardial contractility and improves diastolic function by improving left ventricular diastolic relaxation.
Dosage/administration: Milrinone is administered with a loading dose followed by a continuous infusion.
Loading dose: 50 μg/kg administered through syringe pump over >20 minutes **(Loading doses are generally not given to newborn infants).**
Maintenance dose: 0.25 to 0.5 μg/kg/minute. Titrate dose to effect.
Maximum infusion rate: 1 μg/kg/minute. Usual concentration for infusion is 100 μg/mL. Maximum is 250 μg/mL in NS or dextrose. Central line preferred. **Do not administer through UAC.**
Monitoring parameters: EKG, BP, CBC, electrolytes. Volume expanders may be needed to counteract the vasodilatory effect and potential decrease in filling pressures.

Adverse effects: Thrombocytopenia, arrhythmias, hypotension.

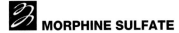 **MORPHINE SULFATE**

Classification: Opiate, narcotic analgesic.
Indication: Analgesia, sedation, treatment of opiate withdrawal.
Dosage/administration: (see Tables A.20, A.21)

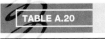

For NAS score	Initial oral dose
8–10	0.32 mg (0.8 mL)/kg/d divided q4h
11–13	0.48 mg (1.2 mL)/kg/d divided q4h
14–16	0.64 mg (1.6 mL)/kg/d divided q4h
>17	0.8 mg (2 mL)/kg/d divided q4h

NAS = neonatal abstinence score; q4h = every 4 hours.

TABLE A.21

For NAS score	Maintenance oral dose
>8 × 3 successive scores	↑ dose by 0.16 mg (0.4 mL)/kg/d divided q4h to max dose
<8 × 3 successive scores	Wean by 10% of the max daily dose. If infant has been weaned too quickly, go back to last effective dose

NAS = neonatal abstinence score; q4h = every 4 hours; ↑ = increasing.

Analgesia/sedation: 0.05 mg/kg/dose intravenously/intramuscularly/subcutaneously every 4 to 8 hours as needed for pain. Administer bolus over >5 minutes on syringe pump.
Continuous intravenous infusion: 0.01 to 0.02 mg/kg/hour. Use only preservative-free formulation.
Concentration for administration: 0.1–to 1 mg/mL in NS or dextrose. **Treatment of opiate withdrawal (Use only 0.4 mg/mL preservative-free morphine concentration)**
If NASs are too low, make sure that the infant is not obtunded because of overdosage. Discontinue when dose is <25% of maximum dose. Administration of oral morphine solution with food may increase bioavailability.
Precautions: Fentanyl is preferred over morphine in neonates with cardiovascular and hemodynamic instability. Morphine causes histamine release leading to increased venous capacitance and suppression of adrenergic tone. Hypotension and chest wall rigidity may occur with rapid intravenous administration. Tolerance may develop following prolonged use (>96 hours).
Contraindications: Increased intracranial pressure. Use with caution in severe hepatic, renal impairment, NEC.
Adverse reactions: Hypotension, respiratory depression, constipation, and urinary retention. Naloxone should be available to reverse adverse effects.

Monitoring: Monitor RR, heart rate, and BP closely; observe for abdominal distention and loss of bowel sounds; monitor input and output to evaluate urinary retention.

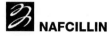 **NAFCILLIN**

Classification: Semisynthetic penicillinase-resistant antistaphylococcal penicillin.
Indications: Primarily active against *staphylococci*. Reserve for penicillin-resistant *S. aureus* infections.
Dosage/administration: (see Table A.22)

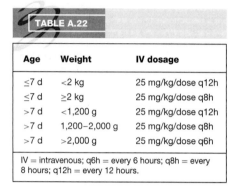

TABLE A.22		
Age	**Weight**	**IV dosage**
≤7 d	<2 kg	25 mg/kg/dose q12h
≤7 d	≥2 kg	25 mg/kg/dose q8h
>7 d	<1,200 g	25 mg/kg/dose q12h
>7 d	1,200–2,000 g	25 mg/kg/dose q8h
>7 d	>2,000 g	25 mg/kg/dose q6h
IV = intravenous; q6h = every 6 hours; q8h = every 8 hours; q12h = every 12 hours.		

Intravenous: Final concentration of 100 mg/mL infused over >30 minutes on syringe pump (see Table A.19).
Precautions: Dosing interval increased with hepatic dysfunction. Oral route not recommended because of poor absorption. Avoid intramuscular administration if possible.
Monitoring: CBC, BUN, creatinine, and LFTs. Observe for hematuria and proteinuria.
Clinical considerations: Better cerebrospinal fluid penetration than methicillin. Decrease dose by 33% to 50% in infants with combined renal/hepatic impairment.
Drug interactions: Blunting of peak aminoglycoside concentration when administered simultaneously with nafcillin.
Adverse reactions: Agranulocytosis hypersensitivity, granulocytopenia, and nephrotoxicity (eosinophilia may precede renal damage). Treat extravasation with hyaluronidase.

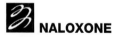 **NALOXONE**

Classification: Narcotic antagonist.
Indications: Used concurrently during neonatal resuscitation for narcotic-induced CNS depression.
Dosage/administration: 0.1 mg/kg bolus intravenously/endotracheally/intramuscularly/subcutaneously. May repeat every 3 to 5 minutes if no response. Multiple doses may be necessary because of its short duration of action. Intravenous or endotracheal tube route preferred, intramuscular or SC route may lead to delayed onset of action.
Contraindications: Use with caution in infants with chronic cardiac disease, pulmonary disease, or coronary disease. Do not administer to newborns of narcotic dependent mothers, as it may precipitate seizures.
Adverse reactions: Will produce narcotic withdrawal syndrome in newborns with chronic dependence. Abrupt reversal may result in vomiting, diaphoresis, tachycardia, hypertension, and tremors.
Monitoring: Heart rate, respiratory rate, BP.

NOREPINEPHRINE

Classification: Adrenergic agonist agent, α-adrenergic agonist, sympathomimetic.
Indications: Treatment of shock which persists after adequate fluid volume replacement; severe hypotension; cardiogenic shock.
Dosage/administration:
Initial: 0.05 to 0.1 μg/kg/minute, titrate to desired effect; maximum dose: 1 to 2 μg/kg/minute Central **venous access is preferred. Do not administer through UAC**.
Precautions: Blood/volume depletion should be corrected, if possible, before norepinephrine therapy; extravasation may cause severe tissue necrosis; do not give to patients with peripheral or mesenteric vascular thrombosis because ischemia may be increased and the area of infarct extended; use with caution in patients with occlusive vascular disease.
Monitoring: BP, heart rate, urine output, peripheral perfusion.
Adverse reactions: Cardiac arrhythmias, bradycardia, tachycardia, hypertension, pallor; Organ ischemia (due to vasoconstriction of renal and mesenteric arteries), ischemic necrosis and sloughing of superficial tissue after extravasation.

 NYSTATIN

Classification: Nonabsorbed antifungal agent.
Indications: Treatment of susceptible cutaneous, mucocutaneous, and oropharyngeal fungal infections caused by *Candida* species.
Dosage/administration:
Oral: Preterm infant: 0.5 mL (50,000 U) every 6 hours. Term infant: 1 mL (100,000 U) every 6 hours. Apply suspension with swab to each side of mouth every 6 hours after feedings.
Topical therapy: Apply ointment or cream to affected area every 6 hours. Continue oral therapy and topical application for 3 days beyond resolution of fungal infection. Breastfeeding mothers should be concurrently treated topically.
Clinical considerations: Combination therapy for candidal perineal infections with oral and topical nystatin is possible because of nystatin's poor absorption in the GI tract and because the GI tract serves as the reservoir for fungi causing perineal infection. Eliminate factors contributing to fungal growth (wet, occlusive diapers and the use of contaminated nipples).
Adverse reactions: Irritation, contact dermatitis, diarrhea, and vomiting.

 OCTREOTIDE

Classification: Antisecretory agent, somatostatin analog.
Indications: Pharmacologic management of persistent hyperinsulinemic hypoglycemia of infancy (nesidioblastosis), adjunct treatment of congenital and postoperative chylothorax.
Dosage/administration: Hyperinsulinemic hypoglycemia : 2 to 10 μg/kg/day initially divided every 12 hours; increase dosage depending upon patient response by either using a more frequent interval (every 6–8 hours) or larger dose.
Maximum dose: 10 μg/kg/dose q6 hours.
Chylothorax: 1 to 7 μg/kg/hour continuous infusion; titrate dose to effect (decreased chyle production).
Precautions: Glucose tolerance; use with caution in patients with renal impairment. suppression of growth hormone with long-term therapy.
Monitoring: Cholelithiasis, blood sugar, thyroid function tests, fluid and electrolyte balance, fecal fat.
Adverse reactions: Hypoglycemia, hyperglycemia, galactorrhea, hypothyroidism, flushing, edema, hypertension, palpitations, CHF, bradycardia, arrhythmias, conduction abnormalities, diarrhea, constipation, fat malabsorption.

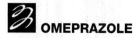

OMEPRAZOLE

Classification: Proton-pump inhibitor; gastric acid secretion inhibitor, GI agent, gastric or duodenal ulcer treatment.

Indications: Short-term (<8 weeks) treatment of documented reflux esophagitis or duodenal ulcer refractory to conventional therapy.

Dosage/administration: 0.5 to 1.5 mg/kg/dose orally, through nasogastric tube, or jejunostomy tube daily for 4 to 8 weeks. Maximum effective dose = 3.5 mg/kg/day divided BID.

Precautions: Mild transaminase elevations have been reported in children who received omeprazole for extended periods of time. Use with caution in infants with respiratory alkalosis due to high content of sodium bicarbonate in the oral suspension; avoid use in infants on sodium restriction.

Contraindications: Hypersensitivity to omeprazole or any component.

Adverse reactions: Tachycardia, bradycardia, palpitations, altered sleeping patterns, hemifacial dysesthesia, fever, irritability, dry skin, rash, hypoglycemia, diarrhea, vomiting, constipation, discoloration of feces, feeding intolerance because of anorexia, irritable colon, urinary frequency, agranulocytosis, pancytopenia, thrombocytopenia, anorexia, leukocytosis, hepatitis, increased LFTs, jaundice, hematuria, pyuria, proteinuria, glycosuria, cough, and epistaxis. Use of H-2 blockade in VLBW infants has been associated with a higher risk of NEC in VLBW infants; omeprazole has not been studied.

Monitoring: Observe for symptomatic improvement within 3 days. Edema, hypertension, weight gain, metabolic alkalosis. Consider esophageal pH monitoring to assess for efficacy (pH >4). Aspartate aminotransferase/ALT if duration of therapy is >8 weeks.

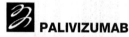

PALIVIZUMAB

Classification: A humanized monoclonal antibody to respiratory syncytial virus (RSV).

Indications: Prophylaxis for the prevention of RSV in high-risk infants; infants <6 months of age with a history of prematurity (<32 weeks' gestational age) or <24 months of age with chronic lung disease (CLD).

Dosage/administration: 15 mg/kg/dose intramuscularly, given every 30 days for up to five doses during the RSV season (i.e., October/November through March/April).

Precautions: History of hypersensitivity related to the use of other immunoglobulin preparations, blood products, or other medications. Efficacy has not been demonstrated in the treatment of established RSV infection. Give with caution to patients with thrombocytopenia or any coagulation disorder. Not recommended for children with cyanotic congenital heart disease.

Adverse effects: Vomiting, diarrhea, rash, rhinitis, and erythema and moderate induration at the injection site.

PANCURONIUM BROMIDE

Classification: Nondepolarizing neuromuscular blocking agent.

Indications: Skeletal muscle relaxation, increased pulmonary compliance during mechanical ventilation, facilitate endotracheal intubation.

Dosage/administration: 0.05 to 0.1 mg/kg/dose intravenously (may be administered undiluted by slow intravenous push) every 1 to 4 hours as needed.

Precautions: Pre-existing pulmonary, hepatic, or renal impairment. In neonates with myasthenia gravis, small doses of pancuronium may have profound effects (may need to decrease dosage).

Monitoring: Continuous cardiac, BP monitoring, assisted ventilation status. Because sensation remains intact, administer concurrent sedation and analgesia as needed. Apply ophthalmic lubricant.

Factors influencing duration of neuromuscular blockade: (see Table A.23)

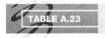

TABLE A.23

Potentiation	Antagonism
Acidosis, hypothermia, neuromuscular disease, hepatic disease, renal failure, cardiovascular disease, aminoglycosides, succinylcholine, hypermagnesemia, and hypokalemia- or potassium-depleting drugs (e.g., amphotericin-B, corticosteroids), diuretics, clindamycin	Pyridostigmine, neostigmine, or edrophonium in conjunction with atropine, alkalosis, epinephrine, theophylline, hyperkalemia

Adverse reactions: Tachycardia, hypertension, hypotension, excessive salivation, rashes, bronchospasm.
Antidote: Neostigmine 0.025 mg/kg intravenously (with atropine 0.02 mg/kg).

PENICILLIN G PREPARATIONS

Classification: Antibiotic.
Indications: Treatment of neonatal meningitis and bacteremia, group B streptococcal infections, and congenital syphilis.
Dosage/administration: Intramuscularly, intravenously (intravenous route is preferred to avoid muscle fibrosis and atrophy). Only aqueous Penicillin G should be used intravenously. Final concentration for intravenous infusion is 50,000 U/mL infused >30 minutes on syringe pump. When treating bacteremia, use the meningitis dose until meningitis is ruled out.
Group B streptococcal infections:
Bacteremia: 200,000 U/kg/day in divided doses every 6 hours.
Meningitis: 400,000 U/kg/day in divided doses every 6 hours.
Infections due to other organisms: (see Table A.24)
Dosages: Bacteremia: 50,000 U/kg/dose; Meningitis: 100,000 U/kg/dose

TABLE A.24

Postmenstrual age	Postnatal age	Frequency
≤29 wk	0–4 wk	q12h
≤29 wk	>4 wk	q8h
30–36 wk	0–2 wk	q12h
30–36 wk	>2 wk	q8h
37–44 wk	0–1 wk	q8h
>45 wk	All	q6h

q6h = every 6 hours; q8h = every 8 hours; q12h = every 12 hours.

Monitoring: Serum potassium and sodium for renal failure and high-dose therapy. Weekly CBC, BUN, creatinine.

Precautions: Dosage adjustment for renal failure. Use only aqueous penicillin G for intravenous administration.

Drug interactions: Blunting of peak aminoglycoside serum concentration if administered simultaneously with Penicillin G preparations.

Test interactions: Positive direct Coombs' test.

Adverse reactions: Bone marrow suppression, granulocytopenia, anaphylaxis, hemolytic anemia, interstitial nephritis, Jarisch–Herxheimer reaction, change in bowel flora (Candida superinfection, diarrhea), CNS toxicity.

 PHENOBARBITAL

Classification: Anticonvulsant, sedative, hypnotic.

Indications: Drug of choice to control neonatal seizures. Management of withdrawal, direct hyperbilirubinemia, cholestasis.

Dosage/administration:

Seizures: Loading dose: 20 mg/kg/dose, administer intravenous loading dose over >15 minutes (<1 mg/kg/minute) on syringe pump. Administer additional doses of 5 mg/kg every 5 minutes until cessation of seizures or a total dose of 40 mg/kg is administered. Use the intravenous route if possible because of unreliable intramuscular absorption. Maintenance therapy: 3 to 5 mg/kg/day intravenously/intramuscularly/orally daily. Begin maintenance therapy 24 hours after loading dose. Parenteral dose preferred for seriously ill neonate.

Cholestasis: 4 to 5 mg/kg/day, intravenously/intramuscularly/orally for 4 to 5 days.

Neonatal withdrawal syndrome: Administer loading dose, then titrate based on NAS. Loading dose: 15 to 20 mg/kg/dose. Closely follow blood levels after stabilization of abstinence symptoms for 24 to 48 hours, decrease the daily dose by 10% to 20%/day (see Table A.25).

TABLE A.25

Neonatal abstinence score	Dosage
8–10	6 mg/kg/d divided q8h
11–13	8 mg/kg/d divided q8h
14–16	10 mg/kg/d divided q8h
>17	12 mg/kg/d divided q8h
q8h = every 8 hours.	

Clinical considerations:

Direct hyperbilirubinemia: More effective in full-term infants.

Neonatal withdrawal syndrome: Avoid using in infants with GI symptoms.

Warnings: Abrupt discontinuation in infants with seizures may precipitate status seizures.

Precautions: Hepatic or renal impairment.

Monitoring: Therapeutic serum concentration: 15 to 40 μg/mL. Obtain trough levels just before the next dose. Monitor respiratory status.

Drug interactions: Benzodiazepines, primidone, warfarin, corticosteroids, and doxycycline. Increased serum concentrations with concurrent phenytoin or valproate.

Adverse reactions: Respiratory depression (with serum concentrations >60 μg/mL), hypotension, circulatory collapse, paradoxical excitement, megaloblastic anemia, hepatitis, and exfoliative dermatitis. Sedation reported at serum concentrations >40 μg/mL.

PHENTOLAMINE MESYLATE

Classification: Extravasation antidote, vasodilator, α-adrenergic blocking agent.
Indication: Local treatment of dermal necrosis caused by extravasation of vasoconstrictive agents (e.g., dopamine, dobutamine, epinephrine, norepinephrine, and phenylephrine).
Dosage/administration: 0.1 mg/kg do not exceed 2.5 mg total. Using a 25- to 30-gauge needle, inject 0.2 mL of solution (made by diluting 2.5–5 mg in 10 mL of preservative-free NS) subcutaneously at five separate sites around edge of infiltration; change needle between each skin entry. Repeat if necessary. Best results if used within 12 hours after extravasation occurrence.
Clinical considerations: Topical 2% nitroglycerin ointment may be used for significantly swollen extremity.
Contraindications: Renal impairment.
Precautions: Gastritis or peptic ulcer.
Monitoring: Assess affected area for reversal of ischemia. Closely monitor BP, heart rate/rhythm.
Adverse reactions: Hypotension, tachycardia, arrhythmias, nasal congestion, vomiting, diarrhea, exacerbation of peptic ulcer.

 PHENYTOIN

Classification: Anticonvulsant.
Indication: Treatment of seizures that are refractory to phenobarbital.
Dosage/administration:
Loading dose: 15 to 20 mg/kg/intravenous infusion on syringe pump over >30 minutes. Dilute to 5 mg/mL with NS. Use a 0.22-μm in-line filter. Start infusion immediately after preparation. Observe for precipitates. **Avoid using in central lines because of the risk of precipitation. If must use a central line, then flush catheter with 1 to 3 mL normal saline before and after administration because of heparin incompatibility**.
Maintenance dose: 4 to 8 mg/kg every 24 hours intravenous infusion on syringe pump over >30 minutes. Maintenance doses usually start 12 hours after loading dose. Avoid intramuscular route because of erratic absorption, pain on injection, and precipitation of drug at injection site.
Precautions: Rapid intravenous administration has resulted in hypotension, cardiovascular collapse, and CNS depression. May cause local irritation, inflammation, necrosis, and sloughing with or without signs of infiltration.
Contraindications: Heart block, sinus bradycardia.
Adverse reactions: Hypersensitivity reaction, arrhythmias, hypotension, hyperglycemia, cardiovascular collapse, liver damage, blood dyscrasias; extravasation may cause tissue necrosis. Treat with hyaluronidase around the periphery of affected site.
Monitoring: Heart rate, rhythm, hypotension during infusion.
Monitoring parameters: Obtain trough level 48 hours after intravenous loading dose. Therapeutic serum concentration: 8 to 15 μg/mL.

 RANITIDINE

Classification: Histamine-2 antagonist.
Indications: Duodenal and gastric ulcers, gastroesophageal reflux, and hypersecretory conditions.
Dosage/administration: Oral dose: 6 mg/kg/day orally divided in three to four doses.
Intravenous dose: 0.5 mg/kg/dose intravenously every 6 hours infused over 30 minutes on syringe pump. Usual concentration for infusion is 1 mg/mL mixed with dextrose or NS. Maximum concentration for intravenous infusion is 2.5 mg/mL.

Continuous intravenous dose: 0.0625 mg/kg/hour. Titrate dose to maintain a gastric pH >4.

Clinical considerations: Because of the absence of possible endocrine toxicity and drug interactions, ranitidine is preferred over cimetidine. Ranitidine effectively increases gastric pH. Increased gastric pH may promote the development of gastric colonization with pathogenic bacteria or yeast.

Precautions: Use with caution in infants with liver and renal impairment. Intravenous formulation contains 0.5% phenol; no short-term toxicity has been reported. Manufacturer's oral solution contains 7.5% alcohol.

Drug interactions: May increase serum levels of theophylline, warfarin, and procainamide.

Monitoring: Monitor gastric pH to assess ranitidine efficacy.

Adverse reactions: GI disturbance, sedation, thrombocytopenia, hepatotoxicity, vomiting, bradycardia, or tachycardia. Use of H-2 blockade in VLBW infants has been associated with a higher risk of NEC.

 SODIUM BICARBONATE

Classification: Alkalinizing agent.

Indications: Treatment of documented or assumed metabolic acidosis during prolonged resuscitation after establishment of effective ventilation. Treatment of bicarbonate deficit caused by renal or GI losses. Adjunctive treatment of hyperkalemia.

Dose/administration:

Replacement: Infuse over >20 to 30 minutes on syringe pump.

Resuscitation: 1 to 2 mEq/kg intravenous slow push over at least 2 minutes.

Correction of metabolic acidosis: HCO_3 needed (mEq) = HCO_3 deficit (mEq/L) × (0.3 × body weight [kg]). Administer half of calculated dose, then assess need for remainder. Usual concentration for infusion is 0.5 mEq/mL; maximum concentration is 1 mEq/mL.

For continuous intravenous infusion: Use 50 mEq sodium bicarbonate (8.4% concentration) and add to 50 mL of appropriate diluent (e.g, dextrose, maximum 10%; NS; or sterile water). Concentration is 0.5 mEq/mL. Maximum infusion rate for continuous intravenous administration is 1 mEq/kg/h.

Precautions: Rapid injection of hypertonic sodium bicarbonate (1 mEq/mL) solution has been linked to cerebral hemorrhage.

Adverse effects: Pulmonary edema, respiratory acidosis, local tissue necrosis, hypocalcemia, hypernatremia, metabolic alkalosis.

Monitoring: Follow acid–base status; arterial blood gases; serum electrolytes, including calcium; and urinary pH. Use hyaluronidase to treat intravenous extravasation.

 SPIRONOLACTONE

Classification: Potassium-sparing diuretic.

Indications: Mild diuretic with potassium-sparing effects. Used in conjunction with thiazide diuretics in the treatment of CHF, hypertension, edema, and BPD when prolonged diuresis is desirable.

Dosage/administration: 1 to 3 mg/kg/day orally divided every 12 hours.

BPD therapy: Chlorothiazide, 20 mg/kg/dose orally every 12 hours for 8 weeks, plus spironolactone 1.5 mg/kg/dose orally every 12 hours for 8 weeks.

Clinical considerations: Offers no additional benefit when included as part of the regimen to treat BPD.

Contraindications: Renal failure, anuria, hyperkalemia.

Monitoring: Serum and urine potassium.

Drug interactions: May potentiate ganglionic blocking agents and other antihypertensive agents.

Adverse reactions: Hyperkalemia, vomiting, diarrhea, hyperchloremic metabolic acidosis, dehydration, hyponatremia.

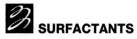 **SURFACTANTS**

Classification: Natural, animal-derived exogenous surfactant agent.
Indications: prophylaxis: Infants with high risk for RDS, defined in clinical trials as a birth-weight <1,250 g, and larger infants with evidence of pulmonary immaturity.
Rescue therapy: Infants with moderate to severe RDS, defined in clinical trials as requirement for mechanical ventilation and fractional concentraton of inspired oxygen (FIO_2) higher than 40%. Treatment of full-term infants with respiratory failure that is due to meconium aspiration, pneumonia, or persistent pulmonary hypertension.
Dosage/administration: (see Table A.26)

 TABLE A.26

Surfactant	Doses	Comments
Beractant (Survanta)	4 mL/kg/dose	Divided into four aliquots, with up to three additional doses (four total), administered q6h if needed
Calfactant (Infasurf)	3 mL/kg/dose	Divided into two aliquots, with up to three additional doses, administered q12h if needed
Poractant alfa (Curosurf)	Initial dose = 2.5 mL/kg/dose Subsequent doses = 1.25 mL/kg/dose	Divided into two aliquots, followed by up to two additional doses of 1.25 mL/kg/dose, administered q12h if needed
q6h = every 6 hours; q12h = every 12 hours.		

Administered intratracheally by instillation into a 5-French end-hole catheter inserted into the infant's endotracheal tube with the tip of the catheter protruding just beyond the end of the endotracheal tube and above the infant's carina.
Prophylactic therapy: Intratracheally as soon as possible after birth.
Rescue therapy: Intratracheally immediately following the diagnosis of RDS.
Clinical considerations: Suction endotracheal tube before administration. Delay suctioning postadministration as long as possible (minimum of 1 hour).
Monitoring: Assess endotracheal tube patency and correct anatomic location before administration of surfactant. Monitor oxygen saturation and heart rate continuously during administration of doses. After administration of each dose, monitor arterial blood gases frequently to detect and correct postdose abnormalities of ventilation and oxygenation.
Precautions: A videotape demonstrating surfactant administration procedure is available from Ross Laboratories and Forest Laboratories and should be viewed before use of their products.
Adverse reactions: Transient bradycardia, hypoxemia, pallor, vasoconstriction, hypotension, endotracheal tube blockage, hypercapnia, apnea, and hypertension may occur during the administration process.

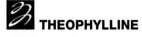 **THEOPHYLLINE**

Classification: Bronchodilator, respiratory stimulant.
Indications: Apnea.
Dosage/administration:
Loading dose: 5 mg/kg/dose orally.

Maintenance dose: 6 mg/kg/day orally, divided every 6 to 8 hours. Start 6 to 8 hours after loading dose. For intravenous use, see Aminophylline.
Contraindications: Uncontrolled arrhythmias, hyperthyroidism.
Clinical considerations: Consider caffeine as first-line agent for apnea of prematurity.
Precautions: Peptic ulcer, hypertension, and compromised cardiac function. Some elixir preparations may contain alcohol.
Drug interactions: Increased theophylline elimination: carbamazepine, isoproterenol, phenytoin, phenobarbital, and rifampin. Decreased theophylline elimination: erythromycin, quinolones, calcium channel blockers, nonselective beta-blockers, and cimetidine.
Monitoring: Heart rate, blood glucose during loading dose, agitation, feeding intolerance. Hold dose if heart rate is greater than 180 beats/ minute.
Therapeutic ranges: Check levels at fifth dose (or before fifth dose if increased number/severity of apnea spells), then every week, or as needed for increased number/severity of apnea spells. Desired serum level in apnea of prematurity is 5 to 15 µg/mL. 1 mg/kg is given for each desired 2 µg/mL increase in serum theophylline level.
Adverse reactions: Vomiting, sinus tachycardia, hyperglycemia, diuresis, dehydration, feeding intolerance, CNS irritability, gastroesophageal reflux, seizures.
Overdosage: Tachycardia, vomiting, seizures, circulatory failure, failure to gain weight, hyperreflexia, encephalopathy.
Theophylline toxicity treatment: Activated charcoal, 1 g/kg slurry through gavage tube every 2 to 4 hours. Sorbitol-containing preparations used for toxicity treatment may cause osmotic diarrhea and should be avoided.

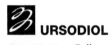

URSODIOL

Classification: Gallstone dissolution agent.
Indications: Facilitates bile excretion in infants with biliary atresia, improves hepatic metabolism of essential fatty acids in infants with cystic fibrosis.
Dosages/administration:
Biliary atresia: 10 mg/kg/dose orally every 12 hours.
Cystic fibrosis: 15 mg/kg/dose orally every 12 hours. Administer with food. Must be refrigerated. Available as a pharmaceutical extemporaneous preparation in concentration of 10 mg/mL or 20 mg/mL oral suspension.
Precautions: Obtain baseline ALT, aspartate aminotransferase, alkaline phosphate, bilirubin.
Contraindications: Use with caution in infants with chronic liver disease.
Adverse reactions: Hepatotoxicity.

VANCOMYCIN HYDROCHLORIDE

Classification: Antibiotic.
Indications: Drug of choice for serious infections caused by methicillin-resistant staphylococci, penicillin-resistant pneumococci, and coagulase-negative *staphylococcus*. The oral route is used for the treatment of *Clostridium difficile*.
Dosage/administration: (see Table A.27)
Intravenous infusion over >60 minutes on syringe pump. Final concentration for infusion is 5 mg/mL. Concentrations >5 mg/mL up to a maximum of 10 mg/mL should be administered centrally. Mix in NS or dextrose.
Precautions: Use with caution in patients with renal impairment or those receiving other nephrotoxic or ototoxic drugs; dosage modification required in patients with impaired renal function.
Adverse reactions: Red neck or red man syndrome (erythema multiform-like reaction with intense pruritus; tachycardia; hypotension; rash involving face, neck, upper trunk, back, and upper arms) usually develops during a rapid infusion of vancomycin or with doses >15 to 20 mg/kg/hour and usually dissipates in 30 to 60 minutes. Lengthening infusion time usually eliminates risk for subsequent doses. Cardiac arrest, fever, chills, eosinophilia,

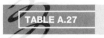

Postnatal age	Weight (kg)	Dose (mg/kg/dose)
<7 d	<1.2 kg	15 mg/kg IV q24h
<7 d	1.2–2 kg	10 mg/kg IV q12h
<7 d	>2 kg	15 mg/kg IV q12h
>7 d	<1.2 kg	15 mg/kg IV q24h
>7 d	1.2–2 kg	15 mg/kg IV q12h
>7 d	>2 kg	10 mg/kg IV q8h

IV = intravenously; q12h = every 12 hours; q24h = every 24 hours; q8h = every 8 hours.

and neutropenia reported after prolonged administration (>3 weeks); phlebitis may be minimized by slow infusion and more dilution of the drug. If extravasation occurs, consider using hyaluronidase around periphery of affected area. Also reported are ototoxicity, enhanced by aminoglycoside therapy and associated with prolonged serum concentration >40 μg/mL, and nephrotoxicity (higher incidence with trough concentrations >10 μg/mL). **Monitoring:** Assess renal function. Therapeutic serum concentrations: Trough 5 to 15 μg/mL. Sample drawn 30 minutes to just before next dose. Peak levels are not clinically significant.

VITAMIN A INJECTION

Classification: Nutritional supplement, fat-soluble vitamin.
Indication: To minimize incidence of CLD in high risk, preterm newborns.
Dosage/administration: 5,000 IU, intramuscularly 3 times/week for 12 doses total. Start within 72 hours of birth in infants with birth weights <1,000 g. Administer with a 25- to 27-gauge needle.
Caution: Do not use concurrently with dexamethasone.
Contraindications: Do not administer intravenously.
Adverse effects: Full fontanel, hepatomegaly, edema, mucocutaneous lesions, bony tenderness.

VITAMIN B₁

Classification: Water-soluble vitamin supplement.
Indications: Treatment of thiamine deficiency (see Table A.28).
Thiamine sources: 1 mL of PolyViSol or ViDaylin supplies 500 μg. Human milk supplies 56 μg/day.
Drug interactions: Thiamine requirements increased with high-carbohydrate diets or high-concentration intravenous dextrose solutions.
Test interactions: Large doses may interfere with spectrophotometric determination of serum theophylline.
Adverse reactions: Allergic reaction, angioedema, and cardiovascular collapse. Severity and frequency of adverse reactions increases with parenteral route of administration.

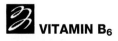

VITAMIN B₆

Classification: Water-soluble vitamin supplement.
Indications: Prevention and treatment of pyridoxine-dependent seizures.

TABLE A.28

Indications	Dosage/administration (for preterm and term infants)
Thiamine RDA	300 mg/d
Thiamine deficiency	Preventive dose 0.5–1 mg/d PO
Thiamine deficiency	Therapeutic dose 5–10 mg/d, divided q6–8h

RDA = recommended daily allowance; PO = orally; q6–8h = every 6 to 8 hours.

Dosage/administration: 50 to 100 mg intravenously over >1 minute, or intramuscularly as a single test dose; followed by 30-minute observation period. Intravenous route is preferred. If response seen, begin maintenance dose of 50 to 100 mg orally every day. The injectable form may be given orally. Mix with feeds if desired.

Monitoring: Electroencephalogram monitoring recommended during initial therapy for pyridoxine-dependent seizures, RR, heart rate, BP.

Precautions: Risk of profound sedation and respiratory depression; ventilatory support may be required.

Adverse reactions: Sedation, increased aspartate aminotransferase, decreased serum folic acid level, allergic reaction. Seizures reported following intravenous administration of very large doses.

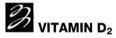 **VITAMIN D$_2$**

Classification: Fat-soluble vitamin.

Indications: Refractory rickets, hypophosphatemia, hypoparathyroidism.

Dosage/administration:

Less than 37 weeks: 10 to 20 μg/day (400–800 IU/day).

37 weeks or more: 10 μg/day (400 IU/day) orally. Administer intramuscularly for fat malabsorption. Ergocalciferol 1.25 mg provides 50,000 IU of vitamin D activity.

Contraindications: Hypercalcemia, evidence of vitamin D toxicity.

Monitoring: Serum calcium, phosphorus, alkaline phosphatase levels. Excessive doses may lead to hypervitaminosis D manifested by hypercalcemia, azotemia, increased serum creatinine, mild hypokalemia, diarrhea, polyuria, metastatic calcification, nephrocalcinosis.

Adverse reactions: Acidosis, polyuria, nephrocalcinosis, hypertension, arrhythmias.

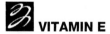 **VITAMIN E**

Classification: Fat-soluble vitamin.

Indications: Prevention and treatment of vitamin E deficiency.

Dosage/administration:

Usual dose: 5 IU orally every day.

Range: 5 to 25 IU orally every day.

Precautions: Aquasol E is very hyperosmolar (3,000 mOsm); a 1:4 dilution with sterile water is required. Poorly absorbed in malabsorption disorders; use water-soluble forms.

Monitoring: Physiologic serum levels for preterm infants are 1 to 2 mg/dL and should be monitored during administration of pharmacologic doses of vitamin E.

Clinical considerations: Requirements for vitamin E increase as the intake of polyunsaturated fatty acids increases.

Adverse reactions: Feeding intolerance, NEC, increased incidence of sepsis.

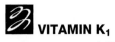 **VITAMIN K₁**

Classification: Fat-soluble vitamin.
Indications: Prevention and treatment of hemorrhagic disease of the newborn, hypoprothrombinemia caused by drug-induced or anticoagulant-induced vitamin K deficiency.
Dosage/administration: Prophylaxis (administered at birth).
Less than 1.5 kg: 0.5 mg intramuscularly/subcutaneously.
1.5 kg or more: 1 mg intramuscularly/subcutaneously.
Warnings: Ineffective in hereditary hypoprothrombinemia or hypoprothrombinemia caused by severe liver disease. Severe hemolytic anemia or hyperbilirubinemia reported in neonates following administration of doses >20 mg. Intramuscular administration not associated with an increased risk of childhood cancer.
Precautions: Despite proper dilution and rate of administration, severe anaphylactoid or hypersensitivity-like reactions (including shock and cardiac/respiratory arrest) have been reported to occur during or immediately after intravenous administration. Intravenous administration is restricted to emergency use, should not exceed 1 mg/minute, and should occur with a physician in attendance. Use with caution in neonates with severe hepatic disease.
Drug interactions: Antagonizes action of warfarin.
Monitoring: Prothrombin time/partial thromboplastin time (PT/PTT) if giving maintenance therapy. Allow a minimum of 2 to 4 hours to detect measurable improvement in these parameters.

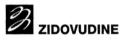 **ZIDOVUDINE**

Classification: Antiretroviral agent, nucleoside analog reverse transcriptase inhibitor.
Indications: Treatment of neonates born to human immunodeficiency virus (HIV)-infected women.
Dosage/administration: May be administered with feeds but manufacturer recommends administration 30 minutes before or 1 hour after feeds. Initiate therapy within 12 hours of birth and continue for 6 weeks, with subsequent therapy dependent on clinical status and results of HIV studies.
Final concentration for intravenous administration: 4 mg/mL.
Dosage/administration: (see Table A.29)

 TABLE A.29

Age	Dose/route	Comment
Term infants	■ Oral: 2 mg/kg/dose q6h ■ IV: 1.5 mg/kg/dose q6h	
GA at birth <30 wk	■ Oral: 2 mg/kg/dose q12h ■ IV: 1.5 mg/kg/dose q12h	Increase interval to q8h at **4** wk of age
GA at birth >30 wk	■ Oral: 2 mg/kg/dose q12h ■ IV: 1.5 mg/kg/dose q12 h	Increase interval to q8h at **2** wk of age
GA = gestational age; IV = intravenously; q6h = every 6 hours; q8h = every 8 hours; q12h = every 12 hours;		

IV dose is administered over >1 hour on syringe pump. Conversion from oral to IV dose: IV dose = 2/3 of oral dose. Do not administer IM.

Clinical considerations: Intravenous dose is two-thirds of oral dose.
Precautions: Use with caution in patients with bone marrow compromise or renal or hepatic impairment.
Adverse reactions: Anemia and neutropenia.
Drug interactions: Acetaminophen, acyclovir (increased toxicity), ganciclovir (increased hematological toxicity), cimetidine, indomethacin, and lorazepam. Coadministration with other drugs metabolized by glucuronidation increases toxicity of either drug and increases granulocytopenia.
Monitoring consideration: Weekly CBC, renal, LFTs, CD4 cell count, HIV RNA plasma levels.

ZINC ACETATE ORAL SOLUTION

Classification: Mineral supplement.
Indication: Prevention and treatment of zinc deficiency states.
Dosage/administration: 0.5 to 1 mg of elemental Zn/kg/day orally every day.
Clinical considerations: May administer with food if GI upset occurs.
Drug interactions: Iron and agents that increase gastric pH (e.g., H-2 blockers, proton pump inhibitors) may decrease zinc absorption.
Monitoring: Periodic serum copper, zinc levels.
Adverse effects: Nausea, vomiting, leukopenia, diaphoresis, GI disturbances. At excessive doses, hypotension, tachycardia, and gastric ulcers.

Suggested Readings

American Heart Association and American Academy of Pediatrics. *Handbook for neonatal resuscitation textbook*, 5th ed. Washington: AHA/AAP, 2006.

Bradley JS, Nelson JD. *Nelson's 2006–2007 pocket book of pediatric antimicrobial therapy*, 16th ed. Baltimore: Lippincott Williams & Wilkins, 2002.

Pickering LK, Baker CJ, Long SS, et al. eds. *Red book: 2006 Report of the committee on infectious diseases*, 27th ed. Elk Grove Village: American Academy of Pediatrics, 2006.

Robertson J, Shilkofski N. *The harriet lane handbook*, 17th ed. Philadelphia: Mosby, 2005.

Taketomo, CK Hodding JH, Kraus DM, eds. *Pediatric dosage handbook*, 14th ed. Hudson, Ohio:. Lexi-Comp, 2007.

Trissel LA. *Handbook of injectable drugs*, 14th ed. Bethesda: Board of the American Society of Health-System Pharmacists, 2006.

Young TE, Mangum B. *Neofax*, 20th ed. Raleigh: Acorn Publishing, 2007.

Zenk KE, Sills JH, Koeppel RM. *Neonatal medications and nutrition*, 3rd ed. Santa Rosa: NICU Ink book Publishers, 2003.

EFFECTS OF MATERNAL DRUGS ON THE FETUS

Camilia R. Martin

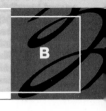

I. INTRODUCTION

A. In most instances, the **risk** of adverse fetal effects from drugs taken by the mother is not known. Properly designed scientific studies cannot be performed ethically, since they would require that women take drugs when they did not need them in order to eliminate the confounding effect of maternal disease or disorder. The current investigational methods (retrospective analysis, cohort studies, and case reports) often cannot differentiate the cause of the malformation or other adverse outcome. When a problem occurs in association with a history of maternal drug ingestion, any of the following can be the cause:

1. The drug itself.

2. The maternal disease state (e.g., diabetes, maternal infection, or environmental toxicity).

3. Preexistent physical disorders (e.g., amniotic bands) producing deformation and disruption.

4. Unrecognized illness (e.g., unrecognized viral illness).

5. An already anomalous pregnancy may have produced symptoms that led to drug ingestion.

6. Genetic aberration.

7. A spontaneous malformation rate of 2% to 3%, a stillbirth risk of 1%, and a spontaneous abortion rate of 25%.

8. Other or unknown cause. In addition, maternal drug histories are extremely unreliable, and findings often depend on how the interview was conducted.

B. Teratogenic effects. Because of tremendous variability in maternal elimination and drug disposition characteristics, very little predictivity comes from knowing the maternal dose. Timing of drug exposure is important. Drugs taken when the embryo is extremely undifferentiated are unlikely to produce physical malformation unless the drug persists in the body or alters the gamete. The most critical period for the induction of physical defects is believed to be 15 to 60 days after conception. Because the timing of this event is rarely known with certainty, however, one cannot exclude the possibility of malformation in any clinical situation. Drugs taken after organogenesis can effect the growth and development of the fetus. The brain, in particular, continues to grow and develop in the latter trimesters and beyond. A drug taken during gestation also can act as a transplacental carcinogen. In short, there is no "guaranteed safe" time for a pregnant woman to take a drug.

C. Even when a drug is associated with a statistically significant increase in the risk of a birth defect, the actual risk may remain low. For example, a birth defect that naturally occurs in 1 and 1,000,000 births may be made 1,000 times more likely by drug exposure and still would be seen in only 0.1% of the drug exposures. A real example of this is with phenytoin exposure. This drug produces a 200% to 400% increase in the risk of common birth defects (cleft lip, heart defects); however, 85% of children born to women who take phenytoin are normal or have minor effects of exposure. Numerical risks cannot be stated with certainty for most drugs because the data have been collected retrospectively. Where a risk is stated, the value should be interpreted with caution. For a given pregnancy, studied risk may not accurately reflect the risk to the fetus; genetic factors may have a strong influence on susceptibility to certain teratogens.

715

TABLE B.1 Effects of Common Maternal Drugs on the Fetus

Class	Drug	Risk category (see Sec. II)	Pharmacokinetics/reported effects on fetus
Analgesics/anti-pyretics and NSAIDs	Acetaminophen	B	Crosses placenta Not implicated as a teratogen When used within dosing recommendations and for short-term use, acetaminophen is considered safe Continuous use, or high-toxic dosages have been associated with: maternal anemia, maternal hepatorenal failure, maternal death, fetal hepatorenal failure, fetal death
	Acetylsalicylic acid (aspirin)	C D—full-dose ibuprofen in third trimester	Crosses placenta Not implicated as an important teratogen No fetal or newborn effects have been shown with *low-dose* aspirin therapy **Full-dose** aspirin associated with delayed onset and prolonged duration of labor (inhibition of prostaglandin synthesis) **Full-dose** ingestion within 5 d of delivery is associated with an increased risk of bleeding in both mother and baby Platelet dysfunction has been described (see Chaps. 26b and d) Association between **full-dose** maternal aspirin near-term and premature closure of the ductus arteriosus (inhibition of prostaglandin synthesis) and the syndrome of pulmonary hypertension in the newborn (see Chap. 24f)
	Ibuprofen	B D—full-dose aspirin in third trimester	Not implicated as a teratogen When used as a tocolytic agent, use is associated with reduced amniotic fluid volume Like aspirin, another prostaglandin synthesis inhibitor, use is associated with delayed onset and prolonged duration of labor, premature closure of the ductus arteriosus, and pulmonary hypertension in the newborn

*Risk Categories are defined at the end of this appendix.

Anesthetic agents used during labor and delivery		
Analgesics/narcotic agents		
Atropine (anesthetic premedication)	C	Parasympatholytic/anticholinergic Rapidly crosses the placenta with fetal uptake May directly effect fetal heart rate When used for premedication at 0.01 mg/kg, no fetal effects on heart rate or variability, and no effects on uterine activity were reported
Benzodiazepines		See psychotherapeutic agents, antipsychotics in the subsequent text
Induction agents		
Ketamine	B	Rapid-acting IV general anesthetic agent Not implicated as a teratogen Rapidly crosses the placenta When used in high doses (1.5–2.2 mg/kg), ketamine is associated with an increase in maternal blood pressure, increased uterine tone and contractions, newborn depression, and increased muscle tone in the infant These maternal/newborn effects were rarely observed with lower doses (0.2–0.5 mg/kg), which are commonly used today
Propofol	B	Hypnotic agent Not implicated as a teratogen Rapidly crosses the placenta Associated with decreased APGAR scores and decreased neurobehavioral scores compared to infants born by spontaneous vaginal delivery

(continued)

*Risk Categories are defined at the end of this appendix.

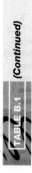

TABLE B.1 *(Continued)*

Class	Drug	Risk category (see Sec. II)	Pharmacokinetics/reported effects on fetus
	Thiopental	C	Rapid and ultrashort-acting IV general anesthetic agent Not implicated as a teratogen Rapidly crosses the placenta Associated with decreased APGAR scores and decreased neurobehavioral scores compared to infants born by spontaneous vaginal delivery
Inhalation agents			
	Enflurane	B	Rapid fetal uptake No adverse effects on APGAR scores or neurobehavioral status in the newborn
	Halothane	C	Associated with uterine muscle relaxation and increased blood loss; however, low-dose halothane (0.5%) not shown to have adverse maternal or newborn effects
	Isoflurane	C	Preferred agent in patients receiving bet-adrenergic therapy because of a reduced incidence of arrhythmias
	Nitrous oxide	?	Short-term use as an obstetric anesthetic is considered safe
Local anesthetics			
	Bupivacaine	C	Long-acting local anesthetic Reports of associated neonatal depression, hypoxia, fetal acidosis, and bradycardia High concentrations may increase forceps delivery rate
	Chloroprocaine	C	

*Risk Categories are defined at the end of this appendix.

Lidocaine	C_B, B_M	Not implicated as a teratogen when used early in pregnancy
		Injection into paracervical tissues or uterine cavity results in fetal heart rate decelerations
		Epidural use associated with maternal hypotension
Ropivacaine	B	Rapidly crosses the placenta
		Use as an obstetric anesthetic is considered safe
Scopolamine	C	Parasympatholytic/anticholinergic
		Used to prevent nausea and vomiting associated with anesthesia and surgery
		Readily crosses the placenta
		Fetal effects may include tachycardia and decreased heart rate variability
		Report of newborn toxicity with fever, tachycardia, and lethargy; symptoms reversed with physostigmine
Skeletal muscle relaxants		
Pancuronium	C	Crosses the placenta in small amounts near term, placenta transfer early in pregnancy has not been reported
Vecuronium		Short-term use has shown no demonstrable adverse effects on the fetus
		Repetitive or large doses have been associated with neonatal depression and transient fetal heart rate changes, which do not seem to correlate or indicate fetal compromise
Anticoagulants		
Heparin	C	Does not cross the placenta
		Not considered a teratogen
		Maternal complications include bleeding
Warfarin and other coumarin derivatives	D_B, X_M	Oral anticoagulants
		Crosses the placenta
		Considered a teratogen

(continued)

---

*Risk Categories are defined at the end of this appendix.
B = Briggs (see Sec. II.B.2); M = Manufacturer (see Sec. II.B.2).

TABLE B.1 *(Continued)*

Class	Drug	Risk category (see Sec. II)	Pharmacokinetics/reported effects on fetus
	Warfarin and other coumarin derivatives (continued)		Fetal effects include: Embryopathy (fetal warfarin syndrome) – growth restriction, blindness, optic atrophy, microphthalmia, nasal hypoplasia, hypoplasia of the extremities, stippled epiphyses, mental deficiency, seizures, hearing loss, congenital heart disease, scoliosis, death Central nervous system defects Spontaneous abortion Stillbirth Prematurity Hemorrhage
	Carbamazepine	D	Crosses the placenta Considered a teratogen Associated with spina bifida, craniofacial defects, fingernail hypoplasia, and developmental delay
Anticonvulsants	Ethosuximide (Zarontin)	C	Used for the treatment of petit mal epilepsy Not well studied making conclusions regarding teratogenicity difficult
	Phenobarbital	D	Some reported newborn associations in a limited number of exposures include: patent ductus arteriosus, cleft lip/palate, mongoloid facies, altered palmar crease, accessory nipple, hydrocephalus Spontaneous hemorrhage in the newborn has been reported Crosses the placenta Considered a teratogen

*Risk Categories are defined at the end of this appendix.

Phenobarbital **(continued)**		No specific phenotype (in contrast to phenytoin) Associated findings: cardiovascular defects, cleft lip/palate, early hemorrhagic disease of the newborn (induction of fetal liver microsomal enzymes depleting vitamin K and suppressing vitamin K–dependent coagulation factors), barbiturate withdrawal, impaired cognitive development
Phenytoin (Dilantin)	D	Crosses the placenta Considered a teratogen, some suggestion that this is dose-related Recognizable pattern of malformations known as *fetal hydantoin syndrome*, features include: broad nasal bridge, wide fontanel, low-set hairline, broad alveolar ridge, metopic ridging, short neck, ocular hypertelorism, microcephaly, cleft lip/palate, abnormal or low-set ears, epicanthal folds, ptosis of eyelids, coloboma, coarse scalp hair, small or absent nails, hypoplasia of distal phalanges, altered palmar crease, digital thumb, dislocated hip, impaired growth, congenital heart defects, CNS malformations, mental deficiency May cause early hemorrhagic disease of the newborn (induction of fetal liver microsomal enzymes depleting vitamin K and suppressing vitamin K–dependent coagulation factors)
Primidone (Mysoline)	D	Structural analog of phenobarbital Considered a teratogen Also may see hemorrhagic disease of the newborn
Valproic acid (Depakene)	D	Readily crosses the placenta Associated fetal/newborn complications include: congenital abnormalities – valproic acid syndrome: neural tube defects, craniofacial, microcephaly, abnormal digits, hypospadias, congenital heart disease, delayed psychomotor development, growth restriction

(continued)

---

*Risk Categories are defined at the end of this appendix.

Class	Drug	Risk category (see Sec. II)	Pharmacokinetics/reported effects on fetus
Antihistamines			
	First-generation		
	Diphenhydramine	B_M	Other – hyperbilirubinemia, hepatotoxicity, transient hyperglycinemia, withdrawal
	Chlorpheniramine	B	No evidence of teratogenicity
	Tripelennamine	B	
	Second-generation		
	Loratadine	B_M	Unknown if crosses the placenta; however with a low molecular weight some passage is expected
			No evidence for teratogenicity
Anti-infectives	**Amebicides**		
	Metronidazole	B	Crosses the placenta
			Although mutagenic and carcinogenic in bacteria and rats, no clear association of these properties in humans
			Most evidence suggests that there is no significant risk to the fetus
	Aminoglycosides		
	Amikacin	C_B, D_M	Rapidly crosses the placenta
			Not considered a teratogen
			Theoretical risk of ototoxicity
	Gentamicin	C	Rapidly crosses the placenta
	Neomycin	D	Not considered a teratogen
	Tobramycin	D	Theoretical risk of ototoxicity

*Risk Categories are defined at the end of this appendix.
B = Briggs (see Sec. II.B.2); M = Manufacturer (see Sec. II.B.2).

Streptomycin	D	Neonatal potentiation of $MgSO_4$-induced neuromuscular weakness has been reported-fetal ototoxicity has been reported
Antibiotics-general		
Chloramphenicol	C	Crosses the placenta at term Not considered a teratogen One report associating cardiovascular collapse (gray baby syndrome) in infants born to mothers receiving chloramphenicol during the latter stage of pregnancy
Clindamycin	B	Crosses the placenta Not considered a teratogen
Erythromycin	B	Crosses the placenta, but in very low concentrations Not considered a teratogen
Pentamidine	C	Antiprotozoal agent
Trimethoprim	C	Folate antagonist May be used alone or in combination with sulfonamides Crosses the placenta Some suggestion that use in the first semester may cause structural defects—cardiovascular defects, neural tube defects
Antifungals		
Amphotericin B	B	Crosses the placenta Not considered a teratogen Drug of choice for the treatment of systemic fungal infections in pregnancy

(continued)

*Risk Categories are defined at the end of this appendix.

Class	Drug	Risk category (see Sec. II)	Pharmacokinetics/reported effects on fetus
	Griseofulvin,	C	Associated with an increased risk of fetal malformations
	Ketoconazole,	C_M	Not recommended for use during pregnancy
	Flucytosine	C_M	
	Miconazole	C	Topical antifungal agent
			No reports documenting associated congenital malformations
	Antiviral —	B	Crosses the placenta
	Acyclovir		No documented reports of adverse effects to the fetus or newborn
	Cephalosporins	B	Cephalosporins as a class of drug is generally considered safe to use during pregnancy
			Many have been shown to cross the placenta
	Moxalactam	C	Some reports of possible cardiovascular malformations and oral cleft defects with cefaclor, ceftriaxone, cephalexin, and cephadrine
	Povidine–iodine (Betadine)	D	Readily crosses the placenta
			May cause transient hypothyroidism
	Penicillins	B	Many penicillin-derivatives have been shown to readily cross the placenta
			As a class of drug, penicillins are not considered teratogenic
	Quinolones, e.g., Ciprofloxacin	C	Unknown for many quinolone-derivatives whether transplacental passage occurs; although the molecule is small enough for this to theoretically be possible
			Norfloxacin and ciprofloxacin have been documented to cross the placenta

*Risk Categories are defined at the end of this appendix.
M = Manufacturer (see Sec. II.B.2).

Norfloxacin	C	Animal evidence suggests association with cartilage damage and arthropathy; although this has never been shown in human studies
		No strong or convincing evidence that quinolone use is associated with congenital abnormalities
		However, some small reports of possible associated birth defects; although a consistent pattern has not been identified
		Most recommend to not use quinolones during pregnancy as safer alternatives exist
Sulfonamides	C	Readily crosses the placenta
	D — if administered near term	When close to term, documented associated toxicities include jaundice (competes with bilirubin for albumin binding sites) and hemolytic anemia
		No strong evidence to suggest an association with congenital abnormalities
Tetracyclines e.g.,	D	Crosses the placenta
Doxycycline		Associated with maternal hepatotoxicity
Tetracycline		Associated with disruption of fetal mineralized structures such as teeth (intense yellow-staining) and bones
		Possible risk for minor fetal anomalies
Urinary germicides	B	Not considered a teratogen
Nitrofurantoin		Caution with use close to term secondary to reports of newborn hemolytic anemia
Antimalarials	C	Crosses the placenta
Chloroquine		Not considered a major teratogen, although a small association to birth defects could not be excluded

(continued)

Risk Categories are defined at the end of this appendix.

Class	Drug	Risk category (see Sec. II)	Pharmacokinetics/reported effects on fetus
	Hydroxychloroquine (Plaquenil)	C	Crosses the placenta It is generally considered safe to use during pregnancy; however, studies and the number of exposures are limited
	Quinine	D_B, X_M	Considered a teratogen Reported associated congenital anomalies including: CNS anomalies, limb defects, facial defects, heart defects, digestive organ anomalies, urogenital anomalies, hernias, and vertebral anomalies Reports of maternal and neonatal thrombocytopenia purpura Reports of neonatal hemolysis in G-6-PD deficient newborns
Antiparasitics	**Crotamiton 10%** (Eurax)	B	No toxicity reported in pregnancy and infants
	Lindane (gamma benzene hydrochloride, Kwell)	B	Possible association with hypospadias Theoretical concern for neurotoxicity, convulsions, and aplastic anemia
	Mebendazole (Vermox)	C	No strong evidence to suggest association with congenital malformations
	Paromomycin	C	No linkage to congenital malformations
	Pyrethrins piperonyl butoxide (A-200, RID, RTC)	C	Little data to assess safety Poorly absorbed so should have minimal potential toxicity
	Thiabendazole	C	No reports of human teratogenicity
Antituberculars	**Ethambutol**	B	Crosses the placenta No reports of associate congenital defects
	Ethionamide	C	One report of increased congenital anomalies

*Risk Categories are defined at the end of this appendix.
B = Briggs (see Sec. II.B.2); M = Manufacturer (see Sec. II.B.2).

		Category*	
	Isoniazid	C	Crosses the placenta No strong association to congenital anomalies Two case reports of association with hemorrhagic disease of the newborn
	Rifampin	C	Crosses the placenta No strong association to congenital anomalies Association with hemorrhagic disease of the newborn
Cardiovascular	**ACE inhibitors** e.g., Captopril Enalapril	C D — if used in second or third trimester	No apparent increased human fetal risk when used in first trimester Second and third trimester use associated with fetal teratogenicity secondary to fetal hypotension and reduced renal blood flow resulting in anuria, renal dysgenesis, and renal failure. Anuria-associated oligohydramnios may result in fetal growth restriction, pulmonary hypoplasia, limb contractures, craniofacial deformation, and neonatal death.
	Antiarrhythmic agents		
	Lidocaine	B	Rapidly crosses the placenta Limited data with use as an antiarrhythmic during pregnancy; the few reports available do not suggest a significant risk to the fetus
	Procainamide	C	Has not been linked to congenital anomalies or adverse fetal or newborn effects
	Quinidine	C_B, B_M	Crosses the placenta Has not been linked to congenital anomalies Report of neonatal thrombocytopenia after maternal use

(continued)

*Risk Categories are defined at the end of this appendix.
B = Briggs (see Sec. II.B.2); M = Manufacturer (see Sec. II.B.2).

TABLE B.1 *(Continued)*

Class	Drug	Risk category (see Sec. II)	Pharmacokinetics/reported effects on fetus
	β-blockers		
	Propranolol	C	Crosses the placenta
		D — if used in second or third trimester	Oxytocic effects
			Multiple reported fetal and neonatal effects: most commonly intrauterine growth restriction, hypoglycemia, and bradycardia
	Calcium channel blockers		
	Diltiazem	C	Suggestion of increased risk for cardiovascular effects
	Verapamil	C	Crosses the placenta
			Has not been linked to congenital anomalies
	Digoxin	C	Transplacental passage and uptake by the fetus increasing with advancing gestational age
			No linkage to congenital anomalies
			Neonatal death has been reported after maternal overdose
	Diuretics		
	Acetazolamide	C	Carbonic anhydrase inhibitor
			No linkage to congenital anomalies in humans
			One report of neonatal sacrococcygeal teratoma, this possible association has not been supported by other reports
	Thiazide diuretics	C	Chlorothiazide, chlorthalidone, hydrochlorothiazide
		D if used in pregnancy induced hypertension (PIH)	

*Risk Categories are defined at the end of this appendix.

		Readily crosses the placenta
		May decrease placental perfusion (use not recommended in PIH due to baseline hypovolemic status)
		Can induce maternal hyperglycemia (infant should be observed for hypoglycemia secondary to hyperinsulinemia response to maternal hyperglycemia)
		Conflicting reports exist regarding association with congenital abnormalities; possible linkage to congenital heart defects with chlorthalidone with first trimester use
		Neonatal thrombocytopenia, hemolytic anemia, and electrolyte imbalances have been reported
Furosemide	C D if used in PIH	Crosses the placenta May decrease placental perfusion (use not recommended in PIH due to baseline hypovolemic status) Associated with increased fetal urine production No strong association to major congenital anomalies; possible associated with an increased risk for hypospadias
Spironolactone	C D if used in PIH	Potassium conserving diuretic Aldosterone antagonist in the distal convoluted renal tubule May decrease placental perfusion (use not recommended in PIH due to baseline hypovolemic status) No strong association to major congenital anomalies; however concern that the anti-androgenic effect caused feminization in male rat fetuses

(continued)

*Risk Categories are defined at the end of this appendix.

Class	Drug	Risk category (see Sec. II)	Pharmacokinetics/reported effects on fetus
Other Antihypertensives			
	Diazoxide	C	Crosses the placenta
			May cause a rapid decrease in maternal blood pressure, decrease placental perfusion, and fetal bradycardia; less effects seen with small doses at frequent intervals
			Uterine relaxant and therefore may inhibit uterine contractions
			Use associated with neonatal hyperglycemia
	Methyldopa	B	Central acting, antiadrenergic agent
			Crosses the placenta
			No association to congenital abnormalities
			Reports of neonatal decreased intracranial volume and reduced systolic blood pressure; neither considered clinically significant
	Nitroprusside	C	Crosses the placenta
			No association to congenital abnormalities
			May see transient fetal bradycardia
			Standard maternal dosing do not appear to increase the risk for excessive cyanide accumulation in the fetus
	Prazosin	C	α1-adrenergic blocking agent
			Crosses the placenta
			No association to congenital abnormalities
Vasodilators			
	Dipyridamole	C	No association to congenital abnormalities
			Increases placental perfusion

*Risk Categories are defined at the end of this appendix.

	Risk Category*	
		Clinical intervention trial suggest benefits of this therapy including reduced incidence of stillbirth, placental infarction, and intrauterine growth restriction
Disopyramide	C	Crosses the placenta
		No association to congenital abnormalities
		Reports of oxytocic effect
Hydralazine	C	Crosses the placenta
		No association to congenital abnormalities
		Reports of fetal arrhythmia
		Neonatal reports of thrombocytopenia and bleeding; however, this may be related to severe maternal hypertension rather than the drug exposure
		One report of lupus-like syndrome developing in mother and baby after exposure resulting in a neonatal death
Nitroglycerin	B_B, C_M	Rapid-onset, short-acting
		Reports, although limited in number, suggest no significant harm to the fetus
		Some reports of fetal bradycardia and loss of beat-to-beat variability in response to a reduction in maternal blood pressure; these fetal cardiac effects are apparently of no lasting clinical significance
Chemotherapy agents		
		Use of antineoplastic agents associated with low birth weight
		Limited exposures with often multiple agents used at once makes final interpretation of observations difficult
		Congenital anomalies of virtually all organ systems have been described

(continued)

*Risk Categories are defined at the end of this appendix.
B = Briggs (see Sec. II.B.2); M = Manufacturer (see Sec. II.B.2).

TABLE B.1 *(Continued)*

Class	Drug	Risk category (see Sec. II)	Pharmacokinetics/reported effects on fetus
Alkylating agents			
	Cytarabine	D	Early use in the first and second trimester is associated with chromosomal and congenital abnormalities
			Pancytopenia in the newborn has been reported with use during the third trimester
	Dactinomycin	C	Limited reports of use during pregnancy
			One report of six exposed pregnancies did not reveal an association with congenital anomalies
	Daunorubicin	D	In one series of 29 exposed pregnancies, newborn complications included anemia, hypoglycemia, electrolyte disturbances, and transient neutropenia
	Doxorubicin	D	Safe use in pregnancy not established–embryotoxic and teratogenic in rats–embryotoxic in rabbits
	5-Fluorouracil	D_B, X_M	Reported association with spontaneous abortions, cleft lip/palate and VSD
	6-Mercaptopurine	D	Neonatal pancytopenia and hemolytic anemia
	Methotrexate	X	Folic acid antagonist
			Crosses the placenta
			Considered a teratogen
			Associated with severe newborn myelosuppression
	Procarbazine	D	Associated with congenital abnormalities
			May produce gonadal dysfunction
	Thioguanine	D	Purine analog interrupting nucleic acid biosynthesis
			Use associated with chromosomal abnormalities, missing digits

*Risk Categories are defined at the end of this appendix.
B = Briggs (see Sec. II.B.2); M = Manufacturer (see Sec. II.B.2).

Drug	Risk Category	Comments
Vinca Alkaloids	D	Antimitotic May produce gonadal dysfunction Associated with chromosomal abnormalities
Drugs of habit or abuse		
Caffeine	B	Crosses the placenta No association with congenital anomalies Moderate to heavy consumption associated with increased risk of late first and second trimester spontaneous abortion In mothers who have experienced a prior loss, even light use has been shown to increase the risk of fetal loss Demonstration of increased fetal breathing and decreased heart rate after caffeine consumption Fetuses of mothers with high caffeine consumption have been shown to have less time in active sleep, and a greater time in arousal High caffeine consumption with cigarette smoking increases the risk for low birth weight than with cigarette smoking alone Newborn cardiac arrhythmias have been described possibly related to caffeine withdrawal
Cocaine	C X if nonmedicinal	See Chap. 19
Ethanol	D X if excessive or prolonged use	see Chap. 19
Marijuana	C	see Chap. 19
Tobacco	C	see Chap. 19

(continued)

*Risk Categories are defined at the end of this appendix.

TABLE B.1 *(Continued)*

Class	Drug	Risk category (see Sec. II)	Pharmacokinetics/reported effects on fetus
Gastrointestinal	**Anti-inflammatory**		
	Sulfasalazine	B	Crosses the placenta
		D — if used near term	No strong linkage to congenital abnormalities; however reports of potential associations including cleft lip/palate, hydrocephalus, VSD, coarctation of the aorta, genitourinary abnormalities
			Caution near term due to the association between sulfonamides and newborn jaundice
	Antilipemic		
	Cholestyramine	B	Resin that binds bile acids
			No linkage to congenital malformations
			One report of fetal subdural hematomas thought to be secondary to vitamin K deficiency caused by the drug or mother's underlying cholestasis
	Antisecretory		
	Cimetidine	B	H$_2$-receptor antagonist inhibiting gastric acid secretion
			Crosses the placenta
			Antiadrenergic activity in animals; although not shown in humans
			No increased risk of congenital malformations
	Ranitidine	B	Like cimetidine, however ranitidine does not shown antiadrenergic activity in animal or human studies

*Risk Categories are defined at the end of this appendix.

Laxative		
Docusate	C	No linkage to fetal toxicity or congenital malformations One report of maternal and neonatal hypomagnesemia thought to be secondary to docusate sodium
Metoclopramide	B	Used in pregnancy for anti-emetic effect and to increase gastric emptying time Crosses the placenta at term
Narcotics		
Butorphanol	C	No linkage to fetal toxicity or congenital malformations See Chap. 19
Meperidine	B	
Pentazocine	C	
Propoxyphene	C for all, D if excessive or prolonged use at term	
Psychotherapeutic agents		
Antipsychotics/ tranquilizers For schizophrenia:		General comments: For drugs in this class that are used for schizophrenia, reports of newborn toxicity when used close to term. Two clinical syndromes described: 1. Syndrome more commonly seen with low-potency agents (e.g., chlorpromazine, prochlorperazine, thioridazine) — neonatal depression, lethargy, gastrointestinal dysfunction, and hypotension. These symptoms may last a few days.

(continued)

---

*Risk Categories are defined at the end of this appendix.

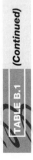

TABLE B.1 *(Continued)*

Class	Drug	Risk category (see Sec. II)	Pharmacokinetics/reported effects on fetus
			2. Syndrome more commonly seen with high-potency agents (e.g., haloperidol) — extrapyramidal signs including tremors, increased tone, spasticity, posturing, arching of the back, hyperactive deep tendon reflexes, and shrill crying. These symptoms may last for several months.
	Chlorpromazine	C	Crosses the placenta Considered safe when used in smaller, anti-emetic dosages When used for analgesia during labor, marked drop in maternal blood pressures have been noted Most studies report no linkage to congenital anomalies
	Haloperidol	C	Conflicting reports regarding an association with limb reduction defects Possible association with cardiovascular defects Use during labor at suggested dosages has not been linked with neonatal effects
	Prochlorperazine, Thioridazine	C	Crosses the placenta Use for nausea and vomiting considered safe Although conflicting results, most suggest that phenothiazines are safe when used in low doses

* Risk Categories are defined at the end of this appendix.

For bipolar disease:		
Lithium	D	Crosses the placenta
		Serum half-life in newborns longer compared to adult values
		Strong association with congenital anomalies, especially cardiovascular defects (Ebstein's anomaly)
		Reported fetal and newborn toxicities including: cyanosis, hypotonia, bradycardia, thyroid depression and goiter, cardiomegaly, and diabetes insipidus
		Most neonatal toxic effects are self-limited
		Most documented to readily cross the placenta with fetal accumulation of levels
Benzodiazepines		
Alprazolam	D	No linkage to congenital anomalies with alprazolam; however, reported associations with other drugs in this class:
Clonazepam	D	Clonazepam — congenital heart defects
Diazepam	D	Diazepam — cleft lip/palate (controversial, no linkage with more recent large cohort and case-control studies), inguinal hernia, dysmorphic features, fetal growth restriction, CNS defects
Lorazepam	D	Lorazepam — anal atresia
		Risk of newborn toxicity and withdrawal especially with increased dosages or prolonged use; described clinical presentation of toxicity and withdrawal include:
		1. "Floppy infant syndrome" — hypothermia, hypotonia, lethargy, sucking difficulties, apnea, cyanosis
		2. "Withdrawal syndrome" — tremors, irritability, inconsolable crying, restlessness, abnormal sleep pattern, hypertonicity, hyperreflexia, seizures, diarrhea, vomiting, vigorous sucking. These symptoms may present up to 3 weeks after delivery and last for several months
		Long-term neurobehavioral consequences controversial and inadequately studied

(continued)

---

*Risk Categories are defined at the end of this appendix.

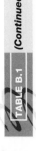

Class	Drug	Risk category (see Sec. II)	Pharmacokinetics/reported effects on fetus
	Tricyclic antidepressants		Crosses the placenta
	Amitriptyline	C	Conflicting reports regarding association with limb reduction defects
	Imipramine	D	Although small number of exposures, possible association with cardiovascular defects with imipramine and nortriptyline
	Nortriptyline	D	The following newborn effects have been described with imipramine and nortriptyline use: periodic apnea, cyanosis, tachypnea, respiratory distress, irritability, seizures, feeding difficulties, heart failure, tachycardia, myoclonus, and urinary retention
			Long-term neurodevelopmental studies lacking, one report of no lasting neurodevelopmental effect (see References, Nulman et al.)
	Selective Serotonin reuptake inhibitors (SSRI)		Recent studies suggest a possible increase in congenital malformations, especially with early, first trimester use (see References, Wogelius et al. and Thormahlen).
	Fluoxetine (Prozac)	C	A neonatal withdrawal syndrome has been described. Onset may occur up to a few days after delivery and last for several months. Symptoms similar to those described for benzodiazepines.
	Fluvoxamine (Luvox)	C	
	Paroxetine (Paxil)	C	
	Sertraline (Zoloft)	B	SSRI exposed infants are also more likely to be low birth weight and experience respiratory distress, including persistent pulmonary hypertension.
	Venlafaxine (Effexor)	C	

*Risk Categories are defined at the end of this appendix.

Thyroid medications

Long-term neurobehavioral data for exposed infants is lacking, one report of no lasting neurodevelopmental effect with Fluoxetine use (see References, Nulman et al.)

Thyroid supplementation

Levothyroxine	A	See Chap. 2B
Antithyroid		
Methimazole	D	see Chap. 2B
Propylthiouracil	D	see Chap. 2B

*Risk Categories are defined at the end of this appendix.

ACE = angiotensin converting enzyme; CNS = central nervous system; IV = intravenous; NSAIDs = nonsteroidal anti-inflammatory drugs; PD = phosphate dehydrogenase; PIH = pregnancy-induced hypertension; SSRI = selective serotonin reuptake inhibitors; VSD = ventricular septical defect.

    D. New information among the effects of drugs and other chemical agents on the fetus. Manufacturer's recommendations and package inserts should be checked before the fetus is exposed to these agents.

II. EFFECTS OF COMMON MATERNAL DRUGS ON THE FETUS (SEE TABLE)

    A. References used to create the summary table are stated at the end of this appendix.

    B. Pregnancy risk category

        1. The Food and Drug Administration has offered a classification system to assign the risk of a particular drug to the fetus during pregnancy. The classification system is as follows:

            a. Category A. Controlled studies show no risk. Adequate, well-controlled studies in pregnant women have not demonstrated a risk to the fetus in the first trimester of pregnancy, and there is no evidence of risk in later trimesters.

            b. Category B. No evidence of risk in humans. Animal studies have not demonstrated a risk to the fetus, but there are no adequate studies in pregnant women; or animal studies have shown an adverse effect, but adequate studies in pregnant women have not demonstrated a risk to the fetus during the first trimester of pregnancy, and there is no evidence of risk in later trimesters.

            c. Category C. Risk cannot be ruled out. Animal studies have shown an adverse effect on the fetus, but there are no adequate studies in humans; or there are no animal reproduction studies and no adequate studies in humans.

            d. Category D. There is evidence of human fetal risk, but the potential benefits from the use of the drug in pregnant women may be acceptable despite its potential risks.

            e. Category X. Contraindicated in pregnancy. Studies in animals or humans demonstrate fetal abnormalities or adverse reaction; reports indicate evidence of fetal risk. The risk of use in pregnant women clearly outweighs any possible benefit to the patient.

        2. The risk category was assigned by referencing the textbook by Briggs et al. or by using the manufacturer's ratings. If Briggs et al. and the manufacturer's ratings differed from one another, both categories were listed (Briggs = subscript B; Manufacturer = subscript M).

        3. Briggs et al. provided additional information beyond that was provided by the manufacturer that is helpful to the reader.

        4. Manufacturer's recommendations and package inserts should be checked before the fetus is exposed to these agents for the most current information.

        5. Additional information can be found at The Pregnancy Environmental Hotline (800-322-5014 or 617-466-8471, fax 617-487-2361) sponsored by the National Birth Defects Center and the Genesis Fund.

Suggested Readings

American Academy of Pediatrics. Use of psychoactive medication during pregnancy and possible effects on the fetus and newborn. Committee on drugs. *Pediatrics* 2000; 105:880–887.

Berkovitch M, Elbirt D, Addis A, et al. Fetal effects of metoclopramide therapy for nausea and vomiting of pregnancy. *N Engl J Med* 2000;343:445–446.

Berlin CM Jr. Effects of drugs on the fetus. *Pediatr Rev* 1991;12:282–287.

Bodendorfer TW, Briggs GG, Gunning JE. Obtaining drug exposure histories during pregnancy. *Am J Obstet Gynecol* 1979;135:490–494.

Boyle RJ. Effects of certain prenatal drugs on the fetus and newborn. *Pediatr Rev* 2002; 23:17–24.

Briggs GG. *Drugs in pregnancy and lactation.* Philadelphia: Lippincott Williams & Wilkins, 2002.

Briggs GG, Freeman RK, Yaffe SJ. *Drugs in pregnancy and lactation: A reference guide to fetal and neonatal risk*, 6th ed. Philadelphia: Lippincott Williams & Wilkins, 2002.

Chambers CD, Hernandez-Diaz S, Van Marter LJ, et al. Selective serotonin-reuptake inhibitors and risk of persistent pulmonary hypertension of the newborn. *N Engl J Med* 2006;354(6):579–587.

Dean JC, Hailey H, Moore SJ, et al. Long term health and neurodevelopment in children exposed to antiepileptic drugs before birth. *J Med Genet* 2002;39:251–259.

Food and Drug Administration. Labeling and prescription drug advertising: content and format for labeling for human prescription drug. *Fed Reg* 1980;44:37434–67.

Holmes LB, Harvey EA, Coull BA, et al. The teratogenicity of anticonvulsant drugs. *N Engl J Med* 2001;344:1132–1138.

Kalter H, Warkany J. Medical progress. Congenital malformations: Etiologic factors and their role in prevention (first of two parts). *N Engl J Med* 1983;308:424–431.

Kalter H, Warkany J. Congenital malformations (second of two parts). *N Engl J Med* 1983;308:491–497.

Koren G, Pastuszak A, Ito S. Drugs in pregnancy. *N Engl J Med* 1998;338:1128–1137.

Koren G, Florescu A, Costei AM, et al. Nonsteroidal anti-inflammatory drugs during third trimester and the risk of premature closure of the ductus arteriosus: A meta-analysis. *Ann Pharmacother* 2006;40(5):824–829.

Levy G. Pharmacokinetics of fetal and neonatal exposure to drugs. *Obstet Gynecol* 1981; 58:9S–16S.

Lusskin SI, Misri S. Infants with antenatal exposure to serotonin reuptake inhibitors (SSRI). In: UpToDate, Feigin RD (Ed), UpToDate, Waltham, MA, 2007.

Moretti ME, Caprara D, Coutinho CJ, et al. Fetal safety of loratadine use in the first trimester of pregnancy: A multicenter study. *J Allergy Clin Immunol* 2003;111:479–483.

Moudgal VV, Sobel JD. Antifungal drugs in pregnancy: A review. *Expert Opin Drug Saf* 2003;2(5):475–483.

Murray L, Seger D. Drug therapy during pregnancy and lactation. *Emerg Med Clin North Am* 1994;12:129–149.

Neubert D, Chahoud I, Platzek T, et al. Principles and problems in assessing prenatal toxicity. *Arch Toxicol* 1987;60:238–245.

Nordeng H, Lindemann R, Perminov KV, et al. Neonatal withdrawal syndrome after in utero exposure to selective serotonin reuptake inhibitors. *Acta Paediatr* 2001;90:288–291.

Nulman I, Rovet J, Stewart DE, et al. Neurodevelopment of children exposed in utero to antidepressant drugs. *N Engl J Med* 1997;336:258–262.

Oberlander TF, Warburton W, Misri S, et al. Neonatal outcomes after prenatal exposure to selective serotonin reuptake inhibitor antidepressants and maternal depression using population-based linked health data. *Arch Gen Psychiatry* 2006;63(8):898–906.

Szeto HH. Maternal-fetal pharmacokinetics and fetal dose-response relationships. *Ann N Y Acad Sci* 1989;562:42–55.

Szeto HH. Kinetics of drug transfer to the fetus. *Clin Obstet Gynecol* 1993;36:246–254.

Szeto HH. Maternal-fetal pharmacokinetics: Summary and future directions. *NIDA Res Monogr* 1995;154:203–217.

Thormahlen GM. Paroxetine use during pregnancy: Is it safe? *Ann Pharmacother* 2006; 40(10):1834–1837.

Ward RM. Maternal-placental-fetal unit: Enique problems of pharmacologic study. *Pediatr Clin North Am* 1989;36:1075–1088.

Ward RM. Drug therapy of the fetus. *J Clin Pharmacol* 1993;33:780–789.

Wogelius P, Norgaard M, Gislum M, et al. Maternal use of selective serotonin reuptake inhibitors and risk of congenital malformations. *Epidemiology* 2006;17(6):701–704.

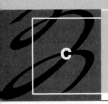

MATERNAL MEDICATIONS AND BREASTFEEDING
Karen M. Puopolo

I. **BACKGROUND.** Questions commonly arise regarding the safety of maternal medication use during breastfeeding. A combination of the biologic and chemical properties of the drug and the physiology of the mother and infant determine the safety of any individual medication. Consideration is given to the amount of drug that is found in breast milk, the half-life of the drug in the infant, and the biologic effect of the drug on the infant.

    A. **Drug properties that affect entry into breast milk.** Molecular size, pH, pKa, lipid solubility, and protein-binding properties of the drug all affect the milk to plasma **(M/P) concentration ratio,** which is defined as the relative concentration of the protein-free fraction of the drug in milk and maternal plasma. Small molecular size, slightly alkaline pH, nonionization, high lipid solubility, and lack of binding to serum proteins all favor entry of a drug into breast milk. The half-life of the medication and frequency of drug administration are also important; the longer the cumulative time the drug is present in the maternal circulation, the greater the opportunity for it to appear in breast milk.

    B. **Maternal factors.** The total maternal dose and mode of administration (intravenous vs. oral) as well as maternal illness (particularly renal or liver impairment) can affect the persistence of the drug in the maternal circulation. Medications taken in the first few days postpartum are more likely to enter breast milk as the mammary alveolar epithelium does not fully mature until the end of the first postpartum week.

    C. **Infant factors.** The maturity of the infant is the primary factor determining the persistence of a drug in the infant's system. Preterm infants and term infants in the first month after birth metabolize drugs more slowly because of renal and hepatic immaturity. The total dose of drug that the infant is exposed to is determined by the volume of milk ingested (per kg of body weight) as well as the frequency of feeding (or frequency of milk expression in the case of preterm infants).

II. **DETERMINATION OF DRUG SAFETY DURING BREASTFEEDING.** A number of available resources evaluate the risk of individual medications to the breastfed infant. Ideally, direct measurements of the entry of a drug into breast milk, and the level and persistence of the drug in the breastfed infant, as well as experience with exposure of infants to the drug, are all used to make a judgment regarding drug safety. Unfortunately, this type of information is available for relatively few medications. In the absence of specific data, a judgment is made on the basis of both the known pharmacologic properties of the drug and the known or predicted affects of the drug on the developing infant. Clinicians providing advice to the nursing mother about the safety of a particular medication should be aware of the following points.

    A. **Resources may differ in their judgment of a particular drug.** Information about some medications (especially newer ones) is in flux, and safety judgments may change over a relatively short period of time. Different resources approach the question of medication use in breastfeeding with different perspectives. For example, *The Physicians Desk Reference* is a compendium of commercially-supplied drug information. In the absence of specific data regarding the entry of a drug into breast milk, drug manufacturers generally do not make a definitive statement about the safety of drugs in breastfeeding. Other resources, such as **Medications in Mother's Milk** (MMM), take the available data and make a judgment about relative safety of the drug.

B. The safety of a drug in pregnancy is often not the same as the safety of the drug during breastfeeding. Occasionally a medication that is contraindicated in pregnancy (e.g., warfarin or ibuprofen) is safe to use while breastfeeding.

C. Definitive data are not available for most medications or for specific clinical situations. There is a need for individualized clinical judgment in many cases, taking into account the available information, the need of the mother for the medication, and the risk to the infant of both exposure to the drug and of exposure to breast milk substitutes. Consultation with the **Breastfeeding and Human Lactation Study Center** at the University of Rochester can aid the clinician in making specific clinical judgments.

III. RESOURCES. Resources listed as items III.A, III.B, III.C, and III.D served as source material for this appendix. Resources III.A–E are used to guide clinical decision making regarding breastfeeding at our institutions.

A. American Academy of Pediatrics (AAP), Committee on Drugs. The Transfer of Drugs and Other Chemicals Into Human Milk. This AAP Pediatrics Policy Statement on medication use and breastfeeding is available through the Internet at http://www.aap.org/policy/0063.html. This statement sites approximately 400 primary references to place >150 substances in six different categories:

1. **Cytotoxic drugs** that may interfere with cellular metabolism of the nursing infant and are contraindicated during breastfeeding.
2. **Drugs of abuse** for which adverse effects on the infant during breastfeeding have been reported and are contraindicated during breastfeeding.
3. **Radioactive compounds** that require temporary cessation of breastfeeding.
4. **Drugs for which the effect on nursing infants is unknown** but may be of concern.
5. **Drugs that have been associated with significant effects** on some nursing infants and should be given to nursing mothers with caution.
6. **Maternal medication** usually compatible with breastfeeding.
7. **Food and environmental agent** effects on breastfeeding are also included in a separate evaluation.

B. Briggs GG, Freeman RK, Yaffe SJ, eds. *Drugs in pregnancy and lactation*, 7th ed. Baltimore:Lippincott Williams & Wilkins, 2005. This book lists primary references and reviews data on over a thousand medications with respect to the risk to the developing fetus and the risk in breastfeeding. For drug use in pregnancy, the book provides a recommendation from 16 potential categories based on available human and animal reproduction data. For drug use in lacation, the book provides a recommendation from six potential categories based on available human and pharmacologic data. In addition, the Food and Drug Administration's pregnancy risk category (PRC) is listed for each drug.

C. Hale T. *Medications and Mother's milk*, 12th ed. Amarillo Texas: Hale Publishing, 2006. This book is a comprehensive listing of hundreds of medications, vitamins, herbal remedies and vaccines, with primary references sited for most. The Food and Drug Administration—assigned PRC and AAP evaluation are provided for each drug. The author's own Lactation Risk Category is as follows:

1. L1: safest.
2. L2: safer.
3. L3: moderately safe. Many drugs fall into this category, which are defined as follows: "There are no controlled studies in breastfeeding women, however, the risk of untoward effects to a breastfed infant is possible, or controlled studies show only minimal, unthreatening effects. Drugs should be given only if the potential benefit justifies the risk to the infant."
4. L4: possibly hazardous.
5. L5: contraindicated.
6. Specific drug updates, erratum and supplemental information for this reference are available on the Internet at http://neonatal.ttuhsc.edu.

D. Lawrence RA, Lawrence RM. *Breastfeeding: A guide for the medical profession*, 6th ed. Philadelphia: Mosby, 2005. This book includes an extended discussion of the pharmacology of drug entry into breast milk. An appendix contains a listing of >600 drugs listed by drug category (analgesics, antibiotics, etc.) with the AAP safety rating, the Hale Lactation Risk Category, and the Weiner Code of Breastfeeding Safety listing, given when available. The appendix also contains extensive pharmacokinetic data for each drug, including values for the M/P ratio and maximum amount (mg/mL) of drug found in breast milk. Primary references published after 1985 are provided.

E. The Breastfeeding and Human Lactation Study Center. The Study Center maintains a drug data bank that is updated monthly. Health professionals may call the phone number listed in the subsequent text to talk to staff members regarding the safety of a particular drug in breastfeeding. The Study Center will provide information immediately by telephone or by e-mail. The Study Center will only take calls from healthcare professionals (not parents). General information about this program can be found at www.usbreastfeeding.org/breastfeeding/compend-bhlsc.htm. Contact information: The Breastfeeding and Human Lactation Study Center, University of Rochester School of Medicine and Dentistry, Department of Pediatrics, Box 777, 601 Elmwood Avenue, Rochester, NY 14642; Telephone: (585) 275–0088, Fax: (585) 461–3614.

F. The Food and Drug Administration's Pregnancy Risk Categories for drugs are detailed at http://www.fda.gov/fdac/features/2001/301_preg.html#categories. A brief summary is as follows:

1. **Category A.** Controlled studies in women fail to demonstrate a risk to the fetus.
2. **Category B.** Either animal-reproduction studies have not demonstrated a fetal risk or, if such a risk was found, it was not confirmed in later controlled studies in women.
3. **Category C.** Either studies in animals have revealed adverse effects on the fetus and there are no controlled studies in women, or studies in women and animals are not available. Drugs should be given only if the potential benefit justifies the potential risk to the fetus.
4. **Category D.** There is positive evidence of human fetal risk, but the benefits from use in pregnant women may be acceptable despite the risk (e.g., in a life-threatening situation or for a serious disease).
5. **Category X.** Studies in animals or human beings have demonstrated fetal abnormalities, and the risk of the use of the drug in pregnant women clearly outweighs any possible benefit.

G. The National Library of Medicine maintains a Drugs and Lactation Database (LactMed) at http://toxnet.nlm.nih.gov/cgi-bin/sis/htmlgen?LACT

IV. INFORMATION ON COMMON MEDICATIONS. Following are tables of medications commonly prescribed to breastfeeding women. They are organized by category and are listed alphabetically within each category, with the Food and Drug Administration PRC, A–D and X; AAP rating (1–6, or NR = not reviewed), the MMM rating (L1–L5).

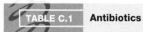

TABLE C.1   **Antibiotics**

Medication	PRC	AAP	MMM
Acyclovir	C	6	L2
Amikacin	C	NR	L2
Amoxicillin	B	6	L1
Amphotericin B	B	NR	L3
Ampicillin/Unasyn	B	NR	L1
Augmentin	B	NR	L1
Azithromycin	B	NR	L2
Aztreonam	B	6	L2
Carbenicillin	B	NR	L1
Cefprozil	C	6	L1
Cephalosporins:			
*List 1:	B	6 or NR	L1
†List 2:	B	6 or NR	L2
Ciprofloxacin	C	6	L3
Clarithromycin	C	NR	L2
Clindamycin	B	6	L2
Doxycycline	D	NR	L3 (acute), L4 (chronic)
Erythromycin	B	6	L3 (<3 months), L1
Famciclovir	B	NR	L2
Floxacillin	B1	NR	L1
Fluconazole	C	6	L2
Gentamicin	C	NR	L2
Griseofulvin	C	NR	L2
Imipenem-cilastatin	C	NR	L2
Isoniazid	C	6	L3
Itraconazole	C	NR	L2
Kanamycin	D	6	L2
Ketoconazole	C	6	L2
Loracarbef	B	NR	L2
Methicillin	B	NR	L3
Metronidazole	B	4	L2
Minocycline	D	NR	L2 (acute), L4 (chronic)
Mupirocin	B	NR	L1
Nafcillin	B	NR	L1
Nitrofurantoin	B	6	L2
Norfloxacin	C	NR	L3
Ofloxacin	C	6	L2
Penicillin G	B	6	L1

(continued)

TABLE C.1 *(Continued)*

Medication	PRC	AAP	MMM
Piperacillin/Zosyn	B	NR	L2
Sulfamethoxazole	C	NR	L3
Trimethoprim	C	6	L2
Valacyclovir	B	NR	L1

AAP = American Academy of Pediatrics;
MMM = Medications in Mother's Milk;
NR = not reviewed; PRC = pregnancy risk category.
*List 1: cefadroxil, cefazolin, cefoxitin, ceftazidime, cephalexin, cephapirin, cephradine.
†List 2: cefaclor, cefdinir, ceftibuten, cefepime, cefixime, cefoperazone, cefotaxime, cefotetan, cefpodoxime, ceftriaxone, cefuroxime, cephalothin.

TABLE C.2 Analgesics

Medication	PRC	AAP	MMM
Acetaminophen	B	6	L1
Aspirin	C/D	5	L3
Butorphanol	B/D	6	L2
Codeine	C	6	L3
Fentanyl	B	6	L2
Hydrocodone	B	NR	L3
Hydromorphone	C	NR	L3
Ibuprofen	B/D	6	L1
Indomethacin	B/D	6	L3
Ketorolac	B/D	6	L2
Meperidine	B	6	L2/L3 (early postpartum)
Methadone	B	6	L3
Morphine	B	6	L3
Nubain	B	NR	L2
Naproxen	B	6	L3/L4 (chronic use)
Oxycodone	B	NR	L3

AAP = American Academy of Pediatrics;
MMM = Medications in Mother's Milk; NR = not reviewed;
PRC = pregnancy risk category.

TABLE C.3   **Antihypertensive and Cardiac Medications**

Medication	PRC	AAP	MMM
Amiodarone	C	4	L5
Atenolol	C	5	L3
Captopril	D	6	L2
Clonidine	C	NR	L3
Digoxin	C	6	L2
Diltiazem	C	6	L3
Dopamine/dobutamine	C	NR	L2
Enalapril	C/D	6	L2
Ephedrine	C	NR	L4
Epinephrine	C	NR	L1
Flecainide	C	6	L3
Hydralazine	C	6	L2
Labetalol	C	6	L2
Magnesium sulfate	B	6	L1
Methyldopa	C	6	L2
Nifedipine	C	6	L2
Nimodipine	C	NR	L2
Procainamide	C	6	L3
Propranolol	C	6	L2

AAP = American Academy of Pediatrics;
MMM = Medications in Mother's Milk; NR = not reviewed;
PRC = pregnancy risk category.

TABLE C.4   Allergy and Respiratory Medications

Medication	PRC	AAP	MMM
Albuterol	C	NR	L1
Beclomethasone	C	NR	L2
Betamethasone	C	NR	L3
Budesonide	C	NR	L2
Cetirizine (Zyrtec)	B	NR	L2
Clemastine (Tavist)	C	5	L4
Cromolyn sodium	B	NR	L1
Dexamethasone	C	NR	L3
Dextromethorphan	C	NR	L1
Diphenhydramine	C	NR	L2
Fexofenadine (Allegra)	C	6	L2
Flunisolide	C	NR	L3
Hydrocortisone (topical)	C	NR	L2
Loratadine (Claritin)	B	6	L1
Methylprednisolone	C	6	L2
Montelukast (Singulair)	B	NR	L3
Phenylephrine	C	NR	L3
Prednisone	B	6	L2
Pseudoephedrine*	C	6	L3/L4
Theophylline	C	6	L3

AAP = American Academy of Pediatrics;
MMM = Medications in Mother's Milk; NR = not reviewed;
PRC = pregnancy risk category.
*Pseudoephedrine can decrease milk production.

| TABLE C.5 | Psychoactive Medications | | |

Medication	PRC	AAP	MMM
Alprazolam	D	4	L3
Amitryptyline	D	4	L2
Bupropion	B	4	L3
Caffeine	B	6	L2
Carbamazepine	C	6	L2
Chloral hydrate	C	6	L3
Chlordiazepoxide	D	NR	L3
Chlorpromazine	C	4	L3
Citalopram (Celexa)	C	NR	L2
Clomipramine	C	4	L2
Clonazepam	C	NR	L3
Clozapine	C	4	L3
Desipramine	C	4	L2
Diazepam	D	4	L3/L4 (chronic use)
Duloxetine (Cymbalta)	C	NR	L3
Fluoxetine (Prozac)	B	4	L3 (neonatal), L2 (older infant)
Gabapentin	C	NR	L3
Haloperidol	C	4	L2
Lithium	D	5	L4
Lorazepam (Ativan)	D	4	L3
Methylphenidate (Ritalin)	C	NR	L3
Midazolam	D	4	L3
Oxazepam (Serax)	D	NR	L3
Paroxetine (Paxil)	C	4	L2
Pentobarbital	D	NR	L3
Phenobarbital	D	5	L3
Phenytoin	D	6	L2
Prochlorperazine	C	NR	L3
Sertraline (Zoloft)	B	4	L2
Valproic acid	D	6	L2

AAP = American Academy of Pediatrics; MMM = Medications in Mother's Milk; NR = not reviewed; PRC = pregnancy risk category.

TABLE C.6	**Gastrointestinal Medications**		

Medication	PRC	AAP	MMM
Bismuth subsalicylate	C/D	4	L3
Cimetidine	B	6	L2
Docusate	C	NR	L2
Domperidone	NR	6	L1
Kaolin-pectin	C	NR	L1
Loperamide	B	6	L2
Metoclopramide	B	4	L2
Nizatidine	C	NR	L2
Omeprazole	C	NR	L2
Ondansetron	B	NR	L2
Ranitidine	B	NR	L2

AAP = American Academy of Pediatrics;
MMM = Medications in Mother's Milk;
NR = not reviewed; PRC = pregnancy risk category.

TABLE C.7	**Medications Contraindicated in Breastfeeding**

Amiodarone

Antineoplastic agents

Bromocriptine

Chloramphenicol

Drugs of abuse

Diethylstilbestrol

Disulfiram

Lithium*

Radioisotopes — usually require only temporary cessation of breastfeeding†

Tamoxifen

Note on oral contraceptives: Estrogen-containing preparations can reduce milk supply. Progestin-only oral contraceptives are safer with respect to milk production.
*Note on Lithium: listed as PRC = D, AAP = 5, MMM = L4. Infant serum lithium levels 30% to 40% of mother's level. Infant must be closely monitored by a pediatrician if used during breastfeeding. Drug has potential effects on infant neurodevelopment, cardiac rhythm, and thyroid function.
†Note: [131]I treatment requires complete cessation of breastfeeding due to the concentration of this agent in the breast and in breastmilk for weeks following completion of treatment.

Suggested Readings

American Academy of Pediatrics (AAP), Committee on Drugs. Transfer of drugs and other chemicals into human milk. *Pediatrics* 2001;108(3):776–789.

Briggs GG, Freeman RK, Yaffe SJ, eds. *Drugs in pregnancy and lactation*, 7th ed. Baltimore: Lippincott Williams & Wilkins, 2005.

Hale T. *Medications and Mother's milk*, 12th ed. Amarillo Texas: Hale Publishing, 2006.

Lawrence RA, Lawrence RM. *Breastfeeding: A guide for the medical profession*, 6th ed. Philadelphia: Mosby, 2005.

INDEX

Note: Page numbers in italics indicate figures; those followed by *t* indicate tables.

AQ1

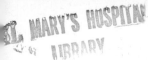

Neonatal Resuscitation (See Chapter 4)

Drug/therapy	Dose/kg	Weight	Volume IV	Volume IT	Method	Indication
Epinephrine 1:10,000 0.1 mg/mL	0.01–0.03 mg/kg	1 kg 2 kg 3 kg 4 kg	0.2 mL 0.4 mL 0.6 mL 0.8 mL	0.5 mL 1.0 mL 1.5 mL 2.0 mL	IV dose preferred Give IV push or intratracheally followed by flush with 1 mL normal saline; do not give into an artery, do not mix with bicarbonate, repeat in 5 min PRN	Asystole or severe bradycardia
Sodium bicarbonate 0.5 mEq/mL	2 mEq/kg	1 kg 2 kg 3 kg 4 kg	4 mL 8 mL 12 mL 16 mL		Give IV over 2 min; do not mix with epinephrine, calcium or phosphate; assure adequate ventilation; do not give intratracheally	Metabolic acidosis
Naloxone (Narcan®) 0.4 mg/mL	0.1–0.2 mg/kg	1 kg 2 kg 3 kg 4 kg	0.25 mL 0.50 mL 0.75 mL 1.0 mL		Give IV push, IM, SQ or IT; repeat PRN 3 times if no response; if maternal narcotic addiction is suspected do not give; do not mix with bicarbonate; see Chap. 19	Narcotic depression
Volume expanders - Normal saline - Whole blood	10 mL/kg	1 kg 2 kg 3 kg 4 kg	10 mL 20 mL 30 mL 40 mL		Give IV over 5 to 10 min Umbilical vein preferred	Hypotension due to intravascular volume loss; see Chap. 17
Cardioversion/ defibrillation	1–4 Joules/kg; increase 50% each time					VT/VF see Chap. 25

Endotracheal tube (ET)	Internal Diameter (mm)	External Diameter (French)	Oral intubation tip of tube to lip distance
<1,000 g	2.5 uncuffed	12	7 cm
1,000–2,000	3.0 uncuffed	14	8 cm
2,000–4,000	3.5 uncuffed	16	9 cm
>4,000 g	4.0 uncuffed	18	10 cm

Laryngoscope blades	
<1,000 g	00 (straight)
1,001–2,000 g	0 (straight)
>2,000 g	1 (straight)

BP, blood pressure; HR, heart rate; IM, intramuscular; IT, intratracheal; IV, intravenous; PRN, as needed; SQ, subcutaneous.